D1576539

OXFORD MEDICAL PUBLICATION

Oxford Desk Reference
Acute Medicine

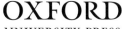

Great Clarendon Street, Oxford, OX2 6DP,
United Kingdom

Oxford University Press is a department of the University of Oxford.
It furthers the University's objective of excellence in research, scholarship,
and education by publishing worldwide. Oxford is a registered trade mark of
Oxford University Press in the UK and in certain other countries

Published in the United States of America by Oxford University Press
198 Madison Avenue, New York, NY 10016, United States of America

British Library Cataloguing in Publication Data

Data available

Library of Congress Control Number: 2013944918

ISBN 978–0–19–956597–9

Printed and bound by
CPI Group (UK) Ltd, Croydon, CR0 4YY

Oxford Desk Reference
Acute Medicine

Edited by

Dr Richard Leach
Consultant Physician and Honorary Reader in
Medicine, Departments of Respiratory and
Critical Care Medicine, Guy's and St Thomas'
Hospital Trust and Kings College,
London, UK

Professor Derek Bell
Professor of Acute Medicine, Faculty of
Medicine, Imperial College London and Chelsea
and Westminster Hospital, London

Professor Kevin Moore
Professor of Hepatology, University College
London Medical School, UCL,
London, UK

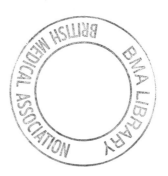

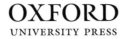

Foreword

Acute and general (internal) medicine is a broad specialty covering a wide spectrum of emergency medical presentations and illnesses, and it is at the forefront of the delivery of acute medical care. Few medical specialties have had to adapt as rapidly to the dramatic improvements in medical care that have become available over the last decade. For many conditions, the improved outcomes are critically dependent on the early phase of management. Consequently, acute physicians, clinical trainees and associated health care workers have had to develop early clinical recognition skills, acquire new theoretical knowledge and implement an increasing number of guidelines and practical requirements.

Acute medical services are under increasing pressure as emergency admissions have increased by 37% over the last decade, whilst acute medical beds have decreased by about a third over the preceding 25 years. Over two thirds of emergency hospital admissions are over 65 years old, and many are frail or suffer with dementia. Recent evidence suggests that for many medical registrars the current emergency, out-of-hours admission work load is unmanageable and will put the delivery of optimal acute medical management at risk. There are no signs that this will fall any time soon.

All acute medical admissions deserve to receive safe, high quality care appropriate to their needs, delivered by caring, compassionate, health professionals. In an era of increasing evidence based medicine, national guidelines, rising workloads and increasing knowledge, the need for text books that provide simple, guideline-based assistance to the busy clinician are ever more important. The Oxford Desk Reference: Acute Medicine brings together the key recommendations found in recent evidence based guidelines and presents them in an easily accessible form so that locating and assimilating the required information is quick and simple. Many of the chapters and specialty sections have been written by recognized national or international leaders in their fields, who have provided the best available advice where guidelines or evidence do not exist.

This eminently practical textbook should be a useful daily resource to all those busy caring for acute medical admissions.

Sir Richard Thompson
President of the Royal College of Physicians (2010–14)

Preface

All of us working as acute and general physicians wish to provide the best care for our acutely unwell patients. The early medical management of such patients is critical and has profound effects on survival and long-term outcomes. One of the major challenges facing the busy general clinician is how to keep abreast of the rapidly changing clinical practice guidelines produced by specialist societies and national organizations. Accessing this information, when it is most needed, is not always easy; and yet, it is in the emergency department or on the post-take ward round where this vital information could make a significant difference to outcome.

Given that most general physicians will be dealing with problems outside their specialist field, it is apparent that we need practice-based textbooks aimed at providing easy access to accredited guidelines, web-based information and details of specialist patient support groups. In the *Oxford Desk Reference of Acute Medicine* we have attempted to produce a practical, comprehensive but brief guide to the management of acute medical emergencies which will enable the acute physician to deliver the best possible early care for their patients, irrespective of the cause or base specialty.

To some extent we have apportioned space according to the frequency with which a clinical problem is likely to be encountered in developed countries, whilst identifying and addressing those emergency presentations, which although rare, require immediate and often life-saving interventions. Key recommendations and evidence-based guidelines have been combined in a uniform and practical format, to enable the reader to quickly locate and rapidly assimilate the key information about a specific topic. Inevitably, in order to produce a succinct, practical and appropriately sized book, some detail is omitted, but much of this can be obtained from the companion specialist Oxford Desk Reference series.

This book is aimed at acute, general and trainee physicians participating in 'unselected' general medical admissions rotas or working in acute medical units. It should also be of interest to acute nurse practitioners, pharmacists participating in 'post-take' ward rounds and to the many specialists and junior clinicians, who at times, may have to deal with acute medical problems. We hope that you will find it a useful, time-saving and reassuring resource in your routine working day.

Dr Richard Leach
Professor Derek Bell
Professor Kevin Moore

Acknowledgements

Development of a new textbook inevitably involves the help and advice of a wide range of people and it is not always possible to acknowledge every contribution. Nevertheless we would like to thank all the chapter authors, from the United Kingdom, United States of America and Europe who, without exception have contributed work of the highest quality. Our thanks are also due to Fiona Goodgame, Katy Loftus, Christopher Reid, and especially Fiona Richardson and Angela Butterworth from Oxford University Press who have guided and supported us throughout, and been instrumental in the production of this book.

Finally, as editors and authors, we owe particular thanks to our partners or wives who between them have provided the essential support, encouragement and patience necessary for the writing and editing process. In particular, RL would like to thank Clare (for her many hours of proofreading and support), Helen, Marc, and Niall.

Contents

Detailed contents

List of contributors

Dr Bhandari Sumer Aditya
Clinical Director and Consultant Physician
Diabetes and Endocrinology Department
Aintree University Hospital NHS Trust
Liverpool

Dr Liju Ahmed
Consultant in Respiratory and General Medicine
Department of Respiratory Medicine
Guy's and St Thomas' Hospital Trust
London

Dr Thomasin C Andrews
Consultant Neurologist
Guy's and St Thomas' NHS Foundation Trust
London

Professor John S Bevan
Consultant and Honorary Professor of Endocrinology
Aberdeen Royal Infirmary
Aberdeen

Dr Sanjay Bhagani
Department of Infectious Diseases and HIV Medicine
Royal Free Hospital
London

Dr Iñaki Bovill
Consultant Physician and Geriatrician/Honorary Senior
Lecturer
Chelsea & Westminster NHS Foundation Trust/Imperial
College School of Medicine
London

Dr Ronan Breen
Consultant in Respiratory and General Medicine
Department of Respiratory Medicine
Guy's and St Thomas' Hospital Trust
London

Dr Andrew Brett
Consultant in Emergency Medicine
Jersey General Hospital
States of Jersey

Dr Stephen Brett
Consultant and Honorary Reader in Critical Care
Medicine
Imperial College Healthcare NHS Trust
London

Professor Christopher Bunker
Consultant Dermatologist/Professor of Dermatology
University College London/Imperial College/Chelsea &
Westminster Hospitals
London

Professor Margaret Callan
Consultant Rheumatologist
Chelsea and Westminster NHS Foundation Trust
London

Dr Arani Chandrakumar
Consultant Dermatologist
Ashford & St Peter's NHS Trust
Ashford

Dr Felix Chua
Consultant in Respiratory Medicine/Honorary Senior
Lecturer
St George's Hospital NHS Trust/St George's University
London

Professor Chris Cooper
Professor of Medicine and Physiology
Departments of Medicine and Physiology
University of California Los Angeles
Los Angeles

Dr Nicola Cooper
Consultant Physician and Honorary Clinical Associate
Professor
Derby Hospitals NHS Foundation Trust
Division of Medical Sciences & Graduate Entry Medicine
University of Nottingham
Nottingham

Dr Alastair Crosswaite
Consultant in Acute Medicine and General Practice
Edinburgh Royal Infirmary
Edinburgh

Dr Mark Dancy
Consultant Cardiologist
Central Middlesex Hospital
London

Dr Andrew Davenport
Consultant Nephrologist and Honorary Senior Lecturer
UCL Centre for Nephrology
Royal Free Hospital and University College Medical School
London

Professor David D'Cruz
Professor and Consultant in Rheumatology
Lupus Unit
King's College/Guy's and St Thomas' Hospital Trust
London

Miss Mandish K Dhanjal
Consultant Obstetrician and Gynaecologist
Honorary Senior Lecturer
Queen Charlotte's and Chelsea Hospital, Imperial
College Healthcare NHS Trust
London

Dr Nicholas Easom
Specialist Registrar Infectious Diseases and General Medicine
Hospital for Tropical Diseases
London

Dr Andrew Elder
Consultant Physician in Acute Medicine for Older People
Weston General Hospital
Edinburgh

Dr Annabel Fountain
Specialist Registrar in Diabetes and Endocrinology
Chelsea and Westminster Hospital
London

Miss Joanna Girling
Consultant Obstetrician and Gynaecologist
West Middlesex University Hospital
Twickenham

Dr Jennifer Gray
Consultant Acute Physician
Forth Valley Royal Hospital
Larbert

Dr Neil Grubb
Consultant Cardiologist
Edinburgh Heart Centre
Edinburgh Royal Infirmary
Edinburgh

Professor David Halpin
Consultant Physician
Department of Respiratory Medicine
Royal Devon and Exeter Foundation Trust
Exeter

Dr Marcus Harbord
Consultant Physician and Gastroenterologist
Chelsea and Westminster Hospital
London

Dr John Harvey
Consultant Respiratory Physician
North Bristol Lung Centre
Southmead Hospital
Bristol

Dr Bernard Higgins
Consultant Respiratory Physician
Department of Respiratory Medicine
Freeman Hospital
Newcastle upon Tyne

Dr Andrew Hodgkiss
Consultant Liaison Psychiatrist/Honorary Senior Lecturer
Kings Health Partners Academic Health Sciences Centre
London

Dr Paul Holmes
Consultant Neurologist
Department of Neurology
Guy's and St Thomas' Hospital Trust
London

Dr Clare Hooper
Consultant Respiratory Physician
North Bristol Lung Centre/University of Bristol
Southmead Hospital
Bristol

Dr Robin Howard
Consultant Neurologist
National Hospital for Neurological Diseases
London

Dr Mike Jones
Acute Physician/Senior Lecturer/SAC Chair Acute Internal Medicine Vice President
University Hospital of North Durham/University of Durham/Royal College of Physicians of Edinburgh

Dr Burhan Khan
Consultant Respiratory Physician
Department of Respiratory Medicine
Darent Valley Hospital
Dartford and Gravesham NHS Trust
Kent

Dr Ramzi Y Khamis
Consultant Cardiologist and Clinical Research Fellow in Cardiovascular Medicine
The Hammersmith Hospital
Imperial College Healthcare NHS Trust
London

Dr John L Klein
Consultant Microbiologist
Guy's and St Thomas' NHS Foundation Trust
London

Professor Michael Koutroumanidis
Consultant Neurophysiologist and Honorary Professor in Clinical Neurophysiology
Department of Neurology
Guy's and St Thomas' Hospital Trust and Kings College
London

Professor Richard Light
Professor of Medicine
Division of Allergy, Pulmonary and Critical Care Medicine
Vanderbilt University Medical Centre
Nashville

Dr Wei Shen Lim
Consultant Respiratory Physician
Nottingham University Hospitals NHS Trust
Nottingham

Dr Donald C Macleod
Consultant in Acute Medicine
Western General Hospital
Edinburgh

Professor Calum Archibald Macrae
Chief of Cardiovascular Medicine and Associate
Professor
Division of Cardiovascular Medicine
Brigham and Women's Hospital and Harvard Medical
School
Boston, USA

Dr Daniel Marks
Wellcome Trust Postdoctoral Clinical Training Fellow
University College Hospital
London

Dr Francis Matthey
Consultant Haematologist
Chelsea and Westminster Hospital NHS Foundation Trust
London

Dr Christopher McNamara
Consultant Haematologist
The Royal Free Hospital
London

Professor Ann B Millar
Professor of Respiratory Medicine/Honorary
Consultant Physician
University of Bristol/North Bristol NHS Trust
Bristol

Professor Alyn Morice
Professor of Respiratory Medicine
Academic Medicine, Hull York Medical School
University of Hull and Castle Hill Hospital
Hull

Mr Neil Morton
Postgraduate Fellow
St Edmund Hall
University of Oxford
Oxford

Professor Catherine Nelson-Piercy
Consultant and Honorary Professor in Obstetric
Medicine
Guy's and St Thomas' Hospital Trust/Queen Charlotte's
Hospital/Imperial College Healthcare NHS Trust
London

Miss Louise Page
Consultant Obstetrician and Gynaecologist
West Middlesex University Hospital
Twickenham

Dr Caroline Patterson
Specialty Trainee in Respiratory Medicine and Medical
Officer RAF
North West Thames Respiratory Training Programme
London

Professor Andrew Peacock
Consultant and Honorary Professor in Respiratory
Medicine
Scottish Pulmonary Vascular Unit and Institute of
Cardiovascular and Medical Sciences
Golden Jubilee National Hospital
Glasgow

Dr Rebecca Preston
Consultant Radiologist
Guy's and St Thomas' NHS Foundation Trust
London

Dr Nicholas Price
Director and Consultant Physician
Directorate of Infection
Guy's and St Thomas' Hospital Trust
London

Dr Alastair Proudfoot
Research Fellow
Royal Brompton & Harefield NHS Foundation Trust
London

Dr Gopinath Ranjith
Consultant Liaison Psychiatrist
Kings Health Partners AHSC
London

Dr Ian Scott
Associate Professor/Director of Internal Medicine and
Clinical Epidemiology
Princess Alexandra Hospital
Brisbane

Dr Kevin Shotliffe
Consultant Endocrinologist
Chelsea and Westminster Hospital
London

Professor Stephen Spiro
Professor of Respiratory Medicine
Royal Brompton Hospital
London

Professor Monica Spiteri
Professor of Respiratory Medicine
Directorate of Respiratory Medicine
University Hospitals of North Midlands NHS Trust
Stoke-on-Trent

Dr Alaisdair Stewart
Consultant Respiratory Physician
Department of Respiratory Medicine
Medway Maritime Hospital
Kent

Dr Anthony Toft
Consultant Physician and past President of the Royal
College of Physicians (Edinburgh)
Royal Infirmary
Edinburgh

Dr Neal Uren
Clinical Director for Cardiac Services
Edinburgh Heart Centre Royal Infirmary
Edinburgh

Dr Louella Vaughan
Senior Clinical Fellow
Nuffield Trust
London

Dr Jananath Bhathiya Wijeyekoon
Consultant Physician and Rheumatologist
Lister Hospital
East and North Herts NHS Trust
Stevenage

Professor John PH Wilding
Professor of Medicine and Honorary Consultant
Physician
Department of Diabetes and Endocrinology
University of Liverpool, University Hospital
Liverpool

Professor Adrian J Williams
Consultant Sleep Physician
Guy's and St Thomas' NHS Foundation Trust
London

Dr Matthew Young
Consultant in Acute Medicine and Diabetes/
Endocrinology
Royal Infirmary
Edinburgh

List of abbreviations

A	ampere	AMS	abbreviated mental state; acute mountain sickness
A-a	alveolar-arterial	AMSAN	acute motor and sensory axonal neuropathy
AA	Alcoholics Anonymous		
AAFB	acid- and alcohol-fast bacilli	AMU	acute medical unit
ABG	arterial blood gas	ANA	antinuclear antibody
ABPA	allergic bronchopulmonary aspergillosis	ANCA	antineutrophil cytoplasmic antibody
ACC	American College of Cardiology	APACHE	acute physiology and chronic health evaluation score
ACCP	American College of Chest Physicians		
ACD	allergic contact dermatitis	APC	activated protein C; argon plasma coagulation
ACE	angiotensin-converting enzyme		
ACE-I	angiotensin-converting enzyme inhibitor	APD	allergic phytodermatitis
AChR	acetylcholine receptor	APH	antepartum haemorrhage
ACR	American College of Rheumatology	APS	antiphospholipid syndrome
ACS	acute coronary syndromes	APTT	activated partial thromboplastin time
ACT	activated clotting time	AR	aortic regurgitation
ACTH	adrenocorticotrophic hormone	ARAS	atheromatous renal artery stenosis
ADC	AIDS dementia complex	ARDS	acute respiratory distress syndrome
ADH	antidiuretic hormone	ARF	acute renal failure
ADL	activities of daily living	ARR	absolute risk reduction
ADP	adenosine diphosphate	ARVC	arrhythmogenic right ventricular cardiomyopathy
A+E	Accident and Emergency		
AED	automated external defibrillator; anti-epileptic drug	ARVD	arrhythmogenic right ventricular dysplasia
		AS	aortic stenosis
AEGN	acute endocapillary glomerulonephritis	ASD	atrial septal defect
AF	atrial fibrillation	ASE	absence status epilepticus
AFB	acid-fast bacilli	ASO	antistreptolysin O
AFE	amniotic fluid embolism	AST	aspartate transaminase
AHA	American Heart Association	ATG	anti-thymocyte globulin
AICD	automated implantable cardioverter defibrillator	ATIN	acute tubulointerstitial nephropathy
		ATLS	Advanced Trauma Life Support
AIDS	acquired immune deficiency syndrome	ATM	atypical mycobacteria
AIP	acute interstitial pneumonitis	ATN	acute tubular necrosis
AKI	acute kidney injury	ATP	adenosine triphosphate
ALF	acute liver failure	ATRA	all-trans retinoic acid
ALI	acute lung injury	AV	atrioventricular; arteriovenous
ALL	acute lymphoblastic leukaemia	AVM	arteriovenous malformation
ALS	advanced life support; amyotrophic lateral sclerosis	AVNRT	atrioventricular nodal re-entrant tachycardia
		AVP	arginine vasopressin
ALT	alanine transaminase	AVRT	atrioventricular re-entrant tachycardia
AMAN	acute motor axonal neuropathy	BAH	bilateral adrenal hyperplasia
AMD	adjustable maintenance dosing	BAL	bronchoalveolar lavage
AML	acute myeloid leukaemia	BAPEN	British Association of Parenteral and Enteral Nutrition
APML	acute promyelocytic leukaemia		

BASDAI	Bath Ankylosing Spondylitis Disease Activity Index
BBV	blood-borne virus
BC	blood culture
BCAA	branched chain amino acid
BCC	basal cell carcinoma
BCG	Bacille–Calmette–Guérin
bd	twice daily
BHL	bihilar lymphadenopathy
BHR	bronchial hyperreactivity
BIPAP	bilevel positive airways pressure
BiVAD	biventricular assist device
BJP	Bence–Jones protein
BMI	body mass index
BMPR	bone morphogenetic protein receptor
BMR	basal metabolic rate
BMT	bone marrow transplant
BNF	British National Formulary
BNP	brain natriuretic peptide
BOOP	bronchiolitis obliterans organizing pneumonia
BP	blood pressure; bullous pemphigoid
bpm	beats per minute
BSD	brainstem death
BTS	British Thoracic Society
Ca^{2+}	calcium ion
CABG	coronary artery bypass graft
CAD	coronary artery disease
CAI	community-acquired infection
CAM	confusion assessment method
cANCA	cytoplasmic ANCA
CAP	community-acquired pneumonia
CAPD	continuous acute peritoneal dialysis
cART	combination antiretroviral therapies
CAVDF	continuous arteriovenous haemodiafiltration
CAVHF	continuous arteriovenous haemofiltration
CBD	corticobasal degeneration; common bile duct
CBF	cerebral blood flow
CBT	cognitive behavioural therapy
CBV	cerebral blood volume
CCB	calcium channel blocker
CCP	cyclic citrullinated peptide
CD	Crohn's disease
CDC	Centers for Disease Control and Prevention
CEA	carotid endarterectomy; carcinoembryonic antigen

CF	cystic fibrosis
CFA	cryptogenic fibrosing alveolitis
CFTR	CF transmembrane conductance regulator
CFU	colony-forming unit
cGMP	cyclic guanosine monophosphate
CHB	complete heart block
CHD	coronary heart disease; congenital heart disease
CHDF	haemodiafiltration
CHF	congestive heart failure
CIDP	chronic inflammatory demyelinating polyradiculoneuropathy
CIWA-Ar	clinical institute withdrawal assessment of alcohol scale-revised
CJD	Creutzfeld–Jakob disease
CK	creatine kinase
CKD	chronic kidney disease
CI	confidence interval; cardiac index
Cl^-	chloride ion
CLD	chronic liver disease
CLL	chronic lymphocytic leukaemia
cm	centimetre
CMR	cardiac magnetic resonance
CMT	Charcot–Marie–Tooth
CMV	cytomegalovirus; controlled mechanical ventilation
CN	cyanide
CNS	central nervous system; coagulase-negative staphylococci
CO	cardiac output; carbon monoxide
CO_2	carbon dioxide
COCPR	compression-only CPR
COHb	carboxyhaemoglobin
COMT	catechol methyltransferase
COP	cryptogenic organizing pneumonia
COPD	chronic obstructive pulmonary disease
CPA	cerebellopontine angle
CPAP	continuous positive airway pressure
CPD	chronic pulmonary disease
CPET	cardiopulmonary exercise testing
CPK	creatine phosphokinase
CPP	cerebral perfusion pressure
CPR	cardiopulmonary resuscitation
CPS	complex partial seizures
CPSE	complex partial status epilepticus
Cr	creatinine
CrAg	cryptococcal antigen
CRF	chronic renal failure; corticotrophin-releasing factor

CRP	C-reactive protein	DM	diabetes mellitus; dermatomyositis
CRT	cardiac resynchronization therapy	DMARD	disease-modifying anti-rheumatic drug
CS	Caesarean section	DMSA	dimercaptosuccinic acid
CSA	central sleep apnoea	DNA	deoxyribonucleic acid
CSF	cerebrospinal fluid	DNACPR	do not attempt cardiopulmonary resuscitation
CSM	Committee on Safety of Medicines	DNR	do not resuscitate
CSS	Churg–Strauss syndrome	DO_2	tissue oxygen delivery
CSW	cerebral salt wasting	DOT	directly observed therapy
CT	computed tomography	DPI	dry powder inhaler
CTA	CT angiography	DPLD	diffuse parenchymal lung disease
CTCL	cutaneous T cell lymphoma	DPT	diffuse pleural thickening
CTD	connective tissue disease	DRESS	drug eruption with eosinophilia and systemic symptoms
CTEPH	chronic thromboembolic pulmonary hypertension	DSA	digital subtraction angiography
CTG	cardiotocography	DsDNA	double-stranded DNA
CTPA	computerized tomography pulmonary angiography	DT	delirium tremens
CVA	cerebrovascular accident	DTH	delayed-type hypersensitivity
CVC	central venous catheter	DU	duodenal ulcer
CVP	central venous pressure	DVT	deep venous thrombosis
CVT	cerebral venous thrombosis	EAA	extrinsic allergic alveolitis
CVVH	continuous venovenous haemofiltration	EAEC	enteroaggregative E. coli
CVVHD	continuous venovenous haemodiafiltration	EBL	endoscopic band ligation
CWP	coal worker's pneumoconiosis	EBUS	endobronchial ultrasound
CXR	chest X-ray	EBV	Ebstein–Barr virus
2D	two-dimensional	ECF	extracellular fluid
3D	three-dimensional	ECG	electrocardiogram
Da	dalton	ECHO	echocardiogram
DAD	diffuse alveolar damage	ECMO	extracorporeal membrane oxygenation
DAH	diffuse alveolar haemorrhage	ED	emergency department
DAT	direct antiglobulin test	EDTA	ethylene-diamine-tetra-acetic acid
DC	direct current	EDV	end diastolic volume
DCM	dilated cardiomyopathy	EEG	electroencephalography
DCT	distal convoluted tubule	EG	ethylene glycol
DDAVP	desmopressin	EHEC	enterohaemorrhagic E. coli
DEXA	dual-energy X-ray absorptiometry	EIEC	enteroinvasive E. coli
DHF	dengue haemorrhagic fever	ELISA	enzyme-linked immunosorbent assay
dHMN	distal hereditary motor neuropathy	EM	erythema multiforme
DHS	drug hypersensitivity syndrome	EMG	electromyography
DI	diabetes insipidus; discriminant index	EMS	emergency medical services
DIC	disseminated intravascular coagulation	EMU	early-morning urine
DIP	desquamative interstitial pneumonia; distal interphalangeal	EN	erythema nodosum
		ENA	extractable nuclear antigen
DKA	diabetic ketoacidosis	EP	electrophysiology; eosinophilic pneumonia
dL	decilitre	EPAP	expiratory positive airways pressure
DLB	dementia with Lewy bodies	EPEC	enteropathogenic E. coli
DLD	diffuse lung disease	ERCP	endoscopic retrograde cholangiopancreatography
DLE	discoid lupus erythematosus		

ESR	erythrocyte sedimentation rate	GM-CSF	granulocyte macrophage-stimulating factor
ESWL	extracorporeal shock wave lithotripsy	GN	glomerulonephritis
ET	endotracheal	GnRH	gonadotropin-releasing hormone
ETEC	enterotoxigenic *E. coli*	G6PD	glucose-6-phosphate dehydrogenase
ETI	endotracheal intubation	GOLD	Global Initiative for Chronic Obstructive Lung Disease
ETS	environmental tobacco smoke		
ETT	endotracheal tube	GORD	gastro-oesophageal reflux disease
EULAR	European League Against Rheumatism	GPI	glycoprotein inhibitor
EWS	early warning scoring	GPS	Goodpasture's syndrome
FDP	fibrin degradation product	GRA	glucocorticoid-remedial aldosteronism
FES	fat embolism syndrome	GRACE	Global Registry of Acute Coronary Events
FEV_1	forced expiratory volume in 1 second	GRV	gastric residual volume
FFP	fresh frozen plasma	GTN	glyceryl trinitrate
FI	faecal incontinence	GU	genitourinary
FiO_2	inspired oxygen concentration	GUM	genitourinary medicine
fL	fluid ounce	GVHD	graft versus host disease
FMD	fibromuscular disease	Gy	gray
FMH	fetomaternal haemorrhage	h	hour
FN	febrile neutropenia	H^+	hydrogen ion
FNA	fine needle aspiration	HAART	highly active antiretroviral therapy
FRC	functional residual capacity	HACE	high-altitude cerebral oedema
FREMEC	Frequent Traveller Medical Card	HACEK	*Haemophilus*, *Actinobacillus*, *Cardiobacterium*, *Eikenella*, and *Kingella*
FRS	Framingham risk score		
FSGS	focal segmental glomerulosclerosis	HADS	HIV-associated dementia syndrome
FSHD	facioscapulohumeral muscular dystrophy	HAE	hereditary angio-oedema
ft	foot	HAI	hospital-acquired infection
FNAB	fine needle aspiration biopsy	HAP	hospital-acquired pneumonia
FTD	frontotemporal lobar degeneration	HAPE	high-altitude pulmonary oedema
FUO	fever of unknown origin	HASU	hyperacute stroke unit
FVC	forced vital capacity	HAV	hepatitis A virus
g	gram	HBsAb	hepatitis B surface antibody
GA	general anaesthesia	HBsAg	hepatitis B surface antigen
GABA	gamma-aminobutyric acid	HBV	hepatitis B virus
GAHS	Glasgow alcoholic hepatitis score	HCA	hyperchloraemic acidosis
GAVE	gastric antral vascular ectasia	HCAP	healthcare-associated pneumonia
GBM	glomerular basement membrane	hCG	human chorionic gonadotrophin
GBS	Guillain–Barré syndrome	HCO_3	bicarbonate
GCA	giant cell arteritis	HCRF	hypercapnic respiratory failure
GCS	Glasgow coma score/scale	HCV	hepatitis C virus
GCSE	generalized convulsive status epilepticus	HDL	high-density lipoprotein
G-CSF	granulocyte colony-stimulating factor	HDN	haemolytic disease of the newborn
GFR	glomerular filtration rate	HDU	high dependency unit
GGO	ground glass opacification	H&E	haematoxylin and eosin
GGT	gamma glutamyl transferase	HELLP	haemolysis, elevated liver enzymes, and low platelets
GHB	gamma hydroxybutyric acid		
GI	gastrointestinal	HES	hydroxyethyl starch
GIT	gastrointestinal tract	HFpEF	heart failure with preserved ejection fraction

HG	hyperemesis gravidarum		IGRA	interferon-gamma release assay
HGV	heavy goods vehicle		IHD	ischaemic heart disease
HHC	hyperosmolar hyperglycaemic coma		IIP	idiopathic interstitial pneumonia
HHT	hereditary haemorrhagic telangiectasia		IJ	internal jugular
HIDA	hepatobiliary iminodiacetic acid		IJV	internal jugular vein
HIT	heparin-induced thrombocytopenia		IL	interleukin
HIV	human immunodeficiency virus		ILCOR	International Liaison Committee on Resuscitation
HLA	human leucocyte antigen		ILD	interstitial lung disease
HMSN	hereditary motor sensory neuropathies		IM	intramuscular
HNIG	human normal immunoglobulin		in	inch
HONK	hyperosmolar non-ketotic diabetic coma		INCAD	Incapacitated Passengers Handling Advice
HP	hypersensitivity pneumonitis		INR	international normalized ratio
HPA	Health Protection Agency		IP	iatrogenic pneumothorax
HPAH	heritable pulmonary arterial hypertension		IPAH	idiopathic pulmonary arterial hypertension
HPT	Health Protection Team		IPAP	inspiratory positive airways pressure
HPV	hypoxic pulmonary vasoconstriction		IPF	idiopathic pulmonary fibrosis
HRCT	high-resolution CT		IPPV	intermittent positive pressure ventilation
HRS	Heart Rhythm Society; hepatorenal syndrome		IRIS	immune restoration inflammatory syndrome
HRT	hormone replacement therapy		ISDN	isosorbide dinitrate
HSAN	hereditary sensory autonomic neuropathy		ISF	interstitial fluid
HSP	hypersensitivity pneumonitis		ISS	injury severity score
HSV	herpes simplex virus		ITP	idiopathic thrombocytopenic purpura
HTLV	human T lymphotropic virus		ITU	intensive therapy unit
HUS	haemolytic uraemic syndrome		IU	international unit
HMWK	high molecular weight kininogen		IUGR	intrauterine growth retardation
Hz	hertz		IV	intravenous
HZO	herpes zoster ophthalmicus		IVCT	*in vitro* contracture test
IAB	intra-aortic balloon		IVIG	intravenous immunoglobulin
IABP	intra-aortic balloon pump		IVU	intravenous urography
IAS	insulin autoimmune syndrome		J	joule
IBD	inflammatory bowel disease		JET	jejunal extension tube
IBM	inclusion body myositis		JME	juvenile myoclonic epilepsy
IBS	irritable bowel syndrome		JVP	jugular venous pressure
ICD	implantable cardiac defibrillators		K^+	potassium ion
ICF	intracellular fluid		kcal	kilocalorie
ICH	intracerebral haemorrhage		KD	Kawasaki disease
ICM	irritant contact dermatitis		kDa	kilodalton
ICP	intracranial pressure; intracerebral pressure		kg	kilogram
ICS	inhaled corticosteroid therapy		kPa	kilopascal
ICT	immunochromatographic test		KS	Kaposi's sarcoma
ICU	intensive care unit		KUB	kidneys, ureters, bladder
IDL	intermediate-density lipoprotein		L	litre
IE	infective endocarditis		LA	left atrium
IFN	interferon		LAD	left axis deviation
Ig	immunoglobulin		LAM	lymphangioleiomyomatosis
IGAN	IgA nephropathy		LAP	left atrial pressure
IGE	idiopathic generalized epilepsies			

LBBB	left bundle branch block	MELAS	mitochondrial encephalomyopathy with lactic acidosis and strokes
LC	lung compliance	MEN	multiple endocrine neoplasia
LCH	Langerhans cell histiocytosis	mEq	milliequivalent
LCMV	lymphocytic choriomeningitis virus	MERRF	mitochondrial encephalomyopathy with ragged red fibres
LD	legionnaires' disease	MF	mycosis fungoides
LDH	lactate dehydrogenase	mg	milligram
LDL	low-density lipoprotein	MG	myasthenia gravis
LFT	liver function test	Mg^{2+}	magnesium ion
LGMD	limb girdle muscular dystrophy	MGN	membranous glomerulonephritis
LHRH	luteinizing hormone-releasing hormone	MGUS	monoclonal gammopathy of undetermined significance
LIP	lymphocytic interstitial pneumonia	mGy	milligray
LMW	low molecular weight	MH	malignant hyperthermia
LMWH	low molecular weight heparin	MHC	major histocompatibility complex
LOS	lower oesophageal sphincter	MI	myocardial infarction
LP	lumbar puncture	MIBG	metaiodo-benzylguanidine
LPB	lipopolysaccharide-binding protein	MIC	minimum inhibitory concentration
LPS	lipopolysaccharide	MIDD	monoclonal immunoglobulin deposition disease
LRT	lower respiratory tract	MILS	manual in-line stabilization
LRTI	lower respiratory tract infection	min	minute
LTOT	long-term oxygen therapy	MIP	maximum inspiratory pressure
LUQ	left upper quadrant	mM	millimole per litre
LUS	lower uterine segment	MMF	mycophenolate mofetil
LUTS	lower urinary tract symptoms	mmHg	millimetre of mercury
LVAD	left ventricular assist device	mmol	millimole
LVEF	left ventricular ejection fraction	MMR	measles, mumps, and rubella; maternal mortality rate
LVH	left ventricular hypertrophy	MMSE	mini-mental state examination
mA	milliampere	MN	malignant hyperthermia
MAC	*Mycobacterium avium* complex	MND	motor neurone disease
MAHA	microangiopathic haemolytic anaemia	MODS	multiple organ dysfunction score
MAO	monoamine oxidase	MOF	multi-organ failure
MAP	mean arterial pressure	mOsm	milliosmole
MASCC	Multinational Association for Supportive Care in Cancer	MPA	microscopic polyangiitis
MCA	Mental Capacity Act	MPGN	membranoproliferative glomerulonephritis
mcg	microgram	MPO	myeloperoxidase
MCGN	mesangiocapillary glomerulonephritis	MR	mitral regurgitation
MCN	minimal change glomerulonephritis	MRA	magnetic resonance angiography
MCP	metacarpophalangeal	MRC	Medical Research Council
M,C&S	microbiology, culture, and sensitivity	MRCP	magnetic resonance cholangiopancreatography
MDE	maternal death enquiry	MRI	magnetic resonance imaging
MDI	metered-dose inhaler	MRSA	meticillin (INN)-resistant *Staphylococcus aureus*
MDM	multidisciplinary team meeting	ms	millisecond
MDMA	methylenedioxy-metamphetamine	MS	mitral stenosis; multiple sclerosis
MDR	multidrug-resistant		
MDRD	Modification of Diet in Renal Disease		
MDT	multidisciplinary team		
MEDIF	Medical Information Form		

MSA	multiple system atrophy		NSTEMI	non-ST segment elevation myocardial infarction
MS-CT	multislice CT		NTM	non-tuberculous mycobacteria
MSLT	multiple sleep latency test		NYHA	New York Heart Association
MSU	midstream urine		OAB	overactive bladder
mSv	millisievert		OCD	obsessive–compulsive disorder
MTB	*Mycobacterium tuberculosis*		OCP	oral contraceptive pill
MTP	massively transfused patient; metatarsophalangeal		od	once daily
MTX	methotrexate		OD	overdose
mU	milliunit		OPMD	oculopharyngeal muscular dystrophy
MUD	matched unrelated donor		OPSI	overwhelming post-splenectomy infection
MuSK	muscle-specific kinase		OR	odds ratio
MUST	Malnutrition Universal Screening Tool		OSA	obstructive sleep apnoea
Mv	minute ventilation		OSAH	obstructive sleep apnoea/hypopnoea
MV	mechanical ventilation		OSF	organ system failure
MVO$_2$	mixed venous oxygen content		OT	oxygen therapy
MW	molecular weight		P	probability
6MW	6-min walk		PA	pulmonary artery; posterior-anterior
Na$^+$	sodium ion		PaCO$_2$	partial pressure of carbon dioxide in arterial blood/arterial carbon dioxide tension
NA	nucleos(t)ide analogue		PACO$_2$	alveolar PaCO$_2$
NAC	N-acetylcysteine		PAH	pulmonary arterial hypertension
nAchR	nicotine acetylcholine receptor		PAI	primary adrenal insufficiency
NCSE	non-convulsive status epilepticus		PAIR	percutaneous-aspiration-injection-re-aspiration
NES	non-epileptic seizures		PAN	polyarteritis nodosa
NF	necrotizing fasciitis		pANCA	perinuclear ANCA
NHS	National Health Service		PaO$_2$	partial pressure of oxygen in blood
NICE	National Institute for Health and Care Excellence		PAO$_2$	alveolar PO$_2$
NIPPV	non-invasive positive pressure ventilation		PAOP	pulmonary artery occlusion pressure
NIV	non-invasive ventilation		PAP	pulmonary artery pressure
NJ	nasojejunal		PASP	pulmonary artery systolic pressure
NK	natural killer		PAVM	pulmonary arteriovenous malformation
nm	nanometre		PAWP	pulmonary artery wedge pressure
NMJ	neuromuscular junction		PBC	primary biliary cirrhosis
NMO	neuromyelitis optica		PBD	post-burn day
nmol	nanomole		PBP	progressive bulbar palsy
NMS	neuroleptic malignant syndrome		PBS	physiologically balanced solution
NNRTI	non-nucleoside reverse transcriptase inhibitor		PCC	prothrombin complex concentrate
NO	nitric oxide		PCD	primary ciliary dyskinesia
NO$_2$	nitrogen dioxide		PCI	percutaneous coronary intervention; prophylactic cranial irradiation
NPV	negative pressure ventilation		PCNSL	primary CNS lymphoma
NRT	nicotine replacement therapy		PCP	pneumocystis pneumonia
NSAID	non-steroidal anti-inflammatory drug		PCR	polymerase chain reaction
NSCLC	non-small cell lung cancer		PCT	proximal convoluted tubule
NSIP	non-specific interstitial pneumonia		PCV	packed cell volume
NSP	non-starch polysaccharide		PCW	pulmonary capillary wedge
NST	nutritional support team			

PCWP	pulmonary capillary wedge pressure	PSA	prostate-specific antigen
PD	Parkinson's disease; peritoneal dialysis	PSC	primary sclerosing cholangitis
PDA	patent ductus arteriosus	PSG	polysomnography
PE	pulmonary embolism	PsNES	psychogenic non-epileptic seizures
PEA	pulseless electrical activity	PSP	primary spontaneous pneumothorax; progressive supranuclear gaze palsy
PEEP	positive end expiratory pressure		
PEF	peak expiratory flow	PSSS	pathology specific scoring system
PEFR	peak expiratory flow rate	PT	prothrombin time
PEG	percutaneous endoscopic gastrostomy	PTE	pulmonary thromboembolism
PEP	post-exposure prophylaxis	PTH	parathyroid hormone
PEPSE	PEP following sexual exposure	PTHrP	parathyroid hormone-related peptide
PET	positron emission tomography	PTLD	post-transplant lymphoproliferative disease
PFO	patent foramen ovale	PTU	propylthiouracil
PFT	pulmonary function test	PUJ	pelviureteric junction
PG	pyoderma gangrenosum	PV	pemphigus vulgaris
PGA	polyglandular autoimmune (disorder)	PVC	peripheral venous catheter
PhNES	physiological non-epileptic seizures	PVE	prosthetic valve endocarditis
PHS	parkinsonism-hyperpyrexia syndrome	qds	four times daily
PHT	pulmonary hypertension	QOL	quality of life
PI	protease inhibitor	RA	rheumatoid arthritis; refractory anaemia
PICC	peripherally inserted central catheter	RAADP	routine antenatal anti-D prophylaxis
PiCCO	pulsion continuous cardiac output monitor	RAAS	renin-angiotensin-aldosterone system
PICH	primary intracerebral haemorrhage	RAEB	refractory anaemia with excess of blasts
PIP	peak inspiratory pressure; proximal interphalangeal	RAP	right atrial pressure
		RAR	rapidly adapting 'irritant' receptor
PLS	primary lateral sclerosis	RAS	renal artery stenosis
PM	polymyositis	RB	respiratory bronchiolitis
PMA	progressive muscular atrophy	RBBB	right bundle branch block
PML	progressive multifocal leukoencephalopathy	RBC	red blood cell
PMN	polymorphonuclear neutrophil	RB-ILD	respiratory bronchiolitis-associated interstitial lung disease
pmol	picomole		
PMR	polymyalgia rheumatica	RCM	restrictive cardiomyopathy
PN	parenteral nutrition; pulmonary nodule	RCMD	refractory cytopenia with multilineage dysplasia
PNP	paraneoplastic pemphigus		
PO	*per os* (oral)	RCT	randomized controlled trial
PO_2	inspired oxygen partial pressure	REM	rapid eye movement
PO_4^-	phosphate ion	RF	respiratory failure
PP	placenta praevia	Rh	rheumatoid; rhesus
PPCI	primary percutaneous coronary intervention	rhAPC	recombinant human activated protein C
		RHC	right heart catheterization
PPD	phytophotodermatitis	RhF	rheumatoid factor
PPE	parapneumonic pleural effusions	RIC	reduced intensity conditioning
PPH	primary post-partum haemorrhage	RIG	rabies immune globulin
PPI	proton pump inhibitor	RNA	ribonucleic acid
PPV	positive pressure ventilation	ROSC	return of spontaneous circulation
PR	pulmonary rehabilitation	RPLS	reversible posterior leukoencephalopathy syndrome
PR3	proteinase 3		
prn	as required	RR	respiratory rate

RRR	relative risk reduction		SPS	simple partial seizures
RSE	refractory status epilepticus		SR	sarcoplasmic reticulum
RSI	rapid sequence induction		SS	serotonin syndrome; Sézary syndrome
RSV	respiratory syncytial virus		SSc	systemic sclerosis
rtPA	recombinant tissue-type plasminogen activator		SSC	Suviving Sepsis Campaign
			SSLR	serum sickness-like reaction
RTA	renal tubular acidosis; road traffic accident		SSPE	subacute sclerosing panencephalitis
RTS	revised trauma score		SSR	serum sickness reaction
RUQ	right upper quadrant		SSRI	selective serotonin reuptake inhibitor
RV	right ventricular; residual volume		SSSS	staphylococcal scalded skin syndrome
RVD	right ventricular dysfunction		STD	sexually transmitted disease
RVF	right ventricular failure		STEMI	ST segment elevation myocardial infarction
RVH	right ventricular hypertrophy		SUI	stress urinary incontinence
RVI	right ventricular infarction		SVCO	superior vena caval obstruction
RVSP	right ventricular systolic pressure		SvO_2	venous oxygen saturation
s	second		SVR	systemic vascular resistance
SA	sinoatrial		SVT	supraventricular tachycardia
sACE	serum angiotensin-converting enzyme		TAL	thick ascending loop
SaO_2	arterial oxygen saturation		TAVI	transaortic valve implantation
SAPS	simplified acute physiology score		TB	tuberculosis
SBP	spontaneous bacterial peritonitis		TBBx	transbronchial biopsy
SBT	Sengstaken–Blakemore tube		TBNA	transbronchial needle biopsy
SC	subcutaneous		TBSA	total body surface area
SCC	squamous cell cancer		TCC	transitional cell carcinoma
SCI	spinal cord injury		tds	three times daily
SCLC	small cell lung cancer		TEG	thromboelastography
SCM	sternocleidomastoid		TEN	toxic epidermal necrolysis
SCV	subclavian vein		TENS	transcutaneous nerve stimulation
SIADH	syndrome of inappropriate antidiuretic hormone		TF	tissue factor
SIMV	synchronized intermittent mandatory ventilation		TGA	transposition of the great arteries; transient global amnesia
SIRS	systemic inflammatory response syndrome		TGF	transforming growth factor
SISS	severity of illness scoring system		Th2	T helper 2
SjO_2	cerebral oxygen saturation		Ti	inspiratory time
SJS	Stevens–Johnson syndrome		TIA	transient ischaemic attack
SLE	systemic lupus erythematosus		TIBC	total iron-binding capacity
SLICC	Systemic Lupus International Collaborating Clinics		TII	toxic inhalational injury
SMA	spinal muscular atrophy		TIPS	transvenous intrahepatic portosystemic shunting
SMR	standard mortality ratio		TIPSS	transjugular intrahepatic portosystemic shunting
SO_2	sulphur dioxide		TLC	transient loss of consciousness
SOF	superior orbital fissure		TIMI	Thrombolysis In Myocardial Infarction
SOFA	sepsis-related organ failure assessment		TINU	tubulointerstitial nephritis and uveitis
SOL	space-occupying lesion		TLC	total lung capacity
SP	secondary pneumothorax		TLE	temporal lobe epilepsy
SpO_2	arterial oxygen saturation		TNF	tumour necrosis factor
spp.	species		TOE	transoesophageal echocardiography

ToF	tetralogy of Fallot		UTI	urinary tract infection
TOF	tracheo-oesophageal fistula		UUI	urge urinary incontinence
TP	traumatic pneumothorax		UV	ultraviolet
tPA	tissue plasminogen activator		V	volt
TPH	thrombophilia		VA	alveolar ventilation
TPMT	thiopurine methyltransferase		VAD	vascular access device
TPN	total parenteral nutrition		VAP	ventilator-associated pneumonia
TR	tricuspid regurgitation		VAS	visual analogue scale
TRALI	transfusion-associated lung injury		VATS	video-assisted thoracoscopic surgery
TRAPS	TNF-alpha receptor-associated periodic syndrome		VC	vital capacity
			VF	ventricular fibrillation
TRH	thyrotropin-releasing hormone		VHF	viral haemorrhagic fevers
TRISS	trauma injury severity score		VKA	vitamin K antagonist
TS	trauma score		VLDL	very low-density lipoprotein
TSH	thyroid-stimulating hormone		VMA	vanillyl mandelic acid
TSS	toxic shock syndrome		VOR	vestibulo-ocular reflexes
TST	tuberculin skin test		VP	ventriculoperitoneal
TT	thrombin time		VPA	valproic acid
TTE	transthoracic echocardiography		V/Q	ventilation-perfusion
TTKG	transtubular potassium gradient		VRE	vancomycin-resistant enterococci
TTP	thrombotic thrombocytopenic purpura		vs	versus
TTR	transthyretin		VSD	ventricular septal defect
Tv	tidal volume		VT	ventricular tachycardia
T2W	T2 weighted		VTE	venous thromboembolism
TXA1	thromboxane A2		VUR	vesicoureteric reflux
U	unit		v/v	volume by volume
UC	ulcerative colitis		vWD	von Willebrand's disease
U&E	urea and electrolytes		vWf	von Willebrand factor
UFH	unfractionated heparin		VZV	varicella-zoster virus
UI	urinary incontinence		W	watt
UIP	usual interstitial pneumonia		WBC	white blood cell
UK	United Kingdom		WCC	white cell count
ULN	upper limit of normal		WG	Wegener's granulomatosis
URTI	upper respiratory tract infection		WHO	World Health Organization
USA	United States of America		WoB	work of breathing
USS	ultrasound scan		ZN	Ziehl–Neelsen

Introduction to acute medicine

Introduction to acute medicine

In the acutely unwell patient, assessment of deranged physiology and immediate resuscitation often precedes diagnostic considerations because the initial history is often incomplete and limited examination and investigations often preclude classification by primary organ dysfunction, specific disease, or primary speciality. This initial diagnostic uncertainty, the requirement for immediate physiological support and/or simultaneous treatment of life-threatening abnormalities, and the need for ongoing modification of the diagnosis as the results of investigations and observed responses to therapy evolve define the speciality of acute medicine.

Many of the conditions causing acute illness will be discussed in detail in the later chapters. Only those aspects relevant to the initial, acute management phase will be discussed in this section.

Recognizing the acutely unwell patient

Early recognition that a patient's condition is deteriorating is essential. It should initiate immediate action to correct abnormal physiology and prevent damage to all vital organs.

Recognition of clinical severity is not difficult when the illness is far advanced and is usually obvious from the end of the bed. Typically, this is the case in patients with:

1. Sudden, catastrophic deterioration (e.g. pulmonary embolism, myocardial infarction).
2. Established severe illness, presenting acutely (e.g. COPD).
3. Advanced, but unrecognized, progressive deterioration on the ward (i.e. post-admission deterioration whilst on a hospital ward has been 'missed' by carers).

In such patients, organ damage may already have occurred, and, although established damage is difficult to reverse, immediate action may prevent progression. It is the failure to recognize progressive deterioration (i.e. 3 in list above), usually manifest as worsening physiological variables, and the subsequent delay in the initiation of preventative action, that is a common and unacceptable cause of morbidity and mortality.

Identification of 'at-risk' patients

Prevention of organ damage is always better than cure. Identifying 'at-risk' patients (e.g. medical and surgical emergencies, the elderly, post-surgical subjects, trauma victims, and those requiring massive blood transfusions) allows complications to be anticipated and prevented.

'At-risk' patients must be monitored, deterioration recognized, and appropriate action initiated early. Six simple physiological parameters, including temperature, oxygen saturation, blood pressure, heart rate, respiratory rate, and conscious level, correlate with mortality. Urine output is also an important and useful physiological variable, but it is not available in all patients and is consequently less useful in 'warning' systems.

Early warning scoring systems, based on these measures, promote early detection and trigger interventions aimed at preventing unnecessary cardiac arrests and critical care admissions. Urine output and disease-specific scoring systems can be used to further assess illness severity and prognosis.

The UK has introduced a validated National Early Warning Scoring system, based on the six physiological measures previously outlined. The national early warning score 'NEWS' (see Figure 1.1) is in common use. Each parameter can have a score from 0 to 3. The scores are summed and, if >4–5 (or single score of 3), require ward

PHYSIOLOGICAL PARAMETERS	3	2	1	0	1	2	3
Respiration rate	≤8		9–11	12–20		21–24	≥25
Oxygen saturations	≤91	92–93	94–95	≥96			
Any supplemental oxygen		Yes		No			
Temperature	≤35.0		35.1–36.0	36.1–38.0	38.1–39.0	≥39.1	
Systolic BP	≤90	91–100	101–110	111–219			≥220
Heart rate	≤40		41–50	51–90	91–110	111–130	≥131
Level of consciousness				A			V, P, or U

A = Alert, V = Voice, P = Pain, U = Unconsciousness
*The NEWS initiative flowed from the Royal College of Physicians' NEWS Development and Implementation Group (NEWSDIG) report and was jointly developed and funded in collaboration with the Royal College of Physicians, Royal College of Nursing, National Outreach Forum, and NHS Training for Innovation.

Figure 1.1 National Early Warning Score (NEWS)* Reproduced from Royal College of Physicians, 'National Early Warning Score (NEWS): Standardising the assessment of acute illness severity in the NHS', Report of a working party, London: RCP, 2012. © Royal College of Physicians 2012. <www.rcplondon.ac.uk/national-early-warning-score>

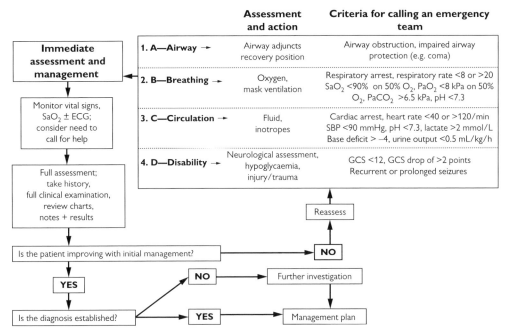

Figure 1.2 Acutely ill patient assessment. SaO_2, saturation; PaO_2, partial pressure of oxygen; $PaCO_2$, partial pressure of carbon dioxide; SBP, systolic blood pressure; GCS, Glasgow coma scale; ECG, electrocardiogram. Data from ALS, ALERT, ATLS, and the 'Care of the Critically Ill Surgical Patient' course.

nursing staff to summon medical assistance from teams composed of senior nurses and doctors familiar with assessment and management of the acutely unwell patient.

Assessment of the acutely ill patient

Figure 1.2 illustrates the immediate assessment and management of acutely ill patients and is based on a number of life support programmes, including the ALS, ALERT, ATLS, and the 'Care of the critically ill surgical patient' course. It is designed to ensure patient safety and survival, rather than establishing a diagnosis which must also be established. Regular reassessment and monitoring is essential to determine the effects of treatment.

At the onset of the assessment, simply asking the patient 'How are you?' or 'Are you alright?' provides important information. A normal response informs you that the patient's airway is patent and the patient is breathing, conscious, and orientated. No response indicates serious illness or unconsciousness. Likewise, a patient having difficulty speaking, or speaking in short gasping sentences, suggests serious breathlessness.

Assessment starts with the detection and simultaneous treatment of life-threatening emergencies. It uses the ABC system: **A**–Airway, **B**–Breathing, **C**–Circulation, in this order, as airways obstruction causes death faster than disordered breathing which, in turn, causes death faster than circulatory collapse due to haemorrhage or cardiac dysfunction. Appropriate lifesaving procedures or investigations are performed (e.g. airway clearance, decompression of tension pneumothorax) during initial assessment and/or examination (i.e. before the next step). Monitoring with pulse oximetry, cardiac monitors, and non-invasive blood pressure monitoring should be used to assist assessment.

Airways obstruction

Airways obstruction is a medical emergency and, unless rapidly corrected, leads to hypoxia, coma, and death within minutes. It may be complete or partial and can occur at any level in the upper respiratory tract from the mouth to the trachea.

- **Complete obstruction** is characterized by absent airflow, accessory muscle use, intercostal recession on inspiration, paradoxical abdominal movement, and absent breath sounds on chest auscultation.
- **Partial obstruction** reduces airflow despite increased respiratory effort. Breathing is often noisy with 'stridor', suggesting laryngeal and 'snoring' nasopharyngeal obstruction.

The causes of obstruction vary according to the site. Thus:

- Oropharyngeal obstruction may be due to aspiration of solid particulate matter, e.g. partially masticated food, coins, teeth, vomit, blood, or gastric fluid.
- Laryngeal oedema is often caused by allergies, burns, or inflammation, and laryngeal spasm is usually due to stimulation by foreign bodies, blood, or secretions.
- Tracheobronchial obstruction may result from bronchospasm, pulmonary oedema, aspiration of particulate matter (e.g. as for oropharyngeal obstruction), or bronchogenic carcinoma.
- The tongue may obstruct the pharynx in the drowsy or sedated patient.

Persistent airways obstruction causes a rapid fall in arterial oxygen tension (PaO_2), progressive hypoxic brain injury, coma, and death. Early recognition is based on the 'look, listen, and feel' approach:

Table 1.1 Clinical features of underlying lung disease

Disorder	Chest wall movement	Percussion note	Breath sounds	Added sounds
Consolidation	↓ on affected side	↓ dull	Bronchial	Coarse crackles
Collapse	↓↓ on affected side	↓ dull	Absent or bronchial	None
Pleural effusion	↓ on affected side	↓↓ stony dull	Diminished	None (± rub)
Pneumothorax	↓↓ on affected side	Normal or hyperresonant	Absent or diminished	None
Asthma/COPD	↓ on both sides Hyperinflation Accessory muscles	Normal or hyperresonant	Vesicular with prolonged expiratory phase	Expiratory wheeze

• **Look.** Is the patient making respiratory effort? Complete airways obstruction causes paradoxical chest and abdominal movement (i.e. during inspiratory effort, the chest moves 'in', instead of 'out', and the abdomen moves 'out', instead of 'in'), increased use of the accessory muscles of respiration (e.g. neck, shoulder), and tracheal tug. Central cyanosis (i.e. hypoxia) is a late sign of airways obstruction. The mouth should be examined for the cause of the obstruction, including foreign bodies and secretions.

• **Listen.** Partial obstruction reduces air entry and is noisy, whereas complete obstruction is silent with no breath sounds. Snoring occurs when the tongue is obstructing the pharynx, and stridor follows partial obstruction at the level of the larynx.

• **Feel** for air movement over the patient's mouth by placing your cheek or hand immediately in front of the patient's mouth.

Aspiration of partially masticated food is the most common cause of acute airways obstruction, giving rise to the 'café coronary'. Following aspiration of a large particle (e.g. food) that completely occludes the larynx or trachea, the subject is unable to speak or breathe and rapidly becomes cyanosed. If a sharp blow to the back of the chest fails to dislodge the particle, the Heimlich manoeuvre should be attempted. The attendant stands behind the patient, with his arms around the upper abdomen, just adjacent to the costal margin, and the hands clenched below the xiphoid process. The hands are pulled sharply backwards, compressing the upper abdomen and lower costal margin. The sudden increase in intrathoracic pressure may dislodge the obstructing particle, which is then exhaled by the patient.

Simple measures to open the airway are all that is required in many patients with acute airways obstruction. These include the chin-lift manoeuvre or insertion of an oropharyngeal (Guedel) airway. If oropharyngeal airway insertion is not possible (i.e. clenched teeth), the use of a soft nasopharyngeal airway may help. Tracheal intubation may be required to establish an airway if these methods fail. This may be performed without medication if the patient is already in extremis (e.g. cardiorespiratory arrest). If the patient is responsive and anaesthetic drugs are required, an anaesthetist or a physician with airways skills must be sought. Whilst awaiting the anaesthetist, simple positioning of the head and oropharyngeal mask ventilation, with 100% oxygen using a bag-valve-mask system, should be used to maintain the airway and ventilate the patient.

As a last resort, an emergency cricothyroidectomy should be attempted. A large bore needle is inserted through the cricothyroid membrane, which is palpable just below the thyroid cartilage. This will only be successful if the obstruction is at the level of the larynx. Oxygen should be fed down the needle or tube, if available. Urgent rigid bronchoscopy and/or thoracic surgery are required to remove the obstruction.

Breathing
The same 'look, listen, and feel' approach is used:

• **Look.** The most useful early sign that breathing is compromised is a respiratory rate <8 or >20/min and indicates the patient is at risk of sudden deterioration. Central cyanosis is usually a late sign. Examine depth, pattern, and symmetry (i.e. equality on both sides) of breathing, increased work of breathing (e.g. accessory muscle use, abdominal breathing), and chest wall expansion. Abnormal expansion, altered percussion note (e.g. hyperresonance), airways noise (e.g. stridor), and breath sounds may determine the cause of underlying lung disease (see Table 1.1). Chest wall deformity, jugular venous pressure (JVP), inspired oxygen concentration (FiO_2), saturation (SaO_2), measured by pulse oximetry, and abdominal distension (that may impede respiratory movement) should be noted.

• **Listen** for airways noise (e.g. rattling secretions), stridor, and wheeze (both with and without a stethoscope). Assess presence and quality of breath sounds to determine the cause of underlying lung disease.

• **Feel** for the position of the trachea to detect mediastinal shift. Assess depth and equality of chest movement, and percuss for hyperresonance (e.g. pneumothorax) or dullness (e.g. pleural fluid, consolidation). Table 1.1 illustrates typical physical signs in respiratory disorders.

Pulse oximetry is a useful measure of oxygenation but provides little information about the adequacy of ventilation, as it does not detect a raised $PaCO_2$ (i.e. SaO_2 normal but $PaCO_2$ high due to poor ventilation). Arterial blood gases (ABG) measure $PaCO_2$, pH, and HCO_3, in addition to PaO_2, and provide information about ventilation as well as oxygenation. The PaO_2 and SaO_2 should be >8 kPa and >90%, respectively, in the acutely ill patient. Respiratory acidosis (pH <7.35, $PaCO_2$ >6.0 kPa) or hypoxaemia, despite high flow oxygen therapy (SaO_2 <90%, PaO_2 <8 kPa), requires urgent intervention.

Specific treatment and management depends on the underlying cause. This, along with the use of oxygen therapy in respiratory failure associated with chronic obstructive pulmonary disease (COPD), is discussed in later sections (see Chapter 5). Initially most critically ill patients should receive oxygen therapy to prevent end-organ damage (see Chapter 5). The aim is to achieve a normal SaO_2 (94–98%), but, if this is not possible, aim for an SaO_2 >90%. To accomplish this, most acutely unwell patients are initially given high flow oxygen therapy (>10 L/min; FiO$_2$ 60–100%) via a reservoir, non-rebreathing mask.

In patients with COPD or type 2 respiratory failure, high oxygen concentrations may precipitate carbon dioxide retention. Nevertheless, hypoxia must still be avoided. Initial O$_2$ therapy (i.e. before blood gas measurements are available) is started at an FiO$_2$ ~35–40% and titrated to maintain the SaO$_2$ at ~88–92%. After blood gas measurement, controlled oxygen therapy with a fixed performance (24–35%) Venturi mask is preferable, aiming for an SaO$_2$ 88–92% (PaO$_2$ ~8 kPa; see Chapter 5). A higher SaO$_2$ has few advantages but may cause or exacerbate hypercapnia and respiratory acidosis. Arterial blood gases must be monitored regularly. If pH falls (<7.35) or if the patient becomes drowsy or fatigued, consider treatment with non-invasive ventilation (NIV).

Circulation
Hypovolaemia should be considered the primary cause of shock until proven otherwise. In surgical patients, haemorrhage, which is not always easily identified (i.e. intraperitoneal haemorrhage), must be considered. Unless there are obvious signs of fluid overload, any patient with cool peripheries and tachycardia should be given intravenous fluid.

As previously discussed, assess the circulation with the 'look, listen, and feel' approach:
- **Look** for cool, pale limbs and digits, peripheral cyanosis, and underfilled veins which indicate poor cardiac output. The capillary refill time (normally <2 seconds) can be assessed by applying cutaneous pressure for 5 seconds on a fingertip held at heart level and measuring the time for the colour to return when the pressure is released. Confusion and reduced urine output are further 'visual' features of poor cardiac output.
- **Listen** for cardiac murmurs, and measure the blood pressure. The initial blood pressure may be normal, as compensatory mechanisms (i.e. increased peripheral resistance) maintain the blood pressure despite a low cardiac output. Cardiac output has to fall by more than 20% (i.e. equivalent to the acute loss of a litre of blood) before blood pressure begins to fall. However, the pulse pressure (i.e. the difference between systolic and diastolic pressure which is normally about 40 mmHg) may narrow during arterial vasoconstriction (i.e. during hypovolaemia or cardiogenic shock), whereas diastolic blood pressure is low during arterial vasodilation (e.g. sepsis).
- **Feel** the peripheral and central pulses for rate, rhythm, and equality. Thready, fast pulses indicate a poor cardiac output, whereas a bounding pulse due to vasodilation, with increased cardiac output, often suggests sepsis (although late sepsis can also be associated with a thready, fast pulse (see Chapter 2)).

Initial stabilization of the circulation will depend on the cause of the circulatory failure. Immediately life-threatening conditions, including haemorrhage, cardiac tamponade, and massive pulmonary embolism, must be detected and treated. The aim is to replace fluid, control bleeding, and restore cardiac output, blood pressure, and tissue perfusion. Good venous access must be established, using wide-bore peripheral and central venous cannulae. In the absence of obvious fluid overload (i.e. failure to detect a raised jugular venous pressure (JVP) or coarse bilateral basal crepitations on lung auscultation), a crystalloid fluid challenge of 0.5–1 L should be given and the response assessed in terms of the pulse rate, blood pressure, and chest auscultation for crepitations.

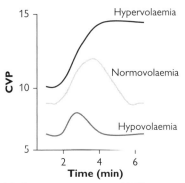

Figure 1.3 Central venous pressure (CVP) response to a 250–500 mL fluid challenge.

The response of the central venous pressure to a fluid challenge (see Figure 1.3) is a more useful measure of the patient's fluid status (i.e. hypovolaemic, normovolaemic, or hypervolaemic). Aim to restore the patient's blood pressure to its normal level (if known), or achieve a systolic blood pressure >100 mmHg.

If no improvement is seen with the initial fluid challenge, the challenge is repeated and the patient reassessed. If continuing fluid resuscitation fails to stabilize the vital signs or the patient develops cardiac failure, alternative means of improving cardiac output and tissue perfusion must be considered (i.e. inotropes, vasopressors). If large volumes of fluid are required, then ongoing reassessment for the cause of fluid loss is essential. If haemorrhage is the cause or suspected, send blood for cross-matching and repeat routine investigations, including full blood count, biochemistry, and clotting profiles.

Disability
Rapid assessment of the neurological status is performed by examining the pupils and by determining whether the patient is alert, responds to voice or to pain, or is unresponsive (AVPU). Patients with reduced conscious levels (i.e. Glasgow coma scale (GCS) <8) should be managed on HDU or ICU.

Hypoglycaemia must be excluded with a dextrostix or glucometer. If below 3 mmol/L, laboratory glucose should be taken and dextrose administered orally or intravenously, depending on clinical condition. Severe or refractory hypoglycaemia (e.g. sulfonylurea or insulin overdose) may require hydrocortisone therapy, and these patients must be admitted for blood sugar monitoring (± glucose infusions). Box 1.1 illustrates common causes of unconsciousness. It is

Box 1.1 Common causes of unconsciousness

Hypoglycaemia
Hypoxia (e.g. cardiac arrest, shock, respiratory failure)
Drugs (e.g. opiates, alcohol, sedatives)
Metabolic (e.g. liver failure, hypothermia, hypothyroidism, thiamine deficiency)
Vascular (i.e. stroke), including intracranial haemorrhage or infarction
Inflammation (e.g. cerebral vasculitis)
Cerebral tumour
Head trauma
Hypercapnia

essential the whole body is examined for evidence of injury, ischaemia, or trauma (e.g. an unrecognized fractured hip in the unconscious subject).

Unconscious patients with spontaneous ventilation and circulation should be nursed in the lateral recovery position, as they are at risk of developing airways obstruction. In addition, protective airway reflexes may be insufficient to prevent inhalation of secretions or vomit. If there is any risk of cervical injury, the patient should be left supine, with constant medical attention to ensure airway patency. If the patient has to be turned, they should be 'log-rolled' into the lateral recovery position by several members of staff.

Full patient assessment

When the cardiorespiratory system has been stabilized, the patient is improving and assistance has been summoned, a full assessment is required. Review the patient's notes and charts (including the drug chart); take a full history; perform a complete clinical examination, and review the results of investigations. If the diagnosis has not been satisfactorily established, further history and investigations should be undertaken. If the diagnosis is clear, the management plan must be communicated to the medical team, including nursing and ancillary staff, and documented in the notes.

Management of the acutely unwell patient frequently involves several teams (e.g. medicine, surgery, critical care), but care should be a 'seamless' process, in which cooperation, communication, and patient interests are foremost. Treatment should occur in clinical areas where staffing and technical support are matched to patient needs (as discussed in the next section).

Organization of acute medical admission wards

Acute medical units (AMUs) provide staffing, monitoring and treatment for patients with potentially reversible, life-threatening conditions that may not be available on general wards. Patients should be managed and moved between clinical areas where the staffing and technical support match the severity of illness and clinical needs of the patient. Five types of ward area are described:

- **Level 3** (e.g. intensive care units (ICU)). Level 3 patients usually have multi-organ failure, requiring inotropic support and/or renal replacement therapy, and may require mechanical ventilation.
- **Level 2** (e.g. high dependency units (HDU), AMU, emergency resuscitation rooms, post-operative recovery areas). Level 2 patients need intensive nursing or invasive monitoring (i.e. central or arterial lines), non-invasive ventilation, and inotropic support. Some level 2 units may provide renal replacement therapy.
- **Level 1** (e.g. AMU, coronary care units). Level 1 patients usually require non-invasive monitoring (e.g. ECG, saturation, BP) and close observation. There is often overlap between level 1 and 2 areas.
- **General or specialist wards** (e.g. chest or surgical wards).
- **Self-care wards** (e.g. 'hotel' accommodation).

Acute medicine encompasses the initial resuscitation, monitoring, investigation, diagnosis, and treatment of acutely unwell patients (including levels 1 and 2), usually for the first 24–48 hours of care, and 40–50% are discharged home within this period, following diagnosis and initial treatment. Subsequent follow-up and management continue in the community or outpatient setting. If ongoing inpatient therapy is required, the patient is transferred to a specialist ward when clinically stable.

Admission and discharge guidelines

Admission and discharge guidelines facilitate efficient use of resources and ensure patients receive appropriate treatment. For example, aggressive hospital treatment may be inappropriate in advanced disease, and patients should be treated in a setting (e.g. hospice) appropriate to their needs. Resuscitation status should always be documented.

Factors determining admission criteria include the primary diagnosis, illness severity, likely success of treatment, comorbid illness, life expectancy, potential quality of life post-discharge, and the patient's (and relatives') wishes. Age alone should not be a contraindication to admission, and each case is judged on merit. If there is uncertainty, the patient should be given the benefit of the doubt and active treatment continued until further information is available.

Discharge from the AMU occurs when the patient is physiologically stable and independent of monitoring and support. Overnight transfers and discharges should be avoided, if possible. The ongoing carer (e.g. medical ward team, general practitioner, family physician, care home nurses) must be fully appraised at verbal handover or in writing.

In patients with no realistic hope of recovery, and after family consultation, withdrawal of therapy may be appropriate. If possible, organ donation should be tactfully discussed with the relatives. In this situation, ongoing care must remain positive to ensure death with dignity.

General supportive care

Optimal care is best delivered by a multi-skilled team of doctors, nurses, occupational therapists, physiotherapists, and pharmacists, as acute illness predisposes to a wide range of potential secondary complications. Many of these can be prevented or alleviated by early prophylactic intervention. They include:

- Fluid and electrolyte imbalance (e.g. Na^+, K^+, Ca^{2+} depletion).
- Respiratory (e.g. atelectasis).
- Venous thromboembolism.
- Hospital-acquired infections (e.g. *C. difficile*).
- Neurological (e.g. muscle wasting).
- Endocrine (e.g. glucose intolerance).
- Constipation.
- Pressure sores.
- Cardiovascular (e.g. autonomic failure).

The importance of skilled nursing and ancillary therapy in the management of these patients cannot be overemphasized. Assessment, continuous monitoring and intervention, nutrition, drug administration, comfort (e.g. analgesia, toilette), reassurance, psychological support, assistance with communication, advocacy, skin care, positioning and physiotherapy (e.g. to prevent aspiration, atelectasis, pressure sores), feeding, and early detection of clinical complications (e.g. line infection) are all vital interventions which have a profound effect on outcome.

Severity of illness scoring systems

Severity of illness scoring systems (SISS) were developed to calculate mortality risks in comparable groups of critically ill hospital patients. They facilitate descriptions of case mix, allow stratification for clinical trials, and aid comparison of predicted and observed outcomes. However, at present, they are not sufficiently accurate to allow outcome prediction in individual patients. EWS scores are in common use in AMUs. SISS scores are used in level 2 and 3 intensive care units (ICUs) and less commonly in AMUs.

Physiological SISS that have been validated include:

- **The acute physiology and chronic health evaluation score (APACHE) II.** This has been demonstrated to predict hospital mortality in specific diagnostic cohorts of hospital patients. It is not designed for, and should not be used to assess, the outcome in individual patients. It is rarely used outwith intensive care units. Scoring is based on:
  - Primary disease process—50 diagnostic categories.
  - Physiological reserve, including age and chronic health history (e.g. chronic cardiovascular, respiratory, renal, liver, and immune conditions).
  - Severity of illness, determined from the worst values observed in the first 24 hours of 12 acute physiological variables, including rectal temperature, mean blood pressure, heart rate, respiratory rate (RR), arterial PaO_2, pH, serum sodium, potassium and creatinine, haematocrit, white cell count, and Glasgow Coma Score (GCS).

Predicted mortality, by diagnosis, has been calculated from large databases. It has been less useful in narrow diagnostic groups (e.g. trauma, AIDS) which were not a major part of the original database. The score allows individual ICUs to compare their performance against reference ICUs, using standard mortality ratio (SMR = observed mortality ÷ predicted mortality) for each diagnostic group. A high SMR (>1.5) should prompt investigation and management changes for specific conditions.

APACHE III is an upgraded version of the APACHE II score, based on a larger reference database, and uses 17 physiological variables and 78 diagnostic categories.

- **The simplified acute physiology score II (SAPS II)** is similar to APACHE II but does not use diagnostic groupings. It has equivalent accuracy and is the most commonly used scoring system in European ICUs. SAPS II uses 12 physiological variables and identifies specific chronic health conditions (e.g. AIDS, haematological malignancy, cirrhosis, and metastases). The probability of death can be calculated from logistic regression equations, based on acute physiology scores and chronic health weightings.
- **Organ failure scores** use the number and duration of five potential organ system failures (OSFs) to determine the probability of mortality. A single OSF lasting 1 day has a mortality of 30%; two OSFs for 1 day have a mortality rate of 60%, and three or more OSFs lasting 3 days have a mortality rate of 90%. Increasing age increases mortality risk. The multiple organ dysfunction score (MODS) is based on six organ systems (respiratory, renal, neurological, cardiovascular, hepatic, and haematological) and takes account of grades of dysfunction and supportive therapy to produce a first-day score (maximum 24) which correlates with mortality.

A number of pathology specific scoring systems (PSSS) have been validated in specific (usually surgical or trauma) patient groups.

- **Trauma score (TS)** assesses triage status, based on RR, respiratory effort, systolic blood pressure, capillary refill, and GCS. A high score indicates the need for transfer to a trauma centre. The revised TS (RTS) uses only GCS,

Table 1.2 Glasgow coma score

Eyes	Open	Spontaneously	4
		To verbal command	3
		To pain	2
		No response	1
Best motor response	Verbal command	Obeys	6
		Localizes pain	5
	Painful stimuli	Flexion—withdrawal	4
		Flexion—decorticate	3
		Extension—decerebrate	2
		No response	1
Best verbal response		Orientated, converses	5
		Disorientated, converses	4
		Inappropriate words	3
		Incomprehensible sounds	2
		No response	1
Total			3–15

Eye opening, best motor and best verbal responses are scored (as shown in the table) and then summed to achieve the Glasgow coma score of 3–15.

Reprinted from *The Lancet*, 304, G Teasdale and B Jennett, 'Assessment of coma and impaired consciousness: a practical scale', pp. 81–84, Copyright 1974, with permission from Elsevier.

respiratory rate, and systolic blood pressure, with improved prognostic reliability, but is less suitable for triage.

- **Injury severity score (ISS)** assesses the extent of anatomical injury. A value of 1 (minor injury) to 6 (unsurvivable) is given to each of six body regions and incorporates a modification for blunt and penetrating injury. The sum of the squares of the injury value in the three most severely damaged body regions correlates with mortality. The maximum score will be 75 (i.e. $5^2 + 5^2 + 5^2 = 75$), as the highest regional score is 5 (i.e. 6 is unsurvivable). A score >16 is defined as severe trauma and correlates with a mortality >10%.
- **Trauma injury severity score (TRISS)** combines ISS and RTS to improve outcome prediction.
- **Glasgow coma score (GCS)** quantifies the level of consciousness after the first 6 hours of head injury (see Table 1.2). It individually scores best eye opening, verbal and motor responsiveness, providing an overall scale between 3 (profound coma) and 15 (normal alert state). The scoring consistency between observers is good. This allows head injury management protocols to be based on initial presentation scores and decisions to be determined by trends in the score and provides some indication of prognosis when combined with age. The GCS is included in a number of other scoring systems.
- **Sepsis-related organ failure assessment (SOFA)** was originally developed to monitor sepsis. It assesses six organs (brain, respiratory, cardiovascular, hepatic, kidney, and coagulation) and scores organ function from 0 (normal) to 4 (extremely abnormal). Although useful for tracking change, it was not designed to assess outcome probability.

The hypotensive patient and 'shock'

Hypotension (i.e. low blood pressure) is a common problem. It is often preceded by warning signs of tachycardia (or bradycardia), nausea, and cold 'clammy' sweating. Most people have experienced these symptoms as a precursor to fainting (i.e. vasovagal hypotension). In general, hypotension is a late sign of a compromised circulation, as

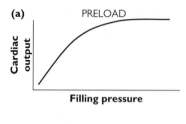

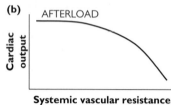

Figure 1.4. Cardiac output response of the normal heart to preload and afterload.

compensatory mechanisms (i.e. increased peripheral resistance) tend to maintain blood pressure despite a low cardiac output. However, prolonged hypotension results in poor perfusion and potential damage to the major organ systems (e.g. brain, kidneys). It should be regarded as an emergency requiring immediate intervention and detection of the cause.

Systemic blood pressure is determined by the cardiac output and the systemic vascular resistance (SVR). A reduction in either cardiac output and/or SVR can cause hypotension. Three factors determine cardiac output:

- **Preload** is the 'filling pressure' on the right or left sides of the heart and reflects the amount of blood returning to the right ventricle from the tissues or to the left ventricle from the pulmonary circulation. The relationship between preload and cardiac output is shown in Figure 1.4. If the filling pressure falls, so will the cardiac output. Hypovolaemia due to fluid loss (e.g. haemorrhage, diarrhoea, vomiting, burns) is the commonest cause of decreased preload. However, reduction of SVR (i.e vasodilation) and/or altered distribution of the circulating blood volume can cause a 'relative' hypovolaemia and a fall in cardiac output. This may be due to sepsis, allergic reactions, drugs, or epidural analgesia.
- **Contractility** is a measure of the strength of cardiac contraction. If contractility is reduced and the heart is unable to pump effectively, cardiac output will fall. Reduced cardiac contractility can be due to myocardial infarction, severe sepsis, valve dysfunction, pulmonary embolism, arrhythmias (which can also affect preload), or cardiac tamponade.
- **Afterload** is the resistance to ejection of blood from the heart and approximates to the 'vascular resistance'. If SVR increases, cardiac output will fall (see Figure 1.4b). However, in practice, hypotension is rarely due to an increase in SVR. In contrast, a fall in SVR often causes hypotension and is usually associated with an increase in cardiac output. Sepsis and allergy are the commonest causes of a fall in SVR and initially cause hypotension with a high cardiac output. Reductions in sympathetic nervous stimulation (i.e. tone) will also reduce SVR, e.g. in high spinal cord damage or with drugs.

Oxygenation is dependent on the flow of blood to tissues. Most organs require a mean arterial blood pressure (BP) >55–65 mmHg to maintain adequate perfusion (i.e. where mean BP = diastolic BP + (systolic BP − diastolic BP/3)). In individual organs, hypotension has the following effects:

- **Kidney.** If mean renal blood pressure falls to <60 mmHg, glomerular filtration decreases and urine production falls. Consequently, urine output is a good indicator of renal perfusion. A urine output below 0.5–1 mL/kg/h indicates poor renal perfusion. Oliguria (<0.5 mL/kg/h) for more than 2 hours indicates the need for immediate intervention if renal damage (acute tubular necrosis) is to be prevented.
- **Cerebral.** Falling conscious level (i.e. a decrease in GCS >2 points) suggests reduced cerebral perfusion pressure and the need for an immediate increase in the blood pressure.
- **Heart.** Coronary blood flow depends on diastolic blood pressure. Hypotension reduces coronary artery filling, causing myocardial ischaemia (or infarction) and a reduction in cardiac contractility.
- **Skin.** A fall in blood pressure reduces skin perfusion (i.e. cold, clammy skin).
- **Gastrointestinal tract.** Reduced gut perfusion may lead to splanchnic ischaemia, with bacterial translocation and subsequent sepsis.

Shock

Shock is discussed in detail in Chapters 2 and 4, and only the essential features will be considered in this section.

Definition

Shock is a loosely defined term used to describe the clinical syndrome that occurs with hypotension and acute circulatory failure. It causes inadequate or inappropriately distributed tissue perfusion. The resulting failure to meet tissue metabolic demands results in generalized cellular hypoxia (with or without lactic acidosis) and tissue damage.

The causes of shock and associated hypotension can be classified into six categories:

- **Hypovolaemic shock** due to major reductions in circulating blood volume caused by haemorrhage, plasma loss (e.g. burns, pancreatitis), or extracellular fluid loss (e.g. diabetic ketoacidosis, trauma).
- **Septic shock** that occurs with infection or septicaemia (e.g. E. coli, Candida). Vasodilation, arteriovenous shunting, and capillary damage cause subsequent hypotension and maldistribution of flow.
- **Cardiogenic shock** is due to severe heart failure (e.g. myocardial infarction, acute mitral regurgitation).
- **Obstructive shock** occurs in response to circulatory obstruction (e.g. pulmonary embolism, cardiac tamponade).
- **Neurogenic (spinal) shock** follows high traumatic spinal cord lesions (above T6). Interruption of sympathetic outflow causes vasodilation, hypothermia, and bradycardia. Unopposed vagal stimulation (e.g. pain, hypoxia) may cause profound bradycardia.
- **Anaphylactic shock** is due to allergen-induced vasodilation (e.g. bee sting, peanut, and other food allergies).

Clinical features

The general features of shock include systolic hypotension (<90 mmHg), tachycardia (>100 beats/min), oliguria (urine output <0.5 mL/kg/h), rapid respiration (>30/min), and drowsiness, confusion, or agitation. Specific clinical features depend on the underlying cause (e.g. haemorrhage, sepsis, pulmonary embolism) and associated severity. Typically, shock presents as one of two clinical patterns, depending on the cause, stage, or severity:

- **'Warm and dilated' shock** is seen in early septic and anaphylactic shock. It is associated with warm peripheries, flushing (i.e. skin vasodilation), bounding pulses, and a high cardiac output due to reduced SVR.
- **'Cold and clammy' shock** is characteristic of hypovolaemic, cardiogenic, and obstructive shock. It is also seen in late or severe septic or anaphylactic shock. It is associated with cold peripheries (i.e. skin vasoconstriction), weak pulses, and evidence of low cardiac output (e.g. oliguria, peripheral cyanosis, confusion).

Investigations
These should include routine blood tests, arterial blood gases, cardiac enzymes, lactic acid measurement, and blood cross-matching if haemorrhage is suspected. Vital signs must be monitored, including temperature, blood pressure, respiratory rate, urine output, and SaO_2.

Circulatory assessment may require measurement of central venous pressure (CVP), intra-arterial blood pressure, echocardiography, and ECG monitoring. Additional measurements are occasionally necessary, including cardiac output, pulmonary capillary wedge pressure (PCWP), SVR, and central venous oxygen saturation (SvO_2).

Chest or abdominal radiographs may be required. In sepsis microbiological examination of blood, sputum, and urine samples is required.

Clinical assessment
The clinical features, CVP, and SVR define the cause of shock. Measurement of CVP, PCWP, and SVR are useful when clinical signs are difficult to interpret. For example:

- **CVP** is reduced in hypovolaemic and anaphylactic shock and elevated in cardiogenic and obstructive shock. In sepsis and septic shock, the CVP may be low, normal, or high at various stages.
- **SVR** is high in cardiogenic shock, with sympathetic-mediated vasoconstriction (i.e. 'cold, clammy' patient), and low in septic vasodilation due to release of inflammatory mediators (i.e. 'warm, dilated' patient).

Consequently, simple haemodynamic patterns may aid diagnosis in the acutely unwell, hypotensive patient:

Hypovolaemic shock: low CVP/PCWP + low CO + high SVR

Cardiogenic shock: high CVP/PCWP + low CO + high SVR

Septic shock: low CVP/PCWP + high CO + low SVR

Complications
Shock with circulatory failure and tissue hypoxia leads to multi-organ failure, including acute respiratory distress syndrome (ARDS), systemic inflammatory response syndrome (SIRS), acute kidney injury with acute tubular necrosis (ATN), disseminated intravascular coagulation (DIC), hepatic failure, and mucosal ulceration.

A cycle of increasing 'oxygen debt' and 'shock-induced' tissue damage develops with reduced myocardial contractility and hypoxaemia (e.g. due to ARDS), further impairing oxygen delivery and tissue oxygenation.

Ischaemic damage to the intestinal mucosa causes bacterial and toxin translocation into the splanchnic, and subsequently systemic, circulation, causing further organ impairment and sepsis. Eventually, 'refractory' shock develops, with irreversible tissue damage and death.

General management
The aims are to correct the underlying cause, reverse the tissue 'oxygen debt', and prevent progressive organ damage. Treatment of cardiogenic, hypovolaemic, obstructive (e.g pulmonary embolism), septic, and allergic/anaphylactic shock are discussed in subsequent chapters. However, the management of shock has a number of common features:

1. **Identify the cause** (e.g. obstructive, septic).
2. **Early treatment is essential.** Mortality increases if shock lasts for more than 1 hour, giving rise to the concept of 'the golden hour' and emphasizing the importance of immediate action.
3. **Correct hypoxaemia** with high flow supplemental oxygen. In the absence of lung disease, severe shock will cause hypoxia due to reduced pulmonary blood flow, ventilation-perfusion (V/Q) mismatch, and a low SvO_2.
4. **Resuscitation** requires appropriate fluid management and is dependent on the cause of shock and the time course of the illness. For example, in hypovolaemic shock with a low CVP, fluid replacement is required. In contrast, in cardiogenic shock due to left-sided heart failure (i.e. with a raised CVP), diuretic therapy with fluid restriction may be indicated. To complicate matters further, cardiogenic shock due to right-sided heart failure (i.e. also with a raised CVP) may require fluid administration to ensure adequate filling of, and cardiac output from, the left side of the heart! The time course of the disease is also important. For example, at the onset of septic shock, fluid replacement is essential, but, if acute respiratory distress syndrome develops later, fluid restriction is necessary to prevent pulmonary oedema.
5. **Inotropic support** is required when hypotension (i.e. mean arterial pressure <60 mmHg) or tissue hypoxaemia (e.g. oliguria) persists, despite adequate fluid replacement, or when fluid resuscitation is contraindicated (e.g. cardiogenic shock). The type of inotropic support will depend on the cause of the shock. For example:
   - **In septic shock** (i.e. 'warm, dilated' patient), the cardiac output is high, but vasodilation (i.e. low SVR) may cause hypotension, inadequate tissue perfusion, and organ hypoxia, with oliguria and confusion. In this situation, noradrenaline, a peripheral vasoconstrictor (alpha-receptor agonist), increases the SVR, restoring blood pressure and tissue perfusion.
   - **In cardiogenic or late septic shock** (i.e. 'cold, clammy' patient), the cardiac output is low due to poor myocardial contractility and a high SVR due to sympathetic vasoconstriction. Treatment with dobutamine, which increases myocardial contractility and causes vasodilation (i.e. reduces SVR), results in increased blood pressure and cardiac output.
6. **Remove circulatory obstructions.** For example:
   - Thrombolysis may be required in massive pulmonary embolism.
   - Drainage of a tension pneumothorax that is compressing the heart and preventing right ventricular filling.
   - Drainage of a pericardial effusion that is causing cardiac tamponade.
   - Correction of disseminated intravascular coagulation to prevent microcirculatory obstruction.
7. **Intubation and ventilation.** The indications for intubation and mechanical ventilation include:
   - Progressive hypoxaemia (PaO_2 <8 kPa on >40% O_2).
   - Hypercapnia ($PaCO_2$ >7.5 kPa).

- Respiratory rate >35 breaths/min.
- Respiratory or metabolic acidosis (pH <7.2).
- Cardiac or respiratory arrest.
- Physical factors (e.g. exhaustion, impaired consciousness, confusion, airways protection).

In obtunded patients, the high risk of aspiration necessitates a low threshold for intubation. Ventilatory support reduces work of breathing, improves cardiac function, and increases tissue oxygen delivery. Non-invasive ventilation (e.g. CPAP) may avoid the need for intubation.

8. **Correction of severe acidosis** which can impair cardiac contractility. Sodium bicarbonate infusion is controversial but may be considered when pH is <7.1 with a normal $PaCO_2$ (i.e. negative base excess >—8).

The 'blue (cyanosed) and breathless' patient

Hypoxia (i.e. inadequate tissue oxygen for normal metabolism) occurs within 4 minutes of failure to deliver oxygenated blood to the organs and tissues (e.g. cardiac or respiratory arrest), as local oxygen reserves in tissues are small. The causes are:

1. Respiratory failure due to inadequate gas exchange.
   - **Type 1 respiratory failure** describes failure of oxygenation and occurs when blood bypasses or is not fully oxygenated in the lungs, causing hypoxaemia (PaO_2 <8.0 kPa or SaO_2 <90%). The $PaCO_2$ is normal (~5.3 kPa) or low because ventilation is unchanged or increased. The causes include ventilation-perfusion (V/Q) mismatch (see section on ventilation-perfusion (V/Q) mismatch), right-to-left shunts, diffusion defects, and low inspired oxygen (FiO_2) levels (hypobaric) as occurs at high altitudes. In these circumstances, oxygenation can usually be improved by re-expanding ('recruiting') collapsed alveoli, oxygen therapy, and reducing V/Q mismatch. This will not be possible if there is a large right-to-left shunt.
   - **Type 2 respiratory failure** is due to inadequate ventilation with associated alveolar hypoventilation. A fall in alveolar ventilation (VA) due to a reduction in respiratory rate or a fall in tidal volume increases $PaCO_2$. This is because $PaCO_2$ is inversely proportional to VA (i.e. $PaCO_2 = 1/VA$) such that, if alveolar ventilation doubles, $PaCO_2$ halves and, if alveolar ventilation halves, $PaCO_2$ doubles.

   The relationship between $PaCO_2$ and alveolar PO_2 (PAO_2) is described by the alveolar gas equation (see Box 1.2). Hypoventilation (see section on hypoventilation) is the commonest cause of type 2 respiratory failure. This causes failure of alveolar carbon dioxide clearance and subsequent arterial hypercapnia ($PaCO_2$ >6–6.5 kPa), with or without hypoxaemia. With hypoventilation, it would be expected that the alveolar-arterial oxygen difference would be <1 kPa, which assists in differentiating it from other causes of hypoxaemia (see next section).

2. **Failure of oxygen transport** is due to reduced blood flow, anaemia, or haemoglobinopathy. In low output cardiac states, high concentration oxygen therapy (FiO_2 >60%) only marginally improves oxygenation because the haemoglobin is fully saturated and the solubility of oxygen in blood is low. These patients require early restoration of tissue blood flow (e.g. blood transfusion or an increase in cardiac output). In carbon monoxide poisoning,

---

Box 1.2 Alveolar oxygen tension and alveolar-arterial oxygen tension difference

Alveolar oxygen tension: as derived from the simplified alveolar gas equation

$$PAO_2 = PIO_2 - (1.25 \times PaCO_2)$$

Where:

$PIO_2 = FiO_2 \times (\text{barometric} - \text{water vapour pressure})$

Thus when breathing air: $PIO_2 = 0.21 \times (101 - 6.2) = 19.9$ kPa

$$PAO_2 \text{ (breathing air)} = 19.9 - (1.25 \times 5.3)$$
$$= \sim13.3 \text{ kPa}$$

Alveolar-arterial oxygen tension difference

$$P(A\text{-}a)O_2 = PAO_2 - PaO_2$$
$$= \sim13.3 - \sim13 = <1.0 \text{ kPa (breathing air)}$$

PaO_2, arterial oxygen tension; $PaCO_2$, arterial CO_2 tension; PAO_2, alveolar oxygen tension; PIO_2, inspired oxygen tension; FiO_2, fractional concentration of oxygen in inspired air; P(A-a) O_2, alveolar-arterial oxygen tension difference.

---

high-dose oxygen therapy (or hyperbaric oxygen) is essential, despite a normal PaO_2, to reduce carboxyhaemoglobin half-life (see Chapters 5 and 18).

3. **Failure of tissue oxygen utilization** occurs during sepsis or poisoning (e.g. cyanide) and is due to failure of cellular (mitochondrial) utilization despite good oxygen delivery.

Clinical features

Successful therapy requires early recognition of tissue hypoxia. The clinical features are often non-specific, including altered mental state, dyspnoea, hyperventilation, cyanosis, arrhythmias, and hypotension, and are often missed or attributed to an alternative cause.

Cyanosis describes the 'blue' discoloration in the skin, lips, or tongue which occurs when the blood passing through these tissues contains more than 1.5 g/dL of reduced (deoxygenated) haemoglobin, which causes the blood to change colour from bright red to deep blue. Cyanosis can be peripheral or central.

- Peripheral cyanosis describes a 'blue discoloration' of the peripheries (e.g. hands and feet) whilst the tongue and lips remain 'pink'. It occurs when the blood flow in the peripheral circulation is slow or reduced (i.e. with heart failure, hypovolaemia, or cold) which allows increased time for the tissues to extract oxygen from blood, increasing the concentration of deoxygenated blood and causing the tissue to appear blue.
- Central cyanosis causes 'blue discoloration' of the tongue and lips as well as the peripheral tissues. It is usually due to a reduction in PaO_2 (or SaO_2). Common acute causes include pneumonia, pulmonary oedema, acute embolism, severe asthma, and pneumothorax. Chronic causes include right-to-left shunts, polycythaemia, COPD, and fibrotic lung disease.

Polycythaemic patients have raised haemoglobin levels and almost always have more than 1.5 g/dL of deoxygenated haemoglobin, and so appear cyanosed, although they may not be hypoxic. In contrast, anaemic patients are less likely to generate 1.5 g/dL of deoxygenated haemoglobin and rarely appear cyanosed, although they may be profoundly hypoxic. Consequently, cyanosis does not always indicate the patient is hypoxic.

Causes of a fall in PaO_2 with associated central cyanosis are:

1. Hypoventilation.
2. Ventilation/perfusion (V/Q) mismatch in the lungs.
3. Impaired gas transfer in the lungs.
4. Right-to-left intracardiac shunts.

Most of the conditions that can cause hypoxaemia (e.g. pulmonary oedema, pulmonary embolism, pneumonia, etc.) will be discussed in later chapters. Similarly, oxygen therapy is discussed in Chapter 5 and is not repeated in this section.

Hypoventilation
The causes of hypoventilation include respiratory muscle weakness (e.g. myasthenia gravis), chest wall deformity (e.g. kyphoscoliosis), impaired respiratory drive (e.g. opioid overdose, CNS disease), and excessive work of breathing (e.g. exhaustion, COPD, pulmonary oedema, and, rarely, asthma). Hypoventilation is characterized by an increased alveolar and arterial blood carbon dioxide concentration ($PACO_2$ and $PaCO_2$, respectively). As $PaCO_2$ rises, PAO_2, and consequently PaO_2, will fall (see Box 1.2). In this situation, hypoxaemia can be corrected with higher inspired oxygen concentrations (FiO_2). However, to correct the elevated $PaCO_2$, alveolar ventilation (VA) must be improved by:

1. Providing additional ventilatory support (e.g. non-invasive ventilation or mechanical ventilation).
2. Reversing drug-induced CNS depression (e.g. naloxone for opiate overdosage).
3. Reducing airways resistance (e.g. bronchodilation in obstructive airways disease or secretion clearance).
4. Decreasing work of breathing (e.g. reinflating collapsed alveoli).
5. Improving lung compliance (e.g. lung stiffness can be reduced in heart failure by treating pulmonary oedema).

6. Ensuring good chest wall positioning (i.e. optimizing the mechanical advantage of respiratory muscles).

Ventilation-perfusion (V/Q) mismatch
Under normal circumstances, ventilation (V) and blood flow (Q) are matched, which ensures almost complete saturation of haemoglobin with oxygen as it passes through the lungs. In patients with pneumonia, areas of consolidated lung are poorly ventilated, whereas blood flow may be maintained, resulting in failure of blood to be oxygenated in these areas. Blood that fails to be oxygenated, as it passes from the right side to the left side of the heart, is termed 'shunt', and, in a normal patient, the shunt is <2–3% of total blood flow. The effect of V/Q mismatch is to 'shunt' more blood through the lungs (or heart septal defects), resulting in a reduction in blood oxygenation and arterial hypoxaemia. V/Q mismatch is the commonest cause of arterial hypoxaemia and occurs in most acute respiratory diseases (e.g. pneumonia, ARDS, asthma, COPD, and pulmonary oedema).

The specific treatment will depend on the cause. Initially, supplemental oxygen is given to achieve an SaO_2 >90% (PaO_2 >8 kPa), aiming for 94–98% in the absence of known type 2 respiratory failure. As the shunt increases (termed shunt fraction), increasing inspired oxygen concentration (FiO_2) is less effective at correcting arterial hypoxaemia. Shunts greater than 30% are always associated with a degree of hypoxaemia (see Figure 1.5a). Similarly, the type of shunt affects the response to supplemental oxygen, and Figure 1.5b illustrates the effect of a few areas of marked V/Q mismatch (i.e very reduced ventilation with almost complete shunt), compared to many areas of relatively mild V/Q mismatch (i.e. some alveolar oxygenation). In patients with V/Q mismatch, the alveolar-arterial oxygen difference ($PAO_2 - PaO_2$) would be expected to be greater than 1 kPa and will assist in differentiating it from hypoventilation (see Box 1.2).

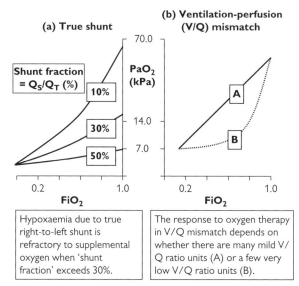

(a) True shunt

(b) Ventilation-perfusion (V/Q) mismatch

Shunt fraction = Q_S/Q_T (%)

10%

30%

50%

PaO_2 (kPa)

70.0

14.0

7.0

A

B

0.2   1.0
FiO_2

0.2   1.0
FiO_2

Hypoxaemia due to true right-to-left shunt is refractory to supplemental oxygen when 'shunt fraction' exceeds 30%.

The response to oxygen therapy in V/Q mismatch depends on whether there are many mild V/Q ratio units (A) or a few very low V/Q ratio units (B).

Figure 1.5 Effect of (a) true shunt (Q_S/Q_T) and (b) V/Q mismatch on the PaO_2 and inspired oxygen fraction (FiO_2) relationship.

When the shunt fraction is high, treatment aims to reduce the shunt. Thus, in obstructive airways diseases like COPD and asthma, relieving bronchospasm with bronchodilators improves ventilation, and the reduction in V/Q mismatch, in conjunction with other mechanisms, aids correction of associated hypoxaemia. Similarly, draining a pneumothorax will restore ventilation to the collapsed lung and rapidly corrects V/Q matching. In pneumonia, antibiotic therapy treats consolidation and, over a longer period, will restore V/Q.

Techniques, such as continuous positive airways pressure (CPAP), non-invasive ventilation, or mechanical ventilation may be required to re-expand collapsed alveoli and improve V/Q matching. In addition, changes in posture can improve oxygenation because V/Q matching is not uniform throughout the chest, with lower V/Q ratios occurring in more dependent regions due to gravity effects.

Impaired gas transfer

The amount of oxygen diffusing across the alveolar capillary membrane is inversely proportional to its thickness and proportional to the pressure across the membrane. In pulmonary oedema and pulmonary fibrosis, the transfer of oxygen from the alveolar air to the capillary haemoglobin may be slowed by interstitial or alveolar fluid and fibrous tissue.

This is rarely a significant cause of hypoxaemia, unless the transit time through the alveolar capillary is substantially shortened as, for example, during exercise. As with V/Q mismatch, the alveolar-arterial oxygen difference would be expected to be >1 kPa with impaired diffusion (see Box 1.2).

Supplemental oxygen partly reverses hypoxaemia due to poor diffusion by increasing the concentration gradient across the membrane, but, when a reversible cause can be corrected like pulmonary oedema, this must be treated.

Right-to-left cardiac shunts

These occur in patients with either congenital cardiac defects or those with acquired defects (e.g. post-myocardial infarction). In this situation, a proportion of the blood bypasses the lungs completely, carrying unoxygenated blood from the right to the left side of the heart. It is an extreme form of V/Q mismatching (i.e. true shunt), and oxygen therapy in these patients is ineffective (see Figure 1.5a).

The oliguric patient

Poor or deteriorating urine output (i.e. <0.5 mL/kg/h) is often an early sign that a patient's clinical condition is deteriorating, and the cause must be identified and corrected quickly. Acute renal failure is discussed in Chapter 11, and only the essential features will be considered in this section. In normal circumstances, urine output is ~1 mL/kg/h and is dependent on:

- Appropriate blood pressure and renal blood flow.
- Healthy, normally functioning kidneys.
- No obstruction to urine flow.

Oliguria describes production of less than 400 mL of urine daily and anuria indicates no urine production. Management of the oliguric patient is summarized in Figure 1.6. The causes of poor urine output include:

1. **'Pre-renal' (volume-responsive) disease** due to reduced renal blood flow or hypotension.
2. **'Renal' (or intrinsic) renal disease** due to kidney disease, including nephrotoxic damage due to drugs (e.g. non-steroidal anti-inflammatory agents), acute tubular necrosis or tubulointerstitial disease, and glomerulonephritis.

1. Palpate the abdomen for a distended bladder. Check drug chart for nephrotoxins, and stop them

2. Insert a urinary catheter or flush catheter if already *in situ*

3. Send urine sample for osmolality and sodium analysis

4. If no urinary obstruction, give fluid challenge

5. If fluid challenges fail to maintain systolic BP >90 mmHg, consider CVP line and inotropes

6. If oliguria persists, consider cautious use of diuretics, BUT remember that these can cause further renal impairment

8. If hypotension or oliguria persist, call for senior assistance

Figure 1.6 Management of oliguria.

3. **'Post-renal' renal disease** due to urinary tract obstruction.

Oliguria due to pre-renal disease

Between mean arterial blood pressures (MAP) of 60 and 160 mmHg, autoregulation ensures a constant renal blood flow of about 1–1.5 L per minute (i.e. ~30% of cardiac output). If the MAP falls below the lower limit of autoregulation or cardiac output decreases, renal blood flow and perfusion decrease rapidly, and autonomic and endocrine responses are activated, including the release of adrenaline, antidiuretic hormone (ADH), and aldosterone, to restore blood pressure. ADH and aldosterone increase renal salt and water retention, increasing circulating blood volume and renal blood flow. This results in a reduced volume of highly concentrated urine (i.e. increased osmolality), with low salt (i.e. sodium) content (see Table 1.3).

If oliguria is pre-renal (i.e. due to hypotension or reduced cardiac output), it may be reversible. The aim is to restore mean arterial pressure (systolic blood pressure >100 mmHg or MAP >65 mmHg), cardiac output, and renal blood flow. This is achieved by increasing cardiac filling pressures with fluid administration. Initially, administer a fluid challenge with 0.5–1 L of crystalloid fluid (e.g. Hartmann's solution), and reassess the blood pressure, filling pressures (e.g. CVP), and urine output. Aim for a urine output >0.5 mL/kg/h. In the

Table 1.3 Urine analysis in patients with pre-renal (volume-responsive) and renal (intrinsic) oliguria

	Normal	Pre-renal	Renal
Urine osmolality (mOsm/kg)	400–500	>500	<400
Urinary sodium (mmol)	10–20	<20	>40
Urine:plasma creatinine ratio	20–40	>40	<20

more severely unwell, CVP monitoring should be undertaken to optimize fluid resuscitation.

Even patients with heart failure and oliguria should receive small boluses of fluid (~250 mL), with careful monitoring to assess whether hypovolaemia is the cause.

If the patient has been adequately fluid-resuscitated, but blood pressure remains inadequate (i.e. cardiac failure, sepsis), inotropes (e.g. dobutamine) and vasopressors (e.g. noradrenaline) may be required to increase the mean arterial blood pressure and restore urine output.

Oliguria due to renal disease
Poor urine output, with elevated urea and creatinine levels, may be due to intrinsic renal disease (e.g. glomerulonephritis), rather than poor renal perfusion. The commonest cause of acute oliguria is acute tubular necrosis (see Chapter 11). This is usually due to delayed or inadequate treatment of renal hypoperfusion and hypotension, although previous administration of nephrotoxins may also be responsible.

Drug charts should be reviewed for any of the commonly used drugs that may potentially cause kidney damage, including non-steroidal anti-inflammatory agents, contrast media, antibiotics (e.g. aminoglycosides, penicillins, cephalosporins, amphotericin), angiotensin-converting enzyme inhibitors, and furosemide (especially with gentamicin), and these stopped, if possible.

In renal disease and acute tubular necrosis, the osmolality of urine will be similar to that of plasma (~280 mOsm/L), and urinary sodium concentration is high due to loss of kidney concentrating ability (see Table 1.3). However, in acute glomerulonephritis, the renal tubules continue to function well and produce urine with a high osmolality and low sodium concentration (<20 mmol/L).

Patients with oliguria due to renal impairment require diagnosis and treatment of the underlying disorder (e.g. glomerulonephritis) whilst continuing to ensure adequate renal perfusion by maintaining blood pressure and cardiac output. Simply maintaining urine output with drug therapy (e.g. furosemide) is not recommended, and diuretics can be nephrotoxic, causing interstitial nephritis.

Oliguria due to post-renal urinary tract obstruction
Urinary tract obstruction may cause acute anuria or oliguria. Initially, palpate the abdomen for a distended bladder which suggests urethral obstruction. In men, the commonest cause of acute urethral obstruction is benign prostatic hypertrophy. Urethral obstruction is less common in women and may be due to malignancy. A urinary catheter should be inserted into the bladder and a sample of urine sent for analysis. If a catheter is already in place, exclude catheter obstruction by flushing with saline. If there is no urinary flow following insertion of a urinary catheter, a renal

ultrasound should be arranged to exclude ureteric obstruction (e.g. renal stones) and to examine the kidneys.

Hyperkalaemia, metabolic acidosis, and fluid overload will develop if the oliguria persists and renal disease progresses. It is essential to monitor serum potassium and acid-base balance (i.e. serum bicarbonate, arterial blood gases) and assess fluid balance carefully.

Hyperkalaemia (K^+ >6.5 mmol/L) is corrected with insulin-dextrose infusions, preceded by intravenous calcium, if the ECG is abnormal, to prevent cardiac arrhythmias. However, as renal impairment progresses, toxin accumulation (e.g. creatinine), hyperkalaemia, and fluid overload will eventually necessitate renal replacement therapy with dialysis or haemofiltration (see Chapter 11).

The 'obtunded' patient with acutely disordered conscious level
Many acutely unwell patients become confused, disorientated, and 'obtunded', with a reduced level of consciousness. A reduction in conscious level is associated with potential airways obstruction, loss of the gag and cough reflexes, and an increased risk of aspiration of upper airways secretion and gastric contents. There are many potential causes for a reduced conscious level (see Table 1.4), including metabolic, hypotensive, temperature-related, drug-induced, cerebral, or traumatic disorders. Impaired conscious level should always be regarded as serious.

The Glasgow coma scale (see Table 1.2) assesses conscious level, with a total maximum score of 15 indicating a fully alert and responsive patient and the lowest score of 3 indicating a completely unresponsive patient. The score is best measured following treatment of hypotension and hypoxaemia, as these will have a considerable effect on the

Table 1.4 Causes of acute confusion and coma

1. *Metabolic disorders*
   - Respiratory
     - Hypoxia: PaO_2 <45 mmHg
     - Hypercapnia: $PaCO_2$ >60 mmHg
   - Renal and hepatic
     - Na^+ <120 or >155 mmol/L
     - Glucose <3 or >30 mmol/L
     - Ca^{2+} <1.7 or >3.0 mmol/L
     - Raised urea, ammonia
   - Alcohol withdrawal (2–5 days post-admission)
   - Nutritional deficiency (e.g. Wernicke's encephalopathy)
   - Endocrine (e.g. thyrotoxicosis, myxoedema)
   - Hypothermia/hyperthermia
2. *Infection*
   - Pneumonia, sepsis, urinary tract infection
3. *Drug/toxin ingestion*
   - Alcohol, sedatives, illicit drugs
4. *Neurological causes*
   - Epilepsy (i.e. ictal/post-ictal phase)
   - Non-convulsive status epilepticus
   - Dementia (+ superimposed illness)
   - Infective (e.g. meningitis, encephalitis)
   - Structural/traumatic (e.g. tumours, raised ICP)
5. *Vascular causes*
   - Stroke (e.g. embolic in atrial fibrillation)
   - Cardiac (e.g. myocardial infarction with hypotension)
   - Hypertensive encephalopathy

result. Patients with a score less than 8–9 may require endotracheal intubation, as airways reflexes will be significantly impaired with the risk of aspiration. A formal anaesthetic induction will be required, and a doctor experienced in airways management should be summoned.

In a patient with abnormal conscious level, the blood glucose, sodium, and arterial blood gases should be assessed and abnormalities treated appropriately.

Hypoxia, hypercapnia, and hypotension all decrease conscious level and may exacerbate cerebral injury and oedema. They must be treated urgently. Other causes of impaired conscious level should be considered, including toxicology, thyroid and liver function tests, blood cultures, including appropriate Imaging and lumbar puncture.

Airway, breathing, and circulation must be secured (as previously described) and the patient given high-dose supplemental oxygen (i.e. FiO_2 >60%). Use intravenous fluids to correct hypotension. When appropriate (i.e. not when a cervical cord injury is suspected), the patient should be positioned in the left lateral decubitus position to protect the airway and prevent aspiration. Patients with the potential for raised intracranial pressure are normally nursed 30° head up, but, in the acute situation, the horizontal recovery position (avoid head down) is still preferred to reduce the risk of aspiration. Drug-induced CNS depression should be reversed (e.g. naloxone for opiate overdosage).

The pupils may provide important clues as to the cause of the reduced conscious level.

- Bilateral pupil dilation occurs with sympathetic drugs (e.g. tricyclic antidepressants, adrenaline) and when there is sympathetic overactivity (e.g. anxiety).
- Pupillary constriction occurs with opiate drugs and following brainstem (usually pontine) infarcts.
- Unilateral, unreactive pupil dilation indicates a space-occupying lesion, like a haematoma, abscess, or tumour, and is a medical emergency requiring rapid intervention. Appropriate neurosurgical assistance should be sought.

When an intracerebral bleed, space-occupying lesion, or raised intracranial pressure is suspected, a CT scan is indicated, but the patient has to be able to lie flat and still for at least 10 minutes. Patients with an unprotected airway should be intubated and monitored (i.e. blood pressure, ECG) for the duration of the scan.

Ongoing management of the acutely ill patient

Management of the acutely ill patient requires a multidisciplinary team approach. Good communication with other teams of doctors and nurses, careful documentation in the notes, leadership, decision-making, and clear objective plans are essential. Try to obtain appropriate help in a timely fashion. Considerate and honest communication with relatives is essential and must be consistent between caregivers.

The ethics of acute medical illness, decisions relating to 'do not resuscitate' (DNR) orders, and the aspects of withholding and withdrawal of treatment are all major issues in the management of these patients and are discussed in later chapters.

Further reading

Anderson ID (1997). Care of the critically ill surgical patient courses of the Royal College of Surgeons. *British Journal of Hospital Medicine*, **57**, 274–5.

Dellinger RP, Carlet JM, Masur H, et al. (2008). Surviving Sepsis Campaign guidelines for management of severe sepsis and septic shock. *Critical Care Medicine*, **32**, 858–73.

Gao H, McDonnell A, Harrison DA, et al. (2007). Systematic review and evaluation of physiological track and trigger warning systems for identifying at risk patients on the ward. *Intensive Care Medicine*, **33**, 667–79.

Hemmila MR and Napolitano LM (2006). Severe respiratory failure: advanced treatment options. *Critical Care Medicine*, **34**, S278–90.

Hillman K, Chen J, Cretikos M, et al. (2005). Introduction of the medical emergency team (MET) system. A cluster randomised controlled trial. *Lancet*, **365**, 2091–7.

Knaus WA, Wagner DP, Draper EA, et al. (1991). The APACHE III prognostic system. Risk prediction of hospital mortality for critically ill hospitalized adults. *Chest*, **100**, 1619–36.

National Institute for Health and Clinical Excellence (2007). Acutely ill patients in hospital. NICE clinical guideline 50. <http://www.nice.org.uk/CG050>.

Smith GB, Osgood VM, Crane S (2002). ALERT™ - a multiprofessional training course in the care of the acutely ill adult patient. *Resuscitation*, **52**, 281–6.

Subbe CP, Kruger M, Rutherford P, et al. (2001). Validation of a modified early warning score in medical admissions. *QJM*, **94**, 521–6.

Vincent J and Gerlach H (2004). Fluid resuscitation in severe sepsis and septic shock; an evidence-based review. *Critical Care Medicine*, **32**, S451–4.

Chapter 2

Fluid management and nutrition

Assessment of the circulation

The cardiovascular system will be discussed in detail in later chapters, but assessment of the circulation is an essential clinical skill and an integral part of fluid management and is, therefore, discussed briefly in this section. Circulatory assessment can be difficult during acute illness and depends on evaluation of both cardiac and circuit factors. The main aims are to maintain cardiac output (CO) and blood pressure (BP) and ensure adequate tissue blood supply to satisfy metabolic demands. Figure 2.1 summarizes the effects of cardiac filling, venous return, and contractility on CO.

Circulatory assessment must address:

1. **Cardiac function.** The aim is to evaluate cardiac filling, cardiac contractility, and CO to exclude heart failure. CO (mL/min) is the product of heart rate (beats/min) and stroke volume (mL) where stroke volume is determined by:

   • **Preload**. This is determined by ventricular end diastolic volume (EDV, i.e. ventricular filling) and is governed by the volume and pressure of blood returning to the heart (see Figure 2.1). Loss of intravascular volume due to sepsis, haemorrhage, or anaphylaxis and raised intrathoracic pressures (e.g. severe asthma) are the most common causes of inadequate ventricular preload (i.e. filling).

   • **Afterload**. This is the load, resistance, or 'impedance' against which the ventricle has to work. Afterload is increased by aortic stenosis, hypertension, high systemic vascular resistance (SVR), low intrathoracic pressures, and ventricular dilation.

   • **Myocardial contractility**. This is the heart's ability to perform work independently of pre- or afterload. Heart failure may be due to either inadequate systolic ejection (systolic dysfunction) or poor diastolic filling (diastolic dysfunction).

   Systolic dysfunction may be due to either reduced contractility (e.g. ischaemia, cardiomyopathy, sepsis) or increased impedance (e.g. hypertension, aortic stenosis). Increasing ventricular EDV (i.e. cardiac dilation) will maintain stroke volume (i.e. by the Frank-Starling relationship), provided myocardial reserve is adequate (see Figure 2.1); otherwise, stroke volume will fall, and inotropic agents will be required to maintain CO and BP.

   Diastolic dysfunction is characterized by reduced ventricular compliance and impaired diastolic filling (i.e. a stiff ventricle). It may be due to mechanical factors (e.g. restrictive cardiomyopathy) or due to the impaired relaxation that occurs during myocardial ischaemia or severe sepsis. This results in an elevated end diastolic pressure and pulmonary venous congestion which manifests clinically as 'flash' pulmonary oedema.

   In addition, CO is reduced by both bradycardia and tachycardia. In tachycardia, this is due to inadequate ventricular filling time. Tachycardia may also reduce contractility because myocardial perfusion occurs during diastole which is reduced in tachycardia, causing myocardial ischaemia.

2. **Circuit factors.** Although frequently overlooked, circuit factors are as important as myocardial contractility in determining CO because venous return determines ventricular filling (i.e. EDV; see Figure 2.1). Arterial 'conducting' vessels contain ~20% of the blood volume and mean arterial pressure is determined by force of

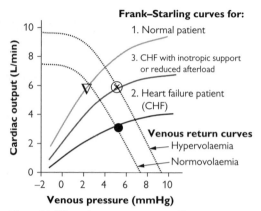

Figure 2.1 Effect of venous return on cardiac output. Cardiac output (CO) is determined by the intersection of the Frank–Starling and venous return curves (∇). In heart failure (2), for the same venous return curve, CO falls despite a higher filling (venous) pressure (●). CO can be returned almost to normal (3) with fluid filling ± inotrope or afterload reduction (⊗).

myocardial ejection and the downstream impedance (i.e. systemic vascular resistance). The venous 'capacitance' system contains ~70% of total blood volume and acts as a physiological reservoir ('unstressed volume'). When circulatory demand rises, sympathetic tone increases, causing reservoir contraction, and the resultant 'autotransfusion' ('stressed volume') can increase venous return by up to 30%. Other complex neurohormonal factors contribute to this circulatory response (e.g. renin-aldosterone, vasopressinergic, and steroid systems), and are modulated by local tissue factors (e.g. endothelin, nitric oxide).

Disruption of peripheral vascular regulation, usually due to reduced responsiveness to sympathetic stimulation (e.g. sepsis, spinal anaesthesia, anaphylaxis), results in circulatory failure due to venous pooling and the inability to generate a 'stressed' volume. Circulatory management usually tends to focus inappropriately on arterial factors when often the problem is mainly due to impaired venous return.

Clinical assessment

Initially, inspect the patient for features of poor perfusion and reduced CO, including cool and pale limbs, peripheral cyanosis, and prolonged capillary refill time (i.e. >2 s for colour to return to an area of skin previously subjected to pressure). Confusion and reduced urine output also indicate poor CO.

Measure the BP, and listen to the heart for leaking valves. Initially, compensatory mechanisms (e.g. tachycardia, increased SVR) maintain BP, and CO has to fall by >20%, equivalent to 1 L of acute blood loss, before the BP will fall. Pulse pressure narrows during arterial vasoconstriction (e.g. hypovolaemia, cardiogenic shock), and, in vasodilated patients (e.g. during sepsis), the diastolic BP is often particularly low.

Palpate the peripheral and central arterial pulses for heart rate, rhythm, and equality. Thready, fast pulses indicate a poor CO, whereas bounding pulses suggest sepsis.

Fluid challenges

A 'fluid challenge' (~0.25 L of fluid given intravenously over <20 min) is a useful, and frequently used, technique to assess the adequacy of circulatory filling (i.e. preload) and need for fluid replacement. It measures the response to a bolus of fluid in terms of heart rate, BP, and central venous pressure (CVP), if available (see Figure 2.2). A transient increase in CVP and/or BP suggests the need for further fluid. A sustained increase in CVP and/or BP indicates that the heart is operating on the flat part of the Starling curve and further fluid administration risks pulmonary oedema. If there is only a transient response to the initial fluid challenge, the challenge is repeated and the patient reassessed.

Although a fluid challenge is clinically useful, it is not always reliable, as it is influenced by venous tone, does not have a linear relationship with CO, and lacks sensitivity/specificity.

In most patients, clinical assessment and fluid challenges are sufficiently reliable to ensure successful circulatory management. However, invasive measurement of physiological variables (e.g. CO, SVR, pulmonary capillary wedge pressure) may be required in acutely or critically ill patients to optimize circulatory performance.

Haemodynamic monitoring

Continuous haemodynamic monitoring aims to ensure early detection of clinical instability, assess progress, and measure response to therapy. Nevertheless, regular clinical examination is essential, as simple physical signs, like appearance (e.g. pallor), peripheral perfusion, and conscious level, may be as important as parameters displayed on a monitor.

When clinical signs and monitored parameters disagree, assume that clinical assessment is correct until potential errors from monitored variables have been excluded (e.g. blocked CVP lines, incorrect calibration of equipment). Trends are generally more important than single readings.

Use non-invasive techniques, if possible, as invasive monitoring is associated with risks (e.g. line infection) and complications (e.g. pneumothorax). Review the need for 'invasive techniques' regularly, and replace them with 'non-invasive' measures as soon as possible. Alarms are a crucial safety feature (e.g. to detect asystole). They are set to physiological safe limits and should never be disconnected. Frequently used monitoring techniques include:

• **Blood pressure (BP)**, which is usually measured intermittently with an automated sphygmomanometer. Continuous intra-arterial BP monitoring may be necessary in severely ill patients. The BP does not reflect CO, and a normal or high BP can be associated with a low CO in patients with marked peripheral vasoconstriction (i.e. high SVR). Conversely, vasodilated, 'septic' patients (i.e. low SVR) may be hypotensive despite a high CO.

• **Central venous pressure (CVP).** This reflects the right atrial pressure (RAP) and is measured through an internal jugular or subclavian vein catheter. It is a useful means of assessing circulating blood volume and aids assessment of the rate at which fluid should be administered. A high CVP can indicate 'fluid overload', impaired myocardial contractility, or high right ventricular afterload. Occasionally, increased venous tone can act to maintain CVP and mask volume depletion during hypovolaemia or haemorrhage. In this situation, CVP is not as important as the response to fluid challenges (see Figure 2.2).

• **Pulmonary capillary wedge pressure (PCWP).** This reflects the left atrial pressure (LAP). Normally, LAP is ~5–7 mmHg greater than RAP, but, in IHD or severe illness, there is often 'disparity' between left and right ventricular function. Thus, LAP may be high, despite a low RAP in left ventricular dysfunction, and a small increase in RAP can cause a large increase in LAP which may precipitate pulmonary oedema. In these patients, PCWP (i.e. LAP) is monitored using a pulmonary artery (PA) catheter. PCWP is normally 6–12 mmHg but may be >25–35 mmHg in left ventricular failure. Provided the pulmonary capillary membranes are intact (i.e. not 'leaky'), a PCWP of ~15–20 mmHg ensures good left ventricular filling and optimal function without risking pulmonary oedema. PA catheters also measure CO, mixed venous saturation, and right ventricular ejection fraction (see Chapter 19).

• **Cardiac output (CO).** Thermodilution techniques for CO measurement (e.g. PA catheter, pulsion continuous CO monitor (PiCCO)) are considered the 'gold standard', but error is at least 10%. Non-invasive techniques of CO monitoring utilize dye/lithium dilution, transoesophageal Doppler ultrasound, echocardiography, or impedance methods.

• **Electrocardiogram (ECG).** Rate and rhythm are displayed by standard single-lead ECG monitors, but ST segment changes can be monitored in patients with IHD.

Management of the circulation

Circulatory management includes fluid replacement, control of bleeding, and restoration of heart rate, CO, BP, and tissue perfusion. Good venous access must be established using wide-bore peripheral and central venous cannulae. Circulatory support utilizes a hierarchy of management:

1. **Diagnosis.** This determines treatment (e.g. fluid restriction in left heart failure vs fluid resuscitation in hypovolaemia). Life-threatening conditions (e.g. haemorrhage, cardiac tamponade) must be detected and treated rapidly.

2. **Rate and rhythm.** Both tachyarrhythmias (>180 beats/min) and bradycardia (e.g. vagal tone) can reduce cardiac output. Restoring sinus rhythm and heart rate rapidly improve BP and CO. Electrolyte concentrations must be optimized (K^+ >4.5 mmol/L, Mg^{2+} >1.2 mmol/L) and arrhythmogenic drugs (e.g. salbutamol) withdrawn. Antiarrhythmic drugs, cardioversion, or pacemakers may be required.

3. **Fluid therapy.** This aims to optimize cardiac preload and maintain BP and CO whilst minimizing potential complications (e.g. pulmonary oedema). Fluid management and choice of fluids for resuscitation (e.g. crystalloid vs colloid)

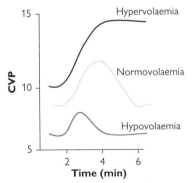

Figure 2.2 Central venous pressure (CVP) response to a 250 mL fluid challenge.

is discussed in Fluid management. In general, crystalloid solutions are used first, or the fluid that is lost is replaced (e.g. blood during haemorrhage). Recent evidence indicates that the benefit of colloids is limited, and they may cause harm, suggesting they should be used with caution and after careful consideration. Large volumes of maintenance fluid suggest ongoing loss, and a cause should be sought. If haemorrhage is suspected, send blood for cross-matching.

4. *Inotropic and vasopressor drugs*. If fluid resuscitation fails to achieve an adequate circulation or precipitates cardiac failure, alternative means of improving CO and tissue perfusion, including inotropic or vasopressor drugs and mechanical ventricular support devices, must be considered.

Further reading

Bradley RD (1977). *Studies in acute heart failure*. Edward Arnold, London.

Goodwin J (1995). The importance of clinical skills. *BMJ*, **310**, 1281–2.

Palazzo M (2001). Circulating volume and clinical assessment of the circulation. *British Journal of Anaesthesia*, **86**, 743–6.

Task Force of the American College of Critical Care Medicine (1999). Practice parameters for haemodynamic support in adult patients with sepsis. *Critical Care Medicine*, **27**, 639–60.

Fluid management

Daily fluid assessment, prescription, and administration are essential daily tasks on most medical and surgical wards. It is a complex task and requires considerable clinical acumen. When done well, it is the hallmark of an outstanding physician. Unfortunately, both under- and overhydration are common due to poor understanding of the basic principles involved. This causes significant morbidity and mortality, although the extent of the problem is difficult to quantify, as it is often multifactorial and under-reported. Nevertheless, it is well recognized by both senior medical and surgical staff.

Post-operatively, overhydration occurs in 17–54% of patients and is reported to prolong hospital stay, increase morbidity (e.g. pulmonary oedema, tachyarrhythmias), and it has been estimated to contribute to about 9,000 deaths annually in the USA. Indeed, up to 50% of patients, especially the elderly, have been documented to develop at least one fluid-related complication related to post-operative overhydration.

Three key issues have consistently been identified as contributing to poor fluid management.

1. **Poor understanding of the principles of fluid balance.** Several studies have demonstrated no relationship between the fluid balance information available (e.g. serum electrolyte data, input/output charts, and daily weights) and the subsequent fluid prescriptions. In addition, few junior medical staff received formal education or were given guidelines on fluid and electrolyte prescribing, and <10% of staff were aware that regular weighing is one of the best serial measures of fluid balance.

2. **Poor fluid chart documentation.** The National Confidential Enquiry into Perioperative Deaths (NCEPOD) in 1999 reported that poor documentation of fluid balance contributed to both morbidity and mortality. Further studies have demonstrated that less than half of fluid balance sheets are complete (i.e. no record of oral intake or urine output) and that intravenous fluids are often administered at incorrect rates. Indeed, the accuracy of fluid rates was not considered important!

3. **Prescription by the most junior member of the team.** Fluid prescription is often delegated to the least experienced members of the medical team. Junior staff are responsible for 80% of perioperative fluid prescriptions. The NCEPOD Report ascribed many of the errors in fluid and electrolyte management to inadequate knowledge and training of junior medical staff. This is reflected in audit evidence suggesting that less than 50% of junior doctors know the sodium content of normal saline.

The British consensus guidelines on intravenous fluid therapy for adult surgical patients and the NICE guideline 'Intravenous fluid therapy in adults in hospital' Clinical Guideline 174 (Dec 2013) are significant steps towards addressing some of the issues of fluid prescription on surgical and medical wards. However, further guidance and support will be required to aid physicians with appropriate medical fluid management.

Fluid is best delivered by oral or nasogastric routes, but intravenous fluid administration may be necessary in patients who are:

- Acutely unwell and requiring large quantities of fluid for resuscitation.
- Unable to drink (e.g. unconscious, unsafe swallow reflex (e.g. following strokes), faciomaxillary injury).
- Unable to absorb adequate quantities of water (e.g. vomiting, paralytic ileus, diarrhoea).
- Losing excessive quantities of fluid (e.g. diarrhoea, haemorrhage, burns).

The principal aims of fluid administration are to:

- Replace normal fluid and electrolyte losses.
- Replenish substantial deficits or complex ongoing losses (e.g. upper and lower intestinal fistulae).
- Provide additional resuscitation fluids to correct for the effects of underlying pathology.
- Maintain an adequate cardiac output, blood pressure, and subsequent peripheral blood flow/distribution of oxygen and other nutrients to satisfy the metabolic needs of body tissues and organs, aid temperature regulation (e.g. sweating), and ensure appropriate removal of carbon dioxide and metabolic waste from the body.
- Ensure a stable cellular and extracellular milieu to preserve cellular transmembrane potentials and normal cellular transport mechanisms for essential ions, respiratory gases, solutes, and waste products.
- Avoid excessive oedema which may impair cellular oxygen and nutrient delivery by increasing capillary-to-cell diffusion distances, especially during hypoxaemia.

Factors affecting fluid and electrolyte balance

Factors that must be addressed when considering fluid administration include:

1. **Fluid and electrolyte compartments.** Water comprises 60% of total body weight, equivalent to ~42 L in a 70 kg man, of which 25 L is intracellular fluid (ICF) and 17 L extracellular fluid (ECF). The ECF is divided into interstitial fluid (ISF) which surrounds the cells (11–14 L) and intravascular plasma (3–4 L), separated by the capillary endothelium which is permeable to low molecular weight (MW) solutes (e.g. sodium) but increasingly impermeable to high MW solutes (e.g. albumin). Compartmental distribution of water is primarily dependent on the 'osmotic pressure' exerted by small diffusible ions.

   - **Osmotic pressure** reflects the ion concentration gradients between compartments created by cellular ion pumps such that sodium (Na^+) and chloride (Cl^-) ions are mainly extracellular and potassium (K^+) and phosphate ions are intracellular. For example, after a saline infusion, the rise in extracellular Na^+ and Cl^- increases the extracellular osmotic pressure, drawing water out of the ICF compartment and into the ECF compartment.

2. **Intravascular volume** is determined by the 'oncotic pressure' of large MW, non-diffusible vascular plasma proteins, the permeability ('leakiness') of the vessels, and circulatory hydrostatic pressure.

   - **Oncotic (colloid) pressure** describes the ability of 'vascular' plasma proteins to 'bind' and retain water in the circulation. Normal plasma 'oncotic' pressure is about 3.4 kPa (26 mmHg), of which albumin accounts for >70%, haemoglobin ~20%, and globulins <5%.
   - **The albumin cycle** (see Figure 2.3). Total body albumin is ~275 g (125 g intravascular, 150 g ISF). One gram of albumin binds 18 mL of water, thus intravascular albumin holds 2.25 L (18 mL × 125 g) of water in the vascular compartment. Normal albumin leakage from blood to the ISF and subsequent return to the vascular compartment via lymphatic drainage is ~125 g/day.

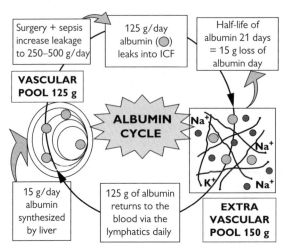

Figure 2.3 Albumin cycle.

The normal 'lifespan' of an albumin molecule in the circulation is about 20 days, after which it is broken down by the reticuloendothelial system and the components recycled in the liver to form new proteins. About 15 g of albumin is broken down daily. To replace this, about 15 g is produced daily by the liver.

During acute illness, albumin production ceases and is replaced by acute phase protein production (e.g. C-reactive protein). Acute phase proteins tend to be smaller molecules with less 'oncotic' potential. Consequently, during prolonged illness, albumin levels fall (e.g. over 10 days, about 150 g of the total albumin pool will be lost (i.e. 10 days × 15 g daily loss)), reducing plasma albumin levels and, as a result, intravascular volume falls due to reduced plasma 'oncotic' pressure.

• **Endothelial permeability** is partly limited by the osmotic effects and high molecular weight of albumin, the barrier function of the endothelial basement membrane (glycocalyx), and because negatively charged albumin molecules are repelled by similarly charged interstitial glycoproteins (e.g. collagen, hyaluronic acid) which trap water to make up the gel-like interstitial matrix.

Permeability is increased in pathological conditions, e.g. surgery and sepsis, where albumin leakage may rise by 100% and 300%, respectively. The resulting fall in plasma albumin reduces intravascular volume, whilst raised ISF albumin increases tissue oedema.

3. **Normal daily fluid and renal function losses** must be replaced in all patients.
   • A normal adult loses 1.5–2.0 L (25–30 mL/kg/day) of water, 70 mmol (1 mmol/kg/day) of sodium (Na^+), and 40–70 mmol (0.5–1 mmol/kg/day) of potassium (K^+) daily. About 0.5 L of 'insensible fluid loss' occurs as lung water vapour and sweat, although during febrile illness and with high ambient temperatures, insensible lung water and sweat losses (with associated electrolytes) can exceed 3 L each day. Loss of skin or mucous membrane barriers (e.g. burns, ulcerative colitis), fluid-losing enteropathies (e.g. diarrhoea), and salt-losing renal failure are also associated with further large fluid and electrolyte losses. When in physiological balance, most of the sodium and potassium lost is excreted, with 400 mmol of urea 'waste' in about 1.7 L (or approximately 1mL/kg/h or 70 mL/h) of urine.
   • Despite wide variations in salt and water intake in normal subjects, the kidneys are able to maintain extracellular Na^+ concentration and osmolality within a narrow range. This is achieved via the osmoreceptors and appropriate changes in vasopressin secretion, affecting urinary concentration and free water clearance.

During salt and/or water depletion, antidiuretic hormone (ADH) secretion increases urine concentration and reduces water clearance, whilst the renin-angiotensin-aldosterone system (RAAS) reduces urinary sodium to <5 mmol/L. In contrast, the response to sodium excess is less efficient. Even normal subjects are slow to excrete a 'sodium load', as this depends on passive suppression of the RAAS, rather than active elimination by natriuretic hormones. In addition, the associated 'chloride ion load' causes renal vasoconstriction, reducing glomerular filtration rate and potentiating sodium retention. Table 2.1 summarizes the causes of sodium and water imbalance.

Table 2.1 Causes of sodium and water loss/retention in acute illness

Sodium and water retention	Sodium and water loss
1. Stress response (ADH release), e.g. surgery, burns, trauma	1. Acute blood loss, e.g. haemorrhage
2. Hyperosmolar states (ADH release), e.g. hyperglycaemia, uraemia	2. Kidney, e.g. diuretics, renal disease, diabetes
3. Reduced ANP with aldosterone release, e.g. dehydration, low Na^+ input, hypovolaemia, excess K^+	3. Skin, e.g. sweating, burns, skin disease
4. Increased capillary permeability with oedema and hypovolaemia, e.g. trauma, burns, sepsis, pancreatitis	4. Gastrointestinal tract, e.g. vomiting, fistula, diarrhoea
	5. Fluid sequestration, e.g. bowel obstruction, ascites, pleural effusions

- Normal daily urine output contains a solute load of 620–840 mOsm. The solute load in urine includes normal losses of sodium and chloride ions, potassium and chloride ions, and 400 mOsm of urea waste. The normal daily urine solute load can be calculated from the equation:

$$((Na^+ \times 2) + (K^+ \times 2) + urea]$$

where $Na^+ \times 2 = Na^+ + Cl^-$ and $K^+ \times 2 = K^+ + Cl^-$

Thus:

$(70 \text{ to } 150 \times 2) + (40 \text{ to } 70 \times 2) + 400 = 620–840 \text{ mOsm}.$

Assuming a urine production of 1.5 L daily, the concentration of waste product in the urine will be 400–560 mOsm per litre of urine. Normal kidneys can achieve a maximum urine concentration of 1,000 mOsm/L. Consequently, the minimum volume of urine to excrete a daily urine solute load of 840 mOsm (assuming normal renal function) would be about 840 mL daily (i.e. ~0.5 mL/kg/h or 35 mL/h).

However, during acute illness, the ability of the kidneys to concentrate urine falls. Thus, during sepsis, the maximum urine-concentrating capacity may be reduced to as little as 500 mOsm/L. In this situation, excretion of the normal daily solute load will require twice the volume of urine (i.e. 1,680 mL or 1 mL/kg/h or 70 mL/h).

Unfortunately, during acute illness, catabolic metabolism increases urea waste production to >1,000 mOsm daily, further diminishing the body's capacity to excrete the total solute load. In addition, during a difficult resuscitation, it is not unusual for a patient to be given 5 L of sodium- and chloride-containing fluids (e.g. normal saline), which represents a large solute load. Normal saline contains 154 mmol/L NaCl or 304 mOsm of solute per litre (i.e. 154 mOsm Na$^+$ and 154 mOsm Cl$^-$) or 1,520 mOsm of solute in 5 L.

The combination of catabolic urea and solutes given during fluid resuscitation often require the kidneys to excrete >3,000 mOsm/daily. With normally functioning kidneys (i.e. concentrating capacities of 1,000 mOsm/L), this would require an increase in urine output to >3 L daily (~2–3 mL/kg/h or 140–210 mL/h). In reality, these demands occur at a time when renal function is impaired (i.e. concentrating capacities of 500 mOsm/L) and urine production is falling. Consequently, solute is retained, and it may take up to 3 days to remove the solute load in 5L normal saline (or other sodium- and chloride-containing solutions). The retained Cl$^-$ causes hyperchloraemic acidosis, renal vasoconstriction, and a further reduction in glomerular filtration.

4. Response to stress. After acute illness or injury, the body retains salt and water. Total fluid retention may be >10 L in some cases. It usually accumulates in the ISF, causing tissue or pulmonary oedema. Causative mechanisms include:

- Antidiuresis and oliguria are mediated by ADH, RAAS, and catecholamines. Fluid may be retained, even in the presence of overload.
- Impaired renal function reduces the ability to excrete free water (as well as the ability to concentrate urine). Free water infusions (e.g. 5% glucose (INN) solution) risk hyponatraemia.
- Increased catabolism and urea production competes with sodium for excretion. The inability of the kidneys to concentrate urine subsequently requires much greater volumes of urine to excrete solutes and leads to further sodium and chloride retention.

- Potassium depletion due to RAAS activity also reduces the ability to excrete a sodium load.
- Hyperchloraemia, associated with saline effusions, subsequently causes renal vasoconstriction, reduces glomerular filtration rate, and further impairs sodium excretion.
- In severely ill patients, impaired energy production may cause intracellular sequestration of sodium and water due to failure of the Na/K ATPase pump, the so-called sick cell syndrome.
- Reduced intravascular volume due to increased capillary permeability and albumin leakage activates RAAS, with further salt and water retention and worsening interstitial oedema.

5. Chronic renal impairment (e.g. glomerulonephritis) and post-renal obstruction (e.g. prostatic hypertrophy) may be associated with either increased or reduced urine output (i.e. polyuric or oliguric renal impairment) and variable ability to excrete solutes (e.g. salt-conserving or salt-losing renal impairment), in addition to impairing metabolic waste excretion. These changes will have a significant effect on fluid management, depending on the associated fluid and electrolyte losses.

6. Cardiac function will also influence fluid management, depending on cardiac contractility, preload (i.e. venous return), and afterload (i.e. vascular resistance or impedance against which the ventricle has to work), as discussed in Assessment of the circulation. However, circuit factors are often overlooked.

- **Circuit factors.** Venous return to the heart is as important as cardiac contractility in maintaining cardiac function, as it determines cardiac end diastolic volumes (and pressures) which subsequently determines cardiac output (see 'Assessment of the circulation', this chapter and Figure 2.3).

Arterial 'conducting' vessels contain ~20% of the blood volume where mean arterial pressure (MAP) is determined by force of myocardial ejection and downstream impedance. In comparison, the venous 'capacitance' system contains ~70% of total blood volume and acts as a physiological reservoir ('unstressed volume'). When circulatory demand increases, venous sympathetic tone increases, causing reservoir contraction, and the resultant 'autotransfusion' ('stressed volume') can increase venous return by up to 30%.

Complex neurohormonal factors control the circulatory response, including systemic adrenergic, renin-aldosterone, vasopressinergic, and steroid systems modulated by local factors (e.g. endothelin, nitric oxide). Disruption of peripheral vascular regulation, usually due to reduced responsiveness to sympathetic stimulation (e.g. spinal anaesthesia, anaphylaxis, sepsis), results in circulatory failure due to venous pooling and the inability to generate a 'stressed' volume.

During resuscitation, management often focuses inappropriately on arterial factors (i.e. systemic vascular resistance, 'afterload'), whereas the problem is often due to impairment of venous return. Fluid loading and manoeuvres to restore effective intravascular volume (e.g. raising the legs and ensuring 'stressed' volumes) should always precede the use of 'vasopressor' drugs.

Assessment of fluid balance

Assessment of fluid balance, and subsequent fluid prescription, is a complex and difficult task. It should not be delegated to the most junior member of the medical team. The key to improvement of fluid management is better training of medical students and junior doctors who must have an

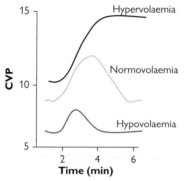

Figure 2.4 Central venous pressure (CVP) response to a 250 mL fluid challenge.

understanding of the issues and the necessary clinical assessment skills. Easily accessible guidelines are now available, and the NICE guideline on intravenous fluid therapy in adults in hospitals was published in December 2013.

Clinical assessment, including review of the National Early Warning Score (NEWS), hourly fluid input (e.g. resuscitation fluids, feed) and output (e.g. urine output, gastrointestinal loss, drainage), monitoring of the circulation, and daily measurements of serum (and occasionally urinary) electrolytes, and urea, is essential to assess fluid balance in acutely unwell patients, particularly those with renal impairment.

The need for accurate fluid balance charts must be emphasized to the nursing staff, as this is frequently neglected on both medical and surgical wards and can result in carers missing gradually progressive over- or underhydration. Daily weights are often very helpful. Day-to-day trends in these parameters guide fluid prescription.

In haemodynamically unstable patients, the cardiovascular (e.g. pulse, blood pressure, central venous pressure (CVP)) response to serial 'fluid challenges' (~250–500 mL over <20 min) is used to determine the need for volume replacement (see Figure 2.4). However, this response is not always reliable, as it is influenced by venous tone, does not have a linear relationship with cardiac output, and lacks sensitivity and specificity. Other measures of inadequate tissue perfusion include an increase in serum lactate and mixed venous saturation (SvO_2) <70%. In more complex cases, non-invasive transoesophageal Doppler or invasive cardiac monitoring may be required to assess cardiac output and filling pressures to determine fluid requirements.

Choice of fluid

Table 2.2 summarizes the electrolyte composition and properties of crystalloid and colloid solutions. With the exception of 5% glucose (INN) solutions, almost all intravenous solutions contain sodium and chloride, some in near physiological concentrations of 140 mmol/L for sodium and 95 mmol/L for chloride, and others in supranormal amounts (e.g. so-called normal saline contains 154 mmol/L of sodium and 154 mmol/L of chloride). Many studies have demonstrated that, in comparison with more physiological solutions, such as Hartmann's, even healthy subjects find it difficult to excrete solutions with a high chloride content, such as normal saline, which can cause hyperchloraemic acidosis and reduced glomerular filtration.

- **Crystalloid solutions** contain low molecular weight salts (e.g. sodium chloride) and sugars (e.g. glucose) which dissolve completely in water and pass freely between the intravascular and interstitial compartments. Although inexpensive and usually isotonic, they redistribute rapidly following intravenous infusion (~1–4 h) from the intravascular to other fluid compartments (e.g. ECF, ICF). Consequently, large volumes are required to maintain intravascular volume, and this may cause interstitial oedema. Low-sodium fluids (e.g. 5% dextrose) disperse throughout the ICF and ECF, with a volume of distribution of 42 L. In contrast, sodium-containing fluids (e.g. normal saline) only distribute within the ECF (because cellular pumps remove ICF sodium), and the smaller volume of distribution (~17 L) means that slightly more will remain intravascular. The use of hypertonic crystalloids (e.g. 7.5% saline), with or without colloids, for initial resuscitation (i.e. to osmotically draw ICF water into the

Table 2.2 Composition of crystalloids and colloids

Fluid	Na (mmol/L)	K (mmol/L)	Cl (mmol/L)	Osmolarity (mosmol/L)	Additions (mmol/L)	
Plasma	136–144	3.5–4	98–105	280–300		
Crystalloids						
glucose (INN) 5%	0	0	0	278	Glucose: 280	
0.45% saline	77	0	77	154		
0.9% saline	154	0	154	308	Nil	
Hartmann's	131	5	111	275	HCO_3 29; Ca 1.8	
Ringer's	130	4	109	273	Ca 2.2	
Colloids					T½ (h)	PVE
Gelofusine®	154	0	125	279	~2	80%
Haemaccel®	145	0	?	300	~1	70%
5% albumin	130–160	0	150	300	days	100%
10% HES	154	0	154	308	12–14 days	145%

T½, approximate effective plasma half-life; PVE, plasma volume expansion (% of volume given); HES, hydroxyethyl starch.

Table 2.3 Properties of colloid solutions

Colloid (MW in Da)	Properties	Disadvantages
Gelatins ~30,000	Cheap and rapidly degraded to water. Maximum volume 1.5–2.0 L daily	Allergic reactions
Dextrans ~40–70,000	~30% intravascular after 24 h. Reduces serum viscosity, so used in PVD and as DVT prophylaxis. Renal and RES clearance	Bleeding risk. Interferes with blood tests. Allergy 5%. Osmotic diuresis and renal impairment
Hydroxyethyl starch ~50–500,000	Plasma volume expansion and long intravascular times. Renal and RES clearance. Use suspended in Europe	Significant renal impairment and potential increase in mortality. Pruritus and bleeding risk
Albumin ~68,000	Few advantages over synthetic colloids. Expensive	Infection risks. Allergic reactions

MW, molecular weight; PVD; peripheral vascular disease; RES; reticuloendothelial system.

ECF) has not improved outcome in general trauma patients. However, associated small fluid resuscitation volumes and hypertonic osmotic effects may reduce cerebral oedema and benefit head trauma patients.

- **Colloid solutions** contain complex, high molecular weight molecules. They are retained in the vascular compartment for longer periods than crystalloid solutions and exert an oncotic pressure determined by the size and structure of the colloid molecule and the permeability of the patients capillaries which expands the intravascular compartment.

It is often quoted that ~3–4 times as much crystalloid is required for the same intravascular volume expansion as a colloid. Consequently, colloids were previously employed for initial resuscitation. However, a recent study demonstrated that the volume ratio of 4% albumin to saline for equivalent resuscitation was 1:1.4. In addition, a meta-analysis has shown no advantage of colloids over crystalloids for initial resuscitation and some colloids may cause significant harm. Consequently colloids should only be used for initial resuscitation after careful consideration.

Both natural (e.g. albumin) and synthetic colloids (e.g. gelatin, dextran) are expensive and have specific properties and side effects which are summarized in Table 2.3. For example, albumin may aid lung water clearance in acute lung injury and may be beneficial in hypoalbuminaemic (<15 g/dL) patients with severe sepsis. Low MW gelatins are rapidly excreted through the kidneys and produce short-term volume expansion but have little benefit over crystalloid fluids for resuscitation. In addition, the European Medicines Agency has recently suspended the marketing authorisation for all hydroxyethyl starch (HES) solutions following the review of recent studies that suggest there is a greater risk of renal impairment (i.e. acute kidney injury) requiring dialysis and an associated increase in mortality. HES solutions vary in molecular weight, degree of branching and pharmokinetic properties but will not be available for use in Europe pending evidence of safety and associated benefit.

In addition to the renal impairment recently demonstrated with HES, other disadvantages of colloids include allergic reactions and clotting abnormalities.

- **Blood** is given to maintain haemoglobin concentration > 70–80 g/L (>7–8 g/dL). However, young patients and those with renal disease, haemoglobinopathies, or chronic anaemia may tolerate lower levels. A haemoglobin of ~100 g/L (~10 g/dL) may improve outcome in cardiac patients.
- **Sodium bicarbonate** (1.26%) is used in patients with metabolic acidosis (pH <7.2) and renal or gastrointestinal losses. Recent acute kidney injury guidelines have advocated the use of 1.26% solutions in renal impairment.

Prescribing fluids

Total fluid requirements should be prescribed daily and adjusted for enteral feeding. When intravenous fluids are required, the type of fluid (i.e. 5% glucose (INN) for water replacement), electrolyte additives (e.g. K^+), route, and rate of infusion should be prescribed, with the date and signature of the issuing physician.

Fluid selection is guided by the underlying condition, extracellular fluid status (e.g. oedema), fluid losses (e.g. diarrhoea), renal function, fluid balance (± weight), and electrolyte concentrations. In the absence of normal homeostatic mechanisms, the fluid prescription should address:

- Basic maintenance fluids to replace normal daily water and electrolyte losses.
- The need for additional replacement and resuscitation fluids to replenish potential fluid deficits and to compensate for the underlying pathology.
- The rate of fluid administration and the time course over which potential fluid deficits should be corrected. This should take into account the rate of development of fluid and electrolyte abnormalities.
- Potential complicating factors, including renal, cardiac, hepatic, and endocrine function.

In general, the fluid that is lost is replaced. Thus, blood is most appropriate for haemorrhagic loss. Replacement fluids should match normal daily losses. However, in more complex situations, it may not be appropriate for the replacement fluid to match the perceived deficit (see section on fluid administration). Thus, in acutely unwell patients and those with renal impairment or complex fluid losses (e.g. burns, fistulae), the selection of replacement fluid (e.g. crystalloid, colloid) should be dictated by speciality guidelines (e.g. diabetic ketoacidosis, sepsis).

Fluid administration

General principles of fluid administration
The principles of fluid administration include:

1. **Normal maintenance fluid.** In a euvolaemic patient unable to take oral fluids (e.g. impaired consciousness), the aim is to replace the normal daily water and electrolyte losses. Ideally, 2.0 L of water (~25–30 mL/kg/day), 70 mmol (1 mmol/kg/day) of sodium, and 40–70 mmol (0.5–1 mmol/kg/day) of potassium should be prescribed intravenously daily. Minimum urine output should be maintained at >0.5 mL/kg/h or 35 mL/h. Ideally, 50–100 g/day of intravenous glucose is required to prevent starvation ketosis.

2. **Replacement and resuscitation fluids.** The aim is to estimate and replace potential fluid deficits and maintain an effective circulation (i.e. blood pressure, cardiac output, and blood distribution) by compensating for potential pathological defects (e.g. profound vasodilation and maldistribution in sepsis). In many cases, rapidly replacing the lost fluid is the best strategy. Consequently, haemorrhage is best corrected with packed red cells, and diarrhoea with balanced electrolyte solution.

However, rapidly replacing the 'lost fluid' is not always the correct response. This is best illustrated by considering the situation that arises following severe water deprivation over several days in a hot climate. In this situation, insensible 'pure water' loss can be considerable and is often associated with profound serum hypernatraemia and a hyperosmolar state due to the kidneys' attempts to preserve salt and water. It would appear logical to rapidly replace the lost 'water' with 5% glucose (INN), but this may result in severe transmembrane electrolyte imbalance and central pontine demyelination which is potentially life-threatening. Longstanding experience has demonstrated that slowly replacing the fluid deficit using a salt-containing solution to minimize potential electrolyte imbalance (e.g. hypernatraemia) is associated with better survival and less morbidity.

Vomiting causes hypokalaemic alkalosis due to excessive hydrogen ion loss. The resulting hypokalaemia is due to the excretion of potassium ions in exchange for hydrogen ions in the kidney (i.e. H^+/K^+ exchanger) which is the normal physiological mechanism used to correct alkalosis. Thus, in patients with significant vomiting, large quantities of potassium (e.g. >150 mmol K^+/day) may have to be prescribed to maintain serum potassium levels and aid correction of the alkalosis. Correcting the complex electrolyte losses associated with fistulae, burns, and trauma can be even more challenging and requires constant monitoring of fluid balance and electrolyte levels.

The volume of resuscitation fluid will depend on the underlying condition. For example, in severe sepsis with endothelial permeability, persistently high-volume infusions may be required to maintain intravascular filling and MAP despite the associated solute retention, electrolyte imbalance, and peripheral oedema. Subsequent correction of this fluid, solute and electrolyte imbalance may take many days to correct following recovery from the septic state. Fluid challenges with 250–500 mL boluses of fluid often help determine the volume of resuscitation fluid required.

3. **Assess how rapidly fluid deficits should be corrected.** The rate of fluid administration depends on the underlying condition. In general, if fluid is lost rapidly, it can usually be replaced rapidly. In contrast, slow fluid depletion often requires gradual correction because time allows cellular membranes to equilibrate the intra- and extracellular milieu. For example, the large fluid deficits and acute electrolyte imbalances associated with diabetic ketoacidosis can be corrected rapidly because the onset and progression of the disease process is rapid. In contrast, hyperosmolar non-ketotic diabetic coma (HONK) requires slow correction of the equally large fluid deficits and associated electrolyte abnormalities because it is a slow progressive disease process which allows intracellular equilibration with extracellular changes. In these patients, a sudden change in established electrolyte abnormalities (e.g. hypernatraemia in HONK, hyponatraemia after prolonged diarrhoea) can have serious consequences, including central pontine demyelination.

4. **Assess complicating factors.** Patients with renal impairment have a reduced ability to excrete solutes and often water. These patients may require a reduction in daily water, sodium, and potassium administration. Careful monitoring of fluid balance, including daily weights, and serum electrolytes is required to determine appropriate fluid and electrolyte administration. Similarly, normal water and electrolyte balance is disrupted in the acutely unwell patients (as discussed previously) and requires careful monitoring and subsequent correction due to stress and inflammatory response.

Fluid administration: specific situations

In many cases, fluid and electrolyte imbalances can be complex, and addressing one aspect of the imbalance may exacerbate another aspect. These situations cause fluid and electrolyte accumulation in the body tissues, commonly the interstitial space. The previous concept of a 'third space', including peritoneum, pleural, and pericardial spaces, for storage of this excess fluid is probably erroneous, according to recent evidence. Typically, this excess fluid and electrolyte load is excreted, following correction of the causative pathology, and is associated with a diuretic phase during recovery.

In some patients, particularly those with renal impairment, large volumes of crystalloid or colloid engender large solute loads (e.g. sodium, chloride) which can be difficult to excrete and may precipitate hyperchloraemic acidosis (HCA) due to high chloride (Cl^-) levels in some fluids (see Table 2.1). In these circumstances, when crystalloid resuscitation or replacement is required, physiologically balanced solutions (PBS) with low Cl^- content (e.g. Hartmann's, Ringer's lactate) are preferred and should replace 0.9% saline, except in cases associated with hypochloraemia (e.g. vomiting). These PBS cause less HCA and the associated nausea, confusion, and oliguria, compared to other fluids (e.g. saline 0.9%).

Solutions, such as 5% glucose (INN) and 4%/0.18% glucose (INN)/saline, are important sources of free water for maintenance. They should be used with caution if fluid requirements exceed maintenance requirements, as excessive amounts may cause hyponatraemia, especially in the elderly. These solutions are not, therefore, appropriate for resuscitation or replacement therapy, except in conditions of significant free water deficit (e.g. diabetes insipidus).

The management of specific clinical scenarios is illustrated in the following examples:

- **Maintenance fluid.** Stable, euvolaemic patients with normal renal function who cannot drink require 2–2.5 L (25–30 mls/kg/day, 1–1.5 mL/kg/h, 100 mL/h) water, 70–150 mmol sodium (Na^+), and 40–70 mmol potassium (K^+) each day. This equates to 0.5–1 L of saline 0.9% (Na^+ 154 mmol/L) and 1–2 L of 5% glucose (INN) (water), with 20 mmol K^+ added to each litre of 5% glucose (INN). If there is significant hypernatraemia ($\uparrow Na^+$, $\uparrow Cl^-$) or hyponatraemia ($\downarrow Na^+$, $\downarrow Cl^-$), additional 5% glucose (INN) or saline 0.9% are used, respectively, as required.

- **Post-major surgery.** If hypovolaemia occurs, despite normal maintenance fluid administration (i.e. 1–1.5 mL/kg/h), increase the infusion rate to 2–3 mL/kg/h using a PBS (e.g. Hartmann's which reduces Cl^- load). Consider 0.5 L Gelofusine® 'fluid challenges' to support the circulation if crystalloid fluid volumes become excessive, although there is little evidence to support this practice. Maintain haemoglobin (Hb) >7–8 g/dL in stable patients, and >10 g/dL in unstable cardiac patients (e.g. heart failure). Remember that large fluid requirements may indicate internal bleeding.

- **Major haemorrhage** usually requires urgent control of bleeding and restoration of circulating volume. Occasionally, aggressive fluid resuscitation before surgery increases blood loss due to dilutional coagulopathy, acidosis, and hypothermia (e.g. ruptured aortic aneurysm). In these patients, the priority is early surgery, with restoration of circulating volume after surgery. Blood is the ideal resuscitation fluid but requires time to prepare. Whilst awaiting blood, fluid replacement starts with 20–30 mL/kg Hartmann's solution. Consider giving 1–1.5 L

Gelofusine® to support the circulation if crystalloids are inadequate alone. Infusion rate is determined by repeated clinical assessment. Ongoing resuscitation includes plasma and platelets.

- **Sepsis and septic shock** cause interstitial (i.e. 'third space') fluid accumulation due to increased vascular permeability. Assessment of associated intravascular hypovolaemia is difficult and may require repeated 'fluid challenges' and close monitoring (e.g. urine output (UO), lactate, CVP, SvO$_2$). Fluid replacement follows the Surviving Sepsis Guidelines and should start immediately in hypotensive patients or if lactate is raised. Initially, give 20–40 mL/kg Hartmann's in aliquots of 0.5–1 L, based on clinical re-sponse. If hypotension or lactate elevation persists, in-sert a CVP line, and continue resuscitation with Gelofusine® 1–1.5 L, aiming for a CVP 8–12 mmHg, MAP >65 mmHg, urine output >0.5 mL/kg/h, mixed venous saturation (SvO$_2$) >70%, and Hb 7–9 g/dL. Further details are available in Chapters 2 and 6.
- **Head injury.** Hyponatraemia, hypoxia, hypotension, and hyperthermia worsen brain oedema. A degree of hypernatraemia may be beneficial, and saline 0.9% is recommended as fluid resuscitation (see Chapter 18). Except with associated diabetes insipidus, 5% glucose (INN) should be avoided.
- **Acute kidney injury** (AKI) is associated with increased morbidity and mortality during acute illness. Inadequate fluid replacement may place a patient at risk of AKI secondary to hypovolaemia. Treatment of hypovolaemia in patients with AKI follows similar principles to those outlined for patients with normal renal function. However, it should be recognized that these patients have a reduced ability to excrete excess fluid and electrolytes and are at significant risk of fluid and sodium overload and associated hyperkalaemia. In general, balanced electrolyte solutions containing potassium can be used cautiously in closely monitored patients with AKI, but, if hyperkalaemia develops, non-potassium-containing crystalloid solutions (e.g., 4%/0.18% glucose (INN)/saline) should be used.

In established oliguric or anuric renal failure, fluid replacement is restricted to insensible loss (0.5–1 L daily) to avoid fluid overload. Electrolytes are monitored daily and sodium and potassium intake restricted. Calcium exchange resins, insulin with glucose (INN), or renal replacement therapy may be required to treat hyperkalaemia.

As reported above, hydroxyethyl starches (HES) have been demonstrated to increase the risk of AKI in critically ill patients with sepsis and are associated with increased mortality. The European Medicines Agency has suspended their marketing authorizations in Europe.

- **Rhabdomyolysis** has many causes, including direct muscle injury and compartment syndrome. Cell lysis results in the release of myoglobin which is freely filtered by the kidneys and, in the setting of hypovolaemia and acidosis, can cause AKI. Effective management requires aggressive fluid resuscitation with an isotonic crystalloid solution. There is limited evidence to support the common practice of alkalinizing the urine through the administration of sodium bicarbonate.
- **Hypotension and oliguria following recovery from critical illness.** This is a common problem and one that illustrates how an understanding of fluid management can improve patient care. Patients discharged from critical care units are often relatively hypotensive, with a poor urine output despite profound tissue oedema, including potential pulmonary oedema. It is not uncommon for these patients

to be treated with fluid and diuretic therapy, in a futile attempt to improve the blood pressure and urine output, with little effect other than to further exacerbate the already severe peripheral (± pulmonary) oedema. Closer inspection will reveal that many of these patients are severely hypoalbuminaemic (e.g. albumin <15 g/dL) due to failure of normal liver production of albumin during the period of critical illness and ongoing natural breakdown of older albumin (as discussed previously). In addition, these patients are often relatively anaemic (e.g. haemoglobin ~8 g/dL).

The combination of both hypoalbuminaemia and anaemia reduces intravascular colloid oncotic pressure and consequently intravascular volume. The low intravascular volume results in hypotension and stimulates the kidneys to conserve salt and water (i.e. reducing urine output). Any fluid given to these patients will rapidly leak out of the circulation into the peripheral tissues due to the lack of colloid pressure, adding to the oedema but having little effect on blood pressure or urine output.

In this situation, the aim should be to facilitate correction of the reduced colloid oncotic pressure (although this will occur naturally over time due to liver production of albumin). Occasionally intravenous albumin supplements are given to increase plasma colloid oncotic pressure as this will attract and bind water in the intravascular compartment, increasing intravascular volume. This corrects the hypotension, stimulates the kidneys to produce larger quantities of urine, and consequently leads to correction of the peripheral oedema. However, intravenous albumin solutions are blood products with all the associated risks and must be used with caution.

Summary

Optimum intravenous fluid prescription is dependent on a sound understanding of the basic principles of physiology as well as the pathophysiology of disease processes. When undertaken thoughtfully, this, often neglected, clinical skill is likely to significantly enhance a patient's chances of making a good recovery and avoiding iatrogenic complications.

Further reading

Arieff AI (1999). Fatal postoperative pulmonary edema: pathogenesis and literature review. *Chest*, **115**, 1371–7.

Awad S, Allison SP, Lobo DN (2008). Fluid and electrolyte balance: the impact of goal directed teaching. *Clinical Nutrition*, **27**, 473–8.

Callum KG, Gray AJG, Hoile RW, *et al.* (1999). Extremes of age: The 1999 report of the National Confidential Enquiry into Perioperative deaths. The National Confidential Enquiry into Perioperative Deaths, London.

Chappell D, Jacob M, Hofmann-Kiefer K, Conzen P, Rehm M (2008). A rational approach to perioperative fluid management. *Anaesthesiology*, **109**, 723–40.

Committee on Medical Aspects of Food Policy, Department of Health (1991). Dietary reference values for food energy and nutrients for the United Kingdom. COMA report on Health and Social Subjects No 41. HMSO, London.

Dellinger RP, Levy MM, Rhodes A, *et al.* (2012). Surviving sepsis campaign: international guidelines for the management of severe sepsis and septic shock. *Critical Care Medicine*, **36**, 296–327.

Edelman I and Leibman J (1959). Anatomy of body water and electrolytes. *American Journal of Medicine*, **27**, 256–77.

European Medicines Agency. PRAC (Pharmacovigilance Risk Assessment Committee) recommends suspending marketing authorisations for infusion solutions containing hydroxyethyl starch. <http://www.ema.europa.eu/ema/>.

Gosling P (2003). Salt of the earth or a drop in the ocean? A pathophysiological approach to fluid resuscitation. *Emergency Medicine Journal*, **20**, 306–15.

Lobo DN, Stanga Z, Simpson JAD, Anderson JA, Rowlands BJ, Allison SP (2001). Dilution and redistribution effects of rapid 2-litre infusions of 0.9% (w/v) saline and 5% (w/v) dextrose on haematological parameters and serum biochemistry in normal subjects: a double-blind cross-over study. *Clinical Science*, **101**, 173–9.

Myburgh JA, Finfer S, Bellorno R, *et al.* (2012). Hydroxyethyl starch or saline for fluid resuscitation in intensive care. *New England Journal of Medicine*, **367**, 1901–11.

National Institute for Health and Clinical Excellence (CG174: 2013). Intravenous fluid therapy in adults in hospital. https://www.nice.org.uk/guidance/cg174

National Institute for Health and Clinical Excellence (CG169; 2013). Acute kidney injury: Prevention, detection and management of acute kidney injury up to the point of renal replacement therapy. <https://www.nice.org.uk/guidance/cg169>.

Perner A, Haase N, Guttormsen HB, *et al.* (2012). Hydroxyethyl starch 130/0.42 versus Ringers' acetate in severe sepsis. *New England Journal of Medicine*, **367**, 124–34.

Powell-Tuck J, Gosling P, Lobo DN, *et al.* (2011). British consensus guidelines on intravenous fluid therapy for adult surgical patients. <http://www.bapen.org.uk/pdfs/bapen_pubs/giftasup.pdf>

Reid F, Lobo DN, Williams RN, Rowlands BJ, Allison SP (2003). (Ab) normal saline and physiological Hartmann's solution: a randomised double-blind crossover study. *Clinical Science*, **104**, 17–24.

Roberts I, Alderson P, Bunn F, Chinnock P, Ker K, Schierhout G (2004). Colloids versus crystalloids for fluid resuscitation in critically ill patients. *Cochrane Database of Systematic Reviews*, **4**, CD000567.

Rooker JC and Gorard DA (2007). Errors of intravenous fluid infusion rates in medical inpatients. *Clinical Medicine*, **7**, 482–5.

Skellett S, Mayer A, Durwood A, Tibby SM, Murdoch IA (2000). Chasing the base deficit: hyperchloraemic acidosis following 0.9% saline fluid resuscitation. *Archives of Disease in Childhood*, **83**, 514–16.

The Renal Association (2011). Acute kidney injury. <http://www.renal.org/clinical/guidelinessection/AcuteKidneyInjury.aspx>.

Walsh SR, Cook EJ, Bentley R, *et al.* (2008). Peri-operative fluid management: prospective audit. *International Journal of Clinical Practice*, **62**, 492–7.

Walsh SR and Walch CJ (2005). Intravenous fluid associated morbidity in postoperative patients. *Annals of the Royal College of Surgeons of England*, **87**, 126–30.

Wilcox CS (1983). Regulation of renal blood flow by plasma chloride. *Journal of Clinical Investigation*, **71**, 726–35.

Shock states

Definition and classification of shock states

Shock can be defined as any clinical situation where tissue perfusion has become inadequate. If uncorrected, it results in progressive organ dysfunction, multi-organ damage and, ultimately, death. In the early stages of shock, a patient may be relatively asymptomatic, as compensatory mechanisms, including sympathetically driven tachycardia and vasoconstriction, attempt to maintain a near normal blood pressure. As the degree of shock worsens, compensatory mechanisms fail; blood pressure falls, and organ hypoperfusion results. At this stage, the patient will be symptomatic, with abnormal haemodynamic findings, cool peripheries, and a prolonged capillary refill time. Restlessness, agitation, and confusion are evidence of compromised cerebral perfusion while oliguria indicates renal hypoperfusion.

The mortality rate for shock still exceeds 50%, and successful treatment demands prompt recognition of physiological abnormalities, together with an awareness of the potential underlying differential diagnosis. The following aetiological classification should be considered:

Hypovolaemic (oligaemic) shock

This category comprises any clinical state that results in reduced circulatory volume.

Haemorrhage is a common cause, and, while this may be due to obvious trauma or overt gastrointestinal bleeding, covert blood loss (from the gastrointestinal tract or into the peritoneum or retroperitoneal space, e.g. a leaking aortic aneurysm) should also be considered.

Fluids, other than blood, may be lost:

- Gastrointestinal fluid from diarrhoea, vomiting, or both.
- The osmotic diuresis associated with diabetic emergencies.
- Pathological salt and/or free water loss from the kidney, as seen in primary renal disease (e.g. post-obstructive uropathy) or endocrine conditions, such as Addison's disease or diabetes insipidus.
- Severe fluid loss from skin pathology, including desquamative skin rashes and extensive burns.

Cardiogenic shock

Failure of the heart to maintain adequate systemic blood flow can be due to several causes, and subclassification is useful because of potential specific therapeutic interventions:

- Myocardial ('pump') failure commonly arises from the reduced systolic function that accompanies myocardial infarction. It can also complicate acute myocarditis or cardiomyopathy.
- Mechanical failure from acute mitral regurgitation, papillary muscle rupture, or from ventricular septal defect. These acute events are usually sequelae of myocardial infarction but can relate to infection or inflammation.
- Obstructive (extracardiac) shock is exemplified by pericardial tamponade, massive pulmonary embolism, or severe pulmonary hypertension.

Distributive shock

Septic shock is the most common example. A detailed discussion follows and includes reference to the 'Surviving Sepsis Campaign'. Any infective organism may cause septic shock, and individual clinical findings are generally non-discriminative for a particular pathogen—the characteristic skin rash of meningococcal septicaemia being an exception.

Anaphylactic and *neurogenic* subtypes of shock are also best classified in the 'distributive' category.

There is considerable overlap within the categories of shock. In sepsis, for example, the distributive element of shock caused by vasodilatation is compounded by hypovolaemia due to third space fluid loss as well as myocardial dysfunction from a direct toxic effect of sepsis. Each of these three pathophysiological contributors to reduced tissue perfusion can predominate at different stages of septic shock. Typically, vasodilatation (both arterial and venous) is the initial dominant factor, followed by fluid shift as a result of 'leaky' capillaries, and, finally, the clinical picture becomes complicated by the development of myocardial dysfunction.

Pathophysiology of shock states

A fundamental concept to grasp is that, while changes in systemic perfusion are invariably present in shock, tissue oxygen delivery is not always reduced. Indeed, in sepsis, oxygen delivery is commonly increased, but utilization at a tissue level is compromised.

Hypovolaemic and cardiogenic shock

Tissue oxygen delivery (DO_2) is reduced in hypovolaemic and cardiogenic shock states. In hypovolaemia, reduced cardiac preload is responsible, whereas, in cardiogenic shock, it is impaired myocardial contractility. Systolic dysfunction is the result of reduced effective myocardial contractility from whatever cause, but cardiac output may also be compromised by diastolic dysfunction. This may result from reduced ventricular compliance or from increased resistance to ventricular filling during diastole.

As DO_2 falls in the early stages of hypovolaemia or cardiogenic shock, the body tissues compensate by extracting more oxygen from their reduced blood supply. This is the phase of 'supply-independent oxygen uptake', which results in a fall in the mixed venous oxygen content (MVO_2) of blood returning to the heart. It follows that change in the calculated arterial to mixed venous oxygen difference is a useful arbiter of changes in cardiac output. However, when DO_2 falls below a critical level (commonly defined as 8–10 mL/kg/min), compensatory mechanisms fail, and, as oxygen uptake in the tissues falls, a stage of 'supply-dependent oxygen uptake' supervenes. The severity of the ensuing tissue hypoxia is proportional to the measured elevation in plasma lactate, provided there is sufficient tissue perfusion to 'wash out' the accumulated lactate. Note that a falsely low plasma lactate can mislead the clinician during early resuscitation of shock, as profound hypoperfusion impairs tissue lactate removal.

Distributive shock states

Septic shock

The sequence of events in septic shock is different. The precipitating event is the presence of microbial components that stimulate the release of pro-inflammatory and anti-inflammatory cytokines (tumour necrosis factor (TNF) alpha and various interleukins are examples). These activate the complement and coagulation cascades, promote platelet aggregation, and stimulate the synthesis of reactive oxygen species and nitric oxide. The net outcome of this complicated series of events is, first, vasodilatation and, secondly, reduced intravascular volume as a result of increased capillary permeability, leading to extravascular fluid leakage.

These events combine to reduce cardiac preload. A sympathetically driven attempt to increase cardiac output (through positive inotropic and chronotropic effects) follows, but, unfortunately, this can occur when myocardial function is itself compromised through the effects of sepsis.

The effects on DO_2 are complicated. At first, DO_2 is increased, largely as a result of increased cardiac output. However, tissue oxygen uptake climbs simultaneously because of increased tissue metabolism, and, even at DO_2 levels above the critical 8–10 mL/kg/min, oxygen supply is inadequate to meet increased demand, and lactate accumulates. This is probably a combination of abnormal tissue perfusion in the microcirculation, together with a deleterious effect of sepsis on mitochondrial function that disrupts cellular oxygen utilization.

In shock, anaerobic cellular metabolism leads to:

- Depletion of adenosine triphosphate, with consequent failure of the cell membrane sodium-potassium pump.
- Progressive lactic acidosis.
- Abnormal mitochondrial function that disrupts cellular function, with an adverse effect on myocardial contractility.

Anaphylactic shock
Anaphylaxis is a severe allergic reaction that follows re-exposure to a foreign allergen (commonly, a drug, food, foreign serum, or venoms) to which a patient has been previously sensitized and developed specific IgE. Re-exposure to the allergen allows linkage of the foreign allergen with IgE attached to mast cells and basophils. This stimulates the release of histamine and other mediators, including platelet-activating factor, interleukins, and prostaglandins. Mediator release results in vasodilatation, smooth muscle contraction in other sites (e.g. bronchial wall and gut), increased glandular secretion, and increased capillary permeability. Shock can be the end result of this process, with other clinical features, including bronchospasm, upper airway obstruction, facial and tongue swelling, generalized or localized urticaria, angioneurotic oedema, and abdominal pain.

Neurogenic shock
Neurogenic shock is uncommon and results from the loss of peripheral vasomotor tone that can complicate spinal cord injury and epidural or general anaesthesia. It can also follow administration of autonomic blocking agents. In these situations, peripheral blood pooling results in diminished cardiac preload, with subsequent reduction in tissue perfusion.

Clinical aspects of shock states
Clinically, shock manifests itself in one of two basic patterns of presentation, depending on whether the cardiac index is decreased (hypodynamic presentation) or increased (hyperdynamic presentation).

Hypodynamic presentation
A low cardiac index is usually seen in hypovolaemic and cardiogenic shock. The patient is poorly perfused, with cool, clammy peripheries with a slow capillary refill time. Tachycardia is the norm because of an agonal chronotropic response, and tachypnoea is common as a response to metabolic acidosis. Reduced cerebral and renal perfusion occurs and results in some degree of mental confusion and oliguria, respectively.

If the cause of hypovolaemia is abnormal renal tract losses, as a result of intrinsic renal pathology or endocrine disease (as discussed previously), urine output can continue at an inappropriately high level despite hypovolaemia.

Central venous pressure is low in hypovolaemic shock and commonly (but not always) elevated in cardiogenic shock. It is best, however, to consider CVP in response to dynamic challenge, rather than as a static measure.

A compensatory sympathetic response can successfully maintain systemic blood pressure in the early stages of hypovolaemic shock, usually in young and previously fit individuals where blood pressure is sustained through progressive systemic vasoconstriction. The clinical clue to this compensatory mechanism is a rising diastolic blood pressure in association with a stable systolic pressure—in other words, a diminishing pulse pressure. This finding on the blood pressure chart of young adults with continuing blood loss should raise concern but is often missed. It is important because compensatory mechanisms can fail suddenly with catastrophic consequences. This adaptive response to hypovolaemia is often blunted or absent in the elderly or infirm.

In cardiogenic shock, clinical and radiographic signs of heart failure may be present, and the central venous pressure is variable. A third or fourth heart sound or a summation gallop is often audible, and there may be obvious cardiac dyskinesia on palpation of the precordium.

Hyperdynamic presentation
The cardiac index is usually, but not always, high in distributive shock. The diagnosis of septic shock requires, by definition, the following combination of clinical factors.

- Proven source of infection.
- A MAP of <65 mmHg, despite fluid resuscitation, or the requirement of pharmacologic vasopressor agents to maintain a normal MAP.
- Two or more of the following manifestations of systemic inflammation:
  - Tachypnoea.
  - Tachycardia.
  - A white cell count that is either elevated or depressed.
  - A body temperature that is either high or low.
- Dysfunction of at least one end organ.

The hyperdynamic state often results in warm peripheries, with 'bounding' peripheral pulses, and, hence in the early stages, the examination findings differ from hypovolaemic and cardiogenic shock.

Reduced cerebral oxygen delivery is common and is a contributing factor to mental confusion.

The characteristic purpuric and non-blanching rash of meningococcal septicaemia suggests a specific infective diagnosis. However, the rash is often minimal at onset and may be confined to pressure areas, such as buttocks and the backs of the thighs—areas often overlooked during routine examination.

An approach to investigations
1. If sepsis is a possible diagnosis, blood cultures and other appropriate samples for culture are mandatory. They should be collected, if possible, before antibiotics are given but must not delay commencing antibiotic therapy.
2. In addition (and modified, according to the likely cause of shock), some basic blood tests are required. These include:
   - Full blood count, including differential white cell count and platelet count. Septic shock can cause a high or low white cell count. The latter is associated with a poor prognosis.

- Clotting screen to exclude disseminated intravascular coagulation (DIC).
- Serum creatinine, urea and electrolytes, including chloride and bicarbonate.
- Liver function tests.
- Troponin level.
- C-reactive protein, a marker of sepsis.
- Arterial blood gases and analysis of acid-base balance and calculation of the alveolar-arterial oxygen difference.
- Plasma lactate (as discussed further in list).

3. Electrocardiograph and chest X-ray (perhaps abdominal X-ray).
4. The following investigations and clinical points should also be considered:
   - Echocardiography is useful to assess left ventricular function. It also detects pericardial and valvular heart disease and may assist in diagnosing pulmonary embolism and the potential need for thrombolysis in submassive pulmonary embolism. Transthoracic echocardiography may not detect small vegetations in bacterial endocarditis, and, if suspected, transoesophageal echocardiography is a more sensitive test.
   - DIC is diagnosed by the combination of prolonged clotting, thrombocytopenia, and a reduced fibrinogen level.
   - Plasma lactate is elevated in most cases of shock and indicates failure to utilize oxygen at a cellular level. In general, lactate levels correlate with the severity of shock and prognosis as well as guiding the success or failure of therapeutic interventions. Plasma lactate should be measured promptly in all cases of suspected shock, recognizing that, in severe tissue hypoperfusion, lactate levels may be artificially low during the early stages of resuscitation.
   Plasma lactate level or/and base excess can be used to predict outcome in patients admitted to a critical care unit.
- Computerized tomography pulmonary artery scanning (CTPA) is pivotal in confirming the diagnosis of pulmonary embolism and assessing the severity of disease by providing additional pathophysiological information related to myocardial function and 'clot load'. It may also guide the need for thrombolysis.

Table 2.4 Invasive haemodynamic measurements available with a pulmonary artery occlusion catheter and potential differences in various categories of shock

	Hypovolaemic shock	Cardiogenic shock	Septic shock
Cardiac Index	Low	Low	High
PA occ. Press	Low	High	Normal or Low
CVP	Low	Normal or High	Normal or Low
SVR	High	High	Low
DO₂	Low	Low	High

PA occ. Press, pulmonary artery occlusion (or wedge) pressure; CVP, central venous pressure; SVR, systemic vascular resistance; DO$_2$, tissue oxygen delivery.

- CT scanning of the abdomen if intra-abdominal pathology is suspected as the cause for shock. A perforated viscus, infarcted bowel, abdominal aortic aneurysm, and pancreatitis are potential causes.
- Pulmonary artery occlusion catheters have fallen out of favour. Measurements may be of potential value in differentiating between the three major causes of shock (see Table 2.4) and may guide fluid replacement (optimizing cardiac preload) and evaluating the effects of pharmacologic inotropic and vasopressor support.

Clinical management of shock states

Generic principles of management are that:
- Shock is a medical emergency, and resuscitation must commence immediately, and in parallel with (rather than subsequent to), investigation of the specific diagnosis.
- Basic supportive management procedures apply, regardless of the category of the shock state.
- Specific therapeutic interventions are indicated, according to the particular diagnosis. For example, in suspected sepsis, antibiotics should be given immediately.
- If the patient is shocked, consider sepsis as the possible cause, and, if the patient is septic, question whether they are shocked. Early diagnosis and management are crucial to securing a favourable outcome in this condition.

General (supportive) management

Ventilatory support and oxygen therapy
In shock, a fundamental aim is to optimize tissue oxygen delivery. High flow oxygen should be administered to all patients to maximize arterial oxygen saturation.

Work of breathing is usually increased in shock states and results in an increased demand for oxygen from the muscles of the respiratory pump. Tachypnoea (a virtually constant feature of severe shock) is a contributing factor, but various pathological processes that accompany shock (such as pulmonary oedema, acute respiratory distress syndrome, or infective pulmonary consolidation) also contribute, as they reduce pulmonary compliance and add significantly to the work of breathing.

For these reasons, early mechanical ventilatory support may be needed.

Fluid resuscitation
The approach to fluid resuscitation is encapsulated in the adjectives 'prompt', 'appropriate', and 'monitored'. The aim is to optimize cardiac preload by prompt restoration of circulating volume with appropriate fluids. If fluid resuscitation is delayed, then tissue hypoperfusion will be prolonged unnecessarily. Logic dictates that the fluid chosen to correct any deficit should reflect the type of fluid lost. In practice, assessment of a patient's fluid balance is difficult, and careful monitoring is essential, whether by continuous clinical reappraisal or by invasive haemodynamic monitoring.

In haemorrhagic shock, blood transfusion is indicated to restore euvolaemia. Two ancillary points are worthy of mention:
- Anaemia is common in intensive care patients, and studies in this population (excluding those with acute coronary syndrome) have demonstrated that a haemoglobin level of 7–9 g/dL is associated with a lower mortality risk than replacement to 10–12 g/dL. This applies to Hb level—the maintenance of euvolaemia is still paramount.
- Current evidence argues against the use of blood substitutes (e.g. cross-linked haemoglobin—DCLHb), as these appear to have a worse clinical outcome.

Prompt replacement of fluid loss cannot be overemphasized, and large-bore peripheral cannulae must be used.

Monitoring of fluid replacement is vital. Prompt restoration of cardiac preload is crucial, but overloading the shocked patient is a constant threat, particularly in the elderly and those with a history of ischaemic heart disease. The indications for invasive haemodynamic measurement remain an area of considerable debate:

- Insertion of a central line in a patient who is severely hypovolaemic is not easy, and early resuscitation often requires intensive, multitasked activity, rather than a myopic emphasis on neck line insertion.

That said, initial resuscitation in the severely shocked patient should usually be guided by scientifically measurable haemodynamics, and a central line is commonly required, with reassessment after fluid challenge. If all else were equal, then pulmonary artery occlusion catheters would be used exclusively, as they reflect left ventricular filling more accurately. All else is not equal, however, as these catheters incur significant risk, and use is based on individual need. Other less invasive systems can now be used, such as oesophageal Doppler.

The 'crystalloid-colloid' debate

There are certain salient points in the ongoing debate.

First, because of compartmental fluid distribution, colloids have been suggested to restore circulating fluid volume more efficiently than crystalloids (it is often quoted that approximately three times more crystalloid is required to achieve the same haemodynamic improvement). It is, therefore, popular to commence fluid resuscitation with a colloid solution until MAP is >65 mmHg and to continue with crystalloids thereafter. However, there is no trial-based evidence to support this, and crystalloid solutions are cheaper.

Secondly, the safety of some colloid replacement fluids has been questioned. A meta-analysis, published by the Cochrane Injuries Group Albumin Reviewers, included 24 studies, with a total of 1,419 patients with hypovolaemia, hypoalbuminaemia, and burns. This meta-analysis suggested a 6% increase in the absolute risk of death when albumin-containing fluids were used. A subsequent meta-analysis of 55 trials involving 3,504 patients found no significant increase in the risk of death with albumin-containing fluids in a 'general population' of critically ill patients.

Conflicting results, such as these, prompted the 'Saline versus Albumin Fluid Evaluation' (SAFE) study in 16 intensive care units in Australia and New Zealand. The trial found no difference in 28-day mortality from any cause when intravascular resuscitation with 4% albumin was compared with 0.9% sodium chloride in intensive care patients.

Other resuscitating fluids are increasingly available, but roles are not confirmed:

- The safety of the synthetic colloid hydroxyethyl starch (MMW-HES-200 kDa) has been questioned. In this regard, the European Medicines Agency has recently suspended the marketing authorization of hydroxyethyl starch (HES) solutions pending further review of recent studies suggesting greater risk of renal impairment requiring dialysis and an associated increase in mortality.
- High molecular weight hydroxyethyl starch (HMW-HES-450 kDa) is also reported to be associated with abnormal clotting and a higher propensity for bleeding.
- There has been a vogue for using hypertonic crystalloids (e.g. 7.5% sodium chloride, with or without dextran 70) in the initial resuscitation of shocked patients, especially in major trauma. Most studies have failed to show a clear benefit. Certain subgroups of patients (specifically, those with severe head injury) may have an improved outcome.

This is interesting because there are reports that large volumes of isotonic crystalloid can worsen cerebral oedema in this situation.

Inotropic support

Hypovolaemic shock

Fluid replacement alone should be sufficient to resuscitate the hypovolaemic patient.

Cardiogenic shock

Fluids are only indicated in cardiogenic shock in those patients who are volume-deplete or are overdiuresed. It is mandatory to monitor fluids carefully, preferably with central venous pressure monitoring.

Vasoactive and inotropic drugs are used in cardiogenic shock, but the physician should be aware that inotropic drugs will increase myocardial oxygen demand and may well compound the primary pathologic process. In some cases, intra-aortic balloon pumps or left ventricular devices are used to bridge myocardial failure.

In cardiogenic shock, cardiac output and blood pressure are typically low while systemic vascular resistance is increased. It follows that a vasodilator and inotropic drug may help, but only if it does not compromise MAP. Drugs of choice include dobutamine or milrinone.

If hypotension is prominent, a vasoconstricting inotrope, such as adrenaline or high-dose dobutamine, will be preferable. An alternative approach is to administer dobutamine for its inotropic effect, with noradrenaline which produces additional vasoconstriction.

Dopamine in high dose is vasoconstricting and inotropic and provides an alternative therapeutic option. However, it has a number of side effects, including adverse effects on pituitary function, intestinal mucosal perfusion, and renal medullary oxygen delivery.

If adrenaline is used, it can cause hyperglycaemia and hypokalaemia and may result in hyperlactataemia. The first two are of therapeutic relevance, and the third demands caution in interpreting subsequent lactate levels.

Septic shock

Aggressive fluid replacement is fundamental in the management of septic shock, and vasoactive drugs may be required to maintain adequate tissue perfusion.

In septic shock, cardiac output is typically high while blood pressure is low, as a result of increased peripheral vasodilatation and compartmental fluid shift. Fluid administration is the first priority to restore cardiac preload and, when achieved, a vasopressor inotrope, such as noradrenaline, may be required if the patient fails to improve. A complicating factor is the adverse effect of sepsis on myocardial function, and this may require concurrent administration of dobutamine.

Specific treatment considerations in individual shock states

Hypovolaemic shock

In all situations, appropriate and prompt fluid replacement is the cornerstone of management. Surgery, interventional radiology, and endoscopy each have a role in controlling haemorrhage. Other sources of continuing fluid loss should be treated appropriately.

Intra-abdominal crises, other than haemorrhage, may result in shock. Visceral perforation, intestinal obstruction, and bowel ischaemia are examples where surgery may be indicated. Effective and prompt collaboration between the surgical and critical care teams can improve patients' outcome post-operatively.

Cardiogenic shock

Cardiogenic shock secondary to acute myocardial infarction (MI) has a high mortality. In this situation, angiography with a view to invasive coronary intervention should be considered.

An intra-aortic balloon pump is useful in supporting myocardial function prior to surgery in the setting of papillary muscle rupture and ischaemic ventricular septal defect. It may be of benefit in the wider setting of post-MI cardiogenic shock, in conjunction with other interventions, such as angioplasty, stenting, and coronary artery bypass grafting.

Septic shock

Sepsis is a common reason for admission to intensive care units. In the early 1990s, the concept of the 'systemic inflammatory response syndrome' (SIRS) was adopted and a more precise series of definitions developed to categorize the degree of sepsis more accurately:

- Sepsis, as suspected, or microbiologically proven infection, together with SIRS (clinical features as detailed previously).
  - Mortality 10–15%
- Severe sepsis as sepsis together with sepsis-induced organ dysfunction.
  - Mortality 17–20%
- Septic shock as sepsis-induced hypotension persisting despite adequate fluid resuscitation.
  - Mortality 43–54%

In 2002, the Surviving Sepsis Campaign (SSC) was launched as an international collaboration.

The evidence base supporting the SSC recommendations derived largely from a single study that reported the benefit of 'early goal-directed therapy' in septic patients, showing that the early use of a standardized method of resuscitation in septic shock resulted in significantly reduced mortality. This has now been the subject of three large international trials. The SSC promoted a standardized approach by promulgating two care bundles.

The first was to guide the first 6 hours' management of a patient with sepsis in the emergency department (ED) or acute medical unit (AMU).

The second, a 24-hour care bundle, was intended to guide continuing management, if needed.

The SSC has been successful in emphasizing the need to manage sepsis in a timely and scientific manner, but a number of aspects of the original (2002) care bundles are controversial:

- The specificity of serum lactate as a guide to tissue hypoxia and adequacy of resuscitation has been questioned.
- The Rivers study has yet to be reproduced. For example, the practicality of comprehensively delivering the resuscitation bundles in the UK has been questioned.
- It is unclear how strictly the care bundles need to be adhered to in order to improve clinical outcome. Partial compliance has been reported to have significant impact on mortality in UK patients with sepsis. In Australia, in the absence of an accepted early goal-directed strategy, an initial resuscitation in ED has reported low mortality rates.

In 2008 and 2012, Dellinger et al. published updates to the original SSC clinical management guidelines, based on consensus conferences. They employed the 'grades of recommendation, assessment, development, and evaluation' (GRADE) system to guide the assessment of quality of evidence from high (A) to very low (D). In addition, a strong recommendation (1) from this expert group reflects the fact that evidence suggests an intervention's desirable effects outweigh its undesirable effects (risk, cost, etc.) or vice versa. Weak recommendations (2) indicate that the distinction between desirable and undesirable effects is less clear.

The salient recommendations of the guidelines are summarized in Box 2.1 (Resuscitation care bundle—within first 6 hours of care) and Box 2.2 (Management care bundle—within first 24 hours of care).

Initial resuscitation and infection

Early goal-directed resuscitation is recommended during the first 6 hours after diagnosis of the septic patient. From a practical point of view, it is crucial to have a high index of suspicion of sepsis. Appropriate, early antibiotic therapy is fundamental to the management of septic shock, and the need for pre-treatment cultures, when possible, is unequivocal. The practical issues of antibiotic administration are vital as is the choice of antibiotic and include:

- Adequate dosing.
- Adequate frequency of dosing.
- Ensuring that antibiotics are given on time.
- Measuring drug levels, if necessary, to ensure appropriate plasma levels.

Although broad-spectrum antibiotics will often be appropriate, initially, this must be tempered by an intelligent choice of drugs to cover likely organisms and may vary according to the clinical setting, e.g. urosepsis, community-acquired pneumonia, intra-abdominal sepsis, or neutropenic sepsis.

Expert microbiological assistance is invaluable. Initial incorrect antibiotic approach is associated with a less favourable outcome.

Vasopressors

If hypotension does not respond to fluid resuscitation, then vasopressors should be used, with a target MAP of ≥65 mmHg. Dellinger et al. recommend noradrenaline or high-dose dopamine (note previous concerns about dopamine).

There is good evidence against the use of low-dose dopamine for 'renal protection'.

Box 2.1 SSC International care bundles updates

- Solid bullet denotes strong recommendation
  - Open bullet is a weaker recommendation, a 'suggestion'

Resuscitation care bundle—within the first 6 hours of care

CARE BUNDLE ELEMENT 1:
Serum lactate measured
- Resuscitate immediately if hypotension or serum lactate >4. *Do not wait for ICU admission* (1C)

CARE BUNDLE ELEMENT 2:
Blood cultures obtained prior to antibiotic administration
- Obtain appropriate cultures before starting antibiotics (to include at least one percutaneous blood culture, one blood culture from each vascular device in place >48 hours, and culture other sites as indicated (1C)

CARE BUNDLE ELEMENT 3:
Broad-spectrum antibiotics to be administered within 3 hours for ED admissions and 1 hour for non-ED intensive care unit admissions—from the time of presentation
- Prompt imaging studies to seek source for infection (1C)
Antibiotic therapy
- Commence antibiotics as soon as possible and always within 1 hour of diagnosis of severe sepsis (1D) and septic shock (1B)

- Use broad-spectrum agents with good tissue penetration into likely site of infection **(1B)**
- Reassess appropriateness of antibiotic policy daily **(1C)**

Source identification and control

- Identify anatomic site of infection as rapidly as possible **(1C)**
- Formally consider the feasibility of source control measures (e.g. abscess drainage or tissue debridement) **(1C)**
- Implement source control as early as possible after resuscitation **(1C)**, with the exception of infected pancreatic necrosis where surgical intervention is best delayed
- Remove intravascular access devices if potentially infected **(1C)**

CARE BUNDLE ELEMENT 4:
If hypotension and /or lactate >4 mmol/L:

1) **Administer an initial minimum of 30 mL/kg of crystalloid (or colloid equivalent)**
2) **Administer vasopressors for hypotension not responding to initial fluid resuscitation to maintain mean arterial pressure >65 mmHg**

Fluid therapy

- Resuscitate using crystalloids or colloids **(1B)**
- Target CVP > or = 8 mmHg (12 mmHg if mechanically ventilated) **(1C)**
- Employ a fluid challenge technique for as long as haemodynamic improvement accrues with 1,000 mL crystalloids or 300 mL colloids over 30 min. More rapid administration may be necessary if there is evidence of tissue hypoperfusion **(1D)**
- Reduce rate of fluid administration if cardiac filling pressures increase in the absence of haemodynamic improvement **(1D)**

Vasopressors

- Maintain MAP ≥65 mmHg **(1C)**
- Noradrenaline and dopamine, centrally administered, are the vasopressors of choice **(1C)**
- Do not use low-dose dopamine for renal protection **(1A)**
- An arterial catheter is indicated if vasopressors are used **(1D)**
  - Neither adrenaline nor vasopressin should be first choice in septic shock **(2C)**
  - Vasopressin (0.03 units/min) may be added to noradrenaline with anticipation of an effect equivalent to noradrenaline alone
  - Adrenaline may be used as an alternative if blood pressure is poorly responsive to noradrenaline or dopamine **(2B)**

Inotropes

- Dobutamine should be used in patients with myocardial dysfunction, as manifested by elevated cardiac filling pressures but poor cardiac output **(1C)**
- Do not increase cardiac index to predetermined supranormal levels **(1B)**

CARE BUNDLE ELEMENT 5:
If hypotension and/or lactate >4 mmol/L despite fluid resuscitation:

1) **Achieve central venous pressure of >8 mmHg**
2) **Achieve central venous oxygen saturation of >70%**

- Resuscitation goals **(1C)**:

  CVP 8–12 mmHg
  MAP ≥65 mmHg
  Urine output ≥0.5 mL/kg/h
  Central venous (superior vena cava) O_2 saturation ≥70% or mixed venous ≥65%

  - If venous oxygen saturation target not achieved, consider:

    Administering more fluid
    Transfusing packed red cells to achieve a haematocrit of ≥30%
    Commencing dobutamine infusion to a maximum infusion rate of 20 micrograms/kg/min **(2C)**

Data from RP Dellinger et al., 'Surviving sepsis campaign: international guidelines for management of severe sepsis and septic shock: 2012', *Critical Care Medicine*, **41**, 2, pp. 580–637.

Box 2.2 24-hour care bundle elements

Management care bundles—within the first 24 hours of care
CARE BUNDLE ELEMENT 1:
Administer low-dose steroids for septic shock in accordance with a standardized ICU policy.
Steroids

- Consider intravenous hydrocortisone for adult septic shock if hypotension responds poorly to fluids and vasopressors **(2C)**
- ACTH stimulation test is not required to identify a subset of adults with septic shock who should receive hydrocortisone **(2B)**
- Hydrocortisone is preferable to dexamethasone **(2B)**
  - Hydrocortisone dose should not exceed 300 mg/day **(1A)**
  - Corticosteroids should not be used to treat sepsis in the absence of shock, unless there is an endocrine reason to do so or a previous history of steroid administration **(1D)**

CARE BUNDLE ELEMENT 2:
Glucose control maintained > lower limit of normal, but <180 mg/dL (10 mmol/L).

CARE BUNDLE ELEMENT 3:
Inspiratory plateau pressures maintained <30 cmH₂O for mechanically ventilated patients.

Data from RP Dellinger et al., 'Surviving sepsis campaign: international guidelines for management of severe sepsis and septic shock: 2012', *Critical Care Medicine*, **41**, 2, pp. 580–637.

Inotropes

Dobutamine should be used if the patient has evidence of myocardial dysfunction—as indicated by elevated cardiac filling pressures in the presence of a low cardiac output.

There is no evidence to 'push' cardiac index to predetermined supranormal levels. These studies did not specifically target patients with severe sepsis or the first 6 hours of resuscitation when the approach to management may need to be different.

Corticosteroids

A French multicentre trial investigated patients with septic shock unresponsive to fluids and vasopressor therapy and showed significant shock reversal and reduced mortality in patients with relative adrenal insufficiency detected by ACTH stimulation. Two smaller randomized controlled trials (RCTs) have also reported beneficial effects.

In contrast, a recent large European multicentre study (CORTICUS) did not show mortality benefit with steroid therapy, although resolution of shock was faster in those patients who received steroids. ACTH testing (undertaken to differentiate responders from non-responders) did not predict a faster resolution of shock. The French trial exclusively enrolled shocked patients who were unresponsive to fluids and vasopressors. CORTICUS, on the other hand, included patients, regardless of their blood pressure response to vasopressors.

The consensus is that intravenous hydrocortisone should be given exclusively to those patients whose blood pressure is unresponsive to fluid resuscitation and vasopressor therapy. This balances the evidence that, although steroids do appear to speed shock reversal, there is no accompanying benefit on mortality. In addition, steroids have side effects, including infection and steroid-induced myopathy. Further studies are needed.

High doses of corticosteroids, equivalent to >300 mg hydrocortisone daily, should not be used in septic shock, as it is ineffective and may be harmful.

It should be noted that some septic patients may have an absolute reason for corticosteroid administration, e.g.

coexisting Addison's or adrenal suppression secondary to previous steroid administration, and this must be detected and treated.

Recombinant human activated protein C

Activated protein C is an endogenous protein that promotes fibrinolysis and inhibits thrombosis and inflammation. In health, an inactive form of the protein is converted to the active form under the stimulation of thrombin bound to thrombomodulin. In sepsis, this conversion is impaired as a result of downregulation of thrombomodulin by inflammatory cytokines.

The initial evidence regarding the benefit of recombinant human activated protein C (rhAPC) in adults with sepsis was based primarily on the PROWESS and the ADDRESS trials, both of which were criticized for the use of subgroup analysis. In a recently completed clinical trial (PROWESS-SHOCK trial), rhAPC failed to show a survival benefit. Results, based on preliminary analyses of the trial that enrolled 1,696 patients, showed a 28-day all-cause mortality rate of 26.4% (223/846) in rhAPC-treated patients, compared to 24.2% (202/834) in placebo-treated patients, for a relative risk of 1.09; 95% CI (0.92, 1.28) and P-value = 0.31. Currently, there is no justification to use rhAPC in septic shock patients assessed to be at lower risk of death, as its use is associated with an increased risk of serious bleeding.

Vasopressin

Vasopressin secretion from the posterior pituitary is an important part of the homeostatic mechanism to restore blood pressure in shock. Studies show that vasopressin levels are elevated in early septic shock, but, as the shock state continues for 24–48 hours, levels fall within normal range in most patients but in the presence of hypotension. As vasopressin levels should remain elevated, this has been termed 'relative vasopressin deficiency'.

Vasopressin may be capable of elevating blood pressure in patients refractory to other vasopressors as well as having other physiological benefits. The recent VASST trial compared the use of noradrenaline alone with noradrenaline and low-dose vasopressin (0.03 units/min) and found no difference in outcome.

The Surviving Sepsis Campaign International Guidelines state vasopressin should not be administered as the initial, or sole, vasopressor in septic shock. Vasopressin at low-dose (0.03 units/min) may be subsequently added to noradrenaline, with the expectation that it will have an effect equivalent to noradrenaline alone.

Glucose control

Early SSC guidelines recommended tight glycaemic control in ICU, using intravenous insulin and a glucose calorie source, as appropriate, to maintain blood glucose at <8.3 mmol/L. However, a recent large, international randomized trial disagrees with this advice. The NICE-SUGAR Investigators reported a higher mortality rate in adults on intensive care units who received intensive blood sugar control. Specifically, they identified a lower mortality in patients whose blood glucose target was 10.0 mmol/L or less, rather than those who were intensively maintained at a glucose level of 4.5–6.0 mmol/L. This debate continues but the most recent 2012 SSC care bundle revision recommends avoiding hyperglycaemia and a target blood glucose <10mmol/L (<180mg/dL).

Other supportive therapies in severe sepsis

High-volume haemofiltration

Haemofiltration is a recognized therapeutic manoeuvre for managing severe metabolic acidosis as well as renal failure in shocked states. In septic shock, haemodynamic parameters often improve, following commencement of haemofiltration, thought to be due to cytokine elimination in the ultrafiltrate. A randomized trial to compare intensive renal replacement therapy with less intensive renal replacement therapy (consisting of haemodialysis 3 times per week) in critically ill patients with acute renal failure and associated failure of at least one non-renal organ or sepsis failed to find any benefits. However, the two treatment limbs in this study involved comparison of renal replacement as different intensities of haemodialysis, and not haemofiltration.

Nitric oxide synthase inhibitors

The initial results of trials of a non-selective nitric oxide synthase inhibitor appeared promising. However, subsequent studies have shown an increased mortality, and this seems to be related to increases in both systemic and pulmonary vascular resistance, leading to cardiac failure.

Anaphylactic shock

Airway management and fluid resuscitation are central to the management of anaphylactic shock. Colloids are commonly preferred for fluid replacement, but there is no strong evidence base.

Adrenaline is the main treatment and should be given intramuscularly at a dose of 0.3–0.5 mg (0.3–0.5 mL of 1:1,000 dilution, every 10–20 min). The intramuscular route is superior to the subcutaneous route.

In severe shock, associated with compromised muscle blood flow, intravenous injection of adrenaline should be substituted but at a reduced dose (e.g. 1 mL of 1:1,000 dilution in 500 mL 5% dextrose at a rate of 0.5–5.0 mcg/min, i.e. 0.25–2.5 mL/min).

Nebulized beta–2 agonists may be necessary for uncontrolled bronchospasm.

Corticosteroids are commonly administered in anaphylactic shock despite a paucity of evidence. In severe anaphylaxis, the data on benefit of antihistamines is inconclusive but they are routinely used. Antihistamines are also of documented value in angioneurotic oedema.

Neurogenic shock

Fluid resuscitation, with or without noradrenaline infusion, is the mainstay of therapy. Correction of the underlying cause and ventilatory support are other aspects of management.

Prognosis of shock states

Provided the source of blood or other fluid loss can be controlled, the prognosis of hypovolaemic shock is better than septic or cardiogenic shock. Prompt recognition and treatment is the mainstay of management.

The Surviving Sepsis Campaign has succeeded in advertising the need for urgent recognition and promotes a systematic approach. However, severe sepsis and septic shock continue to be major problems worldwide. Despite heightened awareness, the mortality rate remains 25% or higher. Moreover, it appears that the incidence of both severe sepsis and septic shock may be climbing.

The mortality rate in cardiogenic shock is poor (>50%), with significant morbidity for those who survive. Prompt diagnosis and specialist intervention, including invasive angiographic procedures, offer the best hope for a successful outcome.

Further reading

Annane D, Sebille V, Charpentier C, et al. (2002). Effect of treatment with low doses of hydrocortisone and fludrocortisone on mortality in patients with septic shock. *JAMA*, **288**, 862–71.

Boyd O, Grounds RM, Bennett ED (1993). A randomised clinical trial of the effect of deliberate perioperative increase of oxygen delivery on mortality in high-risk surgical patients. *JAMA*, **270**, 2699–707.

Dellinger RP, Levy MM, Carlet JM, *et al.* (2008). Surviving Sepsis Campaign: International guidelines for management of severe sepsis and septic shock. *Critical Care Medicine*, **36**, 296–327.

Dellinger RP, Levy MM, Rhodes A, *et al.* (2013). Surviving Sepsis Campaign: International guidelines for management of severe sepsis and septic shock: 2012. *Critical Care Medicine*, **41**, 580–637.

Gao F, Melody T, Daniels D, *et al.* (2005). The impact of compliance with 6-hour and 24-hour sepsis bundles on hospital mortality in patients with severe sepsis: a prospective observational study. *Critical Care*, **9**, R764–70.

Gattinoni L, Brazzi L, Pelosi P, *et al.* (1995). A trial of goal-oriented hemodynamic therapy in critically ill patients. *New England Journal of Medicine*, **333**, 1025–32.

Herbert PC, Wells G, Blajchman MA, *et al.* (1999). A multicentre, randomized, controlled clinical trial of transfusion requirements in critical care. *New England Journal of Medicine*, **340**, 409–17.

Mellemgard K (1966). The alveolar-arterial oxygen difference: its size and components in normal man. *Acta Physiologica Scandinavica*, **67**, 10.

Rivers E, Nguyen B, Havstad S (2001). Early goal-directed therapy in the treatment of severe sepsis and septic shock. *New England Journal of Medicine*, **345**, 1368–77.

Sharshar T, Blanchard A, Paillard M, *et al.* (2003). Circulating vasopressin levels in septic shock. *Critical Care Medicine*, **31**, 1752–8.

Smith I, Kumar P, Molloy S, *et al.* (2001). Base excess and lactate as prognostic indicators for patients admitted to intensive care. *Intensive Care Medicine*, **27**, 74–83.

The NICE-SUGAR Investigators (2009). Intensive versus conventional glucose control in critically ill patients. *New England Journal of Medicine*, **360**, 1283–97.

The SAFE Study Investigators (2004). A comparison of albumin and saline for fluid resuscitation in the intensive care unit. *New England Journal of Medicine*, **350**, 2247–56.

Vincent JL and De Backer D (2001). Pathophysiology of septic shock. *Advances in Sepsis*, **1**, 87–92.

SIRS, sepsis, severe sepsis, and septic shock

Definitions

The term sepsis usually implies infection accompanied by systemic inflammatory manifestations such as fever, tachycardia, and elevated white cell count (WCC). Unfortunately, the systemic changes are often indistinguishable from those of non-inflammatory conditions (e.g. burns, pancreatitis), and, in cases attributed to 'severe sepsis', a potential infective cause is only detected in 65% and blood cultures are positive in less than 25%.

Over the last 20 years, the terminology used to describe varying degrees of sepsis severity has been redefined by consensus conference to avoid confusion. Table 2.5 presents the current terminology used to describe systemic inflammatory response syndrome (SIRS), sepsis, severe sepsis, and septic shock.

- Severe sepsis implies sepsis with sepsis-induced acute organ dysfunction or tissue hypoperfusion.
- Septic shock specifies sepsis with persistent sepsis-induced hypotension not reversed despite adequate fluid resuscitation.

Epidemiology

Sepsis causes significant morbidity and mortality. It is more common at the extremes of age, in patients with diabetes mellitus, renal or hepatic failure, following trauma, surgery, invasive procedures (e.g. endoscopy) or with intravenous lines, and in the immunocompromised (e.g. HIV infection, steroid therapy, malignancy, post-splenectomy).

Table 2.5 SIRS and sepsis definitions

Infection	Invasion of sterile host tissue by micro-organisms
Bacteraemia	Viable bacteria in the blood
Systemic inflammatory response syndrome (SIRS)	An inflammatory response to infective and non-infective conditions (e.g. pancreatitis, trauma, burns) defined as ≥ 2 of four criteria: (1) Temperature >38 or <36°C (2) Heart rate >90/min (3) Respiratory rate >20/min, $PaCO_2$ <32 mmHg (4) WCC >12,000 or <4,000 cells/mm^3 or >10% immature (band) forms
Sepsis	SIRS due to infection
Severe sepsis	Sepsis plus sepsis-induced organ dysfunction or tissue hypoperfusion (i.e. hypotension, ↑ lactate, ↓ UO). Where sepsis-induced hypotension is defined as SBP <90 mmHg or MAP <70 mmHg or SBP fall of >40 mmHg
Septic shock	Sepsis-induced hypotension persisting despite adequate fluid resuscitation (i.e. shock, inadequate organ perfusion)
Multiple organ dysfunction	Development of impaired organ function in SIRS. Multiple organ failure may follow

Reproduced from 'American College of Chest Physicians/Society of Critical Care Medicine Consensus Conference: Definitions of sepsis and organ failure and guidelines for the use of innovative therapies in sepsis', *Critical Care Medicine*, **20**, 6, Copyright 1992, with permission from Wolters Kluwer and the Society of Critical Care Medicine.

The incidence of 'sepsis' and 'severe sepsis' has been increasing by about 8% each year for 10–20 years. In the USA, about 750,000 patients ($275/10^6$ population), with an average age of 55–65 years old and a male predominance, are currently admitted to hospital with sepsis annually. In 2003, 'severe sepsis' accounted for 44% of all cases of sepsis ($132/10^6$ population), and was the leading cause of multiple organ failure, acute respiratory distress syndrome (ARDS), acute renal failure (ARF), and late death following trauma.

Since 1987, Gram-positive organisms have been the main cause of sepsis (50–60%; *Staphylococcus* spp., pneumococci, enterococci), followed by Gram-negative bacteria (30–40%; *Escherichia coli*, *Klebsiella* spp., *Pseudomonas* spp.) and fungi (3–5%; especially *Candida* spp.). Although infection is often community-acquired, it is increasingly contracted in hospital, and nosocomial infection rates are 5–10 times higher on intensive care units (ICU) than on general wards. At any one time, about half of critically ill ICU patients are on antibiotics, with 50% acquiring the infection during admission.

Pathophysiology

The host response, which is, at least partly, genetically determined (i.e. mortality is greater in TNF B_2 homozygous individuals), rather than the infecting organism, often determines the severity of the infection. However, the status of the host's defence mechanisms, which are often impaired during acute illness, and the organism (i.e. virulence, pathogenicity, size of the inoculum) are also important factors.

The host's immune response is stimulated by invasive microorganisms or bacterial endotoxins. Initial cytokine release (e.g. TNF-alpha) activates polymorphs, macrophages, endothelium, platelets, complement, and coagulation pathways. The activated white cells adhere to and damage vascular endothelium, allowing fluid and cells to leak into the interstitial space and microcirculatory thrombosis to impair tissue oxygen delivery. Vasodilation follows the release of inflammatory mediators, including nitric oxide (NO) from the vascular endothelium. Myocardial dysfunction is due mainly to the negative inotropic effects of NO and inflammatory mediators, although hypotension may be associated with reduced coronary perfusion. Tissue oxygen utilization is impaired by sepsis-mediated cellular enzyme inhibition.

In Gram-negative infections, endotoxin (LPS) triggers the systemic inflammatory response and binds to a specific lipopolysaccharide-binding protein (LBP) in the plasma. The LPS-LBP complex binds to macrophage CD14 receptors which present the LPS to the signal-transducing, transmembrane Toll-like receptor protein (TLR4) which activates macrophages, causing the production and release of a potent array of cytokines (e.g. TNF-alpha, IL1, IL6, IL8). These interact with other cells or proteins, releasing adhesion molecules, prostaglandins, and leukotrienes to activate the inflammatory response.

In Gram-positive infections, the whole of the Gram-positive organism and its cell wall components (e.g. peptideglycans, lipoteichoic acids) can trigger sepsis when presented to CD14 receptors and then to Toll-like receptors (TLR2) due to massive cellular cytokine release. Some staphylococcal and streptococcal bacteria produce superantigens (e.g. staphylococcal toxic shock syndrome toxin-1) which can induce T cell proliferation without regard for their antigenic specificity and subsequently trigger the sepsis mechanisms.

The systemic inflammatory response is associated with:

- **Reduced systemic vascular resistance** (SVR), which causes hypotension despite an increase in cardiac output (CO). It is mainly due to NO production, but other mediators (e.g. beta-endorphins, decreased C3 complement, histamine) and impaired catecholamine responsiveness as a consequence of adrenocortical insufficiency are also implicated. Refractory hypotension due to persistent vasodilation occurs in most non-survivors of sepsis. Large increases in venous capacitance, due to increased NO production and associated venodilation, aggravate the hypotension. Initially, pulmonary vascular resistance is normal but rises in late sepsis.

- **Increased capillary permeability** involves both the systemic and pulmonary circulations, with loss of fluid from the intravascular compartment and subsequent hypovolaemia. The mechanism is probably multifactorial, but expression of adherence molecules by the endothelium and subsequent endothelial-leucocyte interaction are thought to play an important role. Severe sepsis increases albumin leakage by up to 300%. This reduces plasma oncotic pressure and further impairs intravascular filling.

- **Coagulopathy** with disseminated intravascular coagulation (DIC). The initial consumptive coagulopathy causes microvascular thrombosis and tissue ischaemia. Subsequent depletion of clotting factors (e.g. antithrombin III) may have anticoagulant effects, with increased risk of haemorrhage.

- **Myocardial dysfunction**, which is associated with increased mortality. Both TNF-alpha and interleukin-1-beta can cause myocardial dysfunction in sepsis and non-infectious SIRS. Despite this, most septic patients initially have a normal or an increased CO.

- **Increased blood lactate**. This may be due to inadequate tissue oxygen delivery or utilization (e.g. impaired mitochondrial function), although increased glycolysis, hypermetabolism, and glycogenolysis have also been implicated. In sepsis, decreased oxygen extraction from blood is a common finding and may result from arteriovenous shunting due to redistribution of blood flow or impaired cellular metabolism limiting the cells' ability to utilize oxygen. The finding of a fall in whole body oxygen extraction, despite an increase in splanchnic oxygen extraction, supports the concept of impaired blood distribution.

Clinical presentation

The clinical features of sepsis are either general or related to the source of the infection. At presentation, the differential diagnosis can be extensive, including other causes of shock (e.g. pulmonary embolism) and systemic inflammatory responses (e.g. pancreatitis). The general clinical features of sepsis include:

- Fever, which occurs in 90% of cases, with hypothermia in 10% of patients, especially the elderly.

- Tachypnoea, which is associated with hypoxia and cyanosis in severe cases. Occasionally, acute respiratory distress syndrome (ARDS) may occur.

- Tachycardia, hypotension, and widespread vasodilation. The characteristic clinical picture of a hyperdynamic, high-output, 'warm/dilated' shock, with a flushed appearance, bounding pulses, increased cardiac output, and warm peripheries, usually occurs in early sepsis. As sepsis progresses or in more severe cases, the clinical pic-

ture changes to one of low-output, 'cold/clammy', vasoconstricted shock, with 'thready' pulses and peripheral shutdown due to myocardial depression.

- Progressive reduction in urine output (oliguria) suggests impaired renal perfusion due to hypotension. It may lead to acute tubular necrosis and acute renal failure with anuria.

- Metabolic acidosis with increased lactate production is due to impaired cellular metabolism or failure of normal blood flow distribution. Associated splanchnic ischaemia may lead to paralytic ileus, gastrointestinal bleeding, and liver dysfunction.

- Raised white cell count (WCC $>9 \times 10^9$/L). The WCC is occasionally reduced ($<4 \times 10^9$/L) in overwhelming sepsis or the elderly.

- Coagulation disorders are due to procoagulant consumptive, and subsequent anticoagulant, effects. They may occur with thrombocytopenia, purpura, bruising, prolonged bleeding (e.g. from venepuncture sites), and DIC. Early recognition of the characteristic 'purpuric' rash of meningococcal septicaemia can be lifesaving.

- Agitation, delirium, and confusion are common and may progress to coma in severe cases. Primary cerebral infection must be excluded (i.e. CT scan, lumbar puncture).

- Increased capillary permeability and albumin leakage lead to peripheral oedema and intravascular fluid depletion.

- Rhabdomyolysis may occur, and critical illness polyneuropathy follows prolonged illness.

Meningococcal septicaemia (see Chapter 6) is a common cause of community-acquired sepsis and results in a characteristic illness, with fever, malaise, myalgia, and the development of a non-blanching rash, proceeding to hypotension and DIC. Symptoms and signs of meningitis may, or may not, be present.

Common sites of infection and appropriate investigations

- Lower respiratory tract infections (e.g. pneumonia, empyema) may be either community- or hospital-acquired and cause 34–45% of sepsis cases. Diagnosis is usually established on chest radiography or, occasionally, CT scan. The causative organism is established by culture and examination of sputum or bronchial washes and aspirates.

- Urinary tract infections are common (~15–20%). Ultrasound scans may establish renal tract obstructions, and midstream urine (MSU) examination for WCC, blood, and organisms confirms the diagnosis and may identify the causative organism.

- Intravascular lines that have been *in situ* for over 3–4 days, particularly central venous catheters, are a common cause of bacteraemia and sepsis. Blood and line tip cultures confirm the diagnosis. Early line removal is usually necessary.

- Abdominal infections are a common source of sepsis, including abscesses, diverticulitis, perforations, cholecystitis, and pancreatitis. Ultrasound and CT scans may establish the source of the infection, and aspirations or samples obtained at laparotomy determine the causative organism.

- Gastrointestinal infections are usually associated with abdominal pain and diarrhoea, and diagnosis is established from stool examination and culture or measurement of *Clostridium difficile* toxin.

- Meningitis is a less common cause of sepsis and is established by examination of cerebrospinal fluid obtained at lumbar puncture.
- Upper respiratory tract infections of the sinuses, ears, or retropharyngeal space may be sources of sepsis and are detected by clinical examination, radiographs and CT scans, and culture of local samples.
- Endocarditis is a rare cause of sepsis but should be suspected in high-risk groups (e.g. drug addicts, heart valve disease). Echocardiography and serial blood cultures usually establish the diagnosis and causative organism.
- Joint, bone, and skin infections are sometimes missed. Skin infections can usually be detected by careful clinical examination. Bone scans and radiographs are required to establish the diagnosis of orthopaedic infections.
- 'Toxic shock syndrome' (see Chapter 6) is a rare cause of sepsis, usually due to retained tampons in young females. It is confirmed at vaginal examination. Endotoxins produced by *Staphylococcus* or *Streptococcus* spp. cause a characteristic illness, with fever, vomiting, diarrhoea, skin desquamation, hypotension, and multi-organ failure.

Examination
This may detect a focus of infection or provide diagnostic clues (e.g. meningococcal rash, splinter haemorrhages in endocarditis). Chest infection is the commonest source of sepsis, and typical clinical signs of pneumonia, chest abscess, or empyema may confirm the diagnosis. Urine should be tested for blood, protein, and nitrites.

Diagnosis
- **Source identification and control.** A specific anatomic site of infection should be identified as rapidly as possible and within the first 6 hours of presentation. This informs subsequent source control measures (e.g. antibiotic choice, abscess drainage, tissue debridement, infected line removal) which should be implemented as soon as possible after initial resuscitation. In particular, potentially infected intravascular devices should be removed rapidly. An exception is infected pancreatic necrosis in which surgical intervention is often best delayed.
- **Routine investigations** include standard blood tests, C-reactive protein, plasma lactate, coagulation profile, arterial blood gases (ABG), central (mixed) venous blood saturation (ScvO$_2$), urinalysis, CXR, and ECG.
- **Monitor** vital signs, biochemistry, ABG, and central venous pressure (CVP). In severe sepsis, haemodynamic measurements of continuous intra-arterial blood pressure, cardiac output, and SVR may be useful to guide fluid (± inotropic) therapy. Urine output should be carefully monitored, and, in severe sepsis, a urethral catheter may be required to monitor hourly urine output.
- **Cultures** of blood, sputum, urine, CSF, and wound pus must be taken before starting antibiotics, providing this does not delay therapy. Obtain at least two blood cultures, of which at least one must be drawn percutaneously and one through each intravascular access device greater than 48 hours old. Culture other sites, as clinically indicated.
- **Specific investigations** depend on the suspected cause (e.g. ultrasonography in abdominal sepsis) and patient mobility (e.g. CT scans).

Management of severe sepsis
'The Surviving Sepsis Campaign' published updated guidelines for sepsis management in 2008 and 2012. These apply to all acute medical and surgical wards. As in MI, the speed and quality of initial therapy influences outcome.

Initial resuscitation (first 6 hours) and antibiotic therapy
- 'Protocol'-guided fluid resuscitation must start immediately in patients with hypoperfusion (i.e. lactate >4 mmol/L, reduced ScvO$_2$) or hypotension. Fluid therapy should aim to achieve the following resuscitation goals:
  - CVP ≥8 mmHg. A higher CVP of 12–15 mmHg is recommended during mechanical ventilation or with pre-existing decreased ventricular compliance.
  - MAP ≥65 mmHg.
  - Urine output ≥0.5 mL/kg/h.
  - ScvO$_2$ ≥70%.
  If the ScvO$_2$ target is not achieved, consider further fluid resuscitation, packed red cell transfusion to a haematocrit ≥30%, and/or a dobutamine infusion (max 20 mcg/kg/min) to increase oxygen delivery and hence ScvO$_2$. Reduce fluid administration if CVP increases without haemodynamic improvement to avoid potential pulmonary oedema.
- **Initial fluid resuscitation** is with crystalloids and should use a fluid challenge technique. Whilst monitoring haemodymanic parameters (i.e. CVP, blood pressure), assess the response to fluid challenges of 0.5–1 L of crystalloid given over 30 min (aiming for at least 30ml/kg). Larger volumes at shorter intervals may be required in severe sepsis-induced tissue hypoperfusion. Albumin (4-5% solution) may be considered for resuscitation in patients with severe sepsis requiring substantial amounts of crystalloids. Previous meta-analysis has shown no difference between crystalloid or colloid resuscitation, although resuscitation with crystalloid required more fluid to achieve the same endpoints. Hydroxyethyl starches are associated with renal impairment and increased mortality and are not recommended. Reduce the rate of fluid administration if the CVP increases without concurrent haemodynamic improvements.
- **Antibiotic therapy** is started as early as possible and always within the first hour of recognizing severe sepsis or septic shock. Therapy is initially empiric, using one or more broad-spectrum agents active against the most likely causative pathogens (bacterial or fungal) and with good penetration into infected tissues.

Antibiotic selection depends on the clinical features, whether community- or hospital-acquired, the site of primary infection, and local antibiotic resistance patterns. About 50% of hospital-acquired staphylococcal infections are due to methicillin-resistant *Staphylococcus aureus* (MRSA). Antibiotic therapy should be reviewed daily to optimize efficacy, prevent resistance, avoid toxicity, and minimize cost. Stop antibiotic therapy if a non-infectious cause is found. Suitable empiric antibiotic choices in the absence of an obvious focus of infection are:

- **Community-acquired sepsis:** second- or third-generation cephalosporins (e.g. cefotaxime) or a penicillin with a beta-lactamase inhibitor (e.g. co-amoxiclav).
- **Hospital-acquired sepsis:** antipseudomonal penicillin with a beta-lactamase inhibitor (e.g. piperacillin with tazobactam) or a carbenopenem (e.g. meropenem) or ceftazidime and/or an aminoglycoside (e.g. gentamicin) and an antistaphylococcal drug effective against MRSA (e.g. vancomycin).

Combination therapy is recommended in neutropenic patients and those infected with *Pseudomonas*. Microbiological results and antibiotic sensitivities guide ongoing therapy, and unnecessary antibiotics should be stopped/de-escalated when results are known (i.e. reduce to antibiotic monotherapy after 3–5 days).

Limit treatment to 5–10 days unless due to MRSA or resistant *Pseudomonas* or if the focus of infection cannot be drained or the patient is immunocompromised when longer courses (e.g. 14–21 days) may be justified.

Ongoing haemodynamic support

Vasopressor and inotropic drugs are used to maintain MAP ≥65 mmHg if initial fluid resuscitation is unsuccessful. Below a critical MAP, autoregulation in some vascular beds (e.g. brain) is lost, and perfusion is linearly dependent on pressure. Drug dose is titrated to specific endpoints (e.g. urine output, lactate, MAP) to maintain tissue blood flow. Thus, MAP may need to be higher in uncontrolled hypertensive patients. These drugs must be given through a central line and require an arterial line for continuous blood pressure monitoring.

- **Vasopressors.** Noradrenaline (norepinephrine), an alpha-adrenergic vasoconstrictor, is the first-line vasopressor agent of choice in severe sepsis and septic shock. In some cases, vasopressin (0.03 units/min) may be added to noradrenaline (norepinephrine) to raise MAP or decrease noradrenaline dose. Adrenaline (epinephrine), which has both vasopressor and inotropic properties, is the best alternative (i.e. second-line agent) in septic shock when blood pressure is poorly responsive to noradrenaline. Dopamine is used as an alternative vasopressor agent to noradrenaline in highly selected cases (e.g. patients with low risk of tachyarrhythmias or bradycardia). Do not use low-dose dopamine for renal protection.
- **Inotropes.** Dobutamine, a vasodilator inotrope, is the first-line inotrope for patients with low cardiac output despite adequate filling pressures (i.e. CVP). Although it effectively increases CO, it may lower MAP due to its vasodilator properties and is often combined with a vasopressor (e.g. noradrenaline). Targeting supranormal oxygen delivery levels is not beneficial.

There are two typical clinical scenarios:

1. **In mild or early sepsis**, widespread vasodilation (i.e. low SVR) causes hypotension and relative hypovolaemia. Reduced left ventricular afterload increases CO, but impaired distribution and a low MAP (with failure of autoregulation) can cause regional (i.e. splanchnic, cerebral) ischaemia. At this stage, a vasopressor agent (e.g. norepinephrine or dopamine) with alpha-receptor agonist properties increases SVR, MAP, and organ perfusion pressure.

2. **In severe or late sepsis**, toxic myocarditis impairs myocardial contractility and reduces CO. At this stage, fluid administration produces only small increases in CO and may precipitate pulmonary oedema, whilst increasing SVR with a vasopressor agent alone may decrease CO. In this situation, an inotropic agent is required to increase cardiac contractility and improve CO. Dobutamine is the agent of choice, but it may cause hypotension, in addition to increasing CO (as discussed previously). Consequently, it is often used in combination with small doses of norepinephrine to maintain the MAP. If the blood pressure remains poorly responsive, epinephrine is the best alternative, as it has both inotropic and vasoconstrictor properties.

Adjunctive therapy

- **Steroids.** Relative adrenocortical insufficiency may occur in severe sepsis, and low-dose hydrocortisone (8 mg/h) should be considered if hypotension is refractory to fluid and vasopressor support. A pre-treatment ACTH stimulation test to identify the patients most likely to benefit is not recommended. The total hydrocortisone dose should be <300 mg/day, and treatment can be weaned when vasopressors are no longer required. Hydrocortisone is preferred to dexamethasone. Do not use steroids in the absence of shock, unless the patient is on long-term steroids or has an associated endocrine disease.
- **Activated protein C** (APC) is an endogenous protein that promotes fibrinolysis and inhibits thrombosis and inflammation. Initial studies suggested that it improved outcome in patients with severe sepsis by preventing microcirculatory thrombosis and subsequent organ damage. However, the PROWESS SHOCK trial in 2011 showed no benefit of APC in patients with septic shock (mortality 26.4% with APC and 24.2% with placebo) and the drug has been withdrawn from use and is no longer available.

Supportive therapy

- **General measures** include oxygen therapy and nutrition.
- **Haemoglobin** should be maintained between 7 and 9 g/dL and blood given below 7 g/dL (70 g/L). A higher haemoglobin is recommended for ischaemic heart disease, hypoxaemia (± lactic acidosis), and acute haemorrhage.
- **Glycaemic control** recommendations for severe sepsis were adjusted in 2009, following the NICE-SUGAR trial. The current aim is to keep the blood glucose <10 mmol/L (180 mg/dL), using a validated insulin protocol. A glucose calorie source should be provided and glucose levels monitored regularly.
- **Respiratory support** with non-invasive or mechanical ventilation (MV) may be required in patients with acute lung injury or ARDS. Low tidal volumes, limited plateau pressures (<30 cmH$_2$O), positive end expiratory pressure, and conservative fluid management strategies should be used. MV patients should be nursed semi-recumbent (30–45°).
- **Renal support** with either haemodialysis or haemofiltration.
- **Thromboembolism prophylaxis** with low molecular weight or unfractionated heparin and/or mechanical prophylactic devices.
- **Stress ulcer prophylaxis** with proton pump inhibitors or H2 blockers.
- **Prevention of sepsis** requires good infection control (e.g. handwashing), appropriate use of prophylactic antibiotics (e.g. for invasive procedures), and prompt management of suspected infection.

Some therapies are not associated with significant benefit in severe sepsis, and may cause harm. These include anti-endotoxin and anti-TNF therapies, interleukin receptor antagonists, anti-prostaglandins (e.g. ibuprofen), ketoconazole (thromboxane synthetase inhibitors), growth hormone, nitric oxide inhibitors, antioxidants (e.g. acetylcysteine), vasopressin, and pentoxifylline (e.g. phosphodiesterase inhibitors)

Prognosis

Gram-negative sepsis has a mortality rate of ~35%, and Gram-positive sepsis has a slightly lower rate of about 15%, but these rates are dependent on factors, such as age and pre-existing illness. Prognosis deteriorates with age, lactic acidosis, low white cell count, cytokine elevation, reduced systemic vascular resistance (SVR), number of organ failures, and female sex. About 20% of patients with sepsis and 37% of cases with severe sepsis die. Overall, the number of deaths has increased each year. Many die from the underlying disease or disorder, but up to half of deaths are directly attributable to the infection itself. Sepsis survivors usually make a complete recovery, but the length of hospital stay is often prolonged

Further reading

American College of Chest Physicians/Society of Critical Care Medicine Consensus Conference (1992). Definitions for sepsis and organ failure and guidelines for the use of innovative therapies in sepsis. *Critical Care Medicine*, **20**, 864–74.

Angus DC, Linde-Zwirble WT, Lidicker J, et al. (2001). Epidemiology of severe sepsis in the United States: analysis of incidence, outcome and associated costs of care. *Critical Care Medicine*, **29**, 1303–10.

Dellinger RP, Levt MM, Carlet JM, et al. (2008). Surviving sepsis campaign: international guidelines for management of severe sepsis and septic shock. *Critical Care Medicine*, **36**, 296–327.

Dellinger RP, Levy MM, Rhodes A, et al. (2013). Surviving Sepsis Campaign: International guidelines for management of severe sepsis and septic shock: 2012. *Critical Care Medicine*, **41**, 580–637.

Dombrovskiy VY, Martin AA, Sunderram J, et al. (2007). Rapid increase in hospitalization and mortality rates for severe sepsis in the United States: a trend analysis from 1993–2003. *Critical Care Medicine*, **35**, 1414–15.

Finfer S, Chittock DR, Su SY, et al. (2009). Intensive versus conventional glucose control in critically ill patients. *New England Journal of Medicine*, **360**, 1283–97.

Kanji S, Perreault MM, Chant C, et al. (2007). Evaluating the use of drotrecogin alfa activated in adult sepsis: a Canadian multicenter observational study. *Intensive Care Medicine*, **33**, 517–23.

Martin GS, Mannino DM, Eaton S, et al. (2003). The epidemiology of sepsis in the United States from 1979–2000. *New England Journal of Medicine*, **348**, 1546–54.

NICE-SUGAR Study Investigators (2009). Intensive versus conventional glucose control in critically ill patients. *New England Journal of Medicine*, **360**, 1283–1297.

Nguyen HB, Corbett SW, Steele R, et al. (2007). Implementation of a bundle of quality indicators for the early management of severe sepsis and septic shock is associated with decreased mortality. *Critical Care Medicine*, **35**, 1105–12.

Organized Wisdom. Sepsis. <http://www.organizedwisdom.com/Sepsis>.

Ranieri MV, Thompson TB, Barie PS, et al. (2012). Drotrecogin Alfa (activated) in adults with septic shock. *New England Journal of Medicine*, **366**, 2055–2064.

Surviving Sepsis Campaign. <http://www.survivingsepsis.org>.

Wiener RS, Wiener DC, Larson RJ (2008). Benefits and risks of tight glucose control in critically ill adults: a meta-analysis. *JAMA*, **300**, 933–44.

Vasopressor and inotropic therapy

Inotropes and vasopressors may be required to provide additional haemodynamic support if optimal fluid resuscitation and heart rate control fail to correct circulatory failure. The aim is to achieve adequate tissue perfusion, rather than a specific blood pressure (BP) which differs between subjects (e.g. a hypertensive patient may require a higher BP).

It is essential to recognize that vasoactive drugs are relatively ineffective in volume-depleted patients and that an adequate circulating volume has to be achieved before using these drugs. Likewise, acidosis (pH <7.1) and electrolyte derangements (e.g. hypokalaemia, hypomagnesaemia) impair the actions of inotropic and vasopressor drugs and should be corrected to ensure effective therapy.

Monitoring. Vasopressor and inotropic effects cannot be predicted in an individual, and the response must be monitored and titrated to specific and effective endpoints (e.g. MAP 65–70 mmHg, urine output >0.5 mL/kg/h). These agents are usually administered through central lines. This ensures rapid distribution, as they have a short half-life, enables delivery at high concentration, and within a narrow safety margin, and avoids tissue necrosis in the event of peripheral extravasation.

In general, haemodynamically unstable patients receiving vasoactive drugs require continuous intra-arterial BP monitoring, ideally using larger arteries (e.g. femoral), as smaller arteries (e.g. radial) tend to underestimate low systemic pressures. However, in practice, the radial artery, which is easily accessible, is preferred. Volume status is most conveniently assessed with a central venous catheter and 'fluid challenges', but, in complex cases, haemodynamic monitoring of cardiac output (CO), systemic vascular resistance (SVR), left-sided filling pressures, and lung water may be necessary to maintain tissue perfusion.

Selection of appropriate vasopressor therapy requires an understanding of the cardiovascular properties of each agent, a knowledge of the adrenergic receptor distribution (and the actions of these receptors), and an accurate assessment of the underlying haemodynamic disturbance. Table 2.6 presents the pharmacological properties of individual agents. Activation of different receptors has specific effects. Thus:

- **Alpha-receptors** cause mainly peripheral vasoconstriction.

- **Beta-1-receptors** are chronotropic (i.e. increase heart rate) and inotropic (i.e. increase the force and velocity of myocardial contractility and consequently BP and CO).
- **Beta-2-receptors** cause vasodilation and bronchodilation.

A specific drug may activate several receptors, but the balance of receptor effects can vary between individual agents. For example, adrenaline has alpha, beta-1, and beta-2-receptor properties, with a significant contribution from the alpha-receptors. In comparison, dobutamine also has alpha, beta-1, and beta-2 properties, but the beta-1 and beta-2 effects are greater than alpha properties. Ideally, a single drug should be used, but, occasionally, the correct balance of receptor stimulation may require combinations of vasopressor and inotropic agents.

Both vasopressin and low-dose steroids (e.g. hydrocortisone 8 mg/h) have been shown to have a 'catecholamine-sparing' effect, particularly in septic shock.

Opinion as to optimal therapy in specific situations differs considerably between institutions and countries, and the following treatment regimes are recommended in the absence of conclusive evidence:

- **In septic shock**, profound vasodilation causes hypotension despite a high CO. An increasing body of evidence supports the initial use of noradrenaline (norepinephrine) (± adrenaline (epinephrine)), which are primarily alpha-vasoconstrictors and act mainly to maintain BP and organ perfusion (without significantly reducing CO). However, prolonged sepsis may eventually impair cardiac contractility, requiring the addition of a beta-1 inotropic agent to maintain CO (e.g. dobutamine).
- **In myocardial ischaemia**, the beta-1 properties of dobutamine increase cardiac contractility without increasing myocardial oxygen consumption, an important property in patients with myocardial ischaemia. In addition, the beta-2 vasodilator properties reduce 'afterload' and increase CO, although, occasionally, this necessitates the use of small doses of noradrenaline (norepinephrine) to offset beta-2-mediated hypotensive effects.
- **Cardiogenic shock.** In systolic heart failure, most catecholamines (e.g. dopamine, noradrenaline (norepinephrine)) effectively support the circulation and allow the myocardium time to recover from post-ischaemic

Table 2.6 Properties of inotropic drugs

Vasoactive agent	Receptors (bold = main action)	Mid-range dose effects		
		Inotrope contractility	Chronotrope	Vasoconstrictor
Inoconstrictors				
Adrenaline (epinephrine)	α, β₁, β₂	++++	+++	++
Dopamine	α, β₁, β₂	+++	++	– to ++
Inodilators				
Dobutamine	(α), β₁, β₂	+++	+	– to ±
Milrinone	PDI/↑ cAMP	+++	0	– –
Enoximone	PDI/↑ cAMP	+++	0	–
Vasoconstrictor				
noradrenaline (norepinephrine)	α, β₁	+/++	0	++++
Phenylephrine	α, β₁	+	0	++++

PDI, phosphodiesterase inhibitor; cAMP, cyclic adenosine monophosphate.

stunning. Phosphodiesterase inhibitors (e.g. milrinone, enoximone) have a role for diastolic dysfunction and catecholamine resistance.

- **'Renal protection'.** Augmentation of MAP may prevent or ameliorate renal failure and this is an important use of inotropes. It can be achieved with several catecholamines (e.g. dopamine, noradrenaline). However, there is no evidence to support the use of low-concentration 'renal dose' dopamine to increase renal blood flow by stimulating dopaminergic receptors, and it is no longer recommended.

Other circulatory support techniques include cardiac pacemakers and ventilatory support to reduce cardiorespiratory work and pulmonary oedema. Intra-aortic balloon pumps are valuable in the failing heart as a bridge to transplantation. They are sited in the descending aorta above the renal arteries. Diastolic balloon inflation enhances coronary and systemic perfusion pressures, whilst systolic deflation increases CO by reducing afterload. Complications include renal and mesenteric ischaemia, infection, and aortic dissection. Other left ventricular assist devices are also being developed.

Further reading

Gillies M, Bellomo R, Doolan L, Buxton B (2005). Bench-to-bedside review. Inotropic drug therapy after adult cardiac surgery—a systemic literature review. *Critical Care*, **9**, 266–79.

Holmes CL (2005). Vasoactive drugs in the intensive care unit. *Current Opinion in Critical Care*, **11**, 413–17.

Nutrition

Malnutrition is both a cause and consequence of disease and affects about 3 million people in the UK. Although often unrecognized and untreated, it is associated with increased risk of poor health, complications during illness, increased mortality, delayed recovery, and increased healthcare costs. Table 2.7 reports the effects and potential consequences of malnutrition on health.

The excess cost of malnutrition in the UK National Health Service (NHS) has been estimated to be £13 billion, and better nutritional care has been identified as the fourth largest potential source of savings in the NHS. Similarly, improvements in nutrition and hydration have been identified as one of eight 'high impact' clinical areas.

Malnutrition has been recognized as a significant problem in hospital patients since 1976 when it was reported to affect 44% and 50% of medical and surgical patients, respectively. In 1994, further investigation revealed that 40% of patients were malnourished, or at risk of malnourishment, on admission, and nutritional status deteriorated in 78% during their hospital stay.

The most recent surveys suggest that 20% of patients in general hospitals are malnourished, as defined by a body mass index (BMI) less than 18.5, or thin and losing weight, or both. The National Screening Survey by the British Association of Parenteral and Enteral Nutrition (BAPEN, 2007) revealed malnutrition in all areas of healthcare delivery, in all age groups, and all types of disease and this malnutrition usually originated in the community. However, older hospital patients are at particular risk, with malnutrition in 34% of those over 80 years old and a 'high risk' of malnutrition in 33% of patients on elderly care and stroke wards.

Factors contributing to poor nutrition in hospital include loss of appetite, difficulty swallowing, malabsorption, and inadequate intake due to catering limitations. Failure to detect and treat hospital patients presenting with, or developing, malnutrition during admission results in delayed recovery and worse outcomes in these patients.

In severely ill patients, there is no clear evidence of benefit for nutritional support, as randomized controlled trials of no feeding, compared to any form of nutritional support, in patients with little or no oral intake would be difficult to support on ethical grounds. Nevertheless, a good case can be made. The US National Institute for Health, the American Society for Parenteral and Enteral Nutrition, and the American Society for Clinical Nutrition recommend that nutritional support should be started in critically ill patients unlikely to regain oral intake within 7–10 days, on the basis that dangerous depletion of lean tissue occurs after 14 days of starvation.

In general, most clinicians agree that the maximum acceptable delay before starting nutritional support in a patient unable to tolerate oral intake is 5–7 days. Earlier feeding may be justified if the patient is malnourished or if there has been a period of inadequate intake before the acute illness.

Principles of nutritional care

- All patients should be screened for malnutrition in all specialities and care settings.
- Those identified to be 'at risk' of malnutrition should be offered assessment by dietitians or other specifically trained health professionals (e.g. nurses) to arrange individualized nutritional care plans and ongoing review. It is essential that other healthcare professionals should be able to undertake these assessments and instigate agreed care plans, as there will never be enough dietitians to address all the cases identified at routine screening. Dietitian referral should be restricted to the more complex cases.
- All care staff should be suitably trained to understand the importance of identifying and treating risks related to malnutrition.
- Organizations providing care should have multidisciplinary committees and management structures to ensure and audit nutritional care/support.

NICE/BAPEN standards of nutritional care

- Information on healthy living and the importance of healthy weight should be available in all care settings.
- Prevention of malnutrition should be an integral part of preventative healthcare.
- Nutritional screening (including height and weight) should be undertaken in all hospital inpatients at admission and also weekly (especially if there is clinical concern). Screening should also occur in all healthcare services including outpatients, GP surgeries and care homes.
- Nutritional assessment should be undertaken and recorded in all patients identified as being at risk of malnutrition on screening.
- Individuals confirmed to be malnourished or at risk should have an appropriate nutritional care plan (including social measures like meals on wheels and/or modified menus) which must be recorded and integrated with pharmacotherapy, surgery, and other aspects of acute care and follow-up. Outcome should be monitored (e.g. nutrient intake, weight).
- Nutritional information must be efficiently transferred between care settings (e.g. hospital to care home).
- All heath care professionals should receive appropriate training in the importance of nutritional care, how to screen for malnutrition, basic nutritional care measures, and indicators for onward referral for nutritional assessment and support.
- Appropriate multidisciplinary teams should be available to ensure that appropriate care pathways are available, followed, and audited.

Table 2.7 Effects of malnutrition

Effect	Examples of consequences
Inactivity	Oedema, pressure sores, venous thromboembolism
Impaired immune response	Impaired ability to fight infection
Reduced muscle strength	Inactivity, falls, weakness, fatigue, poor cough
Loss of temperature regulation	Hypothermia
Poor wound healing	Infection, un-united fractures, delayed healing
Impaired fluid and salt balance	Over- and underhydration
Specific nutrient deficiency	Anaemia, tiredness, scurvy
Poor psychosocial functioning	Depression, self-neglect, loss of libido
Impaired menstrual regulation	Impaired reproduction
Impaired child development	Retarded growth, rickets, poor neurocognitive development, increased lifetime osteoporosis risk

Nutritional assessment

There are two principal issues in the assessment of nutritional status in patients admitted to hospital.

1. Recognition of malnutrition.

2. When and how to provide nutritional support.

Recognition of malnutrition in hospital patients

Despite the frequency of malnutrition and the availability of effective, validated screening tools, it is undiagnosed in up to 70% of patients. Between 70–80% of malnourished patients enter and leave hospital without specific attempts to minimize or treat their nutritional risks and without the diagnosis of malnutrition appearing as a comorbidity on their discharge summary.

Clinical evaluation of malnutrition (e.g. weight loss, poor diet, subcutaneous fat loss, muscle wasting, gastrointestinal symptoms) is more effective than objective measures (e.g. skinfold thickness) or laboratory features (e.g. transferrin, albumin levels, lymphocyte counts) which are independently reduced by acute illness. However, the presence of peripheral oedema or ascites alone should not be viewed as a clinical indicator of malnutrition, as they are not usually seen, even in severely starved individuals. These features tend to occur as a complication of an inflammatory response, usually to overt or hidden superinfection.

In 2003, BAPEN developed a simple scoring system, the 'Malnutrition Universal Screening Tool' (MUST) that allows healthcare providers to identify adults at risk of malnutrition. Its use is illustrated in Figure 2.5. The score is sensitive, specific, and able to predict mortality in older hospitalized patients.

In 2006, the National Institute for Health and Clinical Excellence (NICE) recommended that all hospital patients should be screened and monitored regularly for malnutrition. Unfortunately, this standard has been poorly implemented, as most hospitals have had no dedicated healthcare staff to oversee the delivery of either normal food provision or artificial feeding. However, since early 2010, the Care Quality Commission have also recognized the importance of nutrition in delivering high-quality, effective treatment and have made nutritional care a cross-speciality theme. They have also demanded that all individuals in all NHS and social care settings should have nutritional screening, and this is likely to result in much better implementation of the NICE standards on nutritional screening and treatment.

When and how to provide nutritional support

Benefits of treating malnutrition

Meta-analyses have confirmed the clinical benefits of improving nutritional status in malnourished patients in terms of weight gain, improved quality of life, and performance scores in a wide spectrum of diseases (e.g. emphysema, colon cancer, other malignancies, gastrointestinal disorders). Furthermore, the use of oral nutritional supplements or enteral tube feeding in those at risk of malnutrition has been shown to reduce complication rates by 70% and mortality by 40% in a meta-analysis of studies conducted in hospitals, primarily in post-surgical cases. Improvements in mental and functional ability have also been documented in better nourished patients and are associated with reduced lengths of hospital stay, greater independence, and lower rates of nursing home use.

Potential benefits associated with early nutrition support have also been reported in some acutely ill patients. For example, early nutritional support reduced mortality in head-injured patients when compared to underfeeding.

Nutritional support teams

Nutritional support teams (NSTs) have been demonstrated to be an effective means of implementing the NICE guideline nutritional goals in the UK and aid detection and delivery of nutritional support to 'at-risk' patients. In addition, they have had a significant impact on reducing intravenous catheter-related infections, an important quality issue. Unfortunately, many hospitals still have no dedicated staff or funding for nutritional support, and malnutrition remains a significant and untreated problem.

Nutritional support

In malnourished, post-operative, or acutely unwell patients, who are identified as requiring nutritional support (i.e. unable to take adequate food orally), the timing, route (e.g. enteral, parenteral), and nutritional requirements must be assessed. Adjustments may be necessary for specific disease categories (e.g. respiratory, liver, or renal failure), and the risk of potential complications, which may be either general (e.g. refeeding syndrome) or specific to the type of nutrition (i.e. enteral, parenteral), must be considered.

- **Timing of nutritional support**

Nutritional support is unnecessary in previously well nourished patients who are unable to eat for <5 days. Although early nutritional support may reduce protein catabolism and improve markers of nutritional status (e.g. lymphocyte counts, plasma proteins), there is little evidence that specific regimes improve outcome, and complications often outweigh the benefits.

In general, early nutritional support is recommended for pre-existing malnutrition, hypermetabolic states, and protracted illness. Current guidelines recommend that nutritional support should be started in previously well-nourished patients who are unlikely to regain oral intake (e.g. post-operative, acutely unwell) within 5–10 days.

- **Nutritional route**

If a patient is unable to take food orally, enteral nutrition is usually preferred to total parenteral nutrition (TPN), as it is cheaper and may reduce infective complications in some patients groups (e.g. abdominal trauma by protecting intestinal mucosa and/or by reducing TPN line-related sepsis). Similarly, in acute pancreatitis, jejunal (i.e. transpyloric) feeding has been demonstrated to reduce sepsis and mortality.

However, enteral feeding is often associated with delay in establishing adequate nutrition (e.g. due to reluctance to increase feed rates) or underprovision of nutrients (e.g. due to failure of gastrointestinal absorption), which may worsen outcome. In addition, patients are exposed to the frequently underrated side effects of enteral nutrition without receiving the benefits. Use of protocols to start and maintain feeding usually improves delivery (see Figure 2.6). Table 2.8 lists the complications that occur with both enteral and total parenteral nutrition.

- **Assessment of nutritional requirements**
  - **Energy expenditure (calories)** can be measured by indirect calorimetry, the Fick principle (i.e. pulmonary artery catheter measurements), or predictive equations which calculate basal metabolic rate (BMR). Indirect calorimetry (i.e. measurement of O_2 consumption and CO_2 production) is the gold standard for the measurement of resting energy expenditure. It is now feasible in ventilated ICU patients, following the introduction of reliable commercial devices.

    In most ward settings, however, measurements of energy requirements are not practical, and so predic-

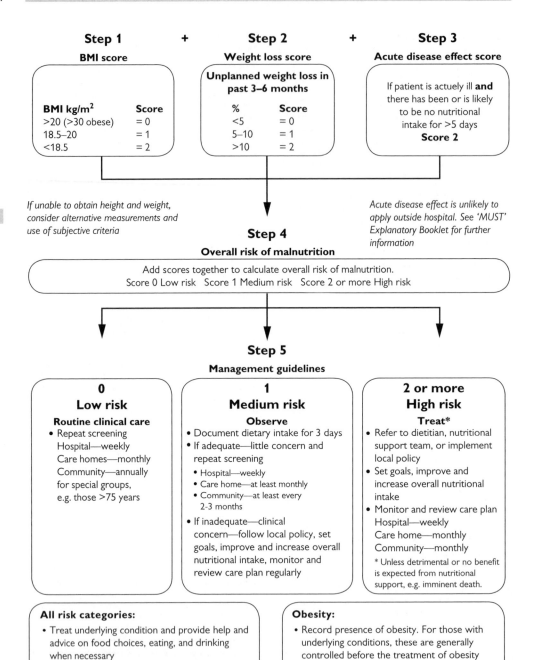

Step 1 + **Step 2** + **Step 3**

BMI score

BMI kg/m²	Score
>20 (>30 obese)	= 0
18.5–20	= 1
<18.5	= 2

Weight loss score

Unplanned weight loss in past 3–6 months

%	Score
<5	= 0
5–10	= 1
>10	= 2

Acute disease effect score

If patient is actuely ill **and** there has been or is likely to be no nutritional intake for >5 days
Score 2

If unable to obtain height and weight, consider alternative measurements and use of subjective criteria

Acute disease effect is unlikely to apply outside hospital. See 'MUST' Explanatory Booklet for further information

Step 4
Overall risk of malnutrition

Add scores together to calculate overall risk of malnutrition.
Score 0 Low risk   Score 1 Medium risk   Score 2 or more High risk

Step 5
Management guidelines

0
Low risk

Routine clinical care
• Repeat screening
  Hospital—weekly
  Care homes—monthly
  Community—annually
  for special groups,
  e.g. those >75 years

1
Medium risk

Observe
• Document dietary intake for 3 days
• If adequate—little concern and repeat screening
  • Hospital—weekly
  • Care home—at least monthly
  • Community—at least every 2-3 months
• If inadequate—clinical concern—follow local policy, set goals, improve and increase overall nutritional intake, monitor and review care plan regularly

2 or more
High risk

Treat*
• Refer to dietitian, nutritional support team, or implement local policy
• Set goals, improve and increase overall nutritional intake
• Monitor and review care plan
  Hospital—weekly
  Care home—monthly
  Community—monthly
* Unless detrimental or no benefit is expected from nutritional support, e.g. imminent death.

All risk categories:
• Treat underlying condition and provide help and advice on food choices, eating, and drinking when necessary
• Record malnutrition risk category
* Record need for special diets and follow local policy

Obesity:
• Record presence of obesity. For those with underlying conditions, these are generally controlled before the treatment of obesity

Reassess subjects identified at risk as they move through care settings
See *The 'MUST' Explanatory Booklet* for further details and *The 'MUST' Report* for supporting evidence.

Figure 2.5 The 'Malnutrition Universal Screening Tool' ('MUST') is reproduced here with the kind permission of BAPEN (British Association for Parenteral and Enteral Nutrition). For further information on 'MUST' see <www.bapen.org.uk>.

Initially, feed at 30 mL/h
Check gastric aspirates 4-hourly

If GRV <200 mL, increase
feed to 60 mL/h
Check gastric aspirates 4-hourly

If GRV <200 mL, increase
feed to 75 mL/h or target volume
Check gastric aspirates 4-hourly

Feed with target volume for 20 h
Daily rest period 4 h
Check gastric aspirates 4-hourly
until feeding established

Figure 2.6 Typical starter feeding regimen. GRV, gastric residual volume.

Table 2.8 Complications of enteral nutrition (EN) and total parenteral nutrition (TPN)

Complications common to both EN and TPN

Metabolic complications (mainly TPN (~5–10%)) over the first 24–48 h
- Hyperglycaemia
- Hypoglycaemia (i.e. if feeding stops abruptly. Replace with 10% glucose infusion)
- Hypokalaemia, hypomagnesaemia, hypophosphataemia
- Metabolic acidosis

Complications of EN	Complications of TPN
• **Aspiration/ventilator pneumonia:** prevented by avoiding gastric distension + 30° elevation of the head of the bed	• **Catheter-related** (e.g. line infection, sepsis, thrombosis, phlebitis, air embolism, occlusion)
• **NG tube problems:** sinusitis, tube obstruction, aspiration, perforation + ulceration	• **Fluid overload + electrolyte abnormalities** (e.g. ↓ K+, ↓ Mg, ↓ PO4 especially in the first 24 h)
• **Impaired gastric emptying + feeding 'intolerance'** (i.e. >300 mL/h residual volume) causes gastric + abdominal distension, vomiting, and ileus	• **Hyperchloraemic metabolic acidosis** is due to amino acid solutions with a high Cl– content. Replace Cl– with acetate in the TPN solution
• **Bacterial overgrowth** due to pH-neutralizing effects of EN in stomach. Predisposes to chest and GIT infections	• **Hepatobiliary:** abnormal liver function tests in ~90% (± jaundice), liver fatty infiltration, intrahepatic cholestasis, cholecystitis
• **Diarrhoea (35%)** is not always due to EN (e.g. *C. difficile*, antibiotic colitis, drugs, malabsorption, prokinetic agents). Reduced using fibre-containing feeds	• **Intestinal:** mucosal + villous atrophy, bacterial translocation
• **Faecal impaction** is rare and due to fibre in feed	• **Trace element + vitamin deficiency** (e.g. zinc, iron and vitamins K, B1, folate)
	• **Refeeding syndrome** (see text)
	• **Bone pain** with prolonged TPN

tive equations tend to be used to estimate resting energy expenditure. Many units then make adjustments for stress and activity. The Schofield equation, an update of the Harris–Benedict equation, is in common use and predicts BMR on the basis of age, sex, and weight (Table 2.9 (1a)). The BMR is then adjusted for potential stress (Table 2.9 (1b)), and, finally, a factor (i.e. percentage) is added for activity-and diet-induced thermogenesis (Table 2.9 (1c)). Further adjustments may be required for specific medical conditions, including starvation, COPD, and hepatic failure (as discussed further).

However, this type of additive approach often leads to very high estimates of energy needs, frequently exceeding those assessed by indirect calorimetry, and, hence in clinical practice, many clinicians either calculate BMR and add about 20% (Table 2.9 (2)), or simply aim to deliver 25–30 kcal/kg/day (Table 2.9 (3)). The use of indirect calorimetry or calculations, using the Fick principle, offers little or no additional benefit.

- **Protein.** Daily nitrogen provision of 0.15–0.2 g/kg/day (equivalent to 1–1.25 g protein/kg/day) is usually adequate, but 0.3 g/kg/day (2 g protein/kg/day) may be required in patients with specific additional direct protein loss (e.g. those with severe burns). Net protein loss can be determined from 24-hour urinary urea nitrogen losses, but such measures are not really helpful in determining nitrogen provision.

Table 2.9 Calculations of nutritional energy (calorie) requirements

1a. Determine BMR from Schofield equation

BMR in kcal/day by age and gender

Age (yrs)	Female	Male
15-18	13.3W +690	17.6W+656
18-30	14.8W +485	15.0W+690
30-60	8.1W +842	11.4W+870
>60	9.0W +656	11.7W+585

Where W = weight in kg, BMR=basal metabolic rate

1b. Adjust for BMR stress

Partial starvation (>10% weight loss)	- 0-15%
Mild infection, IBD, post-operative	+ 0-13%
Moderate infection, long bone #	+ 10-30%
Severe sepsis, multiple trauma	+25-50%
Burns 10-90%	+10-70%

= fractures, IBD = inflammatory bowel disease

1c. Correct for activity + diet-induced thermogenesis

Bed-bound, immobile	+10%
Bed-bound, mobile/sitting	+20%
Mobile around the ward	+25%

2a. Determine BMR from Schofield equation
2b. Add 20%.
2c. Start feeding at 50% of this value.

This is the commonest approach to the calculation of nutritional energy requirements

3. Alternatively calculate energy requirement from **lean body weight:** normally **25-30 kcal/kg/day**, increasing to >60 kcal/kg/day in severe stress (e.g. burns). Non-protein sources supply ~80% of calories (e.g. carbohydrate 30-70%, fat 15-30%).

• **Vitamins and micronutrients.** Requirements of vitamin A, K, thiamine (B1), B3, B6, C, and folic acid increase in severe illness. Vitamin K, folic acid, and thiamine are prone to deficiency during total parenteral nutrition. Deficiencies of zinc (i.e. energy metabolism, protein synthesis), copper (i.e. collagen cross-linking), iron (i.e. oxidative phosphorylation, haematopoiesis), manganese (i.e. neural function, fatty acid synthesis), and selenium (i.e. fat metabolism, antioxidant) have all been reported. Cholestatic liver disease may cause deficits of fat-soluble vitamins. Liver cirrhosis (particularly if caused by alcohol) is frequently accompanied by multiple deficiencies of water-soluble vitamins, particularly of folate, vitamin C, and the B group, including thiamine. Renal replacement therapy is also accompanied by water-soluble vitamin losses.

• **Basal water and electrolytes requirements** are water 30 mL/kg/day (i.e. 70 kg man = $30 \times 70 = 2,100$ mL/day), sodium 1 mmol/kg/day, potassium 0.7–1 mmol/kg/day, magnesium 0.1 mmol/kg/day, calcium 0.1 mmol/kg/day, and phosphorus 0.4 mmol/kg/day, but requirements vary considerably.

• **Refeeding syndrome**

This occurs when food intake or nutritional support is resumed or initiated after a period of starvation. As glucose is reintroduced, increased insulin promotes cellular ion uptake, resulting in severe hypophosphataemia, hypokalaemia, hypomagnesaemia, and metabolic acidosis. Depletion of ATP and 2,3-DGP (± thiamine) causes tissue hypoxia and metabolic inhibition which manifest as cardiorespiratory failure, paraesthesiae, and seizures. Thiamine supplements are essential prior to refeeding in patients with prolonged malnutrition.

• **Disease-specific nutritional requirements**

Specific nutritional requirements are required in many diseases and clinical conditions.

• **Starvation.** Refeeding syndrome occurs after prolonged starvation, as discussed previously. In addition, electrolyte depletion (PO_4^-, K^+, Mg^{2+}) and glucose intolerance can impair cardiac contractility and respiratory muscle function, and early correction is essential.

• **Chronic obstructive pulmonary disease** is often associated with malnutrition, and the increased work of breathing in respiratory failure is associated with high energy expenditure. It has been suggested that overfeeding with carbohydrate increases CO_2 production, exacerbating established respiratory failure or precipitating CO_2 retention due to poor alveolar ventilation. Ideally, feeds should, therefore, contain less carbohydrate and more fat, as fat oxidation produces 30% less CO_2. However, the evidence for benefit is limited, and it is probably more important simply to avoid overfeeding, with consequent unnecessary increases in O_2 demands and CO_2 production.

• **Liver failure.** Both enteral and parenteral nutrition must contain less sodium and volume due to aldosterone-induced water retention in liver failure. Hypoglycaemia is common due to reduced gluconeogenesis. Protein restriction may be required in chronic hepatic encephalopathy. This is, in part, due to the depletion of branched chain amino acids (BCAA), permitting increased cerebral uptake of aromatic amino acids which produce inhibitory neurotransmitters. In protein-intolerant patients, the use of BCAA (instead of aromatic amino acids) may allow increased protein uptake without impairing mental status. However, such measures are rarely of great help, and, in acute hepatic encephalopathy, overall clinical outcomes are significantly better with nutrition support that provides more generous protein provision, compared to a restricted protein intake. In chronic liver failure, fat metabolism is also impaired.

• **Renal failure.** High-energy 'renal' feed are used (i.e. 2 kcal/mL) to reduce volume. In TPN, essential amino acids may stimulate protein synthesis and reduce urea by recycling nitrogen into non-essential amino acids. Low sodium, potassium, and phosphate feeds, with supplemental vitamins, may be required.

• **Acute pancreatitis.** In the past, parenteral nutrition was used to minimize pancreatic stimulation, but recent studies suggest that jejunal, or even intragastric, feeding (if gastric emptying permits) are safe and associated with fewer infective complications. Elemental feeds and pancreatic enzyme supplements may be required if malabsorption is a problem, and PN may still be needed in patients with ileus, and especially those who have needed surgery.

Enteral nutrition

In the acutely unwell patient, enteral nutrition is known to have a number of potential advantages. These include:

• Increased splanchnic perfusion (i.e. protection against bowel ischaemia).
• Prevention of stress ulceration.
• Preserved mucosal integrity which protects against bacterial translocation (± sepsis).
• Increased gut-associated lymphoid tissue, enhancing immunity.
• Better delivery and absorption of complex nutrients (e.g. fibre, medium chain fatty acids).
• Enhanced gall bladder emptying, preventing stasis and secondary gall bladder infection.
• Promotion of insulin secretion by the pancreas (i.e. reduces hyperglycaemia), gastrin (± other gut hormones), and pancreatic secretions.

Access and administration of enteral nutrition

In the acutely unwell patient, a wide-bore (12–14F) nasogastric tube allows aspiration and assessment of gastric residual volumes at 4-hourly intervals. Correct positioning of the tube is achieved by aspirating and confirming the presence of gastric contents by pH testing. If there is any doubt (i.e. difficulty aspirating gastric contents or cough if in the tracheobronchial tree), a chest radiograph is performed.

Once feeding is established, the large-bore tube is replaced with a more comfortable fine-bore nasogastric tube. Stylets are required to stiffen these tubes to aid insertion. Even with a fine-bore tube, gastric aspiration to check tube position is usually achievable, especially if you try repositioning the patient. However, if this proves impossible, a chest radiograph may be required. Fine-bore tube misplacement is not uncommon, but it is essential that attempts to correct this never entail reinsertion of the wire stylet if any part the tube is still within the patient.

Orogastric tubes are uncomfortable and rarely required, except in patients with basal skull fractures, significant sinus infection, and during complex faciomaxillary surgery.

Nasojejunal tubes are preferred in pancreatitis and may be useful in patients with impaired gastric emptying refractory to prokinetic agents. They do not reduce the risk of aspiration. Spontaneous passage through the pylorus is rare but may be encouraged by administration of erythromycin as a prokinetic. In practice, endoscopic or radiological assistance is required for reliable transpyloric placement.

Patients who require long-term enteral feeding may benefit from a percutaneous gastrostomy, which is usually performed endoscopically. In the acutely unwell patient, percutaneous endoscopic gastrostomy is associated with complications (e.g. infection) and a high 30-day mortality rate and is best avoided until the patient is stable. Percutaneous jejunal access is achieved by gastrostomy, radiological replacement, or at laparotomy.

Enteral nutrition is usually given as a continuous infusion. A daily 4-hour feeding rest period prevents stomach bacterial overgrowth by allowing restoration of normal gastric pH (<7.1) and may reduce the risk of aspiration-related pneumonia. In general, enteral nutrition can be achieved in most patients despite abdominal distension, absence of bowel sounds, or diarrhoea. Figure 2.6 illustrates a typical starter feeding regimen. Contraindications to enteral nutrition include intestinal obstruction, ischaemia, and anatomical disruption. Complications are reported in Table 2.8. Blockage of fine-bore tubes is common. Instillation of pancreatic enzyme supplements into the tube with 'dwell times' of at least an hour may aid clearance of blockages.

Failure to establish enteral nutrition
Gastric aspirates are measured every 4 h at the onset of enteral nutrition. Gastric residual volumes (GRV) >400 mL may increase the risk of pulmonary aspiration, although there is no direct evidence of this. However, in this situation, feeding should be stopped and reintroduced at a lower infusion rate. Gastric residual volumes that are consistently >200 mL are treated with prokinetic agents (initially intravenous metoclopramide (10 mg 8-hourly), a dopamine antagonist, and then intravenous erythromycin (250 mg 12-hourly), a motilin receptor agonist), to stimulate gastric emptying. In refractory cases, an endoscopically placed nasojejunal tube (or surgical jejunostomy) often permits successful enteral nutrition, as small bowel function often recovers earlier than gastric emptying.

Feeding formulas
Standard commercial feeds provide 1–1.5 kcal/mL (~45% carbohydrate, ~25% lipid) and most electrolytes and micronutrients. The proportion of non-protein calories, provided as carbohydrate, is usually about two-thirds. They are isotonic, polymeric (i.e. complex protein, fat, and carbohydrate molecules), and gluten-/lactose-free, which reduces the potential for diarrhoea. Elemental diets (i.e. amino acids, oligosaccharides) require minimal digestion (e.g. chronic pancreatitis) and may be useful when small bowel absorption is impaired (e.g. pancreatic insufficiency) or after prolonged starvation.

Parenteral nutrition

Long-term parenteral nutrition is required in a small proportion of patients due to irreversible gastrointestinal damage (e.g. Crohn's disease, bowel ischaemia) or following bowel resection (e.g. after severe bowel ischaemia). In these patients, parenteral nutrition is a life-sustaining treatment and requires expert support in specialized centres.

However, in most cases, parenteral nutrition is a temporary requirement in acute illness associated with reversible gastrointestinal failure (e.g. ileus, intractable diarrhoea) or when there are contraindications to enteral nutrition (e.g. bowel obstruction). In some of these cases, gastrointestinal failure is obvious, but, in others, it only becomes apparent after considerable effort to establish enteral nutrition has failed. Although meta-analyses have shown no benefit of parenteral nutrition in the acutely ill patient, the studies comparing clinical outcomes using parenteral nutrition against either no nutrition support or other means of nutrition support have specifically excluded patients who could only be fed via the intravenous route (i.e. all patients in whom parenteral nutrition is usually used), on ethical grounds. The study results, therefore, have little relevance to usual clinical practice.

Access and delivery of parenteral nutrition
The major issue associated with central venous access for parenteral nutrition is the prevention of infection. The following factors affect central line infection rates:

- Operator expertise and appropriate assistant support (e.g. nurse to help maintain sterility) during line insertion.
- Skin sterility during insertion. The most effective skin cleansant is 2% chlorhexidine.
- Use of sterile technique with mask, cap, gown, and gloves substantially reduces line infection rates. The use of sterile technique outside the ICU is relatively poor.
- Appropriate post-insertion line care, including the use of permeable polyurethane transparent dressings.
- Site of insertion is important, with subclavian and internal jugular lines associated with lower infection rates. Tunnelled and long lines may reduce infection rates and are often used for long-term parenteral nutrition (e.g. PICC lines). The use of PICC lines for medium-term parenteral nutrition is routine in many units.
- Antimicrobial or silver-impregnated catheters may reduce the risk of bacterial line infections.
- Change the catheter when the insertion site becomes inflamed or inflammatory markers begin to rise. Scheduled changes do not reduce infection rates. Use of a guidewire to change a line at the same site is associated with an increased risk of line infection.
- Use of a dedicated parenteral nutrition lumen in the central catheter and daily changes of the infusion sets may reduce line infection.

Parenteral nutrition solutions are nutritionally adequate but irritant and often hyperosmolar. Most solutions are prepared aseptically in hospital pharmacies as a single bag which is infused continuously over 24 hours through the dedicated lumen of a central venous catheter. Pre-prepared solutions are available that can be modified to individual requirements under sterile conditions. Parenteral nutrition can be given into a peripheral vein, but large volumes with low glucose concentrations are necessary to reduce osmolality-induced phlebitis. Nevertheless, new peripheral line sites may be required at 2–3 day intervals due to discomfort or thrombosis in the veins used. Complications associated with parenteral nutrition are reported in Table 2.8. Liver dysfunction is reduced by avoiding overfeeding and, if persistent, by reducing fat content.

Energy is provided as a combination of carbohydrate and lipid. About 35% of non-protein energy is given as lipid. Concentrated glucose solutions are the preferred source of carbohydrate, but exceeding the body's capacity to metabolize glucose can lead to hyperglycaemia, CO_2 production, and lipogenesis. Some patients require additional insulin if hyperglycaemic, but most do not if overfeeding is avoided. Addition of insulin to the parenteral nutrition solutions is strongly discouraged (although it may be considered in ICU where glucose levels are closely monitored).

Lipid infusions provide a more concentrated energy source. Unfortunately, lipid infusions impair neutrophil function and may be immunosuppressive. Nitrogen is supplied as amino acids, but glutamine, cysteine, and tyrosine are unstable and absent. Vitamins and trace element preparations are added to TPN solutions, but thiamine, folic acid, and vitamin K are susceptible to depletion, and additional doses may be required.

Immunonutrition

Immunonutrition uses compounds that, although unproven, may improve metabolic and immune responses in critical illness. Typically, these include:

- Glutamine, an amino acid and primary energy source for enterocytes, may help preserve antioxidant capacity via glutathione and intestinal integrity.
- Arginine is a non-essential amino acid that stimulates immune (e.g. T cell) function and nitrogen balance.
- Omega-3-polyunsaturated fatty acids from fish oils are anti-inflammatory agents and immune modulators.

Other adjuncts to feeding solutions that may be beneficial include medium chain triglycerides that are less dependent on pancreatic enzymes for absorption and are more rapidly metabolized when infused intravenously. The nucleotides, purine, and pyrimidine are precursor molecules in DNA and RNA synthesis and may enhance cell-mediated immunity.

Further reading

Bistrian BR, Blackburn GL, Vitale J, Cochran D, Naylor J (1976). Prevalence of malnutrition in general patients. *JAMA*, **253**, 1567–70.

Convinsky KE, Martin GE Beyth RJ, Juctice AC, Sehgal AR, Landefeld CS (1999). The relationship between clinical assessments of nutritional status and adverse outcomes in older hospitalised medical patients. *Journal of the American Geriatrics Society*, **47**, 532–8.

Dintinjana RD, Guina T, Krznaric Z, et al. (2008). Effects of nutritional support in patients with colorectal cancer during chemotherapy. *Collegium Antropologicum*, **32**, 737–40.

Elia M (2003). Screening for malnutrition: a multidisciplinary responsibility. Development and use of the malnutrition universal screening tool (MUST) for adults. Malnutrition advisory group (MAG), a standing committee of BAPEN. BAPEN, Redditch.

Henderson S, Moore N, Lee E, Witham M (2008). Do the malnutrition universal screening tool (MUST) and Birmingham nutrition risk (BNR) score predict mortality in older hospitalised patients? *BMC Geriatrics*, **8**, 26–31.

Kelly IE, Tessier S, Cahill A, et al. (2000). Still hungry in hospital: identifying malnutrition in acute hospital admissions. *QJM*, **93**, 93–8.

Lean M and Wiseman M (2008). Malnutrition in hospitals. *BMJ*, **336**, 290.

Leach RM, Brotherton A, Stroud M, Thompson RPHT (2013). Nutrition and fluid balance must be taken seriously. *BMJ*, **346**, 801–804.

McWhirter JP and Pennington CR (1994). Incidence and recognition of malnutrition in hospital. *BMJ*, **308**, 945–8.

National Institute for Health and Clinical Excellence (2006). Nutrition support in adults. Clinical guideline no. 32. <http://guidance.nice.org.uk/CG32>.

Patel MD and Martin FC (2008). Why don't elderly hospital inpatients eat adequately? *Journal of Nutrition, Health and Aging*, **12**, 227–31.

Reilly JJ, Hull SF, Albert N, Waller A, Bringardener S (1988). Economic impact of malnutrition: a model system for hospitalised patients. *Journal of Parenteral and Enteral Nutrition*, **12**, 372–6.

Russel CA and Elia M (2008). Nutritional screening survey and audit of adults on admission to hospital, care homes and mental health units. BAPEN, Maidenhead.

Woodcock NP, Zeigler D, Palmer MD, et al. (2001). Enteral versus parenteral nutrition: a pragmatic study. *Nutrition*, **17**, 1–12.

Working Party of the British Association of Parenteral and Enteral Nutrition (1999). Current perspectives on enteral nutrition in adults. BAPEN, Maidenhead.

Lifestyle modification

Healthy nutrition

Food provides the nutrients essential for metabolism, growth, and repair of body tissues. No single food contains all the essential nutrients, and, consequently, a variety of food products must be consumed. Individual foods contain carbohydrates, fats, proteins, vitamins, non-starch polysaccharides (NSP; commonly referred to as fibre), salts (e.g. sodium, potassium, iron, calcium), and trace elements, including magnesium and zinc in differing quantities. It is recognized that prolonged excess of some of these components or an increased proportion in relation to the overall intake can be detrimental to health. For example, excess carbohydrate, fat, or salt can cause obesity, cardiovascular disease, and increased risk of cancer. Consequently, a balanced diet is essential for good health.

A balanced diet is based on the five commonly accepted food groups in the following proportions:

- Bread, cereal, and potatoes: ~33% of total diet.
- Fruit and vegetables: ~33% of total diet.
- Milk and dairy products: ~14%.
- Meat, fish, and alternatives (e.g. beans): ~14%.
- Foods containing fat and sugar (e.g. cakes): ~5%.

Encouraging people to choose a variety of foods from the first four groups every day will ensure that they obtain the wide range of nutrients that their bodies require to remain healthy and function normally. Foods in the fifth group, which contain fat and sugar, are not essential to a healthy diet but add choice and palatability. The main nutrients provided by each food group are as follows:

- Bread, cereal, and potatoes include foods like breakfast cereals, rice, pasta, noodles, maize, beans, pulses, and cornmeal. They contain mainly carbohydrate (starch), fibre (i.e. NSP), vitamin B, and some calcium and iron.
- Fruit and vegetables include fresh, frozen, dried and canned fruit and vegetables, beans and pulses, and fruit juices. They contain vitamin C, folates, carotenes, starch (i.e. NSP), and relatively little carbohydrate.
- Milk and dairy products include cheese, yogurt, and fromage frais. It does not include cream, butter, or eggs. They contain protein, calcium, and vitamins A, D, and B12.
- Meat, fish, and alternatives which include eggs, bacon, salami, sausages, canned fish, fish fingers, poultry, nuts, beans, and pulses. They contain protein, iron, vitamins B and B12, zinc, and magnesium. Aim to eat at least one portion of oily fish (e.g. mackerel) each week for vitamin D.
- Foods containing fat include butter, margarine, low fat spreads, oils, salad dressings, cream, chocolate, crisps, biscuits, cakes, puddings, rich sauces, and ice cream. Foods containing sugar include soft drinks, jams, cakes, and ice cream. Some essential fatty acids, minerals, and vitamins are obtained from these products, but they often contain excess salt and sugar.

People differ in the amount of energy (i.e. calories) they need each day which affects the amount of food an individual requires. However, the relative proportions of food (as discussed previously) should remain the same.

Food energy is measured in calories. For example, a banana has ~80 calories and a piece of bread ~80 calories, but, with butter and jam, this increases to ~160 calories. A small, sedentary individual may require as few as 1,200 calories daily, whereas a manual labourer may require as many as 4,500 calories daily. The factors that affect overall energy requirement are:

- **Gender:** women tend to need less energy than men.
- **Age:** older adults need less energy than the young.
- **Physical activity:** active people need more energy.
- **Obesity:** less calories should be consumed to achieve a healthy weight (a body mass index of >18 to <24).

Fluid intake is important, and everybody should drink 6–8 cups, mugs, or glasses of fluid a day. Drinks containing sugar, fruit juices, and carbonated drinks should be taken in moderation because they can contribute to tooth decay. The regular use of fluoride toothpaste helps protect teeth. Vitamin and mineral supplements are not usually necessary if a healthy diet is consumed.

Food requirements may differ in some groups:

- Children under 2 years old differ because they need full fat milk and dairy products.
- Older people may need extra vitamin D, calcium, and iron.
- Young women may need iron supplements to replace losses related to heavy menstruation.
- Women who intend to become pregnant, or who are pregnant, need extra folic acid and sometimes iron.
- People under medical supervision and those with gastrointestinal disorders (e.g. chronic pancreatitis, inflammatory bowel disease, short bowel syndrome) may need tailored diets and dietary supplements.

The key messages for a healthy diet

These are based on eight guidelines for a healthy diet:

- Enjoy your food.
- Eat a variety of different foods.
- Eat the right amount to be a healthy weight.
- Eat plenty of fruit and vegetables.
- Eat plenty of foods rich in starch and fibre.
- Eat less food containing fat.
- Reduce sugary food and drinks.
- Drink alcohol in moderation.

Practical tips for a healthy diet

- Eat lots of wholemeal, wholegrain, or high-fibre foods.
- Avoid fried food, high-fat foods, cream, and rich sauces or dressings.
- Eat at least five portions of fruit and vegetables daily. Fruit juice and pulses or beans account for only one portion, no matter how much you drink or eat. Avoid adding butter or sauces (fatty or sugary) to fruit and vegetables.
- Use low-fat foods, whenever possible (e.g. skimmed or semi-skimmed milk, low-fat yogurts, or cheese). Remove fat from meat and skin from poultry, and eat fish without batter. Beans and pulses are good alternatives to meat, as they contain protein and are naturally very low in fat.
- Eat foods containing fat sparingly, and use low-fat alternatives.
- Eat less foods and drinks containing sugar. They should be eaten mainly at mealtimes to reduce the risk of tooth decay.

Further reading

Food Standards Agency. <http://www.foodsatndards.gov.uk>

Food Standards Agency. The balance of good health. Food Standards Agency, Department of Health. Factsheet: FSA/0008/0604 100k.

World Health Organization (2006). Obesity and overweight. Factsheet no 311. WHO, Geneva.

Obesity

Obesity and related diseases place a significant burden on healthcare services, and this is expected to increase as the prevalence of obesity rises. Worldwide, 1.9 billion people are overweight and 600 million are obese. Simultaneously, there has been an associated increase in the prevalence of comorbidities, including type 2 diabetes mellitus and obstructive sleep apnoea. In England, 25% of adults are obese, and, by 2050, 60% of adult males, 50% of adult females, and 25% of children will be obese.

Public health interventions, including 'The Change for Life' campaign in the UK, have been implemented. Strategies to prevent obesity include:

- Individual long-term behavioural changes aimed at healthy diet and increased physical activity.
- Family-focused education to improve diet and activity.
- Workplace-related changes aimed at encouraging healthy food options and limiting vending machines.
- Institutional education (e.g. school) from an early age may influence long-term behaviour.
- Healthcare-managed detection and early lifestyle intervention in overweight individuals.
- Community and regional changes to improve access to healthy leisure activities and lifestyle information. Management of transport facilities to encourage walking.
- National factors include healthcare and socio-economic strategies and action to target the food industry and media.
- International intervention aimed at agriculture and food distribution and factors such as smoking and alcohol.

Assessment

Careful assessment of obesity is essential. Secondary causes and contributory factors must be considered, including endocrine (e.g. acromegaly, hypothyroidism), rare genetic causes (e.g. Prader–Willi syndrome, leptin deficiency), neuroendocrine causes (e.g. hypothalamic obesity), and drugs (e.g. insulin, hypoglycaemic agents, anticonvulsants, antipsychotics, steroids, oral contraceptives). Details of family history, changes in lifestyle (e.g. divorce, unemployment), and psychosocial factors are important. Assess dietary habits, physical activity, and obesity-related comorbidities. Details of previous weight loss attempts, causes of failure, barriers for change, and reasons for wanting to lose weight may influence the level of intervention.

Management

Effective obesity management requires a multidisciplinary team of physicians, specialists (e.g. endocrinologists), nurses, dietitians, psychologists, therapists, and bariatric surgeons.

Lifestyle interventions

Education about lifestyle, healthy diets, and eating habits is an essential component of all weight loss therapies.

- *Diets* and dietary intervention-based programmes (e.g. very low calorie diets, high-protein diets) are popular, and, although effective in the short term, they have been shown to be ineffective long-term. In addition, short-term programmes involving significant calorie restriction can be harmful without appropriate monitoring. Adherence to long-term healthy dietary changes with modest calorie restrictions are more likely to be successful and avoids all-or-nothing yo-yo dieting.

- *Physical activity* is as important as energy restriction in obesity prevention and long-term weight loss programmes. In addition, increased daily activity has independent beneficial effects on cardiovascular and comorbid conditions (e.g. diabetes, hypertension). Moderate intensity physical activity for 30 minutes daily or 45–60 minutes three times a week is recommended.

- *Behavioural therapy* can improve outcome when combined with lifestyle, medical, or surgical therapies. Self-monitoring, record-keeping, stimulus control, stress management, problem solving, social support, and cognitive restructuring may help address the problem of compliance which is often associated with modification of lifestyle-based weight loss programmes. Eating disorders (e.g. bulimia, binge eating) may require prolonged and individualized cognitive behavioural therapy and are best managed by psychologists.

Obesity pharmacotherapy

Weight loss drugs should only be used in combination with lifestyle education and careful monitoring.

- In the UK, only orlistat is licensed for prolonged use. **Orlistat** (120 mg tds as prescription or 60 mg tds over the counter) inhibits pancreatic and intestinal lipases and prevents absorption of ~30% of dietary triglyceride. It also modestly reduces blood pressure and cholesterol and contributes to improved glycaemic control in diabetics. Gastrointestinal side effects may prevent use, and it should not be used in patients with malabsorption or cholestasis. About 39% achieve 10% weight loss. It can be used for up to 48 months, but there is the risk of weight regain on completion of therapy.

- **Lorcaserin**, a selective 5HT-receptor agonist, was licensed in 2012 in the USA as a prescription-only drug for obesity management. Its efficacy and potential side effects continue to be assessed.

- In the US, the Food and Drug Administration (FDA) has approved **Qsymia** (phentermine and topiramate extended-release), **Belviq** (lorcaserin hydrochloride; a selective 5HT receptor agonist), **Contrave** (naltrexone hydrochloride and bupropion hydrochloride extended-release tablets) and more recently **Saxenda** (liraglutide (rDNA origin) injection at a higher dose of 3 mg per day) as treatment options for chronic weight management. Some of these may become available in Europe in the near future but the data to prove longterm efficacy and safety of these agents is awaited.

- In the European Union and many other countries (e.g. Canada, India, Australia), **Sibutramine** (10–15 mg daily), a centrally acting inhibitor of serotonin and noradrenaline reuptake which reduces food intake by enhancing natural satiety, has been withdrawn by the licensing authorities due to concerns about potential cardiovascular side effects (i.e. strokes, myocardial infarction) and limited efficacy. In the USA it has been withdrawn from the market by the manufacturer. However, it is still available in some countries (e.g. Russia) and over the last five years it has been detected in several 'herbal' products used for weight loss in countries where it has been withdrawn from use.

In countries where sibutramine is in use (e.g. Russia), considerable caution is recommended in patients with cardiovascular disease. Blood pressure and heart rate should be monitored and the drug stopped if either increases. In addition to cardiovascular disease, it should not be used in patients with renal/liver impairment, psychiatric illness, hypertension, heart failure, thyrotoxicosis, severe eating disorders, or in combination with antidepressants or antipsychotic agents.

In people with other longterm chronic conditions such as type 2 diabetes, using weight-friendly medication options (such as GLP1 analogues and SGLT2 inhibitors) should be considered rather than agents that cause weight gain.

Surgical management

In recent years, the use of minimally invasive laparoscopic surgery has drastically reduced the incidence of perioperative complications and mortality associated with surgical treatments for obesity, which is now considered a cost-effective option for severe obesity. The NICE guidelines recommend surgery for people with a body mass index (BMI) >40 (or >35 in those with serious comorbidity) if other weight loss measures have failed or as first-line intervention in those with a BMI >50, although, in practice, higher thresholds are often used due to lack of resources.

Surgical procedures are best classified by the mechanism they employ to achieve weight loss. In general, malabsorptive procedures cause more weight loss than restrictive procedures but have a higher morbidity and mortality risk.

Sustained weight loss for up to 15 years and improvements in diabetes, dyslipidaemia, obstructive sleep apnoea, cardiorespiratory function, fertility, psychosocial performance, mobility, quality of life, and cancer risks are reported.

- **Restrictive** (e.g. laparoscopic adjustable gastric banding (see Figure 3.1), gastroplasty, gastric balloon) achieves excess weight loss of 46% and diabetic remission in 57%, which, although less than malabsorptive procedures, is associated with lower operative mortality (0.06%). Post-operative band slippage, pouch dilation, infection, erosion, and leakage may occur. Nutritional deficiencies are uncommon, but reoperation and failure rates are higher. It is fully reversible, but the success of this procedure is dependent on the patient's ability to stick to a healthy lifestyle.

- **Restrictive with some malabsorption** (e.g. Roux-en-Y gastric bypass (see Figure 3.2)) achieves excess weight loss of 60% and diabetic remission in 80% but has a higher mortality rate (0.16%). Post-operative complications include strictures, obstruction, stomal ulcers, hernia and anastomotic leaks, chronic nausea, diarrhoea, 'dumping' syndrome, gallstones, hair loss, and nutritional deficiencies (e.g. iron, vitamins D and B12, copper, zinc, magnesium, etc.). Close monitoring is required by a multidisciplinary team. The risk of weight regain is 10%, especially in those who do not follow dietary advice, and requires intensive lifestyle modification, behavioural therapy, and, occasionally, revision surgery.

Sleeve gastrectomy is an increasingly popular surgical weight loss procedure, usually performed laparoscopically, in which the stomach is reduced to about 25% of its original size by surgical removal of a large portion of the stomach along its greater curve. It was originally performed as the first part of a two stage gastric bypass operation (bilio-pancreatic diversion with duodenal switch (see further text)) in extremely obese subjects in whom the risk of performing gastric bypass was considered too great. The initial sleeve gastrectomy performed in these cases (before the gastric bypass) was so effective it has since been used as a stand-alone procedure for weight loss. It has also been shown to have weight loss independent benefits on glucose homeostasis. The mechanisms that produce these benefits are unknown.

- **Malabsorptive** (e.g. bilio-pancreatic diversion with duodenal switch) achieves excess weight loss of 64% and diabetic remission in 95% of cases. It has the highest complication rate and operative mortality (1.1%). A sleeve gastrectomy is performed, leaving a gastric reservoir of 150–200 mL. The duodenum is closed, 2 cm distal to the pylorus, and a duodenoileal anastomosis is performed. The short common limb (75–100 cm), in which food in the alimentary tract mixes with pancreatic juices, results in significant malabsorption and weight loss. There is a high incidence of long-term gastrointestinal side effects, severe nutritional deficiencies, and protein

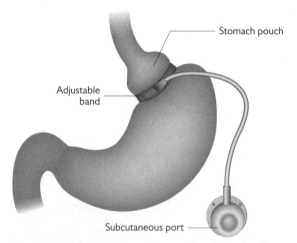

Figure 3.1 Laparoscopic adjustable gastric band. This is a restrictive procedure which involves placing an adjustable band in the upper part of the stomach, just distal to the gastro-oesophageal junction. The amount of restriction can be altered by injecting or withdrawing saline from the band through a subcutaneous port.

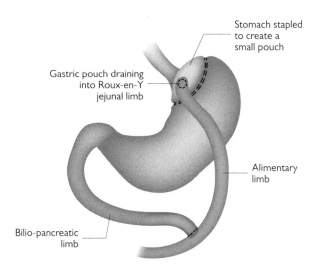

Stomach stapled
to create a
small pouch

Gastric pouch draining
into Roux-en-Y
jejunal limb

Alimentary
limb

Bilio-pancreatic
limb

Figure 3.2 Laparoscopic Roux-en-Y gastric bypass. This is a common procedure and relies mainly on restriction of food intake with a degree of malabsorption. The stomach is reduced to a small gastric pouch which drains into a Roux-en-Y limb of proximal jejunum (75–150 cm long).

malnutrition, particularly in patients who are unable to follow the strict dietary changes that are required.

Genetic research, the development of new drugs, and improved surgical procedures offer the possibility of safer, and more effective, therapies in the future. Several pharmacological therapies are currently been developed, including centrally acting agents, such as serotonin-noradrenaline-dopamine reuptake inhibitors (e.g. tesofensine), selective serotonin receptor agonists, and combination treatments with analogues of peripherally acting satiety signals like amylin, leptin, and glucagon-like peptide-1 which may enhance medical management options. Endoscopic restrictive procedures like balloon insertion and gastric partitioning and laparoscopic procedures like sleeve gastrectomy are currently being studied, with encouraging results.

Further reading

Adams TD, Gress RE, Smith SC, *et al.* (2007). Long-term mortality after gastric bypass surgery. *New England Journal of Medicine*, **357**, 753–61.

Aditya BS and Wilding JPH (2009). Modern management of obesity. *Clinical Medicine*, **9**, 617–621.

Astrup A, Madsbad S, Breum L, *et al.* (2008). Effect of tesofensine on bodyweight loss, body composition, and quality of life in obese patients: a randomised, double-blind, placebo-controlled trial. *Lancet*, **372**, 1906–13.

Buchwald H, Estok R, Fahrbach K, *et al.* (2009). Weight and type 2 diabetes after bariatric surgery: systemic review and meta-analysis. *American Journal of Medicine*, **122**, 248–56.

Dansinger ML, Gleason JA, Griffith JL, Selker HP, Schaefer EJ (2005). Comparison of the Atkins, Ornish, Weight Watchers, and Zone diets for weight loss and heart disease risk reduction: a randomised trial. *JAMA*, **29**, 43–53.

Foresight (2007). Tackling obesities: future choices–project report. Stationery Office, London.

National Institute for Health and Clinical Excellence (2006). Obesity: the prevention, identification, assessment and management of overweight and obesity in adults and children. National Institute for Health and Clinical Excellence, London.

Sjöstrom L, Rissanen A, Andersen T, *et al.* (1998). Randomised placebo-controlled trial of orlistat for weight loss and prevention of weight regain in obese patients. European Multicentre Orlistat Study Group. *Lancet*, **352**, 167–72.

World Health Organization (2006). Obesity and overweight. Factsheet no 311. WHO, Geneva.

Smoking cessation

Worldwide, over a billion people smoke, and 5.4 million deaths occur annually due to smoking. Tobacco kills one person every 6 seconds and remains the most important cause of preventable morbidity and early mortality in the world today. It is the only legal consumer product that can harm everyone exposed to it, and it kills up to half of those who use it. In the last century, the tobacco epidemic has killed 100 million people globally.

In the UK, about 6.3 million people have died from smoking in the period from 1950 to 2000. Currently, 24% of adults in the UK smoke, but overall prevalence has remained static over the last 10 years. Every year, there are 120,000 deaths, 365,000 hospital admissions, and 1.2 million GP consultations, all related to tobacco. Smoking reduces a smoker's life expectancy by an average of 10 years or about 12 minutes for every cigarette smoked.

Smoking prevalence is highest amongst young adults (32% of 20–24 year olds in the UK smoke in comparison to the national average of just under 20%), adults in manual occupations, socio-economically deprived people, and men of South Asian descent. Chinese and Indian women are least likely to smoke. In 2006, 24% of 15-year-old girls and 16% of boys were regular smokers, despite the fact that it is now illegal to sell tobacco to people under the age of 18-years-old. On average, these 15-year-olds smoke 42 cigarettes each week. In the age group of 11–15 years old, 10% of girls and 7% of boys smoke at least one cigarette a week. Overall, 82% of smokers started as teenagers. Factors encouraging children to smoke include family members who smoke, being in a one-parent family, a poor academic record, and being exposed to tobacco advertising. Smoking early in life increases lung cancer risk independently of the amount and duration of smoking.

In developed countries, including the USA, there is early evidence of a decrease in tobacco consumption. In contrast, there has been a substantial increase in smoking in developing countries, as tobacco companies focus their attention on new markets and economies, targeting hundreds of millions of potential new smokers. Thus, although tobacco-related deaths are projected to decline by 9% between 2002 and 2030 in high-income countries, they are to double from 3.4 million to 6.8 million in low- and middle-income countries.

Tobacco, in all its forms, is harmful (i.e. cigarettes, cigars, bidis, water pipes, etc.) and adversely affects nearly every part of the body. Tobacco smoking accounts for 90% of lung cancer cases and approximately 30% of all cancer deaths (i.e. oral, nasal cavity, nasal sinus, pharynx, larynx, oesophagus, stomach, pancreas, liver, urinary tract, uterine cervix, myeloid leukaemia) in developed countries. Smoking morbidity and mortality is also due to COPD, coronary heart disease, peripheral vascular disease, stroke, and peptic ulcer disease. There is unequivocal evidence of the harmful effects of tobacco, whether it be first-, second- or third-hand.

The relative risk of developing lung cancer in a long-term smoker, compared to a lifelong non-smoker, is increased by 10–30 fold. Risk is dependent on dose (i.e. number of cigarettes/day, depth of inhalation, and number of years smoked), age of onset, race (e.g. African-Americans are at greater risk), and pattern of smoking (i.e. a quit period reduces subsequent risk on restarting smoking).

Tobacco smoke is made up of 'sidestream smoke' from the burning tip of the cigarette and 'mainstream smoke' from the filter or mouth end. It is the 'sidestream smoke' that makes up the majority (85%) of environmental tobacco smoke (ETS) and contributes to passive (involuntary or second-hand) smoking. In a meta-analysis of 37 studies, non-smokers who lived with smokers had a 24% (95% CI 13–36%) increased incidence of lung cancer. The risk is 16–19% in those exposed to ETS in the workplace. In the UK, it is estimated that there are 12,000 deaths each year that are attributable to ETS, and 500 of these are due to ETS exposure in the workplace.

Passive smoking is also harmful to children and increases respiratory disease, asthma attacks, cot deaths, and middle ear infections. In the UK, over 30% of children live with at least one adult smoker, and, among low-income families, this increases to 57%. Smoking during pregnancy is associated with increased risk of spontaneous abortion, preterm birth, low birthweight, and stillbirth. In 2005, 32% of women smoked before, or during, pregnancy and 17% throughout pregnancy. These figures were 48% and 29%, respectively, in lower socio-economic groups.

Smoking cessation reduces the risk of developing lung cancer by up to 90%. However, the risk of developing lung cancer is always higher than in lifelong non-smokers and is dependent on the number of cigarettes smoked, age at smoking cessation, and the number of years since smoking cessation. The British Doctors study found that, for every year smoking cessation was postponed after 40 years of age, life expectancy was reduced by 3 months. Smoking cessation results in increased appetite, caloric intake, and weight gain lasting for 6–12 months.

Why is smoking addictive?

All varieties of tobacco contain nicotine, an alkaloid that mediates its effects by the release of the reward neurotransmitter dopamine in the brain's mesolimbic system. Cigarettes are particularly popular because they are efficient nicotine delivery devices, rapidly achieving high brain nicotine levels, as the transit time from the alveoli to the brain, via the bloodstream, is only 7–20 seconds.

After repeated ingestion of nicotine, the motivational system is altered to create a 'drive' similar to hunger, except for cigarettes. This drive is experienced as a 'need to smoke' and develops over the time since the last cigarette. It is influenced by triggers, reminders, stress, and distractions. It usually reduces over weeks of not smoking but can re-emerge unexpectedly. After repeated nicotine exposure, abstinence results in unpleasant withdrawal symptoms, including depression.

Despite tar and carbon monoxide levels being 10 times higher, nicotine is the main barrier to smoking cessation due to the associated physical and psychological dependence. Nicotine exerts its effects through brain and muscle nicotine acetylcholine receptors (nAchR). Activation of brain nAchR stimulates the release of many neurotransmitters, including noradrenaline (arousal, appetite reduction), serotonin (mood regulation), vasopressin (memory improvement), and beta endorphin (anxiety reduction). Most importantly, it stimulates dopamine-secreting neurones in the nucleus accumbens of the mesolimbic dopamine system (brain reward pathway) which elicits pleasurable sensations and is associated with the development of addictive behaviour. Repeated exposure to nicotine desensitizes nAchR, and, despite a 300% increase in receptor numbers, the response to nicotine decreases and natural brain dopamine levels fall, requiring increased nicotine stimulation for equivalent effect. These changes are the basis for the addictive effect of nicotine.

Nicotine substitution can relieve some of the 'need to smoke' by raising the tonic depression of nicotinic acetylcholine activity without being addictive and is the basis for nicotine replacement therapy in smoking cessation programmes.

How is nicotine metabolized?
Nicotine metabolism to cotinine and nicotine N'-oxide occurs mainly in the liver but also in the lung and brain. Cotinine has a long half-life (14 to 20 hours), in comparison to nicotine (2 hours), and is used as a marker of nicotine intake and is used in research studies to evaluate the success of smoking cessation.

Smoking cessation
The majority of smokers would like to stop smoking, but as few as 1% can stop without help, and more than 70% of adult smokers have made at least one attempt. Over 70% of smokers see a physician each year, a time when they are most likely to be receptive and motivated, but only 20% are encouraged to stop smoking! Brief opportunistic advice, even as little as 60 seconds, from a medical professional may trigger a 'quit attempt' in 40% of cases. Consequently, smoking cessation should be encouraged by every healthcare professional at every point of contact. All healthcare workers should be able to offer accurate advice on all forms of assistance available, including medications, help lines, self-help materials, and specialist services. They should encourage smokers to use effective forms of assistance and refer to the smoking cessation service, whenever possible.

In order to use consultation time effectively, it is necessary to understand the natural history of quitting and utilize the use of smoking cessation services appropriately, alongside the correct use of pharmacotherapy. The ability to match individual characteristics that predict success in smoking cessation is important, as this helps to match smokers with the most effective cessation strategies and identifies those who might need more intensive treatment in order to optimize healthcare resources.

The predictors of smoking cessation include:
- **Gender.** Men appear to have better long-term outcomes. This may be due to other factors, including less concern about weight gain and associated depression. Women are more likely to use smoking as a means of handling negative emotions.
- **Age at smoking initiation.** Early exposure to tobacco could detrimentally affect the developing brain, leading to greater nicotine dependence later in life. Those who start smoking before they are 14 years old are more likely to become heavy smokers than those who start after the age of 20 years old.
- **Depression.** The association between nicotine dependence and affective disorders, especially depression, is well recognized. However, a history of depression is not a barrier to smoking cessation. This group of patients experience intense withdrawal symptoms and may benefit from intensive pharmacological treatment and use of antidepressant medication. The presence of depression can be ascertained from validated questionnaires, but the simple question 'Did you feel 'down' during most days of the past 2 weeks?' has also been found to be valid.

- **Nicotine dependence.** The severity of nicotine dependence is inversely proportional to successful cessation and is usually assessed by means of the Fagerström test for nicotine dependence (see Table 3.1) where severe dependence scores >7. This measurement identifies smokers who require high-dose pharmacotherapy, as they are likely to experience more intense withdrawal symptoms, subsequent early relapse, and may require multiple 'quit' attempts. The two most important questions are time to first cigarette in the morning and number of cigarettes smoked daily, albeit the first question alone can be used as a proxy. Those who smoke their first cigarette within 1 hour of waking and smoke more than 10–15 cigarettes per day are significantly addicted to nicotine.
- **Alcoholism.** This is a negative prognostic factor, and stopping drinking is likely to increase successful smoking cessation. In these cases, intense smoking cessation programmes, including behavioural therapy, have been shown to be effective.
- **Motivation.** Assess willingness by asking 'How important is it for you to give up smoking?' and perceived self-efficacy by asking 'If you were to decide to stop smoking, how confident are you that you would succeed?' If readiness to quit is high, but self-efficacy low, treatment and support are critical for success. If self-efficacy is high, but willingness is low, effective health education is needed. If both variables are high, a quit date should be set imminently.

Table 3.1 Fagerström test for nicotine dependence

Question	Response	Score
1. How soon after you wake up do you smoke your first cigarette?	Within 5 min	3
	6–30 min	2
	31–60 min	1
	After 60 min	0
2. Do you find it difficult to refrain from smoking in places where it is forbidden?	Yes	1
	No	0
3. Which cigarette would you hate most to give up?	The first one in the morning	1
	Any other	0
4. How many cigarettes per day do you smoke?	≤10	0
	11–20	1
	21–30	2
	≥31	3
5. Do you smoke more frequently during the first hours after waking than during the rest of the day?	Yes	1
	No	0
6. Do you smoke if you are so ill that you are in bed most of the day?	Yes	1
	No	0

Total score (0–10)

Reproduced from Heatherton TF et al., 'The Fagerström Test for Nicotine Dependence: A revision of the Fagerström Tolerance Questionnaire', *British Journal of Addictions*, 86, 9, pp. 1119–1127, 1991, Copyright © 2006, John Wiley and Sons, with permission from Society for the Study of Addiction and Wiley.

Table 3.2 The 5 As

	Action	Strategy
1. Ask	Identify all tobacco users at every visit	Vital signs should be expanded to include tobacco use
2. Advise	Strongly urge all smokers to quit	Advice should be: Clear Strong Personalized
3. Assess	Identify smokers willing to make a quit attempt	If patient motivated to attempt quitting, provide assistance. If not willing to make a quit attempt, provide motivational intervention
4. Assist	Help the patient with a quit plan	Encourage NRT Set a quit date Inform family, friends, and co-workers Prepare the environment Review previous quit attempts Anticipate challenges
	Key advice	Total abstinence from smoking is essential Alcohol is associated with relapse The presence of other smokers in the household reduces success rates
5. Arrange	Schedule follow-up contact	Follow-up visit soon after quit date If smoking has recurred, review the circumstances and identify problems to anticipate in future quit attempts

Reprinted with permission from AHRQ: Treating Tobacco Use and Dependence: Quick Reference Guide for Clinicians. April 2009. Agency for Healthcare Research and Quality, Rockville, MD. <http://www.ahrq.gov/professionals/clinicians-providers/guidelines-recommendations/tobacco/clinicians/references/quickref/index.html>.

- **Previous cessation attempts.** The previous history of cessation attempts can predict smoking cessation success. Those with previous attempts lasting >5 days are more likely to succeed. Moreover, exploring previous relapses helps to identify ways to prevent future relapses.
- **Social/family environment.** Occupational social class, number of smokers in the household, marital status, and level of support from family members are important predictors. Those married to non- or ex-smokers, and with supportive spouses, are more likely to be successful.

Behavioural techniques and pharmacotherapy

Both behavioural and pharmacological therapies aid smoking cessation. Success rates are low if a smoker's attempt to quit is unaided but doubled if they use a drug.

Behavioural strategy

Simple clinician counselling stimulates patients to think about quitting. Although quit rates are only 1–3%, com-

pared to controls, every health professional should address smoking cessation at every opportunity. Counselling should include the 5As (see Table 3.2):

- **A**sk how much a person smokes, and document pack years.
- **A**dvise how to stop smoking and what help and treatment is available.
- **A**ssess willingness to quit smoking and determine risk of continued smoking, and inform the patient.
- **A**ssist with behavioural support or replacement therapy.
- **A**rrange follow-up.

Individual or group counselling sessions and setting a 'quit date' result in about 20% abstinence at 1-year follow-up. Telephone follow-up, web-based support, and multiple ongoing interviews (i.e. intensive behavioural support) can all improve cessation rates. Evidence for benefit with hypnosis or acupuncture is weak, but these may be helpful following previous failed attempts.

Pharmacotherapy

Pharmacotherapy, in conjunction with behavioural intervention, is the cornerstone of treatment for tobacco dependence. It includes nicotine replacement therapy (NRT), bupropion, and second-line treatments like varenicline. Except in the presence of contraindications, these drugs should be used in almost all patients attempting to quit smoking.

1. **Nicotine replacement therapy (NRT)** ameliorates nicotine withdrawal symptoms, including insomnia, irritability, anger, anxiety, poor concentration, and increased appetite. It is safe, even in patients with known cardiovascular diseases. The Lung Health Study in COPD did not find an increased incidence of cardiovascular disease in smokers who had used nicotine gum for as long as 5 years. This study demonstrated that intensive smoking cessation support, combined with NRT, achieved 1-year abstinence rate of 35% vs 9% with usual care. Nicotine is available as transdermal patches, gum, sublingual tablets, nasal sprays, and inhalers. A 22 mg patch raises blood nicotine levels equivalent to that of one and a half pack of cigarettes. A meta-analysis has shown that all forms of NRT are equal (odds ratio of 1.77; 95% CI of 1.66–1.88). However, the addition of gum or lozenges to the patch helps to overcome breakthrough urges, improving long-term success. The NICE guidelines recommend the use of combination NRT with a patch to maintain 'background' nicotine levels and a second NRT (e.g. gum, inhalator) to produce 'peaks of nicotine' to combat smoking urges.

2. **Antidepressants** may be particularly useful in those with depression, but smokers who are not depressed also benefit from this approach which corrects the low dopamine levels due to nicotine dependence.

   - **Bupropion**, a dopamine uptake inhibitor, is a non-competitive inhibitor of neuronal nAchR activity. It is started 1–2 weeks before stopping smoking and is given for 8 weeks. Prolonged treatment may improve long-term success. In a meta-analysis of 31 studies, smoking cessation was doubled (OR 1.94; 95% CI 1.72–2.14). Combination with nicotine patches has been examined in many trials but is not always beneficial. Bupropion is contraindicated in epilepsy and pregnancy and should be used cautiously in those with other risk factors for seizures (e.g. theophylline, sedating antihistamines, tramadol). The risk of seizures is 1 in 1,000.

• **Nortriptyline**, a tricyclic antidepressant with noradrenergic properties, though not licensed, is an effective second-line agent.
• **Selective serotonin uptake inhibitors** have no long-term benefit.

3. **Varenicline** is a new partial agonist of the alpha-4-beta-2 subunit of nAChR. It reduces craving and withdrawal and, as a partial agonist, decreases the reward and reinforcement effects of smoking. A 12-week course is recommended, and it should be commenced 1–2 weeks before the 'quit date'. Studies show that it is more effective than placebo (OR 3.22), bupropion, and probably nicotine replacement. The 12-week quit rates in two major studies, comparing varenicline, bupropion, and placebo, were 45%, 30%, and 18%, respectively, and, at 12 months, were 23%, 16%, and 9%, respectively. All studies combined behavioural therapy with varenicline, and this may be the best appropriate approach for smoking cessation.

Relapse is common with all drugs, and ongoing support is required. Longer courses of NRT, bupropion, and varenicline should be considered. An additional 12-week course of varenicline reduced smoking relapse by 30% 6 months after the end of all treatment, compared to placebo. Other second-line agents with some efficacy include mecamylamine (nicotine antagonist), clonidine, and ascorbic acid aerosol (mimics the sensory feel of cigarettes).

New pharmacological agents are currently being developed.
• **Cytisine**, a natural insecticide and a partial nicotinic receptor agonist, has been used for several decades in East and Central European countries.
• **Nicotine vaccines** that work by producing antibodies that bind to nicotine and prevent it from crossing the blood–brain barrier. It was hoped that they would prevent relapse in recent ex-smokers as well as helping current smokers to quit. Although phase II trials of two vaccines NicVAX (Nabi, Florida, USA) and NicQb (Cytos, Zurich, Switzerland) suggested benefit, Phase III trials of NicVAX did not show any benefit over placebo.
• **Biomarkers** measure smoke products or by-products in body tissues that provide an objective indication of the extent of smoke intake over a defined period. They can serve as motivational and monitoring tools.

Further reading

American National Cancer Institute. <http://www.cancer.gov>.

British Lung Foundation. <http://www.lunguk.org>. Tel: 0845 850 5020.

Cahill K, Stead LF, Lancaster T (2007). Nicotine receptor partial agonists for smoking cessation. *Cochrane Database of Systematic Reviews*, **1**, CD006103.

Cancer Research UK. <http://www.cancerresearchuk.org>. Helpline tel: 0800 800 4040.

Cancer Research UK (2007). Statistical Information Team, Cancer Stats Mortality, UK.

Doll R, Peto R, Boreham J, Sutherland I (2004). Mortality in relation of smoking: '50 years' observations on male British doctors. *BMJ*, **328**, 1519.

Fagerström KO (2003). Time to first cigarette; the best single indicator of tobacco dependence. *Monaldi Archives for Chest Disease*, **59**, 95–8.

Hackshaw AK, Law MR, Wald NJ (1997). The accumulated evidence on lung cancer and environmental tobacco smoke. *BMJ*, **315**, 980–8.

Hays JT and Ebbert JO (2008). Varenicline for tobacco dependence. *New England Journal of Medicine*, **359**, 2018–24.

Heatherton TF, Kozlowski LT, Frecker RC, Fagerström KO (1991). The Fagerström Test for Nicotine Dependence: a revision of the Fagerström Tolerance Questionnaire. *British Journal of Addiction*, **86**, 1119–27.

Hughes JR, Stead LF, Lancaster T (2007). Antidepressants for smoking cessation. *Cochrane Database of Systematic Reviews*, **1**, CD000031.

Lung Cancer Alliance. <http://www.lungcanceronline.org>.

Macmillan Cancer Support. <http://www.macmillan.org.uk>. Tel: 0808 808 0000.

Mathers CD and Loncar D (2006). Projections of global mortality and burden of disease from 2002 to 2030. *PLOS Med*, **3**, e442.

National Institute for Health and Clinical Excellence (2002). Guidance on the use of nicotine replacement therapy (NRT) and bupropion for smoking cessation. NICE technology appraisal no. 39.

National Institute for Health and Clinical Excellence (2006). NICE public health intervention guidance–brief interventions and referral for smoking cessation in primary care and other settings. Public Health Intervention Guidance no.1.

National Institute for Health and Clinical Excellence (2008). Smoking cessation services in primary care, pharmacies, local authorities and workplaces, particularly for manual working groups, pregnant women and hard to reach communities. NICE public health guidance 10.

NHS SmokeFree: Smoking—advice to help you stop smoking. <http://smokefree.nhs.uk/>.

Peto R, Darby S, Deo H, et al. (2000). Smoking, smoking cessation, and lung cancer in the UK since 1950: combination of national statistics with two case-control studies. *BMJ*, **321**, 323–9.

Roy Castle Lung Cancer Foundation. <http://www.roycastle.org>. Tel: 0800 358 7200.

Silagy C, Lancaster T, Stead L, Mant D, Fowler G (2004). Nicotine replacement therapy for smoking cessation. *Cochrane Database of Systematic Reviews*, **3**, CD000146.

Stopping Smoking <http://www.ash.org.uk/>.

Taioli E and Wynder EL (1991). Effect of the age at which smoking begins on frequency of smoking in adulthood. *New England Journal of Medicine*, **325**, 968–9.

Tønnesen P, Carrozzi L, Fagerström KO, et al. (2007). ERS taskforce: smoking cessation in patients with respiratory diseases: a high priority, integral component of therapy. *European Respiratory Journal*, **29**, 390–417.

West R, McNeill A, Raw M (2000). Smoking cessation guidelines for health professionals: an update. *Thorax*, **55**, 987–99.

World Health Organization (2008). The WHO report on the global tobacco epidemic 2008. World Health Organization, Geneva.

Chapter 4

Cardiac diseases and resuscitation

Symptoms, signs, and diagnostic investigations in cardiac disease

Chest pain

Chest pain is a common reason for referral and self-referral to secondary care. Rapid recognition of acute coronary syndromes (ACS) is clearly important, but equally relevant is the early identification of patients whose symptoms do not reflect cardiac disease. In this regard, however, a blunt negative discharge diagnosis such as 'Chest pain: troponin negative' is unhelpful.

Ischaemic chest pain

Patients often find the symptoms of myocardial ischaemia difficult to describe. A careful history is necessary to establish the common key features (see Table 4.1).

In women and the elderly, ischaemic symptoms may be misleadingly atypical: burning in nature, nauseating in quality, or arising predominantly at sites of radiation.

The functional impact and severity of stable angina gain some objectivity if the Canadian Cardiovascular Society grading scale is applied (see Table 4.2).

The cardiovascular risk factor profile (e.g. age, sex, hypertension, cholesterol levels, diabetes, smoking status, family history etc.) is valuable in weighting the history and is an essential component of ACS risk scoring systems (e.g. TIMI (Thrombolysis In Myocardial Infarction trials) and GRACE (Global Registry of Acute Coronary Events) are ACS risk and mortality calculators which also assess ECG and cardiac enzyme changes, aspirin use, frequency of chest discomfort, comorbid conditions etc.). Pre-existing vascular disease (peripheral vascular disease, stroke) is a powerful adverse indicator. In the context of stable symptoms, the likelihood of coronary artery disease (CAD) may be predicted from the history and clinical data (see NICE clinical guideline CG95).

Table 4.1 Characteristic features and symptoms of the pain associated with myocardial ischaemia

Site	Retrosternal/parasternal
Character	Oppressive, constrictive
Intensity	Severe in ACS
Radiation	Arms: left more commonly than right, neck or throat, back
Duration	Prolonged in ACS
Associated features	Breathlessness, anxiety, nausea, sweating
Precipitating factors	Exercise, anxiety, or emotion
Relieving factors	Rest, sublingual nitrate (rapid)

Table 4.2 Canadian Cardiovascular Society grading scale

Class I	Angina during strenuous or prolonged physical activity
Class II	Angina during vigorous physical activity
Class III	Angina with activities of daily living
Class IV	Angina with any activity, angina at rest

Reproduced from L Campeau, 'Letter: Grading of angina pectoris', *Circulation*, 54, 3, pp. 522–523, copyright 1976, with permission from American Heart Association and Wolters Kluwer

Pericarditis

In the younger adult, retrosternal chest pain of pleuritic character, relieved by sitting forward, perhaps against a background of malaise, is highly suggestive of acute viral pericarditis. Episodes are self-limiting, but approximately one in five patients will experience a recurrence. Other causes of pericarditis should be considered, including malignancy, connective tissue disease, and post-myocardial infarction or surgery, depending on the background and other presenting features.

Thoracic aortic dissection

Sudden, severe, tearing chest pain, either radiating or arising posteriorly (interscapular), usually with a silent ECG, raises the possibility of aortic dissection. Typically, older hypertensive males are affected.

Non-cardiac chest pain

Alternative forms of chest pain include gastro-oesophageal reflux disease and musculoskeletal discomfort. Both are common, often relatively prolonged, and subjectively severe and are, therefore, a source of diagnostic confusion. However, neither has a consistent relationship with exercise nor is associated with ECG evidence of ischaemia. Risk factors for these conditions and for coronary artery disease should be included in the history.

Breathlessness

The possibility of heart failure in a breathless patient is a frequent source of concern and referral.

Acute pulmonary oedema

The dramatic breathlessness of pulmonary oedema, often associated with anxiety and diaphoresis, may be accompanied by a distressing sensation of constriction or choking, suggestive of myocardial ischaemia. ECG evidence of ACS should be sought in all cases, but pulmonary oedema usually reflects existing left ventricular systolic dysfunction, rather than a novel ischaemic event. Frequently encountered precipitants include atrial fibrillation, non-cardiac illness (e.g. sepsis, acute kidney injury, anaemia), and lack of concordance with prescribed medication.

Chronic heart failure

Symptomatic heart failure can be difficult to distinguish from the limiting breathlessness of chronic lung disease. The two often coexist in the acute medical population. A previous history of ischaemic heart disease with episodes of infarction supports a clinical diagnosis of left ventricular systolic dysfunction. Similarly hypertension and (type 2) diabetes mellitus, in combination, carry an increased liability to symptomatic heart failure, often influenced by the presence of chronic kidney disease. Primary heart muscle disease (dilated cardiomyopathy, hypertrophic cardiomyopathy) affects all ages, while degenerative heart valve disease is a feature of the ageing population.

The New York Heart Association Functional Classification is a well-recognized assessment tool and should be used to document the burden of symptoms and to guide evidence-based treatment (see Table 4.3).

Evidence of paroxysmal nocturnal dyspnoea or orthopnoea should be sought, as these may suggest a more chronic problem, but peripheral oedema in the absence of other features is a poor predictor of heart failure.

Palpitation

Awareness of heartbeat is a common symptom and a common source of patient alarm. A careful history must first establish whether or not subjective alteration in heart

Table 4.3 New York Heart Association Functional Classification

Class I	Symptom-free, including ordinary physical activity[1]
Class II	Mild symptoms, slight limitation of ordinary physical activity
Class III	Marked limitation, including less-than-ordinary physical activities,[2] comfortable only at rest
Class IV	Severely limited, symptoms at rest, frequently bed-bound

[1] Walking, climbing stairs; [2] Walking short distances (20–100 m).

Reproduced from Heart Failure Society of America. Copyright 2002.

rhythm is indeed the issue, as opposed to episodes of anxiety, for example. Second, typical features of benign cardiac rhythm disturbance (missed or pausing heartbeat, powerful heartbeat, and not truly rapid, relatively brief duration, occurring at rest) may be rapidly elicited in order to offer reassurance. Third, patients providing a clear description of frequent intermittent tachycardia (>1–2 episodes per week, estimated heart rate >150), perhaps with abrupt onset and offset, may be offered high-yield screening by means of ambulatory ECG monitoring. Lastly, but importantly, the possibility of malignant ventricular rhythm disturbance should be considered in those experiencing rapid palpitation associated with syncope and/or a history of recent myocardial infarction, cardiac surgery, percutaneous intervention, or device implantation. Likewise, the development of sustained rapid palpitation in patients with established left ventricular systolic dysfunction or heart muscle disease may reflect ventricular tachycardia.

Syncope

Complete or incomplete syncope frequently leads to referral. In contrast to vasovagal (vasodepressor) syncope, transient loss of consciousness due to primary cardiac rhythm disturbance is uncommon.

The constellation of symptoms, either volunteered or elicited, in vasovagal syncope usually allows a confident clinical diagnosis. A short prodrome, incorporating light-headedness and apprehension, feeling either unpleasantly hot or cold, perspiration, nausea, and diminishing sound and vision, is typical. The patient is usually standing or seated erect at the outset, and the observer may describe pallor preceding diminishing responsiveness. Pain and emotion may be precipitants. Loss of consciousness is brief, followed by rapid alert recovery, sometimes interrupted and delayed by attempts to assist the individual to an upright position.

Cardiac syncope is the result of either bradycardia (profound sinus bradycardia, sinus arrest, Mobitz II, or higher degree atrioventricular block) or tachycardia (ventricular tachycardia, rarely polymorphic ventricular tachycardia/ventricular fibrillation, supraventricular tachycardia with excessive ventricular rates, e.g. atrial flutter with 1:1 AV conduction, pre-excited atrial fibrillation). Syncope due to supraventricular rhythm disturbance is relatively rare. Atrial fibrillation with normal antegrade conduction, regardless of rapid ventricular rates, rarely accounts for impaired consciousness.

The presentation of cardiac syncope may be unhelpfully similar to vasovagal syncope, but suspicious features include abrupt onset, episodes whilst supine, flushing on recovery, a relevant cardiac history, including the use of rate-limiting

medication, and certain resting ECG abnormalities (e.g. tri-fascicular block, pre-excitation).

Clinical signs

In a climate of rapid access to a wide array of diagnostic investigations, clinical examination may add little to the immediate management of the cardiac patient, particularly if the underlying pathophysiology is ischaemic heart disease. Nonetheless, core traditional clinical signs should be sought and recorded.

Arterial pulses

Rate, rhythm, and regularity: atrial fibrillation is common. The BP should be measured in both arms initially. Peripheral pulses, including bruit, should be documented in all patients.

Venous pulse

Elevation of the jugular venous pressure in a patient appropriately positioned is an important sign in those with systolic dysfunction, valvular heart disease or pericardial disease, and in chronic lung disease. The clinical impression does not usually rest on the precise detail of the waveform.

Auscultation

In developed countries, the incidence and prevalence of rheumatic heart disease has declined. Murmurs in the developed world's general medical population are typically systolic and reflect either degenerative heart valve disease, aortic stenosis or mitral regurgitation, or mitral regurgitation secondary to left ventricular systolic dysfunction. Subtleties of auscultation and interpretation have become less imperative in view of the widespread availability of transthoracic echocardiography, but the careful documentation of murmurs, particularly if new or developing, is fundamental clinical practice.

Essential diagnostic investigations

Electrocardiography

Resting, exercise, and ambulatory ECG recordings are readily performed standard investigations but only acquire diagnostic value in the context of carefully applied clinical information.

The 12-lead ECG is core to the assessment and management of suspected ACS and should be repeated as symptoms evolve or recur. ST segment deviation is a well-characterized marker of pathophysiology and clinical risk, whereas T wave changes may be non-specific. Left bundle branch block limits ECG interpretation to rate and rhythm. A contemporaneous 12-lead ECG is the gold standard for the documentation of cardiac rhythm disturbance and of myocardial ischaemia if a patient has chest pain. It is a facility offered by the newer generation of telemetry systems.

Concerns regarding the applicability, sensitivity, and specificity of treadmill exercise testing in the assessment of chest pain are not new. It is long recognized that this investigation is flawed in younger women and in relation to atypical symptoms. Also, exercise testing is not recommended in the early management of unstable presentations. The role of exercise testing in the investigation of coronary artery disease (CAD) has been revisited in recent guidelines, which propose that it should be restricted to the re-evaluation of patients with previously documented obstructive coronary disease, particularly those with a history of percutaneous or surgical intervention. There is some consensus, however, that exercise testing remains useful in a one-stop environment where history, examination, and exercise performance and findings can be evaluated sequentially.

Ambulatory ECG monitoring is commonly requested as a means of investigating palpitation or syncope. In palpitation, the diagnostic yield is clearly dependent upon the frequency of symptoms, and current systems allow longer periods of acquisition. By nature, syncope is difficult to capture. Screening patients is better justified if the collateral evidence is supportive, e.g. syncope interspersed with recurrent presyncope, or an abnormal resting ECG (sinoatrial disease, first-degree AV block, Mobitz I AV block, bi-/trifascicular block).

Radiography
Cardiac and pericardial disease is best assessed by echocardiography or more complex imaging, but the CXR is a simple, rapidly available investigation, which provides valuable information in the assessment of chest pain and breathlessness. Cardiac and respiratory diseases often coexist in the acutely ill patient, and it is important that both processes are evaluated.

Transthoracic echocardiography
In virtually all patients, transthoracic echocardiography (TTE) can offer clinically useful information regarding cardiac anatomy and function. Doppler techniques allow accurate assessment of valvular stenosis and regurgitation and estimation of right heart pressures.

Two common reasons for requesting an echocardiogram are that symptoms appear consistent with heart failure and to screen for endocarditis. In patients provisionally diagnosed with heart failure, if there are no murmurs and the ECG is free of major abnormalities, left ventricular systolic dysfunction is unlikely. Endocarditis remains a clinical diagnosis, supported by microbiological evidence, and cannot be excluded by transthoracic imaging alone.

In younger stroke patients without carotid disease, paradoxical embolus is a potential cause. The interatrial septum can be scanned for evidence of an atrial septal defect or patent foramen ovale and further interrogated for a right-to-left shunt, using injected agitated saline, combined with a Valsalva manoeuvre (a right heart contrast 'bubble' echo).

Complex imaging
Transoesophageal echocardiography
Detailed images of all four valves can be obtained by means of transoesophageal echocardiography (TOE). Accordingly, if there is a high pre-test likelihood of endocarditis and TTE is non-diagnostic, TOE should be performed. There is less consensus regarding the use of TOE as a routine investigation in staphylococcal bacteraemia of uncertain source.

Other cardiac structures well visualized at TOE are the interatrial septum and the left atrial appendage. Although the ascending aorta, arch, and descending thoracic aorta can be imaged by TOE, CT and MRI provide superior images and have logistic advantages.

Stress and contrast echocardiography
A stress-induced left ventricular regional wall motion abnormality is both sensitive and specific for underlying coronary heart disease. TTE can be performed before and after treadmill exercise testing, but supine bicycle ergometry allows real-time image acquisition. Alternatively, the patient is studied during pharmacologic stress delivered by intravenous dobutamine, supplemented by atropine if necessary; pre-specified endpoints include ST segment deviation, tachycardia, and a rise in blood pressure.

Suboptimal endocardial definition can be improved by chamber opacification, achieved by injecting a left ventricular contrast agent. Changes in myocardial (contrast) perfusion may be observed in these studies but not as consistently or reproducibly as with scintigraphy.

The role of right heart contrast echocardiography using agitated saline is referred to in the previous section on transthoracic echocardiography.

Myocardial perfusion scintigraphy
The presence of underlying CAD is reliably detected non-invasively by myocardial perfusion scintigraphy with single photon emission computed tomography (MPS SPECT). MPS SPECT can be performed before and after graded exercise, but conventional practice is to use pharmacologic stress: intravenous dobutamine to induce ischaemia, or adenosine to elicit heterogeneous blood flow distribution. Traditionally, MPS SPECT is useful in patients unable to exercise or with a pre-existing ECG abnormality, typically left bundle branch block. A widely accepted role is in women with an inherently low risk of underlying CAD and a high risk of a false positive treadmill exercise test.

CT calcium scoring and CT coronary angiography
The progressive development and increasing availability of multislice CT scanning (MS-CT) has provided an alternative non-invasive means of interrogating and imaging the coronary circulation. Optimal imaging requires ECG gating at stable sinus rates of <65 and a 20 s breath hold. If necessary, oral or intravenous metoprolol, or a rate-limiting calcium channel blocker (verapamil, diltiazem), is administered to reduce the heart rate.

Rapid non-enhanced scans (MS-CTCS) generate a calcium score indicative of the extent of obstructive coronary artery disease. Outcome studies have confirmed the favourable prognosis associated with a calcium score of 0, but significant adverse cardiac event rates apply to scores exceeding 400. MS-CTCS has a particular role in the assessment of the low clinical risk symptomatic patient. Screening of asymptomatic individuals is not currently recommended.

For patients at moderate clinical risk, contrast-enhanced CT coronary angiography (MS-CTCA) provides anatomic detail comparable to conventional angiography without the procedural risks and requirements of arterial catheterization but, equally, without the option of direct percutaneous intervention.

At a given level of clinical risk, the logistic advantages and apparent simplicity of cardiac CT must be balanced against the patient's potential benefit from an invasive strategy and the degree of radiation exposure; MS-CTCA delivers at least equivalent dosage (5–6 mSv) to diagnostic coronary angiography.

Cardiac MRI
Cardiac structure and function, the pericardium, and the anatomy of the great vessels are accurately and dynamically displayed by ECG-gated MRI. Wall motion abnormalities, reflecting myocardial infarction, are readily visualized, and myocardial perfusion studies with dobutamine stress and gadolinium contrast may demonstrate areas of reversible ischaemia. It is of increasing use in cardiomyopathies as a routine investigation.

Further reading
ACCF/AHA (2007). Clinical expert consensus document on coronary artery calcium scoring by computed tomography in global cardiovascular risk assessment and in evaluation of patients with chest pain. *Journal of the American College of Cardiology*, **49**, 378–402.

Antman EM, Cohen M, Bernink PJLM, *et al.* (2000). The TIMI risk score for unstable angina/non–ST elevation MI: a method for prognostication and therapeutic decision making. *JAMA*, **284**, 835–42.

Fox KAA and McLean S (2010). NICE guidance on the investigation of chest pain. *Heart*, **96**, 903–6.

GRACE Scoring System. <http://www.outcomes-umassmed.org/GRACE>.

National Institute for Health and Clinical Excellence (2010). Chest pain of recent onset: assessment and diagnosis of recent onset chest pain or discomfort of suspected cardiac origin. <http://www.nice.org.uk/guidance/CG95>.

Roberts WT, Bax JJ, Davies LC (2008). Cardiac CT and CT coronary angiography: technology and application. *Heart*, **94**, 781–92.

Scottish Intercollegiate Guidelines Network (2007). SIGN 96. Management of stable angina. A national clinical guideline. <http://www.sign.ac.uk/pdf/sign96.pdf>.

Adult cardiopulmonary resuscitation

Introduction

Cardiopulmonary resuscitation (CPR) is important. Coronary heart disease (CHD) and other forms of cardiovascular disease account for 40% of all-cause mortality under the age of 75 years old in the developed world. Almost two-thirds of all CHD deaths are due to cardiac arrest. Up to a third of patients with an acute myocardial infarction die within an hour of symptoms, usually following the development of ventricular fibrillation (VF) or pulseless ventricular tachycardia (VT).

The annual incidence of out-of-hospital cardiopulmonary arrests attended by the emergency medical services (EMS) approaches 40/100,000 in Europe, VF being the initial rhythm in approximately 30% of cases. Early mortality is high, but ~ 20% survive to hospital discharge following EMS-treated VF arrest, compared to ~ 10% for all other rhythms.

In-hospital cardiac arrest is more frequent, 1–5/1,000 admissions, reflecting the acuity, comorbidity, and age of the population. Survival-to-discharge figures vary, according to the initial rhythm: 44% for VF/VT, compared to <10% for non-VF/VT. The only effective treatment for VF and pulseless VT is defibrillation, and, in the absence of CPR, the likelihood of success diminishes by 10% each minute.

The principles of resuscitation and ethical considerations, including the 'Do Not Attempt Cardiopulmonary Resuscitation Order' (DNACPR), are important for all practising clinicians. Competency in CPR is achieved through the satisfactory completion of an accredited advanced life support training course.

Guidelines

In 2010, fifty years after Kouwenhoven's landmark paper on closed cardiac massage, updated Resuscitation Council (UK) and European Resuscitation Council guidelines were published, following an established review process led by the International Liaison Committee on Resuscitation (ILCOR). The scientific basis for the new guidelines was drawn from the 2010 International Conference on Cardiopulmonary Resuscitation and Emergency Cardiovascular Care Science with Treatment Recommendations (CoSTR). In the UK, the revised Advanced Life Support (ALS) manual and amended educational material became available on Resuscitation Council (UK) ALS courses from 2011.

2010 Guidelines: changes and new recommendations
Basic Life Support/AEDs

The call for help should include a request for an AED (automated external defibrillator). AEDs are now more widely distributed and available in public access areas, reflecting decreasing costs and acceptance of their safe usage by the lay rescuer. Shock advisory devices rely on ECG analysis software but may incorporate an override facility for healthcare personnel trained in rhythm recognition. The availability of an AED should not compromise good-quality CPR.

CPR (± AED deployment) continues until normal breathing is accompanied by signs of life. Although CPR with ventilation remains the gold standard, compression-only CPR (COCPR) is acceptable for the untrained or unskilled rescuer.

Pre-hospital cardiac arrest

The potential of telephone-advised CPR is well recognized. COCPR may be preferable in this context, as it is simpler to convey, understand, and perform. The untrained bystander may be more willing to participate in resuscitation if ventilation is not involved. COCPR may have advantages over conventional CPR when EMS response times are short (<5 min). In unwitnessed cardiac arrest, it is no longer recommended that a specific period of CPR be performed prior to attempted defibrillation. If ALS-trained EMS personnel are unable to secure the return of spontaneous circulation at the scene, the probability of survival is very poor. Accordingly, in the UK, ambulance paramedics may abandon resuscitation if all the following apply:

- Elapsed time >15 min.
- No CPR administered prior to arrival of the ambulance.
- No suspicion of drowning, hypothermia, poisoning/self-poisoning, pregnancy.
- Asystole present for >30 s on ECG monitoring.

Advanced Life Support: defibrillation

The precordial thump is reserved for witnessed monitored cardiac arrest in VF/VT when a defibrillator is not immediately available. In line with the general emphasis on minimally interrupted chest compressions, chest compressions should continue in a ratio of 30:2 (breaths) while the defibrillator is charging. In the specific circumstances of VF/VT occurring in the cardiac catheter laboratory or in the immediate post-operative period following cardiac surgery, up to three 'stacked' shocks may be delivered in rapid sequence (equivalent to the first shock of the universal algorithm). Biphasic defibrillators have largely replaced monophasic devices and are either biphasic truncated exponential or rectilinear biphasic in design. Regardless of the biphasic waveform, the recommended initial shock energy is now 150 J. If a monophasic defibrillator is in use, initial and subsequent shocks should all be at 360 J.

Advanced Life Support: drugs

Intraosseous drug administration is endorsed in place of the tracheal route when rapid, satisfactory venous access cannot be obtained. In VF/VT cardiac arrest, in order not to delay defibrillation, intravenous (IV) adrenaline 1 mg is given, following the third shock, rather than before, and every 3–5 min thereafter. Amiodarone IV 300 mg is also given after the third shock. Atropine is no longer recommended in asystole or pulseless electrical activity (PEA).

Advanced Life Support: airway

Endotracheal intubation is still considered optimal but should only be attempted by skilled personnel, and either achieved or abandoned within 10 s so as not to compromise CPR. In addition to standard clinical observations, e.g. direct visualization of the cords and auscultation, waveform capnography is a sensitive and specific means of confirming and monitoring correct tube placement and is becoming more widely practised. Supraglottic devices, such as the laryngeal mask airway and i-gel, are technically easier to insert, usually without interrupting chest compressions. There are no outcome data to favour either approach. Circumstances and competency are the principal determining factors. Supraglottic devices may, however, be the preferred option if waveform capnography is not available.

Advanced Life Support: ultrasound

In appropriately skilled hands, ultrasound may assist the recognition of reversible causes of cardiac arrest, e.g. cardiac tamponade, pulmonary thromboembolism, myocardial ischaemia, aortic dissection, but is technically challenging and relies on images captured during a 10 s interruption of CPR.

Core concepts in cardiopulmonary resuscitation

The chain of survival
The aphorism of a chain only being as strong as its weakest link remains relevant to cardiopulmonary resuscitation (see Figure 4.1).
- Out of hospital, early recognition reinforces the importance of chest pain, while, in hospital, identifying the deteriorating patient through early warning scoring systems is a priority.
- Bystander CPR greatly improves the likelihood of survival, following VF arrest out of hospital. However it is performed in less than a third of all community arrests. In hospital, CPR should commence immediately and only be interrupted briefly to allow defibrillation or rhythm assessment.
- Out of hospital, if appropriate, the first shock should be delivered by the EMS within 5 min of arrival. Early defibrillation in the community is being promoted also by the availability of AEDs in public access areas. In hospital, the goal is for all first responders to be trained in defibrillation.
- Good-quality post-resuscitation care must commence with the return of spontaneous circulation (ROSC) in order to maintain and stabilize cardiorespiratory parameters and best preserve cerebral function. This will usually entail transfer to an increased level care environment.

Assessment and communication
The generic ABCDE approach is a valuable means of rapid assessment in the peri-arrest or arrest situation.
- **A—Airway.** Assess and manage airway obstruction, and commence oxygen, if appropriate.
- **B—Breathing.** Assess breathing, respiratory rate, and chest expansion. Record arterial oxygen saturation (SaO$_2$), if possible. Examine the chest for relevant conditions, e.g. asthma, pneumothorax, pulmonary oedema. Administer oxygen, if required, and consider bag-valve-mask or non-invasive ventilation.
- **C—Circulation.** Assess circulation, including capillary refill time (normal <2 s), peripheral and central pulses, heart rate (may require auscultation), and blood pressure. In hypotension, consider precipitating causes e.g. haemorrhage, and insert an intravenous cannula to allow volume replacement. Arrange a 12-lead ECG.
- **D—Disability.** Having performed the ABC manoeuvres, consider other potential causes of collapse, e.g. prescribed and non-prescribed drugs, hypoglycaemia, an intracranial process.
- **E—Exposure.** Fully examine the patient.

The ABCDE approach (see also Chapter 1) should be adequately documented and supported by collateral information, including the patient's medical history, and may indicate the appropriate level of care.

Rapid, accurate, and structured conveyance of clinical information is as important in cardiopulmonary resuscitation as it is in any form of patient handover. The SBAR tool is an example.
- **S—Situation.** Identify yourself and the patient, and summarize the clinical picture.
- **B—Background.** Convey relevant collateral information.
- **A—Assessment.** General observations, ABCDE details, and Early Warning Score (see next section), if recorded.
- **R—Recommendation.** State clearly what current management involves and how you see it progressing.

It will be evident that SBAR, and other similar processes, represents a useful opportunity for case evaluation and discussion.

Prevention and prediction
In the community setting, the importance of symptom recognition has been mentioned, and described previously. Chest pain is commonly cited, but breathlessness and wheeze in an individual with obstructive airways disease or asthma, or in the context of an allergic reaction, would equally prompt an EMS alert. For those with established vascular disease, including coronary heart disease, stroke, and peripheral vascular disease, secondary preventative strategies should be in place. These include both medication, e.g. antiplatelet agents and statins, and education of patients and relatives. Secondary prevention may also extend to device therapy in the form of an automated implantable cardioverter defibrillator (AICD) in patients with either an acquired, usually reflecting heart failure, or genetic predisposition to ventricular arrhythmia.

Prediction or anticipation of cardiac arrest in acute receiving areas and inpatient wards, including higher level care, pivots on illness severity recognition and clinical risk assessment. In this regard, Early Warning Scoring (EWS) systems have been widely adopted (Chapter 1). Cardiopulmonary arrest in hospital is frequently preceded by a period, perhaps several hours, of physiological deterioration. The systematic recording of physiological and related variables, typically SaO$_2$, respiratory rate, temperature, heart rate, blood pressure, and conscious level, is used to generate a score predictive of adverse events, allied to an escalation policy, intrinsic to which is senior review within a specified timescale. The principle of EWS is of particular relevance out of hours and at weekends when staffing levels decline and clinical management is fragile.

Do Not Attempt Cardiopulmonary Resuscitation (DNACPR)
Consistent with good medical practice, a DNACPR order should be considered when serious, often irreversible, medical comorbidity means that cardiopulmonary resuscitation would either be unsuccessful or would unnecessarily prolong life at the expense of dignity. If a competent patient has expressed a wish not to be resuscitated, perhaps in the form of an advanced directive, a DNACPR order must be in place to respect that wish. For any given patient, a decision not to attempt resuscitation should not compromise good clinical care.

Advanced Life Support (ALS) algorithm
Central to cardiac arrest management is the ALS algorithm (see Figure 4.2). The standardized sequence of actions displayed in the algorithm allows the assembled team to proceed confidently and effectively with resuscitation. Good-quality, minimally interrupted CPR is emphasized and should continue until stable ROSC is achieved or resuscitation is abandoned.

The important distinction is between 'shockable' rhythms (VF and pulseless VT where attempted defibrillation is appropriate) and 'non-shockable' rhythms (pulseless electrical activity (PEA) and asystole). During resuscitation, particularly in PEA/asystole, the algorithm prompts

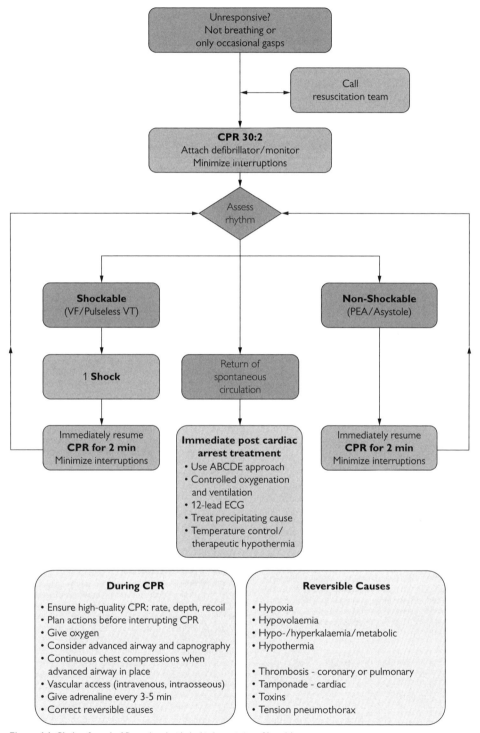

Figure 4.1 Chain of survival Reproduced with the kind permission of Laerdal.

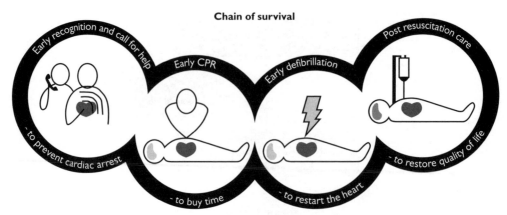

Figure 4.2 ALS algorithm Reproduced with the kind permission of the Resuscitation Council (UK).

consideration of potentially reversible causes of cardiac arrest.

The 4 Hs

- Hypoxia.
- Hypovolaemia.
- Hypo-/hyperkalaemia (+ metabolic disturbance).
- Hypothermia.

The 4 Ts

- Thrombosis (pulmonary or coronary).
- Tamponade.
- Toxins (including prescribed/non-prescribed drugs).
- Tension pneumothorax.

Although trial evidence in man is lacking, regular IV adrenaline 1 mg is recommended, as is IV amiodarone 300 mg, following the third shock in VF/pulseless VT.

Special circumstances

Drowning/hypothermia

Drowning is an important cause of accidental death, typically involving children, adolescents, and young adults, and hypothermia is a common associated feature. The primary event in drowning is hypoxia, and ideally ventilation should be commenced during retrieval of the victim. Thereafter, conventional CPR, rather than COCPR, is essential. With hypothermia, there is an increased risk of ventricular arrhythmia due to myocardial irritability, and adrenaline should be withheld until rewarming has resulted in a temperature ≥30°C. Prolonged cardiopulmonary resuscitation is warranted in both circumstances. In hypothermia, resuscitation is difficult to abandon before achieving a core temperature of 35°C, hence the aphorism 'not dead until warm and dead'.

Pregnancy

Cardiac arrest in pregnancy is rare. In addition to cardiac disease and pulmonary thromboembolism, specific underlying conditions include psychiatric disorders, eclampsia, haemorrhage, and amniotic fluid embolism. A particular issue in resuscitation is gestational age, as, from 20 weeks, the gravid uterus compromises venous return and cardiac output in the collapsed mother. Initial measures include manual displacement of the uterus and left lateral tilt, but

the priority is emergency Caesarean section. At gestational age of 20–23 weeks, this is solely to facilitate successful resuscitation of the mother, whereas, after 24 weeks, there is the potential for both maternal and fetal survival. This is a highly demanding situation, as delivery should be achieved within 5 min. Accordingly, in pregnant arrest, the call for help must include the emergency obstetric service.

Electrocution

Adult cardiac arrest as a consequence of electrocution usually reflects exposure to a high-voltage alternating current in the workplace. In comparison, lightning strikes (direct current) are rare. Electrical current is readily conducted by neurovascular bundles and may cause sudden death due to cardiorespiratory failure. VF is the commonest initial rhythm and should be managed with attempted defibrillation as soon as possible. An important principle in resuscitation from electrocution is rescuer safety. Power sources should be isolated against the possibility of direct transmission and arcing. In following the ABCDE approach, it should be borne in mind that apparently superficial electrical burns may conceal substantial deep tissue injury, leading to compartment syndrome.

Other special circumstances

For information on cardiac arrest in asthma, pulmonary thromboembolism, anaphylaxis, and poisoning, refer to the relevant speciality chapters.

Peri-arrest arrhythmias

Various forms of arrhythmia, either tachyarrhythmia or bradycardia, may occur before, or during recovery from, cardiac arrest. Two important principles apply, both of which influence management. First, in relation to any form of cardiac rhythm disturbance, the patient should be assessed for symptoms and signs reflecting haemodynamic compromise, e.g. chest pain, breathlessness, syncope, excessive tachycardia or bradycardia, evidence of heart failure, and hypotension. Second, in relation to bradycardia, the risk of asystole should be considered, i.e. recent transient asystole, Mobitz II atrioventricular block, broad complex complete heart block, and ventricular pauses >3 s.

For guidance on the management of cardiac rhythm disturbance, in general, refer to the relevant sections in this chapter.

Post-resuscitation care
Although return of spontaneous circulation (ROSC) is pivotal in cardiopulmonary resuscitation, post-resuscitation care must secure cardiopulmonary and metabolic stability in order to improve eventual functional outcome. An important part of this process is transfer to an appropriate care environment, followed by rapid comprehensive reassessment, including previous and collateral medical history, thorough clinical examination, laboratory investigations, 12-lead ECG, CXR, and other imaging, as appropriate. Patients recovering from immediately treated VF/VT arrest may need little adjunctive care, but a period of intensive support is more common. Central venous and intra-arterial pressure monitoring and non-invasive cardiac output measurement may all be required. In post-arrest ventilated patients, hyperoxaemia may be as detrimental as hypoxaemia. It is recommended that ventilation with end-tidal CO_2 monitoring should aim for normocarbia and normoxaemia, with SaO_2 maintained at 94–98%.

Specific interventions
Primary percutaneous coronary intervention/intra-aortic balloon counterpulsation
If the 12-lead ECG following ROSC demonstrates ST elevation myocardial infarction (STEMI), reperfusion therapy is indicated. Ideally, primary percutaneous coronary intervention (PPCI) is performed. If PPCI is not available or cannot be delivered within 90 min, a thrombolytic, such as single bolus tenecteplase (30–50 mg adjusted for body weight, IV over 10 s), should be administered; CPR, even if prolonged, is not a contraindication. The deployment of an intra-aortic balloon pump (IABP) may be beneficial in the adjunctive management of STEMI or in cardiogenic shock post-arrest by improving coronary perfusion.

Seizures
Some form of seizure activity occurs in up to 40% of cardiac arrest survivors, predominantly in those who remain comatose. Treatment options include benzodiazepines, phenytoin, and sodium valproate. Clonazepam may be more effective for myoclonus. Conventional practice is to continue with maintenance therapy, pending functional recovery.

Therapeutic hypothermia
The current consensus is that therapeutic hypothermia (32–34°C) should be considered for any patient requiring invasive ventilation post-arrest. Techniques include external cooling, ice-cold IV fluids, intravascular heat exchange, e.g. femoral vein, and cardiopulmonary bypass.

Glycaemic control
Both hyper- and hypoglycaemia are associated with adverse outcomes post-arrest. Strict glycaemic control (4–6 mmol/L) is not recommended, but blood glucose should be maintained at ≤10 mmol/L, whilst avoiding hypoglycaemia.

Post-cardiac arrest syndrome
The post-resuscitation phase is often complicated by hypoxic brain injury and, regardless of the primary pathology, transient left ventricular dysfunction. Also, multiorgan failure, not dissimilar to sepsis, may result from widespread tissue ischaemic-reperfusion injury.

Prognostication and organ donation
Neurological death is the principal source of mortality in out-of-hospital cardiac arrest patients admitted to intensive care. Following in-hospital arrest, the figure is 25%. Although muscle relaxants and sedation must be taken into consideration, the absence of corneal and pupillary light reflexes at 72 hours is a consistent adverse prognostic indicator, applicable also to those managed with hypothermia. There is no evidence base as yet for brain imaging, neurophysiological parameters, or cerebrospinal fluid markers as predictors of outcome.

Given the prevalence of neurological death in the post-arrest population, the potential for organ donation should not be neglected.

Further reading
American Heart Association (2014). Heart disease and stroke statistics-2014 update. *Circulation*, **129**, e28-e292.

Koster RW, Baubin MA, Caballero A, *et al.* (2010). European Resuscitation Council Guidelines for Resuscitation 2010. Section 2. Adult basic life support and use of automated external defibrillators. *Resuscitation*, **81**, 1277–92.

Kouwenhoven WB, Jude JR, Knickerbocker GG (1960). Closed-chest cardiac massage. *JAMA*, **173**, 1064–7.

Nolan JP, Hazinski MF, Billi JE, *et al.* (2010). International Consensus on Cardiopulmonary Resuscitation and Emergency Cardiovascular Care Science with Treatment Recommendations. Part 1: Executive summary 2010. *Resuscitation*, **81** (Suppl 1), e1–25.

Rea TD, Fahrenbruch C, Culley L, *et al.* (2010). CPR with chest compressions alone or with rescue breathing. *New England Journal of Medicine*, **363**, 423–33.

Resuscitation Council UK (2011). Advanced Life Support (6th edn). <http://www.resus.org.uk>.

Resuscitation Council UK (2014). Consensus paper on out-of-hospital cardiac arrest in England. <https://www.resus.org.uk/pages/OHCA_consensus_paper.pdf>.

Cardiovascular risk assessment

Cardiovascular (CV) risk assessment refers to the evaluation of a patient's risk of death and/or future CV events. It is based on the evaluation of clinical risk factors combined, where appropriate, with results of ancillary tests. Clinical risk prediction tools serve several functions:

- To aid clinical decision-making, in particular identifying patients at high or low risk who benefit most or least from specific interventions.
- To assist patient counselling in initiating discussion about risk factor modification, therapy adherence, and end-of-life issues.
- To enhance quality of care by predicting which patients may be discharged early or require specialized care.

Risk assessment may apply to any patient presenting to acute medical units with: (1) symptom complexes, including non-specific chest pain, syncope, dyspnoea, or palpitations that may indicate CV disease, but where non-cardiac disease is favoured as the provisional diagnosis; (2) known clinically manifest CV disease, even if the current clinical presentation appears unrelated; and (3) one or more cardiovascular risk factors in the absence of overt disease and no suggestive symptoms. The assessment of patients presenting with clinical findings more typical of acute cardiac disease (such as acute myocardial infarction or decompensated heart failure) are dealt with elsewhere.

Predicting future risk of death or CV events needs to be distinguished from screening for established disease in asymptomatic persons. The former involves estimating the absolute probability of an event over a future time period, based on validated risk prediction tools. The latter involves detection of subclinical disease using screening tests, such as exercise stress ECG or myocardial stress imaging for detecting coronary artery disease. However, in some instances, the results of screening tests can be used to predict future event risk.

Clinicians' intuitive estimates of future CV risk can be inaccurate and misleading, with overtreatment of lower risk patients and undertreatment of higher risk patients. Having a more objective risk estimate, better informs the management plan with respect to the intensity of risk factor modification, evidence-based therapies, and patient counselling. Given the burden of mortality and morbidity associated with CV disease and its high prevalence, every opportunity should be taken to assess risk and reinforce healthy lifestyles and adherence to recommended preventive and therapeutic care.

In the following discussion, preference has been given to CV risk prediction tools that: (1) are validated in contemporary cohorts of unselected patients; (2) have adequate discriminative ability (c-statistic or area under the receiver operating characteristic (ROC) curve >0.7); and (3) have the capacity to generate absolute risk estimates, using clinician-friendly nomograms, scoring systems, or prediction rules.

---

[1]Reprinted from American Heart Journal, 151, 1, Baggish et al., 'A validated clinical and biochemical score for the diagnosis of acute heart failure: The ProBNP Investigation of Dyspnea in the Emergency Department (PRIDE) Acute Heart Failure Score', pp. 48-54, copyright 2006, with permission from Elsevier.

Risk prediction in patients presenting with atypical clinical syndromes which may be related to cardiovascular disease

Patients presenting with undifferentiated chest pain are common in acute medical units, and failure to diagnose acute coronary syndrome (ACS) can be as high as 6.4%. Clinical findings that substantially increase the probability of ACS are:

- ST deviation or Q waves on the ECG, elevated cardiac enzymes.
- Pain radiating to both right and left arms.
- Pain that is pressing or burning in nature.
- Presence of a third heart sound and/or hypotension. Findings that decrease the probability of ACS include:
- A normal ECG.
- No elevation in cardiac enzymes.
- Chest pain that is pleuritic, sharp, or stabbing, and reproduced by palpation or varies, according to position.

The probability of future CVD events in such patients can be estimated using the Framingham risk score (FRS), based on traditional risk factors of age, sex, serum cholesterol, blood pressure, smoking status, and presence of diabetes and left ventricular hypertrophy. Simple risk matrices have been developed by Jackson and colleagues that integrate values for each of these factors in computing absolute 5-year risk of CV events. These risk estimates, combined with clinical findings, can help to determine whether further investigations to rule out coronary disease are warranted.

Several scoring systems and prediction tools for identifying patients with chest pain who are safe for early discharge have been evaluated, but all suffer from the problem of less than 100% sensitivity for detecting ACS. The Vancouver Chest Pain Rule, yet to be validated, shows 99% sensitivity in ruling out ACS, based on a decision tree that integrates prior history of angina or myocardial infarction, age, chest pain characteristics, and ECG changes and results of cardiac enzymes after a 2-hour period of observation. More recent scores such as HEART and ADAPT have been suggested as being even more accurate and easier to use in ruling out ACS. The GRACE score, derived from a cohort of patients with ACS, also appears superior to clinical evaluation in predicting a diagnosis of ACS. Requests for provocative testing, such as exercise ECG, dobutamine stress echocardiography, or stress thallium, will depend on the level of clinical suspicion that chest pain may be cardiac, informed by the previously described risk prediction tools, and the local availability of testing facilities. Many acute medical units have on-site treadmill testing that can provide considerable reassurance to both patient and clinician if the test is normal.

In patients with **syncope** with no obvious cause, the San Francisco rule predicts risk of 30-day and 12-month outcomes (death, cardiac arrhythmia, pulmonary embolism, stroke, or subarachnoid haemorrhage) and identifies patients at low risk (<1%) who can be discharged if they have none of the following features:

- Abnormal ECG.
- Dyspnoea.
- Systolic blood pressure <90 mmHg.
- Haematocrit <30%.
- History of congestive heart failure (CHF).

The OESIL score is also simple to use and relies on only four findings in predicting high mortality risk within 12 months: age >65 years, history of CV disease, syncope without prodromal symptoms, and abnormal ECG. The EGSYS score has been validated in predicting higher frequency of cardiac syncope on the basis of abnormal ECG and/or history of heart disease, palpitations prior to syncope, syncope during effort or in supine position, absence of autonomic prodromes, and absence of predisposing and/or precipitating factors.

In patients with **dyspnoea**, a common diagnostic dilemma is whether this reflects CHF or pulmonary thromboembolism (PTE). The PRIDE score is an accurate method for diagnosing or excluding CHF, based on eight criteria[1]:

• Elevated brain natriuretic peptide (BNP).
• Interstitial oedema on CXR.
• Orthopnoea.
• Absence of fever.
• Loop diuretic use.
• Age >75 years.
• Crackles on chest examination.
• Absence of cough.

The Wells and Geneva rules are validated prediction rules for estimating probability of PTE and are discussed in Thromboembolic disease.

In patients with **palpitations**, no prediction tools currently exist that reliably estimate the chance of palpitations representing benign ectopics and anxiety-related symptoms versus sustained arrhythmias which may be potentially serious. However, a careful history and physical examination, combined with a resting 12-lead ECG, can, in most cases, distinguish between the two and avoid unnecessary referral for Holter monitoring or electrophysiological study. Patients in whom clinical assessment suggests a true arrhythmia or a high risk of ventricular arrhythmia or who remain anxious, despite reassurance, are candidates for further investigation.

Risk prediction in patients with known cardiovascular disease presenting with clinical syndromes unrelated to cardiovascular disease

In patients discharged following **acute coronary syndrome (ACS)**, the risk of death at 6 months can be estimated using the GRACE risk prediction tool, based on age, history of heart failure and previous myocardial infarction, serum creatinine, in-hospital use of percutaneous coronary intervention, and heart rate, blood pressure, ST deviation, and elevation in cardiac biomarkers at the time of presentation.

For patients hospitalized with **congestive heart failure (CHF)**, death at 30 days and 1 year can be estimated using the EFFECT prediction rule, based on age, comorbidities of dementia, chronic obstructive pulmonary disease, liver cirrhosis, cancer, and cerebrovascular disease, and clinical parameters at time of initial presentation: systolic blood pressure, respiratory rate, and sodium, urea, and haemoglobin. In ambulant elderly patients with chronic heart failure, 1-year mortality can be estimated, based on age, coronary artery disease, dementia, peripheral vascular disease, systolic blood pressure, serum sodium, and serum urea. A more sophisticated scoring system also considers the impact of multiple comorbidities, such as cancer, diabetes, chronic obstructive lung disease, renal insufficiency, atrial fibrillation, and anaemia as well as concurrent therapies (ACE inhibitors and beta-blockers) and clinical indices of heart failure severity (NYHA class and left ventricular ejection fraction).

In patients with **atrial fibrillation**, the risk of thromboembolic stroke can be predicted using the CHADS$_2$ score, which is available in Gage et al. (2004). The CHADS$_2$VASc score is a newer modification which provides more accurate estimation of stroke risk in patients with CHADS$_2$ score of 1 or 2.

In the absence of a past history of stroke or TIA, previous myocardial infarction or diabetes, no current angina or treatment for hypertension, and systolic blood pressure <140 mmHg, the risk of stroke is the same as for patients with no atrial fibrillation, and anticoagulant therapy can be withheld.

In patients with **recent TIA**, the ABCD2 score may assist in differentiating between those at low, moderate, or high risk of stroke within the next 2 days, based on age, blood pressure, clinical findings (speech impairment, weakness), duration of symptoms, and presence of diabetes.

Risk prediction in persons with no known cardiovascular disease presenting with clinical syndromes unrelated to cardiovascular disease

The previously mentioned FRS is the method that underpins most CV risk prediction models applied to asymptomatic persons. However, FRS-based models have been criticized as: (1) having limited application to ethnic groups (black and other minorities), having been derived from a cohort of mainly white US citizens; and (2) being potentially inaccurate by not including other risk factors, such as family history of premature CV disease or chronic kidney disease. More recently, the QRISK2 risk prediction tool has been validated in 2.3 million UK residents and incorporates all known clinical risk factors as well as ethnicity, socio-economic disadvantage (Townsend deprivation score), treatment for hypertension, atrial fibrillation, and rheumatoid arthritis. However, this risk algorithm is yet to be transformed into a nomogram or matrix for use in routine practice.

While numerous ancillary laboratory tests (or biomarkers), either singly or as multimarker panels (including C-reactive protein, homocysteine, fibrinogen, D-dimer, lipoprotein(a), and troponin), have been proposed as adding predictive value to clinical prediction models, none has shown better discriminative ability after adjustment for traditional risk factors, compared to FRS-based models alone.

For patients who are able to exercise, improved predictive accuracy is possible, using a multivariate model based on results of stress ECG testing (exercise time, extent of ST deviation, provocation of chest pain), combined with clinical risk factors (age, sex, diabetes, smoking status). Coronary artery calcium scores, as calculated using computed coronary tomography, may also provide more accurate estimates of CV risk, and coronary angiography is being used as a screening test increasingly. Based on cost exposure to ionizing radiation, these tests should be reserved for patients with intermediate risk of CV events, based on FRS scores >5% but <10% probability at 5 years (the latter being the currently accepted threshold for initiating medical treatments) or who have an abnormal resting ECG.

Most of the risk prediction tools cited can be accessed free with Excel calculator files at <http://www.medal.org>.

Further reading

Baggish AL, Siebert U, Lainchbury JG, et al. (2006). A validated clinical and biochemical score for the diagnosis of acute heart failure: the ProBNP Investigation of Dyspnea in the Emergency Department (PRIDE) Acute Heart Failure Score. *American Heart Journal*, **151**, 48–54.

Budoff MJ, Shaw LJ, Liu ST, *et al.* (2007). Long-term prognosis associated with coronary calcification: observations from a registry of 25,253 patients. *Journal of the American College of Cardiology*, **49**, 1860–70.

Camm AJ, Lip GY, De Caterina R, *et al.* (2012). 2012 focused update of the ESC Guidelines for the management of atrial fibrillation: an update of the 2010 ESC Guidelines for the management of atrial fibrillation. *European Heart Journal*, **33**, 2719–47.

Christenson J, Innes G, McKnight D, *et al.* (2006). A clinical prediction rule for early discharge of patients with chest pain. *Annals of Emergency Medicine*, **47**, 1–10.

Colivicchi F, Ammirati F, Melina D, *et al.* (2003). Development and prospective validation of a risk stratification system for patients with syncope in the emergency department: the OESIL risk score. *European Heart Journal*, **24**, 811–19.

Del Rosso A, Ungar A, Maggi R, *et al.* (2008). Clinical predictors of cardiac syncope at initial evaluation in patients referred urgently to general hospital: the EGSYS score. *Heart*, **94**, 1620–6.

Friedmann PD, Brett AS, Mayo-Smith MF (1996). Differences in generalists' and cardiologists' perceptions of cardiovascular risk and the outcomes of preventive therapy in cardiovascular disease. *Annals of Internal Medicine*, **124**, 414–21.

Gage BF, van Walraven C, Pearce L, *et al.* (2004) Selecting patients with atrial fibrillation for anticoagulation: stroke risk stratification in patients taking aspirin, *Circulation*, **110**, 2287–92.

Gage BF, Waterman AD, Shannon W, *et al.* (2001). Validation of clinical classification schemes for predicting stroke: results from the National Registry of Atrial Fibrillation. *JAMA*, **285**, 2864–70.

Hippisley-Cox J, Coupland C, Vinogradova Y, *et al.* (2008). Predicting cardiovascular risk in England and Wales: prospective derivation and validation of QRISK2. *BMJ*, **336**, 1475–82.

Huynh BC, Rovner A, Rich MW (2006). Long-term survival in elderly patients hospitalized for heart failure: 14-year follow-up from a prospective randomized trial. *Archives of Internal Medicine*, **166**, 1892–8.

Johnston SC, Rothwell PM, Nguyen-Huynh MN, *et al.* (2007). Validation and refinement of scores to predict very early stroke risk after transient ischaemic attack. *Lancet*, **369**, 283–92.

Larsen TB, Lip GY, Skjøth F, *et al.* (2012). Added predictive ability of the CHA2DS2VASc risk score for stroke and death in patients with atrial fibrillation: the prospective Danish Diet, Cancer, and Health cohort study. *Circulation: Cardiovascular Quality and Outcomes*, **2012**, 335–42.

Lauer MS, Pothier CE, Magid DJ, Smith SS, Kattan MW (2007). An externally validated model for predicting long-term survival after exercise treadmill testing in patients with suspected coronary artery disease and a normal electrocardiogram. *Annals of Internal Medicine*, **147**, 821–8.

Lee DS, Austin PC, Rouleau JL, *et al.* (2003). Predicting mortality among patients hospitalized for heart failure: derivation and validation of a clinical model. *JAMA*, **290**, 2581–7.

Lip GY, Nieuwlaat R, Pisters R, *et al.* (2010). Refining clinical risk stratification for predicting stroke and thromboembolism in atrial fibrillation using a novel risk factor-based approach: the Euro heart survey on atrial fibrillation. *Chest*, **137**, 263–72.

New Zealand Guidelines Group (2003). Assessment and management of cardiovascular risk. New Zealand Guidelines Group, Wellington. <http://www.health.govt.nz/publication/assessment-and-management-cardiovascular-risk>.

Quinn J, McDermott D, Stiell I, *et al.* (2006). Prospective validation of the San Francisco Syncope Rule to predict patients with serious outcomes. *Annals of Emergency Medicine*, **47**, 448–54.

Senni M, Santilli G, Parrella P, *et al.* (2006). A novel prognostic index to determine the impact of cardiac conditions and comorbidities on one-year outcome in patients with heart failure. *American Journal of Cardiology*, **98**, 1076–82.

Than M, Cullen L, Aldous S, *et al.* (2012). 2-Hour accelerated diagnostic protocol to assess patients with chest pain symptoms using contemporary troponins as the only biomarker: the ADAPT trial. *Journal of the American College of Cardiology*, **2012**, 2091–8.

van Walraven C, Hart RG, Wells GA, *et al.* (2003). A clinical prediction rule to identify patients with atrial fibrillation and a low risk for stroke while taking aspirin. *Archives of Internal Medicine*, **163**, 936–43.

Visser A, Wolthuis A, Breedveld R, Ter Avest E (2014). HEART score and clinical gestalt have similar diagnostic accuracy for diagnosing ACS in an unselected population of patients with chest pain presenting in the ED. *Emerg Med J*, 2014 Sep 12. pii: emermed-2014-203798. doi: 10.1136/emermed-2014-203798. [Epub ahead of print.]

Wu EB, Hodson F, Chambers JB (2005). A simple score for predicting coronary artery disease in patients with chest pain. *QJM*, **98**, 803–11.

Heart failure

Introduction

Heart failure is a syndrome characterized by inadequate end-organ perfusion, reduced cardiorespiratory reserve, and compensatory expansion of extracellular volume. The major symptoms and signs of heart failure reflect these physiologic abnormalities, with diminished functional capacity, impaired renal function, pulmonary or splanchnic congestion, and peripheral oedema. Each element may be present to a varying extent in any given patient, possibly representing the distinct contributions in each individual of impaired myocardial contractility, slowed myocardial relaxation, systemic or pulmonary vascular responses, and other cardiac or vascular abnormalities, such as valvular disease, shunting, or arrhythmia.

This chapter complies to guidelines from the National Institute for Health and Clinical Excellence (NICE, UK) and the American College of Cardiology (ACC)/American Heart Association (AHA) guidelines, developed with the International Society for Heart and Lung Transplantation.

Epidemiology

The incidence and prevalence of heart failure continue to increase in the developed and developing worlds. These trends appear to reflect improving survival from myocardial infarction and other forms of coronary artery disease, as well as an increased prevalence of other major predisposing factors, including hypertension and diabetes. As many as 10% of those over 80 years will have the diagnosis, but the prevalence of heart failure is 0.1% in those under 50 years of age. There is emerging evidence of an aetiological relationship between atrial fibrillation and heart failure, with each predicting the subsequent occurrence of the other. This may reflect a shared biology in many patients. Heart failure is less common in females, but their longer lifespan results in women constituting approximately 50% of all cases. Heart failure affects 1 million individuals in the UK and over 5 million in the US and accounts for 5% of all hospital admissions and 2–3% of all healthcare costs.

Several clinical classifications for heart failure exist. Despite the limitations intrinsic to the application of general descriptors to a heterogeneous disorder, these have proven useful clinically and in randomized controlled trials.

Heart failure classification schemes
NYHA symptom level[1]:
- I—No limitation.
- II—Symptomatic only, with moderate activity.
  - Annual mortality 5–10%.
- III—Symptomatic, except when at rest.
  - Annual mortality 10–20%.
- IV—Symptomatic at rest.
  - Annual mortality ~50%.

Despite recent major advances in therapy, the prognosis from heart failure, therefore, remains poor.

Definitions

Heart failure escapes a simple definition because, by the time it is recognized, the primary processes have often given way to a rather non-specific final common pathway. At clinical presentation, normal physiologic reserves are substantially compromised. Inadequate cardiac output often results in exertional limitation or fatigue, rather than in symptoms related to the dysfunction of a specific organ or organs. Elevated filling pressures, associated with the compensatory responses to reduced organ perfusion, are the most commonly recognized clinical features. Three broad syndromes exist, and typically in any individual, all are present to some extent.

- Right heart failure is the presence of elevated right atrial pressure which, if persistent, leads to associated peripheral oedema.
- Left heart failure is the presence of elevated left atrial pressure and is usually associated with increased pulmonary interstitial fluid pressure or pulmonary oedema and is the classic symptom of orthopnoea.
- Diastolic dysfunction is simply defined as heart failure with preserved systolic function. While diastolic dysfunction is almost always present when systolic dysfunction exists, isolated diastolic abnormalities are also seen.

Pathogenesis

The heart failure syndrome is the 'final common pathway' for a host of underlying disorders that affect the myocardium, valves, pericardium, systemic and pulmonary vasculature, or even peripheral organs. There is tremendous variation in the propensity to develop heart failure after a given insult, which is thought, in part, to represent inherited differences in myocardial, renal, or endocrine responses. Most commonly, myocardial injury will lead to increased workload for the remaining myocytes, with consequent cellular hypertrophy and increased myocardial mass. While initially adaptive, in most disorders the remodelling pathways eventually become maladaptive, with secondary effects on systolic or diastolic function and progressive structural or functional changes in the ventricles and vasculature. Relatively late in the evolution of heart failure, paracrine, endocrine, or neurohormonal pathways play a significant role, and the sympathetic nervous system becomes activated. The most common forms of systolic heart failure represent a type of progressive myocardial dystrophy that result from the injury itself or from maladaptive responses. It is this dystrophic process that predisposes the heart to many of the longer-term consequences of heart failure, such as arrhythmia, conduction disease, or sudden death.

Causes of systolic heart failure
- Myocardial ischaemia—acute or chronic.
- Shock.
  - Sepsis.
  - Other causes of hypoperfusion.
- Dilated cardiomyopathy.
  - Inherited.
  - Metabolic.
  - Endocrine.
- Chronic pressure overload.
  - Hypertension.
  - Stenotic valvular disease.
- Chronic volume overload.
  - Regurgitant valvular disease.
  - Shunting—intra- or extra-cardiac.
- Structural heart disease.

---

[1] Reproduced from Heart Failure Society of America. Copyright 2002.

- Obstructive valve disease.
- Regurgitant valve disease.
- Shunts.
- Coarctation.
- Arrhythmias.
  - Chronotropic incompetence.
  - Tachycardia-related cardiomyopathy.
- High-output heart failure.
  - Hyperthyroidism.
  - Chronic anaemia.
  - Nutritional.

Pathophysiologic mechanisms

The pathophysiology of heart failure is complex and, in most instances, has features of a multisystem disease. Elements of the syndrome can be broadly categorized in terms of:

Systolic function

Myocardial injury occurs in many ways. Irrespective of the mode of the primary mechanism, there is also a component of the response to injury that leads to less effective systolic contraction through changes in myocardial biology and the geometry of the ventricles. While this process has been conceived of in many ways, as an effort to normalize wall stress or to restore peripheral organ perfusion, the precise regulation remains obscure. The final outcome is consistent with reduced stroke volumes at higher filling pressures.

Diastolic function

Impaired filling is now recognized as a contributor to the higher filling pressures and the energy inefficiencies seen in all forms of heart failure. As part of the remodelling process in typical myocardial disease or as an independent feature of fibrotic or infiltrative pathologies, the ventricles may become stiff. This impairs ventricular filling and may become a limiting factor in cardiac physiology. Pure pericardial constraint or constriction may cause diastolic dysfunction, with a broad range of specific pathologies affecting the visceral or parietal pericardium. In acute forms of myocardial disease with ventricular dilatation, there may be an element of pericardial constraint with a normal pericardium.

Preload

Apparent heart failure can result from primary changes in extracellular fluid volume, as in renal and hepatic failure. However, the elevated filling pressures seen in heart failure are attributable to a vicious cycle of impaired ventricular emptying, abnormal ventricular filling, reduced cardiac output, and impaired organ perfusion with secondary salt and water retention. This expansion in extracellular fluid volume leads to pulmonary or systemic venous congestion, with potential additional perturbation of myocardial and peripheral organ physiology.

Afterload

Primary changes in myocardial afterload may result from hypertension or from valvular heart disease. An acquired increase in afterload is a typical feature in most forms of heart failure, as a result of neurohormonal activation with prominent sympathetic tone, especially in the decompensated state. Very low afterload conditions, e.g. with major arteriovenous fistulae or nutritional disorders, can result in high-output heart failure.

The traditional framework for discussing heart failure is dominated by the major elements of the haemodynamic model listed previously. While this conceptual outline has proven useful, it is clear that the myocardium changes progressively after any form of injury and that many of the core features of heart failure represent the effects of reactivation of developmental gene programmes or other molecular pathways. These changes in the myocardial phenotype result in fundamental effects on many aspects of myocardial physiology, including energetics, susceptibility to stress and electrophysiology that affect the entire heart and contribute to the final heart failure syndrome.

Diagnosis

The diagnosis of heart failure is made on the basis of typical symptoms, such as:

- Dyspnoea.
- Exercise intolerance or fatigue.
- Fluid retention.

These symptoms are non-specific but should prompt consideration of heart failure. A careful attempt should be made to identify orthopnoea and to obtain a semi-objective functional baseline (NYHA). In many instances, subtle chronic limitation can be detected by comparison of performance with peers or previous years. Less common presentations, especially in younger individuals, include positional cough or wheeze (an orthopnoea equivalent), palpitations, or unexplained rapid weight gain. Young individuals with dilated cardiomyopathy often do not present until there is acute right heart failure with hepatic congestion. This can be accompanied by systemic symptoms and fever, which must be distinguished from a true viral syndrome with myocardial involvement. A comprehensive history, seeking reversible causes of heart failure and any inherited predisposition, should be completed.

Initial physical exam may detect clinical evidence of left or right ventricular dilatation or hypertrophy, as well as evidence of low or high output states. Third or fourth heart sounds and murmurs, which may reveal a primary valvular cause, should be actively sought. Elevated right-sided venous pressures and peripheral oedema are usually obvious, but a careful evaluation of the entire vascular tree, pulmonary pathology, skeletal muscle function, and endocrine state will often aid in the identification of the underlying cause of the heart failure.

Basic assessment should include an ECG and measurement of natriuretic peptide levels, since heart failure is unlikely if these are normal. Transthoracic echocardiography is recommended. Subsequent or parallel tests to assess contributing factors or alternative diagnoses include:

- Chest X-ray.
- Biochemical profile.
- Liver function tests.
- Fasting lipids and glucose.
- Thyroid function tests.
- Assessment of iron stores.
- Urinalysis.
- Pulmonary function testing.

If there is no echocardiographic abnormality, then heart failure is unlikely, and alternative diagnoses should be sought before contemplating referral for evaluation of possible diastolic heart failure (see further text). If the echocardiogram is abnormal, then treatable underlying causes should be explored. Clinical or non-invasive imaging evidence of coronary artery disease should prompt consideration of coronary angiography. Endomyocardial biopsy has a role when giant cell myocarditis or an infiltrative process is suspected.

Clinical syndromes

Heart failure usually presents with one or more features dominating the clinical picture. In practice, the management of each of these syndromes is closely related, and multiple components require to be treated simultaneously. Nevertheless, it has proven useful to distinguish these clinical entities as a guide for management principles.

Right heart failure

The most common cause of right heart failure is left heart failure. Left-sided abnormalities lead to elevations of pulmonary venous pressure and associated regional pulmonary vasoconstriction. Depending on the pace of the underlying condition, the effects of these changes in afterload on right ventricular function are often precipitous.

Causes of right heart failure

• Left heart failure from any cause.
• Cor pulmonale (COPD).
• Primary pulmonary hypertension.
• Secondary pulmonary hypertension, e.g. pulmonary embolism.
• Right-sided valve disease.
• Isolated right ventricular disease (uncommon).

In the absence of any of the above, pericardial disease should be excluded

History will usually be dominated by symptoms of functional limitation and lower extremity oedema, but, occasionally, other features are prominent. Splanchnic congestion may lead to gastrointestinal symptoms, with diarrhoea, malabsorption, and even protein-losing enteropathy. In a small subset, cardiac cirrhosis, with the consequent additional stimulus to secondary hyperaldosteronism, is a feature, and ascites is more notable than peripheral oedema. In the presence of severe lung disease, the incremental effects of posture on diaphragmatic efficiency can cause orthopnoea and mimic biventricular failure.

Physical examination reveals elevated jugular venous pressures, peripheral oedema, and right-sided third or fourth heart sounds. Chronic right ventricular overload may result in a parasternal heave. The manifestations of pulmonary arterial hypertension may be quite focal, and a 'PA tap' should be sought, even if an accentuated pulmonary component of the second heart sound is not obvious.

The management of right heart failure is typically focused on diuresis, but every opportunity to maximize right ventricular output should be explored. Not uncommonly, a degree of chronic elevation of right heart pressure must be tolerated, particularly in the context of truly isolated right-sided disease, as excessive diuresis may reduce left ventricular preload to the point where there is systemic hypotension.

Primary or secondary pulmonary arterial hypertension is a major cause of right heart failure. When pulmonary hypertension is persistent, despite the treatment of any left heart failure, response to vasodilators should be assessed (ideally with right heart catheterization) early in the clinical course.

Acute right heart failure may represent the decompensation of any number of chronic cardiac processes, but acute pulmonary embolism should always be considered. Isolated right heart failure can also result from pericardial disease. Considerable effort is expended on the distinction between constriction and restriction or between tamponade and effuso-constrictive physiology. Ultimately, the most important determinant of prognosis is the underlying process, and, in most cases, a tissue diagnosis is needed.

Left heart failure and pulmonary oedema

Left heart failure is dominated by pulmonary congestion, with orthopnoea, evidence of reduced cardiopulmonary reserve, and later frank dyspnoea. The temporal course of left heart failure ranges from subtle changes in chronic limitation due to dietary indiscretion, through to florid pulmonary oedema in the context of an acute myocardial infarction or other stepwise changes in cardiac function. Chronic elevations in pulmonary venous pressure are remarkably well tolerated.

The management of left heart failure and pulmonary oedema is outlined in the section on management. It is useful to discriminate between decompensation resulting from changes in loading conditions and changes in extracellular volume status as management plans are refined.

Diastolic heart failure

Diastolic heart failure has emerged as a significant problem, with the increase in high-quality non-invasive imaging. While case definitions vary with the resolution of objective evaluation, the concept of heart failure with preserved ejection fraction (HFpEF) is probably the most practical. Unfortunately, the diagnosis is often made without objective assessment of left heart filling pressures or formal indices of ventricular relaxation. Usually, the diagnosis is based on acute or subacute dyspnoea, often with peripheral oedema, in the context of a normal echocardiographic evaluation of left ventricular function. Misdiagnosis is common, as, in large case series, only a small fraction of those in whom the diagnosis is made on clinical criteria have true evidence of isolated diastolic abnormalities.

Ventricular relaxation is abnormal in virtually all conditions in which systolic dysfunction is found. Pure diastolic dysfunction is less common.

The epidemiology of HFpEF is notable for the prominence of current or prior hypertension, female gender, age, and diabetes. Poorly controlled hypertension in this context raises the possibility of renal artery stenosis. Reversible ischaemia, episodic hypertension, and occult pulmonary disease should be excluded. However, before an extensive evaluation is undertaken, objective documentation of cardiac failure should be sought.

Causes of diastolic heart failure

• Misdiagnosis.
  ◦ Inaccurate cardiac assessment.
  ◦ Transient systolic dysfunction, e.g. ischaemia.
  ◦ Valvular heart disease.
  ◦ Pulmonary disease.
  ◦ Obesity.
  ◦ Hypertensive crises.
• True diastolic dysfunction.
  ◦ Hypertrophy.
  ◦ Infiltrative disorders.
  ◦ Storage disorders.
  ◦ Endomyocardial disease.
  ◦ Pericardial disease.

Diastolic heart failure has a similar prognosis to systolic heart failure. There are no definitive studies of management, but the focus is on aggressive treatment of hypertension, heart rate control, and diuretics.

Management aims

The goals of management in heart failure are:

- Improved symptoms and quality of life.
- Improved survival.

These goals are achieved through a systematic approach to the diagnosis and management of heart failure, emphasizing: (1) early diagnosis; (2) efficient treatment of correctable causes; and (3) the introduction of a series of therapies demonstrated in large randomized controlled trials to improve mortality and morbidity, irrespective of the aetiology. Key physiologic goals are the maximization of cardiac output and reduction in congestion, but the latter may become limiting if diuresis is unduly aggressive. As a result, the earliest emphasis should be on optimizing cardiac loading conditions, while fine-tuning of the diuretic requirement can often be completed as an outpatient. This also allows changes in absorption that may result from dramatic reduction in splanchnic venous pressures to be accommodated.

Finally, in the context of any inherited form of heart failure, it is important to identify others at risk. There are few empiric data on which to base this screening, but the availability of therapies proven to be effective in presymptomatic disease (ACE inhibitors) is a major advantage.

Management of stable heart failure

This is an area of active investigation, and numerous guidelines exist.

Pharmacologic

- Diuretics: traditionally have been the mainstay of heart failure therapy and undoubtedly help in reducing symptoms of pulmonary or peripheral congestion. Care must be exercised not to overemphasize diuretics, as their use is associated with neurohormonal activation, and overdiuresis may limit the use of maximal doses of ACE inhibitor or beta-blocker. Ideally, a loop diuretic should be used, with care to avoid hypokalaemia.
- ACE inhibitors: reduce symptoms, reduce hospitalizations, and prolong survival in heart failure, compared to placebo. While higher doses are not clearly associated with better outcomes, the majority of randomized controlled trials have used high target doses. ACE inhibitor doses can be rapidly ramped up until optimal or target dose is reached. Renal function should be followed closely until stable doses are attained, especially in the context of peripheral vascular disease or high-dose diuretic. ACE inhibitors should be avoided in the context of unevaluated renal failure, hyperkalaemia, or critical valve disease without specialist supervision.
- Beta-blockers: have been shown (for some class members) to reduce hospitalization and mortality in heart failure. The best evidence is for carvedilol, bucindolol, and slow-release metoprolol. Beta-blockers should be introduced more cautiously after diuretic and ACE inhibitors are established.
- Aldosterone antagonists: the potassium-sparing diuretics spironolactone and eplerenone reduce mortality in NYHA class III or IV heart failure when added to a loop diuretic and an ACE inhibitor. Care should be exercised if creatinine or potassium is elevated.
- Digoxin: has not been demonstrated to affect symptoms or mortality in randomized controlled trials but does have some benefits in heart failure, reducing the frequency of hospitalization and preventing deterioration in maximal exercise performance. There may be subgroups of heart failure patients in whom digoxin is more beneficial, e.g. atrial fibrillation.
- Angiotensin receptor blockers: reduce symptoms and mortality in heart failure when used as the primary form of vasodilator. No additive effect with ACE inhibitors has been demonstrated.
- Anticoagulation: warfarin is only definitively indicated in heart failure with atrial fibrillation. It should be considered in those with heart failure and a history of thromboembolism, ventricular aneurysm, or a large anterior MI.
- Aspirin: should be prescribed in standard doses for those with heart failure and atherosclerosis.
- Statin: while there may be some evidence that statins have effects in heart failure unrelated to their effects on atherosclerosis, currently they should be prescribed for standard criteria, including dyslipidaemia and vascular disease.
- Hydralazine/nitrate: this combination of vasodilators has been shown to improve mortality in those who cannot tolerate ACE inhibitors.
- Positive inotropes: (such as dobutamine or milrinone) have been found useful in decompensated chronic heart failure. They do not have any long-term effects on the underlying syndrome.
- Newer agents, such as the next generation of endothelin antagonists, natriuretics, and calcium sensitizers, are currently under investigation.

Non-pharmacologic

There are several non-pharmacologic interventions of proven use in heart failure, but the majority require optimization of cardiac function prior to their initiation.

- Exercise training: heart failure may result in a catabolic state, with deconditioning, or even a cachectic syndrome mediated by humoral factors. Several forms of exercise have been shown to improve symptoms, exercise performance, and quality of life.
- Rehabilitation: is known to be effective in coronary heart disease, but there are limited data supporting efficacy in heart failure per se. In the absence of rigorous data, simple aerobic or resistive exercise regimens are recommended.
- Smoking cessation: the known effects of tobacco consumption support immediate abstinence.
- Reduction or cessation of alcohol: since heavy alcohol consumption may cause a cardiomyopathy that is completely reversible with alcohol cessation, limitation of alcohol is recommended for all heart failure patients. Alcohol may precipitate volume overload, atrial fibrillation, or other arrhythmias, irrespective of the aetiology of the failure.
- Outpatient supervision: structured management programmes, with careful monitoring of weight gain, diuretic doses, and comorbidities, have been shown to reduce readmission rates and improve symptoms and quality of life in heart failure patients. Economic data suggest that, in some health economies, such programmes are highly cost-effective.
- Vaccination: currently, inoculation against both influenza and pneumococcal disease are recommended for heart failure patients.

Invasive therapies

- Coronary revascularization: should be considered if heart failure occurs in the context of three-vessel or left main coronary artery disease. A key component of the prediction of a net benefit for surgical revascularization is evidence on nuclear imaging, stress echo, or MRI of substantial volumes of hypocontractile, but viable, myocardium. Percutaneous revascularization has not been demonstrated to be effective in this context.
- Valve surgery: should be considered immediately for stenotic lesions where ventricular function is preserved. In the presence of impaired ventricular function, care should be exercised and chronicity assessed, as ventricular dilatation and contractile failure may be irreversible.
- Implantable cardioverter defibrillators: improve survival in those with ejection fractions less than 0.40, irrespective of a history of ventricular arrhythmias.
- Cardiac resynchronization therapy: has been found to improve symptoms, reduce hospitalizations, and improve survival in individuals with class IV heart failure, low ejection fraction (<0.35), and QRS duration of >120 ms. Recent data suggest that similar benefits may be seen in class II and III heart failure.
- Remote monitoring: using improved functionality of permanent pacemakers or defibrillators as well as dedicated implantable devices, is emerging as a tool for the management of heart failure. Outputs, such as derived autonomic indices, respiration rate monitoring, and thoracic impedance, are currently available, but measurement of pressure or flow may be feasible.
- Ultrafiltration: may be used for reduction in extracellular fluid volume in diuretic-resistant individuals with severe heart failure. The role of this technology is evolving rapidly.
- Ventricular assist devices remain experimental as a 'destination' therapy but can be used acutely (see further text) or as a bridge to transplantation.
- Transplantation: has reached relatively stable use patterns but is limited by the availability of donor organs. While there are no randomized trials, quality of life and length of life are substantially improved in carefully chosen recipients, despite the morbidity of long-term immunosuppression and allograft vasculopathy.
- Radiofrequency ablation of atrial fibrillation: although there is often a diffuse atrial myopathy in heart failure, there are some individuals who appear to benefit anecdotally for prolonged periods from pulmonary vein isolation for their atrial fibrillation. Currently, trials of radiofrequency ablation for atrial fibrillation in heart failure are underway. True tachycardia-induced cardiomyopathy is unusual. Most purported cases likely reflect a common myopathic substrate, underlying atrial arrhythmias and ventricular contractile dysfunction.

Lifestyle recommendations

- Diet and nutrition: play a role in heart failure, but data are limited. Weight loss, salt and fluid restriction are all recommended.
- Sexual activity is feasible if exercise levels of 5 or more metabolic equivalents (METS) can be attained. This is the equivalent of climbing two or more flights of stairs.
- Driving competency is not affected in the absence of syncopal events. In the presence of syncope, driving certification is determined by the underlying mechanism of loss of consciousness.

- Air travel exposes those with heart failure to the risks of relative hypoxaemia, but this should only be an issue in those who are minimally compensated. In practice, those with class IV heart failure should not fly without medical support.

Management of comorbidities

Coronary artery disease is the commonest cause of heart failure. Surgical revascularization has been shown to improve systolic function in selected individuals. Specialist assessment, including evaluation of myocardial viability, is associated with the best outcomes. As noted, valve disease should be approached with care, as surgical therapy in the context of heart failure is high risk. When atrial fibrillation and heart failure coexist, as they often do, anticoagulation is indicated, but aggressive attempts to achieve sinus rhythm have not been proven of benefit. In the setting of renal failure, close cooperation between cardiac and renal specialists is required to optimize the management of heart failure. Complex cases of heart failure, with unusual aetiologies or systemic medical problems, should be referred early for specialist management.

Pharmacologic management of systolic heart failure

Acute heart failure presents several distinctive challenges for management. See Figure 4.3 for the management of acute heart failure. Even in extreme cases, it is usually feasible to avoid intubation, but this may prove necessary in some patients. Diuretic therapy is often overemphasized for historical reasons. The most likely acute precipitants for pulmonary oedema are abrupt changes in afterload, myocardial ischaemia, or a paroxysmal arrhythmia, rather than stepwise changes in extracellular fluid volume status.

Non-pharmacologic

- Oxygen: rapid institution of oxygen therapy will not only improve myocardial supply:demand mismatch but alleviate the tremendous sympathetic activation that accompanies acute pulmonary oedema.
- Continuous positive airway pressure (CPAP): may be used to avoid intubation *in extremis* but should not be used in those with diminished conscious level.
- Intubation and mechanical ventilation: should be avoided, if possible, as a result of the associated haemodynamic effects and the relative risks. However, it may not be possible to prevent this outcome with acute myocardial infarction.

Pharmacologic

Drug absorption and metabolism may be substantially impaired as a result of splanchnic congestion and reduced hepatic or renal blood flow.

- Opiates: small doses of parenteral opiates have been used, to great effect, in acute pulmonary oedema. There is rapid reduction of ventricular afterload, sympatholysis, and direct inhibition of pulmonary interstitial afferents.
- Intravenous nitrates: have been compared to intravenous diuretics in small trials and are at least as effective, with more rapid relief. They are most effective when there is high afterload and high preload but can be used cautiously, even when systolic pressures are low, if there is no preload dependence.
- Inotropes or inodilators: including dobutamine and milrinone, can be useful in the acute setting. Vasoconstrictors must be used with care, as the failing ventricle is extremely

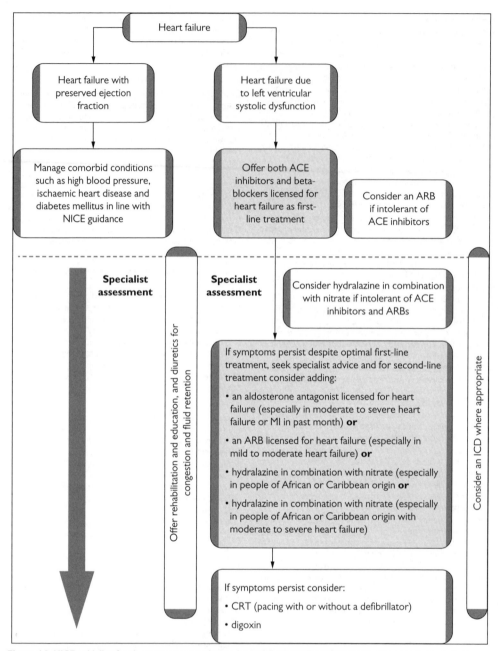

Figure 4.3 NICE guideline for the management of acute heart failure. NICE guidelines for the management of acute heart failure. National Institute for Health and Clinical Excellence (2010) Adapted from 'CG 108 Chronic heart failure: management of chronic heart failure in adults in primary and secondary care'. London: NICE. Available from <http://guidance.nice.org.uk/CG108>. Reproduced with permission.

sensitive to increased afterload. It is important to focus on optimizing cardiac output and end-organ perfusion, rather than systolic blood pressure.

Invasive procedures

- Percutaneous intervention is only effective therapy for heart failure in the context of myocardial salvage during acute coronary syndromes. Late percutaneous intervention (up to 72 hours post-MI) has been shown to be of benefit in cases with cardiogenic shock. It is important to discriminate between these situations and heart failure with incidental chronic coronary artery disease where the procedural risks outweigh any benefits.
- Left ventricular assist devices (LVADs) or biventricular assist devices (BiVAD) should be considered in severe and intractable heart failure in the context of a potentially reversible cause or if heart transplantation is feasible. Implantation of such devices has proven lifesaving in younger individuals with myocarditis, and complete recoveries have been reported. In the pre-transplant patient, the effects of ventricular support on overall physiologic function may reduce the risk of transplantation.
- Cardiac surgery may be required urgently in the setting of acute mechanical causes of heart failure. Ruptured chordae or torn cusps may precipitate torrential regurgitant lesions that can only be addressed using surgical techniques.

Further reading

American Heart Association HeartHub for Patients. <http://www.hearthub.org/hc-heart-failure.htm>.

Hunt SA, Abraham WT, Chin MH, *et al.* (2009). Focused update incorporated into the ACC/AHA 2005 Guidelines for the Diagnosis and Management of Heart Failure in Adults. *Circulation*, **119**, e391–479.

Mann DL (2012). Pathophysiology of heart failure. In RO Bonow, *et al.*, eds. *Braunwald's heart disease*, pp. 485–505. WB Saunders, Philadelphia.

Mann DL (2012). Management of heart failure with reduced ejection fraction. In RO Bonow, *et al.*, eds. *Braunwald's heart disease*, pp. 543–69. WB Saunders, Philadelphia.

National Institute for Health and Clinical Excellence (2010). National clinical guideline for the diagnosis and management of chronic heart failure in adults in primary and secondary care. <http://www.nice.org.uk/nicemedia/live/13099/50514/50514.pdf>.

National Institute for Health and Clinical Excellence (2014). Acute heart failure: diagnosing and managing acute heart failure in adults. Clinical guideline 187. <http://www.nice.org.uk/guidance/cg187/resources/guidance-acute-heart-failure-pdf>.

Patient UK. <http://www.patient.co.uk/health/Heart-Failure.htm>.

Redfield MM (2012). Management of heart failure with normal ejection fraction. In RO Bonow, *et al.*, eds. *Braunwald's heart disease*. pp. 586–601. WB Saunders, Philadelphia.

Scottish Intercollegiate Guideline Network for Patients. Chronic heart failure. <http://www.sign.ac.uk/pdf/pat95.pdf>.

Yancy CW, Jessup M, Bozkurt B, *et al.* (2013). 2013 ACCF/AHA Guideline for the management of heart failure. A report of the American College of Cardiology Foundation/American Heart Association Task Force on practice guidelines. *Circulation*, **128**, e240–e327.

Acute coronary syndromes

Epidemiology

Unstable angina accounts for over 115,000 acute hospital admissions annually in the UK, about 200 admissions per 100,000 population. This compares with an estimated 260 myocardial infarctions per 100,000 people. The ratio of male to female patients is about 1.7:1. About 50% of patients with acute coronary syndromes will require revascularization within 6 months of presentation.

Before the advent of modern interventional practice and antiplatelet drugs, the in-hospital mortality of unstable angina was 5%, with an MI rate of 15%. More recent data (PRAIS-UK registry) show in-hospital mortality for unstable angina of 1.6%, with 4% sustaining an in-hospital myocardial infarction and 3.5% developing refractory ischaemia. By 6 months, 6% had died, 13% had recurrent ischaemia, and 4% sustained a non-fatal MI. The GRACE registry suggests similar 6-month mortality for unstable angina of 5% and for NSTEMI of 9.5%. Importantly, a year after the unstable episode, the risk returns to that of a stable patient with a similar risk factor profile.

Definitions

The term 'acute coronary syndrome' (ACS) describes the collection of ischaemic conditions which occur through coronary plaque rupture and includes:

- Unstable angina (UA; troponin/cardiac enzyme negative ischaemic chest pain).
- Non-ST segment elevation MI (NSTEMI; tropinin/cardiac enzyme positive ischaemic chest pain but without persistent ECG ST-segment elevation; previously non-Q wave MI/subendocardial MI).
- ST segment elevation MI (STEMI; tropinin/cardiac enzyme positive ischaemic chest pain with sustained ECG ST-segment elevation; formerly Q wave myocardial infarction/transmural MI).

Unstable angina and NSTEMI are similar in mode of presentation and are only distinguished by the presence of raised cardiac enzymes (CK-MB or troponin) after presentation. In the non-ST segment elevation MI group, this indicates that the ischaemia has caused myocardial injury. On ECG, UA/NSTEMI do not exhibit persistent ST-segment elevation but may show persistent or transient ST-segment depression or T-wave inversion, flat T waves, or no ECG changes at presentation. Depending on the definition of a myocardial infarction, NSTEMI and STEMI present with a ratio of at least 2:1. Unstable angina means that the patient presents with chest pain, with the quality of typical angina, but the episodes are more severe and prolonged, may occur at rest, or may be precipitated by less exertion than was previously necessary. STEMI is addressed in a separate chapter and this section will focus on UA/NSTEMI.

Pathophysiology

Several simultaneous processes contribute to the reduction in oxygen supply at the time of a vulnerable plaque fissure. Angiographic studies have demonstrated complex eccentric morphology, consistent with ruptured plaque and superimposed thrombus. Vulnerable plaques which fissure or rupture have large eccentric lipid pools, with foam cell infiltration, and tend to rupture at the border of the fibrous cap and adjacent normal intima. The weakness to the integrity of the plaque is initiated by matrix metalloproteinases, secreted by macrophages, and ultimately occur due to acute changes in wall shear stress. Intravascular ultrasound studies show that unstable coronary plaques are associated with more expansive arterial remodelling, compared to stable lesions. This may imply a marked recent progression in the extent and severity of plaque at the site of rupture/erosion.

The lipid core is a potent substrate for platelet-rich thrombus formation, with the initiation of the coagulation cascade through the interaction of tissue factor with factor VIIa. Platelet adhesion to subendothelial collagen through the release of tissue factor and expression of the vitronectin (av-beta-3) receptors leads to platelet activation and aggregation through the expression of the glycoprotein IIb/IIIa receptor. This event creates platelet-rich thrombus, associated with cyclical reductions in coronary blood flow and additional coronary vasoconstriction with the endothelial disruption and increased thromboxane A2 (TXA2) and serotonin production with reduced nitric oxide (NO) generation. Inflammatory acute phase proteins, cytokines, and systemic catecholamines stimulate the production of tissue factor, procoagulant activity, and platelet hypercoagulability.

There is a strong association with unstable plaques generating thrombus and, in a secondary role, contributing to intermittent complete occlusion. However, the thrombus load is less important in an unstable plaque than in a ruptured plaque, leading to persistent coronary occlusion, given the lack of benefit with thrombolytic drugs and even the positive harm possible in unstable angina or NSTEMI. Recent studies suggest plaque erosion, rather than rupture, may explain the differences between UA/NSTEMI and STEMI. Rapid conformational changes in a coronary lesion may occur through rapid proliferation of smooth muscle cells resulting from endothelial injury. This decreases the lumen area, and may be exacerbated by erosion of the plaque surface alone.

Risk stratification

The management of unstable angina and non-ST segment elevation myocardial infarction differs from the acute treatment of ST segment elevation myocardial infarction.

In STEMI, the use of aspirin and a thrombolytic drug has an immediate effect on the acute coronary occlusion but little effect on subsequent complications, such as reinfarction and recurrent ischaemia. In contrast, the treatment of UA/NSTEMI by medical therapy has limited impact on mortality but leads to a reduction in subsequent infarction. At presentation, it may be difficult to differentiate myocardial infarction from unstable angina. As there is such heterogeneity of patients presenting with UA/NSTEMI, assessment of risk is central to deciding on a conservative or invasive strategy. This decision should be made on presentation of the patient to hospital. Most patients stabilize with aggressive anti-anginal therapy, but 50–60% of patients still go on to 'failure' of therapy, defined as further ischaemia at rest or on early exercise testing.

Certain characteristics indicate the likelihood of failure of medical therapy: reversible ST segment change, previous angina, prior aspirin use, family history of premature coronary disease, and age. If all of these characteristics are present, medical failure occurs in 90% of cases, compared to 38% if none are present. Current evidence suggests an early invasive strategy is associated with an improved clinical outcome in high- and intermediate-risk patients.

In unstable angina, the following parameters are adverse prognostic variables for myocardial infarction or death: age, persistent rest pain, abnormal basal ECG, e.g. ST segment depression, reduced LV function, intracoronary thrombus/

complex coronary morphology or multivessel disease, renal impairment (<60 mL/min creatinine clearance) and raised troponin I/T and/or highly sensitive C-reactive protein (CRP) levels. These parameters allow the patient to be defined as high-, intermediate-, or low-risk. Another important element in prognosis is the speed of the clinical course (relating to the short-term risk of events) and the likelihood of surviving an ischaemic event. The patient's history, the nature of symptoms, a prior history of coronary disease, age, sex, and the number of traditional risk factors present all indicate that the chest pain at presentation is likely to be due to myocardial ischaemia.

The risk associated with an acute coronary syndrome (UA/NSTEMI) may be defined, using the TIMI (Thrombolysis in Myocardial Infarction Study Group) risk score. The score allows the definition of low risk (score 0–2), intermediate risk (score 3–5), and high risk (score 6–7). A large prospective observational registry of 43,810 patients—GRACE (Global Registry of Acute Coronary Events)—has refined outcome scoring further, using eight weighted risk factors (<http://www.outcomes.org/grace>) to predict death/MI in-hospital and at 6 months (see Table 4.4). The GRACE registry has been extended to STEMI risk stratification.

Diagnosis

This is based on the clinical history, including risk factors, a 12-lead ECG, cardiac biomarkers, and coronary angiography. A diagnosis of cardiac chest pain is considered likely if the patient is male, pain radiates to the neck or left arm, there is nausea/sweating, or the patient has a history of previous MI, angina, percutaneous coronary intervention (PCI), or coronary artery bypass grafting (CABG). These features are particularly relevant if the patient has a normal ECG.

ECG

The 12-lead ECG is the first investigation. The presence of new ST segment elevation indicates that the pain is likely to be due to acute myocardial infarction. Conversely, a completely normal ECG during pain significantly reduces the likelihood that the pain is cardiac.

Transient ST segment changes (≥0.5 mm) that develop with symptoms at rest and resolve with the resolution of symptoms strongly suggest ischaemia. In UA/NSTEMI presentation (i.e. excluding STEMIs), on average, 20% have ST segment depression; 26% have T wave inversion; 11% have a non-diagnostic ECG (bundle branch block, paced rhythm), and 43% have a normal initial ECG. With age less than 60 years at an odds ratio of 1.0, risk increases to 2.1 between 60 and 70 years and 2.8 for those over 70 years. The presence of heart failure increases risk by 1.9, similar to the two-fold risk of being male. The risk of death or MI at 1 year with a normal ECG, T wave inversion, ST elevation, ST depression, and both ST depression and elevation is 8%, 13%, 15%, 17%, and 25%, respectively. In UA/NSTEMI, 1-year mortality is 16.7% and 23.2% in cases with refractory ischaemia (ischaemic symptoms with ECG changes for at least 10 min despite treatment), respectively, compared to 7.6% and 11.9% with non-refractory ischaemia and 6.0% and 9.2% with no recurrent ischaemia.

Biochemical markers

The troponin complex is a sensitive and specific marker of minor myocardial damage. This complex is an integral part of the cardiac myofibril and is released, following damage to myocardium. Two components troponin I and T, released by myocardial microinfarction, are detectable. In myocardial infarction, troponin levels rise about 4 hours

Table 4.4 Risk score in ACS

GRACE score (score 1)

- Age
- Heart rate
- Systolic blood pressure
- Plasma creatinine
- Killip acute heart failure class
- Cardiac arrest at admission
- ST segment deviation
- Elevated cardiac biomarkers (troponin)

Reproduced by permission of the GRACE Coordinating Center, Center for Outcomes Research, University of Massachusetts Medical School.

after the onset of chest pain in 30–50% of patients, with 100% of infarct patients being positive at 12 hours. A strong relationship exists between the peak level of plasma troponin at 12–24 hours from the onset of pain, and the extent of myocardial damage and the clinical outcome, such as death and MI over the short and medium term.

In an early trial in unstable angina, death/MI was 30% in patients with an elevated troponin (>0.2 mcg/L), compared to 2% in the remainder. In the FRISC (Fast Revascularisation during Instability in CAD) study, cardiac death or myocardial infarction occurred in 5%, 9%, and 13% of patients with a maximum troponin level of 0.06 mcg/L, 0.06–0.2 mcg/L, and >0.2 mcg/L at 12 hours, respectively. A combination of the two variables (troponin level and ST segment depression) predicted adverse outcome in 1% of low-risk, 7% of intermediate-risk, and 20% of high-risk patients.. Thus, there must be an effective assessment for all patients in terms of admission to a cardiology ward and to an early invasive strategy when troponin levels are raised. Troponin-positive patients have most to gain from specific antiplatelet therapies.

Management of acute chest pain

On admission, the history, examination, 12-lead ECG, and cardiac markers assign the patient to one of four categories (ACC/AHA guidelines):

- Non-cardiac pain,
- Chronic stable angina,
- Possible unstable angina (a recent episode of chest pain at rest not entirely typical of ischaemia, but pain-free when initially evaluated, with a normal ECG and a negative troponin level), and
- Definite unstable angina (recent episode of ischaemic chest discomfort that is either new-onset or severe or exhibits an accelerating pattern, particularly if at rest or within 2 weeks of MI, even if the ECG and troponin levels are initially normal).

The goal from the initial assessment in a monitored environment is to decide whether ischaemia is present or absent and to characterize it as unstable angina or non-ST elevation myocardial infarction. The subsequent management plan should be defined within a period of 6–12 hours. Patients with definite or possible acute coronary syndrome, but with a normal ECG and negative cardiac biomarkers (e.g. UA), should be observed in a monitored environment where repeat ECG and blood tests can be obtained 6–12 hours later. If normal, i.e. low-risk, an exercise stress test or stress myocardial imaging should be performed, either as an inpatient or early after discharge as an outpatient. Patients with a possible acute coronary syndrome and negative cardiac markers who cannot exercise or who have resting ECG abnormalities should have a pharmacological stress test.

Patients with definite acute coronary syndrome and ongoing pain, new ST segment change, new deep T wave inversion, haemodynamic abnormalities, or a positive stress test should be admitted to a cardiology unit for invasive management. Patients with an acute coronary syndrome who develop ST segment elevation should go for immediate reperfusion therapy, i.e. percutaneous coronary intervention where available.

Once patients are admitted to a cardiology unit, if they are pain-free, with unchanged or normal ECGs, and haemodynamically stable with normal cardiac markers, the need to make a definitive diagnosis may still be present. Further symptoms despite therapy, ECG changes, and a rise in troponin/CK-MB levels or haemodynamic decompensation will require early angiography, based on increasing risk.

Initial management of UA/NSTEMI

- Bed rest, with the option for continuous ECG monitoring by telemetry.
- Glyceryl trinitrate (GTN), initially sublingual, followed by intravenous therapy for the relief of symptoms if no hypotension is present. Also effective for treatment of pulmonary oedema.
- Opiate analgesia where symptoms are not quickly relieved by GTN or where pulmonary oedema supervenes. Care regarding dosing is important in patients with hypotension.
- Early beta-blockade, which may be given intravenously if the patient remains in pain, followed by oral therapy.
- Non-dihydropyridine calcium channel blockade, e.g. verapamil or diltiazem, when beta-blockade is contraindicated.
- Aggressive antiplatelet therapy with aspirin, clopidogrel, and glycoprotein IIb/IIIa receptor inhibition, as appropriate.
- Anti-thrombotic therapy, such as fondaparinux or enoxaparin.

It is imperative that a decision is made regarding the need for early coronary angiography and intervention. In patients with severe continuing ischaemia or frequent ischaemia, despite intensive medical therapy or haemodynamic instability, intra-aortic balloon counterpulsation may be used before or after coronary angiography.

Drug therapy
Anti-ischaemic therapy
The aim of oral and intravenous anti-anginal therapy is to reduce myocardial oxygen demand and improve symptoms.

Nitrates are used to reduce chest pain in unstable patients through a reduction in myocardial oxygen demand (preload and afterload reduction). In addition, nitrates increase coronary collateral blood flow and reduce coronary vasoconstriction. They are of no prognostic benefit. If sublingual nitrate fails to relieve symptoms completely, the patient should receive intravenous therapy, either GTN starting at a dose of 10 mcg/min (0.6 mg/h), increasing every 20–30 min to a maximum dose of 4 mg/h, or isosorbide dinitrate (ISDN) at a starting dose of 1 mg/h to a maximum of 10 mg/h. The aim should be to relieve symptoms, with a reduction of the mean arterial pressure by 10%. This therapy tends to lose effect within 24 hours, as tolerance develops.

Beta-blockers reduce myocardial oxygen demand effectively, and, although no individual study has demonstrated prognostic benefit in unstable angina, meta-analysis suggests a reduction in MI rate of 13%. Although it is recommended

that intravenous metoprolol is given in 5 mg increments every 5 min, up to 15 min prior to oral therapy, oral beta-blockade with atenolol or bisoprolol is the standard. It is important to monitor for hypotension, the development of acute heart failure, or bronchospasm.

Calcium channel blockers are used to control ischaemia-related symptoms in patients receiving adequate doses of beta-blockade and nitrate, or patients intolerant of either of these drugs, and patients with variant angina. Diltiazem or the dihydropyridine calcium channel blockers (nifedipine, nicardipine) may be added to beta-blockers as additional anti-anginal medication. Because of the tendency to reflex tachycardia through arterial vasodilatation, nifedipine or nicardipine should not be used as monotherapy. Second-generation dihydropyridines (amlodipine, felodipine) have not been studied in unstable angina. Verapamil and diltiazem have the benefit of inhibiting the sinus node. Verapamil can be used as an alternative to beta-blockade, but the combination with beta-blocker can depress left ventricular function.

Antiplatelet therapy
Aspirin should be administered immediately on presentation with unstable symptoms and continued indefinitely. Aspirin inhibits the cyclo-oxygenase enzyme in platelets, leading to the formation of thromboxane A2, a potent stimulus to platelet activation. From a meta-analysis of antiplatelet studies, a 35% reduction in vascular events occurred over 20 months with aspirin. Aspirin is started at a dose of 300 mg in patients not already receiving aspirin, with subsequent daily dosing of 75 mg. Aspirin only inhibits one pathway of platelet activation, and platelets are also activated by adenosine diphosphate (ADP), thrombin, and collagen.

Clopidogrel is a thienopyridine derivative, which blocks ADP-mediated platelet aggregation irreversibly. The CURE (Clopidogrel in Unstable Angina to Prevent Recurrent Events) trial confirmed the additive value of clopidogrel, in addition to aspirin. Benefits occurred within 24 hours, with a 20% reduction in death/MI/CVA (primary endpoint), largely driven by a reduction in MI from 6.7% to 5.3%. This was irrespective of revascularization. Of interest, in CURE, the benefit with clopidogrel appeared to occur, in addition to any use of glycoprotein IIb/IIIa inhibitors.

Clopidogrel is given as a 600 mg loading dose, then 75 mg daily for a median of 9 months after UA/NSTEMI presentation. The Triton TIMI-38 trial confirmed that compared to clopidogrel, another theinopyridine, prasugrel, had a more predictable effect on platelet inhibition and produced better results with a greater reduction in subsequent myocardial infarction, particularly in the diabetes subgroup. Most recently, the PLATO trial compared ticagrelor with clopidogrel and demonstrated a mortality benefit (i.e. death from vascular causes, myocardial infarction, and stroke reduced by 16%) with ticagrelor 90 mg bd over a period of 1-year follow-up with an increase in non-procedure-related bleeding.

Potent inhibition of the final pathway of platelet activation/aggregation can be achieved using the **glycoprotein IIb/IIIa inhibitors (GPIs)**. There is considerable data on the use of the chimeric antibody fragment abciximab and the synthetic small molecules tirofiban and eptifibatide. These agents are used in advance of, and during, PCI and in patients with high-risk UA/NSTEMI, with dose adjustment for patients with renal failure. Data from several trials, including CAPTURE, PRISM-Plus, and ESPRIT, have established GPIs in UA/NSTEMI management, with a potential reduction in 30-day mortality of 12%. The AHA/ACC recommends that a GPI should be given if coronary angiography and PCI are planned in NSTEMI, although, in practice, GPIs are focused particularly on troponin-positive high-risk patients.

In a meta-analysis of randomized trials designed to study the clinical efficacy and safety of GPIs in patients with UA/NSTEMI not routinely scheduled to undergo early coronary revascularization at 30 days, a 9% reduction in the odds of death or myocardial infarction was seen with GPIs, compared with placebo or control. Current data suggest GPI therapy may be considered in patients early after admission and especially in high-risk groups and then continued until a decision about early coronary revascularization has been made. Their use is contraindicated in patients with recent or active bleeding, severe hypertension, any haemorrhagic stroke or recent stroke within 2 years, and in thrombocytopenia.

Anti-thrombotic therapy
Enoxaparin, a low molecular weight heparin, is now routinely used in patients with UA/NSTEMI. Most recently, however, LMWH has been replaced by fondaparinux, a synthetic pentasaccharide which, unlike direct factor Xa inhibitors, mediates its effects indirectly through antithrombin III but, unlike heparin, is selective for factor Xa. OASIS-5 (Organization to Assess Strategies for Ischaemic Syndrome) compared subcutaneous fondaparinux (2.5 mg daily) or enoxaparin (1 mg/kg twice daily) for a mean of 6 days and evaluated death, myocardial infarction, or refractory ischaemia at 9 days (primary outcome) and 6 months. The primary outcome events were similar, although there was a trend towards better outcome in the fondaparinux group. However, the rate of major bleeding at 9 days was 52% lower with fondaparinux than with enoxaparin. Fondaparinux was associated with a significantly reduced mortality at 30 days.

Statins
Statin therapy is well established in the primary prevention of coronary heart disease and in the secondary prevention of further events in patients with angina and previous unstable angina or infarction. There is evidence to support their role as adjunctive therapy in acute coronary syndromes. The rationale is based on their pleiotropic effects, such as a positive effect on endothelial function, a reduction in platelet aggregability, and an anti-inflammatory effect, manifest as a reduction in the CRP. Recent studies using atorvastatin have shown mortality reduction when used in patients with acute coronary syndromes.

Revascularization strategy
Invasive coronary angiography, leading on to percutaneous coronary intervention (PCI), has become the dominant treatment for UA/NSTEMI. The adjunctive use of intracoronary stents and glycoprotein IIb/IIIa receptor antagonists has diminished the procedural risk and improved the outcome associated with PCI. The in-hospital mortality is now less than 1%, with indicators of infarction risk well-defined in clinical and angiographic terms.

Historically, in UA/NSTEMI, coronary artery bypass grafting (CABG) has an operative mortality of up to 4%, with predictors of risk being poor left ventricular function, the need for pre-bypass intra-aortic balloon pumping and previous CABG. There is up to a 10% incidence of perioperative myocardial infarctions and 16% incidence of a low cardiac output immediately after coronary surgery. With successful hospital discharge, the 5-year survival is 90%, with the greatest relative benefit in those with reduced left ventricular function—in patients with a left ventricular ejection fraction less than 50%, the 3-year mortality was 6.1% after surgery, compared to 17.6% in medically treated patients.

The FRagmin & Fast Revascularization during Instability in Coronary artery disease (FRISC-II) compared early invasive with a conservative strategy in patients with unstable angina. Angiography was performed within 7 days in 96% of the invasive group, compared to 10% of the conservative group. Revascularization (55% PCI, 45% CABG) was performed within 10 days in 71% of the invasive group, compared to 9% of the conservative group.

PCI was performed in FRISC-II if one or two flow-limiting lesions were identified. In the invasive group, 522 patients had intervention, with a stent rate of 61% and an abciximab usage of 10%. There was no in-hospital death. Coronary artery bypass surgery was performed if three flow-limiting lesions or left main stem disease was identified. There was an in-hospital death rate of 1.2%, with a 30-day mortality of 2.1%. The mean time to surgery was 7 days (range 5–13), compared to a mean of 28 days in the crossover group.

At 6 months, the invasive group had a 22% reduction in the composite endpoint of death/MI through a reduction in the rate of MI. Furthermore, there was a reduction in readmission rate by 44% and a 36% reduction in the presence of angina, compared to the conservative group. At 12 months, this effect was sustained, with a reduction in readmission rates and a 70% reduction in the need for further PCI (P <0.001), and an 80% reduction in CABG (P <0.001). The primary endpoint of death or MI was reduced by 38% in the invasive group. Invasive treatment was of greatest advantage in the elderly, men, longer duration of angina, chest pain at rest, and ST segment depression, consistent with the recent AHA/ACC guidelines on the management of unstable angina.

In TACTICS-TIMI (Treat Angina with aggrastat and determine the Cost of Therapy with Invasive or Conservative Strategy - Thrombolysis In Myocardial Infarction) studies, patients with UA/NSTEMI were all treated with aspirin, heparin, and the glycoprotein IIb/IIIa inhibitor tirofiban. They were randomly assigned to an early invasive strategy, which included routine catheterization within 4 to 48 hours and revascularization as appropriate, or to a more conservative (selectively invasive) strategy. At 6 months, death/MI/repeat hospitalization was 15.9% with use of the early invasive strategy and 19.4% with use of the conservative strategy (odds ratio 0.78; 95% confidence interval 0.62–0.97; P = 0.025). The rate of death or non-fatal myocardial infarction at 6 months was similarly reduced (7.3% vs 9.5%; odds ratio 0.74; 95% confidence interval 0.54–1.00; P <0.05). These data support a policy involving broader use of the early inhibition of glycoprotein IIb/IIIa in combination with an early invasive strategy in such patients.

In the RITA-3 (Randomized Intervention Trial of unstable Angina) trial (median of 5 years' follow-up), 16.6% of patients with intervention treatment and 20.0% with conservative treatment died or had non-fatal myocardial infarction, with a similar benefit for cardiovascular death or myocardial infarction. The benefits of an intervention strategy were mainly seen in patients at high risk of death or myocardial infarction (P = 0.004).

Invasive management of UA/NSTEMI patients is the standard for many patients; however, the timing is equally important. Recent data suggest that the greatest benefit occurs with PCI without delay, particularly in high-risk patients.

Specific clinical situations

- Diabetes mellitus. Diabetes is an independent risk factor for coronary events and is an important part of the initial risk stratification of patients. Diabetics have more extensive disease, more unstable lesions, other comorbidities, and less favourable results from revascularization, especially PCI. Should these patients undergo PCI, benefit is seen with abciximab.

- Post-CABG patients. These patients account for 20% of unstable patients and are at a higher risk, with more extensive disease and left ventricular dysfunction. Saphenous vein graft degeneration increases over time and is the highest risk substrate for PCI in grafts older than 5 years.
- Elderly patients. This group has more atypical presentations, more comorbidities, less definitive ECG stress tests, and variable responses to drug therapy. Outcomes from revascularization are less good, but PCI may be a reasonable strategy, even in diffuse disease, given the lower morbidity/mortality, compared to CABG. The general medical and mental status of the patient, as well as anticipated life expectancy, should be considered when planning treatment.
- Variant angina. This is a specific form of unstable angina, characterized by transient ST segment elevation caused by focal coronary artery spasm at the site of significant endothelial dysfunction and hypersensitivity. It is important to differentiate this clinical presentation from the early stages of acute myocardial infarction due to plaque rupture that is far more common. Coronary spasm responds to sublingual nitrates, long-acting nitrates, and calcium channel blockade, and the latter should be given at high doses, e.g. verapamil 480 mg/day or nifedipine 120 mg/day, as maintenance therapy. Coronary angiography is indicated in patients with episodic chest pain and ST segment elevation. In such patients, where a non-obstructive lesion is demonstrated, provocative testing, e.g. with ergometrine (INN) or acetylcholine, is appropriate.

Post-discharge care

Patients admitted with UA/NSTEMI require follow-up determined by their initial risk and mode of therapy. Low-risk patients treated medically and revascularized patients should be reviewed within 6 weeks. Patients treated conservatively who subsequently develop unstable symptoms or significant stable symptoms of angina on exercise (<400 m) should have immediate coronary angiography.

All patients with clinical or echocardiographic evidence of left ventricular dysfunction should receive an ACE inhibitor. All appropriate risk factors, such as LDL cholesterol level, hypertension, and hyperglycaemia in diabetics, weight, and smoking habit should be modified, according to guidelines.

Further reading

Antman EM, Cohen M, Bernink PJ, et al. (2000). The TIMI risk score for unstable angina/non-ST elevation MI: a method for prognostication and therapeutic decision-making. *JAMA*, **284**, 835–42.

Boersma E, Harrington RA, Moliterno DJ, et al. (2002). Platelet glycoprotein IIb/IIIa inhibitors in acute coronary syndromes: a meta-analysis of all major randomised clinical trials. *Lancet*, **359**, 189–98.

Cannon CP, Weintraub WS, Demopoulos LA, et al. (2001). Comparison of early invasive and conservative strategies in patients with unstable coronary syndromes treated with the glycoprotein IIb/IIIa inhibitor tirofiban. *New England Journal of Medicine*, **344**, 1879–87.

Carruthers KF, Dabbous OH, Flather MD, et al. (2005). Contemporary management of acute coronary syndromes: does the practice match the evidence? *Heart*, **91**, 290–8.

Collinson J, Flather MD, Fox KA, et al. (2000). Clinical outcomes, risk stratification and practice patterns of unstable angina and myocardial infarction without ST elevation: Prospective Registry of Acute Ischaemic Syndromes in the UK (PRAIS-UK). *European Heart Journal*, **21**, 1450–7.

ESC/EACTS Guidelines on myocardial revascularization (2014). The Task Force on Myocardial Revascularization of the European Society of Cardiology and the European Association for Cardio-Thoracic Surgery. *European Heart Journal*, **35**, 2541–2691.

Fox KAA, Dabbous OH, Goldberg RJ, et al. (2006). Prediction of risk of death and myocardial infarction in the six months after presentation with acute coronary syndrome: prospective multinational observational study (GRACE). *BMJ*, **333**, 1091–4.

Fox KAA, Poole-Wilson P, Clayton TC, et al. (2005). 5-year outcome of an interventional strategy in non-ST-elevation acute coronary syndrome: the British Heart Foundation RITA 3 randomised trial. *Lancet*, **366**, 914–20.

Lindahl B, Andrén B, Ohlsson J, Venge P, Wallentin L and the FRISC study group (1997). Risk stratification in unstable coronary artery disease: additive value of troponin T determinations and predischarge exercise tests. *European Heart Journal*, **18**, 762–70.

Mehta SR, Granger CB, Boden WE, et al. (2009). Early versus delayed invasive intervention in acute coronary syndromes. *New England Journal of Medicine*, **360**, 2165–75.

National Institute for Health and Clinical Excellence (2014). Acute coronary syndromes (including myocardial infarction). Quality standard 68. <http://www.nice.org.uk/guidance/qs68/resources/guidance-acute-coronary-syndromes-including-myocardial-infarction-pdf>.

Peterson ED, Pollack CV Jr, Roe MT, et al. (2003). Early use of glycoprotein IIb/IIIa inhibitors in non-ST-elevation acute myocardial infarction: observations from the National Registry of Myocardial Infarction 4. *Journal of the American College of Cardiology*, **42**, 45–53.

Pursnani S, Korley F, Gopaul R, et al. (2012). Percutaneous coronary intervention versus optimal medical therapy in stable coronary artery disease: a systematic review and meta-analysis of randomized clinical trials. *Circulation: Cardiovascular Interventions*, **5**, 476–90.

The Platelet Receptor Inhibition in Ischemic Syndrome Management in Patients Limited by Unstable Signs and Symptoms (PRISM-PLUS) Study Investigators (1998). Inhibition of the platelet glycoprotein IIb/IIIa receptor with tirofiban in unstable angina and non-Q-wave myocardial infarction. *New England Journal of Medicine*, **338**, 1488–97.

Stone PH, Thompson B, Zaret BL, et al. (1999). Factors associated with failure of medical therapy in patients with unstable angina and non-Q wave myocardial infarction: a TIMI-IIIB database study. *European Heart Journal*, **20**, 1084–93.

Wallentin L, Lagerqvist B, Husted S, Kontny F, Ståhle E, Swahn E (2000). Outcome at 1 year after an invasive compared with a non-invasive strategy in unstable coronary-artery disease: the FRISC II invasive randomised trial. FRISC II Investigators. Fast Revascularisation during Instability in Coronary artery disease. *Lancet*, **356**, 9–16.

Wallentin, L, Becker RC, Budaj A,Cannon CP, Emanuelsson H, Held C, et al. for the PLATO Investigators (2009). Ticagrelor versus clopidogrel in patients with acute coronary syndromes. *New England Journal of Medicine*, **361**, 1045–1057.

Wiviott SD, Braunwald E, McCabe CH, Montalescot G, Ruzyllo W, Gottlieb S, et al. for the Triton TIMI-38 investigators (2007). Prasugrel versus clopidogrel in patients with acute coronary syndromes. *New England Journal of Medicine*, **357**, 2001–15.

Yusuf S, Mehta SR, Chrolavicius S, et al. (2006). Comparison of fondaparinux and enoxaparin in acute coronary syndromes (OASIS-5). *New England Journal of Medicine*, **354**, 1464–76.

Yusuf S, Zhao F, Mehta SR, et al. (2001). Effects of clopidogrel in addition to aspirin in patients with acute coronary syndromes without ST-segment elevation. *New England Journal of Medicine*, **345**, 494–502.

ST segment elevation myocardial infarction

Epidemiology
Coronary heart disease mortality data for 2006 estimated that there were 87,000 heart attacks in men per annum and 59,000 in women, giving a total of 146,000 cases annually in the UK. The World Health Organization MONICA (monitoring trends and determinants in cardiovascular disease) project collected data on the incidence of heart attack in 35 populations in 21 countries. Results showed that incidence rates in the two UK populations included in the study, Belfast and Glasgow, were among the highest in the world, particularly in women. The case fatality rate of myocardial infarction was 50%, with half of the deaths occurring within the first 2 hours. Although this has changed little over time, the mortality for diagnosis to in-hospital management has steadily diminished from as high as 30% prior to coronary care units in the 1960s to 4–6% in the current era due to prompt ambulance response times, thrombolysis, antiplatelet strategies, and, most recently, primary (immediate) percutaneous coronary intervention (PCI).

Definitions
The term ST segment elevation myocardial infarction (STEMI) is used to describe the clinical presentation of a patient with characteristic ECG changes in the context of an acute coronary occlusion. Although the term acute coronary syndrome (ACS) is an umbrella term for the triad of clinical presentations (a history compatible with coronary artery disease), electrocardiographic (ECG) changes, and biochemical cardiac markers, STEMI is usually considered as a separate clinical entity from NSTEMI and unstable angina due to its acute nature and demands a different clinical approach from the management of other causes of ACS.

In STEMI (formerly known as transmural or Q wave myocardial infarction (MI)), the diagnosis is defined by the presence of ≥1 mm ST elevation in at least two adjacent limb leads, ≥2 mm ST elevation in at least two contiguous precordial leads, or new-onset bundle branch block (usually left). The diagnosis is confirmed with the measurement of cardiac enzymes, such as creatine kinase (CK), and specifically its MB isoform (CK-MB) or troponin I/T within 3–4 hours of the index event, with peak values occurring at 12 hours from the onset of chest pain.

Pathophysiology
Most STEMIs occur due to coronary atherosclerotic plaque rupture, with complete occlusion of an epicardial coronary artery. This occurs in so-called vulnerable plaques which may not necessarily be severe or flow-limiting and hence can be the first clinical manifestation of coronary artery disease and may be associated with sudden cardiac death. Vascular inflammation is an important driver for the development of a vulnerable plaque(s). Increased cellular and enzymatic activity in the intimal plaque leads to the development of a lipid-rich pool below a thin fibrous cap at the luminal surface. This thin fibrous cap is susceptible to shear stress within the vessel which can increase at times of increased beta-adrenergic stimulation. This, along with increased hypercoagulability and platelet activity in the early hours of the day may explain the higher incidence of STEMI at this time, as well as during physical and emotional stress. Following exposure of tissue factor and subintimal collagen to blood, an acute thrombus develops at the site of plaque rupture, driven by platelet activation. This leads to thrombin formation and the production of fibrin strands which bind the platelet-rich thrombus together. Once there is complete occlusion, with inadequate collateral supply, myocardial necrosis starts within 15 minutes, spreading from the subendocardium to the subepicardium. At the time of thrombosis, there is associated coronary vasospasm, with activation of the endogenous fibrinolytic system, such that, at the time of initial angiography, up to 30% of vessels have reopened with restoration of coronary flow.

Diagnosis and immediate assessment
A well-functioning and integrated regional system of care, based on pre-hospital diagnosis by paramedics, with immediate triage to the most appropriate facility to deliver (primary) PCI is now the key to the success of treatment.

The diagnosis is based on the clinical history of sudden onset of central chest discomfort, usually lasting at least 30 minutes, associated with characteristic 12-lead ECG changes. The chest pain may radiate to the neck and jaw or left arm; there is usually a sensation of nausea (which may lead to vomiting) and sweating. The patient may have a history of previous MI, angina, PCI, or coronary artery bypass graft (CABG). On occasion, the pain may be epigastric or interscapular. In the elderly population, the presence of chest pain may be less prevalent, with symptoms of acute dyspnoea, fatigue, or collapse as the initial presentation. In an STEMI which affects a significant area of myocardium, the patient will show signs of reduced cardiac output or haemodynamic instability, such as pallor, cold extremities, and possible cerebral hypoperfusion. The treatment for STEMI is time-critical and requires immediate clinical assessment.

In the early hours of infarction, the 12-lead ECG may be equivocal with non-specific changes. It is important to repeat the ECG and compare it with previous records, if possible, particularly in the context of a stuttering presentation. Additional posterior or right chest leads should be considered to exclude or confirm a true posterior or right ventricular infarction. Continuous ECG monitoring should be initiated to detect significant dysrhythmias. Two-dimensional echocardiography can be used where the clinical diagnosis is uncertain, as a regional wall motion abnormality will be detected with major myocardial injury, although the presence of previous infarction or significant reversible ischaemia limits diagnostic interpretation. Importantly, normal biventricular function excludes significant myocardial infarction and suggests a different cause for the acute chest pain.

For risk stratification, the GRACE STEMI (see Table 4.4) score is currently the most accurate method for assessment, with increasing age, higher Killip class score (indicating left ventricular failure), tachycardia, hypotension, and anterior wall infarction having the highest predictive accuracy for early mortality.

Acute management of STEMI
Immediate care
At first medical contact with the diagnosis of STEMI, stabilization of the patient along with pain relief is a priority. Relief of pain and anxiety dampens the increased sympathetic nervous system activation which drives tachycardia and systolic/diastolic blood pressure and may place an increased workload on the heart. Intravenous opiate analgesia should be given, along with antiemetic medication. Opioids can

contribute to hypotension and respiratory depression and should be administered with care and monitoring of vital signs. Supplemental oxygen (by nasal prongs or mask) should be given in patients who are breathless or hypoxaemic, or have heart failure or cardiogenic shock.

A proportion of patients do not survive the initial presentation of a myocardial infarction due to ventricular fibrillation and cardiac arrest. It is imperative to respond quickly to haemodynamically significant ventricular tachydysrhythmias with defibrillation. Patients are more likely to receive appropriate evidence-based therapies when treated by cardiologists than by general physicians. It is unclear whether this benefit is attributable to the specialist physician in isolation or reflects the overall care and treatment of patients within a specialist cardiology service. A systematic review suggests that this increase in evidence-based therapy is associated with improved clinical outcomes, including mortality.

Reperfusion therapy

The indications for reperfusion therapy are based primarily upon the meta-analysis of the Fibrinolytic Therapy Trialists' Collaboration (FTTC group). They reported that electrocardiographic predictors of mortality that benefit from fibrinolytic therapy were the presence of ST segment elevation or new-onset bundle branch block. They did not distinguish between left and right bundle branch block, although several guidelines and trials specifically stipulate left bundle branch block only. Importantly, registry data of acute myocardial infarction show that right bundle branch block is as common as, and has a higher mortality than, left bundle branch block.

Primary PCI

A comprehensive systematic review and meta-analysis of randomized controlled trial data have shown that primary PCI is superior to thrombolysis for the treatment of patients with STEMI. Compared with thrombolysis, primary PCI reduces short- and long-term mortality, stroke, reinfarction, recurrent ischaemia, and the need for CABG surgery as well as the combined endpoint of death or non-fatal reinfarction. This benefit was consistent across all patient subgroups and independent of the thrombolytic agent used. The greatest benefit was in patients treated within 12 hours of symptom onset. After 12 hours of the index event, there is no firm consensus regarding the benefit of PCI in the absence of ongoing ischaemia, infarction, or shock. All patients in cardiogenic shock should undergo immediate PCI, with intervention to all significant lesions.

The benefit of primary PCI over thrombolysis is time-dependent. The difference between the delivery of the two reperfusion therapies is described as the 'PCI-related delay'.

The European Society of Cardiology (ESC) Guidelines recommend that patients should be taken to a PCI-capable hospital (with a 24-hour/7-day service), where possible, and that the time from first medical contact to balloon inflation should be within 90 minutes and within 2 hours of symptoms, or within 2 hours in all-comers. If PCI is not possible within 2 hours of symptoms, then patients should receive intravenous thrombolysis, ideally pre-hospital.

Thrombolysis

Prior to primary PCI, the evidence for intravenous thrombolysis was well established, with 30 early lives saved per 1,000 patients treated and 20 lives saved per 1,000 patients at 7–12 hours. The benefit of thrombolysis is directly time-related and most effective within 2 hours of symptom onset which has encouraged pre-hospital thrombolysis. It is likely that there is no mortality benefit comparing very early thrombolysis with primary PCI, although the latter is a more cost-effective strategy with a reduction in subsequent MI, need for intervention and stroke, and re-hospitalization.

Thrombolysis is associated with a small, but significant, increase in stroke (1%), with most strokes being haemorrhagic and within 24 hours. There is an excess of non-cerebral bleeding that is mainly procedure-related. Fibrin-specific thrombolytics are the therapy of choice, e.g. accelerated tissue plasminogen activator (tPA) or weight-adjusted TNK-tPA (tenecteplase) which is associated with equivalent mortality benefit but fewer strokes, compared to tPA, and, as a single bolus, is preferable, particularly pre-hospital. Absolute contraindications to thrombolysis are:

- Any previous haemorrhagic stroke or stroke of uncertain origin.
- Ischaemic stroke within the last 6 months.
- Major surgery.
- Head injury with in the last 3 weeks.
- Gastrointestinal bleeding within 4 weeks.
- Bleeding diathesis and aortic dissection.

Because of the prothrombotic state which occurs after fibrinolysis, anticoagulation should be given for the duration of in-hospital stay, with evidence of a reduction in reinfarction after fibrin-specific agents. Anticoagulation regimens include intravenous heparin 60 U/kg bolus, then 12 U/kg (up to 1000 U/h) for up to 48 hours or enoxaparin 30 mg intravenous bolus, followed by 1 mg/kg subcutaneously given every 12 hours, adjusted for age and renal function or fondaparinux 2.5 mg intravenous bolus, followed by 2.5 mg subcutaneously daily, adjusted for severe renal impairment.

Angiography during initial hospital admission

If thrombolysis is successful, based on resolution of ST segment elevation, resolution of chest pain or perfusion dysrhythmia, early angiography is recommended within 3–24 hours. This is to avoid the immediate prothrombotic period after treatment and to prevent early re-occlusion.

In asymptomatic STEMI patients presenting at 12–48 hours from symptom onset, PCI is associated with an increase in myocardial salvage (but not early clinical outcome benefits).

Rescue PCI

Rescue PCI describes intervention in patients who have not undergone successful reperfusion with thrombolysis. This is defined as <50% resolution in the highest ST segments at initial presentation at 90 minutes from intravenous treatment. In the REACT trial (n = 427), a strategy of rescue PCI within 12 hours of symptom onset was shown to be associated with a higher event-free survival than repeat thrombolysis or no treatment.

Aspirin

All patients with STEMI should receive standard oral aspirin (150–325 mg) which should be chewed (although the taste may not be pleasant), unless the patient has known hypersensitivity or has active gastrointestinal bleeding. When given within the first 12 hours of acute myocardial infarction, aspirin reduces the combined endpoint of death, reinfarction, or stroke—an absolute risk reduction (ARR) of 4%, a relative risk reduction (RRR) of 28%. It should be continued at a dose of 75 mg daily.

Clopidogrel

The CLARITY-TIMI 28 (clopidogrel 300 mg stat and 75 mg daily) and COMMIT/CCS (n = 45,852; clopidogrel 75 mg daily) trials demonstrated an increased patency rate of the infarct-related artery and reduced mortality when comparing combination aspirin and clopidogrel therapy with aspirin alone in patients with STEMI (with thrombolysis as the reperfusion therapy). In CLARITY, the composite endpoint of cardiovascular death, recurrent MI, or urgent revascularization at 30 days was reduced by 20%. In patients undergoing primary PCI, clopidogrel 600 mg should be given at first medical contact to achieve maximum platelet inhibition, with a dose of 75 mg daily for a finite period.

Glycoprotein IIb/IIIa receptor inhibitors
These agents block the final common pathway of platelet aggregation. Most studies in STEMI have used abciximab, rather than the small molecule inhibitors tirofiban and eptifibatide. Systematic reviews of intravenous abciximab, delivered periprocedurally to STEMI patients with aspirin and heparin, is associated with a 32% reduction in 30-day mortality, with no excess in bleeding. In general, all patients undergoing primary PCI should receive a glycoprotein IIb/IIIa receptor inhibitor both during and after the procedure.

Antithrombotic drug therapy (primary PCI)
Unfractionated heparin is given to patients undergoing PCI at a dose of 60–100 U/kg, the dose dependent on whether or not the patient is also receiving a glycoprotein receptor inhibitor (GPI). Bivalirudin, a direct thrombin inhibitor, has been used with provisional GPI, in comparison to a GPI/heparin combination, and this appears to give additional benefits.

Antithrombotic drug therapy (post-thrombolysis)
The use of the low molecular weight heparin (LMWH) enoxaparin for up to 7 days after tenecteplase is associated with a reduction in reinfarction and refractory ischaemia, compared with heparin. Given pre-hospital, however, it was associated with an excess of intracranial haemorrhage in the elderly which led to a lower dose being used in patients over 75 years and those with renal impairment. In OASIS-6, the synthetic anti-factor Xa drug fondaparinux was also associated with reduced mortality and reinfarction, compared to heparin.

Antithrombotic drug therapy (no reperfusion therapy)
In patients who present 12 hours after STEMI where immediate reperfusion therapy is not mandated, aspirin, clopidogrel, and antithrombotic therapy (LMWH or fondaparinux) should be administered. All such patients should undergo coronary angiography prior to discharge.

Beta-blockers
Prior to the development of reperfusion therapy for STEMI, beta-blockers were used in the immediate care of STEMI. The ISIS-1 trial described an early (7-day) benefit in cardiovascular mortality of intravenous beta-blocker therapy in patients with myocardial infarction, with a 15% relative risk reduction (0.68% ARR). These benefits were of borderline significance and appeared to be mediated through a reduction in cardiac rupture. This trial is, therefore, only of relevance in patients not undergoing reperfusion therapy. More recently, the COMMIT/CCS trial (n = 45,852 STEMIs receiving thrombolysis) demonstrated no benefits from beta-blockade (immediate intravenous metoprolol 5–15 mg, followed by oral metoprolol 100 mg bd) on death or the combined endpoint of death, reinfarction, or cardiac arrest.

In summary, there is no robust evidence in the modern era for the routine use of intravenous beta-blockade in STEMI. Any potential benefit from oral beta-blockade is likely to occur in patients with significant myocardial injury from STEMI.

Angiotensin-converting enzyme inhibitors/angiotensin receptor blockers
ACE inhibitors should be given to patients with a left ventricular ejection fraction <40% or who have heart failure in the early phase of STEMI (GISSI-3, ISIS-4). A small mortality benefit has been shown in the first 6 weeks post-event when started within the first 24 hours of the STEMI in the absence of contraindications, such as hypotension.

Based on current data, there is no indication for the routine use of calcium channel blockers, oral nitrates, intravenous magnesium, or glucose-insulin infusion post-STEMI with regard to survival benefit.

Management of pump failure/shock
Heart failure is usually due to myocardial damage but may also be caused by valvular dysfunction (acute mitral regurgitation), ventricular septal defect (VSD), or dysrhythmia. It is associated with a poorer prognosis, related to the Killip classification[1]:
- Class 1: no basal lung crepitations or added heart sounds.
- Class 2: pulmonary congestion, with crepitations over <50% of the lung fields or a third heart sound.
- Class 3: pulmonary oedema, with crepitations over >50% of the lung fields.
- Class 4: cardiogenic shock.

The most important diagnostic tool is echocardiography which allows the immediate assessment of myocardial and valvular function and the demonstration of an acquired VSD. A variable degree of non-functioning or poorly functioning myocardium at echocardiography may be stunned but still viable with the potential for recovery after the acute insult. The extent of viable and non-viable myocardium may be assessed by cardiac magnetic resonance imaging (MRI) once the patient is haemodynamically stable.

Killip class 2
All patients should receive supplemental oxygen, with pulse oximetry monitoring. In the absence of hypotension, intravenous GTN (0.25 mcg/kg/min) should be given and titrated against the blood pressure, with intermittent intravenous use of loop diuretic, as required. An ACE inhibitor or angiotensin receptor blocker should be considered within the first 24 hours in the absence of hypovolaemia or renal impairment.

Killip class 3
In addition to oxygen and regular monitoring of blood gases, if needed, continuous positive airways pressure (CPAP) should be instituted. If CPAP fails or the patient is demonstrating respiratory exhaustion, intubation and mechanical ventilation should be considered. If blood pressure permits, intravenous GTN should be used and titrated to avoid dropping the systolic blood pressure below 100 mmHg. The vogue for additional inotropic support has diminished with the routine use of invasive mechanical support (see next paragraph), but both intravenous dobutamine (5–20 mcg/kg/min) and dopamine (5–15 mcg/kg/min) may be considered in patients with hypotension and renal hypoperfusion.

Killip class 4
Cardiogenic shock is defined as tissue hypoperfusion occurring through pump failure with a systolic blood pressure

---

[1]Reprinted from The American Journal of Cardiology, 20, 4, Killip T and Kimball JT, 'Treatment of myocardial infarction in a coronary care unit: A Two year experience with 250 patients', pp. 457–464, Copyright 1967, with permission from Elsevier.

<90 mmHg and a pulmonary capillary wedge pressure >20 mmHg, or a cardiac index (CI) <1.8 L/min/m². It is also implied when inotropes and/or mechanical support are required to maintain an SBP >90 mmHg or a CI >1.8 L/min/m². The diagnosis is based on extensive left ventricular injury, in the absence of hypovolaemia, electrolyte imbalance, tamponade, or dysrhythmia, but may be contributed to by acute mitral regurgitation or VSD or significant right ventricular infarction in its own right.

The primary management strategy is the insertion of an intra-aortic balloon counterpulsation pump (IABP) by the femoral route, with additional support of inotropic drugs to maintain a CI >2 L/min/m². To optimize left ventricular filling (particularly in the context of right ventricular infarction), an intrapulmonary balloon catheter may be used to maintain a left ventricular filling pressure of at least 15 mmHg. If post-primary or rescue PCI has not taken place, urgent revascularization should be considered, including coronary artery bypass grafting (CABG) where appropriate. In the SHOCK trial, the in-hospital mortality of cardiogenic shock was reduced from 63% to 36% with an early revascularization strategy and maintained at follow-up. Novel cardiac support devices inserted percutaneously, such as the Impella device, which sits in the left ventricle across the aortic valve, can contribute as much as 2 L/min to the cardiac output and may improve outcome in severe cardiogenic shock until myocardial recovery can occur.

Mechanical complications

Although the majority of patients with free wall rupture die immediately, around 25% have a subacute wall rupture where the outflow of blood is sealed by pericardium or thrombus. It is associated with sudden decompensation, often with chest pain and further ST segment elevation and transient or sustained hypotension. There is often cardiac tamponade. Echocardiography confirms the diagnosis, and immediate cardiac surgery should be considered.

Acute VSD is associated with the development of a loud pansystolic murmur with clinical deterioration and is confirmed by echocardiography. The insertion of an IABP is the most effective immediate therapy, and intravenous GTN may be considered in the absence of hypotension. The timing of surgery is controversial, and surgical VSD closure is associated with a high surgical mortality. In stable patients, there has been a vogue to delay IABP support, as the ruptured myocardial tissue is very friable in acute infarction, diminishing successful early repair. Percutaneous VSD repair is available in some interventional centres but is usually reserved for patients considered too high risk for conventional surgery.

Acute mitral regurgitation may occur through papillary muscle dysfunction in inferior myocardial infarction or by rupture of the papillary muscle tip/trunk itself. In patients with significant myocardial injury and early ventricular dilatation, it can develop as a result of annular ring dilatation. Partial or complete muscle rupture usually occurs in the posteromedial muscle and is associated with sudden haemodynamic decompensation and acute pulmonary oedema, often with a low-intensity pansystolic murmur. The diagnosis is confirmed by echocardiography, and the left atrium is usually of normal size which excludes pre-existing significant regurgitation. As with acute VSD, patients benefit from IABP insertion and early cardiac surgery with valve replacement, rather than repair, the predominant strategy.

Acute rhythm management

Life-threatening dysrhythmias, such as ventricular fibrillation (VF), sustained ventricular tachycardia (VT), or complete atrioventricular block, may be the first manifestation of acute ischaemia and account for a significant number of sudden cardiac deaths during STEMI. In this setting, the dysrhythmia may be driven by continued ischaemia, pump failure, electrolyte imbalance, hypoxia, acidosis, and autonomic overactivity. The priority is to restore the patient to a haemodynamically stable rhythm and correct reversible factors.

Ventricular dysrhythmias

Ventricular fibrillation is associated with increased in-hospital mortality. The incidence of VF in the first 48 hours is reducing with optimal reperfusion therapy (primary PCI) and early beta-blockade. However, it is still important to correct hypokalaemia and hypomagnesaemia.

Non-sustained VT, lasting less than 30 seconds, or an accelerated idioventricular rhythm (heart rate <120 bpm) usually indicate successful reperfusion and are rarely associated with the development of early VF. Sustained and/or haemodynamically significant VT requires immediate DC cardioversion as a definitive strategy and prophylactic anti-dysrhythmic therapy, such as an intravenous amiodarone bolus (300 mg) followed by an infusion (900 mg over 24 hour), to reduce recurrence. In patients resistant to cardioversion on anti-dysrhythmic therapy, transvenous pacing termination of monomorphic VT should be considered.

Polymorphic VT, occurring with a normal QT interval, may be treated with intravenous amiodarone, intravenous lidocaine (0.5–0.75 mg/kg bolus), or beta-blockade (2.5–5 mg metoprolol over 2 minutes, up to three boluses; or esmolol 500 mcg/kg bolus and 50–200 mg/kg/min infusion) if left ventricular function is good. In the presence of VT with a prolonged or uncertain QT interval, consideration should be given to the immediate correction of electrolyte imbalance (particularly hypomagnesaemia) and the use of intravenous isoprenaline (0.5–2.0 mcg/kg/min) to reduce the QT interval and/or overdrive pacing.

Supraventricular dysrhythmias

Atrial fibrillation occurs in up to 20% of patients with STEMI and is common in the elderly and those with severe LV dysfunction. Although often well-tolerated and usually managed with medical therapy, when associated with haemodynamic instability or significant ischaemia, DC cardioversion and/or rate control with intravenous beta-blockade or even amiodarone should be considered. Patients in atrial fibrillation should be fully anticoagulated, given the increased risk of stroke.

Bradydysrhythmia

Sinus bradycardia can occur early after inferior STEMI and should only be treated if symptomatic or of haemodynamic significance. Atrioventricular (AV) block occurs in 7% of STEMI patients, with persistent bundle branch block occurring in 5%. It is associated with a higher in-hospital and late mortality, as it often correlates with the extent of myocardial injury. AV block associated with inferior STEMI is usually transient and associated with a narrow complex escape rhythm. When AV block occurs with anterior STEMI, it is often infranodal, with an unstable, wide QRS morphology from extensive myocardial damage. Similarly, new left bundle branch block is usually associated with extensive injury, with a high likelihood of AV block and pump failure. Although intravenous atropine (500 mcg bolus, up to 2 mg in total) may be effective in transient sinus bradycardia or in second/third degree AV block, temporary pacing is often required.

Management of infarction in specific situations

Right ventricular infarction
Infarction of the right ventricle (RVI) may manifest as cardiogenic shock, although the management is different from pump failure secondary to LV dysfunction. It is often diagnosed where the patient is hypotensive but with clear lung fields and a raised jugular venous pulse in the context of an inferior STEMI. 12-lead ECG may have Q waves, with ST segment elevation in leads V1–3 and in lead V4R. Right ventricular dysfunction may be confirmed by echocardiography. The mainstay of therapy is volume loading to maintain RV preload and avoidance of vasodilating drugs. Atrial fibrillation, which is often associated with RVI, should be corrected quickly. Prompt restoration of coronary flow by PCI in the infarct-related vessel is the optimal strategy.

Diabetes
Diabetic patients with STEMI have double the mortality of non-diabetic patients. Insulin infusion, followed by multiple-dose insulin administration, improves long-term mortality, compared to oral antidiabetic therapy. It is recommended that plasma glucose levels are kept between 5.0 and 7.8 mmol/L, taking care to avoid hypoglycaemia.

Post-STEMI management
The in-hospital management of the STEMI patient depends on the extent of myocardial injury and the general health of the patient, including comorbidities. Uncomplicated patients post-primary PCI with minor myocardial injury may go home within 48 hours, whereas those with significant infarction and/or complications may require a longer in-hospital stay.

Deep venous thrombosis
This is now a rare complication and is avoided by early ambulation and prophylactic LMWH.

Intraventricular (mural) thrombus
This is usually found at echocardiography in large anterior myocardial infarctions and mandates oral anticoagulation with warfarin for a minimum of 3 months.

Pericarditis
This is an unpredictable complication of infarction which manifests as positional or pleuritic chest pain, associated with an audible rub. It is best treated with NSAIDs. Rarely, a haemorrhagic effusion develops which requires pericardiocentesis if clinical evidence of tamponade develops.

Late ventricular dysrhythmias
Unlike ventricular dysrhythmias within the first 24–48 hours, those which occur later are associated with an increased risk of sudden death. Left ventricular dysfunction and electrolytic abnormalities should be treated aggressively. No randomized evidence exists to suggest that myocardial revascularization (if not already performed) reduces VT/VF post-STEMI. Where LV ejection fraction is <40%, implantation of an automatic cardioverter defibrillator (ICD) is associated with a reduction in mortality. Patients with haemodynamically significant sustained polymorphic VT or resuscitated VF outside the first 24–48 hours of STEMI should also undergo ICD implantation.

Sustained monomorphic VT occurs in a lower-risk subgroup where ICD therapy can be considered to avoid side effects of long-term drug therapy. Non-sustained VT does not require specific treatment unless symptomatic. With the exception of beta-blockers, anti-dysrhythmic drug therapy does not alter clinical outcome in patients after STEMI with life-threatening ventricular dysrhythmias.

Oral amiodarone in patients with NYHA class III heart failure and low ejection fraction (<35%) is harmful.

Post-infarction angina
Angina or evidence of recurrent myocardial ischaemia is an absolute indication for coronary angiography and PCI. Planned PCI in otherwise well patients 3–28 days after STEMI in the absence of symptoms, complications, or ischaemia is not indicated. In patients with extensive multivessel disease or severe left main stem stenosis, particularly with left ventricular impairment, CABG may be the best form of revascularization.

The assessment of risk
In the primary PCI era, the risk assessment for subsequent events is made easier by knowledge of the coronary anatomy with the infarct-related artery (and often other vessels) revascularized. Echocardiography is usually performed during the index admission to assess left ventricular function which helps to inform drug therapy. LDL and HDL cholesterol should be checked on admission, along with random glucose and renal function.

Regional left ventricular wall dysfunction after STEMI can be due to necrosis, stunning of viable myocardium, and subsequent hibernation of viable myocardium to accommodate a reduced myocardial blood flow. In patients with significant LV dysfunction, it is imperative to assess the extent of viability, as revascularization may stimulate recovery of viable, but hibernating, myocardium. Stunned myocardium usually recovers within 2 weeks of the initial insult. Myocardial viability can be assessed by myocardial perfusion scan, dobutamine stress echocardiography, or magnetic resonance imaging with gadolinium enhancement.

The assessment of risk for sudden cardiac death is pertinent for patients with reduced LV function (LVEF <40%) where the presence of non-sustained VT, clinical heart failure, and sustained monomorphic VT at electrophysiologcal testing indicate patients at high risk who would benefit from ICD implantation.

Rehabilitation and secondary prevention
In addition to the early revascularization of STEMI patients and appropriate drug therapy, early rehabilitation during the hospital phase is important to support a return to normal daily activities and should be continued for the weeks following the index event. An explanation of the nature of the illness, with reassurance to both the patient and the relatives, is important to reduce anxiety and the potential for depression. Appropriate advice about a graded return to exercise and a return to work, as well as lifestyle advice should be reinforced. Undertaking an exercise test as a means of reassuring the patient and encouraging them to exercise within their general level of fitness is of value in the rehabilitation process.

The following secondary prevention measures should be initiated in-hospital and continued in the community:
- **Smoking cessation.**
- **Diet and weight reduction.** The goal is to reduce body weight below 30 kg/m^2 with a diet based on low saturated fat and low salt intake. An increased consumption of oily fish to increase omega-3 fatty acid intake should be recommended.

- **Physical activity.** Meta-analysis suggests that there is a mortality benefit from regular exercise.
- **Antiplatelet therapy.** The Antiplatelet Trialists Collaboration suggested a 25% reduction in reinfarction and mortality in men using a dose of 75–325 mg daily of aspirin.
- **Beta-blockade.** In the modern era, the strongest evidence for beta-blockade post-STEMI is in patients with heart failure. The long-term use of beta-blockade is recommended in all patients post-STEMI.
- **ACE inhibitors/ARBs/aldosterone blockade.** ACE inhibitors reduce mortality in patients with an LVEF <40%, and there is a strong argument to start them in all patients with acute heart failure. The benefit is less in the presence of normal LV function. ARBs may be used as an alternative. In post-STEMI patients with an LVEF <40% and heart failure or diabetes, eplerenone is associated with a 15% relative reduction in mortality. Monitoring for hyperkalaemia is important.
- **Statin therapy.** A recent meta-analysis of intensive lipid lowering confirmed a mortality reduction of up to 25% in acute coronary syndromes, compared to standard therapy. The current LDL cholesterol treatment target 2.0 mmol/L.
- **Cardiac resynchronization therapy.** Once stunning of viable myocardium has been excluded, patients with an LVEF <35% with LV dilatation, sinus rhythm, and a wide QRS complex (>120 ms) may be considered for biventricular pacing.
- **Prophylactic ICD implantation.** ICD implantation as a primary preventative strategy can be considered in patients with an LVEF <40%, with spontaneous non-sustained VT and monomorphic VT induced at an electrophysiological study, and in patients with an LVEF <30% with a STEMI at least 40 days earlier in the presence of heart failure. The evaluation of the need for an ICD should be deferred for 3 months after revascularization to allow for myocardial recovery.

Further reading

ACCF/AHA Guideline for the Management of ST-Elevation Myocardial Infarction (2013). A Report of the American College of Cardiology Foundation/American Heart Association Task Force on Practice Guidelines. *Circulation*, **127**: e362–e425. <http://circ.ahajournals.org/content/127/4/e362.full>.

Baigent C, Collins R, Appleby P, Parish S, Sleight P, Peto R (1998). ISIS-2: 10 year survival among patients with suspected acute myocardial infarction in randomized comparison of intravenous streptokinase, oral aspirin, both, or neither. The ISIS-2 (Second International Study of Infarct Survival) Collaborative Group. *BMJ*, **316**, 1337–43.

Boersma E (2006). Does time matter? A pooled analysis of randomized clinical trials comparing primary percutaneous coronary intervention and in-hospital fibrinolysis in acute myocardial infarction patients. *European Heart Journal*, **27**, 779–88.

COMMIT collaborative group (2005). A randomized placebo-controlled trial of adding clopidogrel to aspirin in 45,852 patients with acute myocardial infarction. *Lancet*, **366**, 1607–21.

ESC/EACTS Guidelines on myocardial revascularization (2014). The Task Force on Myocardial Revascularization of the European Society of Cardiology and the European Association for Cardio-Thoracic Surgery. *European Heart Journal*, **35**, 2541–2691.

Fibrinolytic Therapy Trialists' (FTT) Collaborative Group (1994). Indications for fibrinolytic therapy in suspected acute myocardial infarction: collaborative overview of early mortality and major morbidity results from all randomized trials of more than 1000 patients. *Lancet*, **343**, 311–22.

Fox KAA, Dabbous OH, Goldberg RJ, *et al.* (2006). Prediction of risk of death and myocardial infarction in the six months after presentation with acute coronary syndrome: prospective multinational observational study (GRACE). *BMJ*, **333**, 1091–4.

Gershlick AH, Stephens-Lloyd A, Hughes S, *et al.* (2006). Rescue angioplasty after failed thrombolytic therapy for acute myocardial infarction. *New England Journal of Medicine*, **353**, 2758–68.

Go AS, Rao RK, Dauterman KW, Massie BM (2000). A systematic review of the effects of physician specialty on the treatment of coronary disease and heart failure in the United States. *American Journal of Medicine*, **108**, 216–26.

GUSTO Investigators (1993). An international randomized trial comparing four thrombolytic strategies for acute myocardial infarction. *New England Journal of Medicine*, **329**, 673–82.

Josan K, Majmudar SR, McAlister FA (2008). The efficacy and safety of intensive statin therapy: a meta-analysis of randomized trials. *Canadian Medical Association Journal*, **178**, 576–84.

Keeley EC, Boura JA, Grines CL (2003). Primary angioplasty versus intravenous thrombolysis for acute myocardial infarction; a quantitative review of 23 randomized trials. *Lancet*, **361**, 13–20.

National Institute for Health and Clinical Excellence (2013). NICE clinical guideline 167. Myocardial infarction with ST-segment elevation: The acute management of myocardial infarction with ST-segment elevation. <https://www.nice.org.uk/guidance/cg167>.

Sabatine MS, Cannon CP, Gibson CM, *et al.* (2005). Addition of clopidogrel to aspirin and fibrinolytic therapy for myocardial infarction with ST segment elevation. *New England Journal of Medicine*, **352**, 1179–89.

Steg PG, Bonnefoy E, Chabaud S, *et al.* (2003). Impact of time to treatment on mortality after pre-hospital fibrinolysis or primary angioplasty; data from the CAPTIM randomized clinical trial. *Circulation*, **108**, 2851–6.

Stone GW, Witzenbichler B, Guagliumi G, *et al.* (2008). HORIZONS-AMI Trial investigators. Bivalirudin during primary PCI in acute myocardial infarction. *New England Journal of Medicine*, **358**, 218–30.

Van't Hof AW, Ten Berg J, Heestermans T, *et al.* (2008). ONTIME2 study group. Pre-hospital initiation of tirofiban inpatients with ST segment elevation myocardial infarction undergoing primary angioplasty: a multi-centre, double-blind, randomized controlled trial. *Lancet*, **372**, 537–46.

Arrhythmias

Introduction

Arrhythmias account for 25% of cardiological problems seen in medical clinics and may occur in up to 10% of acute medical admissions. Arrhythmias are a heterogeneous collection of conditions characterized by abnormal conduction or automaticity of cardiac tissue, leading to bradycardia or tachycardia.

Clinical presentations range from benign, asymptomatic rhythm disturbances to cardiac arrest and sudden death. An understanding of arrhythmia mechanisms is the key to understanding appropriate treatments. While antiarrhythmic drug therapies have not advanced significantly in the past 20 years, major developments have occurred in the field of interventional electrophysiology, such as catheter ablation therapy and implantable cardiac defibrillators.

Several general and specific guidelines have been published. The National Institute for Health and Care Excellence (NICE, UK), European Society of Cardiology, and the American College of Cardiology/American Heart Association/Heart Rhythm Society (AHA/ACC/HRS) have all produced guidance on management of arrhythmia and implantable device therapy. There are some variations in detail, but the core recommendations are consistent and reflected in this chapter.

Investigation of suspected arrhythmia

Patients with arrhythmias may present without symptoms, where the arrhythmia is found incidentally, or with palpitation, dizziness, syncope, or cardiac arrest. Arrhythmias are often intermittent and may not be evident at the time of assessment. A 12-lead ECG may indicate the presence of structural heart disease (e.g. evidence of previous MI) or electrical disease (e.g. AV block, QT interval prolongation) but is often normal between episodes. Ambulatory ECG monitors can be used to capture the ECG during episodes and can be used continuously for up to 7 days. For less frequent episodes, a patient-activated ECG recorder may be required to establish a diagnosis. In cases of very infrequent presyncope or syncope, an implantable ECG (loop) recorder, which resembles a small pacemaker, can be used to document the cardiac rhythm for up to 3 years.

Extrasystoles

Atrial and ventricular extrasystoles are common in healthy individuals and do not require treatment. They may cause a sensation of a thump or pause in the chest. Frequent atrial extrasystoles may reflect sinoatrial disease and are associated with a risk of atrial fibrillation. Frequent ventricular extrasystoles (>50 per hour) warrant investigation, as they may be a sign of underlying ischaemic heart disease or cardiomyopathy.

Tachyarrhythmias

Tachyarrhythmias are arbitrarily defined as rhythms with a ventricular rate greater than 100 bpm. They may be asymptomatic or associated with palpitation and light-headedness and sometimes aggravate angina or heart failure symptoms in susceptible patients. Syncope often accompanies malignant ventricular arrhythmias.

Atrial fibrillation

Atrial fibrillation (AF) is the most common tachyarrhythmia encountered in clinical practice. Its prevalence increases with age, affecting 1.5% of individuals aged over 60 years

and 8% of those aged over 80 years. Atrial fibrillation is important to diagnose and treat, as it affects effort tolerance and has a recognized risk of stroke and other thromboembolic events.

Pathophysiology

Atrial fibrillation is characterized by a complex set of electrophysiological disturbances within the atria, including rapid automatic firing, multiple interacting re-entry circuits, and autonomic influences. This results in a very rapid (>300 bpm) and complex atrial rhythm. The AV node limits the number of depolarizations reaching the ventricles, and patients typically develop an irregular ventricular rhythm of 120–180 bpm at the onset of an episode. AF is predominantly a left atrial arrhythmia, and, in most cases, the right atrium is driven passively. It is more likely to occur in patients with enlarged or diseased atria, so conditions which cause left atrial stretch are especially likely to cause AF. Common causes of atrial fibrillation are shown in Box 4.1.

The initiating event in AF is usually rapid automatic ectopic firing, which initiates re-entry in the left atrium. In many cases, this occurs in, or near, the pulmonary veins as they enter the left atrium. Sleeves of conducting tissue may extend several centimetres into the pulmonary veins. In young patients with 'lone' AF (i.e. atrial fibrillation occurring in an otherwise normal heart), pulmonary vein ectopy is nearly always the initiating mechanism, whereas, in older patients with structural heart disease, ectopy can arise either from the pulmonary veins or areas of diseased atrial tissue.

Atrial fibrillation is more likely to become sustained if there is potential for re-entry to occur. Enlarged atria and atria with diseased, slowly conducting zones are more likely to accommodate re-entry (see Figure 4.4). Autonomic factors are also known to affect propensity to atrial fibrillation, probably because of their effects on automaticity and atrial refractoriness.

When AF persists for more than 24 hours, mechanical stasis can result in thrombus formation within the left atrial appendage. This is especially likely to occur in patients with left atrial dilatation and in older patients. Thrombus can embolize and cause TIA, stroke, or a peripheral embolism. Risk stratification and anticoagulation strategies are therefore essential.

Symptoms

Symptoms occur because AF has several effects on cardiovascular efficiency. Loss of coordinated atrial contraction results in impaired diastolic filling. This is especially deleterious in patients with heart failure or left ventricular hypertrophy where the atrial contribution to cardiac output is proportionately greater. The resting heart rate usually increases significantly, although some elderly patients with

---

Box 4.1 Common causes of atrial fibrillation

Hypertension
Mitral valve disease (especially stenosis)
Coronary heart disease
Cardiomyopathies
Congenital heart disease
Thyrotoxicosis
Acute chest infection
Alcohol misuse
Pulmonary embolism

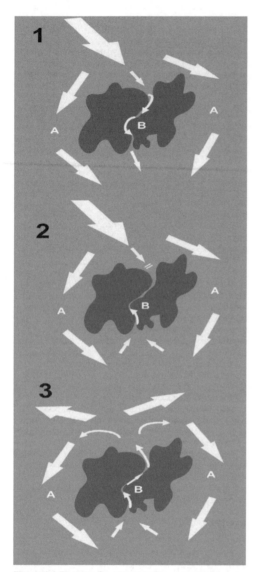

Figure 4.4 Re-entry. Re-entry normally occurs around an anatomical barrier (e.g. scar, vein, valve ring) and is initiated by an ectopic beat. Conduction block in one limb of the circuit causes unidirectional conduction. (A) Illustrates an ectopic beat passing around but blocked through the scar. Re-entry will only occur if the refractory period of tissue in the circuit is shorter than the circuit time. (B) Illustrates the re-entry circuit of the tachycardia. Thus, larger circuits (e.g. in dilated chambers) or circuits with zones of slow conduction (e.g. involving diseased tissue) are more likely to sustain re-entrant arrhythmias. Reproduced from Punit Ramraka and Jonathan Hill, *Oxford Handbook of Cardiology*, second edition, 2012, Figure 11.1, page 547, with permission from Oxford University Press.

atrial fibrillation have a normal heart rate without treatment because of age-dependent slowing of AV node conduction. Furthermore, heart rate tends to increase disproportionately with exercise, causing fatigue and dyspnoea. In susceptible patients, angina and heart failure symptoms may be aggravated by poor rate control. Finally, the irregular ventricular rhythm causes palpitation which many patients find disturbing and uncomfortable.

Patients with AF are divided into three categories:

- Paroxysmal.
- Persistent.
- Permanent.

Paroxysmal AF comprises usually short episodes of AF which self-terminate. Persistent AF does not self-terminate but can be terminated by antiarrhythmic drugs, electrical cardioversion, or catheter ablation. Permanent AF does not respond to any of these manoeuvres. As interventional electrophysiology techniques evolve, the proportion of patients classified with permanent AF is reducing.

Electrocardiographic features

The ECG (see Figure 4.5) is characterized by the absence of P waves and the presence of low-amplitude, irregular waves known as 'F waves' or fibrillation waves. QRS complexes are normally narrow, unless the patient has pre-existing or rate-dependent bundle branch block. The ventricular rhythm is irregularly irregular. The irregularity of the rhythm can be difficult to appreciate when the ventricular rate is very high. When atrial fibrillation occurs in association with complete AV block, P waves are absent, but the ventricular rhythm is slow and regular because of regular firing of a junctional or ventricular escape focus (see Figure 4.6).

Management of new-onset AF

It is unusual for AF to be associated with serious haemodynamic compromise, unless there is associated significant left ventricular dysfunction or valve disease or a major concomitant non-cardiac illness, such as sepsis. When compromise occurs, AF should be managed, in accordance with European Resuscitation Council guidelines on peri-arrest arrhythmias.

If there is a *clear* history of AF of less than 24 hours' duration, then pharmacological cardioversion can be attempted. This can only be done safely if continuous ECG and non-invasive BP monitoring are available and staff are familiar with arrhythmia management.

Flecainide, 2 mg/kg IV over 30 min (to a maximum of 150 mg total), is effective at terminating acute AF in approximately 80% of cases. This drug should not be given to patients known to have impaired ventricular function or heart failure because of the risk of proarrhythmia (a new or more frequent occurrence of a pre-existing arrhythmia, paradoxically precipitated by antiarrhythmic therapy). Proarrhythmia is also more common in patients with coronary heart disease. An alternative is amiodarone 5 mg/kg over 30 min, followed by 1.2 g over 24 hours, via a central venous catheter or peripherally inserted central catheter (PICC) line. Amiodarone can cause serious thrombophlebitis and should not be given via a peripheral venous cannula other than as an emergency. If pharmacological cardioversion is unsuccessful or contraindicated, electrical cardioversion can be performed under general anaesthesia.

If AF is of uncertain duration or known to be of greater than 24 hours' duration, cardioversion should not be performed because there is a risk that atrial thrombus may be present. Restoration of atrial mechanical contraction can cause embolization within 48 hours if cardioversion is

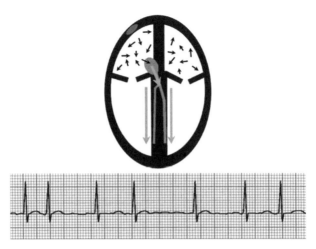

AF. Irregular QRS complexes. No obvious discrete P wave activity, although it is not unusual to see more organized activity in lead V1 with sharp bumps every 4–6 small squares. Black arrows indicate a compulsory part of the rhythm/circuit, grey arrows indicate bystander (non-participating) pathways.

Figure 4.5 Atrial fibrillation. P waves are absent, and low-amplitude fibrillation waves are visible. QRS complexes are usually narrow, and the ventricular rhythm is rapid and irregular. Reproduced from Saul G. Myerson, Robin P. Choudhury, and Andrew R. J. Mitchell, *Emergencies in Cardiology*, 2006, p. 141, with permission from Oxford University Press.

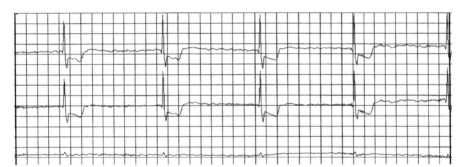

Figure 4.6 Atrial fibrillation with third-degree atrioventricular block. P waves are absent. Here, the ventricular rhythm is slow and regular because the ventricular rhythm is driven by a slow escape focus in the ventricles. Reproduced from Hung-Fat Tse, Gregory Y.H. Lip, and Andrew J. Stewart Coats, *Oxford Desk Reference: Cardiology*, 2011, Figure 3.1.5, p. 60, with permission from Oxford University Press.

performed inappropriately. The patient should be anticoagulated with warfarin, aiming for an international normalized ratio (INR) of 2.5. AV node-blocking drugs should be used for rate control. Beta-blockers (e.g. metoprolol 25–100 mg twice daily) are more effective than digoxin at providing rate control during exercise. Digoxin (125-375 micrograms daily) can be added if beta-blockade alone fails to control the ventricular rate. Verapamil (120–360 mg daily in divided doses) is an alternative if beta-blockers are contraindicated or poorly tolerated but should never be co-prescribed with a beta-blocker. A target resting heart rate of 50–80 bpm is appropriate. Patients should be considered either for rate or rhythm control, as described in the following section.

Management of persistent/permanent AF
The two approaches to long-term management of continuous AF are the **rate** and **rhythm control** strategies. The rate control strategy assumes that atrial fibrillation is permanent and utilizes AV node-blocking drugs to limit the ventricular rate. The rhythm control strategy utilizes antiarrhythmic drugs, cardioversion, and sometimes catheter ablation to restore sinus rhythm.

Rate control strategy
AV node-blocking drugs are used, as described in the previous section. In rare cases where rate control cannot be achieved or drugs are poorly tolerated, a permanent pacemaker can be implanted and AV nodal conduction eliminated using catheter ablation (the 'pace and ablate' strategy). Patients with rheumatic mitral valve disease should be prescribed warfarin (target INR 2.5) unless known contraindications. Patients with non-rheumatic atrial fibrillation should be risk-stratified, using the CHADS-2 scoring system (available in Gage *et al.* 2004).

Box 4.2 Risk factors for recurrence of atrial fibrillation after cardioversion

Mitral valve disease
Heart failure or left ventricular impairment
Hypertension
Left ventricular hypertrophy
Left atrial enlargement
Increasing age

Rate control is appropriate for patients with risk factors for recurrence of AF—principally elderly patients and those with significant structural heart disease (see Box 4.2).

Rhythm control strategy
Cardioversion is performed a minimum of 3 weeks after therapeutic anticoagulation is achieved. Beta-blockers promote maintenance of sinus rhythm after cardioversion. There is little evidence that sotalol is superior to conventional beta-blockers (e.g. metoprolol, bisoprolol) in maintaining sinus rhythm, and the risk of proarrhythmia is greater. For patients in whom atrial fibrillation occurs or recurs despite beta-blockade, consideration should be given to the addition of flecainide OR propafenone OR amiodarone (see Table 4.5) before cardioversion.

Cardioversion is ideally performed using a short-acting general anaesthetic, although it is possible using conscious sedation with appropriate monitoring and staff training. An initial 200 J biphasic shock should be used. There is no advantage in using lower shock energies. Cardioversion restores sinus rhythm in 95% of cases, but AF will recur in approximately half of cases within 6 months. In these cases, either rate control or, if symptomatic, catheter ablation need to be considered. FAQ1 addresses the need for post cardioversion anticoagulation.

Pharmacological management of paroxysmal AF
Patients with paroxysmal AF, associated with minimal or no symptoms, do not require antiarrhythmic therapy. Consider anticoagulation if prolonged (>12 hour) episodes occur. In patients with significant symptoms, antiarrhythmic drug therapy should be considered (see Table 4.5). Beta-blockers are effective first-line agents.

Flecainide or propafenone can be used if breakthrough symptoms occur or if beta-blockers are contraindicated or not tolerated. These agents should always be co-prescribed with an AV node-blocking drug (beta-blocker or rate-limiting calcium channel blocker) when used for AF prophylaxis because some patients will develop atrial flutter with a relatively slow atrial rate (250 bpm). If no AV node blockade is given, 1:1 AV conduction can occur, causing haemodynamic collapse. Amiodarone is used as a last resort for prophylaxis. Although it is very effective, side effects can limit its use. Dronedarone has shown promise in recent trials and may be useful in preference to amiodarone in some younger patients. Sotalol, which has class III (potassium channel-blocking) action, is not significantly more effective than pure class II agents and can be proarrhythmic, especially if used with other drugs which prolong the QT interval (see Table 4.5).

As an alternative to regular antiarrhythmic prophylaxis, the 'pill in pocket' approach can be used where patients self-administer either oral flecainide (200–300 mg) or propafenone (300–600 mg). This approach is only suitable for patients who do not have structural or coronary heart disease.

Catheter ablation of AF
Radiofrequency catheter ablation has been developed as a treatment for AF. In patients with paroxysmal AF, the objective of ablation is to electrically isolate or obliterate triggering foci within, and around, the ostia of the pulmonary veins. Pulmonary vein isolation is effective at preventing AF in 75–85% of patients without significant structural heart disease, although some need a repeat procedure. Ablation for persistent AF involves a more extensive procedure, with a lower procedural success rate. Complications include tamponade (1–2%), stroke (<0.5%), AV nodal block (0.5%), and rarely pulmonary vein stenosis, phrenic nerve paralysis, and atrio-oesophageal fistula. Iatrogenic arrhythmias, such as atrial tachycardias and left atrial flutter, sometimes complicate ablation. Catheter ablation is normally reserved for patients with drug refractory symptoms and is preferable to long-term amiodarone therapy in younger patients.

FAQ 1 I have had a successful cardioversion for atrial fibrillation. Why do I need to take warfarin afterwards and for how long?

It takes some weeks for the atria to recover their function after a successful cardioversion, and, during this time, there is a continued risk of clot formation and stroke. Also, there is a risk that AF might recur. Most cardiologists recommend continuing warfarin for at least 1 and ideally 3 months after cardioversion.

Atrial flutter

Atrial flutter is a 'macro re-entrant' arrhythmia, involving a single large re-entry circuit in one of the atria. It is characterized by rapid, regular atrial depolarization and is usually associated with a rapid ventricular rhythm.

Pathophysiology
Most cases of atrial flutter are caused by re-entry in the right atrium. Right atrial flutter is characterized by depolarization around the tricuspid annulus (see Figure 4.7). Importantly, the flutter circuit funnels through the 'cavotricuspid isthmus' between the tricuspid annulus and the inferior vena cava. This isthmus forms a target for radiofrequency ablation. Atypical atrial flutter (i.e. flutter not involving the cavotricuspid isthmus) occurs in patients after cardiac surgery, after closure of atrial septal defects, and after ablation of AF. Atrial flutter is initiated by atrial ectopic beats and, like atrial fibrillation, is more likely to occur in enlarged or diseased atria. Thus, the same conditions which predispose to atrial fibrillation also predispose to atrial flutter.

The atrial rate in atrial flutter is normally around 300 bpm. In patients with intact AV nodal conduction, this can produce a regular ventricular rhythm at 150 bpm because of 2:1 block at AV node level. Slower and more irregular ventricular rhythms can also occur, mimicking AF. In young patients or patients in whom the atrial rate is relatively slow (around 250 bpm) or if an accessory pathway is present, 1:1 AV conduction may occur. This generates a paradoxically very rapid ventricular rate and may precipitate haemodynamic collapse. Class Ic antiarrhythmic drugs slow the atrial rate and can trigger this arrhythmia. Thus, they should be avoided in atrial flutter.

Table 4.5 Antiarrhythmic drugs (Vaughn Williams classification)

Drug class*	Examples	Other agents	Main uses	Notes
I—sodium channel blockers				
Ia—'intermediate' sodium channels	Disopyramide 300–800 mg daily (divided doses)	Quinidine* Procainamide* Ajmaline*	- AF prophylaxis - (Rarely) ventricular arrhythmias - Ventricular arrhythmias	Lidocaine only administered IV. Caution in heart failure/ventricular impairment.
Ib—'fast' sodium channels	Lidocaine IV 50–100 mg bolus; 1–4 mg/min for up to 24 hours	Mexiletine*	- AF prophylaxis (co-prescribed with class II or IV—see text)	Do not use if heart failure, ventricular impairment, or coronary heart disease as proarrhythmia common.
Ic—'slow' sodium channels	Flecainide 50–150 mg twice daily Propafenone 150–300 mg twice daily		- SVT prophylaxis - Ventricular arrhythmias	Flecainide IV 2 mg/kg, up to maximum of 150 mg, can be used for cardioversion of new-onset AF.
II—beta-blockers	Metoprolol 25–100 mg twice daily	Bisprolol Atenolol Propranolol	- AF and SVT prophylaxis - Rate limitation in AF/flutter - Prevention of ventricular arrhythmias in coronary heart disease and cardiomyopathies	Avoid in acute heart failure, asthma/COPD, and critical limb ischaemia. Esmolol IV 50–200 micrograms/kg/min is an ultra short-acting beta-blocker, useful for rate control in AF and for arrhythmia prophylaxis in the ICU setting.
III—potassium channel blockers	Amiodarone 200–400 mg daily after loading dose Dronedarone 400 mg twice daily Sotalol 40–160 mg twice daily	Dofetilide* Ibutilide*	- AF/flutter prophylaxis - Prevention of ventricular arrhythmias	Amiodarone causes photosensitivity, thyroid, liver, and lung dysfunction. Amiodarone IV 5 mg/kg over 30 min; up to 1.2 g in 24 hours can be used for cardioversion of new-onset AF and for ventricular arrhythmias. Several class III antiarrhythmics may cause liver dysfunction. Monitoring of liver function required. Most class III agents are contraindicated in persistent atrial fibrillation, heart failure or if left ventricular dysfunction. Indicated for prophylaxis of atrial fibrillation only. Sotalol and most class III agents prolong the QT interval. However, sotalol is more likely to cause torsades than amiodarone. Class III agents also have multiple drug interactions (<http://www.crediblemeds.org/healthcare-providers/practical-approach/>)
IV—calcium channel blockers	Verapamil 80–240 mg twice daily	Diltiazem	- Rate control in AF - SVT prophylaxis	Avoid in heart failure/LV impairment. May aggravate dependent oedema, particularly in women.

Some drugs (e.g. digoxin, atropine, adenosine) are not covered by this schema. More complex classifications can be used, according to ion channel physiology (Task Force 1991). Doses given are for oral administration unless otherwise stated (italics for IV doses). * Not widely used/available in Europe.

Data from Vaughan Williams EM. Classification of antiarrhythmic drugs. In: *Symposium on cardiac arrhythmias*. Sandoe E, Flensted-Jensen E, Olesen KH, eds. Sodertalje: AB Astra, 1970: 449–72.

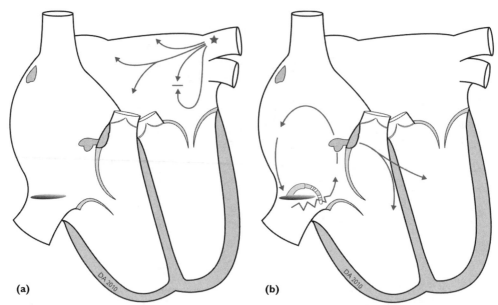

(a)   (b)

Figure 4.7 Atrial flutter and atrial fibrillation mechanisms. (a) Atrial fibrillation: ectopic beats arising from the pulmonary vein ostia initiate re-entry in the left atrium. Multiple interacting re-entry circuits maintain the arrhythmia. (b) Atrial flutter: a single large re-entry circuit maintains the arrhythmia, normally in the right atrium, with the critical isthmus of slowed conduction (zigzag arrow) between the inferior vena cava and tricuspid valve (note: ablation at this site blocks the re-entry circuit). Reproduced from Punit Ramraka and Jonathan Hill, *Oxford Handbook of Cardiology*, second edition, 2012, Figure 11.6, page 565, with permission from Oxford University Press.

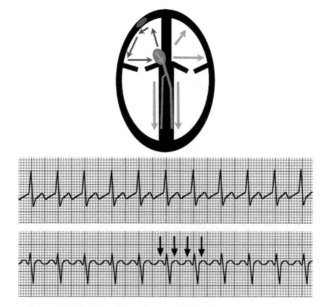

Atrial flutter. Regular QRS complexes, typically at 150 bpm. Rapid, regular atrial activity usually between 280 and 320 bpm (one flutter wave every large square). During 2:1 AV conduction alternate flutter waves may be hidden in QRS complexes. Lead V1 is often a good lead for spotting atrial activity (arrows). In typical flutter the flutter waves are negative in leads II, III and aVF (sawtooth pattern). Black arrows indicate a compulsory part of the rhythm/circuit, grey arrows indicate bystander (non-participating) pathways.

Figure 4.8 ECG of atrial flutter. Sawtooth flutter waves are seen, and the ventricular rhythm may be either regular or irregular. Lead V1 is good for spotting atrial activity (arrows), as in this illustration. Reproduced from Saul G. Myerson, Robin P. Choudhury, and Andrew R. J. Mitchell, *Emergencies in Cardiology*, 2006, p. 145, with permission from Oxford University Press.

Electrocardiographic features

The ECG (see Figure 4.8) shows 'sawtooth' flutter waves of high amplitude. QRS complexes are normally narrow as in AF. The ventricular rhythm may be regular or irregular, depending on AV nodal conduction. Flutter waves may be difficult to appreciate if there is 2:1 or 1:1 AV conduction because they may be obscured by QRS complexes or T waves.

Management of atrial flutter

Emergency management is similar to that of AF. Intravenous amiodarone or DC cardioversion can be used in cases of sustained atrial flutter of less than 24 hours' duration. Since patients with atrial flutter are quite likely to maintain sinus rhythm after cardioversion and have the option of catheter ablation with a good prospect of success, a rhythm control strategy is normally adopted. The same guidance for warfarin anticoagulation applies as for AF.

Pharmacological management

Rate control is more difficult in atrial flutter than in atrial fibrillation. A beta-blocker OR rate-limiting calcium channel blocker can be used, adding digoxin, if necessary. For prophylaxis in paroxysmal atrial flutter or after cardioversion, either a beta-blocker or amiodarone can be prescribed. Class Ic drugs should be avoided.

Catheter ablation of atrial flutter

Catheter ablation is a very effective treatment for atrial flutter. It is effective in more than 90% of cases of typical flutter. It is less likely to be successful for atypical flutter variants. Complications are uncommon but include tamponade and iatrogenic AV nodal block. AF occurs in 40% of treated patients within 5 years of ablation because the two arrhythmias share the same aetiologies. Catheter ablation should be considered as first-line treatment in all patients with persistent or recurrent symptomatic atrial flutter.

Supraventricular tachycardia

Supraventricular tachycardia (SVT) is a term used to describe a family of rapid, regular rhythms which produce a similar appearance on the surface ECG. These are the most common tachycardias seen in patients less than 40 years. The prevalence of SVT is 1 in 500 adults.

Pathophysiology

SVT is caused by one of three mechanisms: atrioventricular re-entrant tachycardia (AVRT—50% of cases), AV nodal re-entrant tachycardia (AVNRT—40%), and atrial tachycardia (10%). AVRT is caused by an accessory (atrioventricular) pathway, which allows re-entry to occur retrogradely from the ventricles to the atria. In half of cases, the pathway conducts rapidly and antegradely in sinus rhythm, distorting the QRS complex and giving rise to the classic short PR interval and delta wave of Wolff–Parkinson–White syndrome (see Figure 4.9). In the remainder of cases, the pathway only conducts retrogradely, and the ECG is normal in sinus rhythm ('concealed' accessory pathway).

AVNRT is caused by re-entry between the AV node and right atrium, via two right atrial input pathways. The inferior ('slow') pathway can be targeted during catheter ablation. Atrial tachycardia is caused either by automatic firing or re-entry within one of the atria.

Symptoms

Symptoms may begin in infancy or early childhood but, more often, start in teenagers and young adults. Episodes of SVT cause sudden, rapid palpitation, sometimes associated with light-headedness and chest discomfort. The palpitation is regular. Episodes may be felt to terminate abruptly or gradually (sinus tachycardia often ensues after an episode). Trivial actions, such as coughing or bending, may precipitate SVT. In some patients, specific triggers, such as alcohol or exercise, are identified. Contrary to common teaching, it is quite uncommon for caffeine to be a precipitating factor. Patients often learn that breathing manoeuvres and relaxation can help terminate an episode.

Electrocardiographic features

The ECG usually shows a regular, narrow QRS tachycardia, with a rate of 140–240 bpm (see Figure 4.10). P waves may be obscured by the QRS complex but are sometimes visible in the ST segment. P waves are often visible during atrial tachycardia, but the morphology differs to that in sinus rhythm. Wide QRS complexes can occur during SVT because of: (i) pre-existing bundle branch block; (ii) rate-dependent bundle branch block (aberrancy); or (iii) pre-excitation (e.g. antidromic AVRT where antegrade conduction is through the accessory pathway and retrograde conduction through the AV node. This is uncommon.).

Acute management

Patients should be taught to use the Valsalva manoeuvre at onset. Carotid sinus pressure can be used but should not be used in patients with a history of stroke or TIA, or with carotid bruit. IV adenosine is very effective at terminating SVT caused by AVRT or AVNRT. As it has an extremely short half-life, adenosine is administered by rapid bolus into a large antecubital vein in a raised arm, followed by a saline flush. The initial dose is 3 mg, and, if this fails to terminate tachycardia, incremental doses at 6 and 12 mg can be used. Before administration, patients should be warned that adenosine causes unpleasant flushing and chest tightness for a few seconds. Note that patients taking dipyridamole are extremely sensitive to small amounts of adenosine (use 0.5–1 mg only), while patients taking theophylline may be adenosine-resistant. Adenosine should not be used in patients with active asthma.

For patients with frequent or disabling SVT, catheter ablation is normally recommended. Pharmacological prophylaxis can be used but commits a young person to long-term medication. FAQ 2 addresses the risk of SVT and management options in pregnancy.

Catheter ablation of SVT

Catheter ablation is curative in 95% of cases of SVT. Recurrences occur in around 5% of cases, necessitating a second procedure. Serious complications are uncommon, as with atrial flutter. The risk of iatrogenic AV nodal block depends on the proximity of the culprit tissue to the AV node but is typically less than 0.5%. Patients can resume normal activity and work within a few days of the procedure.

Pharmacological management

Drugs are normally reserved as a bridge to catheter ablation or for patients where ablation has failed or been abandoned because of risk of AV block. Beta-blockade (e.g. metoprolol 25–100mg twice daily) or verapamil (120–360

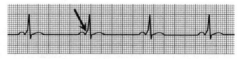

Sinus rhythm and pre-excitation. There is a short PR interval and delta wave at the beginning of the QRS (arrow). Black arrows indicate a compulsory part of the rhythm/circuit, grey arrows indicate bystander (non-participating) pathways.

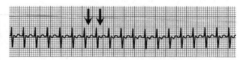

Orthodromic tachycardia. A rapid, regular rhythm. The circuit goes from atrium to ventricle through the AV node and bundle branches so the delta wave disappears and the QRS is narrow (unless there is bundle branch block aberrancy); then from ventricle to atrium through the accessory pathway. The retrograde P wave occurs after the QRS (arrows). Black arrows indicate a compulsory part of the rhythm/circuit, grey arrows indicate bystander (non-participating) pathways.

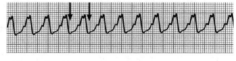

Antidromic tachycardia. Much less common. A rapid, regular rhythm. The circuit goes from atrium to ventricle through the accessory pathway so the ventricle is totally pre-excited and the QRS is very wide; then from ventricle to atrium through the bundle branches and AV node. The retrograde P wave occurs at the end of the QRS (arrows). Black arrows indicate a compulsory part of the rhythm/circuit, grey arrows indicate bystander (non-participating) pathways.

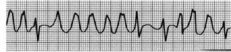

Pre-excited AF. AF is conducted to the ventricles through a combination of the AV node (narrow complexes) and the accessory pathway (wide, pre-excited complexes). The accessory pathway tends to dominate producing a very rapid ventricular rate. Black arrows indicate a compulsory part of the rhythm/circuit, grey arrows indicate bystander (non-participating) pathways.

Figure 4.9 ECG features of Wolff–Parkinson–White syndrome. The PR interval is short, and a triangular 'delta wave' precedes the main body of the QRS complex (arrow). Reproduced from Saul G. Myerson, Robin P. Choudhury, and Andrew R. J. Mitchell, *Emergencies in Cardiology*, 2006, p. 153, with permission from Oxford University Press.

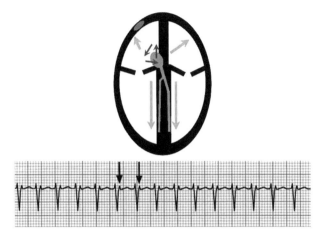

AV nodal re-entrant tachycardia. A rapid, regular tachycardia. Usually narrow complex (unless bundle branch aberrancy occurs). Retrograde P wave occur during the QRS complex and are difficult to see, although typically appear as a 'pseudo-R wave' in lead V1 (arrows). Black arrows indicate a compulsory part of the rhythm/circuit, grey arrows indicate bystander (non-participating) pathways.

Figure 4.10 Supraventricular tachycardia. The QRS complexes are classically narrow and regular, and P waves are often obscured (arrows). Reproduced from Saul G. Myerson, Robin P. Choudhury, and Andrew R. J. Mitchell, *Emergencies in Cardiology*, 2006, p. 151, with permission from Oxford University Press.

mg daily) can be used as first-line prophylaxis. Flecainide (50–100 mg twice daily) or propafenone (150–300 mg twice daily) are particularly effective in Wolff–Parkinson–White syndrome because these agents preferentially block accessory pathway conduction. Amiodarone should never be used for SVT prophylaxis other than in the palliative setting.

> **FAQ 2** I have SVTs. Is it safe to become pregnant?
>
> It is very uncommon for SVT to cause harm during pregnancy, and most patients go through it without significant problems. However, SVT episodes may be triggered by pregnancy and are uncomfortable and tiring. While beta-blockers can be used, they are avoided early in pregnancy, as they can slow fetal growth. It is sensible to consider catheter ablation therapy before planning pregnancy.

Ventricular tachycardia

'Ventricular tachycardia' (VT) refers to a family of tachyarrhythmias arising from the ventricles. VT causes understandable concern among clinicians because of its association with haemodynamic collapse and cardiac arrest.

Electrocardiographic features
Monomorphic VT is characterized by a regular, wide complex (QRS duration >120 ms) rhythm, rate 120–250 bpm (see Figure 4.11). SVT can be associated with a similar ECG appearance, and diagnosis can sometimes be difficult. The clinical context is important; the rhythm is more likely to be SVT in a young, healthy patient and more likely to be VT in an elderly patient with heart failure. AV dissociation is diagnostic of VT, as are capture and fusion beats (which are caused by intermittent conduction of sinus beats into the

ventricles during VT). Other features favouring VT are a very wide QRS complex (>150 ms), extreme axis deviation, and concordance of QRS direction in the chest leads.

Polymorphic VT is a rapid rhythm comprising multiple QRS complex morphologies, usually associated with a heart rate >200 bpm. It can complicate acute myocardial infarction. Torsades de pointes VT (see Figure 4.12) is a variant of polymorphic VT in which the QRS complexes appear to rotate around the baseline as the axis shifts. It is associated with QT interval prolongation during sinus rhythm. See further text for precipitating factors.

Management of VT
Pulseless VT or VT associated with significant haemodynamic compromise should be managed with prompt cardioversion, according to current resuscitation guidelines (see 'Adult cardiopulmonary resuscitation' earlier in this chapter). Management of stable VT depends on its substrate or context. Not all forms of VT are malignant.

VT in structural/ischaemic heart disease
Here, VT occurs because of the presence of a scar substrate. Re-entry around scar is initiated by ventricular ectopy. This may be either be sustained or non-sustained. By far, the most common example is VT after myocardial infarction, although it can occur in cardiomyopathies, hypertension, congenital heart disease, or aortic valve disease.

Acute management
Post-infarction VT is more likely to cause haemodynamic collapse or to degenerate into ventricular fibrillation in patients with conducting system disease (e.g. those with left bundle branch block) or poor left ventricular function. Acute management is with intravenous amiodarone 5 mg/kg over 30 min, followed by 1.2 g over 24 hours, via a central catheter or PICC line.

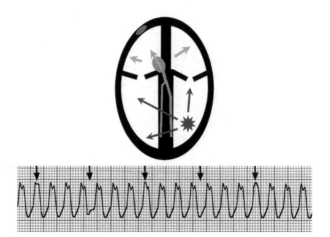

Monomorphic ventricular tachycardia. A regular, wide complex tachycardia. The QRS shape is constant although may be distorted by the independent P wave activity if there is visible AV dissociation (arrows). Black arrows indicate a compulsory part of the rhythm/circuit, grey arrows indicate bystander (non-participating) pathways.

Figure 4.11 Monomorphic VT. The QRS complexes are broad and regular, and AV dissociation (arrows), capture and fusion beats may be present. Reproduced from Saul G. Myerson, Robin P. Choudhury, and Andrew R. J. Mitchell, *Emergencies in Cardiology*, 2006, p. 157, with permission from Oxford University Press.

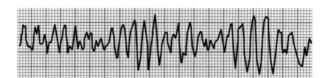

Torsade de Pointes. An irregular, broad complex tachycardia. The QRS axis twists around the baseline.

Figure 4.12 Torsades de pointes VT. The QRS axis twists around the baseline, and the ventricular rate is extremely rapid. Reproduced from Saul G. Myerson, Robin P. Choudhury, and Andrew R. J. Mitchell, *Emergencies in Cardiology*, 2006, p. 160, with permission from Oxford University Press.

IV lidocaine 100 mg, followed by an infusion of 1–2 mg/min, can be used but should be avoided in patients with hypotension or left ventricular failure. In resistant cases, synchronized DC cardioversion (150 J biphasic shock) is used. Overdrive pacing, using a temporary pacing catheter, is occasionally useful.

Prevention and long-term management
Left ventricular function is the major determinant of risk in patients with coronary heart disease. Coronary revascularization and rigorous application of secondary prevention therapies, particularly beta-blockade, significantly reduce the risk of VT and VF after myocardial infarction.

If symptomatic VT occurs, despite beta-blockade, amiodarone (200–400 mg daily after loading) can be used for prophylaxis. Class Ic antiarrhythmic drugs are contraindicated after myocardial infarction and in patients with significant ventricular dysfunction.

Implantable cardiac defibrillators (ICDs)
ICDs are implantable devices used to terminate life-threatening ventricular arrhythmias. They have all of the functions of a permanent pacemaker (for bradycardia prevention) but also

terminate malignant ventricular arrhythmias, either by 'overdrive pacing' or by delivering a shock through the heart. ICDs are implanted in the pectoral position and deliver therapy via a lead placed in the right ventricle. Cardiac resynchronization therapy (CRT) defibrillators can be used to treat patients with heart failure who exhibit evidence of dyssynchrony. ICDs do not prevent VT or VF and should be regarded as complementary to drug therapy, rather than an alternative.

ICDs can be implanted for secondary prevention (i.e. in patients who have already experienced a serious ventricular arrhythmia) or primary prevention (in patients at high risk of future arrhythmia). Some guidelines allow for primary prevention ICD implantation in selected patients with dilated cardiomyopathy. ICD therapy is not appropriate for patients whose life expectancy is significantly curtailed by other comorbid conditions. The indications for ICD insertion, according to NICE, are listed as follows:

Secondary prevention
Patients who present, in the absence of a treatable cause, with:

• Cardiac arrest due to either VT or VF.

- Spontaneous sustained VT, causing syncope or significant haemodynamic compromise.
- Sustained VT associated with LV ejection fraction <35% and no worse than NYHA class III heart failure.

Primary prevention
- Patients with a history of previous (> 4 weeks) MI, and **Either**
  - LVEF <35% and no worse than NYHA class III heart failure, **and**
  - Non-sustained VT on ambulatory ECG monitoring, **and**
  - Inducible VT on electrophysiological (EP) testing. **Or**
  - LVEF <30% and no worse than NYHA class III heart failure, **and**
  - QRS duration of equal to or more than 120 ms.
- Patients with a familial cardiac condition with a high risk of sudden death, including long QT syndrome, hypertrophic cardiomyopathy, Brugada syndrome, or arrhythmogenic right ventricular dysplasia (ARVD), or have undergone surgical repair of congenital heart disease.

Patients presenting with a suspected ICD shock should be seen as soon as possible at the nearest implanting centre. ICD shocks can be painful and traumatic, and patients may require a short hospital admission until the ICD is interrogated and necessary changes in therapy initiated. Anxiety is common among patients with ICDs, and education and psychological support are extremely important. Many patients benefit from contact with an ICD support group. FAQ3 reports when a patient can legally drive following implantation of an ICD.

'Normal heart' VT
VT is occasionally seen in young individuals with no evidence of structural or coronary heart disease. Exercise stress testing, echocardiography, and cardiac magnetic resonance imaging are required to establish the diagnosis. These forms of VT usually have an automatic mechanism and normally arise from the outflow tract of the right ventricle. Repetitive short episodes of monomorphic VT are seen. 'Fascicular VT' is another variant, arising from Purkinje fibres in the left ventricle.

Acute management
Unless the patient is confirmed by a cardiologist to have a normal heart VT variant, it is safest to follow the protocols in the previous section for acute management (e.g. amiodarone). In patients with known outflow tract or fascicular VT, IV beta-blockade (e.g. IV metoprolol 5 mg over 2 min, repeated every 5 min to a maximum of 15 mg) is effective. Other antiarrhythmics (e.g. IV verapamil or flecainide) should not be given without first consulting with a specialist.

Prevention/long-term management
These VT variants usually respond well to beta-blockade. Verapamil (normally contraindicated in VT) can also be used, but specialist opinion should be sought before initiating treatment. Catheter ablation is an effective treatment.

Torsade de pointes VT
This malignant VT variant is associated with QT interval prolongation (see Figure 4.12). Episodes are often initiated by R-on-T ventricular ectopy. Torsade is dangerous because it can lead to ventricular fibrillation and sudden cardiac death. Predisposing factors include electrolyte disturbance (hypokalaemia, hypomagnesaemia, hypocalcaemia), myo-

cardial ischaemia, drugs (e.g. methadone, lithium, sotalol, amiodarone, flecainide, antihistamines, quinine-based antimalarials, phenothiazines, and some antidepressants—see <http://www.crediblemeds.org/healthcare-providers/practical-approach/> for a comprehensive list), and the familial long QT syndrome.

Acute management
Torsades associated with haemodynamic collapse should be treated with an immediate unsynchronized DC shock. In an otherwise stable patient with episodes of torsades, cardioversion is inappropriate because, until the underlying cause is treated, the arrhythmia is likely to recur. Electrolyte disturbance should be corrected promptly. Drug induced torsades should be managed with IV magnesium sulfate (2 g over 10–15 min). Torsades can be effectively suppressed by artificially increasing heart rate, which leads to rate-dependent shortening of the QT interval. IV isoprenaline (isoproterenol) (40–200 mcg/min) or temporary atrial pacing can be used.

VT in inherited heart disease
VT and VF are manifestations of several inherited arrhythmia conditions. Syncope, palpitation, or cardiac arrest may be the mode of presentation. Risk stratification of affected individuals and screening of first-degree relatives requires specialist input, usually from an electrophysiologist and cardiac geneticist.

Long QT syndrome
This family of conditions is caused by mutations in cardiac sodium and potassium channel genes. The phenotypic manifestation is QT interval prolongation, which predisposes the patient to torsades de pointes VT (see Figure 4.12). Not all affected individuals are at high risk. Low-risk patients may require no treatment or simple beta-blockade. High-risk patients may require ICD implantation to prevent sudden death. Patients should avoid drugs which prolong the QT interval (see section on torsade de pointes VT). Hypokalaemia may also precipitate arrhythmia.

Brugada syndrome
The ECG in Brugada syndrome is characterized by right bundle branch block and convex ST segment elevation in leads V1–V3. Patients may present with syncope or cardiac arrest. Affected individuals usually require ICD implantation.

Arrhythmogenic right ventricular cardiomyopathy (ARVC)
This inherited cardiomyopathy commonly causes ventricular ectopy and VT. In early stages, it may not be obvious with echocardiography, but magnetic resonance imaging may reveal right ventricular dilatation, aneurysms, and scar. The ECG may be normal or may show T wave inversion in leads V1–V3 or 'epsilon waves'—small deflections which follow the QRS complex. Antiarrhythmic drugs are often ineffective, and ICD implantation is often required. Additionally, catheter ablation or right ventricular isolation surgery may be required to prevent arrhythmia episodes.

Reversible causes of VT/VF
Ventricular arrhythmias may be precipitated by many other factors. Acute myocardial ischaemia/infarction, mechanical trauma, and mechanical irritation (e.g. thoracic tumour, surgical drain) are all causes. Additionally, hypokalaemia, hypomagnesaemia, hypocalcaemia, and some drugs can predispose to QT interval prolongation and torsades de pointes VT. IV isoprenaline or atrial overdrive pacing artificially shorten the QT interval and are effective short-term treatments for drug-induced torsades.

Ventricular fibrillation

See Adult cardiopulmonary resuscitation.

Bradyarrhythmias

Bradyarrhythmias are arbitrarily defined as rhythms with a ventricular rate less than 60 bpm. These can be asymptomatic or produce symptoms of low cardiac output—fatigue, light-headedness, and syncope. Indeed, many bradyarrhythmias are benign and physiological, e.g. sinus bradycardia and nocturnal Mobitz type I AV block in young or athletic individuals.

Sinus bradycardia and junctional bradycardia

Sinus bradycardia is the most commonly encountered bradyarrhythmia. Causes are given in Table 4.6. Asymptomatic sinus bradycardia requires no treatment.

Acute treatment

Symptomatic patients should be treated with IV atropine (0.6–1.2 mg) and underlying causes corrected. Resistant cases can be treated with IV isoprenaline (isoproterenol) (40–200 mcg/min). Temporary pacing is rarely required.

Electrocardiographic features

The ECG in sinus bradycardia exhibits a regular rhythm, with normal P wave axis, rate <60 bpm, usually a normal PR interval, and narrow QRS complexes. If the sinus rate falls below the intrinsic rate of the AV node, *junctional bradycardia* occurs. This rhythm is characterized by a regular, narrow QRS rhythm and P waves, either masked by the QRS complex or dissociated from it. The key to distinguishing junctional bradycardia with AV dissociation from third-degree AV block (see section on atrioventricular block) is that the atrial rate is slower than the ventricular rate, and some sinus P waves conduct normally to the ventricles. This is an important distinction because third-degree AV block rarely responds to atropine and may require temporary pacing because of the risk of asystole.

Sinoatrial disease and long-term treatment

Sometimes referred to as 'sick sinus syndrome', this pathology not only affects sinoatrial node function but also conduction and automaticity throughout both atria. As a result, it can produce both atrial tachyarrhythmias, such as atrial tachycardia and atrial fibrillation, and bradyarrhythmias, such as sinus bradycardia, junctional bradycardia, and sinus arrest.

Since arrhythmia episodes are intermittent, the diagnosis is usually made with ambulatory ECG monitoring. Daytime sinus pauses >3 s and night-time pauses >4.5 s are associated with significant risk of syncope. In some patients, a combination of tachycardic and bradycardic episodes is seen.

Permanent pacemaker implantation is the only effective treatment for symptomatic patients with bradycardia caused by sinoatrial disease. A single chamber atrial pacemaker can be used to prevent sinus bradycardia, but, because some patients subsequently develop AV block, dual chamber pacemakers are implanted in many centres. These systems have a lead placed in the right atrium and right ventricle so that the ventricles can be paced if AV conduction subsequently fails.

Atrioventricular block

Atrioventricular conduction can be affected by drugs and by any disease or process affecting the electrical pathways which connect the atria and ventricles. Thus, blocks, either

Table 4.6 Causes of sinus bradycardia

- Drugs (e.g. beta blockers, calcium channel blockers, digoxin, amiodarone)
- Hypoxia
- Hypothermia
- Hypothyroidism
- Pain (may also cause tachycardia)
- Acute myocardial infarction
- Pericardial tamponade
- Sick sinus syndrome
- Severe obstructive jaundice
- Adrenal insufficiency
- Pleural/peritoneal stimulation
- Raised intracranial pressure (with irregular breathing + wide pulse pressure)
- Rarely infection (e.g. typhoid)

in the atrioventricular node or more distally in the conducting pathways (His–Purkinje system), can cause failure of sinus impulses to activate the ventricles.

Pathophysiology

AV block can be caused by any of the factors listed in Box 4.1 (Common causes of atrial fibrillation). Sinoatrial disease can affect AV nodal conduction, and up to 25% of affected patients develop AV node disease later in life. AV block can complicate acute myocardial infarction. It usually resolves after inferior MI, where it reflects AV nodal ischaemia, but is a sinister sign in anterior MI because it reflects widespread damage to the ventricles and His–Purkinje system. Other causative pathologies include congenital AV block, aortic valve disease, endocarditis, dilated cardiomyopathies, myocardial infiltration (e.g. sarcoidosis), and Lyme disease. AV block may complicate cardiac surgery and catheter ablation procedures.

Electrocardiographic features

First-degree AV block is associated with constant PR interval prolongation (>200 ms) and almost never causes symptoms and does not require treatment (see Figure 4.13a).

Second-degree AV block is characterized by intermittent failure of conduction of sinus P waves to the ventricles. Block at AV nodal level causes Mobitz type I (Wenckebach) AV block, in which the PR interval progressively lengthens until a sinus P wave fails to conduct, after which the PR interval resets and the process repeats (see Figure 4.13b). Mobitz type I AV block rarely causes symptoms and is usually benign. It may be caused by high vagal tone and is a common nocturnal/rest finding on ambulatory monitoring in physically fit young people.

Block at His/Purkinje level causes Mobitz type II AV block and is associated with a normal PR interval and intermittent sudden failure of AV conduction (see Figure 4.13c). Mobitz type II block is usually pathological, may reflect myocardial disease, and can be associated with asystolic episodes. In patients with 2:1 AV block, it is not possible to determine the level at which conduction block is occurring.

Third-degree AV block is characterized by complete failure of P waves to conduct to the ventricles and dissociation of atrial and ventricular activity. The atrial rate is normal, and a slow, regular 'escape' rhythm is seen (see Figure 4.13d). Narrow QRS escape rhythms arise from the AV junction, with a rate of 40–50 bpm. Broad QRS escape rhythms arise from the ventricles, with a rate of 30–40 bpm. Third-degree AV block is associated with risk of asystole, especially if associated with a slow, wide QRS escape rhythm.

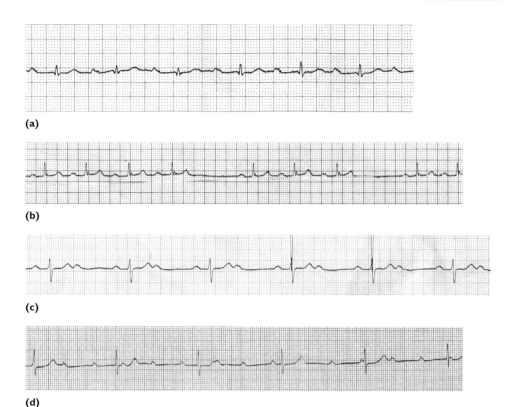

(a)

(b)

(c)

(d)

Figure 4.13 (a) First-degree AV block. (b) Mobitz type I second-degree AV block. (c) Mobitz type II second-degree AV block. (d) Third-degree AV block. Reproduced from Hung-Fat Tse, Gregory Y.H. Lip, and Andrew J. Stewart Coats, *Oxford Desk Reference: Cardiology*, 2011, Figure 3.1.1, 3.1.2, 3.1.3, 3.1.4, pp. 59–60, with permission from Oxford University Press.

Atrial fibrillation can occur with complete AV block. Fibrillation waves are seen associated with one of the above regular escape rhythms (see Figure 4.6).

Acute management

Symptomatic second- or third-degree AV block may respond to IV atropine if increased vagal tone is a contributing factor (e.g. in vasovagal syncope or myocardial infarction). IV isoprenaline can be administered if this fails, but temporary pacing is normally required until either the underlying cause is treated or a permanent pacemaker is implanted. Asymptomatic AV block (type I and usually type II) does not require acute treatment. Patients with persistent third-degree AV block should be admitted for monitoring and assessment.

Long-term management

Permanent pacemaker implantation is generally indicated in Mobitz type II AV block and in third-degree AV block (even if asymptomatic). In rare cases of symptomatic Mobitz type I AV block, pacemaker implantation may be needed. It is usual to wait at least 2 weeks after myocardial infarction for AV block to resolve before committing the patient to permanent pacing. Permanent pacing is also indicated in some patients with neurocardiogenic syncope associated with sinus bradycardia or AV block (e.g. malignant vasovagal syndrome) if other measures fail.

A dual chamber pacemaker is normally implanted. This allows sensing of sinus P waves and sequential pacing of the ventricles. In patients with atrial fibrillation and complete AV block, a single chamber ventricular pacemaker is used.

FAQ 3 Can I drive if I have a pacemaker or ICD?

In the UK, driving is allowed 1 week after permanent pacemaker implantation if symptoms have resolved. The same applies for patients who have an ICD implanted purely on prophylactic (primary prevention) grounds. Patients treated with an ICD for secondary prevention cannot drive for a minimum of 6 months, and only then if the ICD has not delivered a shock or symptomatic antitachycardia pacing.

Further reading

ACC/AHA Task Force on Practice Guidelines (2002). ACC/AHA/NASPE 2002 Guideline Update for Implantation of Cardiac Pacemakers and Antiarrhythmia Devices: Summary Article. *Circulation*, **106**, 2145–61.

ACC/AHA/ESC Task Force (2006). ACC/AHA/ESC 2006 guidelines for management of patients with ventricular arrhythmias and the prevention of sudden cardiac death–executive summary. *European Heart Journal*, **27**, 2099–140.

AHA/ACC/HRS (2014). Guideline for the Management of Patients With Atrial Fibrillation: Executive Summary. *Journal of the American College of Cardiology*, **64**, 2246–2280.

Antzelevitch C, Pollevick GD, Cordeiro JM, *et al.* (2007). Loss-of-function mutations in the cardiac calcium channel underlie a new clinical entity characterized by ST-segment elevation, short QT intervals, and sudden cardiac death. *Circulation*, **115**, 442–9.

Arrhythmia Alliance. <http://www.heartrhythmcharity.org.uk/>.

Atrial Fibrillation Association. <http://www.atrialfibrillation.org.uk/>.

British Heart Foundation. <http://www.bhf.org.uk>.

CredibleMeds. Overview of long QT syndrome and torsades de pointes. <http://www.crediblemeds.org/healthcare-providers/practical-approach/.

Ellinor PT, Milan DJ, MacRae CA (2003). Risk stratification in the long-QT syndrome. *New England Journal of Medicine*, **349**, 908–9.

Gage BF, van Walraven C, Pearce L, *et al.* (2004) Selecting patients with atrial fibrillation for anticoagulation: stroke risk stratification in patients taking aspirin. *Circulation*, **110**, 2287–92.

Mant J, Hobbs FD, Fletcher K, *et al.* (2007). Warfarin versus aspirin for stroke prevention in an elderly community population with atrial fibrillation (the Birmingham Atrial Fibrillation Treatment of the Aged Study, BAFTA): a randomised controlled trial. *Lancet*, **370**, 493–503.

National Institute for Health and Clinical Excellence (2006). Arrhythmia—implantable cardioverter defibrillators (ICDs) (review). <http://guidance.nice.org.uk/TA95>.

Sen-Chowdhry S, Syrris P, McKenna WJ (2007). Role of genetic analysis in the management of patients with arrhythmogenic right ventricular dysplasia/cardiomyopathy. *Journal of the American College of Cardiology*, **50**, 1813–21.

Sicilian Gambit (2001). New approaches to antiarrhythmic therapy, Part I: emerging therapeutic applications of the cell biology of cardiac arrhythmias. *Circulation*, **104**, 2865–73.

Syncope Trust And Reflex anoxic Seizures (STARS UK). <http://www.stars.org.uk/>.

Task Force of the Working Group on Arrhythmias of the European Society of Cardiology (1991). The 'Sicilian Gambit': A new approach to the classification of antiarrhythmic drugs based on their actions on arrhythmogenic mechanisms *European Heart Journal*, **12**,1112–31.

van Walraven C, Hart RG, Singer DE, *et al.* (2002). Oral anticoagulants vs aspirin in nonvalvular atrial fibrillation: an individual patient meta-analysis. *JAMA*, **288**, 2441–8.

Hypertension and hypertensive emergencies

In the management of acutely unwell patients, the physician will recognize that hypertension can present in three ways:

- Hypertensive emergencies: acute life-threatening presentations with a BP ≥180/120 mmHg, with obvious end-organ damage. In pregnancy, blood pressure > or = 140/90 mmHg, associated with proteinuria, is termed pre-eclampsia and also requires urgent treatment.
- Hypertensive urgencies: defined as acute elevation in systolic or diastolic BP ≥160/100 mmHg, without evidence of end-organ damage.
- Hypertension as a common chronic condition and a recognized risk factor for developing cardiovascular, cerebrovascular, and renal disease. In this context, the hypertension is often already being treated. This is probably the most common finding in acute care. Target blood pressures for treatment are 140/90 mmHg for most but, in diabetics and patients with chronic renal disease, 130/80 mmHg, at most, and some authorities now aim for 125/75 mmHg.

For the purposes of this section, the diagnosis and treatment of hypertensive emergencies will be discussed. These require prompt assessment and subsequent treatment of the blood pressure although not necessarily to normal levels. The term hypertensive emergency includes so-called malignant or accelerated hypertension. Patients with a hypertensive emergency should be managed in a fully monitored environment and may require intensive care.

In contrast, hypertensive urgencies can usually be treated over 24–48 hours, and oral therapy is usually sufficient.

Hypertensive emergencies

Patients presenting with high blood pressure and clear evidence of acute end-organ damage are suffering from a true medical emergency that requires urgent treatment of the blood pressure as well as measures to treat the presenting problem. Often, this will require parenteral treatment.

Examples of this include:

- Hypertensive encephalopathy (malignant hypertension).
- Acute myocardial infarction and acute coronary syndrome.
- Acute pulmonary oedema.
- Acute aortic dissection.
- Acute renal failure.
- Acute cerebral infarction or haemorrhage.
- Eclampsia, pre-eclampsia, and HELLP.
- Microangiopathic haemolytic anaemia.

Pathophysiology

The pathophysiology is not fully understood. There is a failure of autoregulation that normally maintains tissue perfusion at a constant level, preventing the high pressure being transmitted to smaller arterioles. As autoregulation fails, systemic vascular resistance increases, with damage to the arterioles and capillaries, associated with a cycle of endothelial damage characterized by local activation of the clotting cascade, fibrinoid necrosis of small vessels, and release of local vasoconstrictors.

Most patients presenting with a hypertensive emergency will have single-organ involvement, but a smaller proportion of patients will have two- or three-organ damage.

Clinical presentations

There are a variety of clinical presentations associated with a BP ≥180/120 mmHg and acute end-organ damage. These

are often in patients with previously poorly controlled blood pressure or recent discontinuation of treatment. Common secondary causes of hypertension, including renal artery stenosis, primary hyperaldosteronism, and intrinsic renal disease, should be considered as part of the differential diagnosis. A full clinical examination is essential, including fundoscopy.

All patients require routine investigations as well as disease-specific investigations. Routine investigations should include serum urea, creatinine and electrolytes estimations, full blood count and blood film, ECG, chest X-ray, and urinalysis for blood and protein. In addition, disease-specific investigations will also be required.

Hypertensive encephalopathy

This develops as a result of cerebral oedema and is characterized by gradual onset of headache, nausea, and vomiting, the development of non-focal neurological symptoms, including confusion, agitation, and ultimately fits and coma, if untreated. Papilloedema is commonly but not universally present. CT or MRI of the head is often used to exclude other neurological causes. MRI has the advantage, as it may show evidence of white matter oedema (T2-weighted images) of the parieto-occipital regions (posterior leukoencephalopathy syndrome) which is also sometimes seen in the pons.

Intravenous labetalol, a combined alpha- and beta-blocker, is most commonly used as an infusion at a rate of 0.5–2 mg/min to treat this presentation.

Acute myocardial infarction or acute coronary syndrome

These conditions are treated, according to standard protocols (see 'Acute coronary syndromes'). The presence of severe hypertension is a contradiction to immediate thrombolysis, and, as such, primary coronary intervention may be more attractive. Intravenous nitrates and beta-blockers will often have been used, but, if the hypertension persists, a labetalol infusion should be considered. Intravenous nicardipine may also be of benefit in controlling the hypertension, improving the ischaemia, and can be easily continued as an oral medication once the need for intravenous therapy has passed.

Acute pulmonary oedema

In the context of a hypertensive emergency, standard therapy for pulmonary oedema is indicated, with diuretics and nitrates. Morphine and CPAP are used as needed (see 'Heart failure'). If the blood pressure fails to respond to treatment, then expert cardiology input, including urgent echocardiography, should be obtained to assess left ventricular ejection fraction and systolic and diastolic function. If standard therapy, as already outlined, is not successful, then it is possible to use intravenous nitroprusside, an arteriolar and venous dilator, at a starting infusion rate of 0.25–0.5 mcg/kg/min increasing to a maximum of 8–10 mcg/kg/min. The use of nitroprusside is now rare in the UK. Cyanide toxicity prohibits prolonged use, and the risk is greater in renal failure. It is contraindicated in pregnancy.

Acute aortic dissection

Aortic dissection can affect the thoracic aorta or abdominal aorta. Surgical review is essential, usually after the diagnosis is confirmed, by imaging with CT scan and/or echocardiography. In addition to analgesia, a labetalol infusion should be started and titrated to lower BP within the first 30 min of presentation.

Acute renal failure

In the context of a hypertensive emergency, these patients will have haematuria and proteinuria at presentation, in association with elevation of serum urea and creatinine. In addition to full supportive measures for acute renal failure (see Chapter 11), the hypertension is best treated with fenoldopam, a selective post-synaptic dopaminergic (DA1) receptor agonist with weak alpha-2 antagonistic properties. Fenoldopam is a natriuretic agent that has a potent vasodilator activity, affecting primarily the renal vasculature. At a dose of 0.2–0.5 mcg/kg/min, fenoldopam decreases BP to desired levels within 5 to 40 min.

Acute cerebral infarction or haemorrhage

Elevated blood pressure is a common clinical finding at presentation. For ischaemic stroke, there is no evidence for treating blood pressure acutely, and antihypertensive agents are withheld. National guidelines suggest treating if BP exceeds 220 mmHg systolic or 120 mmHg diastolic. If eligible for thrombolysis, then a systolic of 180 mmHg or diastolic 110 mmHg is the recommended cut-off for treatment. Labetalol or nicardipine should be considered. Lowering blood pressure too aggressively may lead to further tissue hypoperfusion.

Eclampsia, pre-eclampsia, and HELLP

Standard treatment for this is discussed in Chapter 21. HELLP (haemolysis (H), elevated liver enzymes (EL), and low platelets (LP)) is a microangiopathic syndrome, associated with pre-eclampsia or eclampsia in up to 20% of cases. Blood pressure limits are >140/90 mmHg, with associated proteinuria. Target pressures on treatment should be a systolic pressure <160 mmHg and diastolic <110 mmHg. If platelet count is low, then treatment targets are 10 mmHg lower. All patients should receive intravenous magnesium to prevent or treat seizures.

A labetalol infusion is most commonly used to control blood pressure.

Microangiopathic haemolytic anaemia (MAHA)

MAHA may complicate malignant hypertension and reflects the degree of endothelial damage that has occurred with associated fibrin deposition. Treatment of the underlying hypertension remains very important and requires intravenous therapy, often with intravenous labetalol as described previously. As the blood pressure is controlled, the red cell destruction also tends to resolve.

Goals of treatment

When antihypertensive therapy is initiated in a hypertensive emergency, the aim is to lower the diastolic pressure to about 100–105 mmHg over a 2–6-hour period. It must be recognized, however, that patients must be continually monitored to ensure the clinical condition is improving, as there is a risk of aggravating tissue hypoperfusion by too rapid or over-aggressive lowering of the blood pressure. Once the blood pressure is controlled, the patient can be changed to oral therapy, dictated by disease, age, and ethnicity.

Further reading

Haas AR and Marik PE (2006). Current diagnosis and management of hypertensive emergencies. *Seminars in Dialysis*, **19**, 502–12.

Thromboembolic disease

Pulmonary embolism

Pulmonary embolism (PE) is a common illness, with an age- and sex-adjusted incidence of around 100–300 cases per 100,000 person years, rising sharply after the age of 60 years old. While mortality rates are under-appreciated (10–15% in the first 3 months after diagnosis), they are less than 10% if PE is diagnosed and treated promptly. In around 25% of cases, the initial clinical manifestation is death. More than half of patients with PE remain undiagnosed.

The iliofemoral veins are the source of most clinically recognized PE. The majority of PE cases manifest as multiple, lower lobe emboli.

Large thrombi may cause haemodynamic compromise due to both anatomical obstruction of blood flow and release of humoral factors. The extent of the haemodynamic compromise depends on the size of the embolus, coexistent cardiopulmonary disease, and the neurohormonal effects.

Clinical approach

Clinical presentation is extremely heterogeneous and non-specific. PE is, therefore, a common differential diagnosis, and a high index of suspicion is required to make the diagnosis. The symptoms, signs, and abnormal routine investigations are of limited value in confirming PE. The use of a validated probability scoring system and D-dimer testing has allowed senior clinicians to make a more accurate assessment of clinical probability to guide and potentially rationalize ongoing investigative modalities.

Risk factors

Patients with PE usually have identifiable risk factors for the development of venous thrombosis at the time of presentation.

Major risk factors (5–20x risk)

- Surgery.
- Late pregnancy.
- Major orthopaedic trauma.
- Immobility.
- Hospital admission.
- Previous PE or DVT.
- Varicose veins.

Minor risk factors (2–4x risk)

- Cardiovascular disease.
- Oral contraception.
- Hormone replacement therapy.
- Obesity.
- Travel (>5–6 hours).
- Thrombophilia (inherited or acquired).

Malignancy is eventually detected in 17% of patients who have recurrent 'idiopathic' venous thromboembolism and is uniformly associated with a poor prognosis. Occult cancers can usually be detected by a combination of careful clinical assessment, routine blood tests, and chest radiography alone. Recent guidance advises further investigation in unprovoked PE in those >40 years with an abdomino-pelvic CT scan ± mammography.

History and examination

Although up to 90% of emboli arise from the lower limbs, the majority of patients have no leg symptoms at the time of diagnosis. The most common presenting symptoms are dyspnoea (73%), pleuritic pain (66%), cough (37%), and haemoptysis (13%). The most common signs are tachypnoea (70%), crepitations (51%), tachycardia (30%), and a fourth heart sound (24%). Fever (>38.9°C) occurs in 14% of patients.

Probability scoring

Clinical probability assessment is an essential component of optimal PE management. Its use encourages good clinical assessment, allows better interpretation of imaging results, and, in combination with D-dimer assays, can reduce the need for further radiological investigation.

Several clinical probability scores exist. The most extensively validated are the Wells and the Geneva scores (see Table 4.7); both classify patients as low, intermediate, or high risk and have demonstrated similar accuracy. A dichotomous version of the Wells clinical decision rule (likely vs unlikely) is equally accurate and may be more pragmatic in clinical practice. The use of a particular score will vary, according to the physician's familiarity, the type of D-dimer assay used, and local prevalence of PE. The proportion of patients with confirmed PE can be expected to be 10%, 30%, and 65% in low, intermediate, and high probability categories respectively. When the dichotomous classification is used, PE will be confirmed in about 12% of the 'PE-unlikely' group.

Investigations

Baseline investigations

ECG is often abnormal but is insensitive and non-specific. The most common abnormalities are tachycardia, non-specific ST segment, and T wave changes. S1Q3T3 pattern, atrial arrhythmias, and complete right bundle branch block are also seen, and, whilst their diagnostic value is limited, they may be associated with a poor prognosis.

Chest X-ray is interpreted as 'normal' in only 12% of patients with confirmed PE. The most frequent radiographic abnormalities are atelectasis or a pulmonary parenchymal abnormality. Pleural effusion is evident in up to 47% of patients, although this is non-specific.

Arterial blood gases do not appear to have a major role in excluding or establishing the diagnosis of PE. Similarly, pulse oximetry is of little diagnostic value. Both may have a role in prognostication.

D-dimer assay is only useful as an exclusion test for pulmonary embolism when results are negative. Positive results are highly non-specific. Increasing age, malignancy, recent hospitalization, pregnancy, infection, and peripheral vascular disease will cause elevation, irrespective of the presence of venous thromboembolism. Higher levels may be associated with a poorer prognosis.

Guidelines suggest that a negative, quantitative D-dimer reliably excludes PE in patients with low or intermediate clinical probability (>95% negative predictive value); such patients have an estimated 3-month risk of VTE of 0.14% (if anticoagulation is withheld) and do not need further imaging for PE. A negative D-dimer should never be used as a stand-alone prognostic strategy. Patients with high clinical probability should not undergo D-dimer assessment and should proceed to further radiological assessment.

CT pulmonary angiography (CTPA)

This is now the main diagnostic imaging modality to evaluate suspected PE. It is superior to isotope scanning, is quick to perform, available out of hours, and, when negative, often allows an alternative diagnosis to be made. Newer

Table 4.7 Clinical prediction rules for PE.

Items	Clinical decision rule points	
Wells rule	**Original version**	**Simplified version**
Previous PE or DVT	1.5	1
Heart rate ≥100 b.p.m.	1.5	1
Surgery or immobilization within the past four weeks	1.5	1
Haemoptysis	1	1
Active cancer	1	1
Clinical signs of DVT	3	1
Alternative diagnosis less likely than PE	3	1
Clinical probability		
Three-level score		
Low	0–1	N/A
Intermediate	2–6	N/A
High	≥7	N/A
Two-level score		
PE unlikely	0–4	0–1
PE likely	≥5	≥2
Revised Geneva score	**Original version**	**Simplified version**
Previous PE or DVT	3	1
Heart rate		
75–94 b.p.m.	3	1
≥95 b.p.m.	5	2
Surgery or fracture within the past month	2	1
Haemoptysis	2	1
Active cancer	2	1
Unilateral lower limb pain	3	1
Pain on lower limb deep venous palpation and unilateral oedema	4	1
Age >65 years	1	1
Clinical probability		
Three-level score		
Low	0–3	0–1
Intermediate	4–10	2–4
High	≥11	≥5
Two-level score		
PE unlikely	0–5	0–2
PE likely	≥6	≥3

Reproduced from Konstantinides SV et al., '2014 ESC Guidelines on the diagnosis and management of acute pulmonary embolism', *European Heart Journal*, 2015, 35, 43, pp. 1–48, by permission of the European Society of Cardiology.

multidetector CT scanners have increased the detection rate of subsegmental PE, virtually eliminating non-diagnostic studies.

The PIOPED II study found that, in patients with a low or intermediate clinical probability of PE (using the Wells score), normal findings on CTPA had a high negative predictive value for PE (96% for patients with a low probability and 89% with an intermediate probability), whereas the nega-tive predictive value was only 60% in patients with a high probability before testing. Conversely, the positive predictive value of abnormal findings on CTPA was high (92% to 96%) in patients with an intermediate or high clinical probability but much lower (58%) in patients with a low likelihood of PE. Clinical assessment should, therefore, be included in the diagnostic work-up of PE to allow for an adequate interpretation of test results (see Figure 4.14).

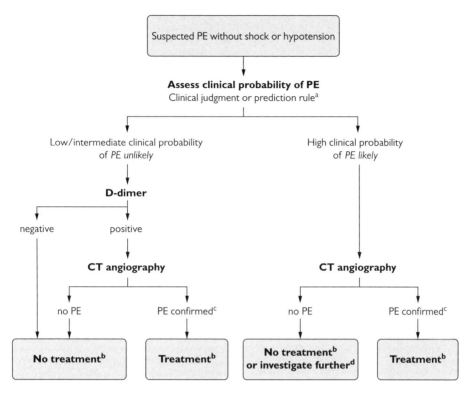

CT = computed tomographic; PE = pulmonary embolism.

[a]Two alternative classification schemes may be used for clinical probability assessment, i.e. a three-level scheme (clinical probability defined as low, intermediate, or high) or a two-level scheme (PE unlikely or PE likely). When using a moderately sensitive assay, D-dimer measurement should be restricted to patients with low clinical probability or a PE-unlikely classification, while highly sensitive assays may also be used in patients with intermediate clinical probability of PE. Note that plasma D-dimer measurement is of limited use in suspected PE occurring in hospitalized patients.

[b]Treatment refers to anticoagulation treatment for PE.

[c]CT angiogram is considered to be diagnostic of PE if it shows PE at the segmental or more proximal level.

[d]In case of a negative CT angiogram in patients with high clinical probability, further investigation may be considered before withholding PE-specific treatment.

Figure 4.14 Proposed diagnostic algorithm for patients with haemodynamically stable PE. Reproduced from Konstantinides SV et al., '2014 ESC Guidelines on the diagnosis and management of acute pulmonary embolism', *European Heart Journal* 2015, 35, 43, pp. 1–48, by permission of the European Society of Cardiology.

Clinicians should be wary of results that are discordant with their clinical judgement. Normal results on CTPA should be interpreted as ruling out PE only in patients with unlikely clinical probability. CTPA assessment of right ventricular dysfunction and clot load may also offer additional prognostic information (comparable to echocardiography). The addition of CT venography of the lower limbs to CTPA may be of use in complex cases.

V/Q scanning
Given its limitations and restricted out-of-hours availability, V/Q scanning has largely been replaced by CTPA. It may have a role in the investigation of PE in pregnancy due to its potentially lower radiation dosage. This also applies to patients with severe contrast allergy, and those with significantly impaired renal function, although lower limb

Doppler should be performed initially in all these patient groups.

Lower limb Doppler USS
This should be utilized as the initial investigation in those patients presenting with signs and symptoms of both DVT and PE, or those with equivocal or discordant CTPA imaging, and patients with a contraindication to CTPA (as discussed in the previous paragraph).

Transthoracic echocardiography
This has a low sensitivity for diagnosing PE; 30% to 40% of patients with PE have abnormalities of right ventricular (RV) size or function. It may have a role in intermediate-risk PE as a prognostic test; registries and cohort studies have demonstrated an association between echo parameters of

RV dysfunction and a poor in-hospital outcome. However, standardized prognostic criteria and user dependence may limit its clinical utility.

Pulmonary angiography
This is the reference method for the diagnosis of PE. Its use is now uncommon, as it is an invasive procedure with limited availability. It is generally safe and well tolerated, with a mortality of less than 2% and morbidity of around 5%.

Magnetic resonance angiography
This has been limited by respiratory and cardiac motion artefacts, suboptimal resolution, complicated blood flow patterns, and magnetic susceptibility effects from the adjacent air-containing lung. Technologic advances offer promise for an expanded role of MRA and simultaneous MR venography of lower limbs.

Thrombophilia screening
This is controversial and, with the exception of lupus anticoagulant and antithrombin screening, does not generally alter management in most cases, so it is no longer recommended as routine. It may be considered in those with unprovoked VTE who wish not to receive lifelong anticoagulation.

Cardiac biomarkers
Serum levels of cardiac biomarkers, in particular troponin and brain natriuretic peptide (BNP), have been proposed as risk stratification tools in normotensive patients. Troponin I and T have a negative predictive value of 98% for mortality and in-hospital morbidity, following PE, and are, therefore, particularly useful for the identification of low-risk patients. Whilst data suggest elevations in troponin and BNP are associated with poor outcome, their use as a tool to justify aggressive therapy in intermediate-risk PE is limited due to their poor specificity and positive predictive value. Current ACCP guidance suggests that cardiac biomarkers (as well as echo and CT assessment of RV function) should not be measured routinely. Highly sensitive troponin assays and heart-type fatty acid binding protein (H-FABP) show promise in terms of improved prognostic performance, as may combinations of blood-borne biomarkers and imaging (see section on thrombolysis for details on PEITHO trial).

Outpatient management of PE
Clinical risk scores, such as PESI (see Jiménez et al. 2010) and sPESI, have facilitated the identification of a low-risk group, with a mortality less than 1.5% who may be suitable for early discharge or outpatient management. A recent meta-analysis, comparing 14 (mostly cohort) studies with a combination of early discharge and inpatient management studies, found no difference in recurrent VTE, major bleeding, or all-cause mortality. The addition of biomarkers (e.g. highly sensitive troponin) to clinical scores may maximize their sensitivity and negative predictive value.

Treatment
General approach
In patients with a high clinical suspicion of PE, an empiric therapeutic dose of heparin, usually low molecular weight heparin (LMWH), should be given immediately after the decision has been made that anticoagulation is appropriate and safe. Given the high incidence of mortality due to recurrent PE in untreated patients (approximately 30%), the risk of empirical treatment in those patients with suspected but unconfirmed PE, outweighs the risk of major bleeding (less than 3%).

If clinical suspicion is low, empiric anticoagulation should be considered on a case-by-case basis. In cases where there is a high clinical suspicion of PE, but a contraindication to anticoagulation, e.g. active bleeding, diagnostic imaging should be expedited so that alternative therapies, such as inferior vena caval filters, may be considered. In patients with idiopathic thromboembolic disease, there is a 15–20% risk of recurrence within 2–3 years.

Heparins
- **Low molecular weight heparin** is the current anticoagulant of choice in haemodynamically stable patients with PE. It reduces recurrent thrombotic events, decreases thrombus size, and results in less major bleeding than intravenous unfractionated heparin.
- Monitoring is not necessary except in those with a creatinine clearance less than 30 mL/min, obese patients, and pregnant patients. If required, an anti-Xa assay, 4 hours following administration, is advised with appropriate dosage titration. LMWHs should be continued for a minimum of 5 days (see section on warfarin).
- **Unfractionated heparin (UFH).** Given the superiority of LMWH, UFH is only advised in patients with persistent hypotension due to PE (i.e. massive PE where thrombolysis is not considered) and patients who have a creatinine clearance of less than 30 mL/min or who are at risk of bleeding or are perioperative.

Warfarin
Long-term treatment with warfarin is effective in preventing recurrent PE.

Treatment duration
- Patients with a first episode of PE who have a reversible or temporary risk factor (e.g. immobilization, surgery, or trauma) should receive anticoagulation for 3 to 6 months.
- Patients who have an idiopathic PE should be treated for 6 to 12 months. Lifelong anticoagulation should be offered, particularly if the event was life-threatening in males <50 years old; benefit should be balanced against the small, but ongoing, risk of bleeding (7.4% risk of recurrence vs 0.25% risk of bleeding per annum). Measurement of D-dimer levels 1 month after cessation of warfarin may refine the recurrence risk.
- Patients with PE and an irreversible risk factor (e.g. antithrombin deficiency) should be treated for at least 6 to 12 months. Lifelong anticoagulation may be considered.
- Patients who have two or more episodes of idiopathic PE (or DVT) should receive lifelong therapy.

Target INR
A target INR of 2.5 is the default target for prevention of PE. Thrombosis rates at 4 years are 2.5%, with a target INR of 2.5; 7.5% with a target INR of 1.5–1.9/2.0; and 20% without warfarin, with no significant difference in bleeding between the warfarinized groups. Of note, a recent meta-analysis (>6,000 patients) of home monitoring suggested efficacy, cost efficiency, and safety.

Risks
- Less than 3% of patients will develop major haemorrhage.
- The antithrombotic effect of warfarin (irrespective of INR) is delayed for 72 to 96 hours. LMWH should, therefore, be prescribed for a minimum of 5 days and INR should be therapeutic for at least 48 hours.
- Drug interactions are common.
- Warfarin-induced skin necrosis in patients with known protein C deficiency.

Newer anticoagulants

New oral anticoagulants (NOACs) may overcome issues with current anticoagulants, including subcutaneous administration, variable dosing, need for monitoring, and heparin-induced thrombocytopenia. Several have been evaluated in phase III trials, meaning that fixed-dose therapy without monitoring has become a reality in the treatment of PE (and DVT). All are contraindicated in renal failure (CrCl <15 mL/min). Improved bleeding profiles may also enable safer life-long anticoagulation in idiopathic PE. Practical recommendations for the use of NOACs and management of their bleeding complications have been published by the European Heart Rhythm Association (see Heidbuchel *et al.* 2013).

Direct thrombin inhibitors (dabigatran)

These have several advantages over heparins, including the inhibition of fibrin-bound thrombin, a more predictable dose response, and less potential to produce immune thrombocytopenia. The RE-COVER trials showed non-inferiority of dabigatran 150 mg bd in the treatment of VTE, with no increase in bleeding rates. Dabigatran requires 5 days of initial LMWH.

Factor Xa inhibitors (rivaroxaban, apixiban, fondaparinux)

Recent trials have demonstrated non-inferiority of rivaroxaban and apixaban, compared to standard therapy. Neither requires an initial period of parenteral injections; the risk of early VTE recurrence is overcome by a higher dose during the initial phase of therapy. Fondaparinux, once daily, subcutaneously is an effective and safe therapy for the treatment of PE; its application is limited by subcutaneous administration.

Aspirin

Emerging data suggest aspirin may have a role as alternative continuation therapy in those patients at high risk of recurrent VTE, intolerant of full anticoagulation.

Thrombolysis

Despite no large study or meta-analysis demonstrating a survival advantage, compared to heparin therapy alone, current international guidelines (BTS, ACCP, and ECS) recommend that thrombolysis be administered in the event of cardiac arrest where suspicion of PE is high and in patients with persistent hypotension or shock (systolic BP <90 mmHg or a decrease in systolic BP by >40 mmHg from baseline). Compared with heparin alone, thrombolysis produces:

- More rapid clot lysis.
- Improved pulmonary perfusion.
- Reductions in RV and pulmonary artery pressures.

A suggested regimen is outlined in Box 4.3. Overall risk of haemorrhage is reported to be about 10%. Intracerebral haemorrhage has an incidence of 0.9%, based on recent epidemiological data.

Thrombolysis for other situations, including haemodynamically stable PE with evidence of right ventricular dysfunction (RVD) or severe hypoxaemia, remains

---

Box 4.3 Thrombolysis regimens

Alteplase 100 mg over 2 h
- Once aPTT <80 s, start IV heparin (without bolus)
Accelerated Alteplase regimen
- Alteplase 0.6 mg/kg over 15 minutes
Tenecteplase weight adjusted IV bolus over 5 s (30–50 mg, with a 5 mg step every 10 kg from 60 to 90 kg)

---

controversial. Risk stratification and the putative benefits of thrombolysis in haemodynamically stable patients with RVD was recently addressed in the PEITHO trial. This multicentre, double-blind, randomized controlled trial (1,006 patients) compared thrombolysis (tenecteplase) with an infusion of unfractionated heparin. Recruited patients had confirmed PE with an abnormal RV (echo or CT parameters) and positive troponin (T or I). There was a reduction of 56% in the primary endpoint (circulatory collapse or death from any cause) in the thrombolysis group (2.6% vs 5.6%, P = 0.015). However, this was at the expense of increased bleeding (6.3% vs 15%, P <0.001). The treatment effect was magnified in those patients <75 years who also had only a 1.1% incidence of CVA. The study was also designed to assess 6-month and 24-month effects on progression to chronic thromboembolic pulmonary hypertension, which currently has an incidence of around 4%; these data are currently unavailable.

The PEITHO trial, therefore, supports the use of thrombolysis in selected patients (<75, low bleeding risk, absence of renal disease) at high risk of clinical deterioration, defined by a combination of troponin and imaging. The administration of local, endovascular thrombolysis, combined with ultrasound energy or half-dose fibrinolysis, may offer an advance in the field by overcoming issues with haemorrhage while achieving physiological improvements in right heart function. Given the inherent risks, thrombolysis should be prescribed on a case-by-case basis, following risk/benefit assessment and informed patient consent.

Vena caval filters

These are an important alternative when anticoagulation is contraindicated. Filters function effectively in the prevention of pulmonary embolism (2–4% symptomatic PE). However, strong evidence that they reduce mortality is not currently available. Temporary/retrievable filters allow short-term avoidance of anticoagulation and avoid the long-term complications of filter placement, in young patients at high risk of haemorrhage, including pregnancy.

Filters may also be considered in patients with PE despite therapeutic anticoagulation. Alternative options, such as long-term high-intensity anticoagulation therapy (INR target 3.5) or LMWH, should be considered prior to filter placement.

Surgical embolectomy

A case series of 47 patients suggests that embolectomy is effective in patients with centrally located thrombi with an adverse prognosis (96% survival at 27 months). It can also be applied in patients with persistent right heart thrombi who have failed thrombolysis, but, in either case, it should be performed as an emergency in specialist centres with clinical expertise.

PE in pregnancy

Investigations

None of the investigations available for PE are validated in pregnancy, and the most widely validated probability score, the Wells score, excludes pregnant patients. D-dimer levels increase with gestational age and pregnancy-related complications, such as pre-eclampsia. Consequently, they have a limited role in pregnancy. It may, however, maintain its negative predictive value.

Despite its limitations, given the absence of radiation exposure, bilateral leg Doppler should be the initial investigation of PE in pregnancy.

No clear consensus exists regarding further imaging when Doppler USS scanning is negative but in general imaging (including CTPA) should not be withheld (see Chapter 22). Data on radiation exposure differences between CTPA and V/Q scanning is variable, and consideration needs to be given to both mother and fetus. Informed consent should be obtained, and the protocol should be modified to minimize radiation dose.

The baby should have thyroid function tested within a week of birth to exclude contrast-induced hypothyroidism.

Treatment
LMWH is safe and efficacious in pregnancy. A twice-daily dosage regimen is recommended. Therapy should be continued throughout pregnancy and usually requires at least 6 months of therapy; warfarin should then be administered for at least 6 weeks post-partum.

Close liaison between local obstetricians, haematologists, and physicians is recommended.

Deep vein thrombosis
The incidence of DVT is underestimated but stands at 80 cases per 100,000 persons annually.

Virchow's triad, i.e. venous stasis, vessel wall injury, and hypercoagulable state, is the primary mechanism for the development of DVT. Death is attributable to fatal PE; accurate diagnosis and prompt therapy are, therefore, crucial. The risk of symptomatic or 'silent' PE with proximal vein thrombosis is approximately 50%.

History and examination
Symptoms and signs are non-specific. Symptoms of DVT include swelling, pain, and discoloration in the involved extremity. Signs include a thrombosed vein, oedema, warmth, and superficial venous dilation. Homan's sign is non-specific and is no longer recommended as a clinical sign due to the potential risk of dislodging clot. In addition, risk factors (as per PE) should be sought and probability score documented to assist interpretation of diagnostic testing.

Investigations
Given the inaccuracy of clinical diagnosis and the potential implications of missed diagnosis, further testing is generally indicated.

D-dimer should be utilized as an exclusion test, linked to clinical probability score in the same manner as PE.

A negative quantitative D-dimer, in conjunction with a low clinical probability of DVT, is useful and cost-effective in excluding DVT without the need for an ultrasound examination.

Doppler ultrasound is the diagnostic test of choice in suspected DVT with a (Wells) probability score >2 and/or positive D-dimer analysis.
- Sensitivity and specificity for proximal DVT are more than 95%.
- Imaging of the calf veins is not routinely performed, as sensitivity is only around 70%, with a positive predictive value of only 80%.
- If the initial study is negative and clinical probability high, a repeat study should be obtained at 5 to 7 days.

Venography is the gold standard diagnostic test. Given its technical difficulties and patient discomfort, its use should be reserved for patients with highly suggestive clinical signs or symptoms but negative results on ultrasonography.

Treatment
Outpatient anticoagulation is safe. Studies show more than 80% of patients can be treated without hospitalization. Outpatient treatment is unsuitable for patients with extensive thrombosis, significant comorbidities, or a high risk of haemorrhage (post-surgical or hepatorenal disease). Warfarin should be instituted as for PE, with similar treatment durations and target INRs.
- **Vena caval filters** should be considered in patients that have a contraindication to anticoagulation or those in whom treatment has failed.
- **Compression stockings** are recommended for two years post-event to minimize post–thrombotic syndrome.
- **Thrombolysis** can be considered to restore venous patency in limb-threatening thrombosis.

In-hospital prophylaxis
Prophylaxis for venous thromboembolism is underprescribed in hospitalized patients.

Certain inpatient populations are at particularly high risk for DVT and PE; these include:
- Total hip or knee replacement patients.
- Trauma and spinal cord injury patients.
- Acute medical patients (15% increased risk).
- Patients with stroke or congestive heart failure.

Anticoagulant prophylaxis is proven to reduce the risk of asymptomatic DVT and proximal DVT in hospitalized patients. Fondaparinux or LMWH should be administered to acutely ill medical patients with at least one risk factor for VTE and no tendency towards haemorrhage. Patients with renal failure (CrCl <30 mL/min) should receive UFH. Daily review of the need for continuation of therapy should be undertaken, and, where risk is low, prophylaxis should be avoided altogether.

Newer oral anticoagulants (as discussed previously) should be considered as an efficacious and safe alternative to LMWH in orthopaedic patients, based on numerous phase III trials. LMWH, UFH, or fondaparinux should be used in general surgical patients. Pneumatic compression devices, with or without stockings, should be used where bleeding risk is high or in low-risk patients.

The optimal timing for post-operative administration of thromboprophylaxis is between 4 and 12 hours, with due consideration of bleeding risk. The optimal duration of therapy remains unclear, but extended out-of-hospital prophylaxis may be warranted in patients undergoing major orthopaedic surgery.

All hospitalized patients should be assessed for the need for prophylaxis on admission. All hospitals should formulate written guidelines, and, in the UK, this should conform to NICE guidance.

Fat embolism syndrome (FES)
FES remains a diagnostic challenge. Mortality ranges from 10-15%.

History and examination
- Most frequently associated with long bone and pelvic fractures (90%), closed rather than open.
- Also associated with acute pancreatitis, burns, liposuction, sickle cell crises, and steroid therapy.
- The classic triad of hypoxaemia, neurological abnormalities, and a petechial rash (head, neck, axillae, subconjunctivae) typically occurs 12 to 72 hours after the initial insult.
- A syndrome similar to that of ARDS may develop, followed by an acute confusional state or seizures.

Investigations
FES is primarily a clinical diagnosis, with a compatible history and the triad of clinical signs.

- Chest X-ray is normal in the majority but may progress to bilateral infiltrates.
- CT thorax may show areas of ground glass opacification with interlobular septal thickening.
- Bronchoalveolar lavage to detect fat droplets in alveolar macrophages may have a future role.

Treatment and prevention
Treatment is supportive, and most patients will recover fully.
- Early immobilization of fractures reduces the incidence of FES; fixation within 24 hours has been shown to reduce the incidence of ARDS fivefold.
- Steroid therapy is controversial; studies have suggested a reduced incidence and severity of FES when given prophylactically. The optimal timing, dose, and duration of therapy remain unclear.

Further reading

Chong LY, Fenu E, Stansby G, Hodgkinson S; Guideline Development Group (2012). Management of venous thromboembolic diseases and the role of thrombophilia testing: summary of NICE guidance. *BMJ*, **344**, e3979.

Guyatt GH, Eikelboom JW, Gould MK, et al. (2012). 9th edn: American College of Chest Physicians Evidence Based Clinical Practice Guidelines. *Chest*, **14** (Suppl 2), e185S–94S.

Heidbuchel H, Verhamme P, Alings M, et al. (2013). European Heart Rhythm Association Practical Guide on the use of new oral anticoagulants in patients with non-valvular atrial fibrillation. *EP Eurospace*, **15**, 625–651.

Jiménez D, Aujesky D, Moores L, et al. (2010). Simplification of the Pulmonary Embolism Severity Index for Prognostication in Patients With Acute Symptomatic Pulmonary Embolism. *Archives of Internal Medicine*, **170**,1383–89.

National Institute for Health and Care Excellence (NICE). Clinical Guideline 92. (2010). Venous thromboembolism: reducing the risk: Reducing the risk of venous thromboembolism (deep vein thrombosis and pulmonary embolism) in patients admitted to hospital. <https://www.nice.org.uk/guidance/cg92>.

Konstantinides SV, Torbicki A, Agnelli G, et al. (2014). 2014 ESC Guidelines on the diagnosis and management of acute pulmonary embolism. *European Heart Journal*, **25**, 3033–3080.

PEITHO trial. Meyer G, Vicaut E, Danyas E, et al. (2014). Fibrinolysis for patients with intermediate risk pulmonary embolism. *New England Journal of Medicine*, **370**(15), 1402–11.

Royal College of Obstetricians and Gynaecologists (2015). Thromboembolic Disease in Pregnancy and the Puerperium: Acute Management. Guideline No 37b. RCOG Press, London.

Stein PD, Fowler SE, Goodman LR, et al. (2006). Multidetector computed tomography for acute pulmonary embolism. *New England Journal of Medicine*, **354**, 2317–27.

Wells P, Anderson DR, Rodger M, et al. (2000). Derivation of a simple clinical model to categorize patients' probability of pulmonary embolism: increasing the models utility with the SimpliRED D-dimer. *Thrombosis and Haemostasis*, **83**, 3, 416–20.

Valvular disease

Introduction

Valves in the heart are passive structures, relying on their flexibility, integrity, and supporting structures to function normally. Conditions resulting from valvular disease usually cause an increased load on the heart, and the resulting presentation depends on the ability of the heart to handle this additional load. Many mild valve diseases or disorders are asymptomatic and discovered because of incidental murmurs. They must be distinguished from the more important conditions with signs of severe valve disease and decompensation.

Epidemiology

Valve diseases may be congenital/genetic or acquired. Congenital lesions may be associated with other cardiac malformations, such as septal defects, and may only be detected in later life.

Common congenital/genetic lesions include:
- Bicuspid aortic valve (1% of population).
- Mitral valve prolapse (4% of population).
  Acquired causes include:
- Rheumatic fever (see section on rheumatic fever).
- Infective endocarditis (see section on infective endocarditis).
- Myocardial infarction disrupting papillary muscles.
- Fibrosis and calcification.
- Stretching of the valve ring.

Assessment of valve lesions

The severity of a valve lesion is assessed by a combination of symptoms, signs, and the results of investigations. Understanding the haemodynamic effects of different lesions helps with the evaluation of symptoms and signs. The heart is able to compensate for many lesions, but, if too great a load is placed on a chamber acutely or chronically (after many years), the resultant pressure changes produce a step change in symptoms and signs which is evidence of decompensation and heart failure.

The most important test of valvular function is the echocardiogram which highlights valve dysfunction in a number of ways:
- Wall motion can be normal, reduced, or hyperdynamic.
- Regional wall motion abnormalities (typically coronary artery disease).
- Wall thickness may be increased with hypertrophy.
- Valve(s) may look abnormal. Planimetry is a validated technique used to assess the area of a heart valve orifice, by the tracing out of the open valve on a still image obtained during echocardiography.
- Filling rate may be reduced (e.g. mitral stenosis).
- Estimation of abnormal pressure gradients (pulsed wave Doppler).
- Abnormal turbulence (colour flow Doppler).

Cardiac catheterization may be necessary to confirm the echo estimate of the severity of a valve lesion and document the coronary anatomy prior to surgery.

Individual valve lesions

Mitral stenosis

Mitral stenosis is rare in western populations but remains common in other parts of the world, particularly the Middle East. It is almost universally due to rheumatic fever, although many patients are unaware they have had rheumatic fever

(also see Chapter 6). It results in characteristic echocardiographic appearance of thickened valve leaflets, sometimes involving the chordae which can become matted (see Figure 4.15). From the fourth decade, calcification contributes to the stiffening.

Haemodynamics

Stiffening of the valve results in progressive restriction to flow from left atrium to left ventricle. Rising pressure in the left atrium causes dilatation and, ultimately, atrial fibrillation. Left ventricular filling is highly dependent on heart rate because available filling time in diastole shortens as heart rate increases. This means that exercise and uncontrolled atrial fibrillation are common causes of breathlessness.

With increasing severity of mitral stenosis, left atrial and pulmonary arterial pressure rise to a point where the patient complains of breathlessness. The rise in pulmonary artery pressure is initially due to the high left atrial pressure, but, in long-standing mitral stenosis, pulmonary vascular resistance increases, and patients may develop very high pulmonary artery pressures, with right heart failure (peripheral oedema, raised venous pressure, and ascites).

As mitral stenosis worsens, the progressive fall in left ventricular filling causes a fall in cardiac output. This may result in weight loss, breathlessness (compounding the breathlessness due to high left atrial pressures), and 'mitral facies'.

Symptoms

Breathlessness is the most prominent symptom. Other presentations include stroke (thromboembolic) and right heart failure.

Signs

The first heart sound is loud due to the mitral valve closing late when left ventricular pressure is rising fast. A palpable first heart sound is sometimes called a 'tapping apex'. The murmur of mitral stenosis comes shortly after the second heart sound and may be preceded by an opening snap from the diseased valve. The murmur is very low-pitched and best heard between the apex and base of the heart, with the patient turned on the left side. The length of the murmur relates to severity, and, if the patient is in sinus rhythm, the murmur may increase in intensity at the end of diastole when the left atrium contracts. There may also be signs of left heart failure (crackles at the lung bases) or right heart failure, as previously discussed.

Investigations

- ECG may show atrial fibrillation and right heart strain. In sinus rhythm, the p wave may be prolonged (p mitrale).
- Chest X-ray may show an enlarged left atrium, enlarged pulmonary artery, calcification in the valve, pulmonary oedema, pulmonary haemosiderosis (long-standing due to pulmonary haemorrhage), and enlargement of the right heart.
- Echo is the main diagnostic test and may show the valve to be thickened and sometimes calcified. The left ventricle may be small, with slow filling and enlarged left atrium. Measurement of the valve orifice area by planimetry may be possible, and, if images are good, it is a reliable indicator of stenosis. 3D echo may be even better. Doppler imaging will show reduced rate of fall of transmitral flow during diastole. Pulmonary hypertension can be estimated from Doppler imaging of tricuspid regurgitation. Transoesophageal echo allows good imaging of the valve and chordal apparatus and can detect thrombus in the left atrial appendage.

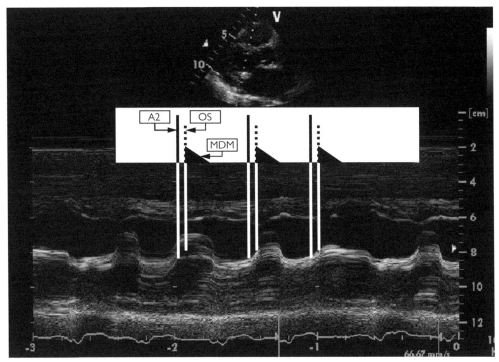

Figure 4.15 M-mode echocardiogram in rheumatic mitral stenosis showing thickened mitral valve leaflets. The patient is in atrial fibrillation, and the auscultatory signs are shown above. A2, aortic component of the second heart sound; OS, opening snap; MDM, mid-diastolic murmur.

• Cardiac catheterization can measure the transmitral gradient by comparing left ventricular pressure with indirect left atrial pressure (pulmonary capillary wedge pressure) or directly by transeptal puncture (echo estimates of mitral valve gradient and calculated mitral valve area are usually reliable). Pulmonary artery pressure can be measured and pulmonary vascular resistance can be calculated by right heart catheterization if the echo data are inadequate or conflicting with clinical evaluation.

Treatment

• **Mild MS.** No treatment needed, unless in atrial fibrillation when warfarin should be given and heart rate optimized with digoxin and/or rate-slowing calcium channel blockers and/or beta-blockers.

• **Moderate MS.** Breathlessness can be improved with diuretics. If the patient is in atrial fibrillation, rate control is very important to prolong diastolic filling time.

• **Severe MS.** If symptoms cannot be controlled by medical therapy, consider valve procedure, as discussed in the following sections.

Procedures for improving mitral valve function

• **Mitral balloon valvuloplasty** can be effective in patients with little calcification and mitral regurgitation. TOE is used to assess the valve and chordal apparatus, and, if suitable, a balloon is passed through the venous system, across the atrial septum, and positioned and inflated in the mitral orifice.

• **Mitral valvotomy** is carried out surgically, usually on bypass ('open') in the UK. The commissures are divided, and limited repair of the valve is possible.

Procedures for replacing the mitral valve

• **Mitral valve replacement** is required in severely stenotic valves with significant calcification or if there is much mitral regurgitation. The left atrial appendage is amputated to reduce the risk of future thromboembolism.

Mitral regurgitation

Mitral regurgitation (MR) is caused by two distinct groups of conditions. Primary MR is due to disease of the valve leaflets or the chordae. Secondary MR is due to changes in the shapes of surrounding structures (especially left ventricular dilatation stretching the valve ring) or abnormalities of papillary muscle function (usually ischaemic).

Mitral valve prolapse is a connective tissue disease in which parts of the valve, and sometimes also the chordae, stretch or rupture. The abnormal part of the valve then prolapses back into the left atrium in systole, disrupting the normal coaptation of the two leaflets. Other causes of MR are:

• **Primary MR:**
  • Marfan's syndrome (similar to mitral valve prolapse, but the clinical picture may be dominated by extracardiac features).
  • Congenital lesions, including clefts of the mitral valve, associated with ostium primum atrial septal defects.

- Infective endocarditis (often on a previously abnormal valve).
- **Secondary MR:**
  - Myocardial infarction interfering with the normal function of papillary muscles.
  - Stretching of the valve ring, secondary to left ventricular dilatation ('functional').

When the mitral valve leaks, left ventricular 'work' is wasted by ejecting blood backwards into the left atrium. The ventricle becomes volume-loaded, and the stroke volume increases to compensate with an increase in the end-diastolic dimension. Ultimately, if the ventricle fails, the end-systolic dimension also rises.

The sudden ejection of blood into the left atrium causes a pressure pulse which may spread into the pulmonary veins. Over time, the left atrium enlarges and may cushion the shock of the systolic pressure wave.

Left atrial pressure increases as a result of both the pressure wave and any rise in left ventricular end-diastolic pressure when the ventricle fails. High left atrial pressures cause breathlessness. Pulmonary artery pressure will also rise but rarely to the levels seen in mitral stenosis.

The assessment of true ventricular function is difficult in mitral regurgitation because there is little resistance to backward flow. This takes the load off the ventricle, making it seem to be more active than it would appear if there was no leak. The timing of intervention is difficult (see further text).

Acute MR

When MR develops gradually, adaptations occur that delay the onset of symptoms (e.g LA dilatation). If MR occurs rapidly (eg infective endocarditis or papillary muscle/chordal rupture), the patient may suddenly develop severe pulmonary oedema. Emergency surgery may be necessary, but aggressive afterload reduction and intra-aortic balloon pumping can stabilize the situation and buy time for antibiotic therapy in cases of endocarditis.

Symptoms of MR

Unless there is comorbid disease (coronary artery or infective endocarditis, for example), the only common symptom is breathlessness due to raised pulmonary venous pressure.

Signs

The patient may be in AF. The left ventricular impulse is hyperdynamic if there is significant volume-loading. On auscultation, there will be a loud pansystolic murmur, usually heard well at the apex, but radiating to the axilla or other places, depending on the direction of the jet. In mild MR due to mitral valve prolapse, there may be only a mid-/late systolic murmur, and one or more mid-systolic clicks. Murmurs in secondary MR are often softer or absent.

Investigations

- ECG will show left ventricular hypertrophy and sometimes AF.
- Chest X-ray shows an enlarged cardiac outline, with features of both left ventricular and left atrial enlargement. There may be pulmonary oedema.
- Echo details the anatomy of the valve and, therefore, the underlying cause of the MR. The changes to left ventricular dimensions and function, atrial size, flow reversal in the pulmonary veins, coupled with estimates of pulmonary artery pressure, help to establish the severity of the haemodynamic disturbance. Colour flow Doppler ultrasound will reveal the direction of the jet and estimate of

the extent of the turbulence in the left atrium. Specific measures, such as jet width and flow convergence, provide further evidence of severity, but the prognostic value is, as yet, unclear. Transoesophageal and 3D echo reveal detail about the disease process to allow the surgeon to plan a repair. Serial echo is particularly valuable in following gradual changes in LV dimensions to give early warning of deterioration in LV function. Practical clinical measures for early contractile dysfunction are a left ventricular end-systolic dimension of >45 mm and an ejection fraction of <60% (MR with good LV function should produce a supranormal ejection fraction). The full degree of dysfunction of the left ventricle may only be revealed after the mitral valve is replaced or repaired. One of the best single measures of left ventricular function is end-systolic dimension which should not exceed 45 mm.

Cardiac catheterization will confirm the echo results and check for coronary artery disease.

Treatment

Treatment consists of management of the valve lesion and its cause. For treatment of endocarditis, see Infective endocarditis. Coexistent coronary artery disease should be treated invasively on its own merits.

- **Mild MR.** Needs no treatment, but patients with systemic hypertension should be treated vigorously.
- **Moderate MR.** Symptoms can be improved by afterload reduction, aiming to reduce the volume of regurgitation by reducing the resistance to outflow through the aorta as well as taking the load off the left ventricle. Many cardiologists treat patients with moderate MR with ACE inhibitors, although there is no clear evidence to support their use, except if additional heart failure or hypertension is present. The condition may remain stable for many years, but close follow-up is important. Decisions about early surgery in asymptomatic, or mildly symptomatic, patients are difficult because of the problems in assessing LV function. Regular echo may be needed to identify early deterioration in LV function or dimensions.
- **Severe MR.** The timing of surgery in patients with significant MR remains one of the most difficult decisions and the decisions about intervention are different between primary and secondary MR. Primary MR has better outcomes and is more likely to be amenable to mitral valve repair, whereas secondary MR is usually associated with adverse ventricular remodelling and worse outcomes. Therefore a higher threshold for surgery is recommended for secondary MR. Surgery is recommended for primary MR if patients are symptomatic or there is evidence of left ventricular deterioration. Apart from the echo criteria suggesting left ventricular dysfunction (as previously discussed), pulmonary artery pressure >50 mmHg or recurrent atrial fibrillation are pointers towards surgery. If the native valve can be repaired, the long-term results are better than if a prosthetic valve is necessary, plus patients do not automatically need warfarin. Where conservative surgery is likely to be possible in a young patient, there is a tendency to operate early to avoid irreversible damage to the LV, but attempts to define reliable indices that predict future deterioration have been fruitless. Conservative surgery carries a lower mortality (1–2%) than mitral valve replacement (5–10%), with better long-term survival partly because the risk of infective endocarditis is less and there is less need for warfarin.

An alternative to surgery is beginning to be used on a trial basis for selected patients. This is carried out percutaneously under ultrasound control when a clip is placed at the tips of the two leaflets, binding them together. The technique remains experimental, and may be overtaken by percutaneous mitral valve replacement which is being developed.

- **Acute severe MR.** When MR develops suddenly, usually due to rupture of part of the valve, chordal apparatus, or papillary muscle, the ventricle does not have time to adapt to the sudden volume load and may fail. Both output and input to the left heart are severely deranged: cardiac output falls, and pulmonary oedema develops. Medical therapy has a limited role to improve the patient's condition prior to surgery. Afterload reduction with ACE inhibitors may be possible if the blood pressure allows. If not, intra-aortic balloon counterpulsation will improve cardiac output and reduce the degree of MR.

Aortic stenosis
Congenital aortic stenosis is rare, but bicuspid valves, which do not usually offer obstruction in the first two decades of life, are common (1% of the population). As they have to stretch to open, they tend to become thickened and eventually calcify, producing obstruction, usually in the fifth or sixth decade. Bicuspid valves can also cause predominant regurgitation because the valve ring and aorta above stretches (post-stenotic dilatation). In later years, the common cause of aortic stenosis is degeneration of the valve in a condition resembling atherosclerosis (but not amenable to conventional treatments for atheroma) which affects the flexibility of all three leaflets. Hypertension may be a factor. Rheumatic heart disease may cause aortic stenosis but usually in combination with mitral stenosis.

In aortic stenosis, blood pressure is usually maintained, but left ventricular pressure rises above aortic systolic pressure by an amount which depends on the degree of stenosis (the transaortic gradient). The left ventricle has to do additional pressure work to maintain cardiac output, causing left ventricular hypertrophy. Left atrial pressure rises due, firstly, to reduced compliance (diastolic dysfunction) and, ultimately, to systolic dysfunction as the ventricle fails. Both forms of left ventricular dysfunction can cause breathlessness.

Increased pressure work for the left ventricle increases myocardial oxygen consumption and can result in effort angina which may be confounded by additional coronary disease.

When the stenosis is sufficiently severe, the most sinister symptom, syncope, may occur or, occasionally, sudden death. Syncope is, therefore, regarded as a major symptom and requires urgent investigation and treatment.

Symptoms
The three common symptoms are, therefore, dyspnoea, chest pain, and syncope.

Signs
The usual evidence of aortic stenosis is an ejection systolic murmur, starting sometimes after an ejection click (evidence of a bicuspid valve) and continuing until the second heart sound. It is louder in the middle of systole when the transaortic pressure gradient and flow are greatest. When the stenosis is significant, additional signs may appear: the slow-rising carotid pulse, narrow pulse pressure, clinical left ventricular hypertrophy, and evidence of left ventricular failure (basal crackles). Importantly, when the left ventricle fails, the rate of ejection falls, and the murmur may become softer or inaudible. Hence, in any patient with unexplained left ventricular failure, critical aortic stenosis must be ruled out (usually by echo).

Investigations
- ECG may show left ventricular hypertrophy or ischaemia.
- Chest X-ray may reveal calcification in the valve, post-stenotic dilatation, cardiomegaly (late), or pulmonary venous hypertension.
- Echo shows a restricted valve, and the number of leaflets can be seen. Left ventricular thickness can be measured and function assessed. Flow velocity across the valve, as measured by Doppler ultrasound, is a useful measure of severity of obstruction, unless the left ventricle is failing. This velocity can be converted into a transaortic pressure gradient, and, with knowledge of the diameter of the outflow tract, an effective valve area can be calculated. Comparison of flow velocity at valve level and above is another useful parameter.
- Stress echo is sometimes used in a particular group of patients who have impaired left ventricular function, low cardiac output, and a small gradient across the aortic valve by Doppler estimate. It answers the question as to whether the aortic valve is moving poorly because of the low cardiac output (pseudo-stenosis) or whether the ventricle is moving poorly because the aortic valve is rigid and stenosed. The response to dobutamine shows no increase in Doppler gradient in pseudo-stenosis because any increase in cardiac output opens the valve wider, whereas, in true stenosis, the Doppler gradient increases in proportion to any increase in cardiac output.
- Cardiac catheterization can confirm the transaortic gradient and define the coronary artery anatomy.

Treatment
AS is a condition that can progress rapidly, and all patients need to be aware of the risk and be assessed regularly. Medical therapy is of limited value.

- **Mild AS** (sometimes confusingly called aortic sclerosis in the elderly which wrongly suggests that it does not progress) usually requires no treatment. Systemic hypertension should be managed aggressively.
- **Moderate AS** (transaortic pressure gradient between 40 and 70 mmHg) can be treated conservatively if the patient has no more than mild symptoms. Patients with syncope need to be investigated for other causes of syncope (e.g. Stokes–Adams attacks) and, if none are found, should be considered for surgery. Breathless patients do not usually improve with diuretics, unless they are in left ventricular failure. Patients managed conservatively should have annual echocardiograms to assess progression.
- **Severe AS** should be treated by surgery in any symptomatic patient (particularly syncope). After the onset of symptoms, average survival is 2 to 3 years. There is controversy around asymptomatic patients with severe AS. Because of the fear of sudden death (rare in truly asymptomatic patients), some cardiologists recommend surgery in younger patients with severe AS. Others recommend exercising the patient to see if they are genuinely asymptomatic. A third group will only recommend operation if the patient admits to symptoms. Available evidence supports the latter approach.

Aortic valve replacement has been the standard treatment for many years and is a very successful operation with low mortality and good long term results. In the last decade a new treatment, transaortic valve implantation (TAVI) has been developed and is being used increasingly. It is carried out percutaneously or transapically using a stent-like artificial valve which is collapsed around a large balloon. The new valve is positioned within the native aortic valve and the balloon inflated to stretch the stenotic native valve and allow the prosthetic valve to deploy once the balloon is removed. Results with this technique have been promising and it is now the treatment of choice for patients with an unacceptably high risk for open heart surgery. Further refinements are likely to see its use in a wider range of patients and it may reduce the number of open valve operations.

No drug treatment has been shown to prolong life, and, in inoperable patients, palliative heart failure treatments are for symptom relief only.

Aortic regurgitation

Aortic regurgitation may be caused by a number of conditions, including:

- Bicuspid aortic valve and post-stenotic dilatation of the aorta (usually with a degree of stenosis as well).
- Aortic root disease, producing enlargement of the aorta and stretching the valve.
- Marfan's syndrome—a more extreme version of the above.
- Aortic root dissection, with extension into the valve ring.
- Endocarditis.
- Rheumatic heart disease (usually, in combination with MS and the aortic valve, is more often stenotic).
- Syphilis.

The leaking valve produces a volume load on the left ventricle. Pressure in the aorta falls more quickly in diastole (lowering diastolic pressure), and the additional volume ejected in systole causes a rise in systolic pressure. Provided the ventricle compensates, the forward flow in the aorta is maintained, but the stroke volume may be significantly increased, reflected by an increase in the end-diastolic volume. As the condition progresses, the ventricle fails, and end-systolic volume also increases. Eventually, left ventricular end-diastolic pressure increases, and the patient develops pulmonary oedema.

The amount of unnecessary work the ventricle has to do is represented by the 'regurgitant fraction' which is the difference between the expected and observed stroke volume. While the ventricle compensates for the volume load, conventional measures of left ventricular function (e.g. ejection fraction) are 'supranormal'. As the ventricle fails, the left ventricular function appears to normalize before deteriorating further.

Symptoms

The main symptoms are dyspnoea and syncope. Syncope, as in aortic stenosis, carries a poor prognosis. Angina is uncommon, unless there is accompanying coronary artery disease.

Signs

- **Mild AR** may produce no detectable effect on blood pressure or evidence of volume-loading of the left ventricle. The main finding will be an early diastolic murmur in the second left intercostal space, beginning when the aortic valve closes (A2) and getting softer as diastole progresses. It is often very soft and high-pitched and best heard with the patient sitting forwards in held expiration.
- **Moderate AR** produces an increase in pulse pressure, as evidenced by the blood pressure and by signs, such as a sharpened carotid pulse. The murmur is more easily heard and may last throughout diastole.
- **Severe AR** produces greater widening of the pulse pressure, with diastolic pressures of 50 mmHg or less. The aortic and left ventricular pressures may equilibrate in

mid-diastole, or earlier, and the murmur, therefore, shortens or, in very severe cases, disappears. The left ventricular impulse (apex beat) is hyperdynamic. The extremely wide pulse pressure is responsible for a number of physical signs: collapsing carotid pulse, waterhammer pulse, Quincke's sign (flashing nail bed capillaries), Duroziez's sign (reversed flow in the femoral arteries in diastole), and pistol shot femoral pulses.

When the heart fails, there may be signs of left, and ultimately right, ventricular failure.

Acute severe AR is a medical emergency, most often caused by endocarditis or aortic dissection. Acutely compensatory mechanisms do not have time to develop, and the associated causes are themselves life-threatening. The patient presents in acute pulmonary oedema. The usual signs of severe AR may be unimpressive with a short, or absent, diastolic murmur but, provided the systolic pressure is maintained, the various signs, e.g. collapsing pulse, may be impressive. The diagnosis is confirmed by echo. Cardiac catheterization may be hazardous. CT or cardiac MR gives excellent images of the aorta. Temporary support may be provided by offloading and positive pressure ventilation, but usually the only remedy is surgery with replacement of the valve and sometimes the aortic root as well.

Investigations for AR

- ECG may show left ventricular hypertrophy.
- Chest X-ray will show cardiomegaly, even if the condition is compensated (compared to AS where the heart only enlarges if it fails), and evidence of pulmonary venous hypertension if the left ventricle fails.
- Echocardiography will show a volume-loaded left ventricle, unless the AR is mild or the ventricle is failing. The aetiology of the AR with aortic root dilatation, a bicuspid valve, or vegetations may be determined. The jet from the AR may close the mitral valve prematurely. Colour flow Doppler reveals turbulence in the left ventricular outflow tract in diastole, and measurements are made of the jet characteristics (see section on mitral regurgitation). An additional measure of severity is the time taken for the diastolic pressure gradient between LV and aorta to fall to half its initial value (the pressure half-time). Defining left ventricular dysfunction is difficult because even patients with 'normal' ejection fractions can have reduced forward flow (stroke volume minus regurgitant fraction). An ejection fraction of <50%, an end-diastolic dimension of >70 mm, or an end-systolic dimension of >50 mm are current criteria used as discriminators. A rising end-systolic dimension is particularly important.
- Other non-invasive imaging modalities: if aortic dissection is suspected, then anatomical extent is important to guide surgery. CT or cardiac magnetic resonance imaging (CMR) gives excellent images, often superior to angiography because of 3D reconstruction. In the future, CMR may become important in assessing left ventricular function and the severity of AR.
- Cardiac catheterization is used to check for coronary artery disease and give further information about the severity of the AR. Left ventricular end-diastolic pressure rises if the ventricle is failing and is influenced by both the degree of regurgitation and overall left ventricular function. Aortography is the traditional way of grading regurgitation and shows the shape of the aortic root. The amount of dye leaking into the left ventricle and rate of clearance (number of beats) can be estimated.

Treatment
- **Mild AR** usually needs no treatment.
- **Moderate AR** is usually well tolerated for many years, but patients must be followed up with regular echocardiography to detect progressive symptoms or evidence of the ventricle failing. Although reduction of aortic pressure (afterload reduction) has the potential to reduce the amount of regurgitation, and hence reduce the work of the left ventricle, there is no evidence to support its use.
- **Severe AR** may be well tolerated for many years but is likely, ultimately, to need surgery with valve replacement. The development of symptoms or evidence of an enlarging heart on echo would be indications for surgery. As discussed previously, medical treatment with afterload-reducing agents is logical but not supported by evidence. Medical treatment does not offer a long-term solution, as heart failure with severe AR has a poor prognosis without surgery.

Tricuspid regurgitation (TR)
Isolated tricuspid valve disease (primary TR) is uncommon in adults, except in infective endocarditis. Tricuspid endocarditis is usually found in intravenous drug abusers (see 'Infective endocarditis'). It causes pure TR associated with volume loading of the right ventricle.

In young patients, the commonest cause is Ebstein's anomaly.

More commonly, TR is caused by pulmonary hypertension, either due to increased pressure on the valve or enlargement of the right ventricle and stretching of the tricuspid valve ring (secondary TR). The impact of TR on the right ventricle depends partly on the degree of valvular or ring disruption and partly on the pulmonary artery pressure.

A number of rare conditions are associated with TR, and their management is peculiar to the condition (e.g. rheumatoid arthritis, carcinoid, radiation, and anti-obesity drugs like fenfluramine). Some congenital (Ebstein's anomaly, cleft tricuspid valve) and acquired cardiac diseases (eosinophilic cardiomyopathy, constrictive pericarditis) also cause TR.

Physical signs
The pressure pulse during right ventricular ejection is transmitted through the right atrium and vena cavae in systole, and the jugular pulse may display a prominent systolic wave. The rise in right atrial and venous pressures generally causes disruption to flow in a number of organs. The liver enlarges and may be pulsatile. Ascites and peripheral oedema may develop. Renal impairment may occur.

Cardiac signs may be subtle: often, there is little, or no, murmur (pansystolic), and the detection of right ventricular volume overload is difficult (right ventricular heave).

Investigations
- ECG may show right ventricular hypertrophy.
- Echocardiography will show an overloaded right ventricle and any associated enlargement. Reversed septal motion may be seen. Doppler will estimate pulmonary artery pressure, and colour flow will provide information about the severity of the regurgitation. (Note many normal tricuspid valves show a minor degree of TR on Doppler imaging, and this should not alarm the medical staff or the patient).
- CMR may be valuable to assess the volume overload, as it provides accurate 3D images of the right ventricular cavity.

Treatment
TR is often well tolerated for many years. Medical treatment with diuretics may relieve symptoms of oedema but does not influence the course of the condition. Where TR is primarily due to pulmonary hypertension, treatment should initially be aimed at the cause of the pulmonary hypertension (e.g. left heart disease, especially MS, pulmonary valve stenosis, recurrent pulmonary embolism, primary pulmonary hypertension, cor pulmonale). If severe TR continues, despite efforts to lower pulmonary artery pressure, or if the TR is primary, surgery may be considered. This may take the form of valve repair, replacement, and/or tricuspid annuloplasty. Tricuspid valve replacement has a high mortality between 7 and 40%.

Tricuspid stenosis (TS)
Tricuspid stenosis is caused by rheumatic fever and is almost always associated with left-sided valve disease which is usually the dominant lesion. Signs are similar to mitral stenosis but with evidence of raised right atrial pressure (JVP), hepatic congestion and peripheral oedema.

Echo is the investigation of choice, although measures for assessing severity are less well established. 3D echo offers the potential to planimeter the valve (i.e. measure the area of the tricuspid valve orifice).

If intervention is required, balloon valvuloplasty can be used, but there is limited experience, and surgery is occasionally necessary.

Pulmonary valve disease
The pulmonary valve is rarely affected by the conditions that afflict other cardiac valves (rheumatic fever, endocarditis). Congenital pulmonary stenosis is sometimes seen in adults but rarely causes problems. If severe, it is associated with reduced exercise tolerance due to dyspnoea or angina. Echo will accurately assess the degree of stenosis. It is rare for any treatment to be advised, unless the gradient across the valve is 40 mmHg or greater. Treatment, if necessary, is by balloon valvuloplasty (preferable) or valve replacement.

Non-cardiac surgery in patients with valve disease
Patients who are discovered to have valve disease, while being assessed for non-cardiac surgery, require full assessment of the severity of the valve disease. If surgery is not essential, consideration should be given to correcting the cardiac problem first.

Significant risk is attached to surgery in patients with severe symptomatic valve disease or the following conditions:
- MS with pulmonary artery pressures over 50 mmHg.
- AR or MR with evidence of impaired left ventricular function.

Further reading
Nishimura RA, Otto CA, Bonow RO, et al. (2014). 2014 AHA/ACC Guideline for the management of patients with valvular heart disease. A Report of the American College of Cardiology/American Heart Association Task Force on Practice Guidelines. *Journal of the American College of Cardiology*, **63**, e57–e185. doi:10.1016/j.jacc.2014.02.536.

Vahanian A, Baumgartner H, Bax J, et al. (2007). Guidelines on the management of valvular heart disease. The Task Force on the management of valvular heart disease of the European Society of Cardiology. *European Heart Journal*, **28**, 230–68.

Infective endocarditis

Infective endocarditis (IE) is an uncommon condition with a high mortality and morbidity, in which heart valves or related structures become infected by blood-borne spread of the infective organism. It commonly affects hearts or valves that are already abnormal, but, increasingly, it affects previously normal hearts. The infection may have devastating effects due to destruction of affected structures, embolization of infected products, or the systemic effects of infection.

Epidemiology

IE has an incidence of 3.6 per 100,000 population per year in studies reported between 1993 and 2003. The nature of the infection has changed over the last 50 years from being a condition largely affecting patients with rheumatic or congenital heart disease, to the current situation where degenerative valve disease, intravenous drug abuse, and prosthetic valve infections are more common. The organisms responsible for infection have also changed from oral streptococci to staphylococci (with an association to hospital contact) and enteric streptococci (*Streptococcus bovis*), which may be associated with colonic malignancy and a large range of other agents, including fastidious organisms and fungi.

Pathophysiology

Pathogens causing IE are blood-borne. Bacteraemias are not uncommon, but only in specific situations do the organisms attach to the heart and produce infection.

One of the unifying features of IE is that infective lesions tend to appear at sites where there is a high pressure jet. This gives rise to the concept that the jet is responsible for mechanical damage to the endothelium, allowing microbes to attach to the surface. The subsequent infection and disruption of the endothelium exposes extracellular constituents, triggering the coagulation cascade, adhesion of platelets and the beginnings of a vegetation.

Staphylococcal infection, in particular, may result in abscess formation in the lungs when the infection is right-sided, or in and around the aortic root when the aortic valve is affected. These abscess cavities are poorly accessible to antibiotics and may require prolonged treatment with specific antibiotics or surgical drainage.

Infection of the sewing ring of prosthetic valves may cause dehiscence.

Conditions predisposing to IE

Congenital heart disease

Patients with congenital valve disease, septal defects (mainly ventricular) or patent ductus arteriosus are susceptible to IE. Patients may present with a non-specific febrile illness, and a high index of suspicion is needed to make the diagnosis. Patients with common congenital valve disorders, e.g. bicuspid aortic valves, will show changing cardiac murmurs, as the valve is destroyed and becomes progressively regurgitant. The importance of frequent examination for the stigmata of IE and documenting of murmurs cannot be overstated.

Degenerative valve disease

Middle-aged and elderly patients with the two commonest degenerative conditions (mitral valve prolapse and senile aortic valve disease) are susceptible to IE. The clinical picture may be difficult because of multiple comorbidities, unimpressive or absent fever, unusual organisms (including nosocomial infections), immune suppression, and equivocal echocardiograhic findings. These patients are also more likely to have intracardiac devices which are a potential source or repository of infection, often with resistant organisms.

Intravenous drug abusers

The tricuspid valve is affected in >50% of IE patients who infect themselves with unclean needles, impure injectates, and poor skin hygiene. The valve may become grossly regurgitant, but the major morbidity is due to the infection. For example, staphylococcal infection and embolization to the lungs may produce lung abscesses and intractable swinging fevers. These patients may produce copious purulent sputum, as the abscesses discharge spontaneously.

Immune-suppressed patients

Patients with depressed immune systems are at particular risk from intravenous lines and haemodialysis catheters. IE resulting from intravenous lines often affects previously normal hearts. The organisms responsible may be unusual, and appropriate culture techniques are necessary.

Patients with intracardiac devices

Like most foreign materials within the circulation, intracardiac devices are virtually impossible to sterilize once infected and need to be removed. For patients whose device has been implanted recently, it is usually not difficult to remove, but, over time, pacemaker and defibrillator leads become embedded in the heart and may require specialist percutaneous extraction or surgery to ensure all foreign material is removed.

Patients with prosthetic valves

Approximately 150,000 patients in Europe and the USA receive prosthetic valves per year. Prosthetic valve endocarditis (PVE) is a particularly dangerous complication which occurs in 0.3–1% per patient year and accounts for 5–25% of all cases of endocarditis. A large selection of organisms may be responsible, but the commonest is *Staphylococcus aureus*. The infection is described as early (within 60 days of surgery) or late, and the in-hospital mortality is up to 40%.

Clinical features

The diagnosis of IE is frequently difficult, and the best outcomes are achieved in cases identified and treated early. There is a wide variety of presentations, many of which are uncommon. A high index of suspicion is necessary. Depending on the infecting organism, the presentation may vary from acute to indolent.

Signs of infection

Fever is usual, but not invariable, and may be low-grade. Prior treatment with antibiotics may suppress fever without eliminating the infection. Weight loss is common in less acute presentations. Night sweats and rigors may occur. Anaemia is common but difficult to detect clinically. With a prolonged course, clubbing may develop.

Murmurs

Because IE destroys structures, valve infections cause progressive regurgitation. The most significant auscultatory sign is a changing, or new, murmur, and, to make this observation, one needs to examine the patient daily.

Signs of cardiac adaptation and decompensation
If the haemodynamic disturbance is sufficiently great, there will be signs of haemodynamic changes (e.g. fall in diastolic pressure in aortic regurgitation). Overt heart failure is a particularly sinister development and is usually due to overwhelming valve destruction but may be caused by coronary embolism or the development of heart block.

As with changing murmurs, evidence of worsening haemodynamic state may support the diagnosis of IE.

Evidence of immune complex formation
Most of the cutaneous manifestations of IE are due to immune complex deposition. They include splinter haemorrhages under the nail beds, retinal haemorrhages, sometimes in the form of Roth's spots where they have a central pale area, Janeway lesions (purpuric lesions on the palms or soles and sometimes more extensively), Osler's nodes (infarcts in the pulp of the digits).

In other parts of the body, immune complexes can cause a vasculitis, arthritis, or glomerulonephritis with microscopic haematuria; hence, urinalysis is an essential component of routine investigation.

Immune complex formation may continue, even after successful treatment is commenced, and does not necessarily imply that the infection is not under control.

Embolism
Vegetations from the infected area can embolize to any part of the body. As the vegetations contain organisms, they can establish distant infection, resulting in 'mycotic aneurysm' formation. The areas affected (in order of frequency) are brain, spleen, kidneys, lungs, and peripheral vascular, coronary, and ocular vessels. Treatment may allow the vegetations to heal and stabilize, but embolization may occur, even after the disease appears controlled.

Risk of embolization is one of the issues that can advance the decision to operate.

Diagnosing IE

The diagnosis of IE is confirmed if there is evidence of systemic infection and involvement of the endocardium. Positive blood cultures or bacterial DNA detection confirm the infection is 'microbiologically positive'; otherwise, it is 'culture-/microbiologically negative'. The modified Duke's classification is used to define different levels of diagnostic certainty (see Boxes 4.4 and 4.5), but, although it is useful for research and epidemiology, its value in the individual patient is limited.

Tests to support the diagnosis of IE

Haematology
Elevated ESR, often >100 mm in the first hour. Elevated CRP, often >100 mg/L. Normocytic anaemia, neutrophilia.

Blood cultures
The value of growing the culprit organism (or organisms) is incalculable, as it confirms the diagnosis and guides appropriate antibiotic treatment. Blood cultures should be taken, if possible, before antibiotics have been given. If the patient is known to have had antibiotics, the culture medium can be modified to neutralize the effects of antimicrobials. The majority of successful cultures are derived from the first or second samples taken. All samples should be cultured for anaerobic and aerobic organisms.

Cultures can be negative, even in active infection, usually the result of previous antibiotic treatment. Some organisms (e.g. HACEK group (*Haemophilus, Actinobacillus,*

Box 4.4 Definition of terms used in the proposed modified Duke criteria for the diagnosis of infective endocarditis (IE).[1]

Major criteria
Blood culture positive for IE
　Typical microorganisms consistent with IE from two separate blood cultures:
　Viridans streptococci, *Streptococcus bovis*, HACEK group (**H**aemophilus, **A**ctinobacillus, **C**ardiobacterium, **E**ikenella, and **K**ingella), *Staphylococcus aureus*; or
　Community-acquired enterococci, in the absence of a primary focus; or
　Microorganisms consistent with IE from persistently positive blood cultures, defined as follows:
　At least two positive cultures of blood samples drawn 12 h apart; or
　All of three or a majority of >4 separate cultures of blood (with first and last sample drawn at least 1 h apart)
Single positive blood culture for *Coxiella burnetii* or antiphase I IgG antibody titre >1:800
Evidence of endocardial involvement
　Echocardiogram positive for IE (TOE recommended in patients with prosthetic valves, rated at least 'possible IE' by clinical criteria, or complicated IE (paravalvular abscess); TTE as first test in other patients), defined as follows :
　Oscillating intracardiac mass on valve or supporting structures, in the path of regurgitant jets, or on implanted material in the absence of an alternative anatomic explanation; or
　Abscess; or
　New partial dehiscence of prosthetic valve
New valvular regurgitation (clinical evidence of worsening or changing of pre-existing murmur not sufficient)
Minor criteria
Predisposition, predisposing heart condition, or injection drug use
Fever, temperature >38°C
Vascular phenomena, major arterial emboli, septic pulmonary infarcts, mycotic aneurysm, intracranial hemorrhage, conjunctival haemorrhages, and Janeway's lesions
Immunologic phenomena: glomerulonephritis, Osler's nodes, Roth's spots, and rheumatoid factor
Microbiological evidence: positive blood culture but does not meet a major criterion as noted above[*] or serological evidence of active infection with organism consistent with IE

TOE, transoesophageal echocardiography; TTE, transthoracic echocardiography.

[1] Li et al, 2000.

[*] Excludes single positive cultures for coagulase-negative staphylococci and organisms that do not cause endocarditis.

Reproduced from JS Li, et al., 'Proposed Modifications to the Duke Criteria for the Diagnosis of Infective Endocarditis', Clinical Infectious Diseases, 2000, 30, pp. 633–638, by permission of Oxford University Press and Infectious Diseases Society of America.

Cardiobacterium, Eikenella, and *Kingella*)) require prolonged incubation periods (>6 days).

Other cultures
All material excised at surgery should be cultured.

Histopathology
Organisms may be identified histologically from the excised material, including emboli.

Serology
Less common causes of IE can be demonstrated by serology (e.g. *Bartonella, Legionella, Chlamydia,* and *Coxiella burnetii*).

Definite infective endocarditis pathologic criteria

(1) Microorganisms demonstrated by culture or histologic examination of a vegetation, a vegetation that has embolized, or an intracardiac abscess specimen; or

(2) Pathologic lesions; vegetation or intracardiac abscess confirmed by histologic examination showing active endocarditis

Clinical criteria[a]

(1) 2 major criteria; or

(2) 1 major criterion and 3 minor criteria; or

(3) 5 minor criteria

Possible infective endocarditis

(1) 1 major criterion and 1 minor criterion; or

(2) 3 minor criteria

Rejected

(1) Firm alternate diagnosis explaining evidence of infective endocarditis; or

(2) Resolution of infective endocarditis syndrome with antibiotic therapy for <4 days; or

(3) No pathologic evidence of infective endocarditis at surgery or autopsy, with antibiotic therapy for <4 days; or

(4) Does not meet criteria for possible infective endocarditis, as above

[1] Li et al, 2000.

[a] See Box 4.4 for definitions of major and minor criteria.

Polymerase chain reaction (PCR)

Demonstration of DNA from microbes can aid detection of fastidious organisms (i.e. organisms that require specific nutrients for culture). It cannot distinguish between active and treated infection.

Urinalysis

Classical urinalysis in patients with IE shows microscopic haematuria.

Chest X-ray

Chest X-ray may show evidence of an enlarged heart or pulmonary oedema. In tricuspid IE, it may show lung abscesses, with or without fluid levels.

ECG

Conduction disorders may be seen (classically, prolongation of the PR interval, but higher levels of heart block do occur) or evidence of haemodynamic disturbance caused by valve damage (LVH, RVH).

Echocardiography

Echo is the most important single investigation for the diagnosis of IE. Serial echo is valuable to follow the course of the disease. Patients with IE do not always have an abnormal echo, but the majority of cases become abnormal with time, as the vegetations or the degree of regurgitation increase. Common findings are vegetations attached to the valve leaflets or around the sewing ring of a prosthetic valve, Doppler evidence of regurgitation through the affected valve or around the sewing ring, chordal rupture of mitral or tricuspid valve, and abscess formation usually around the aortic valve.

Vegetations are poorly echogenic, or often not extensive at first, but become more echo-dense as time progresses.

Ultimately, they may calcify. It can be difficult to assess if a dense vegetation is new (and infected) or old (and sterile).

A negative, good-quality transthoracic echo in a patient with a low clinical suspicion of IE is strong evidence against the diagnosis. In patients with greater suspicion of IE, transoesophageal echo should be carried out if transthoracic echo is normal. A negative transoesophageal echo is an important finding, with a 68–97% negative predictive accuracy. Transoesophageal echo is very useful for demonstrating complications of IE, such as abscesses, and should be carried out in all patients who require surgery. Where there is doubt about the diagnosis, transthoracic echo should be repeated weekly.

Imaging of vegetations in prosthetic valve endocarditis is difficult due to the solid parts of the valve, and transoesophageal echo often gives greater clarity and allows inspection of the structures around the sewing ring.

Colour flow Doppler is valuable to pinpoint and grade unusual jets, particularly those due to fistulas and fenestrations.

Documentation of left ventricular function is very important in left-sided IE, as failure may be a factor in the timing of valve surgery.

Three particular echo findings are considered major criteria for the diagnosis of IE:

• A mobile echo-dense mass attached to a valve, mural endocardium, or prosthetic material.

• Demonstration of abscesses or fistulas.

• New dehiscence of a prosthetic valve.

Although echo can confirm the diagnosis in up to 90% of cases, it cannot rule out IE.

Cardiac catheterization

Catheterization is usually avoided in IE to minimize embolization. However, in patients who need surgery, it can be important to assess whether they have coronary disease that could be tackled at the same time. Occasionally, cautious coronary angiography may be warranted, provided that the catheter can be kept clear of the vegetations.

Treatment of IE

Prevention and prophylaxis

Patients known to be susceptible to IE (vulnerable native or prosthetic valvular disease or previous IE) must be informed of measures to reduce the chances of infection or reinfection. Good dental hygiene and prompt treatment of bacterial infections elsewhere in the body, particularly staphylococcal, is important. The prophylaxis guidelines have recently been changed in the UK. Previously, antibiotic prophylaxis in situations where bacteraemia might be expected (e.g. before dental or other surgical procedures) was recommended. The reason for the change is partly due to lack of evidence and partly due to evidence of harm. NICE summarizes the reasoning thus:

• There is no consistent association between having an interventional procedure, dental or non-dental, and the development of IE.

• Regular toothbrushing almost certainly presents a greater risk of IE than a single dental procedure because of repetitive exposure to bacteraemia with oral flora.

• The clinical effectiveness of antibiotic prophylaxis is not proven.

• Antibiotic prophylaxis against IE for dental procedures may lead to a greater number of deaths through fatal anaphylaxis than a strategy of no antibiotic prophylaxis, and is not cost-effective.

Other national bodies have issued similar guidance. Given the paucity of evidence in this area, careful monitoring of cases of IE is recommended.

Current NICE guidance suggests:

Antibiotic prophylaxis against infective endocarditis is not recommended:

- **For people undergoing dental procedures.**
- **For people undergoing non-dental procedures at the following sites:**
  - **Upper and lower gastrointestinal tract.**
  - **Genitourinary tract; this includes urological, gynaecological and obstetric procedures, and childbirth.**
  - **Upper and lower respiratory tract; this includes ear, nose and throat procedures and bronchoscopy.**
- **Chlorhexidine mouthwash should not be offered as prophylaxis against infective endocarditis to people at risk of infective endocarditis undergoing dental procedures.**

If there is an independent reason for giving prophylactic antibiotics for a patient undergoing a procedure, then:

- **If a person at risk of infective endocarditis is receiving antimicrobial therapy because they are undergoing a gastrointestinal or genitourinary procedure at a site where there is a suspected infection, the person should receive an antibiotic that covers organisms that cause infective endocarditis.**

The guidelines stress that patients at risk should be aware of the manifestations and dangers of IE so that they seek appropriate help as soon as possible.

Treatment of acute infective endocarditis

The treatment of IE is complex. The emergence of drug resistance, the difficulties of predicting likely organisms in culture-negative IE, and the decisions about when to employ surgical approaches demand a team approach from cardiology, infectious diseases, cardiothoracic surgery, microbiology, and histopathology.

Ideally, treatment for IE is started once the causative organism is identified. However, in some cases, the clinical circumstances require blind antibiotic treatment before blood cultures are available (e.g. severe sepsis or complications). In these cases, three blood cultures should be taken an hour apart and antibiotics then started. In less urgent cases, antibiotics should only be started once the organism is grown. In patients who have been previously treated with antibiotics, it may take three or more days without antibiotics for the organism to become recoverable (plus the time for it to grow on culture).

If cultured, susceptibility testing will help to rule out antibacterials that are likely to be effective or ineffective, and minimum inhibitory concentrations need to be established for the chosen drug.

Antibiotic recommendations

Streptococci are usually sensitive to penicillin; although relative resistance is emerging, it can be overcome by appropriate regimens. Penicillin G 12–18 million units/24 h IV in six doses, combined with an aminoglycoside (usually gentamicin 3 mg/kg/24 h IV in one dose), for 2 weeks, followed by a further 2 weeks of penicillin alone (which, under the right conditions, can be given at home) results in a high cure rate.

Staphylococci are considered resistant to penicillin (90%) but sensitive to meticillin (INN). IE due to staphylococci is a particularly severe, and rapidly destructive, illness. Effective treatment started promptly can be lifesaving. With the exception of early prosthetic valve cases, IE is often due to coagulase-negative staphylococci, particularly *Staphylococcus epidermidis* meticillin-resistant species.

Meticillin (INN)-sensitive *Staphylococcus aureus* can be treated with a penicillinase-resistant penicillin, such as flucloxacillin 12 g/24 h IV in four doses (or vancomycin 30 mg/kg/24 h IV in two doses for patients with genuine penicillin allergy), given for at least 4 weeks, combined with gentamicin 3 mg/kg/24 h (max 240 mg/day), divided into three doses (1 mg/kg 8 hourly) for the first 3–5 days, to reduce continuing bacteraemia.

Endocarditis affecting prosthetic material (valves or intracardiac devices) is particularly difficult to treat, and regimens are longer and more complex. Meticillin (INN)-sensitive infection can be treated with flucloxacillin 12 g IV/24 h, with rifampicin 1,200 mg/24 h in two doses orally or IV for 6 weeks and gentamicin 3 mg/kg/24 h (max 240 mg/day) in two (i.e. 1.5 mg/kg 12 hourly) or three (i.e. 1 mg/kg 8 hourly) doses for 2 weeks. If there is meticillin (INN) resistance, vancomycin 30 mg/kg/24 h IV in two doses, with rifampicin 1,200 mg/24 h IV or orally in three doses, each for at least 6 weeks with gentamicin 3 mg/kg/24 h IV (max 240 mg/day) in three doses (i.e. 1 mg/kg 8 hourly) for 2 weeks may be used.

Enterococci and penicillin-resistant streptococci are resistant to many antibiotics, and each organism is treated, according to its resistance pattern. Microbiological advice is essential. Enterococcal infections are associated with colonic adenoma or carcinoma and should be investigated appropriately.

Q fever and fungi: Valve infection occurs in 10% of all cases of Q fever due to *Coxiella burnetii*. There are no reliable antibiotic cures, and relapses are common, so valve surgery may be necessary for eradication. Antibiotic treatment with doxycycline and rifampicin is used for at least a year after surgery or even lifelong.

Fungal IE is increasingly common in immune-compromised patients. Agents, such as amphotericin or 5-fluorocytosine, are used, but it is often only eradicated by surgery.

Doses and frequency of antibiotic dosing

For optimal treatment, knowledge of the susceptibility of the organism (minimum inhibitory concentration, MIC), the kinetics of the antibiotics chosen, and related toxicity and mode of excretion are important. Drugs, such as gentamicin and vancomycin, need regular monitoring of levels to ensure therapeutic ranges and reduce toxicity. This is best achieved by a multidisciplinary approach and close working with the microbiologists.

Culture-negative IE

At least 5–10% of IE is culture-negative or treatment has to be started prior to microbiological confirmation. Hence treament is blind and based on likely organisms. If an organism subsequently grows, then antibiotics can be altered appropriately.

Patient factors may have a direct bearing on the possible causative organism (e.g. intravenous drug abusers or early prosthetic valve infection) but are insufficiently accurate to allow specific antibiotic choices. Therefore, broad-spectrum drugs are used (see Table 4.8).

Prosthetic valve and intracardiac device IE

Prosthetic IE accounts for up to 25% of all cases of endocarditis. As the number of patients with prosthetic valves or intracardiac devices increases, so will the incidence of infection. About one third of such infections probably relate to hospital attendance, including patients with frequent hospital visits (e.g.

Table 4.8 Empirical antimicrobial therapy in *culture-negative* endocarditis of native valve endocarditis or prosthetic valve endocarditis*

Native valve endocarditis:		
Vancomycin	15.0 mg/kg IV every 12 h[1,2]	4–6 weeks
+ Gentamicin	1.0 mg/kg IV every 8 h	2 weeks
Prosthetic valve endocarditis:		
Vancomycin	15.0 mg/kg IV every 12 h	4–6 weeks
+ Rifampicin	300–450 mg PO every 8 h	4–6 weeks
+ Gentamicin	1.0 mg/kg IV every 8 h	2 weeks

[1] Maximum 2 g/day; for drug level monitoring

[2] Aminopenicillin may be added

* From ESC guidelines on prevention, diagnosis, and treatment of infective endocarditis (see Further reading).

Reproduced from European Society of Clinical Microbiology and Infectious Diseases (ESCMID) and by the International Society of Chemotherapy (ISC) for Infection and Cancer, 'Guidelines on the prevention, diagnosis and treatment of infective echocardits (new version 2009): The Task Force on the Prevention, Diagnosis, and Treatment of Infective Endocarditis or the European Society of Cardiology', *European Heart Journal*, 2009, 30, 19, pp. 2369–2413, by permission of Oxford University Press and the European Society of Cardiology.

for wound care, dialysis) or those hospitalized for over 48 h, probably due to intravenous cannula. In early prosthetic valve or intracardiac device IE, the commonest organism is *Staphylococcus aureus* (23%), followed by coagulase-negative *Staphylococcus* (17%). Surgery may be necessary to control the infection, but some patients are too ill, and mortality is high at 30–50%. In late IE (more than 1 year after surgery), the spectrum of organisms is similar to native valve endocarditis.

Unlike native valve IE, the condition may worsen abruptly due to valve dehiscence or rupture of an abscess. Sterilization of the prosthesis is challenging, and most intracardiac devices have to be removed.

IE in intravenous drug abusers
Direct injection of bacteria into the veins is probably not the sole cause of IE in intravenous drug abusers. The chemicals (solvents, additives, etc.) and the injectate contents play a part in endothelial damage of the tricuspid valve.

Tricuspid IE is not usually as dangerous as left-sided IE, partly because the lung filters emboli and because the function of the tricuspid valve is less crucial. Moderate, or even severe, tricuspid regurgitation may be well tolerated, particularly if the pulmonary artery pressure is low. Surgery to the tricuspid valve is necessary only in 2%, and mortality is less than 5%. Surgery should be avoided, if possible, in addicts because of the potential for reinfection, unless they stop injecting. The cases that develop left-sided IE (50%) have a much worse prognosis.

The commonest organism is *Staphylococcus aureus*. As a result of the difficulties with intravenous treatment in drug addicts and the problems of compliance, short oral treatments with rifampicin and ciprofloxacin for 2 weeks may be sufficient, but management needs to be tailored to the patient. In the 40–90% of patients who also have HIV infection, longer treatments are necessary.

Subsequent course after initiation of antibiotic treatment
In uncomplicated IE with minimal valve damage, treatment for the recommended time with the appropriate antibiotics is all that is necessary. Resolution is usually defined by fever defervescence and normalization of acute phase reactants. In a proportion of cases, complications arise due to failure to control the infection, with embolization or haemodynamic deterioration due to valve destruction or fistula.

Evidence of treatment failure
Daily clinical examination and observations of temperature, heart rate, and weight are the simplest way to record continuing infection or recovery. However, persisting fever may be due to antibiotic sensitivity, and continued cropping of splinter haemorrhages and other immune complex manifestations may occur, even if the infection is controlled. Persistence or changes in these signs should prompt more extensive re-examination for evidence of the effectiveness of treatment. Echo may show a reduction in the size of vegetations, but this can sometimes be due to embolization, rather than resolution.

If it is suspected that continuing fever is due to antibiotic hypersensitivity, changing antibiotics should be considered.

Embolism
The morbidity and mortality from IE is significantly increased by the development of embolism and occurs in up to 40% of cases, although many episodes are unrecognized. The frequency of embolism falls quickly with effective antibiotic treatment.

Embolism, or the risk of embolism, influences the decision to proceed to surgery. Echo appearances can, to a certain extent, predict this. Larger vegetations that are particularly mobile and vegetations on the mitral or aortic valve are more likely to embolize. Certain infections (staphylococci, *Streptococcus bovis*, and *Candida*) give rise to particularly fragile vegetations.

The risk of embolism decreases after 2 weeks of effective treatment.

Embolism results in infarction of the affected organ (stroke, splenic infarction, digital infarction, myocardial infarction, etc.), but sometimes the infection metastasizes, causing local infection ('mycotic' aneurysms in the brain or pulmonary abscesses in the lung).

Surgery
One of the most difficult decisions in patients with IE is to proceed to surgery. Operating on a patient with an indolent infection to implant a prosthetic valve into a potentially infected area requires the conviction that medical therapy alone has a high probability of failure and hence death. Patients with heart failure, left-sided native valve infection, and large vegetations have a poor prognosis with medical treatment, and prognosis is improved by early surgery. Early surgery allows possible repair of the infected valve, particularly if there is a fenestration, and that is preferable to implanting a prosthetic valve into a potentially infected site.

Homografts may be used for the aortic valve in an attempt to prevent the new valve from being colonized and help to reconstruct the perivalvular area if disrupted by abscess formation.

Overall surgical mortality in active IE is 8–16%.

Three principal reasons for operating during the acute illness are:

- Haemodynamic deterioration.
- Risk of embolism (as discussed previously).
- Uncontrolled infection (usually when there is foreign material present or for Q fever).

Haemodynamic deterioration
The objective of surgery in acute IE with haemodynamic compromise is to improve the performance of the affected valve. However, any surgical material (including sutures, rings, grafts, and prosthetic valves) introduced into an infected area risks infection of the foreign material and a potential worsening of the situation. Usually, surgery can be delayed by intensive medical support to allow time for antibiotics to penetrate the infected area. Occasionally, surgery has to proceed in the face of uncontrolled infection (treatment failure or culture-negative). In these circumstances, conservative surgery or the use of homografts may be valuable, and any excised material must be made available for culture, histology, and PCR to identify a target organism or even a second unsuspected organism (e.g. in treatment failures).

Uncontrolled infection
Even if the responsible organism is known and appropriate antibiotics are given, infection may not be controlled, and the patient is at risk from the toxic or destructive effects of the infection. Surgery in this condition is then complex and risky.
    Patients with cerebral embolism are a particularly difficult group. If on warfarin, they should be converted to heparin, so anticoagulation can be reversed quickly, if necessary. Those with cerebral embolism represent a high-risk group for surgery.

Surgery after the infection has been treated
About 50% of patients who develop IE have cardiac surgery at some point. Ideally, surgery is delayed until the infection is eradicated and the risks of cross-infection of the prosthetic valve are reduced.

Prognosis
The mortality of IE remains stubbornly high (22%) despite advances in antibiotics, cardiovascular support, and surgical treatments. One reason is the changing nature of the patients—they are older, with more comorbidities, and they more often have prosthetic valves or intracardiac devices. Along with the change in patient characteristics, there has been a change in the organisms responsible, with streptococci (most often seen in native valve IE, 8% mortality) being replaced by staphylococci (33% mortality or 47% for MRSA). Nosocomial (hospital-acquired) infections account for about 35% of infections, with a mortality of 27%.

There are a number of variables that are associated with higher mortality, including age, gender (higher in women), causative organism, hospital-acquired infection, embolism, heart failure, contraindication to surgery, and prosthetic valve IE.

Optimal management of IE requires close cooperation between cardiologists, microbiologists, and cardiothoracic surgeons, with frequent review of the patient's clinical progress and the results of cardiological and microbiological investigations.

Further reading
Bonow RO, Carabello BA, Chatterjee K, *et al.* (2008). 2008 Focused update incorporated into the ACC/AHA 2006 guidelines for management of patients with valvular heart disease: a report of the American College of Cardiology/American Heart Association Task Force on Practice Guidelines. <http://circ.ahajournals.org/cgi/content/full/118/15/e523>.

Habib G, Hoen B, Tomos P, *et al.* (2009). Guidelines on the prevention, diagnosis and treatment of infective endocarditis (new version 2009). The task force on the prevention, diagnosis and treatment of infective endocarditis of the European Society of Cardiology (ESC). *European Heart Journal*, **30**, 2369–413.

Hill E, Herijgers P, Claus P, *et al.* (2007). Infective endocarditis: changing epidemiology and predictors of 6-month mortality: a prospective cohort study. *European Heart Journal*, **28**, 196–203.

Li J, Sexton D, Mick N, *et al.* (2000). Proposed modifications to the Duke criteria for the diagnosis of infective endocarditis. *Clinical Infectious Diseases*, **30**, 633–8.

National Institute for Health and Clinical Excellence (2008). NICE clinical guideline 64: prophylaxis against infective endocarditis: antimicrobial prophylaxis against infective endocarditis in adults and children undergoing interventional procedures. <http://www.nice.org.uk/CG064>.

Prendergast BD (2006). The changing face of infective endocarditis. *Heart*, **92**, 879–85.

Cardiomyopathies

Introduction

The term cardiomyopathy was originally applied to idiopathic primary heart muscle diseases and was previously a diagnosis of exclusion. As understanding of the underlying disorders has grown, the term cardiomyopathy has been applied to conditions where definitive diagnostic tests are available. The current classification scheme (see Box 4.6) is based on echocardiographic morphology once coronary artery disease (CAD) and valve disease have been excluded. As molecular insights accumulate, newer classifications will emerge.

Family history

The family history is central for the evaluation of anyone with unexplained myocardial disease where sudden death may be the initial mode of presentation.

Affected relatives with chest pain syndromes or fatal arrhythmias have often been mislabelled as 'myocardial infarction', and a careful assessment, ideally of primary clinical data from family members, can be very useful. In some cases, there is overlap with other forms of cardiomyopathy or valve disease diagnosed in first-degree relatives. Ultimately, a definitive diagnosis can sometimes only be made through evaluation of the entire family.

Dilated cardiomyopathy

DCM is defined by the WHO as:
- Reduced ejection fraction.

Box 4.6 Cardiomyopathy classification

Dilated cardiomyopathy (DCM)
   Chamber dilatation—usually bilateral
   Contractile dysfunction
Hypertrophic cardiomyopathy (HCM)
   Unexplained myocardial hypertrophy
   Minority with outflow obstruction
Restrictive cardiomyopathy (RCM)
   Normal wall thickness
   Restrictive physiology
Arrhythmogenic right ventricular cardiomyopathy (ARVC)
   Initial right ventricular dysfunction
   Prominent RV origin arrhythmias
   LV involvement in some
Overlap syndromes
Components of multiple morphologic forms within a single family
One form will usually dominate clinically
Syndromic variants
Emery–Dreifuss syndrome
Atrial standstill and AV block
   Skeletal muscle involvement
   Contractures
Mitochondrial cardiomyopathies
   Usually hypertrophic, may be dilated
Extraocular muscle abnormalities
Diabetes

Reprinted from *Journal of Cardiac Failure*, **15**, 2, Hershberger RE, et al., 'Genetic Evaluation of Cardiomyopathy—A Heart Failure Society of America Practice Guideline', pp. 83–97, Copyright 2009, with permission from Heart Failure Society of America and the Japanese Heart Failure Society, and Elsevier.

- Left ventricular volumes of >110 mL.
- Exclusion of CAD or other causes.

DCM is the final outcome of many types of myocardial injury, but the end-stage pathology is remarkably homogeneous. DCM is a form of myocardial dystrophy, with patchy cardiomyocyte loss, low-grade inflammation, and compensatory hypertrophy of the remaining cardiomyocytes. There may be extensive interstitial and subendocardial fibrosis. Even in myocardial infarction, the pathology of remote segments is similar to DCM, suggesting that ventricular remodelling pathways may be shared by many disease entities.

Epidemiology

DCM is the commonest form of cardiomyopathy, with a prevalence of approximately 37 per 100,000. This may be an underestimate, as DCM is the final diagnosis in 15–20% of those with congestive heart failure. Notably, non-ischaemic heart failure was the aetiology in up to 30% in recent large clinical trials.

Pathogenesis

Virtually any cause of myocardial cell loss will result in DCM. Up to 50% of cases are inherited, and the remainder results from a broad range of myocardial insults:
- Inherited:
  - Autosomal.
  - X-linked.
  - Mitochondrial.
- Inflammatory:
  - Infectious myocarditis (viral, bacterial, fungal, parasitic).
  - Non-infectious (vasculitides, drug reactions).
  - Granulomatous (sarcoidosis, giant cell myocarditis).
- Toxic:
  - Alcohol.
  - Anthracyclines.
  - Nucleosides.
  - Antimetabolites.
  - Tyrosine kinase inhibitors.
  - Heavy metal.
- Endocrine:
  - Thyroid, diabetic.
- Nutritional:
  - Thiamine, carnitine, selenium, calcium, phosphate, magnesium.
- Catecholamines:
  - Cocaine.
  - Phaeochromocytoma.
- Miscellaneous:
  - Peripartum.
  - Haemochromatosis.

Pathophysiology

Reduced cardiac reserve, as a result of impaired contractility or chronotropic incompetence, is the normal presentation. Exertional dyspnoea, orthopnoea, or overt heart failure are common, while atypical chest pain, arrhythmia, or sudden death are less frequent. In younger individuals, who tolerate elevated left heart pressures more readily, presentation with acute right heart failure, accompanied by hepatic congestion, systemic symptoms, and fevers, may mimic a viral syndrome.

Diagnosis

Clinical evaluation should focus on defining possible aetiologies for DCM and the extent of any physiologic decompensation. A careful history (including a complete family history) and full physical examination are essential.

Specific laboratory testing

- ECG.
- Chest X-ray.
- Echocardiogram.
- Biochemistry:
  - Electrolytes, LFTs, CK.
  - TSH, ferritin.
- Haematology.
- Serology:
  - Acute and convalescent titres.
  - ANA, Rh factor, ESR.
  - Specific titres, e.g. Chagas (only required in specific subgroups).
- Exclusion of CAD.
- Endomyocardial biopsy (only required in specific subgroups).

Exclusion of CAD may be difficult using non-invasive tools when there is a very low ejection fraction. Clues to a non-ischaemic aetiology include a family history, extracardiac evidence of a myopathy, and biventricular involvement. Nevertheless, coronary angiography is often required.

Prognosis

The prognosis in DCM varies widely. There is evidence that, in many cases, ventricular function may wax and wane in the face of inflammatory or other insults. In common with other forms of heart failure, left ventricular ejection fraction and NYHA class are powerful predictors of 5- and 10-year survival.

Family history is a poor prognostic factor in its own right, though this may simply reflect the penetrance. The risk of sudden death is difficult to predict and does not always correlate with ejection fraction.

Management aims

The treatment of DCM, as with other forms of cardiomyopathy, is focused on improving symptoms and prolonging survival. It is important to exclude treatable conditions, such as hyperthyroidism, haemochromatosis, and toxic exposure, e.g. alcohol or drugs. Most therapies for heart failure have been tested in DCM patients and, in the absence of specific interventions, should be instituted for conventional indications, based on functional evaluation. These include:

- Angiotensin-converting enzyme inhibitors.
- Angiotensin receptor blockers.
- Beta-blockers.
- Diuretics.
- Spironolactone.
- Implantable cardiodefibrillators.
- Cardiac resynchronization therapy.

In patients with an inherited form of DCM, screening of at-risk family members with ECG and echocardiography is recommended.

Hypertrophic cardiomyopathy

HCM is defined as unexplained myocardial hypertrophy. Several common causes of hypertrophy should be excluded, including: hypertension, obstructive valve disease, and athletic activity. Where such factors exist, they rarely, if ever, result in left ventricular wall thicknesses greater than 16 mm. Wall thicknesses greater than this are almost certainly HCM, and, in the context of a family history or other clues, even intermediate wall thicknesses (11–16 mm) must be regarded with suspicion.

The pathology of HCM is characterized by sarcomere disarray and hypertrophy of individual myocytes, but histology is not useful ante mortem. Myocardial mass is typically greatly increased but may be completely normal despite widespread disarray.

True HCM must be distinguished from a range of rare storage disorders that may cause increased ventricular wall thickness in the absence of true hypertrophy. Importantly, myocyte disarray (i.e. loss of the normal parallel alignment of the myocytes) is often seen in the septum of healthy individuals. Some forms of HCM also exhibit mitral valve abnormalities or endocardial fibrosis.

Epidemiology

Estimates of the prevalence of HCM vary widely. Recent studies suggest the disorder may affect as many as 1 in 1,000.

Pathogenesis

Early descriptions of HCM recognized a substantial inherited contribution to the disease, and, of those diagnosed with HCM, 70–90% have a family history of the disease. The vast majority of inherited cases exhibit autosomal dominant transmission, but penetrance can be variable, and skipped generations are not uncommon.

Molecular genetic studies of large kindreds have identified several sarcomeric contractile protein genes as the cause of HCM. The manifestations of HCM are quite varied, even within a given family, though certain phenotypic features are recognized to be commonly associated with specific genes.

The following clinical features are rare in true HCM: massive LV wall thickness (>30 mm), high-grade atrioventricular block, and ventricular pre-excitation. Molecular genetic studies in such families have identified mutations, not in sarcomeric contractile protein genes, but rather in genes in several metabolic pathways. In these cases, while hypertrophy may coexist, the increase in wall thickness is mainly due to storage abnormalities.

Importantly, in all forms of HCM, there is expression of the mutant proteins outside the heart in skeletal muscle or vascular smooth muscle. This may explain some of the exertional symptoms, vasomotor abnormalities, and other associated features.

Many individuals with HCM will be completely asymptomatic, and, as a result, the familial nature of the disease is often only identified after a clinical event in a family member. Common symptoms include:

- Syncope or presyncope, often with exercise or post-exertion.
- Exertional dyspnoea.
- Atypical chest pain.
- Palpitations or arrhythmias.

Typically, symptoms emerge during the pubertal growth spurt. Unfortunately, sudden death is often the initial presenting feature, and many individuals will require reassurance after the loss of a relative. A small subset of individuals will progress to overt heart failure.

Diagnosis

Clinical evaluation should focus on excluding other causes of myocardial hypertrophy and, in particular, forms of pseudohypertrophy that may be amenable to specific treatment.

A careful history (including a complete family history) and a full physical examination are essential. Typical physical findings, such as a bisferiens pulse, a palpable S4, and variable ejection systolic murmurs, are not always present.

In view of the emerging evidence that Fabry's disease (a rare, genetic, X-linked, lysosomal storage disease due to alpha galactosidase enzyme deficiency) may manifest as isolated HCM, a history of acroparaesthesiae and evidence of renal impairment should be sought.

Specific laboratory testing:
• ECG.
• Chest X-ray.
• Echocardiogram.
• Biochemistry:
  • Electrolytes, urea/Cr, LFTs, CK.
  • TSH, ferritin.
• Haematology.
• Serology.
• 48h ambulatory ECG.
• Exercise testing.
• Exclusion of CAD.
• Tomographic imaging—CTA, MRI.
• Electrophysiology testing.

Evidence of hypertrophy need not be present, but the ECG features (including characteristic 'dagger-like' septal Q waves and diffuse precordial T wave changes/inversion) are usually more sensitive than echocardiography, at least in the context of an extended family. MRI not only identifies unusual focal hypertrophy but also offers insights into tissue abnormalities, including scarring which may ultimately prove useful in risk stratification. Tomographic imaging can be useful in the evaluation of those resuscitated from sudden death where there is still concern for other causes, including arrhythmogenic right ventricular cardiomyopathy (ARVC) and coronary anomalies.

Cardiac catheterization
Usually, the diagnosis of HCM will have been made prior to invasive testing, though occasionally, in the context of chest pain and ECG abnormalities, angiography will be performed acutely.

There is little correlation between haemodynamic findings and symptoms or exercise performance. Coronary angiography may reveal anomalous origins, in which case the course of the coronaries, with respect to the great vessels, should be defined. Severe myocardial bridging (i.e. normally the large coronary arteries lie on top of the heart muscle but in ~5% of patients some parts of the artery can be surrounded by heart muscle, forming a myocardial bridge, with associated arterial compression during myocardial contraction) may result in exertional chest pain or arrhythmias, but less significant bridging is not uncommon.

Electrophysiology evidence is often sought when considering defibrillator implantation. However, inducible arrhythmias in HCM do not predict the risk of sudden death. More recent efforts to characterize the arrhythmic substrate, using multielectrode arrays with systematic assessment of myocardial electrical heterogeneity, have shown some promise. The presence of a bypass tract is an indication for electrophysiologic evaluation.

Prognosis
The main concern with HCM is the risk of sudden cardiac death. This risk is highest during the pubertal growth spurt but remains elevated throughout life. The majority of the risk factors thought to predict sudden death have been studied without regard for the familial nature of the disease, and it can be difficult to discriminate the family-specific risk from the disease-specific risk. Currently, accepted risk factors are:
• Syncope.
• Ventricular ectopy and ventricular tachycardia on monitoring.
• Exercise hypotension.
• Family history of sudden death.
• Extreme LVH (>30 mm).

At present, the best predictor of sudden death in HCM patients is a personal history of cardiac arrest; 59% of individuals with one episode of cardiac arrest have a second one within 5 years. In the absence of a prior cardiac arrest, the criteria for risk prediction become less clear. A personal history of unexplained syncope or a family history of sudden cardiac death has modest additional predictive utility. Caution is necessary in defining the true risk of sudden death within a family. In particular, it can be difficult to estimate the risk of sudden death if there is no reliable assessment of the denominator, i.e. the number of family members with actual HCM.

Management
Most individuals with HCM are asymptomatic and at low risk and do not require any therapeutic intervention. Substantial exertional symptoms, particularly in the presence of an outflow tract gradient, are usually treated with beta-blockers or calcium channel blockers initially. Failure to respond to a combination of these drugs can be approached by adding disopyramide, but this must be monitored for autonomic and proarrhythmic effects (QT). These drugs are thought to reduce myocardial contractility and diminish the outflow tract gradient and its physiologic consequences. Responses are difficult to predict but can be excellent.

In the presence of an outflow tract gradient, failure of medical therapy has led to measures to address the gradient mechanically.

In the presence of significant mitral regurgitation with primary valvular abnormalities, surgical myomectomy and mitral valve replacement/repair have been undertaken with some success. In those at high risk for surgery or who do not wish surgery, controlled iatrogenic myocardial injury, using alcohol septal ablation, has been attempted. Results are similar to surgery, though randomized controlled trials are unlikely ever to be performed.

Atrial fibrillation has a major impact on haemodynamics in HCM, and aggressive efforts are made to maintain sinus rhythm, usually with amiodarone. There are no studies of the utility of pulmonary vein isolation in HCM, but, given the diffuse nature of the underlying myopathy, such interventions might be predicted to be of limited duration. Ablation of the AV node and permanent pacing can be used in extreme circumstances.

ICD implantation is recommended for those who have any malignant arrhythmia or are at high risk for sudden death. Prediction of risk is poor, and the risks and benefits of chronic device implantation have to be carefully weighed for each patient. In those in whom ICD is not feasible or refused, long-term therapy with amiodarone has been used.

Competitive sports and isometric exercise are prohibited, without hard data. Endocarditis prophylaxis is no longer recommended for isolated HCM, though estimates of the incidence of endocarditis in HCM suggest it is close to that in congenital heart disease.

Restrictive cardiomyopathy

Restrictive cardiomyopathies (RCM) demonstrate several rare hereditary variants, including familial idiopathic restrictive cardiomyopathy and hereditary amyloidosis. Familial idiopathic RCM is extremely rare, with reports only in small case series. No gene has yet been identified. Furthermore, in some families with HCM, individual members can show a pattern of restrictive filling, with little or no LV hypertrophy.

Hereditary amyloidosis represents a more common form of heritable RCM and typically involves a genetic defect in the transthyretin (TTR) protein or Apo AI protein, leading to misfolded proteins and infiltration of the myocardium with amyloid fibrils. Inheritance is usually autosomal dominant.

Arrhythmogenic right ventricular cardiomyopathy

ARVC is characterized by myocardial disease, predominantly involving the right ventricle (RV), and associated with ventricular tachycardia arising from this chamber (left bundle branch block morphology), syncope, and sudden death. At autopsy, there is an unusual distribution of fatty and fibrotic tissue within the RV, preferentially affecting three areas: the apex, inflow and outflow tracts. In typical cases, there is a familial trait, but this may only be revealed when relatives are examined directly.

Genetic studies, to date, have established that ARVC is not a single disorder, but a syndrome consisting of multiple entities with discrete clinical features. There is significant variation in the natural history of the underlying diseases, but also substantial pleiotropy of clinical expression of the same single disease gene segregating within individual families. The mutated genes identified so far, strongly suggest that ARVC is the result of perturbation in specialized intercellular adhesion junctions known as desmosomes, and hence mechanistically distinct from either hypertrophic or dilated cardiomyopathy.

Clinical presentation is usually with syncope or sudden death. History may reveal some prior palpitations but often is unimpressive. ECG evidence of right-sided abnormalities may be subtle. Definitive diagnosis requires the demonstration of abnormal RV structure on echo or MRI. Isolated fibrofatty abnormalities on MRI or CT are less specific than previously thought. As more individuals survive, late heart failure is emerging as a problem.

Cases are best managed in centres with extensive expertise in the diagnosis and management of ARVC, ideally with systematic evaluation of the entire family.

Further reading

Hare JM (2012). The dilated, restrictive and infiltrative cardiomyopathies. In RO Bonow, *et al. Braunwald's heart disease*, pp. 1561–81. WB Saunders, Philadelphia.

Hershberger R, Lindenfield J, Mestroni L, Seidman CE, Taylor MR, Towbin J (2009). Heart Failure Society of America. Genetic evaluation of cardiomyopathy: a HFSA Practice Guideline. *Journal of Cardiac Failure*, **15**, 83–97.

Maron BJ (2012). Hypertrophic cardiomyopathy. In RO Bonow, *et al. Braunwald's heart disease*, pp. 1582–94. WB Saunders, Philadelphia.

Seidman JG, Pyeritz R, Seidman CE (2008). Inherited causes of cardiovascular disease. In RO Bonow, *et al. Braunwald's heart disease*, pp. 70–80. WB Saunders, Philadelphia.

Congenital heart disease

Introduction

Congenital heart defects are the most common type of birth defect, affecting 8 of every 1,000 newborns. Each year, more than 35,000 babies in the United States are born with congenital heart defects.

There are many different types of congenital heart disease. These range from relatively common, simple defects with no symptoms to complex defects with severe, life-threatening symptoms.

A small number of babies are born with complex congenital heart defects that need special medical attention soon after birth. Over the past few decades, the diagnosis and treatment of these complex defects has greatly improved. As a result, almost all children with complex heart defects grow to adulthood and can live active, productive lives because their heart defects have been effectively treated. Increasingly, adult physicians will encounter these patients with their often unique pathology and physiology. In all but the most straightforward of circumstances, referral to a specialist is recommended.

The causes of congenital heart defects are incompletely understood, but there are well-established links with intrauterine exposures to toxins and infectious agents. Recent work has implicated a genetic contribution to many forms of congenital heart disease. There appears to be tremendous pleiotropy, with clinical defects representing only the most extreme abnormalities in many instances. Importantly, there is increasing recognition that there are specific contractile and electrical abnormalities associated with many of these syndromes.

This chapter will discuss the common, simple congenital heart defects, most likely to be encountered by the generalist, and illustrative examples of complex defects.

Atrial septal defects

There are many types of atrial septal defect (ASD), classified by anatomic location and their associations.

Patent foramen ovale

A patent foramen ovale (PFO) is the remnant of the fetal channel across the atrial septum, the foramen ovale. PFOs have been found to be slightly more common in individuals with stroke, transient ischaemic symptoms, migraine, and other neurologic symptoms. There is no clear mechanistic link between the interatrial communication and the neurological symptoms, and the association may reflect shared mechanisms. Clinical trials performed to date suggest that PFO closure is not associated with a beneficial outcome in these settings, but more definitive trials are under way.

Ostium secundum atrial septal defect

The ostium secundum ASD is the most common of all congenital cardiac lesions and usually arises from an enlarged foramen ovale, excessive absorption of the septum primum, or inadequate growth of the septum secundum.

Ostium primum atrial septal defect

Abnormal development of the endocardial cushions results in a range of defects in the atrioventricular canal, most commonly a defect in the ostium primum, associated with mitral valve abnormalities and mitral regurgitation.

Sinus venosus atrial septal defect

Defects in the atrial septum that involve the venous inflow tracts (either superior or inferior vena cava) are known as sinus venosus defects. These communications are often associated with anomalous drainage of the right-sided pulmonary veins into the right atrium.

Epidemiology

ASDs are identified in one child per 1,500 live births. PFOs are present in 20% or more of adults and frequently detected incidentally on echocardiography. Overall, ASDs make up 30 to 40% of all congenital heart disease seen in adults.

Pathophysiology

The physiologic effects of simple ASDs are related to shunting of blood across these communications. The relative compliance of the vascular compartments on either side of the defect determines the magnitude of interatrial shunting. Initially, the lower physiologic compliance of the left heart results in left-to-right shunting, with increased pulmonary artery flows, as well as dilatation of the right atrium and ventricle. Pulmonary arterial hypertension will eventually develop in almost 50% of cases. In a minority of patients, atrial arrhythmias, emboli, and right heart failure occur. Eisenmenger syndrome, with reversal of shunting and systemic cyanosis, will complicate 5–10% of ASDs.

Intra-atrial and/or atrioventricular conduction delay is often seen with an ASD. In extended families, the electrical findings or atrial septal aneurysms may be more penetrant than the septal defect. In ostium primum ASDs, marked left axis deviation is also observed, suggesting additional developmental pathology.

Diagnosis

Most individuals with ASDs who present as adults have few, if any, symptoms until their fifth decade when reduced exercise capacity, exertional dyspnoea, and general fatigue are usually seen.

Physical exam typically reveals evidence of right ventricular volume overload. There may be a parasternal heave, a pulmonary flow murmur, and, classically, a fixed splitting of the second heart sound. Later in the course of the disease, there may be evidence of chronic cyanosis, pulmonary hypertension, and right heart failure. Signs of associated conditions, such as heart-hand or Holt–Oram syndromes, should be sought.

The ECG may reveal intra-atrial delay, PR prolongation, or AV block. As previously noted, left axis deviation is seen in ostium primum lesions, and right axis deviation will often supervene in other forms.

Echocardiogram will usually allow a detailed evaluation of the anatomic lesion and its physiologic consequences. On occasions, transoesophageal echocardiography or tomographic imaging is required to fully evaluate associated structural heart disease and potential anomalous connections.

Management aims

The main goal of management in ASD is the prevention of pulmonary hypertension (PHT) and its downstream consequences, including the Eisenmenger syndrome (i.e. reversal of initial left to right shunt across the ASD, to right to left shunt as a consequence of raised right heart pressures due to PHT). ASD closure is recommended for those with significant shunting and associated pulmonary systolic pressures less than 40 mmHg. In older individuals and in those with mildly elevated pulmonary pressures, closure is more controversial. Once Eisenmenger syndrome has developed, closure is contraindicated. Closure is usually surgical, but percutaneous techniques are increasingly common.

Pharmacologic therapy

In those in whom surgery is not possible, pulmonary hypertension can be treated using conventional therapies. However, given the selection of these individuals, responses are less impressive.

Antibiotic prophylaxis is no longer routinely recommended for non-cyanotic ASDs, except in the presence of prosthetic material or in the event of prior endocarditis.

Ventricular septal defects

VSDs are also classified on the basis of their location and associations. These defects are increasingly recognized as abnormalities of ventricular differentiation and growth.

Membranous septum

The most common site for a congenital VSD is the thin, poorly muscularized region of the septum, immediately below the aortic valve. These defects are usually small and often involve surrounding muscular areas of the septum, specifically the infundibular or the inlet areas.

Infundibular septal defect

This type of VSD is located in the septum between the crista supraventricularis and the pulmonary valve.

Inlet septal defects

These VSDs, situated between the mitral and tricuspid valves are rare, but when present, are often associated with other defects in the AV canal.

Muscular septal defects

When abnormal communications arise in the trabeculated part of the interventricular septum, these are often multiple. This type of VSD will often close spontaneously, usually in the first decade of life.

Epidemiology

VSDs are seen in approximately 30% of all cases with congenital heart disease.

Pathophysiology

The physiologic impact of communication at the ventricular level is also determined largely by the extent of shunting. In contrast to ASDs, shunting usually occurs during systole when the gradient between left and right ventricle is highest. Large defects may result in very high flows through the pulmonary circuit, with the development of compensatory right ventricular hypertrophy, pulmonary hypertension, and, in a small minority, the development of Eisenmenger syndrome with reversal of shunting and systemic cyanosis.

Diagnosis

Most individuals with VSDs who present as adults have relatively small defects. Some may have residual patency after surgical closure of a larger defect that was symptomatic, as is typical during childhood. Occasionally, chronically cyanotic individuals with untreated Eisenmenger complex will be seen. Symptoms are typically those of reduced cardiorespiratory reserve and exertional dyspnoea.

Physical exam will usually reveal a rather diffuse ventricular impulse, a variable degree of right ventricular overload, and a systolic murmur. The pulmonary component of the second heart sound will be accentuated in pulmonary hypertension.

ECG evidence of left atrial and left ventricular enlargement may be present, but there are rarely any specific findings.

Echocardiography usually identifies the location and size of the defect using Doppler. Evidence of shunt fraction may be gleaned from chamber enlargement, pulmonary artery pressure, and the presence or absence of right ventricular hypertrophy.

Invasive assessment is reserved for those in whom surgery is being contemplated.

Management aims

The major goals are the improvement of symptoms and survival. Small defects can occasionally lead to complications through involvement of adjacent valvular structures but usually do not require intervention. Surgical management of the Eisenmenger complex is precluded by irreversible elevation of pulmonary vascular resistance. Intermediate lesions with significant shunting should be closed surgically or, in some situations, percutaneously.

Pharmacologic therapy

Pulmonary hypertension, when present, is managed using conventional medical interventions. Success is limited, given the irreversible nature of the pulmonary vascular disease in most of those selected for medical approaches.

Antibiotic prophylaxis is no longer routinely recommended for non-cyanotic VSDs, except in the presence of prosthetic material or in the event of prior endocarditis.

Arrhythmias are commonly seen after surgical correction, but antiarrhythmic prophylaxis has not been proven to be beneficial.

Right ventricular outflow tract obstruction

Right ventricular outflow tract obstruction may occur at several anatomic levels, each with its own specific associations.

- Infundibular stenosis:
  - May be isolated.
- Pulmonary valve stenosis:
  - May be associated with Noonan's syndrome.
- Supravalvular or branch stenoses:
  - May be associated with Noonan's or Williams' syndromes.
- Pulmonary atresia:
  - Typically with VSD.

Pathogenesis

The underlying mechanisms of these defects are poorly understood, but, increasingly, a genetic basis is suspected for many for these disorders.

The most prominent physiologic problems are a result of chronic right ventricular pressure overload, with consequent right ventricular hypertrophy, remodelling, and ultimately, right ventricular failure. Presentation will usually occur, as right ventricular reserve is diminished.

There may be associated myocardial defects, which can complicate the natural history.

Diagnosis

Patients are often asymptomatic until quite late in the pathophysiologic cascade. Typical symptoms include exercise intolerance, presyncope, or even right ventricular angina. Arrhythmias, including ventricular tachycardia, are not uncommon.

Physical exam reveals evidence of right ventricular overload and right ventricular failure. Venous pressures are elevated with a prominent parasternal heave, the murmurs of the primary outflow tract lesion, and secondary tricuspid regurgitation.

ECG evidence of right ventricular hypertrophy and right atrial delay is usually obvious. Echocardiography will, in most instances, confirm these findings and define the anatomic location of the obstructive lesion.

Management

Surgical or percutaneous relief of the obstructive lesion is usually undertaken if there is evidence of right ventricular remodelling. Medical management of right heart failure will also be required once this has supervened.

Left ventricular outflow tract obstruction

This may occur at multiple levels.

- Subaortic membrane:
  - 50% have significant aortic insufficiency.
- Congenital valvular aortic stenosis:
  - Usually bicuspid.
  - May present as calcific aortic stenosis.
  - Associated aortic abnormalities.
- Supravalvular aortic stenosis:
  - Classically Williams' syndrome.
- Aortic coarctation:
  - Associated with bicuspid aortic valves and with coronary disease.

Pathogenesis

The pathophysiology of left-sided obstructive lesions is predictable on the basis of chronic left ventricular pressure overload or fixed cardiac output. Ultimately, overt left heart failure will result. Hypoperfusion syndromes are related to the specific obstruction but include angina and hypertension in the case of aortic coarctation. The capacity of the circulatory system to remodel is evident in the extent to which cardiorespiratory reserves must be compromised before symptoms emerge.

Both bicuspid aortic valve and aortic coarctation (which often occur together) are associated with abnormalities of the proximal aortic segment that may result in dissection or premature coronary disease.

Diagnosis

Presenting symptoms include angina, presyncope, syncope, or those of heart failure. Physical exam will reveal evidence of left ventricular hypertrophy, including a sustained apex beat, a prominent, even palpable, fourth heart sound, as well as the systolic murmur of the obstructive lesion. Asymmetric brachial pressures, intercostal collaterals, and radiofemoral delay are suggestive of coarctation.

The ECG is remarkable for evidence of left atrial delay and left ventricular hypertrophy.

Echocardiography will, most often, confirm the location of the obstruction, though coarctation will not be detectable in those in whom supra-aortic windows are not available.

Chest X-rays may reveal evidence of rib notching from collaterals, but imaging of the aorta, ideally by MRA, allows definitive diagnosis.

Management

Surgical intervention has typically been undertaken in those with transcoarctation gradients of 30 mmHg or more. Percutaneous intervention is usually used for focal stenoses at the site of previous surgery. After age 40, many patients will have persistent hypertension, even after correction of the coarctation while, if the intervention is performed prior to age 5, the incidence is less than 10%.

Complex congenital lesions

Complex lesions are so called because of the constellation of associated defects. However, all forms of congenital heart disease should be treated with circumspection, as there are often subtle structural or functional defects present in even 'simple' lesions.

Tetralogy of Fallot

Tetralogy of Fallot is the most common cyanotic form of congenital heart disease and is characterized by:

- Pulmonary stenosis.
- Ventricular septal defect.
- Aortic override.
- Right ventricular hypertrophy.

The septal defect is perimembranous in the vast majority of cases. Additional structural defects are seen in complex cases, but in most instances it is unclear whether these represent distinctive syndromes.

The severity and location of pulmonary circuit obstruction is the key determinant of the extent and dynamics of right-to-left shunting and thus the major determinant of the physiologic manifestations in a tetralogy patient. This may range from mild stenosis to pulmonary atresia. Typically, activities, such as exercise, that decrease systemic vascular resistance in the face of a fixed pulmonary vascular resistance lead to increased right-to-left shunting. Children rapidly learn to squat, increasing systemic resistance, at the end of exercise. The majority of those who complete puberty will have had a palliative procedure, as native pulmonary perfusion is usually inadequate.

Physical exam is notable for cyanosis, clubbing, evidence of right ventricular hypertrophy, and the absence of a pulmonary component to the second heart sound. Systolic murmurs are usually related to flow across the pulmonary outflow tract and are often a sign that pulmonary obstruction is less severe. Aortic regurgitation is common.

The ECG is notable for right atrial enlargement, right axis deviation, and dominant R waves in V1 and V2. Post-repair, the majority of cases exhibit right bundle branch block. The chest X-ray is classically reported as a 'boot'-shaped heart—a consequence of the upturned hypertrophied right ventricular apex. Echocardiography will define the cardiac lesion, but tomographic imaging is often required to identify associated lesions, such as peripheral pulmonary vascular abnormalities.

As adult tetralogy patients will usually have undergone surgery (typically closure of the VSD and relief of pulmonary obstruction), their presentation is often a result of a residual shunt, pulmonary stenosis, or pulmonary regurgitation. Ventricular arrhythmias arising in the right ventricle are seen as 'late' phenomena, and, though correlated with the QRS duration and attributed to surgical intervention, there is increasing evidence of associated primary myocardial abnormalities.

Transposition of the great arteries

Complete transposition of the great arteries, or TGA, is the second most frequent cyanotic complex lesion, and surgically corrected adults are increasingly common. Typically, the atria and ventricles are located normally, but the aorta arises from the right ventricle and the pulmonary artery from the left ventricle. This anatomy is lethal, unless some form of shunting enables oxygenated blood to mix with the systemic circulation. This may result from a VSD (present in 10–20%), a PDA, or an ASD. Balloon atrial septostomy can be performed as a palliative procedure, but this solution, as well as the original surgical repairs in which left atrial oxygenated blood was redirected with baffles to the right ventricle, fails to alleviate the unnatural systemic load on this latter chamber. A complete arterial switch procedure is now performed to avoid this functional complication.

Physical exam reflects the extent of right ventricular failure in the face of a systemic load. The second heart sound is usually single.

ECG reveals sinus bradycardia or junctional rhythm. Atrial flutter is common. Chest radiology demonstrates right ventricular enlargement. Late complications include atrial arrhythmias, right ventricular failure, baffle complications, or left ventricular outflow tract obstruction.

Further reading

Gatzoulis MA, Webb GD, Daubeney PEF (2007). *The diagnosis and management of adult congenital heart disease.* Churchill Livingstone, Philadelphia.

Heart disease in pregnancy

Introduction

In the UK report 'Saving Lives, Improving Mothers' Care: Confidential Enquiries into Maternal Death 2009–12', cardiac disease remains the commonest cause of maternal death. Ischaemic heart disease is the largest category, reflecting the increasing age, BMI, and prevalence of diabetes mellitus in pregnant women, followed by sudden adult death syndrome and peripartum cardiomyopathy. The re-emergence of rheumatic heart disease as a cause of maternal death reflects the rising number of women born outside the UK. Half of the women who died had substandard care.

Cardiovascular changes during pregnancy

Significant physiological changes occur in the cardiovascular system from the earliest stages of pregnancy. A thorough understanding of these changes is vital for those involved in the management of pregnant women with heart disease.

Peripheral vascular resistance falls by 50% in early pregnancy. Cardiac output increases by a similar amount due to an increase in both stroke volume and heart rate. The rise in stroke volume is due to an increase in ventricular wall muscle mass, myocardial contractility, and ventricular end-diastolic volume.

Arterial blood pressure falls by, on average, 10/15 mmHg to reach a nadir by the end of the first trimester, returning to pre-pregnancy levels late in the third trimester. It should be measured using Korotkoff sound V and in a sitting (and not supine) position.

Blood volume increases by 50%, and there is a 20–40% increase in erythrocyte mass, reducing blood viscosity and causing a physiological dilutional fall in haemoglobin; in pregnancy, anaemia is diagnosed when haemoglobin is less than 105 g/L.

There is minimal change in pulmonary capillary wedge pressure or central venous pressure in pregnancy. Pregnant women are more susceptible to pulmonary oedema (both spontaneous and iatrogenic, following intravenous fluid) due to a reduction in serum colloid osmotic pressure and to endothelial dysfunction, especially in pre-eclampsia.

Venous return is dramatically reduced in the supine position due to the compression of the inferior vena cava by the gravid uterus. The subsequent reduction in cardiac output leads to supine hypotension and can reduce uterine and placental perfusion, which may cause fetal compromise. The left lateral position should replace the supine position in pregnancy.

Intrapartum, the cardiac output rises again, with a 15% rise in the first stage and a 50% rise in the second stage of labour. There is an increase in heart rate as a sympathetic response to the pain of contractions. Stroke volume rises during contractions, as uterine blood is returned to the systemic circulation.

There is a further rise in cardiac output immediately after delivery due to the removal of vena caval compression and autotransfusion (of 500mL) from sustained uterine contraction as the placenta delivers. Women unable to mount or sustain this response, e.g. tight stenotic valve lesions, pulmonary hypertension, or a severely dysfunctional left ventricle, are at greatest risk of developing pulmonary oedema during the second stage of labour and immediately postpartum.

Many of the normal symptoms of pregnancy can mimic symptoms of heart disease. Dyspnoea is a common and subjective sensation in pregnancy of uncertain aetiology, possibly due to the increase in tidal volume needed to support increased ventilation; respiratory rate is usually unchanged, and pulse oximetry, if indicated, is normal. Dependent oedema is virtually universal in pregnant women. The decreased venous return associated with inferior vena caval compression may cause dizziness or presyncope. Palpitations are common, reflecting the normal sinus tachycardia of pregnancy.

Cardiovascular system examination findings are also altered in normal pregnancy. The increase of ventricular wall muscle mass may lead to lateral displacement of the apex. Pronounced splitting of the second heart sound is common, as is a third heart sound due to rapid ventricular filling (in the absence of cardiac failure). An ejection systolic murmur is very common in pregnancy due to the hyperdynamic circulation, with increased flow through the aortic and pulmonary valves.

Chest pain (other than heartburn), haemoptysis, paroxysmal nocturnal dyspnoea, diastolic murmurs, and pansystolic murmurs that radiate over the whole precordium are not typical of normal pregnancy and require investigation.

General principles of care

Pre-conception care and contraception

All women, including teenagers, with significant heart disease should have planned and opportunistic pre-conception care from cardiologists and obstetricians, with an emphasis on contraception, so that pregnancies are planned, ideally for when cardiac status is optimal. For a few women, such as those with pulmonary hypertension, the risk of maternal death may be so high that pregnancy is not recommended. These women need particularly careful and sensitive discussions, which must not alienate them and must allow them to receive support if they choose to conceive,

Pre-conception counselling allows the risks of pregnancy to both the woman and fetus, and of any medication she may be taking, to be outlined. Children born to women with congenital heart disease (CHD) have an increased risk of CHD, and, therefore, a fetal echocardiogram in mid-pregnancy is advisable (see Table 4.9).

Risks vary, depending on the family history of CHD and whether there is an identifiable, non-recurring cause for the

Table 4.9 Likelihood of congenital heart disease (CHD) in offspring if mother has congenital heart disease

Type of maternal congenital heart disease	Risk of congenital heart disease in fetus (%)
None	1
Atrial septal defect	3–10
Ventricular septal defect	6–10
Coarctation of the aorta	4–7
Tetralogy of Fallot	5
Transposition of the great arteries	1
Patent ductus arteriosus	4
Marfan's syndrome	50

pregnant woman's CHD, e.g. *in utero* exposure to anticonvulsants or being offspring of a diabetic woman. When CHD is due to a chromosome deletion, such as 22q–, recurrence risk is 50%.

Multidisciplinary team
Women with cardiac disease should have their pregnancy care managed in a hospital setting by an experienced multidisciplinary team of obstetricians, cardiologists, anaesthetists, midwives, and neonatologists.

Antenatal, intrapartum (labour), and post-natal care
Early in the pregnancy a detailed antenatal care plan should be clearly outlined for the woman and all clinicians involved. Table 4.11 documents the cardiac medications that can be used during pregnancy and breastfeeding. The need for maternal and fetal monitoring will depend on the nature of the cardiac disease, but serial maternal echocardiograms or fetal growth scans should be considered and planned appropriately. A thorough anaesthetic assessment is needed. The optimal place and gestational age for delivery must be determined.

The intrapartum care plan should be distributed to all clinical areas. Vaginal delivery with low-dose epidural analgesia is usually appropriate, although exceptions may be made when the aortic root is >4 cm, for aortic dissection/aneurysm, or warfarin treatment within 2 weeks. An experienced obstetric anaesthetist should site the epidural for women with significant cardiac lesions, since great care is needed to avoid alterations in preload with vasodilatation. For similar reasons, peripartum blood loss should be minimized. Some women may need to have a shortened active second stage of labour, with elective instrumental vaginal delivery, to decrease the maternal expulsive effort and associated changes in cardiac output.

Management of the third stage of labour should be active, rather than passive, to reduce the risk of post-partum haemorrhage. Standard third stage management is a bolus of Syntometrine® (5U oxytocin, 500 mcg ergometrine). Women with significant heart disease should avoid this, since the former can cause hypotension and the latter hypertension. A oxytocin infusion (e.g. 5U over 5 minutes) should be considered.

As many cardiac conditions can deteriorate significantly in the post-partum period, the haemodynamic monitoring commenced in labour should be continued for 24–72 hours. Women with pulmonary hypertension require monitoring for up to 14 days after delivery.

All women should have a post-natal consultation to debrief them on the events of the pregnancy and provide contraceptive advice and pre-pregnancy counselling.

Endocarditis prophylaxis
Women traditionally thought to be at risk of endocarditis in pregnancy are those with prosthetic heart valves, valvular heart disease, structural congenital heart disease, hypertrophic cardiomyopathy, or those with a previous episode of infective endocarditis. Exceptions are women with a repaired patent ductus arteriosus, an isolated ostium secundum atrial septal defect, and those with mitral valve prolapse without regurgitation.

However, National Institute for Health and Clinical Excellence (NICE) guidance (March 2008) suggests that women undergoing obstetric procedures do not need endocarditis prophylaxis, as, although bacteraemia can occur, there is no clear association with the development of infective endocarditis and that women and their babies may be unnecessarily exposed to the adverse effects of antibiotics.

However, if there is suspicion of genital tract infection at the time of the obstetric procedure, antibiotics that include endocarditis prophylaxis should be given to women at risk.

Pregnancy outcome
Women with cyanotic heart disease are at significant risk of miscarriage, fetal growth restriction, and intrauterine death, as the placental gaseous exchange cannot compensate for the maternal hypoxaemia.

Neonates born to mothers with cardiac disease are at increased risk of preterm birth (spontaneous and iatrogenic), low birthweight, respiratory distress syndrome, intraventricular haemorrhage, and death. In some cases, there is an increased likelihood of CHD in the babies.

In general terms, women in New York Heart Association (NYHA) class III or IV are less likely to have a good pregnancy outcome than those women in NYHA class I or II. The NYHA grade, combined with the presence of cyanosis, left heart obstruction, the systemic ventricle ejection fraction, and past history of a cardiovascular event, allows for a more detailed predication of the likelihood of a maternal cardiac event in pregnancy to be made—the Toronto risk predictor score (see Table 4.10).

Investigations and procedures
Chest X-ray
When clinically indicated, a chest X-ray (CXR) should be performed in pregnancy, with abdominal shielding. The radiation dose to the fetus is small: equivalent to 10 days of background radiation in London or one transatlantic flight. Normal CXR changes in pregnancy include an increased cardiothoracic ratio and increased vascular markings.

Electrocardiogram
Normal ECG changes in pregnancy include sinus tachycardia and premature atrial or ventricular beats. T wave inversion and Q waves in lead III may be seen in healthy pregnant women.

Echocardiogram
Transthoracic or transoesophageal echocardiograms are safe in pregnancy and provide extremely useful information on the cardiovascular reserve as well as identifying structural abnormalities, atrial thrombus, or bacterial vegetations. Normal echocardiogram changes in pregnancy include an increase in heart size and left ventricular mass and mild regurgitation in all valves.

Table 4.10 Assessing risk of cardiac event in pregnancy; the Toronto risk predictor score

Total score	Risk of cardiovascular event in pregnancy (%)
0	5
1	27
>1	75

Score 1 for each: NYHA grade ≥2 or cyanosis (SaO$_2$ <90%)

Systemic ventricle ejection fraction <40%

Left heart obstruction

Prior cardiovascular system event (pulmonary oedema, arrhythmia, cerebrovascular accident, transient ischaemic attack)

Reprinted from *Canadian Journal of Cardiology*, 22, 3, Ivanov J, et al., 'The Toronto Risk Score for adverse events following cardiac surgery', pp. 221–227, Copyright 2006, with permission from Canadian Cardiovascular Society and Elsevier.

Table 4.11 Cardiac drugs in pregnancy and breastfeeding

Drug	Pregnancy	Breastfeeding
Digoxin	√[1]	√
Furosemide	√	√
Thiazides	√[2]	√
Nitrates	√	√
Hydralazine	√	√
Angiotensin-converting enzyme inhibitor	x[3]	√
Beta-blockers	√[4]	√
Lidocaine	√	√
Procainamide	√	√
Verapamil	√	√
Amiodarone	x[5]	x[5]
Flecainide	√	√
Adenosine	√	?
Statins	x[6]	?
Warfarin	x[7]	√
Heparin	√	√
Clopidogrel	√[8]	?
Low-dose (75 mg) aspirin	√	√

√ = safe to use, x = not safe to use, ? = not known

An individual risk benefit analysis should be always be made. Wherever possible, changes to medication should be planned prior to conception and short courses (e.g. clopidogrel following angioplasty) completed before pregnancy.

[1] Monitor drug levels: maternal toxicity may be associated with intrauterine death. Digoxin renal clearance is increased in pregnancy, and so the dose may need to be increased

[2] The physiologically increased circulating volume should not be reduced, unless overload is a clinical issue.

[3] Stop prior to conception, or in very early pregnancy, as associated with teratogenesis in 1st trimester, oligohydramnios in 2nd and 3rd trimesters,

[4] High-dose beta-blocker has been linked with intrauterine growth restriction, but this is considered to be a complication of iatrogenic hypotension, rather than the drug itself; in lactation, beta-blockers with high lipid solubility (e.g. labetalol), and therefore high protein binding, are preferred

[5] High iodine may cause congenital goitre, or fetal or neonatal hypothyroidism.

[6] Stop pre-pregnancy or as soon as possible after conception—theoretical concerns of risks to fetal development.

[7] Stop as soon as possible after conception and before 6 weeks' gestation; crosses placenta and should be used only after 1st trimester if risk to mother of thrombosis outweighs risk of fetal haemorrhage.

[8] Safety data limited; risk of bleeding if taken at delivery.

Helpful information:

• Exposure in pregnancy: National Teratology Service 0844 892 0909/<http://www.toxbase.org/exposure-in-pregnancy>.

• Use in breastfeeding: <www.toxnet.nlm.nih.gov/newtoxnet/lactmed>.

Angiography

Coronary angiography ± angioplasty can be used in acute myocardial infarction in pregnancy, with fetal shielding; they allow treatment of both acute coronary artery occlusion and coronary artery dissection. The supine position must be avoided, and, in advanced pregnancy, the gravid uterus may make a femoral approach difficult. If stenting is carried out, the management of anticoagulation is challenging, since there is conflict for the mother. Powerful antiplatelet agents, such as clopidogrel, are important for preventing stent thrombosis but carry a high risk of bleeding from surgical trauma at delivery.

Cardiopulmonary bypass

Occasionally, cardiopulmonary bypass is used in pregnant women. However, if the mother is too sick to withstand a Caesarean section delivery prior to the use of this technique or the gestational age is too early for this to be feasible, the hypothermia and relative hypoxia of bypass are associated with high fetal loss at all stages of pregnancy.

Congenital heart disease

With increasing advances in cardiac surgery and medication, 85% of infants with congenital heart disease now survive to reproductive maturity. The ability of a woman with congenital heart disease to have a successful pregnancy outcome depends on the type of lesion, current haemodynamic status, and previous surgical procedures. The cornerstone is the ability of her cardiovascular system to adapt to the increased cardiovascular workload of pregnancy.

Low-risk lesions (maternal mortality <1%)
Patent ductus arteriosus

Most women with a patent ductus arteriosus (PDA) will have undergone surgical correction in childhood. These women suffer no additional problems during pregnancy. Women with an uncorrected PDA generally have no additional pregnancy problems but are at risk of congestive heart failure.

Atrial septal defect

In the absence of pulmonary hypertension, women with atrial septal defects tolerate pregnancy well. They are at risk of atrial arrhythmias and paradoxical emboli; therefore, heparin prophylaxis should be considered. Vasodilatation following regional anaesthesia or acute blood loss can increase the left-to-right shunt in the intrapartum period that may lead to a reduction in left ventricular output and coronary artery blood flow.

Coarctation of the aorta

Coarctation of the aorta diagnosed in childhood is usually surgically corrected or treated by balloon dilatation or stent implantation. Pregnancy in women with an adequately corrected coarctation is well tolerated. Pre-pregnancy assessment of these women should include a search for re-coarctation, aneurysm at the surgical site, a bicuspid aortic valve, or systemic hypertension. These must be appropriately managed prior to conception.

Women with uncorrected coarctation are at risk of angina, hypertension, congestive cardiac failure, aortic rupture, and aortic dissection during pregnancy. Beta-blockers can reduce these risks by controlling hypertension and decreasing cardiac contractility, leading to a reduction in the haemodynamic load on the aorta.

Aortic stenosis

Aortic stenosis is most commonly congenital and associated with a bicuspid valve. Pregnancy is usually well tolerated if the

woman is asymptomatic, with a normal ECG, exercise tolerance test, and left ventricular function. Women with severe
aortic stenosis (peak transaortic gradient >100 mmHg) are
at increased risk of complications. Warning signs include
tachycardia (as the failing left ventricle is unable to maintain
the raised cardiac output of pregnancy), new dyspnoea,
angina, ischaemic changes on ECG, or a fall in peak valve gradient (the cardiovascular changes of normal pregnancy cause
an increase in cardiac output and increased flow across the
valve and, therefore, an increase in the gradient). Pulmonary
oedema and sudden death can occur in pregnancy.

Hypovolaemia, hypotension, and vasodilatation should
be avoided. If left ventricular function is good, beta-blockers
may be used for symptom control. Women with severe stenosis and left ventricular dysfunction may require aortic balloon valvotomy during pregnancy. If valvotomy is
complicated by acute aortic regurgitation, a failing left ventricle may struggle to cope. Ideally, women with severe aortic stenosis should have valve replacement pre-conception.

Tetralogy of Fallot
The combination of a ventricular septal defect, an overrid-
ing aorta, subpulmonary stenosis, and right ventricular
hypertrophy make up the commonest form of cyanotic
congenital heart disease, Tetralogy of Fallot (ToF).

Women who have had ToF corrected surgically in childhood are no longer cyanotic and generally tolerate pregnancy well, including those with severe pulmonary
regurgitation and a dilated right ventricle. However, paradoxical embolism and thrombotic cerebrovascular accidents can occur. This risk can be reduced by heparin
prophylaxis.

Moderate risk (maternal mortality 1–10%)
Corrected transposition of the great arteries (TGA)
Women currently of reproductive age had this repaired
using the Mustard procedure where the right ventricle
pumps oxygenated blood into the systemic circulation.
Women with an uncomplicated repair usually tolerate pregnancy well but may experience problems with right ventricular dysfunction and/or atrial arrhythmias or sinus node
dysfunction. Women with long-term complications, following their repair, tolerate pregnancy poorly.

Univentricular circulation post-Fontan procedure
Fontan procedures are characterized by the construction of
atriopulmonary connections so that venous blood enters
the pulmonary circulation directly, and then oxygenated
blood is returned to the single ventricle before being
pumped into the systemic circulation. Women who underwent this palliative procedure in childhood for complex
cyanotic heart disease increasingly survive to childbearing
years.

The ability to adjust stroke volume and heart rate may be
compromised in these women. They are at risk of atrial
arrhythmias. If the univentricle has the morphology of a left
ventricle, function is likely to be good and pregnancy well
tolerated; this is less likely if the ventricle is morphologically
right-sided.

Cyanotic heart disease without pulmonary hypertension
Pregnancy in women with persisting cyanosis (e.g. due to
uncorrected TGA, uncorrected ToF with pulmonary steno-
sis/atresia, univentricular heart, tricuspid atresia, and
Ebstein's anomaly with ASD) has a poorer maternal and fetal
outcome. This is proportional to ventricular function, hypoxia, and the associated cyanosis (e.g. maternal haemoglobin
(Hb) <160 g/L, 71% live birth; Hb >200 g/L, 8% live birth).

Cyanosis and hypoxia may deteriorate because of worsening right-to-left shunting, caused by systemic vasodilatation. Polycythaemia increases the risk of thromboembolism:
hydration, mobilization, and compression stockings are
needed. Anticoagulation is not routine, as cyanosis also
increases the risk of haemorrhage. Maternal oxygenation
can be maximized by bed rest (with the use of compression
stockings and intermittent pneumatic compression devices
to reduce the thrombotic risk) and oxygen therapy in an
effort to maintain fetal oxygenation and growth.

High-risk lesions (maternal mortality >10%)
*Primary pulmonary hypertension and Eisenmenger
syndrome*
Pregnancy in women with pulmonary hypertension of any
aetiology carries a very high maternal mortality of 50%.
Women who wish to pursue a pregnancy, regardless of this
risk, need multidisciplinary care by an experienced team of
anaesthetists, cardiologists, and obstetricians. Systemic
vasodilatation worsens the right-to-left shunt, so they must
avoid dehydration and further vasodilatation. Admission for
bed rest, thromboprophylaxis, and oxygen therapy is often
needed in the third trimester.

The intrapartum and post-natal periods provide clinicians
with many management difficulties, and intensive care is
usually needed after delivery. Fatal pulmonary hypertension
can develop up to 2 weeks after delivery. A wide range of
agents, including nitric oxide, prostacyclin, and sildenafil,
have been tried, but the evidence base is weak.

Marfan's syndrome
Women with Marfan's syndrome are at increased risk of
aortic aneurysm in pregnancy, with possible aortic dissection or rupture due to the hyperdynamic circulation and
hormonal effects on smooth muscle and collagen.

The risk of maternal mortality can be stratified, according
to the aortic root diameter, with a risk of 25% when the
aortic root is greater than 4 cm. Ideally, these women
should have aortic arch replacement before pregnancy.

If, during pregnancy, serial echocardiography shows aortic root dilatation, beta-blockers and aggressive control of
hypertension are recommended.

Acquired heart disease
Valvular heart disease
In general, pregnant women with regurgitant valves do not
experience significant cardiovascular problems; those with
valvular stenosis are at greater risk. Worldwide, the major
cause of acquired heart disease is valvular damage by rheumatic fever. In the UK, the incidence in pregnancy is rising
due to the increasing immigrant population. Many may not
have been examined by a doctor before or may experience
symptoms for the first time in pregnancy or the puerperium
due to the increased cardiovascular stress.

Mitral stenosis
Mitral stenosis is the most significant valve problem in pregnancy and the puerperium. When the valve area is less than
1 cm^2, women often experience cardiac problems. The
pressure gradient across the stenotic valve, and therefore
left atrial pressure, is increased in early pregnancy due to the
increased preload and reduced ventricular filling time (secondary to the increase in heart rate). The risk of pulmonary
oedema is increased by this physiological tachycardia and
with infection or exercise. The development or deterioration of symptoms, such as dyspnoea, orthopnoea, paroxysmal nocturnal dyspnoea, and decreased exercise tolerance,
should be taken seriously in women with, or at risk of,

mitral stenosis. Beta-blockers can be used to slow the heart rate and allow more ventricular filling; diuretics can be used for acute relief of pulmonary oedema.

They are also at risk of developing atrial fibrillation, which should be promptly treated with beta-blockers, digoxin, or DC cardioversion. Anticoagulation should be considered, since there is an increased risk of thrombosis with atrial fibrillation, especially if the left atrium is significantly enlarged.

Balloon mitral valvotomy may be performed during pregnancy if symptoms are significant despite maximal medical treatment. Ideally, women with severe mitral stenosis (valve area <1 cm^2) should undergo surgery before conception.

Mitral regurgitation

Mitral regurgitation is usually well tolerated in pregnancy due to the decreased systemic vascular resistance, increased stroke volume, and therefore decreased left ventricular afterload. Symptomatic heart failure in pregnancy can be treated with nitrates, hydralazine, diuretics, and digoxin.

Mitral valve prolapse

Mitral valve prolapse without regurgitation is a benign condition in pregnancy, which does not lead to cardiovascular compromise.

Prosthetic heart valves

The needs of pregnant women with mechanical heart valves conflict with the needs of their fetus, and a successful outcome can be difficult to achieve. The evidence for different management approaches is not strong, and expert opinion and individual care plans are needed. These patients require anticoagulation throughout pregnancy, as they have a significant risk of valve thrombosis and subsequent embolus, or valve dysfunction. However, warfarin in early pregnancy can cause an embryopathy (6%), and, in the 2nd and 3rd trimesters, it anticoagulates the fetus and can (especially when the maternal dose is greater than 5–7 mg) cause life-threatening fetal haemorrhage. Converting to treatment doses of low molecular weight (LMWH) or unfractionated heparin during the period of organogenesis (6–12 weeks) and/or 2nd and 3rd trimesters until labour is approaching (e.g. 35–36 weeks) is associated with an increased risk (4% to 9%) of thrombosis, especially on smaller valves and those in the mitral position, but is safe for the fetus, since neither crosses the placenta.

Regardless of prior anticoagulation, delivery should be managed with the woman off warfarin and LMWH, as they each have long half-lives. Warfarin crosses the placenta, and the fetus may remain anticoagulated for some days after the maternal effect is gone. Unfractionated heparin is the usual anticoagulant of choice, which can be stopped as labour establishes and recommenced after delivery. Warfarin can then be restarted once the risk of primary post-partum haemorrhage and bleeding from surgical sites has passed (usually 3–5 days). Labour may need to be induced to minimize the contrasting risks of valve thrombosis due to prolonged spells off anticoagulation, or haemorrhage due to delivery before anticoagulation is ineffective, but must be timed judiciously to minimize obstetric complications.

Bioprosthetic valves do not usually require anticoagulation but may deteriorate more quickly during pregnancy.

Ischaemic heart disease

Although still uncommon, with advancing maternal age and more obesity and diabetes, the incidence of ischaemic heart disease in pregnant women is rising. Maternal mortality rates from myocardial infarction can be up to 50%, although there were no deaths in a recent prospective study of 25 cases.

The treatment of myocardial infarction in a pregnant woman is the same as outside of pregnancy. Treatment is aimed at maximizing tissue oxygenation and limiting further infarction. Oxygen, aspirin, heparin, beta-blockers, and nitrates may all be used. Coronary angiography and angioplasty are safe. Caution is needed with the use of thrombolysis due to the risk of placental bleeding, but its use is justified in life-threatening acute coronary insufficiency.

Myocardial infarction may be due to atherosclerosis, but other causes, such as coronary artery dissection (21%), coronary artery thrombus (7%) or coronary artery spasm (13%) are more common in pregnancy and should be considered.

If cardiac arrest occurs and output is not achieved after 4 minutes of resuscitation, a perimortem Caesarean section should be performed. This will improve venous return and allow for removal of the left lateral tilt recommended for resuscitation of the pregnant woman, which, in turn, will make external cardiac compressions more effective. It may save the baby.

Aortic dissection

Aortic dissection has a very high mortality rate in pregnancy, even with optimal management. Women presenting with chest pain or intrascapular pain, especially those with systolic hypertension, should have suitable imaging (CXR, CT/MRI chest, transoesophageal echocardiogram) performed and aortic dissection included in the differential diagnosis.

Cardiac arrhythmias

Hormonal changes, changes in autonomic tone, increased haemodynamic demands, and mild hypokalaemia predispose the pregnant woman to cardiac arrhythmias—de novo or by exacerbating pre-existing arrhythmias.

Sinus tachycardia may be seen in normal pregnancy; however, persistent tachycardia over 100 bpm requires investigation to exclude treatable conditions, such as anaemia, hyperthyroidism, hypovolaemia, sepsis, respiratory or cardiac pathology. ECG, 24-hour Holter tape or event monitor, and/or echocardiography may be required.

Atrial and ventricular ectopic beats are common in pregnancy, are benign, and require no investigation or treatment. Supraventricular tachycardia (SVT) is also more common in pregnancy. If simple measures of vagal stimulation do not halt the SVT, adenosine, beta-blockers, or flecainide may be safely used. Definitive treatment of re-entrant tachycardia, such as Wolff–Parkinson–White syndrome, is usually deferred until after delivery.

Atrial fibrillation and atrial flutter are rare and usually occur in women with pre-existing congenital or valvular heart disease. These must be excluded when AF presents for the first time in pregnancy. Early treatment, with cardioversion to sinus rhythm or medical treatment for ventricular rate control plus anticoagulation, is vital.

Ventricular tachycardia is also rare in pregnancy. Women who are haemodynamically stable may be treated with pharmacological agents, such as lidocaine or procainamide. Electrical cardioversion should be used in all women who are haemodynamically compromised by their arrhythmia.

Cardiomyopathy

Hypertrophic cardiomyopathy

The majority of cases of hypertrophic cardiomyopathy (HOCM) are familial, with an autosomal dominant pattern of inheritance. Many women are asymptomatic, having been diagnosed following family screening.

The symptoms of HOCM include chest pain or syncope secondary to left ventricular outflow tract obstruction.

Clinical findings include double apical pulsation, ejection systolic murmur, pansystolic murmur, arrhythmias, or signs of heart failure.

Pregnancy is generally well tolerated in asymptomatic women with HOCM. Beta-blockers can be used in symptomatic women. The hypotension sometimes seen with regional anaesthesia or hypovolaemia can lead to increased left ventricular outflow tract obstruction so should be avoided.

Women with severe symptoms or heart failure pre-pregnancy are at risk of deterioration during pregnancy, with the possibility of new-onset atrial fibrillation, syncope, or maternal death.

Peripartum cardiomyopathy

This is a rare condition specific to pregnancy. Onset is in the last few weeks of pregnancy or, more commonly, post-partum, up to 6 months after delivery. It is more common in older, multiparous women with a multiple pregnancy or those in whom the pregnancy was complicated by hypertension.

Women present with dyspnoea, reduced exercise tolerance, palpitations, and symptoms due to peripheral or cerebral emboli or pulmonary oedema.

Diagnosis is suggested by the findings of a large heart on CXR, and, at echocardiography, global dilatation of all chambers and significantly reduced left ventricular function. All other causes of congestive heart failure should be excluded before the diagnosis is made.

Mortality can be high. Delivery should be arranged if the diagnosis is made antenatally: this will need careful planning and will be determined by obstetric as well as cardiac factors. Pharmacological treatment includes beta-blockers, diuretics, hydralazine, and digoxin. ACE inhibitors can be used post-natally. Anticoagulation should be considered, as the dilated heart chambers predispose to thromboembolism. Some women will not recover completely and will have ongoing left ventricular dysfunction. These women have a high risk of relapse in future pregnancies.

Cardiac transplantation may be necessary in women refractory to conventional treatment.

Conclusion

Cardiac disease is a significant and an increasing contributor to maternal and neonatal morbidity and mortality. In order to reduce the disease burden, women with cardiac disease should aim to have a planned pregnancy that is managed by an experienced multidisciplinary team of clinicians.

Further reading

Bush N, Nelson-Piercy C, Spark P, Kurinczuk JJ, Brocklehurst P, Knight M, UKOSS (2013). Myocardial infarction in pregnancy and postpartum in the UK. *European Journal of Preventive Cardiology*, **20**, 12–20.

Centre for Maternal and Child Enquiries (CMACE) (2011). Saving Mothers' Lives: reviewing maternal deaths to make motherhood safer: 2006–08. The Eighth Report on Confidential Enquiries into Maternal Deaths in the United Kingdom. *BJOG*, **118** (Suppl. 1), 1–203.

Chia P, Chia H, Subramaniam R (2002). A clinical approach to heart disease in pregnancy. Part 1: general considerations in management. *The Obstetrician & Gynaecologist*, **4**, 162–8.

Chia P, Chia H, Subramaniam R (2002). A clinical approach to heart disease in pregnancy. Part 2: specific considerations in management. *The Obstetrician & Gynaecologist*, **4**, 212–16.

Gelson E, Johnson M, Gatzoulis M, Uebing A (2007). Cardiac disease in pregnancy. Part 1: congenital heart disease. *The Obstetrician & Gynaecologist*, **9**, 15–20.

Gelson E, Johnson M, Gatzoulis M, Uebing A (2007). Cardiac disease in pregnancy. Part 2: acquired heart disease. *The Obstetrician & Gynaecologist*, **9**, 83–7.

James DK, Steer PJ, Weiner CP, Gonik B (1999). *High-risk pregnancy—management options*. Saunders, London.

Knight M, Kenyon S, Brocklehurst P, Neilson J, Shakespeare J, Kurinczuk JJ (eds) on behalf of MBRRACE-UK (2014). *Saving Lives, Improving Mothers' Care - Lessons learned to inform future maternity care from the UK and Ireland Confidential Enquiries into Maternal Deaths and Morbidity 2009–2012*. National Perinatal Epidemiology Unit, University of Oxford, Oxford.

National Institute for Health and Clinical Excellence (2008). Prophylaxis against infective endocarditis. <http://publications.nice.org.uk/prophylaxis-against-infective-endocarditis-cg64>.

Nelson-Piercy C (2010). *Handbook of obstetric medicine.*, 4th edn. ISIS Medical Media, London.

Steer PJ, Gatzoulis MA, Baker P (2006). *Heart disease in pregnancy*. RCOG Press, London.

Diseases of arteries and veins

Venous disorders: superficial thrombophlebitis

Symptoms and signs

Superficial thrombophlebitis is characterized by leg pain, with reddening of the skin and swelling along the line of the superficial veins, which feel hard due to *in situ* thrombosis.

Superficial thrombophlebitis may be associated with underlying deep venous thromboembolism, and it is essential this is considered.

Causes

Predisposing factors include varicose veins, immobilization, surgery, trauma, pregnancy and childbirth, active malignancy, oral contraceptives or hormone replacement therapy, and obesity.

Investigation

Whilst this is primarily a clinical diagnosis, Doppler ultrasound should be performed to exclude associated deep venous thrombosis

Treatment

Low molecular weight heparin and non-steroidal anti-inflammatory drugs are the treatments of choice. There is debate over which is best or whether they should be used together.

Antibiotics have no routine role in the management, unless there is clear evidence of sepsis, which is often cannula-associated.

Venous disorders: venous ulceration

Symptoms and signs

Venous ulceration is ulceration of the skin, usually the lower limb, associated with venous eczema, haemosiderin deposition, and venous insufficiency.

Causes

Predisposing factors include previous deep venous thrombosis, cardiac failure, diabetes mellitus, and obesity.

Investigation

It is important to exclude accompanying arterial insufficiency by Doppler ultrasound assessment of arterial pressures and flow.

The size, depth, and wound bed characteristics of the ulcer should be noted to monitor progress.

Routine bacteriological swabbing is not required unless there is clinical evidence of infection.

Treatment

Primary treatment for venous ulceration is elevation. The wound bed should be cleaned with water and debrided or desloughed using a scalpel or hydrolytic dressings. Compression bandaging should be employed once arterial disease has been excluded. Varicose vein surgery may improve healing if compression bandaging alone is insufficient

Antibiotics are not indicated for the management of venous ulceration unless clinically infected.

Venous disorders: venous gangrene

Symptoms and signs

Venous gangrene is often mistaken for acute arterial insufficiency. However, in contrast, the limb is swollen, and the superficial veins are filled. Often, it may be impossible to palpate pulses due to the degree of oedema. Handheld Doppler can usually detect pulse signals.

Causes

Venous gangrene develops due to complete occlusion of the central veins and associated collaterals. It is typically associated with pelvic or intra-abdominal tumours, causing pressure on the iliac veins or inferior vena cava. Other rarer causes include pregnancy, thrombotic disorders, vena caval filters, ulcerative colitis, and, paradoxically, warfarin therapy, particularly in cancer patients.

Investigation

Doppler ultrasound will confirm the occlusion of the venous system and presence of arterial signals. Pelvic ultrasound or CT scanning of abdomen and pelvis should be performed to determine the underlying cause.

Treatment

Primary treatment for venous gangrene is elevation of the affected limb. Patients should receive intravenous unfractionated heparin, maintaining the APTT between 2.0 and 2.5 times normal. Thrombolysis has been used, but there are significant risks associated with bleeding if there is an underlying tumour.

The predisposing cause, once established, should be treated.

If the leg is slow to reperfuse, then tissue loss should be allowed to demarcate and amputation performed at the lowest possible level.

Even if the leg reperfuses, the degree of damage to valves and endothelial integrity make acute complications, such as compartment syndromes, highly likely and chronic post-phlebitic legs almost inevitable.

Arterial disorders: chronic ischaemia

Symptoms and signs

The principal symptom of chronic arterial insufficiency is intermittent claudication, defined as intermittent cramp-like pain on walking. The site of the pain and the presence or absence of peripheral pulses depend on the site of the arterial stenosis. Common sites include the superficial femoral artery, causing calf claudication and absent popliteal and foot pulses, or the aorta and iliac arteries, producing weak or absent femoral pulses and claudication at any level, including thigh or buttock claudication.

Conditions, such as cauda equina and lumbar canal stenosis, sciatica, and other nerve compression syndromes, can be confused with intermittent claudication, but, in most of these cases, the pain is bilateral, the pulses are present, and the pain will come on after standing and is not usually quickly improved by rest.

Causes

Predisposing factors for occlusive peripheral arterial disease include diabetes, hypertension, smoking, and obesity. It is strongly associated with the other atherosclerotic conditions: ischaemic heart disease, cerebrovascular disease, and renal artery stenosis.

Investigation

Duplex arterial scanning is the first-line investigation to quantify the level and degree of arterial disease. Arteriography should be reserved for patients with lifestyle-limiting claudication in whom bypass surgery or angioplasty are being considered. MRI angiography is now common after duplex scanning to allow surgical planning without the risks of unnecessary arterial puncture and the risk of radiographic contrast nephropathy.

If the pulses are normal on resting examination, but intermittent claudication is still suspected, then exercise testing can demonstrate a falling arterial pressure and the onset of pain in patients with arterial ischaemia.

If the arterial tests are normal or if the diagnosis of cauda equina syndrome or lumbar canal stenosis is considered on clinical grounds, then MRI scanning of the spine and spinal cord is indicated.

Treatment
Intermittent claudication should be treated by regular exercise and careful attention to secondary cardiovascular prevention, including smoking cessation, blood pressure control, antiplatelet agents, aspirin or clopidogrel, and statins. ACE inhibitors should be used with caution due to the risk of associated renal artery stenosis.

Angioplasty or surgery should be reserved for those with severely limiting, and reducing, claudication distance, rest pain, or with tissue loss due to localized gangrene.

Arterial disorders: critical limb ischaemia

Symptoms and signs
Critical limb ischaemia develops in the context of chronic occlusive peripheral arterial disease, as opposed to acute limb ischaemia, as described in Arterial disorders: acute ischaemia. Patients with critical limb ischaemia describe decreasing claudication distance and increasing rest pain. Rest pain typically occurs at night when in bed or when the feet are elevated.

Arterial ulceration of pressure points, such as the heel or the toes, may develop, especially in patients with diabetes, leading to localized gangrene and tissue loss.

Investigation
Patients with critical limb ischaemia should be referred for conventional or MRI angiography.

Treatment
Analgesia is the first-line management of rest pain and critical limb ischaemia. This invariably requires opiate level analgesia.

Cardiovascular prevention measures, including smoking cessation, antiplatelet therapy, blood pressure control, and statins, are essential as in chronic limb ischaemia.

Angioplasty or surgical bypass should be considered but may be technically difficult due to multilevel disease and poor run-off vessels, particularly in diabetes patients.

If the arterial disease cannot be treated by surgery or interventional radiology, then amputation may be necessary to relieve pain.

Patients with significant comorbidity who are unfit for amputation will require pain control, and, in some cases, this may be palliative.

Therapies, such as iloprost and sympathectomy, may be considered but are largely outmoded or not licensed in the UK.

Arterial disorders: acute ischaemia

Symptoms and signs
Acute arterial ischaemia can, if complete, result in irreversible life- and limb-threatening tissue damage within 6 hours if circulation is not restored.

The two main signs of complete arterial occlusion requiring urgent surgical intervention are paralysis of muscle function and anaesthesia due to sensory nerve impairment. All other signs, such as the absence of pulses or limb pallor, are less reliable and may also be present in chronic ischaemia. Pain is usually present in complete ischaemia but is often a late finding once muscle necrosis is established.

Causes
The principal cause of acute limb ischaemia is thrombotic occlusion of an existing arterial stenotic plaque.

A third of cases are due to embolic phenomena. These typically arise from the atria in patients in atrial fibrillation. Other sources, such as metal heart valves, proximal aneurysms, especially aortic or popliteal arteries, and atrial myxomas, should be excluded.

Less common causes include:

- Thrombosis *in situ* secondary to reduced cardiac output, hypotension following myocardial infarction, or meningococcal and pneumococcal septicaemia.
- Intra-arterial injection, usually of poorly soluble drugs of misuse, frequently causes peripheral emboli as well as local spasm and thrombosis.
- Fractures and dislocations of the elbow (especially in children) or ankle (adults) are the usual traumatic causes.
- Aortic dissection, particularly the aortic arch, resulting in upper limb ischaemia.
- Thoracic outlet syndrome, more commonly causing recurrent subacute ischaemia, can lead to post-stenotic dilatation of the subclavian artery and then to peripheral emboli.

Investigation
If the diagnosis of complete arterial occlusion is suspected, then investigations should not delay treatment. Emergency vascular surgical referral and, if necessary, perioperative angiography are the best options to reduce tissue damage.

If the limb still has sensation and movement, then the occlusion is more likely to be partial, and there is time to resuscitate the patient and organize an urgent angiogram.

Treatment
The initial medical treatment of patients with acute limb ischaemia is fluid resuscitation and control of metabolic disturbances, including hyperkalaemia and acidosis.

Intravenous unfractionated heparin should be given pending surgery or embolectomy.

Thrombolysis is less successful in large artery thrombosis and ineffective in complete occlusion due to the time taken to work and the degree of tissue damage that can develop while awaiting reperfusion.

Arterial disorders: reperfusion syndromes
The features of reperfusion injury are:
- Acidosis and hyperkalaemia due to the release of H^+ and K^+ ions from ischaemic and dead tissue.
- Myoglobinuria, leading to renal failure.
- ARDS.
- Intestinal capillary leak, leading to fluid sequestration, hypovolaemia, and shock.
- Localized limb swelling due to leakage from damaged endothelium which can cause compartment syndromes.

Arterial disorders: compartment syndrome
The hallmark of compartment syndrome is loss of muscle function and pain on active or passive contraction of muscle. Ultimately, the muscle shortens and develops ischaemic contracture. Urgent compartment monitoring is required with fasciotomy if the compartment pressure rises to within 30 mmHg of the diastolic blood pressure.

Arterial disorders: aortic aneurysm

Symptoms and signs
Over three-quarters of aortic aneurysms are asymptomatic until found at screening, incidentally during abdominal

ultrasound, or when they rupture. In a minority of patients, other symptoms and signs, including non-specific abdominal pain or peripheral embolization, can occur.

Rupture of abdominal aortic aneurysms classically presents as abdominal and/or back pain, hypovolaemic shock, and a palpable abdominal mass. However, pain may be minimal, and the mass may not be detectable by external palpation. Hypotensive patients with vague abdominal pain should be investigated for ischaemic bowel and aortic aneurysm as a matter of urgency, particularly if they have a known diagnosis of abdominal aneurysm.

Causes
Smoking, hypertension, male gender, and a family history are the main predisposing factors for abdominal aortic aneurysm.

Investigation
Ultrasound is the most reliable method of confirming the presence of an aortic aneurysm; however, when the diagnosis is clear on clinical grounds, then immediate surgery should not be delayed for investigations.

CT scanning is often used to determine the extent of an aneurysm pre-elective surgery but has a low specificity for detecting rupture.

Treatment
Emergency surgical repair is the only treatment for a ruptured aortic aneurysm. However, the outcome remains poor, particularly if the patient is elderly, unconscious, and anaemic, or has significant comorbidity. Around 80% will die pre-theatre and around 50% in the peri- and post-operative periods.

Elective surgery is a pre-emptive measure to prevent rupture once the aneurysm is over 55 mm and the patient has no major comorbidities. Endovascular repair is increasing, particularly in patients where open surgery is hazardous.

Diabetes foot ulceration

Symptoms and signs
Foot ulceration is a common complication of diabetes, with a prevalence of around 5% of all diabetes patients. Diabetes foot ulcers are classified by their relative depth (superficial to involvement of bone), the presence of infection, and the degree of ischaemia (see Figure 4.16).

Infection can be difficult to detect clinically and may have few systemic manifestations. However, once present, infection can spread rapidly through a foot, destroying tissue, and may become life-threatening (see Figure 4.17). Patients with foot ulceration may present with pyrexia of seemingly unknown origin, as feet are often overlooked during routine examination, particularly between the toes.

A swollen hot foot in a diabetes patient could also be a Charcot foot, and all suspected cases should be referred to a diabetes foot care team as a matter of urgency.

Causes
Predisposing factors for foot ulceration include sensory neuropathy and/or peripheral arterial insufficiency. Other factors include male gender, living alone, smoking, drinking to excess, lower socio-economic group and poor diabetes control. The presence of other diabetes complications is also associated with an increased incidence of ulceration.

Patients with renal failure or previous transplantation are another very high-risk group.

Investigation
Clinical examination will determine the cause of the ulcer. If pulses are not palpable, then it is important to determine if there is pulsatile arterial flow by Doppler ultrasound.

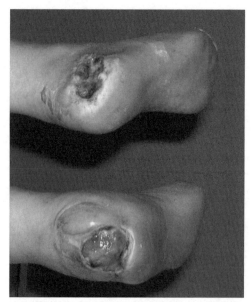

Figure 4.16 Diabetes foot ulceration.

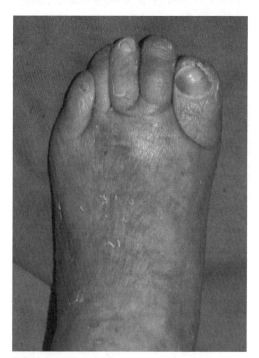

Figure 4.17 Infected diabetes ulceration with associated foot tissue damage.

Probing the ulcer gently will determine its depth. If bone cannot be felt at the base of the ulcer, then osteomyelitis is unlikely. Radiological investigations do not exclude osteomyelitis, as plain films may take several weeks to reveal the extent of bony involvement. If bone is palpable, then many authorities would treat as osteomyelitis and observe with serial X-rays. If it is important to exclude osteomyelitis, then MRI scanning is the most sensitive and specific imaging method.

Routine bacteriological swabbing is not required, unless there is clinical evidence of infection. It is less reliable than tissue samples at detecting pathogens.

Treatment

As an incidental finding

Superficial ulceration, with no clinical signs of infection, can be dressed with a simple foam dressing and referred to the diabetes foot care team for debridement and offloading. Patients should be encouraged to rest the foot as much as possible until suitable offloading is provided. They should not wear their own shoes, as these are the frequent cause of ulceration, but should, however, never walk barefoot or in backless or ill-fitting slippers.

Heel ulceration is a particular problem, and diabetes patients with neuropathy or vascular disease should have heel protectors whilst lying in bed for any significant period of time.

As the reason for admission

If a patient is admitted because of a diabetes foot ulcer, then it is important to determine the degree of infection and vascular compromise. An urgent diabetic foot review is required.

Infection with systemic features will require admission and intravenous antibiotics. Antibiotic regimens vary but must include antistaphylococcal, particularly MRSA, and faecal bacterial cover. Typical prescriptions would be vancomycin and ciprofloxacin, or vancomycin and tazobactam.

Metabolic control, including rehydration and insulin therapy, to ensure good glucose control (blood glucose level below 10 mmol/L at all times) may also be needed.

Vascular insufficiency with rest pain and advancing gangrene may improve with antibiotics and metabolic stabilization. A vascular or orthopaedic surgical opinion, depending on local availability, should be obtained by the diabetes foot care team if there is no improvement. If there is no diabetes foot care team or there is doubt about the viability of the foot (or patient) without operative drainage and surgical removal of the infection, then same-day surgical review is required.

Charcot foot

Symptoms and signs

Charcot neuro-osteoarthropathy is a clinical process characterized by the destruction, dislocation, and fragmentation of bone and joints. Although it can affect any joint, the Charcot process principally affects the foot and ankle of people with diabetes (see Figure 4.18). The Charcot foot is characterized by increased temperature and foot and leg swelling in a diabetic patient with neuropathy. Patients may report some pain in the foot during the active stages, but, in the early phases, deformity is not always present. Although fractures are a key component of the condition, only 50% of patients report an initial injury.

A Charcot joint is frequently misdiagnosed as deep vein thrombosis or cellulitis. However, it should be suspected in any diabetes patient who presents with a hot swollen foot, particularly if they have a history of neuropathy.

Causes

The main predisposing factors for the development of a Charcot joint are sensory neuropathy, autonomic neuropathy with normal or increased blood flow, and local or generalized osteopenia. These are typically found in patients who have had long-standing diabetes and have other diabetic complica-

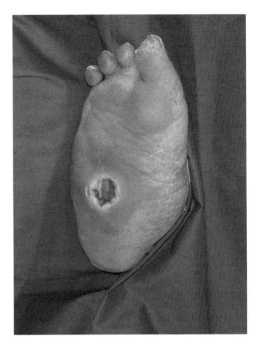

Figure 4.18 Charcot foot: Charcot neuro-osteoarthropathy of the foot with an associated neuropathic ulcer in a diabetes patient.

tions. Diabetes patients post-transplantation are particularly susceptible to developing Charcot joints.

Investigation

The initial investigation of a Charcot joint is plain radiography of the foot. X-rays may be normal at the start of the process, and bone scanning or MRI scanning should be performed to detect increased bone activity or microfractures before deformity sets in.

Treatment

The primary treatment for acute Charcot neuroarthropathy is immobilization, preferably in a below-knee cast, and minimal weight-bearing. Adjunctive treatment with antiresorptive therapies, such as bisphosphonates and calcitonin, are the subject of research.

Once the Charcot process settles, patients with significant deformity are provided with appropriate footwear but still have a high risk of recurrent ulceration, infection, and amputation. Ulceration of a deformed Charcot foot is difficult to treat, and surgical correction of the deformity may be considered by specialist teams experienced in managing this condition.

Further reading

National Institute for Health and Clinical Excellence (2011). NICE clinical guideline 119. Diabetic foot problems: Inpatient management of diabetic foot problems. <https://www.nice.org.uk/guidance/cg119>

Scottish Intercollegiate Guidelines Network (1998). SIGN 26. The care of patients with chronic leg ulcer. SIGN, Edinburgh.

Scottish Intercollegiate Guidelines Network (2001). SIGN 55. Management of diabetes. SIGN, Edinburgh.

Scottish Intercollegiate Guidelines Network (2006). SIGN 89. Diagnosis and management of peripheral vascular disease. SIGN, Edinburgh.

Rheumatic fever

Aetiology

Rheumatic fever is caused by cross-reaction of antibodies formed in response to Lancefield group A beta haemolytic *Streptococcus* infection with the patient's tissues, particularly in the heart. Only about 0.3–3% of patients infected with this group of organisms go on to develop rheumatic fever, suggesting a genetic predisposition. Much research has focused on the culprit antigens, perhaps the M protein in the bacterial cell wall, but no unifying antigen has been found, making the development of a vaccine difficult.

Epidemiology

In the first half of the 20th century, rheumatic fever was common in Europe, and entire hospitals were devoted to its treatment. With improvements in living standards and the widespread use of antibiotics for sore throat, it has become a rare acute condition in developed countries, except where there are severely disadvantaged groups (e.g. aboriginals). In the undeveloped world, it is a major health problem, with an estimated worldwide incidence of rheumatic heart disease of 15.6 million, with 470,000 new cases and 233,000 deaths per year.

Clinical course

Acute rheumatic fever affects mainly 5–15-year-olds and may be a relatively mild or subclinical condition. In more severe forms, it causes fever, florid arthritis, and skin manifestations (erythema marginatum) which can persist for weeks. It occurs 2–3 weeks after the initial streptococcal infection which usually takes the form of a pharyngitis but, in some parts of the world, appears more commonly associated with skin infection or pyoderma (e.g. in aboriginals). The diagnosis is made by the clinical features plus raised inflammatory markers and serological evidence of streptococcal infection (e.g. raised ASO titres). During the acute phase, there may be inflammation of the heart, principally a valvulitis, but also sometimes a pancarditis, and this may lead to chronic rheumatic heart disease.

Recurrent rheumatic fever

Many children suffer recurrent episodes of rheumatic fever, with increasing damage to the heart with each infection. Secondary prevention with antibiotics is very effective in preventing further attacks.

Chronic rheumatic heart disease

Valvulitis initially causes a loss of strength and stretching of leaflets and chordae, causing regurgitation. Later, it results in a chronic scarring condition, causing progressive thickening and contraction of the valve and supporting structures, particularly the chordae tendinae. The valve may ultimately calcify which further reduces its flexibility. Contraction of the valve leads to failure of coaptation and regurgitation, whereas fusion of valve commissures and general rigidity lead to stenosis. The valves tend to be affected in the order mitral > aortic > tricuspid. The pulmonary valve is not affected. The symptoms depend on the particular valve affected and the severity of the haemodynamic disturbance (see 'Valvular disease').

Diagnosis

Acute rheumatic fever

The diagnosis can be difficult but is important because of the potential long-term sequelae. The differential diagnosis includes Still's disease, septic arthritis, connective tissue diseases, Lyme disease, sickle cell anaemia, infective endocarditis, leukaemia, and lymphoma. A system of diagnostic criteria has been developed and modified by Jones and incorporated into the WHO criteria for categorizing the different phases of the disease process. The modified Jones criteria are divided into major and minor.

- Major criteria:
  - Carditis, polyarthritis, subcutaneous nodules, erythema marginatum, chorea.
- Minor criteria:
  - Prolonged PR interval on ECG, raised acute phase reactants (ESR or C-reactive protein), arthralgia, fever.

The diagnosis of acute rheumatic fever is made with supporting evidence of preceding streptococcal infection and either two major criteria or one major and two minor criteria.

The various forms of rheumatic fever have been defined in the 2002–2003 World Health Organization criteria for the diagnosis of rheumatic fever and rheumatic heart disease (based on revised Jones criteria).

Diagnostic categories

Primary episode of rheumatic fever

Two major, or one major and two minor manifestations plus evidence of a preceding group A streptococcal infection.

Recurrent attack of rheumatic fever in patients without established rheumatic heart disease

Two major, or one major and two minor manifestations plus evidence of a preceding group A streptococcal infection.

Recurrent attack of rheumatic fever in patients with established rheumatic heart disease

Two minor manifestations plus evidence of a preceding group A streptococcal infection.

Rheumatic chorea, insidious onset rheumatic carditis

Other major manifestations or evidence of group A streptococcal infection not required.

Chronic valve lesions of rheumatic heart disease (patients presenting for first time with pure mitral stenosis, mixed mitral valve disease, and aortic valve disease)

Do not require any other criteria to be diagnosed as having rheumatic heart disease.

Echocardiography in the diagnosis of rheumatic heart disease

Echocardiography has revolutionized the diagnosis and management of rheumatic heart disease and rheumatic fever, so much so that the echo features are sufficient on their own to make a confident diagnosis of rheumatic heart disease. Because acute rheumatic fever was already rare in developed countries before echo was developed, the experience of the echocardiography in this context is much less, hence the requirement for the corroborating features described previously. In contrast, the lack of echo availability in underdeveloped countries seriously undermines the efforts of those who wish to target patients who have had rheumatic fever for prophylaxis and treatment.

Echo in acute rheumatic fever

Acute valvulitis manifests as leaflet thickening and shortening, with nodules on the body or tip, chordal elongation, mitral annular dilatation, leaflet prolapse, and often evidence of mitral regurgitation. Heart failure is unusual, unless there is severe mitral regurgitation. Lesions may resolve with time.

Echo in chronic rheumatic heart disease

The characteristic appearances of rheumatic mitral valves are thickening, rigidity, shortening, and commissural fusion. The chordal apparatus may become matted and can be a significant cause of mitral obstruction on its own. Doppler flow shows a high velocity sustained through diastole if there is significant mitral stenosis. If the left atrial pressure is increased, the atrium dilates, and the patient may develop atrial fibrillation.

The aortic valve shows similar characteristics, but, being a less complex valve, the lesions are more difficult to distinguish from other causes of aortic valve disease. However, it is rare to find rheumatic aortic stenosis without mitral valve involvement; hence, the diagnosis can be made on the features of the mitral valve.

Tricuspid disease is similar to mitral but causes high right atrial pressures and features of right heart failure (raised venous pressure, oedema, ascites, enlarged liver, and ultimately cirrhosis).

Treatment

Acute rheumatic fever

The acute treatment of rheumatic fever is divided into active elimination of the causative agent, measures to deal with symptoms, and attempts to prevent the development of recurrent attacks.

Antibiotics are the main treatment, and penicillin is the drug of choice. It is most likely to be effective if given early when sore throat is present. In deprived areas, the diagnosis has to be made clinically, based on an exudative tonsillitis and enlarged tender cervical lymph nodes. Early treatment of the sore throat has a 70% success rate in preventing the development of rheumatic fever. Trials of antibiotic therapy in later stages of the condition, when evidence of rheumatic fever is present, have not shown a clear benefit. Amoxicillin and cephalosporins have also been used. In penicillin allergy, erythromycin is often used, although there is evidence of the emergence of resistance to erythromycin.

Efforts to prevent the development of antibiotic resistance discourage the tendency to give antibiotics for non-specific sore throat, and it might be thought that this could give rise to a recrudescence of rheumatic fever in developed countries. However, where rheumatic fever has become a rare disease, it appears that the Lancefield group A beta haemolytic *Streptococcus* has been largely replaced by other organisms that do not cause rheumatic fever.

Measures to deal with symptoms include anti-inflammatory analgesics (especially aspirin), bed rest, corticosteroids, and immunoglobulins. None has been shown to influence the course of the disease, but most evidence is based on poorly designed trials that are 50 years old.

Occasionally, the degree of regurgitation is so severe that valve surgery becomes necessary. As with other regurgitant conditions, conservative surgery is preferable, particularly in younger subjects who may have to be fitted with a small prosthesis, condemning them to a second operation later.

Recurrent rheumatic fever

The prevention of recurrent rheumatic fever represents a major opportunity to save lives in countries where rheumatic fever is common. It relies on identifying patients who have had an episode of acute rheumatic fever and providing them with antibiotic prophylaxis until they are adults. The antibiotic of choice is benzylpenicillin, and it is most effective given as a depot IM injection every 3–4 weeks. Oral therapies appear less effective, perhaps because of compliance.

Prevention of rheumatic fever

Public health measures are effective in reducing the incidence of rheumatic fever. Awareness campaigns, encouraging early presentation and treatment of exudative tonsillitis and more general improvements to living standards, overcrowding, and hygiene, along with education about the condition, are the main measures.

Prophylaxis for recurrent rheumatic fever relies on identifying patients who have had an acute attack. Unfortunately, many acute attacks go undiagnosed, and those patients remain at risk. Screening programmes using echocardiography to detect evidence of rheumatic heart disease are in operation but are difficult to implement where rheumatic fever is most prevalent because of the cost of the equipment and the technical expertise.

Vaccination against the causative group A *Streptococcus* has the potential to make major inroads into the disease but has proved elusive. Human trials of potential streptococcal vaccines (CANVAS; Coalition to advance new vaccines for Group A *Streptococcus*) are currently ongoing.

Further reading

Carapetis JR (2007). Rheumatic heart disease in developing countries. *New England Journal of Medicine*, **357**, 439–41.

Cilliers AM (2006). Rheumatic fever and its management. *BMJ*, **333**, 1153–6.

World Health Organization (2004). Rheumatic fever and rheumatic heart disease: report of a WHO expert consultation, Geneva. WHO, 29 Oct to 1 Nov, 2001. *WHO Technical Report Series*, **923**. WHO, Geneva. <http://www.who.int/cardiovascular_diseases/resources/trs923/en/>.

Pericarditis

Acute pericarditis accounts for up to 5% of emergency department visits with non-ischaemic chest pain. There is a recurrence rate of between 15 and 30% reported in the literature.

Aetiology and causes

Most patients who present with pericarditis in developed countries are given the final diagnosis of idiopathic or viral pericarditis. The controversy of how thoroughly one should investigate the aetiology of an episode of pericarditis remains debated, as this rarely changes the management.

The most common cause of acute pericarditis is viral, accounting for 30–50% in some series. The common viruses are Coxsackie A9, B1-4, Echo 8, mumps, EBV, CMV, varicella, rubella, HIV, and Parvo B19. Bacterial causes account for 5–10% of the aetiology, with pneumococcus, meningococcus, and TB included. Fungi and parasites are rare. Pericarditis is also seen as part of the presentation of systemic autoimmune diseases, such as SLE, rheumatoid arthritis, ankylosing spondylitis, systemic sclerosis, Reiter's syndrome, and familial Mediterranean fever. Type 2 autoimmune reactions, such as in rheumatic fever, account for a small percentage of the cases. Diseases and inflammation in adjacent organs, such as pneumonia and myocardial infarction, can also trigger pericarditis. Neoplastic pericardial disease is usually due to secondary disease, most commonly from lung or breast carcinoma. Metabolic disorders, such as uraemia, Addison's disease, diabetic ketoacidosis, and myxoedema, can be implicated. Finally, traumatic pericarditis, either due to direct or indirect injury or irradiation, is not uncommon.

'Idiopathic', recurrent acute pericarditis may have an immune-mediated origin. The recent finding of serum heart-specific antibodies in patients with recurrent pericarditis seems to support this theory.

HIV manifestations of pericarditis can include infective, non-infective, and neoplastic diseases. Infective pericarditis or myopericarditis can be secondary to direct local HIV infection or other viruses, such as CMV and herpes simplex. Bacterial and fungal co-infections can also occur. Kaposi's sarcoma and other HIV-related malignancies can manifest in the pericardium. Additionally, tuberculous pericarditis is more common in the immunocompromised patients. Treatment with anti-HIV agents can occasionally trigger lipodystrophy, which may result in depots of fat in the pericardial space, triggering pericarditis.

Clinical presentation

Pericarditis often presents suddenly, with mainly substernal or left pericardial pain. This usually radiates to either the left or both trapezius ridges (where the trapezius muscles insert into the clavicles) but can mimic ischaemic pain by radiating to other areas around the shoulders. The quality of pericarditic pain is usually sharp or stabbing, with a dull or oppressive constant background sensation. This is in contrast to the heavy pain of ischaemia. Inspiration usually worsens the pain, and the pain can wax and wane. An important differentiating characteristic of the pain is its worsening on lying flat and improvement on sitting or leaning forwards.

Clinical examination

Auscultation is key in the clinical examination of acute pericarditis. Listening carefully to the left lower sternal edge and the cardiac borders may reveal a pericardial friction rub. If heard, a monophasic, biphasic, or triphasic pericardial rub is virtually diagnostic of pericarditis. It is important to note that pericardial rubs may be transient which means there may be discrepancy in the examination findings amongst consecutive doctors examining the same patient. Perimyocarditis can cause the presence of a new S3 heart sound. In the presence of a pericardial effusion, heart sounds may be quiet. Pulsus paradoxus (a drop of blood pressure on inspiration and increase on expiration) may indicate either constriction or tamponade. Kussmaul's sign (a rise of the JVP with inspiration) occurs in constriction, including effusive-constrictive pericarditis, which can be acute as well as chronic.

Investigations

The European Society of Cardiology guidelines for the diagnosis and treatment of pericardial disease lists electrocardiography, chest X-ray, echocardiography, and basic blood analysis as mandatory investigations. Further targeted investigations should be guided by clinical judgement, according to the suspected aetiology.

Electrocardiography (ECG)

This is usually diagnostic with widespread concave ST elevation at the J point (see Figure 4.19). Classically, the changes occur with initial PR depression when the ECG is observed at an early stage. This is typically followed by the classical anterior and inferior point ST elevation (stage I). As recovery occurs, the ST segments return to baseline, but the PR depression remains (early stage II). Late stage II is when the T waves flatten and invert. Stage III is characterized by generalized T wave inversion, and finally stage IV is when the ECG returns to pre-pericarditis stage. Clearly, these stages have become less common, as treatment with NSAIDs usually aborts the progression in stage I. Early repolarization commonly referred to as 'high take-off' on the ECG can mimic J point ST elevation on the ECG. The absence of symptoms in this group is an important factor in avoiding unnecessary investigations and treatment.

Blood analysis

This should include inflammatory markers (ESR, CRP, LDH, and leucocytes), markers of myocardial insult (troponin I, CK-MB), and renal function markers (creatinine, urea).

Echocardiography

In acute pericarditis, echocardiography is key in identifying the presence of pericardial effusions and assessing the presence of physiological evidence that points towards tamponade or risk of tamponade. Collapse of the right-sided chambers, the duration of diastole and relation with respiration, as well as early diastolic septal bounce and respiratory shift of the ventricular septum can all point towards an effusion that is haemodynamically significant. Furthermore, echocardiography can assess the suitability of a pericardial effusion for needle pericardiocentesis. Doppler examination, including tissue Doppler velocities of the mitral and tricuspid annuli, with colour Doppler of mitral inflow, are added tools that can help in the assessment of the importance of a pericardial effusion. If there is an element of myocardial involvement, echocardiography demonstrates regional wall motion abnormalities.

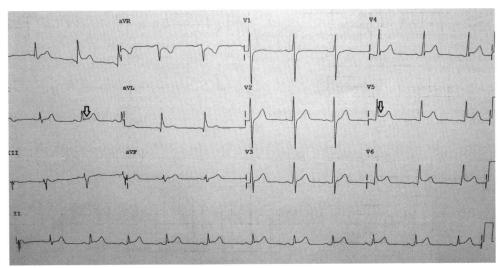

Figure 4.19 Widespread J point ST elevation (black arrows) in a 20-year-old with presumed acute viral pericarditis, following a viral prodrome. aVR displays corresponding ST depression. Note that, in leads III and aVF, there is no ST elevation, which is often the case when the axis in those leads is horizontal or the QRS is of low voltage. V5 and V6 display the typical 'upsloping' ST elevation greater than 25% of the peak of the T wave. There is an element of PR depression in most lateral leads and more clearly in lead II.

Chest X-ray

This may reveal a normal cardiac silhouette in the absence of a significant pericardial effusion. The appearance of a 'water bottle' heart shadow suggests a significant effusion. The chest X-ray in many cases becomes the key investigation, revealing additional serious pulmonary and mediastinal pathology, such as neoplasia, pneumonia, or tuberculosis.

Cardiac CT scanning

This can help in assessing pericardial thickening and calcification, localization and distribution of pericardial effusions, as well as assess the coronary anatomy. Volumetric cine analysis can provide functional evaluation of the myocardium.

Cardiac MRI scanning (CMR)

This has the advantage of being non-invasive and excellent at differentiating the different constituency of fluid within pericardial effusions. The lack of need of an iodinated contrast agent makes it more attractive than CT. CMR can provide valuable information on myocardial involvement, presence of myocardial scar, and regional wall motion abnormalities. In myocarditis, it is a valuable tool in follow-up and establishing progress.

Pericardiocentesis, pericardial biopsy, and pericardioscopy

These are rarely necessary. However, pericardiocentesis is mandatory in cardiac tamponade and if there is a high suspicion of a virulent, tuberculous, or neoplastic aetiology. Large effusions refractory to medical therapy will also require drainage. Pericardial biopsy and pericardioscopy are reserved for use in expert centres where the pericarditis is refractory or diagnostic uncertainty exists in a worsening clinical scenario.

Further blood analysis and serology

These should be targeted carefully. Yield from viral serology rarely alters management and should be selective.

Autoimmune studies may be undertaken in some cases, but routine ANA analysis may be misleading. Frequently, low positive ANA titres are found, leading to a clinical diagnosis in less than 10% of cases.

Treatment

NSAIDs are the mainstay of treatment and should be used at full anti-inflammatory doses until symptoms resolve and inflammatory markers are back to normal levels. Ibuprofen is effective and should be used at 1,600 mg to 3,200 mg daily in divided doses. Aspirin is widely used worldwide and should be given at 2–4 g daily in divided doses.

Colchicine is useful in recurrent cases. Its best use is as an adjunct to other NSAIDs in doses of 0.5 mg bd for several months. There is evidence that it halves recurrence rates when used as an adjunct.

Corticosteroids may induce recurrence and should be limited to cases where NSAIDs are completely contraindicated, such as in severe allergic reactions. When used, low doses with slow tapering are favoured to reduce the added risk of recurrence. Prednisolone 0.2–0.5 mg/kg/day is suggested.

Prognostic factors and sequelae

Most cases of simple acute pericarditis, felt to be 'idiopathic', resolve with little sequelae. Risk factors for complications include high fever >38°C, large pericardial effusion or tamponade, subacute onset, lack of response to NSAIDs after 1 week of therapy, myocarditis, immunosuppression, and trauma.

Myocarditis is usually diagnosed by a troponin or a CK-MB rise. The range of involvement of the myocardium in pericarditis cases varies and should be expressed as myopericarditis when there is some involvement to the myocardium; perimyocarditis when the myocardium is predominantly affected, or, at the extreme, pure myocarditis.

The more severe forms may result in serious sequelae, such as heart failure and arrhythmias. A reduced dose of NSAIDs should be used to minimize the possible harmful effects of NSAIDs to the myocardium. Admission and monitoring are mandatory, and refraining from exercise for 4–6 weeks is recommended.

Further reading

Imazio M, Spodick DH, Brucato A, Trinchero R, Adler Y (2010). Controversial issues in the management of pericardial diseases. *Circulation*, **121**, 916–28.

Maisch B, Seferovic PM, Ristic AD, *et al.*; for the Task Force on the Diagnosis and Management of Pericardial Diseases of the European Society of Cardiology (2004). Guidelines on the diagnosis and management of pericardial diseases. *European Heart Journal*, **25**, 587–610.

Spodick DH (2003). Acute pericarditis: current concepts and practice. *JAMA*, **289**, 1150–3.

Verhaert D (2010). The role of multimodality imaging in the management of pericardial disease. *Circulation: Cardiovascular Imaging*, **3**, 333–43.

Respiratory diseases and respiratory failure

Clinical presentations of respiratory disease

Introduction

Respiratory disease (excluding lung cancer) is the third most common cause of death (after non-respiratory cancer and ischaemic heart disease) in the United Kingdom (UK). It affects one in five people and is responsible for about a million hospital admissions every year. In 2012/13 it cost the NHS an estimated £4.7 billion (APPG Report into Respiratory Deaths 2013). In addition, in 2010, the UK had the worst death rate due to respiratory disease when compared with other OECD countries (UK 104.9, USA 80.2, Finland 31.5, OECD average 66.2 per 100,000 population).

In 2014 there were a total of 501,424 deaths in England and Wales of which 82,455 (15.5%) were due to ischaemic heart disease, 113,068 (22.5%) were due to non-respiratory cancer, and 100,494 (20.0%) were due to respiratory disease (including lung cancer 33,922 (33.7%); COPD/asthma 27,381 (27.2%) and pneumonia/TB 25,463 (25.3%)). Table 5.1 reports respiratory illness as a cause of death in the UK in 2004–5.

Respiratory disease usually presents with one or more of the following symptoms of breathlessness, cough ($\pm$ sputum expectoration), chest pain, haemoptysis, fever ($\pm$ sweats), infection ($\pm$ halitosis), and chest radiograph (CXR) abnormalities.

The pathophysiology, clinical assessment, and general therapeutic approach to management of clinical symptoms is discussed in the following section. Greater detail is presented in sections on the management of individual diseases.

Breathlessness

Dyspnoea derives from the Greek *dys* meaning difficult (or painful) and *pneuma* meaning breath. It describes a variety of sensations experienced when breathing is difficult, uncomfortable, or laboured.

The American Thoracic Society defines dyspnoea as: 'a term used to characterize a subjective experience of breathing discomfort that is comprised of qualitatively distinct sensations that vary in intensity. The experience derives from interactions among multiple physiological, psychological, social, and environmental factors and may induce secondary physiological and behavioural responses'.

Like pain, breathlessness has specific descriptors, referring to different sensations, including chest tightness, the need for deep inspiration, frequency and depth of ventilation. Unfortunately, the 'language of dyspnoea' is not specific, and description by individual patients is dependent on the physiological context, personality, social and ethnic factors. Consequently, a detailed history is invaluable in the assessment of breathlessness.

Dyspnoea is the most frequent symptom experienced by patients with end-stage respiratory disease and twice as common as pain or confusion. In chronic lung disease, breathlessness was reported in 94% during the last year, and 91% during the last week of life, compared to 78% and 69%, respectively, in lung cancer patients.

Mechanisms of dyspnoea

The physiological mechanisms of dyspnoea are poorly understood but may be expressed as:

1. *A central drive or 'urge to breathe'*, that functions to maintain blood gas and acid-base homeostasis by modulating ventilatory activity. This drive incorporates the sensory afferent input from chemoreceptors sensing hypoxaemia and hypercapnia (e.g. medulla, carotid and aortic bodies), mechanoreceptors (e.g. chest wall, lung receptors), and higher cerebral cortex activity (e.g. anxiety, personality).

2. *'Work of breathing'*, associated with ventilation where the 'sense of respiratory effort' is the ratio of the pressure actually generated by the respiratory muscles, compared to the maximum that could be generated.

An attractive unifying theory is that dyspnoea results from a mismatch between central motor activity and incoming afferent information from chemo- and mechanoreceptors. The absence of dyspnoea after prolonged hypoxia or hypercapnia suggests that the medullary respiratory centre may adapt to prolonged stimulation. Alternatively, the drive may be the same whilst there is cortical adaptation to the sensation. Lung and peripheral (e.g. chest wall, facial skin) afferent receptors may also modulate dyspnoea such that blowing cold air on the face may decrease dyspnoea. An individual's emotional state, personality, experience, and cognitive function also influence the perception of dyspnoea, which is worse when it occurs suddenly, unexpectedly, or in inappropriate situations and is often influenced by previous experience of the sensation.

Assessment of dyspnoea
History and examination

Speed of onset frequently suggests the cause of dyspnoea (see Table 5.2). However, duration is often underestimated. Establishing change in exercise tolerance over time is a useful way of assessing onset and progress of breathlessness. Severity and impact on daily activity should be assessed. Exacerbating factors may indicate a cause; thus, orthopnoea suggests left ventricular failure, and trepopnoea, which refers to breathlessness whilst lying on one side, suggests ipsilateral lung disease. Similarly, atopy or occupational exposure may precipitate asthma. Regularly assess associated symptoms, medication, family history, employment, smoking history, illicit drug use, travel, and hobbies. Routine examination should include rate and pattern of breathing, peak expiratory flow rate (PEFR), sputum inspection, signs suggestive of respiratory distress (e.g. accessory muscle

Table 5.1 Deaths from ischaemic heart disease, non-respiratory cancer, and respiratory disease in the UK in 2004–2005

All UK deaths (2004)	587,808
Ischaemic heart disease	106,081
Non-respiratory cancer	122,512
All deaths due to respiratory disease	117,456 (100%)
Pneumonia and TB	35,814 (30.5%)
Lung cancer	34,721 (29.6%)
Progressive (non-malignant)	35,979 (30.6%)
• COPD + asthma	28,859 (24.6%)
• Pulmonary circulatory disease	3926 (3.3%)
• Pneumoconiosis + fibrosis	3,024 (2.6%)
• Cystic fibrosis	139 (0.1%)
• Sarcoidosis	31 (0.03%)
Others (congenital, foreign body)	10,527 (9.3%)

Data from: Office for National Statistics (2005). Mortality statistics by cause. Series DH2 no. 31. The Stationery Office, London, General Register Office (2005) Annual Report 2004. General Register Office for Scotland, General Register Office (2005) Annual Report 2004. Northern Ireland Statistics and Research Agency.

Table 5.2 Causes of dyspnoea, grouped by speed of onset

Rate of onset	Typical causes
Instantaneous	• Pneumothorax • Pulmonary embolism • Inhaled foreign body • Laryngeal spasm
Acute (minutes–hours)	• Airways obstruction (asthma, COPD) • Pneumonia, pulmonary oedema, alveolar haemorrhage • Pulmonary embolus (i.e. large) • Heart disease (tamponade, arrhythmia) • Hyperventilation
Subacute (days)	• As above, with pleural effusion, lobar collapse, acute interstitial pneumonia • Pulmonary embolus (i.e. recurrent small)
Chronic (months–years)	• Some of the above and airways obstruction, diffuse parenchymal disease, chronic thromboembolic disease, primary pulmonary hypertension, hypoventilation (obesity, chest wall deformity), anaemia

use), and paradoxical abdominal movement (e.g. due to diaphragmatic paralysis) and resting/exercise oximetry.

Diagnostic tests
Routine outpatient investigations include full blood count, ESR, C-reactive protein, D-dimers, sputum evaluation, spirometry, and chest radiography (CXR). Biochemical and liver function profiles are often performed but rarely contribute to dyspnoea assessment. Further tests depend on clinical suspicion.
- **Arterial blood gases** (± A-a gradient measurement).
- **Pulmonary function tests** determine lung volumes, gas transfer (DLCO, KCO), response to bronchial challenge, and allergy testing.
- **Imaging techniques** include high-resolution CT (HRCT) scans, angiography, diaphragmatic fluoroscopy, and positron emission tomography (PET). Isotope ventilation-perfusion (V/Q) scans are now less commonly used.
- **Bronchoscopy** with bronchial washings and biopsy.
- **Cardiac evaluation** may require ECG, echocardiography, cardiac angiography, and myocardial perfusion scanning.
- **Other techniques** include sleep studies, oesophageal pH monitoring, and otolaryngoscopy.

Assessment of dyspnoea severity
Aids decision-making and indicates the success of a particular therapy. In general, the simpler the measurement technique, the more likely it is to be used.
- **Simple intensity scales:** are reproducible and rely on numerical scales. The visual analogue scale (VAS) requires the patient to mark a point on a 10 cm line, with no breathlessness and maximum breathlessness at the two ends, so that the length reflects the intensity of the dyspnoea. The Borg scale is a 12-point category scale with extremes of no breathlessness and maximal breathless-

ness, with verbal descriptors such as slight and severe to assist the subject to rate the symptom. Many others are available.
- **Quality of life (QOL) measures:** assess physical, emotional, and social functioning in response to symptoms and disease. Although mainly used in research, these questionnaires assess the impact of respiratory disease on QOL. The chronic respiratory disease questionnaire evaluates dyspnoea, fatigue, and emotional function in a 20-item questionnaire; the St Georges respiratory questionnaire assesses symptoms, activity, and impact of disease on daily life in a 76-item questionnaire, and the pulmonary functional status scale measures mental, physical, and social functioning in COPD patients to assess the effect of respiratory distress on functional activity.
- **Physiological techniques** include:
  - **Simple tests**, which, in practice, should be undertaken in all cases but are also useful in severe lung disease when more complex tests are not possible. These include spirometry and resting oxygen saturation (SaO$_2$). Unfortunately, FEV$_1$ is a poor predictor of dyspnoea, and improvements in breathlessness after bronchodilator therapy do not correlate with FEV$_1$ changes. Nevertheless, spirometry is a useful aid in the assessment of reversible airways disease.
  - **Intermediate tests** aid detection of specific diagnoses and are useful in research settings. They include simple 'corridor' exercise tests (e.g. endurance, six minute or shuttle walking) which can be used to assess dyspnoea and response to therapy, even in severe disease.
  - **Complex tests** are used occasionally when the diagnosis is unclear (i.e. whether breathlessness is due to cardiac or pulmonary disease). It includes formal cardiopulmonary exercise testing, with assessment of both cardiac and respiratory function.
- **Serial chest radiography** is of limited value in severity assessment but may detect reversible problems (e.g. pneumonia).

Treatment of dyspnoea
Most acute illnesses and end-stage respiratory disease are associated with breathlessness. Treatment must address the mechanisms causing dyspnoea and the specific disease process (see individual diseases).
Treatment strategies aim to:
- **Reduce work of breathing.** Optimize bronchodilation (e.g. beta-2 agonists, theophyllines), breathing techniques (e.g. purse-lip breathing), posture (e.g. sit upright or lean forwards), and nutrition. Rest respiratory muscles and counterbalance lung hyperinflation and auto-PEEP (e.g. with non-invasive ventilation; see COPD).
- **Decrease respiratory drive** using pharmacological treatments (e.g. opiates, anxiolytics, oxygen), by encouraging afferent input to the medulla (e.g. facial fans), psychotherapy, and improving CO$_2$ elimination with breathing techniques.
- **Increase muscle strength** (e.g. improve movement efficiency; encourage dyspnoea desensitization) with exercise training and pulmonary rehabilitation. Similarly, the benefits of oral steroid therapy need to be balanced against the disadvantage of muscle wasting.

In end-stage disease, dyspnoea often persists, despite optimal treatment of the underlying disease, and therapy must focus on symptom relief. Determining the point at which active treatment of the underlying disease should give way to symptomatic relief can be difficult. In this context, the risks of respiratory depression with opiates and benzodiazepines have sometimes been overstated.

Specific situations

The breathless pregnant patient

Normal physiological changes cause breathlessness in 75% of pregnant women. Tidal volume and minute ventilation increase due to stimulation of respiratory drive by raised progesterone levels. The associated fall in maternal $PaCO_2$ encourages fetal CO_2 clearance, but, conversely, maternal hypercapnia rapidly causes fetal acidosis. Surprisingly, respiratory rate is not increased in pregnancy, and tachypnoea is often a useful sign that breathlessness is due to an underlying pathological cause.

The diaphragms are raised by the enlarging uterus, reducing functional residual capacity, but vital capacity, peak flow, FEV_1, and oxygen consumption are largely unaffected. PaO_2 may be 2 kPa lower when supine in the third trimester, but A-a gradient is unaffected, except near term. Upper airway oedema, especially in pre-eclampsia, predisposes to obstructive sleep apnoea.

Table 5.3 lists pathological causes of breathlessness in pregnancy. Venous stasis and coagulopathy increase the risk of thromboembolism fourfold, and pulmonary embolism is one of the more common causes of maternal death. Amniotic fluid embolism with subsequent ARDS is a rare cause. Chronic respiratory diseases, of which asthma is the commonest, also cause breathlessness.

Patients with severe interstitial lung disease (VC <1 L) or significant pulmonary hypertension have a poor prognosis and should avoid pregnancy. In cystic fibrosis, successful pregnancies with an FEV_1 of 30–50% predicted are common, but caution is required if the FEV_1 is <30% predicted.

White cell count (WCC), ESR, and D-dimers are raised during pregnancy. CXR should be performed, when necessary, as abdominal shielding limits radiation dose to low levels. V/Q scans are considered safe and, after Doppler ultrasound scans, are often the investigation of choice for

PE in pregnancy. However, this must be balanced against the lack of precision of the V/Q scan and potential delays when compared to the small theoretical risk of the higher radiation dose with CT pulmonary angiogram (CTPA) (see Chapter 21). However, pregnancy-induced hormonal changes do increase the future CTPA-induced risk of breast cancer.

Cardiac output is elevated in pregnancy due to increased heart rate and stroke volume and reduced peripheral resistance. Consequently, previously stable cardiac diseases like mitral stenosis may also deteriorate during pregnancy, causing breathlessness and heart failure (see Chapters 4, 21).

The breathless post-operative patient

Post-operative breathlessness is common, particularly after thoracic or upper abdominal surgery due to:
- Infection and/or atelectasis.
- Acute lung injury or ARDS (non-cardiogenic pulmonary oedema).
- Heart failure or fluid overload.
- Exacerbation of pre-existing lung disease (e.g. COPD).
- Pulmonary emboli (PE).

Important investigations include haemoglobin, renal and liver function tests, arterial blood gases, ECG to exclude myocardial ischaemia, CXR, and occasionally CTPA to exclude PE. Unhelpful investigations include D-dimers, CRP, and WCC which are usually raised post-operatively. Early breathlessness may be related to anaesthetic complications (e.g. aspiration, laryngeal spasm), atelectasis, hypovolaemia, fluid overload, and fat or air embolism. Late causes include PE, ARDS, infection, and myocardial ischaemia.

Distinguishing respiratory from cardiac dyspnoea

In practice, this can be difficult, as heart and lung disease often coexist. B-type natriuretic peptide (BNP) increases with myocardial wall stress and is sensitive and specific for heart failure. A BNP level <50 ng/L is unlikely to be associated with heart failure. A cardiac cause is also unlikely if the ECG is completely normal. Echocardiography may demonstrate heart wall hypokinesia, ventricular enlargement, or a reduced ejection fraction in cardiac disease, although CO and BP may be normal. In the outpatient setting, cardiac catheterization is rarely required to establish the diagnosis.

Causes of dyspnoea with a normal CXR
- Pulmonary: obstructive airways disease (e.g. asthma), early parenchymal disease (e.g. sarcoidosis).
- Infectious: viral, early pneumocystis pneumonia.
- Pulmonary vascular disease: pulmonary embolism, pulmonary hypertension.
- Systemic causes: anaemia, metabolic acidosis (e.g. renal failure), thyrotoxicosis.
- Cardiac causes: arrhythmias, valve disease, intracardiac shunts.
- Other causes: neuromuscular disease, psychological (e.g. hyperventilation syndrome).

Causes of episodic dyspnoea

Episodic dyspnoea typically occurs with asthma, ischaemic heart disease, pulmonary embolism, pulmonary oedema, hypersensitivity pneumonitis, vasculitis, and hyperventilation syndrome.

Cough

Cough is a distressing symptom in many diseases (see Table 5.4). It is uncommon in health (although it frequently

---

Table 5.3 Causes of breathlessness in pregnancy

Pulmonary
Pre-existing lung disease (e.g. asthma)
Pneumonia (bacterial, viral, fungal)
Aspiration pneumonia
Pneumothorax
Ovarian hyperstimulation syndrome

Vascular
Amniotic fluid embolism
Pulmonary embolism
Pulmonary hypertension
Air embolism

Pulmonary oedema
Pre-existing heart disease (e.g mitral stenosis)
Peripartum cardiomyopathy
ARDS (e.g. pre-eclampsia, sepsis)
Inhibition of labour with beta-agonists

Other
Anaemia

Table 5.4 Causes of cough

Respiratory tract
- Upper airways
  - Sinusitis*, post-nasal drip*, URTI*
- Lower airways
  - LRTI (viral/bacterial)*, TB, pertussis
  - COPD*, chronic bronchitis*
  - Asthma*, cough variant asthma*
  - Eosinophilic bronchitis
  - Foreign body, airways irritants (e.g. smoke)
  - Bronchiectasis, ILD, lung cancer, OSA
  - Airway compression (e.g. lymph nodes)
  - Mediastinal masses

Gastro-intestinal tract
- GORD*
- Oesophageal dysmotility or stricture with recurrent aspiration
- Oesophago-bronchial fistula

Drugs
- ACE inhibitors*
- Steroid inhalers*

Other
- Left ventricular failure
- Left atrial enlargement (e.g. mitral stenosis)
- CNS disease with aspiration (e.g. MS, MND)
- Psychogenic, idiopathic

* = common.
U/LRTI, upper/lower respiratory tract infection; TB, tuberculosis; OSA, obstructive sleep apnoea; COPD, chronic obstructive pulmonary disease; ILD, interstitial lung disease; GORD, gastro-oesophageal reflux disease; ACE, angiotensin-converting enzyme; CNS, central nervous system; MS, mitral stenosis; MND, motor neurone disease.

occurs and is not complained about), as mucociliary transport ensures airways clearance. In respiratory disease, this clearance mechanism may be reduced by 50%, and cough acts as a reserve system, increasing clearance by up to 20% (normally ~2.5%). Excessive cough prevents sleep, interrupts communication, and causes social embarrassment. The associated high pressures and rapid airflow may have haemodynamic effects (e.g. syncope, arrhythmias) and cause ruptured vessels (e.g. eyes), urinary incontinence, hernia, headache, pneumothorax, and rib fractures.

Cough classification
1. Acute cough is defined as an episode lasting <3–8 weeks. Most is due to viral upper respiratory tract infections (URTI). Cough occurs in 40–50% of URTI, equating to 48 million cases of acute cough each year, of whom half self-medicate. Of the 12 million who consult doctors, twice as many are women, reflecting the increased cough reflex sensitivity in females. In the absence of significant comorbidity, acute cough is usually benign and self-limiting, but associated absenteeism has a major economic impact. Further investigation is required in patients with haemoptysis, severe systemic illness, or if foreign body inhalation is suspected.
2. Chronic cough is defined as an episode lasting >8 weeks. 'Post-viral coughs' may linger for 8–24 weeks, but, in many cases, the cause of prolonged cough is never established. Sputum production usually indicates primary lung pathology.

The term chronic cough usually refers to a patient with a persistent cough and a normal CXR. In practice, over 90% of these cases are due to: (a) cough variant asthma or eosinophilic bronchitis; (b) gastrooesophageal reflux disease (GORD); and (c) post-nasal drip due to allergic rhinitis or chronic sinusitis. Epidemiologically, chronic cough affects 10–20% of adults. It often impairs QOL and is commoner in women, smokers, asthmatics, and obesity. The cause can be difficult to establish, but specialist clinics, using management protocols, report diagnosis and effective treatment in over 70% of patients (see section on cough management algorithms).

Mechanism of cough
Involuntary cough is initiated by rapidly adapting 'irritant' receptors (RARs) that transmit through fast-velocity myelinated vagal fibres. The larynx, main carina, and tracheobronchial branching points are the most sensitive sites for cough induction. Stimulation of smaller airways and alveoli does not cause cough. RARs respond to chemical (e.g. smoke), inflammatory, and mechanical (e.g. foreign body) stimuli and also cause bronchoconstriction and mucous hypersecretion. Serotonin, opioids, GABA and dopamine receptors in the medulla integrate afferent input and motor output controlling cough, which has therapeutic implications. Conscious cerebral cortex input can bypass these integrative centres to suppress or generate voluntary cough.

Cough assessment
The cause, effectiveness, and impact on QOL should be assessed.
- History can be unhelpful because, although mainly due to asthma, GORD, or post-nasal drip, characteristic symptoms are not always present. The history should include onset, severity, timing, and triggers for the cough. For example, early morning or nocturnal cough or cough after exposure to dust, pollen, or cold suggests asthma, whereas cough after meals or with bending suggests GORD. Associated symptoms (e.g. wheeze, dyspnoea), previous medical history (e.g. childhood whooping cough may cause bronchiectasis), drug therapy (e.g. ACE inhibitors), atopy (e.g. eczema, asthma), sinusitis, smoking history, pets, and occupation may suggest possible causes.
- Examination should focus on sites associated with cough (e.g. nasal passages, larynx, chest, heart). Impact on health status is assessed with VAS and cough-specific QOL questionnaires.
- Routine investigation includes serial PEFR measurements, spirometry, and CXR.

Consider a trial of treatment if a potential cause is identified (e.g. asthma, GORD, or sinusitis), and record the response. If the aetiology is not clear or initial treatment is ineffective, further investigation may be required:
- **Methacholine bronchial provocation tests** detect cough variant asthma. The dose of nebulized methacholine that reduces FEV_1 by 20% (PC_{20}) is determined. A PC_{20} <8 mg/mL suggests asthma (normal PC_{20} >16 mg/mL).
- **Induced sputum** may reveal increased eosinophil counts in asthma and eosinophilic bronchitis.
- **Oesophageal pH and manometry** confirms GORD.
- **ENT examination** (e.g. laryngoscopy, sinus radiology) may detect upper airways pathology.
- **Bronchoscopy** has a low diagnostic yield (1–6%) but is performed if foreign body aspiration is suspected.

- **HRCT scans** provide additional diagnostic information (e.g. bronchiectasis, interstitial lung disease) in 24–48% of patients with a normal CXR and persistent cough (i.e. after initial therapeutic trials), who subsequently undergo further investigation.
- **Cardiac investigations** (e.g. ECG, echocardiography) exclude potential cardiac causes of cough.

Cough treatment

1. **Treat the cause** (e.g. asthma, heart failure, GORD). Smoking cessation abolishes cough in 50% of COPD patients, and nasal decongestants are effective for post-nasal drip.
2. **'Clearance' (protussive) therapy** improves secretion clearance. Techniques include steam inhalations, nebulized saline to loosen tenacious secretions, physiotherapy with forced exhalation, postural drainage, and assisted cough techniques. Pharmacological therapies include aerosolized hypertonic saline to induce cough, beta-agonists (e.g. salbutamol), and cysteine derivatives (e.g. acetylcysteine) to liquefy viscid sputum. Bronchorrhoea (i.e. 0.5–2L sputum/day) may respond to steroids, erythromycin, or inhaled indometacin (INN).
3. **Antitussive therapy** suppresses cough when the cause is not reversible or does not respond to treatment. It is usually used for dry, rather than productive, coughs. There are a number of options:
   - **Opioids** act on the central cough centre. Morphine is most effective but is only used in end-stage disease. Dihydrocodeine (30 mg 4–6-hourly) is useful and causes less constipation and neuropsychological side effects than codeine. Dextromethorphan is often used in 'over-the-counter' medications (see section on cough management).
   - **Local anaesthetics** (e.g. benzocaine lozenges) alleviate upper airway irritation but risk aspiration.
   - **Other antitussive agents** include theophyllines and beta-2-agonists to stimulate mucociliary clearance, and oral or inhaled steroids which reduce inflammatory cough in obstructive or infiltrative (e.g. sarcoidosis) pulmonary disorders. Although largely redundant, sodium cromoglicate (INN) may occasionally be used to reduce atopic cough.
   - **Decongestant** (e.g. pseudoephedrine) and expectorant (e.g. guaifenesin) preparations are available over the counter and have varying, and unproven, efficacy.
   - **Antimuscarinic agents** like hyoscine hydrobromide (0.2–0.4 mg SC) or glycopyrronium bromide (0.2–0.4 mg IM) control the distressing 'chest rattle' associated with loose secretions in terminal lung disease. Antimuscarinic bronchodilators (e.g. ipratropium bromide) reduce secretions without increasing viscosity or impairing mucociliary clearance.

Cough management

1. **Acute cough** may not require prescribed treatment and is often best managed with over-the-counter medications like:
   - **Dextromethorphan:** a pharmacologically effective, non-sedating, long-acting antitussive agent with a dose-dependent effect and maximum efficacy at about 60 mg. Most proprietary formulations deliver subtherapeutic doses, but caution is required with higher doses, as many formulations contain other drugs (e.g. pseudoephedrine, paracetamol).
   - **Menthol:** causes brief cough suppression and is delivered by inhalation or capsules.
   - **Sedative antihistamines:** suppress cough but cause drowsiness.
   - **Codeine and pholcodine:** are opiate antitussives with significant side effects (e.g. constipation, confusion). They are no more effective than dextromethorphan and must be used with caution, particularly in the elderly.

2. **Chronic cough** due to pulmonary disease (e.g. bronchiectasis) is a debilitating symptom, but suppression is contraindicated, especially when sputum clearance is important. If non-productive and associated with a normal CXR, chronic cough is usually 'post-viral' or due to asthma, GORD, or post-nasal drip. The optimal and most cost-effective approach to the management of these patients involves a protocol combining selective diagnostic testing and empirical treatment trials determined by the clinical scenario (see Figure 5.1). Specific chronic cough syndromes include:
   - **Cough variant asthma and eosinophilic bronchitis** represent one end of the asthma spectrum, with isolated cough but minimal airways inflammation or bronchoconstriction. Cough is typically nocturnal, worse in the mornings, after exercise, and in cold air. In cough variant asthma, spirometry may be normal, but bronchial challenge tests are usually positive. Eosinophilic bronchitis is associated with steroid-sensitive cough, airway eosinophilia, but no airway hyperresponsiveness. Negative bronchial challenge tests do not exclude steroid-sensitive cough, and a trial of oral steroids (e.g. prednisolone 30 mg/day for 2 weeks) is recommended in all chronic cough patients. If there is no response, the cough is unlikely to be due to asthma or its cough variants. If the cough responds to steroids, treatment continues with high-dose inhaled steroids, leukotriene receptor antagonists, and antihistamines, but there is no evidence for the use of long-acting beta-2-agonists.
   - **GORD** is reported to account for 5–40% of chronic cough in the British Thoracic Society guidelines and up to 60% in the American College of Chest Physician (ACCP) guidelines. GORD-induced cough may be due to microaspiration of gastric contents or a vagally mediated oesophageal reflex stimulated by lower oesophageal sphincter (LOS) acid reflux or large volume non-acid reflux. Oesophageal dysmotility may contribute to these mechanisms.
   GORD is usually long-standing, typically worse after meals or with bending/sitting, and is associated with daytime cough, intermittent dysphonia, and sore throat. Dyspepsia and reflux are common but not always present. Treatment with proton pump inhibitors (e.g. omeprazole 20 mg twice daily) for 8–12 weeks reduces cough in 40–60% of cases. Prokinetic agents (e.g. metoclopramide) are also helpful. Medications that worsen reflux (e.g. theophyllines) should be stopped. Baclofen increases LOS tone and reduces GORD-related cough resistant to other treatments. Antireflux surgery (i.e. fundoplication) can be effective in carefully selected cases.
   - **Upper airways disease** causes cough associated with nasal congestion, sinusitis, 'recurrent throat clearing', and post-nasal drip syndrome. Treatment is with first-generation antihistamines which have helpful anticholinergic properties, nasal ipratropium bromide, and high-dose nasal steroids for 3 months with an initial 2-week course

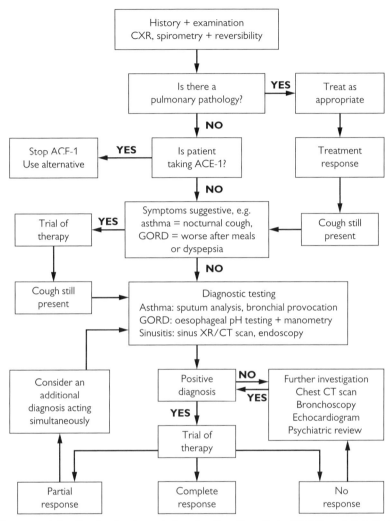

Figure 5.1 Management algorithm for chronic cough. Reproduced from *Thorax*, Morice AH, McGarvey L, Pavord I on behalf of the BTS guideline group, 'British Thoracic Society Guidelines: Recommendations for the management of cough in adults', 61, Supple 1, p. i1–i24, copyright 2006, with permission from BMJ Publishing Group Ltd.

of antibiotic to cover *H. influenzae* (e.g. doxycycline) if sinusitis is suspected.

- **ACE inhibitor cough** occurs in ~10% of people on ACE inhibitors. It occurs within hours or up to a year after starting treatment. Cough is due to bradykinin accumulation in the lung due to failure of normal breakdown by ACE in these patients. When the drug is stopped, the median time to cough resolution is 3–4 weeks but, occasionally, can be much longer. Most patients with ACE inhibitor-induced cough tolerate angiotensin II receptor blockers.
- **Idiopathic or undiagnosed cough.** About 20% of patients with chronic cough are undiagnosed after extensive investigation. In psychogenic cough, cognitive behaviour therapy has proven benefit.

Cough management algorithms

Diagnosis and treatment outcomes in hospital clinics without chronic cough management algorithms are poor. In contrast, specialist clinics report treatment success in >70% of cases. Referral to a specialist clinic should be considered when there has been a failure of empirical treatment for asthma, GORD, and rhinosinusitis or if serious cough complications occur (e.g. syncope, rib fractures).

Chest pain

Chest pain is common in lung disease and exacerbates breathlessness, inhibits secretion clearance, and impairs QOL. Lung parenchyma and the visceral pleura are insensitive to pain which arises from the chest wall, parietal pleura, diaphragm, mediastinum, and major airways. Processes affecting the upper parietal pleura produce pain localized to the chest. The lower parietal pleura and outer diaphragm are innervated by the lower intercostal nerves, and pain is referred to the abdomen. The central diaphragm is innervated by the phrenic nerve (C3–5), and pain is referred to the ipsilateral shoulder. Despite the proximity of many organs and the visceral nature of the discomfort, it is often possible to identify the cause of chest pain by 'pattern recognition'. Nevertheless, investigations, including blood tests, ECG, CXR, CT scans, and, very occasionally, V/Q scans, aid diagnosis. Management depends on identifying and treating the cause.

Musculoskeletal disorders
These are often, but not exclusively, associated with localized tenderness which may also occur in malignant disease and following pulmonary infarction.

- **Rib fractures** due to cough, tumour, or trauma limit chest wall movement and risk hypoventilation and atelectasis. Adequate analgesia can usually be achieved with combinations of oral or intravenous non-opiate and opiate analgesia. Local intercostal nerve blocks using subcostal bupivacaine 0.25% (± adrenaline 1:200,000) efficiently alleviate chest wall discomfort, and, when feasible, thoracic epidural is most effective, but, in practice, these techniques are seldom required. External chest wall stabilization (e.g. sandbagging, fixation) rarely relieves pain and impedes chest wall movement, causing atelectasis.
- **Costochondritis** (Tietze's syndrome) is often due to viral infection, fibrositis, or connective tissue disease (e.g. SLE, rheumatoid arthritis) and causes localized anterior chest wall tenderness. Subcostal pain occurs with muscle strain/fatigue, following prolonged difficult breathing.
- **Spinal, disc, and nerve root pain.** Cervical or thoracic osteoarthritis and associated intercostal radiculitis cause severe discomfort and chest wall hyperalgesia or anaesthesia exacerbated by movement. Neuropathic pains may be due to infections (e.g. shingles/herpes zoster, often associated with immune suppression) or malignant brachial plexus invasion (e.g. Pancoast apical lung tumours).

Pleuropulmonary disorders
Pleurisy describes a characteristic sharp, 'knife-like' pain, associated with deep breathing and due to inflammation of the parietal pleura. There is usually no local tenderness. Sudden onset suggests a pneumothorax, pulmonary embolism, or rib fracture. Development over days often heralds pneumonia or empyema, particularly if associated with fever and rigors. Slow-onset 'boring' chest pain, with weight loss and lethargy, suggests benign pleural disease, mesothelioma, malignancy, or tuberculosis.

The pain of tracheobronchitis is characteristically substernal. It is a sharp, raw, or burning pain, worse with coughing. Pulmonary hypertension (PHT) is often associated with crushing central chest pain which radiates into the neck and arms and is difficult to differentiate from myocardial ischaemia. It has been reported in acute (e.g. massive pulmonary embolus) and chronic (e.g. primary PHT, mitral stenosis) PHT.

Visceral chest pain
Cardiovascular (e.g. ischaemic heart disease, pericarditis), gastrointestinal (e.g oesophagitis, cholecystitis), and psychological disorders (e.g. anxiety, hyperventilation syndrome) present with characteristic chest discomfort and clinical features and are discussed in subsequent chapters. Missed diagnosis and delayed treatment may result in unnecessary discomfort.

Stridor
Obstruction of the larynx or major airways results in a hoarse inspiratory wheeze termed stridor. Airways infection (e.g. epiglottitis, diphtheria), tumours, anaphylactic attacks, aspirated particulate matter, and sputum plugs can obstruct the upper airways.

Immediate management requires an assessment of the cause and removal of any obstructing foreign bodies, including aspirated objects (e.g. food), viscid sputum, blood clots, or dislodged tumour particles that have been coughed into, and obstruct, the upper airways. Physiotherapy and posture may alleviate obstruction, but, occasionally, laryngoscopy, bronchoscopy, and surgery are required to determine the cause and for management.

Inhalation of helium and oxygen (ratio 4:1) reduces airflow resistance and produces temporary improvement. Corticosteroids (dexamethasone 16 mg daily) rapidly reduce obstruction due to inflammatory oedema. Endoscopically placed stents or a tracheostomy to bypass bronchial or laryngeal obstructions are required in some cases.

Recurrent aspiration
Recurrent aspiration may be a significant factor in the development of respiratory failure. Bulbar palsy (e.g. motor neurone disease, multiple sclerosis) and cerebrovascular disease cause recurrent aspiration due to impairment of the complex swallowing reflexes. Repeated micro-aspiration leads to infection, bronchiectasis, and lung scarring. The right main bronchus is the most direct path for aspirated material, and the right lower lobe is most commonly involved. Posture affects susceptibility to aspiration, and nursing in the semi-recumbent position reduces the risk.

Failure to recognize recurrent aspiration is common, but coughing after drinking or eating and crepitations in the right lower lobe are characteristic clues. Dyes (e.g. methylthioninium chloride = methylene blue) added to drinks may be detected in sputum and tracheal aspirates. Recurrent pneumonia and CXR changes of atelectasis or inflammation in the right lower lobe should raise suspicion of repeated micro-aspiration. A barium swallow confirms the diagnosis when contrast enters the bronchial tree. However, an oesophageal-tracheal fistula that requires stenting or surgical intervention is detected occasionally.

If aspiration is suspected, swallowing must be assessed by a speech therapist and strategies for prevention tested, including posture manipulation and thickening of food. If these fail, fine-bore nasogastric feeding or gastric PEG may have to be considered. Pneumonia and atelectasis associated with aspiration are treated with physiotherapy and broad-spectrum antibiotics effective against nasopharyngeal organisms (e.g. including anaerobes).

Haemoptysis
Minor haemoptysis is a common occurrence in many lung diseases (see Table 5.5) but, occasionally, can be a dramatic development. The majority of episodes are mild or moderate and occur in the outpatient setting. Massive haemoptysis, defined as 500–1,000 mL blood/day, accounts for <20% of episodes and is a medical emergency. As such, the acute or general physician must be prepared to initiate resuscitation and appropriate management whilst awaiting specialist aid. Most cases of haemoptysis, particularly in Third World countries, are due to treatable causes, including infection (~80%, e.g. tuberculosis) or bronchiectasis, with less than 20% of cases due to malignancy or irreversible causes.

Table 5.5 Causes of haemoptysis

Common causes	Rare causes
• Bronchial tumours	• Mycetoma
• Benign (e.g. carcinoid)	• Abscess
• Malignant	• Arteriovenous
• Bronchiectasis (mild–	malformations
massive)	• Hereditary haemorrhagic
• Tuberculosis	telangiectasia
• Active	• Severe pulmonary
• Inactive (e.g. mycetoma)	hypertension
• Pneumonia (e.g.	• Mitral stenosis
Pneumococcus, Klebsiella)	• Congenital heart disease
• Vasculitis (e.g. SLE,	• Fungal/parasitic infection
Wegener's)	• *Aspergillus* infection
• Thromboembolic disease	• Aortic aneurysm
• Warfarin and coagulopathy	• Iatrogenic (e.g. lung biopsy)
	• Endometriosis

Small volume haemoptysis

Small volume haemoptysis is usually encountered and safely managed in the outpatient setting. However, beware the sentinel bleed heralding massive haemoptysis. Most cases are due to minor upper or lower respiratory tract infections, but, in a third of cases, the cause is not identified. These patients have a good prognosis, and, in most, the haemoptysis resolves spontaneously without treatment.

Assessment

This requires a good history and examination. The amount, type (e.g. fresh, old, streaks, clots), and time course of bleeding are essential. Exclude nasopharyngeal bleeding and haematemesis, and check for systemic features (e.g. malignancy). The characteristic picture of typical causes (e.g. PE, bronchiectasis) often directs subsequent investigation. Examination of expectorated blood may provide clues. For example, food particles suggest haematemesis, whereas purulent material may indicate bronchiectasis or a lung abscess.

Investigation

In small volume haemoptysis, this includes:
• Sputum microbiology (e.g. AFB, fungi) and cytology.
• Urine testing (e.g. haematuria in vasculitis).
• CXR for mass, abscess, arteriovenous malformation (AVM), and bronchiectasis. Diffuse alveolar shadowing, due to widespread distribution of blood, may obscure the site and cause of bleeding.
• CT scans may be diagnostic (e.g. AVM, bronchiectasis) and also improve diagnostic rates of subsequent bronchoscopy. CTPA is required to exclude PE.
• Bronchoscopy visualizes the airway, localizes the bleeding site and may aid control of bleeding.
  Occasional investigations include:
• Blood tests, including antibodies (e.g. ANA, ANCA, anti-GBM).
• Bronchial angiogram (± bronchial artery embolization) identifies and treats active bleeding sites.
• Echocardiography may identify pulmonary hypertension and cardiac causes of haemoptysis.
• ENT assessment detects upper airways causes.

Massive haemoptysis

Massive, life-threatening haemoptysis is a medical emergency but extremely rare. It usually occurs in the emergency department or in a ward patient with established lung disease (e.g. lung cancer). It can be very distressing for the patient, nursing staff, and relatives. Consequently, it is essential that the attending physician is calm and well trained in the initial management of such an emergency.

Death results from asphyxia due to alveolar flooding, rather than circulatory collapse, and mortality is directly related to the rate and volume of blood loss and the underlying pathology. Haemoptysis of >600 mL within <4 hours is associated with 71% mortality, compared to 45% in patients expectorating the same quantity over 4–16 hours and 5% over 16–48 hours.

In end-stage respiratory disease (e.g. lung cancer), active management of the haemoptysis is not always appropriate. Patients at risk of dying from haemoptysis (i.e. previous episodes) require careful preparation prior to further bleeds (e.g. immediate access to drugs) to ensure optimal management and to prevent distress. Relatives must be informed of the possibility and the planned management discussed. Simple measures include the use of green linen to mask blood, nursing the patient with the affected chest side down, and a controlled, calm environment. Palliative treatment aims to reduce distress using opioid and anxiolytic therapy.

If resuscitation is appropriate, the key aspects of management are:
• Maintain a patent airway, and provide supplemental oxygen. Endotracheal intubation and mechanical ventilation may be required.
• Position the patient slightly head down in the lateral decubitus position, with the 'presumed' bleeding side down to promote drainage and avoid alveolar 'soiling' with reduced gas exchange in the unaffected lung.
• Determine the cause, site, and severity of the bleeding (see next section).
• Correct coagulation abnormalities, and maintain the circulation. Consider nebulized adrenaline (5–10mL of 1 in 10,000) and, in those without renal impairment, oral tranexamic acid (500 mg tds).
• Avoid excessive chest manipulation (e.g. physiotherapy), as this may restart bleeding. Cough suppression with codeine 30–60 mg 6-hourly may be helpful.
• Institute appropriate therapeutic measures, depending on the underlying cause (e.g. antibiotics in bronchiectasis, anticoagulation in PE).

Determine the site and cause of massive haemoptysis

Most episodes of haemoptysis will stop spontaneously, but recurrence is common. Therefore, once the patient has been stabilized, the site and cause of bleeding must be established.

1. Early rigid bronchoscopy under general anaesthesia is the most effective technique for examining the bronchial tree and facilitates adequate suctioning of airway blood. A flexible bronchoscope, inserted through the rigid scope, enables inspection of the upper lobes.
2. If bronchoscopy is unsuccessful and the patient is sufficiently stable, CT scans with contrast may detect the bleeding site, tumours, and other structural abnormalities. In practice, the combination of bronchoscopy and CT scanning has the highest diagnostic yield. Occasionally, radionucleotide scans may be helpful.
3. Bronchial or pulmonary angiograms may be required but are only possible when there is ongoing active bleeding.

Control of massive haemoptysis

Bleeding must be controlled during ongoing investigation and may require temporizing measures or bronchial embolization. When the patient's condition has been stabilized, surgery may have to be considered.

1. *Immediate lavage* of the bleeding site with iced saline and adrenaline (10 mL; 1:10000 dilution) controls 95% of bleeding temporarily. Topical thrombin, balloon catheter tamponade, and intravenous vasoconstrictors (e.g. terlipressin) may also be effective.

2. *Bronchial angiography and embolization* controls 70–100% of early haemoptysis. It is particularly effective in patients with dilated bronchial arteries due to bronchiectasis. Early rebleeding is relatively common after bronchial embolization, but long-term control (>3 months) is reported in 45% of cases. Infarction of the anterior spinal artery and paraplegia occurs in about 5%. Rare complications include bronchial necrosis and arterial dissection.

3. *Surgical therapy* has the best overall outcome in massive haemoptysis, with long-term survival of 82–99% in isolated lesions, compared to 46–68% with conservative management (i.e. if surgery was feasible). Medical therapy may be mandatory in multifocal end-stage lung (FEV_1 <40% predicted) or cardiac diseases and severe bleeding diatheses.

Further reading

Action on Smoking and Health. Stopping smoking. <http://www.ash.org.uk/>.

All Party Parliamentary Group (APPG) on Respiratory Health (2014). Report on Inquiry into Respiratory Deaths. <https://www.blf.org.uk/Page/Report-on-inquiry-into-respiratory-deaths>.

Best Health. Lungs and breathing. <http://besthealth.bmj.com/x/set/topic/condition-centre/15.html>.

British Lung Foundation Breathe Easy Group. <http://www.lunguk.org>.

British Thoracic Society (2006). The burden of lung disease. 2nd edn. <http://www.brit-thoracic.org.uk/SearchResults/tabid/37/Default.aspx?Search=burden+of+lung+disease>.

Chest, Heart & Stroke Scotland. <http://www.chss.org.uk/>.

de Lemos JA, McGuire DK, Drazner MH (2003). B-type natriuretic peptide in cardiovascular disease. *Lancet*, **362**, 316–22.

Edmonds P, Karlsen S, Khan S, Addington-Hall J (2001). A comparison of the palliative care needs of patients dying from chronic respiratory diseases and lung cancer. *Palliative Medicine*, **15**, 287–95.

Emphysema Foundation. <http://www.emphysema.net/>.

Hirshberg B, Biran I, Glazer M, Kramer MR (1997). Hemoptysis: etiology, evaluation, and outcome in a tertiary referral hospital. *Chest*, **112**, 440–4.

Irwin RS, Boulet LP, Cloutier MM, *et al.* (1998). Managing cough as a defence mechanism and as a symptom: a consensus panel report of the American College of Chest Physicians. *Chest*, **114**, 133S–81S.

Irwin RS, Baumann MH, Bolser DC, *et al.* (2006). Diagnosis and management of cough: ACCP evidence-based clinical practice guidelines. *Chest*, **129**, 1S–23S.

Jones KD and Davies RJ (1990). Massive haemoptysis. *BMJ*, **300**, 889–900.

Lung Foundation Australia. The COPD-X plan. Australian and New Zealand guidelines for the management of chronic obstructive pulmonary disease 2012. <http://copdx.org.au/>.

Mahler DA (2000). Do you speak the language of dyspnea? *Chest*, **117**, 928–9.

Maisel AS, Krishnaswamy P, Nowak RM (2002). Rapid measurement of B-type natriuretic peptide in the emergency diagnosis of heart failure. *New England Journal of Medicine*, **347**, 161–7.

Mal H, Rullon I, Mellot F, *et al.* (1999). Immediate and long-term results of bronchial artery embolisation for life-threatening hemoptysis. *Chest*, **115**, 996–1001.

Morice AH, McGarvey L, Pavord I, on behalf of the BTS guideline group (2012). British Thoracic Society Guidelines: Recommendations for the management of cough in adults. <http://www.brit-thoracic.org.uk/Portals/0/Guidelines/Cough/Guidelines/coughguidelinesaugust06.pdf>.

Mukerji B, Mukerji V, Alpert MA, Selukar R (1995). The prevalence of rheumatological disorders in patients with chest pain and angiographically normal coronary arteries. *Angiology*, **46**, 425–30.

NHS SmokeFree: Smoking—advice to help you stop smoking. <http://smokefree.nhs.uk/>.

No authors listed (1995). A controlled trial to improve care for seriously ill hospitalized patients. The study to understand prognoses and preferences for outcomes and risks of treatment (SUPPORT). The SUPPORT Principal Investigators. *JAMA*, **274**, 1591–8.

No authors listed (1999). Dyspnea. Mechanisms, assessment and management. A consensus statement. American Thoracic Society. *American Journal of Respiratory and Critical Care Medicine*, **159**, 321–40.

Office for National Statistics (2000). Mortality statistics by cause. Series DH2 no.26. The Stationery Office: London.

Office for National Statistics. Mortality Statistics (2014). Death Registrations Summary Tables, England and Wales. <http://www.ons.gov.uk/ons/publications/re-reference-tables.html?edition=tcm%3A77-370351>.

Parvez L, Vaidya M, Sakhardande A, *et al.* (1996). Evaluation of antitussive agents in man. *Pulmonary Pharmacology & Therapeutics*, **9**, 299–308.

Patient UK. Chronic obstructive pulmonary disease. <http://www.patient.co.uk/showdoc/23068705/>.

Tan RT, McGahan JP, Link DP, Lantz BMT (1991). Bronchial artery embolisation in management of haemoptysis. *Journal of Interventional Radiology*, **6**, 67–76.

Thompson AB, Teschler H, Rennard S (1992). Pathogenesis, evaluation and therapy for massive haemoptysis. *Clinics in Chest Medicine*, **13**, 69–82.

Wise CM (1994). Chest wall syndromes. *Current Opinion in Rheumatology*, **6**, 197–202.

Assessment of diffuse lung disease

Diffuse lung disease (DLD) describes any widespread pulmonary process. It typically presents with varying degrees of breathlessness (± cough) and bilateral chest X-ray (CXR) changes. Although a common scenario in the acute medical setting, the time course and symptom severity vary considerably which often aids diagnosis. For example, acute interstitial pneumonitis (AIP) causes rapidly progressive dyspnoea, associated CXR infiltration, and death within weeks, whereas sarcoidosis may develop as asymptomatic lung infiltration over many years.

The primary pathological changes associated with diseases that cause DLD may affect the connective tissue fibrous framework of the lung as 'interstitial or diffuse parenchymal lung disease', blood vessels as 'vasculitis', airways as 'bronchiolitis', or airspaces as 'pneumonia'. Usually, several lung components are affected simultaneously. Thus, interstitial lung disease may involve not only the interstitium, but also the airways, vessels, and airspaces. Table 5.6 lists the many potential causes of DLD, according to their rate of progression and mechanism. A systematic approach to diagnosis is essential. Individual DLDs are discussed in later chapters.

Table 5.6 Causes of diffuse lung disease, according to speed of onset and causative mechanism

Acute onset (days to weeks)
- **Infection:** bacterial* (e.g. pneumococcal, TB), viral (e.g. varicella, influenza), fungal (e.g. aspergillosis, PCP), atypical (e.g. mycoplasma)
- **Other acute causes:** ARDS, hypersensitivity pneumonitis, acute interstitial pneumonia

Acute to chronic (weeks to months)
- **Drugs:** cardiac (e.g. amiodarone), immunosuppressants (e.g. methotrexate), cytotoxics (e.g. bleomycin), antibiotics (e.g. nitrofurantoin), illicit (e.g. cocaine inhalation)
- **Vasculitis:** SLE, Goodpasture's syndrome, Wegener's granulomatosis, Churg–Strauss, microscopic polyangiitis
- **Pulmonary venous hypertension:** cardiac pulmonary oedema, pulmonary veno-occlusive disease
- **Toxins:** paraquat, high-concentration oxygen
- **Other causes:** sarcoidosis, cryptogenic organizing pneumonia, eosinophilic pneumonia

Chronic (months to years)
- **Idiopathic interstitial pneumonias:** UIP, NSIP, DIP, LIP, RB-ILD
- **Occupational:** inorganic (e.g. asbestosis, silicosis), organic hypersensitivity pneumonitis (e.g. psittacosis, farmer's lung)
- **Malignancy:** lymphangitis carcinomatosis, bronchoalveolar cell carcinoma
- **CT disease:** SLE, rheumatoid arthritis, scleroderma, Sjögren's syndrome
- **Other causes:** bronchiectasis, amyloidosis, Langerhans cell histiocytosis

* = common.

TB, tuberculosis; PCP, *Pneumocystis jirovecii* pneumonia; ARDS, acute respiratory distress syndrome; SLE, systemic lupus erythematosus; UIP, usual interstitial pneumonia; NSIP, non-specific interstitial pneumonia; DIP, desquamative interstitial pneumonia; LIP, lymphocytic interstitial pneumonia; RB-ILD, respiratory bronchiolitis-interstitial lung disease.

Clinical assessment

History

This is essential and frequently indicates the likely diagnosis. Key features include:

- **Presenting symptoms.** Breathlessness is the most common symptom, and its rate of onset is often helpful diagnostically (see Table 5.6). Wheeze occurs in eosinophilic pneumonia (EP) and Churg–Strauss syndrome. Other causes of episodic breathlessness with associated diffuse CXR changes include hypersensitivity pneumonitis (HSP), pulmonary oedema, vasculitis, allergic bronchopulmonary aspergillosis (ABPA), and cryptogenic organizing pneumonia (COP). Cough may be a prominent symptom in sarcoidosis, lymphangitis carcinomatosis, HSP, COP, and EP. Copious purulent sputum (± haemoptysis) suggests bronchiectasis, whereas bronchorrhoea (>0.5 L sputum/day) occurs in bronchoalveolar cell carcinoma. Haemoptysis with widespread CXR infiltration suggests diffuse alveolar haemorrhage (DAH). Weight loss and fever are usually non-specific.

- **Past medical history.** Immunosuppression, infection, malignancy, and connective tissue diseases are often associated with diffuse CXR abnormalities. If available, comparison with previous CXR may be helpful. Check for systemic manifestations of connective tissue disease, sarcoidosis, and vasculitis (e.g. haematuria, rash, arthritis). Infertility may be associated with cystic fibrosis and bronchiectasis.

- **Drug history** is essential, but CXR changes may be delayed for months or years after starting drug therapy (e.g. amiodarone, methotrexate). Ask about illicit drug use, including route of administration (e.g. intravenous injection of heroin mixed with talc causes CXR changes, and inhaled cocaine may cause DAH, EP, or interstitial pneumonia).

- **Family history.** Potential hereditary DLD include sarcoidosis, rare forms of usual interstitial pneumonia (UIP), non-specific interstitial pneumonia (NSIP), and alpha-1-antitrypsin deficiency.

- **Social assessment** should include smoking history which is associated with increased incidence of respiratory bronchiolitis-associated interstitial lung disease (RB-ILD), desquamative interstitial pneumonia (DIP), Langerhans cell histiocytosis (LCH), and Goodpasture's syndrome. Assess immunocompetency (e.g. sexual history) to exclude opportunistic infections and lymphoma. Lifelong employment history should include exposure to, and protection against, organic and inorganic dusts. Inorganic dusts (e.g. silica, asbestos, tin) cause DLD, whereas organic dusts cause HSP (e.g. Thermoactinomycetes in mouldy hay cause farmer's lung; avian proteins cause bird fancier's lung or psittacosis). Travel history may suggest TB exposure or parasitic disease (e.g. pulmonary eosinophilia in the tropics, histoplasmosis in north and central USA).

Clinical examination

This may reveal clubbing (e.g. UIP, bronchiectasis) and cyanosis. Chest examination may detect fine (e.g. UIP, asbestosis, connective tissue disease, lymphangitis carcinomatosis, etc.) or coarse (e.g. bronchiectasis, pulmonary oedema) lung crackles. Absence of crepitations, despite diffuse CXR infiltration, suggests sarcoidosis, HSP, LCH, or pneumoconiosis. Wheeze occurs in bronchiolitis or vasculitis. Check for systemic, eye, skin, renal (e.g. haematuria), and joint manifestation (e.g. sarcoidosis, rheumatoid arthritis).

Chest imaging

Chest radiography (CXR)

In diffuse lung disease (DLD), the CXR is diagnostic in up to half of cases (see Figure 5.2) but normal in a further ~5–15% (i.e. with proven DLD on HRCT scanning or biopsy). Previous CXR aids assessment of duration and progress.

High-resolution CT (HRCT) scans

HRCT are often diagnostic and are more sensitive and specific than CXR for DLD. It aids assessment of the distribution, extent, and disease activity. Thus, ground glass opacification (GGO) suggests steroid-sensitive inflammation, whereas honeycomb changes indicate treatment-resistant late fibrosis. HRCT scans aid assessment of disease distribution and should always precede biopsy to determine the optimal sites for lung sampling. The distribution, pattern, and specific features on HRCT often aid DLD diagnosis.

Distribution

- **Upper zone involvement** suggests old TB, chronic sarcoidosis, silicosis, HSP, pneumoconiosis, and LCH.
- **Midzone (perihilar) disease** suggests pulmonary oedema, acute sarcoidosis, or PCP.
- **Lower zone involvement** is typical in UIP, asbestosis and, connective tissue disease.
- **Peripheral distribution** is typical of UIP, amiodarone toxicity, COP, and EP. Radiation-associated fibrosis has clearly defined borders.

Patterns

- **Ground glass opacification** (see Figure 5.3): describes a hazy, increased opacity of lung (grey appearance to the

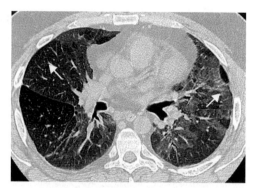

Figure 5.3 HRCT scan showing ground glass opacification (→) and mosaic pattern typical of alveolitis in desquamative interstitial pneumonitis.

lung tissue, compared with air in the bronchi which looks black) through which the vascular and bronchial margins are preserved (i.e. can still be distinguished). It can be artifactual due to inadequate inspiration during the scan or confused with a 'mosaic' attenuation pattern (i.e. well-defined normal lung abutting abnormal lung) that occurs due to variable lung perfusion in chronic thromboembolic disease, small airways disease, or HSP. Ground glass opacification may be patchy or diffuse and due to air-space or interstitial disease. Typical causes include idiopathic interstitial pneumonias (e.g. DIP, RB-ILD, NSIP, see section on diffuse parenchymal lung disease), sarcoidosis, HSP, ARDS, drugs, PCP, bronchoalveolar cell carcinoma, and pulmonary oedema or haemorrhage.

- **Reticular change.** Numerous small linear opacities which overlap each other to produce a fine net-like pattern. It typically occurs in usual interstitial pneumonia (UIP), with a patchy, basal, subpleural distribution (see Figure 5.4) and may be associated with ground glass opacification, loss of secondary pulmonary lobule architecture, honeycombing, and traction bronchiectasis. Reticular change is also seen in sarcoidosis, connective tissue disease, and drug-induced fibrosis. Asbestosis-related reticular change may occur with pleural plaques. Chronic HSP reticulation is associated with expiratory air

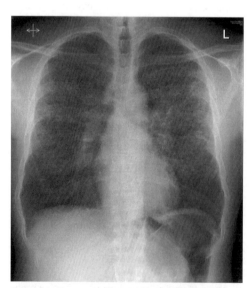

Figure 5.2 Chest radiograph showing diffuse bilateral alveolar infiltration (and bihilar lymphadenopathy). The adenopathy is characteristic of sarcoidosis, but radiological alveolar sarcoid occurs in 10–20% of cases or less.

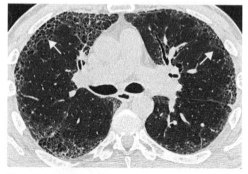

Figure 5.4 HRCT scan showing subpleural, patchy, reticular change (→) and 'honeycombing', typical of usual interstitial pneumonitis (UIP).

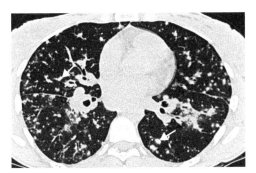

Figure 5.5 HRCT scan showing numerous discrete rounded opacities (→) in sarcoidosis. Nodules are predominantly peribronchovascular and centrilobular. Fissural nodules are characteristic.

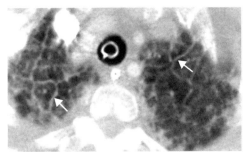

Figure 5.7 HRCT scan showing interlobular septal thickening (→) in acute eosinophilic pneumonia.

trapping, ground glass opacification, and centilobular micronodules.

- **Nodular change** describes numerous discrete rounded opacities (2–10 mm diameter), usually due to interstitial disease processes like sarcoidosis which causes nodule formation in the interlobular septa, around the bronchovascular bundles, and subpleurally (see Figure 5.5). However, airspace diseases (e.g. HSP, miliary TB, metastatic disease, varicella pneumonitis) may also result in affected acini becoming visible as nodules. A micronodule is a nodule less than 3 mm in size.
- **Cystic change** describes well-defined thin-walled airspaces (see Figure 5.6) and occurs in UIP (subpleural honeycombing), LCH (apical, irregularly shaped cysts and nodules), lymphangioleiomyomatosis (LAM; thin-walled cysts in normal lung), lymphocytic interstitial pneumonia (LIP), and PCP. Centrilobular emphysema may mimic cystic disease, but airspaces lack well-defined walls.
- **Interlobular septal thickening** (see Figure 5.7) is due to processes involving lymphatics and venules like pulmonary oedema (smooth thickening), sarcoidosis, UIP, and lymphangitis carcinomatosis (irregular thickening).
- **Consolidation** (airspace shadowing) describes increased attenuation characterized by air bronchograms (i.e. air-filled bronchi superimposed against opacified alveolar

lung tissue), with loss of the visibility of adjacent vasculature. It is due to infiltration and 'filling' of airspaces with fluid, pus, blood, fibrous tissue, or malignant cells during many disease processes, including pneumonia, ARDS, pulmonary oedema (or haemorrhage), COP, drugs, EP, or bronchoalveolar cell carcinoma.

Specific features

Characteristic features, in combination with the distribution and pattern, aid diagnosis.

- Lymphadenopathy occurs in sarcoidosis, lymphoma, infection, silicosis, LIP, and malignancy.
- Pleural involvement/effusion may suggest pulmonary oedema, infection, asbestosis, malignancy, or CT disease.

For example, breathlessness in a young black man with bihilar lymphadenopathy and diffuse upper and midzone reticular and interlobular septal thickening on CXR suggests a diagnosis of sarcoidosis.

Confirmatory investigations

Final diagnosis requires a systematic approach guided by initial radiological findings.

Routine tests

These include:

- **Blood tests.** Full blood count with eosinophils (e.g. PE, HSP), ESR, C-reactive protein, renal function (e.g. impaired in vasculitis), liver function tests, and calcium (e.g. elevated in 10% of sarcoid cases). A raised serum angiotensin-converting enzyme (sACE) may suggest sarcoidosis but is a non-specific and insensitive test. Antineutrophil cytoplasmic antibody (ANCA) and anti-glomerular basement membrane (anti-GBM) antibody (e.g. Goodpasture's syndrome) may indicate an underlying vasculitis. Autoantibodies, including rheumatoid factor or antinuclear antibody, are increased in connective tissue diseases, UIP, or malignancy. Raised serum precipitins (e.g. antibodies to avian antigens) may indicate HSP, but specificity is poor.
- **Urine tests.** Dipstick and microscopic examination (e.g. haematuria, proteinuria) may suggest renal involvement in vasculitis or connective tissue diseases.
- **Sputum examination.** Induced sputum for PCP or TB and cytology for malignancy (e.g. bronchoalveolar cell carcinoma).
- **Electrocardiograms (ECG)** are rarely normal in heart failure and may reveal conduction abnormalities in sarcoidosis.

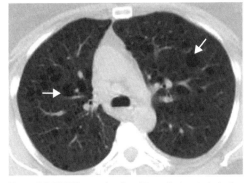

Figure 5.6 HRCT scan showing thin-walled cysts (→) of Langerhans cell histiocytosis.

- **Pulmonary function tests** often reveal a restrictive pattern, with a reduced gas transfer, although obstructive patterns may occur with coexisting COPD, in sarcoidosis, and LCH. Gas transfer increases with alveolar haemorrhage. Normal lung volumes with reduced gas transfer suggests pulmonary vascular disease (e.g. vasculitis, pulmonary hypertension). Disease progression is best assessed with transfer factor and vital capacity.
- **Oxygen saturation/arterial blood gases.** Exercise-induced desaturation often precedes significant clinical and radiographic abnormality.

Specialist tests
Bronchoalveolar lavage
This aids diagnosis of malignancy, EP, DAH, or opportunistic infection (e.g. PCP, fungal pneumonia). Occasionally, differential cell counts may be helpful (e.g. sarcoidosis).

Lung biopsy
This provides histological confirmation of the diagnosis when the cause of DLD is uncertain (e.g. after HRCT scan) and when establishing a diagnosis has therapeutic and prognostic benefit. Characteristic HRCT findings (± clinical picture) may be diagnostic in some situations (e.g. UIP, sarcoidosis). However, biopsy of end-stage fibrosis is unlikely to be helpful. Clearly, the patient's clinical condition and preferences must be taken into account. A pragmatic approach to empirical treatment is often adopted when the diagnosis is probable, but not biopsy-proven, and/or the patient is either too unwell for, or declines, biopsy.

Transbronchial biopsies (TBBx)
These (TBBx x 4–6) are small but have a high diagnostic yield in centrilobular diseases (e.g. sarcoidosis, malignancy, COP). Blind endobronchial biopsies are often diagnostic in sarcoidosis.

Cutting needle percutaneous biopsy
This may establish a diagnosis in well-localized, peripheral or pleural lesions, or dense infiltrates.

Open lung biopsies
These provide larger samples than TBBx and are typically indicated for suspected idiopathic interstitial pneumonia, LCH, vasculitis, lymphangioleiomyomatosis, and lymphoma. They are diagnostic in >90% of cases. Video-assisted thoracoscopic (VATS) biopsy is less invasive than thoracotomy, has a low morbidity, and is most suitable in stable, self-ventilating patients.

Further reading

Devaraj A, Wells AU, Hansell D (2007). Computed tomographic imaging in connective tissue disease. *Seminars in Respiratory and Critical Care Medicine*, **28**, 389–97.

Hansell DM, Bankier AA, MacMahon H, McLoud TC, Müller NL, Remy J (2008). Fleischner Society: glossary of terms for thoracic imaging. *Radiology*, **246**, 697–722.

King TE (2005). Clinical advances in the diagnosis and therapy of the interstitial lung diseases. *American Journal of Respiratory and Critical Care Medicine*, **172**, 268–79.

Lynch DA, Travis WD, Müller NL, *et al.* (2005). Idiopathic interstitial pneumonia: CT features. *Radiology*, **236**, 10–21.

No author listed (2000). Joint statement of the American Thoracic Society (ATS) and the European Respiratory Society (ERS). Idiopathic pulmonary fibrosis: diagnosis and treatment. International Consensus Statement 1999. *American Journal of Respiratory and Critical Care Medicine*, **161**, 646–64.

Pandit-Bhalla M, Diethelm L, Ovella T, Sloop GD, Valentine VG (2003). Idiopathic interstitial pneumonia: an update. *Journal of Thoracic Imaging*, **18**, 1–13.

Ryu JH, Olson EJ, Midthun DE, Swensen (2002). Diagnostic approach to the patient with diffuse lung disease. *Mayo Clinic Proceedings*, **77**, 1221–7.

Hypoxaemia, respiratory failure, and oxygen therapy

Tissue hypoxia occurs within 4 minutes of cardiorespiratory arrest, as tissue, blood, and lung oxygen reserves are small. Oxygen delivery (DO_2) depends on adequate ventilation, gas exchange, and circulatory distribution, but, despite their fundamental importance in mammalian pathophysiology, the mechanisms of oxygen uptake, utilization, and transport to the tissues are relatively poorly understood. Similarly, there are limited data available on the role and optimal use of supplementary oxygen.

As little oxygen dissolves in blood, most is carried attached to the oxygen-carrying protein haemoglobin. The amount of oxygen carried by the blood is often expressed as a percentage of the maximum possible carriage of oxygen by the haemoglobin, the arterial haemoglobin 'saturation' (SaO_2). Figure 5.8 illustrates the relationship between the partial pressure of oxygen in blood (PaO_2) and SaO_2. The key features are that, initially, SaO_2 remains high, despite marked falls in PaO_2, and subsequently that PaO_2 remains relatively stable as SaO_2 declines, factors which optimize oxygen uptake, delivery, and tissue oxygenation. Temperature, pH, and 2,3-diphosphoglycerate can modulate the dissociation curve and, during chronic hypoxia, a rightward shift maintains tissue DO_2.

Definitions of hypoxia

Hypoxaemia refers to a low partial pressure of oxygen in arterial blood (PaO_2). Most authors define hypoxaemia as a PaO_2 <8 kPa (60 mmHg) or an arterial saturation (SaO_2) <90%, as there is no known risk of hypoxic injury above this level in acute illness. Type 1 respiratory failure (RF) is defined as a PaO_2 <8 kPa, with a normal or low $PaCO_2$ (see 'Respiratory failure').

Pathophysiological mechanisms of hypoxia

Tissue hypoxia is either due to hypoxaemia or failure of the oxygen-haemoglobin transport system (see Table 5.7). Mechanisms contributing to arterial hypoxaemia include:

Table 5.7 Causes of tissue hypoxia

Arterial hypoxaemia
- Low inspired partial pressure of O_2 (e.g. altitude)
- Alveolar hypoventilation (e.g. drugs)
- V/Q mismatch (e.g. consolidation)
- Right-to-left shunts (e.g. ASD, PAVM)

Failure of oxygen-haemoglobin transport
- Stagnant hypoxia. Inadequate tissue perfusion
- Anaemic hypoxia. Low haemoglobin concentration
- Reduced O_2 dissociation (e.g. haemoglobinopathies)
- Histotoxic hypoxia. Failure of O_2 utilization (e.g. cyanide poisoning)

O_2, oxygen; V/Q, ventilation/perfusion; ASD, atrial septal defect; PAVM, pulmonary arteriovenous malformation

- **Reduced inspired oxygen partial pressure** (PO_2) or 'hypoxaemic hypoxia'. This occurs at high altitude due to reduced barometric pressure, during fires due to O_2 combustion, and after toxic fume inhalation.
- **Hypoventilation** which results from failure to replace alveolar O_2 as rapidly as it is taken up by blood.
- **Shunt or 'true' shunt.** This describes venous blood that bypasses lung gas exchange (venous admixture) and passes directly into systemic blood (e.g. through a heart defect). Increasing inspired O_2 (FiO_2) has little effect on PaO_2 when 'true' shunt fraction is >30% (see Figure 5.9a).
- **Ventilation/perfusion (V/Q) mismatch.** This is the commonest cause of hypoxaemia. Even in diseases like pulmonary fibrosis, where poor diffusion is expected to predominate, V/Q mismatch is more important than diffusion defect. Figure 5.9b illustrates the effect of V/Q mismatch on PaO_2 from a few severe, and many mild, V/Q mismatch lung units. High V/Q units contribute to deadspace, not hypoxaemia.

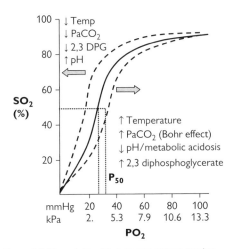

Figure 5.8 The relationship between oxygen tension (PO_2) and haemoglobin saturation (SO_2).

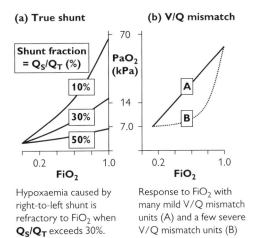

(a) True shunt

Hypoxaemia caused by right-to-left shunt is refractory to FiO_2 when Q_S/Q_T exceeds 30%.

(b) V/Q mismatch

Response to FiO_2 with many mild V/Q mismatch units (A) and a few severe V/Q mismatch units (B).

Figure 5.9 Effect of true shunt (Q_S/Q_T) and V/Q mismatch on the arterial oxygen tension (PaO_2) and inspired oxygen fraction (FiO_2).

- **Impaired diffusion.** This is rarely clinically significant, except when rapid pulmonary capillary blood flow prevents equilibration of alveolar oxygen with the capillary blood (e.g. exercise).
- **Venous admixture.** Venous blood returning to the right heart with a very low SaO_2 usually has little effect on PaO_2 but, in patients with V/Q mismatch or heart failure, may contribute to subsequent hypoxaemia.

Definition of hypercapnia

Hypercapnia is present when the partial pressure of carbon dioxide in the arterial blood ($PaCO_2$) is above the normal range of 4.6–6.1 kPa (34–46 mmHg). Patients are defined as having type II RF (see the following section) when $PaCO_2$ is raised, even if PaO_2 and SaO_2 are in the normal range.

Pathophysiology of hypercapnia

Normally, carbon dioxide levels in the blood are tightly controlled by chemical sensors in the carotid bodies and brainstem. A rise in $PaCO_2$ stimulates an increase in ventilation by activating afferent (i.e. spinal, phrenic, intercostal) nerves and respiratory muscles, increasing lung and, consequently, bloodstream clearance of CO_2. However, this mechanism is less effective in some respiratory diseases, such as COPD, where increased airways resistance and respiratory muscle weakness restrict the normal response. Indeed, any cause of hypoventilation will cause hypercapnia, as $PaCO_2$ is inversely proportional to alveolar ventilation. The three main causes of failure of ventilation are impaired central drive, excessive respiratory workload, and neuromuscular impairment. Table 5.8 illustrates potential causes in each category.

The mechanism by which excess oxygen precipitates hypercapnia and progressive respiratory acidosis with organ dysfunction and coma in patients with COPD, chest wall deformity, or muscle weakness is not fully understood. Although the concept of 'reduced hypoxic ventilatory drive', following an improvement in oxygenation, is still widely held, other mechanisms are probably equally, or more, important.

- **V/Q mismatch.** During air breathing, poorly ventilated 'hypoxic' alveoli, with a low partial pressure of alveolar oxygen (PAO_2), will be poorly perfused due to the protective pulmonary vascular response of hypoxic pulmonary vasoconstriction (HPV). PAO_2 increases with oxygen therapy, reversing HPV and increasing alveolar capillary blood flow. However, despite the increase in

PAO_2, the alveolus remains poorly ventilated, with a high partial pressure of alveolar carbon dioxide ($PACO_2$), and, because more blood is flowing through these poorly ventilated alveoli, $PaCO_2$ will rise. This mechanism is probably more important than 'reduced hypoxic ventilatory drive' as a cause of hypercapnia in COPD (see text below).

- **The Haldane effect.** Deoxygenated haemoglobin has a greater carbon dioxide buffering effect than oxygenated haemoglobin, and consequently improved oxygenation will increase $PaCO_2$.
- **Absorption atelectasis.** This follows absorption of oxygen from alveoli with high PAO_2 beyond obstructed airways, resulting in greater V/Q mismatch. It can occur with an FiO_2 as low as 30–50%.
- **Hypoxic ventilatory drive.** Hypoxaemia increases the drive to breathe, so it is often believed that alleviating hypoxaemia should reduce ventilation. However, an increase in PaO_2 above 8 kPa does not significantly reduce ventilation, and several studies suggest that 'hypoxic drive' makes only a small contribution to oxygen-induced hypercapnia and is unlikely to be a significant factor.

Clinical presentations

Tissue hypoxia and hypoxaemia usually presents with non-specific symptoms, the earliest feature of which is impaired mental state, as the brain is the most sensitive organ to the adverse effects of hypoxia. Dyspnoea, hyperventilation, arrhythmias and hypotension, and coma follow.

- **Central cyanosis** is detected when deoxygenated haemoglobin (Hb) is >1.5 g/dL. However, it is an unreliable indicator of hypoxia because it may be absent in the hypoxic, anaemic patient (i.e. an SaO_2 of 80%, with 5 g/dL Hb, produces 1 g/dL of deoxygenated Hb) but apparent in a normoxic, polycythaemic subject (i.e. an SaO_2 of 90%, with 20 g/dL Hb, produces 2 g/dL of deoxygenated Hb).

Hypercapnia often presents insidiously with fatigue, ankle oedema, morning headache, confusion, and cyanosis. Features of the underlying cause may be present (e.g. dysphagia in MND). Sudden severe respiratory failure and coma requiring ventilation can be precipitated by minor respiratory tract infection if the significance of earlier symptoms is not appreciated. Hypercapnic patients can be difficult to wean from mechanical ventilation.

Measuring oxygenation

Arterial blood gas (ABG) analysis measures PaO_2, the 'tension' driving oxygen into tissues. The normal range is 12–14.6 kPa (90–110 mmHg) in young adults. SaO_2 measures the level of arterial oxygen carriage by haemoglobin as a percentage of maximum carriage. If measured by pulse oximetry, it is termed SpO_2; the normal range is 94–98%. PaO_2 and SaO_2 are the principal measures used to initiate, monitor, and adjust oxygen therapy. However, they can be normal when tissue hypoxia is caused by low cardiac output, anaemia, or failure of oxygen utilization (e.g. sepsis). In these circumstances, mixed venous oxygen saturation (SvO_2) <55–60% (normally >70%) reflects inadequate DO_2 better. The alveolar-arterial (A-a) oxygen gradient ($PA-aO_2$) is a measure of gas exchange efficiency. PAO_2 is determined from the simplified alveolar gas equation (see Figure 5.10), which, by incorporating $PaCO_2$, eliminates hypoventilation and hypercapnia as causes of hypoxaemia (i.e. a high $PaCO_2$ lowers PAO_2). The A-a gradient is increased by shunts, V/Q mismatch, and diffusion

Table 5.8 Causes of ventilatory failure

Increased respiratory load
- Resistive loads (e.g. bronchospasm, secretions, scarring)
- Elastic loads (e.g. oedema, infection, obesity, ascites, atelectasis, pneumothorax, kyphosis)
- Minute ventilation loads (e.g. sepsis, PE, hypovolaemia)

Neuromuscular (NM) failure
- Impaired NM transmission (e.g. myasthenia gravis, Guillain–Barré syndrome, phrenic nerve injury)
- Muscle weakness (e.g. myopathy, fatigue, malnutrition)

Depressed respiratory drive
- Drug overdose (e.g. opioids)
- Central nervous system (e.g. brainstem strokes)
- Endocrine (e.g. hypothyroidism)

Alveolar oxygen tension derived from the simplified alveolar gas equation

$$P_AO_2 = PIO_2 - (1.25 \times PaCO_2)$$

Where

PIO$_2$ = FiO$_2$ × (barometric − water vapour pressure)
Breathing air; PIO$_2$ = 0.21 × (101 − 6.2) = 19.9 kPa

$$P_AO_2 \text{ (breathing air)} = 19.9-(1.25 \times 5.3)$$
$$= {\sim}13.5 \text{ kPa}$$

Alveolar-arterial (A-a) gradient (breathing air)

$$P(A\text{-}a)O_2 = P_AO_2 - PaO_2$$
$$= {\sim}13.5 - {\sim}13 = {<}1.0 \text{ kPa}$$

Figure 5.10 Alveolar oxygen tension and alveolar-arterial (A-a) gradient. P$_A$O$_2$, alveolar oxygen tension; PIO$_2$, inspired oxygen tension; FiO$_2$, fractional concentration of oxygen in inspired air; P(A-a)O$_2$, alveolar-arterial oxygen tension difference; PaO$_2$, arterial oxygen tension; PaCO$_2$, arterial CO$_2$ tension.

impairment. It is normally ~0.2 kPa but increases with age and FiO$_2$. Detecting organ ischaemia is difficult, and most techniques have limitations (e.g. gastric tonometry, near-infrared spectroscopy).

Respiratory failure

Respiratory failure (RF) may be acute, chronic, or acute-on-chronic. It is due to inadequate gas exchange and is defined by a PaO$_2$ <8 kPa, PaCO$_2$ >6 kPa, or both. RF patients must be monitored (e.g. SaO$_2$, respiratory rate) in an area commensurate with clinical need (e.g. high dependency unit) and treatment directed at the underlying cause.

1. **Type I RF is due to failure of oxygenation.** It occurs when blood bypasses, or is not completely oxygenated in the lungs, causing hypoxaemia (as previously discussed). PaCO$_2$ is normal or low because ventilation is unchanged or increased due to breathlessness. There are many causes (see 'Hypoxaemia'), including V/Q mismatch (e.g. pneumonia), right-to-left shunts (e.g. heart defects), low FiO$_2$ (e.g. high altitude), and diffusion impairment (e.g. during exercise in pulmonary fibrosis). PaO$_2$ is usually improved with oxygen therapy (see section on oxygen therapy), but re-expansion or recruitment of collapsed alveoli and reduction of V/Q mismatch may be equally effective. For example, continuous positive airways pressure (CPAP) may improve oxygenation by recruiting collapsed lung in acute lung injury.

2. **Type II RF is due to inadequate ventilation.** Hypercapnia is usually due to hypoventilation (see Table 5.8) which is associated with a normal A-a gradient (i.e. <1 kPa). The PaO$_2$ may be normal or low. Other mechanisms contributing to hypercapnia are as previously discussed and include V/Q mismatch in COPD (i.e. indicated by a large A-a gradient) and inadequate compensatory hyperventilation in severe asthma. Typically, hypoventilation is due to:

   • **Inadequate respiratory drive** due to brainstem abnormality (e.g. strokes, tumours, cerebellar herniation (Arnold–Chiari malformation), syringobulbia), encephalitis, sedative drugs (e.g. opioids), or metabolic alkalosis.

   • **Ineffective ventilation** due to neuromuscular weakness (e.g. MND, Guillain–Barré, myasthenia gravis),

chest wall deformity (e.g. kyphosis, obesity, flail chest), and excessive work of breathing (WoB) due to primary lung disease (e.g. COPD, asthma). The WoB required to ventilate abnormal lungs may increase from normal levels of 5% to >30% of total O$_2$ consumption.

Assessment of respiratory failure
A careful history and thorough examination are essential. Particular attention should be paid to potential neurological and muscular diseases if type II RF is suspected. Specific investigations include blood gases on air (i.e. >20 min without oxygen), calculation of A-a gradient to detect V/Q mismatch, lung function tests to exclude airways obstruction, and supine vital capacity to detect ventilatory failure (i.e. if <1 L). Specific tests (e.g. MRI, EMG, sleep studies) determine the underlying cause of RF.

Management
Arterial hypoxaemia
Oxygen is widely available and commonly prescribed. When given correctly, it is a lifesaving drug, but it is often used without appropriate evaluation of potential benefits and side effects. Published acute oxygen guidelines recommend giving supplemental oxygen to achieve a normal target SaO$_2$ of 94–98% and >90% in acutely ill patients. Higher saturations risk coronary or cerebral vasoconstriction, absorption atelectasis, hypercapnia in those at risk (e.g. COPD), and tissue damage due to reactive oxygen species.

Hypoxaemia is also corrected by treating the underlying cause (e.g. pneumonia) and improving V/Q matching by optimizing ventilation, (e.g. alveolar recruitment with physiotherapy, CPAP, or non-invasive ventilation (NIV)), clearing airways (e.g. sputum clearance, bronchodilation), and maintaining perfusion (e.g. preventing heart failure or pulmonary embolism).

Hypercapnia
If possible, treat the cause of the type II RF (e.g. myasthenia gravis). Bronchodilation and improved lung compliance (e.g. secretion clearance, alveolar recruitment) reduce WoB and improve ventilation. In some neuromuscular disorders, ventilatory mechanics can be improved by sleeping with the whole bed tilted head up by 20° which facilitates descent of the abdominal contents, offloading the diaphragm, and improving ventilation. Elevating the top half of the bed is unhelpful. If hypercapnia and acidosis persist, NIV is often effective and widely available.

Indications for intubation and mechanical ventilation in RF
These include a RR >35/min, PaO$_2$ <8 kPa on >50% FiO$_2$; PaCO$_2$ >7.5 kPa, pH <7.25, decreased conscious level (GCS <8), inadequate secretion clearance, exhaustion, and failure to improve within 1–4h with NIV.

Oxygen therapy
Box 5.1 lists the indications for initiating oxygen therapy. It should be prescribed on the drug chart (i.e. dose, delivery method, duration, target saturation), signed for by the doctor, and documented by the nursing staff at each drug round

---

Box 5.1 Indications for acute oxygen therapy

1. **Cardiac and respiratory arrest**
2. **Hypoxaemia (PaO$_2$ <8 kPa, SaO$_2$ <90%)**
3. **Hypotension (systolic BP <100 mmHg)**
4. **Low cardiac output**
5. **Metabolic acidosis (bicarbonate <18 mmol/L)**
6. **Respiratory distress (respiratory rate >24/min)**

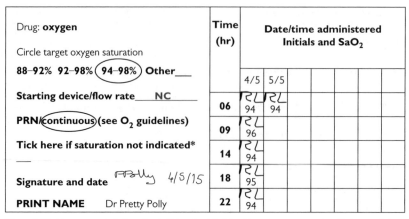

Drug: **oxygen**	Time (hr)	Date/time administered Initials and SaO$_2$					
Circle target oxygen saturation							
88–92% 92–98% (**94–98%**) **Other___**		4/5	5/5				
Starting device/flow rate___ NC___	06	$\mathcal{R}\mathcal{L}$ 94	$\mathcal{R}\mathcal{L}$ 94				
PRN/(**continuous**)**(see O$_2$ guidelines)**	09	$\mathcal{R}\mathcal{L}$ 96					
Tick here if saturation not indicated*	14	$\mathcal{R}\mathcal{L}$ 94					
___	18	$\mathcal{R}\mathcal{L}$ 95					
Signature and date *PPolly* 4/5/15	22	$\mathcal{R}\mathcal{L}$ 94					
PRINT NAME Dr Pretty Polly							

Figure 5.11 Oxygen prescription chart. *Saturation is indicated in most cases, except in palliative terminal care. NC, nasal cannulae.

(see Figure 5.11). The initial SaO$_2$ and associated FiO$_2$ should be recorded. In emergency situations, oxygen is often started without prescription, but therapy should always be documented retrospectively. Immediate airway, breathing, and circulation (i.e. ABC) assessment is essential and confirms airway patency and good circulation.

The therapeutic aims of oxygen therapy depend on the risk of developing hypercapnic RF.

Normal patients
Aim to achieve an SaO$_2$ of 94–98% if aged <70 years and 92–98% if aged >70 years (i.e. wider normal saturation range in the elderly). These ranges are on the plateau of the oxygen-haemoglobin dissociation curve where haemoglobin is fully saturated. Consequently, further increases in PaO$_2$ have no impact on oxygen delivery, as little oxygen is dissolved in plasma.

Patients at risk of hypercapnic respiratory failure
About 10% of breathless patients, mainly COPD, have type II RF, and approximately 40% of COPD patients are at risk of developing type II RF with oxygen therapy. In these patients, the target SaO$_2$ is 88–92%, pending ABG analysis. Higher SaO$_2$ have few advantages but may cause hypercapnia and respiratory acidosis (as previously described).

Initial oxygen dose and delivery method depends on the suspected cause of hypoxaemia:
- **High-dose supplemental oxygen** (>60%) is given during cardiac or respiratory arrests, shock, major trauma, sepsis, carbon monoxide (CO) poisoning, and other critical illness. It is delivered through a non-rebreathing, reservoir mask at 10–15 L/min. Once clinical stability has been restored, the oxygen dose is reduced whilst maintaining an SaO$_2$ of 92–98%. All seriously ill patients, even those at risk of hypercapnic RF (e.g. COPD), are initially treated with high-dose oxygen, pending ABG analysis.
- **Moderate-dose supplemental oxygen** (30–60%) is given in serious illness (e.g. pneumonia), preferably through nasal cannulae (2–6 L/min) or simple face masks (5–10 L/min), aiming for an SaO$_2$ of 92–98% (as previously described). A reservoir mask is substituted if target saturations are not achieved. Patients at risk of hypercapnic RF (e.g. COPD) are managed as described in the following section.

- **Low-dose (controlled) supplemental oxygen** (24–28%) is indicated in patients who are at risk of hypercapnic (type II) RF, for example, in those with COPD, neuromuscular disease, chest wall disorders, morbid obesity, and cystic fibrosis. It is usually delivered through a fixed performance Venturi mask (see Figure 5.12). Long-term smokers who are >50 years old, with exertional dyspnoea and without another cause for breathlessness, are treated as COPD. The target saturation is 88–92% whilst awaiting ABG results. If PaCO$_2$ is normal, SaO$_2$ is adjusted to 92–98% (except in patients with previous hypercapnic RF) and ABG rechecked at 1 hour. If an air compressor is not available, nebulizers are driven with oxygen but only for 6 min (maximum) to limit the risk of hypercapnic RF. A raised PaCO$_2$ and bicarbonate with normal pH on ABG measurements suggests long-standing hypercapnia, and the target SaO$_2$ should be 88–92%, with repeat ABG at 1 hour. If the patient is hypercapnic (PaCO$_2$ >6 kPa) and acidotic (pH <7.35) on ABG assessment, consider non-invasive ventilation (NIV) if the acidosis has persisted for >30–60 min despite appropriate medical treatment. Venturi masks are replaced with nasal cannulae (1–2 L/min) when the patient is stable. An oxygen alert card and Venturi mask should be issued to patients with previous hypercapnic RF to warn future emergency staff of the potential risk.

Oxygen therapy is of little benefit in 'normoxic' patients because the haemoglobin is fully saturated and oxygen solubility is low, even at high PaO$_2$. Early restoration of tissue blood flow is often more important in these cases. Therefore, oxygen therapy is of little value in myocardial infarction, drug overdoses, metabolic disorders, hyperventilation, or during labour in non-hypoxic pregnant women.

Indeed, oxygen may be harmful in normoxic patients with strokes, paraquat poisoning, bleomycin-induced lung injury or acid inhalation, and to the fetus in normoxic obstetric emergencies. However, in carbon monoxide poisoning (see Chapter 18), high-dose oxygen is essential, despite a normal PaO$_2$, as this reduces the carboxyhaemoglobin half-life. Table 5.9 reports the dangers of oxygen therapy. A common, and often serious error, following inadvertent development of oxygen-induced hypercapnia, is the sudden withdrawal of oxygen therapy, as this may cause life-threatening rebound hypoxaemia. Ideally, oxygen should be

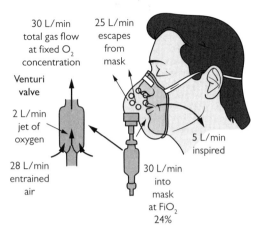

30 L/min
total gas flow
at fixed O_2
concentration

25 L/min
escapes
from
mask

Venturi
valve

2 L/min
jet of
oxygen

5 L/min
inspired

28 L/min
entrained
air

30 L/min
into
mask
at FiO_2
24%

Figure 5.12 'High-flow', low-concentration Venturi face mask. Venturi valves are colour-coded and deliver 24–60% FiO_2.

Table 5.9 Risks associated with high-dose oxygen therapy

1. Carbon dioxide retention
~10% of breathless patients, mainly COPD, have type II RF.
~40–50% of COPD patients are at risk of type II RF.

2. Rebound hypoxaemia
Occurs if oxygen is suddenly withdrawn in type II RF.

3. Absorption collapse
O_2 in poorly ventilated alveoli is rapidly absorbed, causing collapse, whereas N_2 absorption is slow.

4. Pulmonary oxygen toxicity
FiO_2 >60% may damage alveolar membranes, causing ARDS if inhaled for >24–48 h. Hyperoxia can cause coronary and cerebral vasospasm.

5. Paul–Bert effect
Hyperbaric O_2 causes cerebral vasoconstriction + epileptic fits.

6. Fire
Deaths and burns occur in smokers during O_2 therapy.

gradually reduced (± NIV) whilst monitoring SaO_2 and ABG to avoid further complications.

Monitoring. SaO_2 should be measured regularly in all breathless patients and recorded on the observation chart with the oxygen dosage. In unstable patients, SaO_2 is monitored continuously in high dependency areas. SaO_2 should be observed for 5 minutes after starting or changing oxygen dose and adjusted to achieve the target saturation. If possible, an ABG is measured before and within 1 hour of starting oxygen therapy, especially in those at risk of hypercapnic RF, and then at intervals to assess therapeutic response.

Stop oxygen therapy when the patient is clinically stable on low-dose oxygen (e.g. 1–2 L/min) and SaO_2 is within the desired range on two consecutive occasions. Monitor SaO_2 for 5 minutes after stopping oxygen, and recheck at 1 hour. If SaO_2 remains within the desired range, oxygen has been safely discontinued.

Other techniques to improve oxygenation

• **Anaemia.** In anaemic patients, oxygen delivery is best corrected by blood transfusion.

• **Secretion retention.** Physiotherapy, mucolytic agents (e.g. N-acetylcysteine), and bronchoscopy remove impacted sputum plugs and improve alveolar ventilation.

• **Fluid restriction.** Reduces alveolar oedema and improves oxygenation in settings of increased alveolar permeability (e.g. ARDS).

• **Alveolar recruitment.** Oxygenation is improved by reducing V/Q mismatch and shunt. Simple postural changes may improve oxygenation, such as sitting upright. Regular turning and prone positioning may improve secretion drainage and optimizes V/Q matching in supine patients (see Chapter 1). Techniques to increase alveolar pressures and recruitment (e.g. PEEP, CPAP, increased I:E ratio) also improve PaO_2.

• **Ventilatory support**, including NIV and CPAP, improve oxygenation by correcting hypoventilation and associated hypercapnia.

Further reading

Bateman NT and Leach RM (1998). Acute oxygen therapy. ABC of oxygen. *BMJ*, **317**, 798–801.

Denniston AK, O'Brien C, Stableforth D (2002). The use of oxygen in acute exacerbations of chronic obstructive pulmonary disease: a prospective audit of pre-hospital and hospital emergency management. *Clinical Medicine*, **2**, 449–51.

Forkner IF, Piantadosi CA, Scafetta N, Moon RE (2007). Hyperoxia-induced tissue hypoxia: a danger? *Anaesthesiology*, **106**, 1051–5.

Gooptu B, Ward L, Ansari SO, Eraut CD, Law D, Davison AG (2006). Oxygen alert cards and controlled oxygen: preventing emergency admissions at risk of hypercapnic acidosis receiving high inspired oxygen concentrations in ambulances and A&E departments. *Emergency Medicine Journal*, **23**, 636–8.

Murphy R, Mackway-Jones K, Sammy I, et al. (2001). Emergency oxygen therapy for the breathless patient. Guidelines prepared by the North West Oxygen Group. *Emergency Medicine Journal*, **18**, 421–3.

National Institute for Health and Clinical Excellence (2007). Acutely ill patients in hospital. <http://guidance.nice.org.uk/CG50>.

O'Driscoll BR, Howard LS, Davison AG (2008). British Thoracic Society guideline for emergency oxygen use in adults. *Thorax*, **63** (Suppl 6), vi1–68.

Rawles JM and Kenmure AC (1976). Controlled trial of oxygen in uncomplicated myocardial infarction. *BMJ*, **1**, 1121–3.

Pneumonia

Pneumonia is a significant worldwide cause of morbidity and mortality. It is a general term describing several distinct, mainly infective, clinical entities. Correct classification is vital, as the aetiology, infective organisms, antibiotic management, and outcome are determined by how and where the pneumonia was contracted. Early recognition and appropriate treatment improves outcome. This chapter is based on British (BTS, NICE), American, and Canadian guidelines for the management of community-acquired pneumonia and American, Canadian, and NICE guidelines for the management of adults with hospital-acquired pneumonia. The recommended antibiotic therapy differs between guidelines, and these variations are highlighted.

General definition of pneumonia

Pneumonia describes an acute lower respiratory tract (LRT) illness, usually, but not always, due to infection, associated with fever, focal chest symptoms (with or without clinical signs), and new-onset shadowing on chest radiography (CXR; see Figure 5.13). Table 5.10 lists microorganisms and pathological insults that cause pneumonia.

Pneumonia classification

Microbiological classification is of limited value as the causative organism may not always be detected or microbiological diagnosis may take several days. Likewise, anatomical (radiographic) classification as 'lobar' (i.e. consolidation localized to one lobe) or 'bronchopneumonia' (i.e. patchy consolidation affecting ≥1 lobe) gives little practical information about the cause, course, or prognosis of pneumonia.

The following classification is widely accepted:

- **Community-acquired pneumonia (CAP):** describes an acute lower respiratory tract infection (LRTI), occurring prior to hospital admission in patients who have not recently been admitted to hospital and who do not reside in, or currently use (see HCAP below), other healthcare facilities (e.g. nursing homes, haemodialysis clinics). Common causative organisms include *Streptococcus pneumoniae* (20–70%), 'atypical' bacteria, including *Mycoplasma pneumoniae*, *Legionella* spp., and *Chlamydophila pneumoniae* (5–25%), *Haemophilus influenzae* (4–10%), and viral infections, including influenza A (8–12%). In most series, *Klebsiella pneumoniae* (<5%) and *Staphylococcus aureus* (<5%) infection are uncommon and associated with impaired host defences, alcoholism, dia-

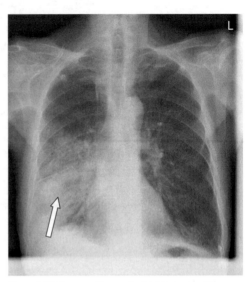

Figure 5.13 Community-acquired pneumonia with consolidation of the right lower lobe (arrow).

betes mellitus (DM), and chronic pulmonary disease (CPD).

- **Hospital-acquired (nosocomial) pneumonia (HAP):** is an LRTI developing >48 hours after hospital admission which was not incubating at the time of admission. Causative organisms differ from those in CAP and include Gram-negative bacilli (~45–70%) or staphylococci (~20%). HAP includes ventilator-associated pneumonia (VAP) which refers to pneumonia developing in patients receiving mechanical ventilation. VAP accounts for 80% of infections occurring in ICUs. Non-ICU HAP probably accounts for ~65% of HAP, but there are few data on these patients, as most studies have been performed in VAP. In the USA, healthcare-associated pneumonia (HCAP) is described and identifies patients who, at admission to hospital, are at immediate risk of pneumonia caused by 'hospital-acquired' type pathogens (i.e.

Table 5.10 Microorganisms and pathological insults that cause pneumonia

Bacterial infections	Atypical infections	Fungal infection
Streptococcus pneumoniae	Mycoplasma pneumoniae	Aspergillus
Haemophilus influenzae	Legionella pneumophila	Histoplasmosis
Klebsiella pneumoniae	Coxiella burnetii	Candida
Pseudomonas aeruginosa	Chlamydophilia psittaci	Nocardia
Gram-negative (E. coli)		

Viral infections	Protozoal infections	Other
Influenza A + B	Pneumocystis jiroveci	Aspiration
Coxsackie	Toxoplasmosis	Lipoid pneumonia
Adenovirus	Amoebiasis	Bronchiectasis
Respiratory syncytial	Paragonomiasis	Cystic fibrosis
Cytomegalovirus		Radiation

Gram-negative), rather than the expected 'community-acquired' pathogens (i.e. *S. pneumoniae*). HCAP includes any patient admitted to hospital for >2 days within 90 days of the current pneumonia, residing in a nursing home, receiving wound or intravenous therapy within 30 days of the current infection, or who attends a hospital or haemodialysis clinic.

* **Aspiration pneumonia:** is due to bacteroides and anaerobic organisms, following aspiration of oropharyngeal contents due to impaired laryngeal competence (e.g. CVA) or reduced consciousness (e.g. alcohol, drugs). The term 'aspiration pneumonia' is commonly applied to patients with risk factors for aspiration presenting with pneumonia, whereas true aspiration pneumonia is likely to be much less common. Periodontal and chronic lung disease (e.g. bronchiectasis) are also associated with anaerobic infections.
* **Opportunistic pneumonia:** occurs in HIV-positive cases or immunosuppressed patients on high-dose steroids or chemotherapy. These patients are susceptible to viral, fungal, and mycobacterial infections, in addition to the normal range of bacterial organisms.
* **Recurrent pneumonia:** is due to aerobic and anaerobic organisms, usually on a background of chronic lung disease (e.g. cystic fibrosis, bronchiectasis).
* **Rare pneumonias:** may be caused by a range of viral, bacterial, or fungal pathogens, including melioidosis, plague, anthrax, tularaemia, and nocardiosis.

Community–acquired pneumonia (CAP)

Epidemiology
Prospective population studies report an annual CAP incidence of 5–11 cases per 1,000 adult population. About 22–44% are hospitalized, and, of these, 1.2–10% require intensive care unit (ICU) admission. Incidence is highest in the very young and elderly (e.g. ~35 cases/year per 1,000 adults aged >75 years old). Mortality is <1% in cases treated at home, 5–12% in hospital, and >30% in ICU patients. In the USA, ~2.5 million cases of CAP cause 0.5 million hospital admissions and 45,000 deaths annually. Seasonal variations include *Streptococcus pneumoniae* and staphylococcal occurrence in winter; *Legionella* spp. infection in September to October and *Coxiella burnetii* in spring. Viral infections are commoner and predispose to CAP in the winter months. The occurrence of mycoplasma pneumonia has a cyclical pattern, with epidemics occurring every fourth year. This increases the normal incidence of mycoplasma pneumonia from ~5% to ~18% of all pneumonic episodes during epidemic years.

Aetiology
Identifying the causative pathogen in CAP is difficult, and study results vary, according to methodology used (e.g. bacterial quantification), geography (e.g. UK, Europe, USA), seasonal timing, severity of illness, site of study (e.g. community, hospital, or ICU), and patient population (e.g. 'atypical' bacteria are more common in the young). In routine care, an infective cause is found in <20% of cases.

* **Streptococcus pneumoniae** (20–70%) is the most frequently identified organism in hospitalized patients. It is a Gram-positive diplococcus with a complex polysaccharide capsule which provides the basis for serotyping. More than 90 serotypes are described, but only about 20 cause most of the infections.
  In the UK, *Streptococcus pneumoniae* antibiotic resistance is uncommon, and there has been no evidence of any

increase in recent years. Currently, ~6% of bacteraemia isolates and 8% of respiratory isolates are penicillin-resistant. Drug resistance rates vary globally and are >20% in some countries (e.g. Japan).

Pneumococcal infection occurs mainly in the winter and spring months. Aerosolized droplet transmission propagates the infection and is encouraged by overcrowding and poor ventilation. *S. pneumoniae* is the commonest cause of influenza-related secondary pneumonia.

Presentation is usually abrupt with fever, followed within hours by cough, dyspnoea, and rusty, mucoid sputum production. Pleurisy occurs in 75% of cases, and ~40% will develop a parapneumonic effusion, but empyema is rare (<1%) since the advent of antibiotics (see 'Pleural effusions').

Extrapulmonary symptoms (e.g. headache, abdominal discomfort) can occur. Unfortunately, the pneumococcus is recovered from sputum Gram stain and culture in <20% of cases. Bacteraemia occurs in about 10% of hospitalized patients and may occasionally cause metastatic infection (e.g. meningitis, endocarditis).

Although *S. pneumoniae* infection is 'classically' associated with 'lobar' pneumonia, 'bronchopneumonic' patterns of infection are equally common and cause corresponding clinical and radiological features. Radiological changes resolve over 4–8 weeks.

The prognosis in healthy young adults is excellent with appropriate antibiotic therapy, but the elderly and those with underlying comorbidity (e.g. cirrhosis) are at much higher risk. Mortality is 15–20% in hospitalized patients with bacteraemic pneumococcal pneumonia, increasing to 20–50% in patients >65 years old. Pneumococcal vaccination and smoking cessation are the major preventative measures.

* **'Atypical' bacterial pathogens** (~5–25%), including *Mycoplasma pneumoniae*, *Legionella* spp., and *Chlamydophila pneumoniae* are important causes of CAP. At presentation, they are indistinguishable from other pneumonias. Initial chest examination may be unremarkable, despite radiological abnormality, and the white cell count can be unexpectedly normal.
  * **Mycoplasma pneumoniae** (5–18%) usually causes URTI (e.g. pharyngitis) in the young and spreads by aerosolized transmission within families and closed communities. Outbreaks occur throughout the year but are more common in autumn. The incubation period is 9–20 days.

  Early symptoms include fever, rigors, cough, headache, with an URTI in ~25–50% of cases. Chest pain, dyspnoea, and myalgia are rare. Within days, the early symptoms resolve, and the patient is left with a low-grade fever (<39°C) and 'hacking', non-productive cough. Not uncommonly, chest examination is normal despite radiographic abnormalities.

  Extrapulmonary features may dominate the clinical and laboratory picture. Pharyngitis and cervical adenopathy affect ~25%, ear infection ~10%, and skin rashes (e.g. urticaria, erythema multiforme) ~25% of patients.

  The white cell count is normal in >75%, and cold agglutinins occur in 50% of cases. Autoimmune haemolysis is confirmed by a positive Coombs' test. Alveolar or interstitial parenchymal infiltrates may be segmental or multilobar on CXR. A microbiological diagnosis is made through PCR of respiratory tract samples or the detection of increased serological titres on acute convalescent

samples. Management of patients on the basis of a single raised titre is unreliable.

Mycoplasma pneumonia is usually a relatively benign, self-limiting disease, but severe complications include meningoencephalitis, fulminant intravascular haemolysis, Stevens–Johnson syndrome, pericarditis, and myocarditis.

Treatment is with tetracyclines, macrolides, or fluoroquinolones. Tetracycline and fluoroquinolones should be avoided in young children and pregnant women.

*   ***Chlamydophila pneumoniae*** (5–15%) is a recognized cause of CAP in college students and nursing home residents, particularly in the USA. It is often preceded by a mild URTI with fever and cough, and a sore throat may occur and resolve in the week before the pneumonia.

Serological tests are widely used, but problems relating to sensitivity and specificity remain. Microimmunofluorescence and whole cell immunofluorescence are used as reference tests.

Young patients usually recover, but fatalities can occur in the elderly with comorbid conditions. Treatment is with tetracyclines, macrolides, or fluoroquinolones.

*   ***Legionella species*** cause sporadic and epidemic outbreaks of CAP (2–15%) and HAP (2–5%). Over fifty *Legionella* species have been identified, some of which cause pneumonia, especially in immunocompromised patients (e.g. *Legionella micdadei* causes Pittsburgh pneumonia). The natural habitat of many *Legionella* species is water, and they are widely distributed throughout natural and synthetic reservoirs. *Legionella pneumophila* serogroup 1 accounts for over 90% of cases of legionnaires' disease (LD) in Europe and the USA. Outbreaks of *L. pneumophila* infection have been linked to air conditioners, water evaporating systems, whirlpool baths, and ultrasonic mist devices.

Infection occurs mainly in adults and is 2–3-fold more common in men. Risk factors include travel and domestic plumbing work.

Most cases affect the lungs, but a self-limiting illness with fever and headache (Pontiac fever) can occur. After an incubation period of 2–10 days, early constitutional symptoms include headache, rigors, lethargy, and myalgia. Pneumonic symptoms of high fever (~30% >40°C), non-productive cough, dyspnoea (~50%), pleurisy (~30%), and haemoptysis (~30%) develop within several days.

Extrapulmonary symptoms are common and may overshadow the respiratory complaint. They include diarrhoea (~50%), abdominal pain (~25%), bradycardia (~60% at the height of the fever), acute renal failure independent of associated shock (~10%), and neurological features of headache, confusion, obtundation, and seizures.

Laboratory findings include hyponatraemia and hypophosphataemia (>50%), raised liver function tests, and leucocytosis. Alveolar infiltrates on CXR lag behind the initial clinical illness but may take months to resolve. Rapid diagnosis of *L. pneumophila* serogroup 1 infection is possible with urinary antigen testing. Treatment with a fluoroquinolone (e.g. levofloxacin 750 mg od) is recommended. This may be combined with a macrolide (e.g. azithromycin or clarithromycin) in severely ill cases. Mortality is over 30% if ventilatory or renal support is required.

*   ***Haemophilus influenzae*** (4–7%) and ***Moraxella (Branhamella) catarrhalis*** (<5%) CAP occur particularly in elderly patients with underlying COPD, alcoholism, malnutrition, malignancy, and reduced immunity.
    *   ***H. influenzae:*** is a small fastidious Gram-negative rod that grows best in CO_2-enriched environments. They are typed (a–f), according to their polysaccharide capsules. However, most isolates that colonize the adult oropharynx do not have a capsule, are nontypable, and cause mild illness, except in the chronically ill or elderly patient. Type b accounts for most pneumonia in children. Transmission is through aerosolized droplets. Presentation and subsequent bronchopneumonia are indistinguishable from other causes of pneumonia, although a subacute onset, with low-grade fever and cough for several weeks, can occur. Both intrathoracic (e.g. empyema, haemoptysis) and extrathoracic (e.g. bacteraemia) complications are rare. Penicillin resistance in different parts of the UK range from 2 to 17%. Serious infections should be treated empirically with cefuroxime, a third-generation cephalosporin or a beta-lactam/beta-lactamase until sensitivities are known. Mortality from *H. influenzae* pneumonia is around 10%, though higher mortality rates (30%) occur in the elderly with underlying disease.
    *   ***M. catarrhalis:*** is a capnophilic, Gram-negative diplococcus. Pneumonia follows several days of dyspnoea and cough. Pleurisy, pleural effusion, and haemoptysis may occur, but extrapulmonary manifestations are rare. Single lobe involvement is most common, and CXR shows both lobar and bronchopneumonic consolidation. Virtually all *M. catarrhalis* is penicillin-resistant, and initial treatment with a beta-lactam/beta-lactamase (e.g. co-amoxiclav), cephalosporin, or quinolone is recommended. Macrolides are alternatives.

*   ***Other causes of CAP:*** include influenza A and other viral infections (8–18%; see Viral pneumonia). *Klebsiella pneumoniae* (<5%), other Gram-negative bacilli, and *Staphylococcus aureus* (<5%) are rare and often associated with other predisposing factors (e.g. compromised host defences, alcoholism, diabetes mellitus, heart failure, chronic pulmonary disease, and residence in nursing homes). Staphylococcal pneumonia often follows influenza and may account for up to 25% of CAP during influenza epidemics.

Risk factors for CAP are listed in Box 5.2. Specific factors include age (e.g. mycoplasma pneumonia is commoner in young adults), occupation (e.g. brucellosis in abattoir workers, *Coxiella burnetii* (Q fever) in sheep workers), environment (e.g. psittacosis with pet birds, tularaemia and erlichiosis due to tick bites), and geographical area (e.g. coccidioidomycosis in southwest USA). Epidemics of *Coxiella burnetti* or *Legionella* spp. infection are often localized. For example, patients with legionnaires' disease may have been exposed to a contaminated air conditioner at a specific hotel.

Diagnosis of CAP

This is inaccurate without a CXR and cannot be confidently made on the basis of the history and clinical findings alone. Similarly, several studies have demonstrated that the causative organism cannot be predicted from clinical features alone. In particular, 'atypical' pathogens (e.g. *Mycoplasma*

Box 5.2 Risk factors for pneumonia

Age: >65, <5 years old
Chronic disease (e.g. COPD, renal)
Diabetes mellitus (DM)
Immunosuppression (e.g drugs, HIV)
Alcohol dependency
Aspiration (e.g. epilepsy)
Recent viral illness (e.g. influenza)
Malnutrition
Mechanical ventilation
Post-operative (e.g. obesity, smoking)
Environmental (e.g. psittacosis)
Occupational (e.g. Q fever)
Travel abroad (e.g. paragonomiasis)
Air conditioning (e.g. *Legionella*)

discoloured sputum, haemoptysis). Signs include cyanosis, tachycardia, and tachypnoea, with focal dullness, crepitations, bronchial breathing, and pleuritic rub on chest examination. In some, especially older patients, non-respiratory features (e.g. headache, confusion, rashes, diarrhoea) may predominate. Complications are shown in Figure 5.14 and include bacteraemia, pleural effusions, and respiratory failure. An infected parapneumonic effusion (empyema) must be drained. Diagnosis is supported by demonstrating a low sugar content, acidic pH, elevated white cell count, and raised lactate dehydrogenase (LDH) in aspirated pleural fluid (see pleural disease section later in this chapter).

Investigation of CAP
This includes:
- **Blood tests:** a raised white cell count (WCC) and C-reactive protein (CRP) indicate infection; low albumin and raised renal function tests (e.g. urea and creatinine) indicate increased disease severity. Haemolysis and cold agglutinins occur in ~50% of mycoplasma pneumonias.
- **Blood gases:** identify respiratory failure.
- **Microbiology (± virology):** are essential but no pathogen is isolated in ~50–85% of cases due to previous antibiotic therapy, inadequate specimen collection, or limitations in microbiological tests. Collect sputum, pleural fluid, and bronchoalveolar lavage (BAL) samples. Appropriate staining (e.g. Gram stain), culture, and assessment of antibiotic sensitivity may determine the pathogen and effective therapy. Viral and atypical

pneumoniae) do not have a characteristic clinical presentation or course. The aims are to:
- **Establish the diagnosis.**
- **Assess severity** which determines the most appropriate ward placement (e.g. ward, HDU, or ICU).
- **Adjust antibiotic therapy** when microbiological results are available.
- **Identify and treat complications.**

Clinical features
Symptoms may be general (e.g. malaise, fever, rigors, myalgia) or chest-specific (e.g. dyspnoea, pleurisy, cough,

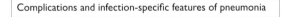

Complications and infection-specific features of pneumonia

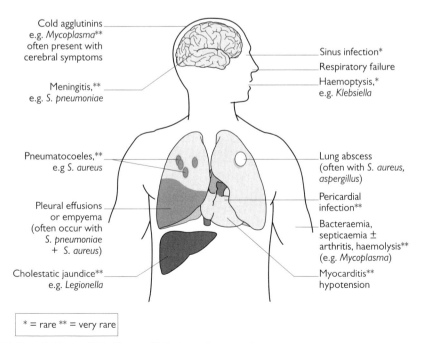

Cold agglutinins e.g. *Mycoplasma*** often present with cerebral symptoms

Meningitis,** e.g. *S. pneumoniae*

Pneumatocoeles,** e.g *S. aureus*

Pleural effusions or empyema (often occur with *S. pneumoniae* + *S. aureus*)

Cholestatic jaundice** e.g. *Legionella*

Sinus infection*
Respiratory failure
Haemoptysis,* e.g. *Klebsiella*

Lung abscess (often with *S. aureus, aspergillus*)
Pericardial infection**
Bacteraemia, septicaemia ± arthritis, haemolysis** (e.g. *Mycoplasma*)
Myocarditis** hypotension

* = rare ** = very rare

Figure 5.14 Complications and infection-specific features of pneumonia.

pathogens (e.g. *Mycoplasma* spp. and *Chlamydophila* spp.) can be identified using PCR techniques.

- **Blood cultures** are positive in ~25% of patients with severe pneumonia.
- **Serology** identifies atypical pathogens (e.g. *Mycoplasma* spp.), but processing time limits practical clinical value.
- **Urinary antigen detection tests** for *Legionella* spp. and *S. pneumoniae* are rapid and specific.
- **CXR** (see Figure 5.13) and **CT scans** confirm the diagnosis, monitor deterioration, indicate severity, and aid the early detection of complications. Resolution of CXR changes is slow (~4–6 weeks), and further radiological investigation is not usually necessary if the patient continues to improve clinically.

Severity assessment

Poor prognostic factors include:

- **Clinical:** age ≥65 years, respiratory rate (RR) ≥30/min, diastolic blood pressure (BP) ≤60 mmHg, new atrial fibrillation, confusion, coexisting disease (e.g. DM, COPD), and multilobar involvement on CXR.
- **Laboratory:** urea >7 mmol/L, albumin <35 g/L, hypoxaemia PO_2 <8 kPa, leucopenia (WCC <4 x 10^9/L), leucocytosis (WCC >20 x 10^9/L), and bacteraemia.

When assessing CAP severity, it is useful to bear in mind that mortality is increased twentyfold in a patient with a RR ≥30/min, low diastolic (≤60 mmHg) BP, and a urea >7 mmol/L.

The CURB-65 score allocates one point to each of the following: confusion; urea >7mmol/L; RR ≥30/min; low systolic (<90 mmHg) or diastolic (≤60 mmHg) BP, and age ≥65 years. The score stratifies patients into mortality groups suitable for different management pathways (see Figure 5.15). Scores of 3–5, 2, and 0–1 are associated with mortalities of >15%, 9%, and <3%, respectively. High scores (4 or 5) indicate the need for ICU. Low scores may allow home management, but caution is required, as patients with CAP can deteriorate rapidly. Severity scoring tools should be employed in conjunction with clinical judgement in all instances.

CAP management

- **Supportive measures:** include high concentration oxygen via a face mask to maintain PaO_2 >8 kPa (SaO_2 <90%); intravenous (IV) fluid (± inotropic support) to maintain a mean BP >65 mmHg and urine output >0.5–1 mL/kg/min. Physiotherapy may aid sputum clearance and sample collection for further microbiology. Nutritional support is important in prolonged illness. Corticosteroids may aid resolution and correct relative adrenocortical insufficiency (e.g. hydrocortisone 8 mg/h) in critically ill patients who require inotropic support for shock.
- **Ventilatory support:** may be required in respiratory failure. The role of non-invasive ventilation (e.g. CPAP, NIPPV) remains equivocal, as early studies were not beneficial and were potentially harmful. Persisting hypoxaemia (i.e. PaO_2 <8 kPa despite a high FiO_2), progressive hypercapnia, severe acidosis (pH <7.2), shock, or depressed consciousness are indications for mechanical ventilation. Alveolar recruitment strategies using positive end expiratory pressure (PEEP) aid oxygenation, and ventilator modes that avoid high peak pressures and alveolar hyperinflation are optimal.
- **Initial 'empirical' antibiotic therapy:** represents the 'best guess', according to severity, likely organisms, and

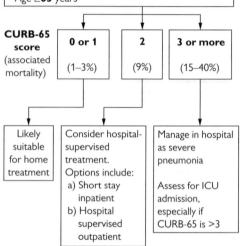

Score 1 point for each of:
- **C**onfusion (mental test score <8)
- **U**rea >7 mmol/L
- **R**espiratory rate ≥30/min
- **B**lood pressure (SBP <90 mmHg, DBP ≤ 60 mmHg)
- Age ≥**65** years

CURB-65 score (associated mortality)	**0 or 1** (1–3%)	**2** (9%)	**3 or more** (15–40%)
	Likely suitable for home treatment	Consider hospital-supervised treatment. Options include: a) Short stay inpatient b) Hospital supervised outpatient	Manage in hospital as severe pneumonia. Assess for ICU admission, especially if CURB-65 is >3

Figure 5.15 Severity scoring in CAP using the CURB-65 score. Reproduced from *Thorax*, Lim WS, *et al.*, 'British Thoracic Society guidelines for the management of community acquired pneumonia in adults: update 2009', 64, sIII, pp. iii1–iii55, copyright 2009, with permission from BMJ Publishing Group Ltd.

local antibiotic resistance patterns. Early antibiotic administration improves outcome, and, in the critically ill patient, treatment should not be unduly delayed for investigations or results. Microbiological findings are not usually available for >36 hours, but therapy is adjusted when results and antibiotic sensitivities are reported. North American and British (IDSA/ATS, BTS, NICE) recommendations for initial antibiotic therapy differ. Reference to the relevant guidelines is recommended.

- **Non-hospitalized patients** with:
  - Less severe illness usually responds to oral (PO) monotherapy therapy with amoxicillin 500 mg tds (BTS, NICE) or a macrolide (e.g. clarithromycin 500 mg bd) (BTS, IDSA/ATS) or doxycycline 100 mg od (after a 200 mg loading dose) (BTS, IDSA/ATS).
  - Risks for drug-resistant *S. pneumoniae* (e.g. recent antibiotics, comorbidity, alcoholism, immunosuppressive illness), in regions with high levels of *S. pneumoniae* resistance are treated with beta-lactams (e.g. high-dose amoxicillin 1 g tds or co-amoxiclav 2 g bd PO) plus macrolide or doxycycline PO; or antipneumococcal fluoroquinolone alone (e.g. levofloxacin 750 mg od PO) (IDSA/ATS).

  Treatment is usually for 7 days.

- **Hospitalized patients.** Antibiotic therapy to cover 'atypical' organisms and *S. pneumoniae*.
  - Low-severity CAP where admission is indicated for reasons other than pneumonia severity can usually be treated with amoxicillin alone (BTS).

- In moderate-severity CAP (i.e. not severe), combined beta-lactam (e.g. amoxicillin) plus a macrolide PO/IV (BTS, NICE) is recommended.
- In high-severity CAP, IV co-amoxiclav 1.2 g tds or a second-/third-generation cephalosporin (e.g. cefuroxime 1.5 g tds IV) plus a macrolide (e.g. clarithromycin 500 mg bd IV) is recommended (BTS, NICE). For patients admitted to ICU, the IDSA/ATS guidelines recommend a beta-lactam (e.g. ceftriaxone) plus either azithromycin or an antipneumoccocal fluoroquinolone PO (e.g. moxifloxacin).

In severe, microbiologically undefined CAP, treatment is usually for ~10 days. Legionella, staphylococcal, and Gram-negative pneumonias are usually treated for 14 21 days.

Treatment failure may be due to incorrect diagnosis (e.g. pulmonary embolism), an unexpected pathogen, slow clinical response in the elderly with secondary complications (e.g. empyema), inappropriate antibiotic, or impaired immunity.

Follow-up

Patients at risk of underlying lung cancer (e.g. smokers aged >50 years) should be reviewed, with a repeat CXR at 4–6 weeks.

Influenza and pneumoccocal vaccination are recommended for patients at risk of developing pneumonia (e.g. patients with COPD, diabetics, nursing home residents). If applicable, smoking cessation should be encouraged.

Hospital-acquired pneumonia

Hospital-acquired pneumonia (HAP), including ventilator-associated pneumonia (VAP), affects 0.5–2% of hospital patients. Pathogenesis, causative organisms, and outcome differ from CAP. Preventative measures and early antibiotic therapy, guided by an awareness of the potential role of multidrug-resistant (MDR) pathogens (see Box 5.3), improves outcome. Definitions: for HAP, VAP, and HCAP are reported earlier.

Epidemiology

HAP is the second commonest nosocomial infection (i.e. after urinary tract infections) and accounts for 15% of hospital-acquired infections in the USA/UK. It is the most important in terms of mortality. It affects 5–10 per 1,000 hospital admissions and lengthens hospital stay by 3–14 days/patient. Incidence is highest on surgical and ICU wards and in teaching hospitals. ICU HAP accounts for 37% of all HAP while VAP accounts for more than 80% of ICU HAP. In ICU, HAP/VAP accounts for 25% of infections and ~50% of all antibiotics used. The risk of developing VAP increases 6–20-fold during mechanical ventilation and occurs in between 9 and 27% of intubated patients. The VAP risk is

---

Box 5.3 Risk factors for multidrug-resistant pathogens causing hospital-acquired pneumonia

- Antimicrobial therapy in the previous 90 days
- Current hospitalization of >5 days
- High frequency of local antibiotic resistance
- Presence of risk factors for HCAP
  - Hospitalization for >2 days in the previous 90 days
  - Home wound care or intravenous therapy
  - Chronic dialysis within 30 days
  - Family member with MDR pathogen
- Immunosuppressive disease and/or therapy

3%/day during the first 5 days of mechanical ventilation, 2%/day during days 5–10, and 1%/day after this. As most mechanical ventilation is short-term, 50% of episodes occur during the first 4 days.

Pathogenesis

Microaspiration, which occurs in ~45% of normal people during sleep, is the main cause. In hospital, oropharyngeal colonization with enteric Gram-negative bacteria occurs in 75% of patients within 48 hours of admission. This is due to antibiotic therapy, immobility, instrumentation (e.g. nasogastric tubes), and poor attendant hygiene with cross infection. In addition, frequent inhibition of gastric acid secretion (e.g. proton pump inhibitors) decreases upper gastrointestinal tract sterility. Subsequent aspiration of oropharyngeal secretions (± gastric contents) is encouraged by supine position, impaired consciousness, difficulty swallowing and leakage past endotracheal tubes (ETT). An infected ETT biofilm with embolization to distal airways, and direct inoculation during airway suctioning introduces potentially infective organisms into the lower respiratory tract. Impaired mechanical, cellular, and humoral host defences and inability to clear secretions (e.g. sedation, postoperative pain) promote ensuing infection. Haematogenous spread from distant infected sites (e.g. central lines) also causes HAP.

Aetiology

HAP is caused by a wide spectrum of bacterial pathogens, and accurate data are limited. Time of onset (i.e. early or late-onset HAP) and risk factors for infection with multidrug-resistant (MDR) organisms determine potential pathogens (see Box 5.3). In general, the core bacterial pathogens implicated in HAP and VAP are similar. Core pathogens include *Streptococcus pneumoniae*, *Streptococcus* species, *Haemophilus influenzae*, *Enterobacteriaceae*, such as *Escherichia coli*, *Klebsiella* species, *Enterobacter* species, *Proteus* species, and *Serratia marcescens*, as well as meticillin-susceptible *Staphylococcus aureus*. Aerobic Gram-negative bacilli (see next section) cause ~45–70% of infections and Gram-positive bacteria (e.g. *Streptococcus pneumoniae* and *Staphylococcus aureus*) ~10–40%. Polymicrobial infection is increasing (~50%) and is especially high in ARDS cases. Isolated anaerobic infection occurs in 25% of cases. Viral and fungal infections are rare in immunocompetent hosts.

Gram-negative bacilliary pneumonia (45–70%)

This refers to infection with *Enterobacteriaceae* (including *Klebsiella*), *Pseudomonadaceae*, and other aerobic, non-fermentative Gram-negative bacilli. It excludes infections with *Haemophilus*, *Legionella*, and anaerobic organisms. Gram-negative bacilli cause 45–70% of HAP/VAP but less than 5% of CAP.

- **Klebsiella pneumoniae (Friedlander's bacillus):** causes ~20% of HAP/VAP, is more common in older (>40 years) men, and is often associated with alcohol abuse, diabetes mellitus, and chronic respiratory illness. The 'classical' presentation is with sudden, severe toxicity, high fever (>39°C), dyspnoea, pleurisy, and cough productive of large volumes of thick, bloody sputum with the consistency of 'redcurrant jelly'. Haemoptysis, prostration, shock, and bacteraemia (>25%) may develop. Clinical and radiological examination demonstrates severe, necrotizing lobar (~50% multilobar) consolidation, affecting mainly the upper lobes (often right) with loss of lung volume and abscess formation (~25%).

Complications are usually local (e.g. cavitation, fibrosis), rather than metastatic, and mortality is ~30–40%. Broad-spectrum, combination antibiotic therapy is required for at least 2 weeks, adjusted according to sensitivities. Surgical resection of infected tissue may be necessary if lobar gangrene develops.

- **Other Enterobacteriaceae**, including *Escherichia* (e.g. *E. coli*), *Serratia, Proteus, Morganella, Enterobacter*, and *Salmonella* cause pneumonia in debilitated or ventilated patients due to aspiration of oropharyngeal secretions. They are not sufficiently characteristic to distinguish individually. Infections are often polymicrobial, and blood cultures are positive in 20–30%. Respiratory features and radiological bronchopneumonia predominate. Mortality is ~40%.

- **Pseudomonas aeruginosa** is a hardy, ubiquitous organism that can use CO_2 and ammonia as its only carbon and nitrogen sources. These properties and its natural resistance to disinfectants encourage hospital survival where it contaminates sinks and vital equipment (e.g. ventilators, bronchoscopes). *Pseudomonas* pneumonia occurs in two distinct forms:

  - **Bacteraemic Pseudomonas pneumonia** affects neutropenic patients with haematological or lymphoproliferative malignancies because polymorphonuclear (PMN) leucocytes are required for organism eradication. Clinical features include severe toxicity, high fever, confusion, dyspnoea. Occasionally, cutaneous haemorrhagic macules develop into necrotic lesions as *P. aeruginosa* invades vascular tissue, causing vasculitis. Clinical and CXR features of bronchopneumonia and associated cavitation are often delayed.

  - **Non-bacteraemic Pseudomonas pneumonia** occurs typically in elderly, debilitated patients with immunosuppression, chronic pulmonary disease, and those requiring mechanical ventilation. Fever and respiratory features dominate the clinical picture. CXR usually demonstrates bilateral basal infiltration, occasionally with secondary abscesses and empyema. Multidrug-resistant organisms are common, and treatment requires aggressive combinations of broad-spectrum antibiotics. Mortality can exceed 40%, even with antibiotic therapy.

- **Acinetobacter species** (e.g. *Acinetobacter baumannii*) can cause a fulminant pneumonia in alcoholics. It occurs in specific geographical areas (e.g. Northern Territories of Australia). Nosocomial infection is usually associated with mechanical ventilation. Mortality is 50–65%.

Staphylococcus aureus (15–30%)

This is a facultative Gram-positive coccus, that causes beta-haemolysis on blood agar. It is responsible for ~15–30% of HAP/VAP but <5% of CAP (except after influenza outbreaks when it may cause ~25% of cases). Pneumonia due to *S. aureus* is more common in diabetics, intravenous drug users, and chronically ill ICU or head trauma patients. In ICU, >50% of *S. aureus* infections are meticillin-resistant (MRSA). The lungs are infected by either oropharyngeal aspiration or haematogenous spread. Nasal colonization occurs in 30–50% of healthy, asymptomatic adults and is greater in healthcare workers. Following oropharyngeal aspiration, respiratory symptoms predominate, whereas, in cases due to haematogenous spread, respiratory features may be absent or overshadowed by the underlying infection (e.g. endocarditis). Lobar consolidation is uncommon. Abscesses, pneumatocele formation, pleural effusions, and

empyema are common. Metastatic infection of joints, skin, kidneys, and brain occurs with haematogenous spread. Mortality is ~30%.

Mortality

The crude mortality rate for HAP is 30–70%. However, many critically ill patients die as a result of their underlying disease, rather than pneumonia. In case-matched VAP studies, 'directly attributable' mortality due to VAP is estimated to be 33–50%. Delayed or ineffective antibiotic therapy, bacteraemia (especially *P. aeruginosa* or *Acinetobacter* species), medical, rather than surgical, illness, and VAP increase mortality.

Early-onset HAP/VAP, defined as occurring within 4 days of hospital admission, is usually caused by antibiotic-sensitive bacteria. It carries a better prognosis than late-onset HAP/VAP, defined as occurring after ≥5 days in hospital, which is associated with MDR pathogens.

However, in early-onset HAP/VAP, prior antibiotic therapy or hospitalization predisposes to MDR pathogens and requires treatment as late-onset HAP/VAP.

Risk factors

These include those that predispose to CAP and factors associated with the development of MDR organisms and HAP pathogenesis (see Table 5.11). Critical risk factors include prolonged (>48 h) mechanical ventilation, duration of hospital or ICU stay, severity of illness (including acute physiology and chronic health evaluation (APACHE) scores), presence of acute respiratory distress syndrome (ARDS), and medical comorbidity. In ventilated patients, prior use of antibiotic therapy appears protective, whereas continuous sedation, cardiopulmonary resuscitation, high ventilatory pressures, upper airway colonization, and duration of ventilation are independent risk factors. **Prevention:** Table 5.11 lists modifiable risk factors that reduce the incidence of HAP.

Diagnosis

Diagnosis of HAP is based on clinical and microbiological assessment. It is difficult, as clinical features are non-specific and may be obscured by concurrent illness (e.g. ARDS). Previous antibiotic therapy limits microbiological evaluation.

- **Clinical criteria** include new radiographic infiltrates (± hypoxaemia) with at least two of three clinical features suggestive of infection (e.g. fever >38°C, purulent sputum, leucocytosis, or leucopenia). Purulent tracheobronchitis may mimic the clinical features of HAP.

- **Diagnostic tests** verify infection and determine the causative organism and antibiotic sensitivity. They include the routine blood and radiographic tests used in CAP, blood cultures, diagnostic thoracocentesis of pleural effusions, and lower respiratory tract cultures, including endotracheal aspirates and BAL in intubated patients. CT scans aid diagnosis and detection of complications, including cavitation, effusions, and haemoptysis (see Figures 5.15 and 5.16).

Management

Early diagnosis and treatment improves morbidity and mortality and requires constant vigilance in hospital patients. Antibiotic therapy must not be delayed whilst awaiting diagnostic and microbiological results.

- **Supportive therapy** includes supplemental oxygen to maintain PaO_2 >8 kPa (oxygen saturation >90%) and intravenous fluids (± inotropes) to maintain a mean blood pressure >65 mmHg and urine output 0.5–1 mL/kg/min. Physiotherapy and analgesia aid sputum clearance

Table 5.11 Risk factors for HAP and VAP

Unmodifiable risk factors	Modifiable risk factors
1. Host-related • Malnutrition • Age: >65, <5 years old • Chronic disease (e.g. renal) • Diabetes • Immunosuppression (e.g SLE) • Alcohol dependency • Aspiration (e.g. epilepsy) • Recent viral illness • Obesity • Smoking **2. Therapy-related** • Mechanical ventilation • Post-operative **3. Epidemiological factors** • Hot/cold water systems (e.g. *Legionella*), note that hospital outbreaks of *Legionella* are mainly due to *Legionella* in hospital water systems	**1. Host-related** • Avoid enteral feeding • Pain control, physiotherapy • Limit immunosuppresive therapy • Posture, kinetic beds • Preoperative smoking cessation **2. Therapy-related** • Adopt semi-recumbent posture (30° head up) • Remove IV lines, ET/NG tubes early • Minimize sedative use • Avoid gastric overdistension • Avoid intubation + re-intubation • Maintain ET cuff pressure >20 cmH$_2$O • Subglottic aspiration during intubation • Change + drain ventilator circuits • ? Sucralfate stress ulcer prophylaxis **3. Infection control** • Hand washing, sterile technique • Patient isolation • Microbiological surveillance

in post-operative and immobile patients. Heavy sedation and paralytic agents which depress cough are avoided. Semi-recumbent nursing, with 30° elevation of the bed head, reduces the risk of aspiration and associated pneumonia. Continuous subglottic aspiration, using specially designed ETTS, reduces early-onset VAP. Frequency of ventilator circuit changes does not alter the incidence of VAP.

• **Blood sugar control.** Hyperglycaemia is associated with poor outcomes in critical illness and current guidelines recommend insulin therapy should aim to maintain serum glucose (SG) levels between 5.5 (100) and 9 (150) mmol/L (mg/dl). These parameters optimize the potential benefits of blood sugar control whilst reducing the risk of potentially harmful hypoglycaemia (SG <4mmol/L (70mg/dl))

• **Stress ulcer prophylaxis** with sucralfate prevents gastric bacterial overgrowth at normal gastric pH and may rep-

resent a lower risk for VAP, compared with proton pump inhibitors.

• **Ventilatory support**, including non-invasive (e.g. CPAP, NIPPV) or mechanical ventilation, may be required in respiratory failure (see 'CAP management').

Antibiotic therapy is empirical whilst awaiting microbiological guidance. The causative organisms and effective antibiotics differ from CAP. The key decisions are, firstly, whether the patient has risk factors for MDR organisms (see Box 5.3) and, secondly, whether the HAP/VAP is early or late-onset, which determines the need for broad-spectrum (i.e. combination) antibiotic therapy. Initial therapy should be intravenous in all patients. The starting empiric treatment regime will need modification in ~50% of cases due to either resistant organisms or failure to respond. Nevertheless, getting antibiotic treatment 'right the first time' is important because mortality is lower in patients receiving effective initial antibiotic therapy, compared to those that require a treatment change. Consequently, local patterns of infection and antibiotic resistance must be used to establish the 'best empiric regimen' for individual hospitals. The ATS guidelines (2005) for initial antibiotic therapy in HAP/VAP is given below (see Figure 5.17). Alternative regimens can be found in the 2008 Canadian clinical practice and 2014 NICE guidelines for HAP/VAP.

• **Early-onset HAP/VAP** (≤4 days in hospital) with no risk factors for MDR organisms is treated with antibiotic monotherapy; either a beta-lactam/beta-lactamase inhibitor (e.g. piperacillin-tazobactam 4.5g qds IV) or a third-generation cephalosporin (e.g. ceftazidime 2 g tds IV) or a fluoroquinolone (e.g. ciprofloxacin 400 mg tds IV)

• **Late-onset HAP/VAP** (≥5 days in hospital) with risk factors for MDR pathogens (see Box 5.3) requires treatment covering MDR Gram-negative bacilli and MRSA using a broad-spectum antibiotic regime, including:

  • An antipseudomonal cephalosporin (e.g. ceftazidine 2g tds IV) or an antipseudomonal carbapenem (e.g. imipenem 0.5–1g qds IV) or a beta-lactam/beta-lactamase inhibitor (e.g. piperacillin-tazobactam 4.5g qds IV).

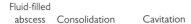

Fluid-filled
abscess   Consolidation   Cavitation

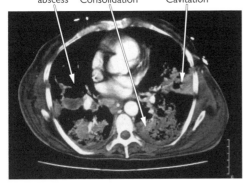

Figure 5.16 CT scan from a patient with HAP showing consolidation, cavitation, and abscess formation.

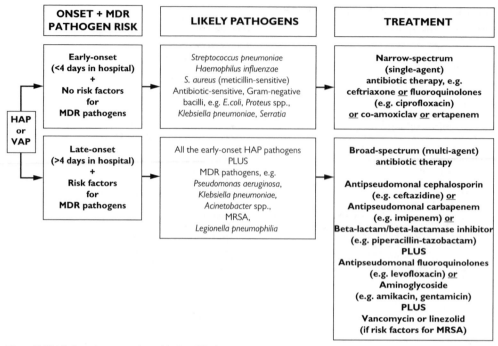

Figure 5.17 Likely pathogens and empirical antibiotic treatment of hospital-acquired pneumonias. Data from Figure 2, Table 3, and Table 4 in the 'American Thoracic Society: Guidelines for the management of adults with hospital-acquired, ventilator-associated, and healthcare-associated pneumonia', *American Journal of Respiratory Critical Care Medicine*, 2005, 171, pp. 388–416.

- *Plus* an antipseudomonal fluoroquinolone (e.g. levofloxacin 750 mg od IV) *or* aminoglycoside (e.g. gentamicin 7 mg/kg od IV; maintain monitored trough levels <1 mcg/mL).
- *Plus* vancomycin 15 mg/kg bd IV (maintain monitored trough levels at 15–20 mcg/mL) *or* linezolid 600 mg bd IV.
- *Adjunctive therapy* with inhaled aerosolized aminoglycosides or polymyxin should be considered in patients not improving with systemic antibiotic therapy or who have VAP due to MDR Gram-negative pathogens and/or carbapenem-resistant *Acinetobacter* species.

If the clinical response is good, a short course of therapy (e.g. 7 days) is appropriate. However, aggressive or resistant pathogens (e.g. *P. aeruginosa*) require treatment for 14–21 days (or longer). Overuse of antibiotics is avoided by tailoring therapy to lower respiratory tract culture results, withdrawing unnecessary antibiotics and shortening treatment duration to the minimum effective period. Sterile cultures, in the absence of new antibiotics in the preceding 72 hours, virtually excludes the presence of HAP (94% negative predictive value for VAP), and withdrawal of antibiotic therapy should be considered. Although there is some evidence for a reduction in ICU-acquired VAP following prophylactic antibiotic administration, routine use is **not** recommended.

Aspiration/anaerobic pneumonia
Bacteroides and other anaerobic infections follow aspiration of oropharyngeal contents due to impaired laryngeal competence (e.g. CVA) or reduced consciousness (e.g. drugs, alcohol). Pure anaerobic infection occurs in 30–60%

of patients, with mixed anaerobic, aerobic, and facultative organisms in the remaining third. The most commonly isolated anaerobic organisms are Gram-negative *Fusobacterium nucleatum* or Gram-positive *Peptostreptococcus* and microaerophilic *Streptococcus* species. *Bacteroides fragilis* occur in 5–20% of cases. The major aerobic and facultative organisms recovered in conjunction with anaerobes are *Streptococcus* species, *S. aureus*, *Pseudomonas*, and other enteric Gram-negative bacilli.

Aspiration syndromes are discussed in the section 'Airways obstruction, aspiration syndromes, and near-drowning' in this chapter. Prevention is essential (i.e. swallowing assessment), as gastric contents are acidic and cause alveolar inflammation and damage within minutes of inhalation. Aspiration may be microscopic, for example, in elderly patients with impaired swallowing, and the onset of pneumonia is often insidious and unrecognized, with coughing during eating or drinking and repeated minor infections. Specific anaerobic coverage in such circumstances is not required in the vast majority of cases. Large aspirations are potentially life-threatening. Tracheal suctioning or bronchoscopy remove large particles but do not prevent or reduce the subsequent alveolitis due to gastric acid aspiration. If ARDS develops, mortality can be as high as 90%. Broad-spectrum antibiotic therapy should include anaerobic coverage (e.g. metronidazole). Lung abscesses are a common complication and may require prolonged oral antibiotic therapy.

Pneumonia during immunosuppression
Patients with HIV, bone marrow transplant, or receiving chemotherapy are susceptible to viral (e.g. cytomegalovirus),

fungal (e.g. aspergillus), and mycobacterial infections, in addition to the normal range of organisms. Severely immunocompromised patients require isolation, barrier nursing, and potential treatment with combined broad-spectrum antibiotic (e.g. piperacillin, vancomycin, metronidazole), antifungal (e.g. amphotericin), and antiviral (e.g. aciclovir) regimes. HIV patients with CD4 counts <200/mm^3 are at high risk of opportunistic infections, including *Pneumocystis jirovecii* pneumonia, toxoplasmosis, and mycobacterial infections.

Recurrent pneumonia

Recurrent pneumonia with predominantly aerobic organisms occurs in cystic fibrosis and bronchiectasis (see section on 'Bronchiectasis and cystic fibrosis' in this chapter).

Rare bacterial pneumonias

Rare bacteria account for <5% of bacterial pneumonias.

* **Streptococci** (other than *S. pneumoniae*) cause <1% of adult pneumonia but account for 10% of empyemas. They include *S. pyogenes* (group A beta-haemolytic streptococcus), which often follows viral URTI and can occur as epidemics (e.g. military camps), and group B streptococci, which occasionally causes pneumonia in debilitated adults but is a major cause in neonates.
* **Psittacosis** is caused by *Chlamydophila psittaci*. It is a systemic infection, but pulmonary manifestations predominate. Over 50% of cases occur in the owners of infected birds (e.g. canaries), but 25% of cases are sporadic. After a 1–2 week incubation period, it presents with an influenza-like illness, including fever, myalgia, headache, and arthragia. This may be followed by inappropriate bradycardia and respiratory symptoms of dry cough, pleurisy, and progressive dyspnoea. Splenomegaly, a pale macular rash (Horder's spots), and CXR bronchopneumonic infiltrates may occur. Complement-fixing antibodies do not distinguish between *Chlamydophila* species. Microimmunofluorescence and PCR techniques are increasingly used for diagnosis. Doxycyline is the treatment of choice. Macrolides and quinolones are also effective.
* **Coxiella burnetii** (Q fever) is a zoonotic, systemic infection that affects a wide range of domestic (e.g. sheep) and wild animals, rodents, and insects. Infected animals usually have no evidence of disease. The organism multiplies in the placenta of infected animals during pregnancy. Humans become infected after inhaling organisms aerosolized at the time of parturition. The organism is resistant to drying and remains infective for months whilst dormant in contaminated soil. It is associated with occupational exposure to farm animals and animal products (e.g. tanneries, wool-processing plants).

  After an incubation period of 2–4 weeks, a self-limiting influenza-like illness develops, but 10–20% of patients develop symptoms of a dry cough, fever, dyspnoea, haemoptysis, and chest pain. Severe cases report neck stiffness, myalgia, and headache. High fever, relative bradycardia, conjunctivitis, and chest crepitations are typical, but rashes are uncommon. Raised liver function tests reflect subclinical granulomatous hepatitis, but the white count is usually normal. Although patients are acutely ill, the disease is rarely fatal and resolves in ~2 weeks. Subacute endocarditis is an important late complication and may develop months after the initial infection.

  A diagnosis is usually made based on a combination of epidemiological and clinical features plus a 4-fold rise in acute convalescent antibody titres. The organism can be cultured, but this requires biosafety level 3 laboratory facilities and is not routinely conducted. Tetracycline is the recommended first-line therapy. Macrolides and quinolones are also effective.

* **Actinomycosis and nocardiosis:** are bacteria that cause insidious chronic chest infections. They may resemble tuberculosis, malignancy, and chronic fungal infections. Nocardiosis is associated with distant haematogenous spread, particularly to the central nervous system (e.g. cerebral abscesses) and skin.
* **Melioidosis:** is caused by *Burkholderia* (previously *Pseudomonas*) *pseudomallei*, which is found in soil, vegetation, and water. It occurs in tropical regions (mainly Thailand) and causes either a fulminant septicaemic pneumonia or indolent cavitary infection, following cutaneous inoculation and haematogenous spread.
* **Pasturella multocida:** an oropharyngeal commensal in animals, may cause pneumonia after a cat or dog bite.
* **Tularaemia:** due to *Francisella tularensis*, is widely distributed in the temperate Northern hemisphere. It causes an acute pneumonic illness after contact with infected tissue from a wild or domestic animal or a bite from an infected tick or deerfly. It classically occurs in hunters and is associated with a painful ulcer and adenopathy at the infection site. Streptomycin is the treatment of choice, but gentamicin and tetracyclines are effective.
* **Plague:** is caused by *Yersinia pestis*, a zoonosis carried by small ground animals (e.g. rats, rodents) and transmitted by fleas. Aerosol-mediated transmission causes pneumonia. Bubonic, septicaemic, and pneumonic forms of plague occur and caused millions of deaths during the pandemics of the 14th and 19th centuries. Plague pneumonia develops 2–7 days after exposure, with fever, chest pain, cough, dyspnoea, and haemoptysis. If pulmonary disease is complicating bubonic plague, painful adenopathy is also present. Shock may occur with septicaemia. Treatment is with streptomycin or tetracycline.
* **Bacillus species:** *Bacillus anthracis* (anthrax) resides in soil, water, and vegetation and usually infects sheep and cows. Occupational exposure to hides and wool is the major cause of human anthrax which is normally cutaneous or gastrointestinal. The inhalational form (woolsorters' disease due to inhaled spores) is rare. A 2-stage illness is evident. The first stage resembles a viral illness. Following a transient improvement, severe pneumonia and shock develop. High-dose penicillin is the treatment of choice. Alternatives are ciprofloxacin or doxycycline.

Viral pneumonia

Viral upper respiratory tract infections are common self-limiting infections, whereas viral pneumonia is an infrequent, but serious, cause of pneumonia. In hospital, viral infections are implicated in between 8 and 12% of adult and ~50% of infant pneumonias.

The influenza virus causes >50% of viral pneumonias in healthy adults, but adenovirus, parainfluenza, respiratory syncytial virus, hantavirus, and measles virus also cause sporadic cases. Immunosuppressed patients are susceptible to cytomegalovirus (CMV), herpes simplex, and varicella zoster infections. Viral pneumonia is difficult to differentiate from bacterial infection, except for measles and varicella zoster which are distinguished by the associated rash. Viral cultures or PCR and serological tests may establish a causative virus.

Treatment is largely supportive, combined with early antiviral therapy in selected infections and antibiotic therapy in secondary bacterial infections. Some cases have a progressive, relentless course, with extensive alveolar and interstitial infiltration, and are fatal despite supportive therapy and mechanical ventilation.

- **Influenza A and B viruses** cause sporadic cases or epidemic/pandemic outbreaks, with significant morbidity and mortality. Viral genetic mutations result in antigenic variation. Consequently, vaccines require constant updating. Healthy adults are often affected, but elderly, immunocompromised, unwell, or institutionalized patients are particularly susceptible. Typical clinical features of infection include an abrupt onset of fever and cough, associated with headache, myalgia, malaise, retrosternal discomfort, and nasal congestion. By the third day of illness, symptoms usually abate. In a minority of patients, progression of respiratory symptoms (especially dyspnoea), hypoxaemia, and CXR infiltrates indicates the development of a primary viral pneumonia. Non-respiratory complications are infrequent and include myocarditis, myositis, and abdominal pain that may mimic appendicitis. Otitis media is common in children. Secondary bacterial pneumonia is common in children and adults and is most frequently due to *S. pneumoniae*, although *S. aureus* accounts for >25% of cases. Vaccination is protective and is indicated for all high-risk subjects, such as the elderly with chronic respiratory diseases. Neuraminidase inhibitors, such as zanamivir and oseltamivir are effective for chemoprophylaxis and treatment against both influenza A and B.
- **Cytomegalovirus** is ubiquitous and harmless in normal adults. However, in the immunocompromised subject, it causes a generalized infection, involving multiple organ systems, of which pneumonia is the most frequently recognized life-threatening event. Diagnosis is usually based on a combination of clinical features, supported by evidence of viraemia (by antigen or PCR testing on blood or BAL fluid) or tissue invasion (i.e. biopsies show 'owl eye' inclusion bodies in infected cells). Effective antiviral agents include ganciclovir and foscarnet.
- **Adenovirus** was recognized as a cause of pneumonia in military recruits. Proven, effective antiviral treatment is not available. Ganciclovir and ribavirin have been tried in severe pneumonic infections.
- **Hantavirus** was first recognized as a cause of acute respiratory illness in healthy young adults in southwestern USA in 1993. It develops following inhalation of the virus from aerosolized rodent urine or faeces. After prodromal fever, myalgia, malaise, and abdominal discomfort, progressive cough and dyspnoea develop due to increased alveolar permeability, which may progress to ARDS. Laboratory testing reveals neutrophilia, thrombocytopenia, mild liver dysfunction, and in some cases, renal impairment. CXR demonstrates pulmonary infiltrates. Treatment is supportive with careful fluid management. Studies assessing ribavirin therapy are inconclusive. Mortality is 30–50%
- **Measles** is rare in adults, but lower respiratory tract infection with reticulonodular infiltrates occurs in up to 50% of cases. Pneumonia occurs in immunocompromised patients, pregnant women, and, rarely, in normal subjects. In-hospital mortality rates are >40%, and secondary bacterial infection occurs in >30%. No antiviral therapy is of proven value, but ribavirin and immunoglobulin have been used.

- **Respiratory syncytial virus** is a major cause of viral lower respiratory tract infection in young children. It is particularly severe in infants <6 months of age, in whom it is the principal cause of bronchiolitis and viral pneumonia. In adults, it causes an unpleasant upper respiratory infection, except in the immunocompromised and those with coexisting disease in whom mortality can be >60% (e.g. bone marrow transplant recipients).
- **Varicella** pneumonia is a rare, and sometimes serious, complication of varicella zoster infection (i.e. chickenpox, shingles) in healthy adults, pregnant and immunocompromised subjects. It presents 1–6 days after the onset of the rash, with fever, tachypnoea, cough, dyspnoea, pleurisy, and haemoptysis. Infected patients are very infectious and require isolation. Radiographs show diffuse nodular infiltrates which resolve, occasionally leaving miliary calcification. Treatment is with aciclovir 10 mg/kg for 7 days. Most cases recover, but mortality may be up to 40% in certain patients (e.g. in pregnancy).
- **Severe acute respiratory syndrome (SARS)** is a rapidly progressive acute respiratory illness that emerged in China in 2002 and rapidly spread worldwide. It is due to a previously unrecognized coronavirus (SARS-CoV). It is spread in aerosolized airways secretions and by person-to-person contact. After an incubation period of 2–10 days, it presents with high fever, headache, and myalgia. A lower respiratory tract infection follows, with watery diarrhoea in about 25% and diffuse CXR infiltrates consistent with pneumonia or ARDS. Treatment is supportive, as there is no active antiviral agent. Overall mortality is 11% but >40% if aged >60 years old.

Fungal respiratory disease

Aspergillus lung disease: *Aspergillus fumigatus* is a ubiquitous fungus which can affect the lung as follows:

- **Atopic allergy and asthma:** due to IgE (type I) mediated allergy to inhaled *Aspergillus* spores, with subsequent airways inflammation. About 10% of asthmatics are skin prick-positive to *Aspergillus* species. Asthmatics with IgE responses to *Aspergillus* can also develop IgG antibodies, blood eosinophilia, and occasionally hyphae in sputum, with mucous plugging and distal consolidation causing flitting CXR infiltrates. Treatment with short courses of oral corticosteroids and an increase in inhaled corticosteroid therapy is usually effective.
- **Allergic bronchopulmonary aspergillosis** is due to type I and type III hypersensitivity to *Aspergillus fumigatus*. Initial bronchoconstriction is followed by more severe airways inflammation which damages bronchial walls, causing bronchiectasis. Patients usually have a long history of asthma, with recent deterioration, including wheeze, dyspnoea, cough, and expectoration of dark mucous plugs. Diagnostic features include raised IgE and IgG, blood eosinophilia, and flitting lung infiltrates and central bronchiectasis on CXR. Acute episodes are treated with courses of corticosteroids, such as prednisolone (30–40 mg). Addition of itraconazole may reduce maintenance steroid requirements and improve exercise capacity.
- **Invasive aspergillus pneumonia** occurs when *Aspergillus* hyphae invade tissue, usually in the lung. Haematogenous spread may occur to any part of the body, mostly in immunosuppressed patients. Presentation is with fever, chest pain, dyspnoea, cough, haemoptysis, and pulmonary infiltrates in a severely neutropenic patient, typically due to chemotherapy, advanced HIV disease, or

immunosuppressive therapy for transplants. Prolonged antibiotics, high-dose steroids, and SLE are also risk factors. Diagnosis is usually based on clinical features, supported by biopsy (e.g. transbronchial) detection of invasive hyphae, or typical X-ray findings (e.g. halo sign, a ring of 'ground glass' shadowing around a denser pulmonary nodule or mass) on thoracic CT scanning. Treatment is with antifungal agents such as intravenous amphotericin (nephrotoxic), lipophilic amphotericin (less nephrotoxic), itraconazole (liver toxicity), voraconizole (oral), or caspofungin.

- **Semi-invasive aspergillosis** (chronic necrotizing aspergillosis) describes a low-grade chronic invasion of *Aspergillus* into airway walls and lung, typically in patients with pre-existing chronic lung disease and mild immunocompromise (e.g. steroid therapy, diabetes mellitus). Patients develop fever and cough, with patchy shadows and small cavities on CXR. The CT scan findings include areas of chronic progressive peripheral consolidation, multiple nodular opacities, tree in bud shadowing, and cavitation. Oral antifungals such as voriconazole and itraconazole are recommended.

- **Aspergilloma/mycetoma** describes a ball of fungus within a pre-existing lung cavity often caused by tuberculosis. Most are asymptomatic, but malaise, fever, weight loss, cough, and chest pain may occur. Up to 75% present with haemoptysis, which may be massive, from blood vessels on the inner wall of the cavity. Most do not require treatment, but antifungals may reduce the tendency to haemoptysis. Occasionally, bronchial angiograms with arterial embolization, surgery, or intracavitary injections of amphotericin paste are required to control life-threatening haemoptysis (see section on 'Haemoptysis' earlier in this chapter).

- **Extrinsic allergic alveolitis (EAA)** is caused by sensitivity to *Aspergillus* spores (e.g *Aspergillus clavatus* in malt workers lung) and is managed as for other EAA (see hypersensitivity pneumonitis in section on 'Diffuse parenchymal (interstitial) lung disease' in this chapter).

Pneumocystis pneumonia

Pneumocystis pneumonia (PCP) is caused by *Pneumocystis jirovecii* (previously termed *Pneumocystis carinii*), a widespread environmental fungi, causing commensal infection in most people. Pathological infection usually occurs in immunocompromised patients with advanced HIV (CD4 <200 x 10^6/L), on treatment with chemotherapy (e.g. fludarabine) or corticosteroids, and in severely malnourished children. It is much less common since the use of prophylactic septrin in high-risk cases. It presents with gradual onset of fever, dry cough, exertional dyspnoea, chest tightness, tachypnoea and rarely pneumothorax. Chest auscultation is often normal. Initial exercise-induced desaturation progresses to resting hypoxaemia. CXR may be normal (~10%), but most show bilateral, perihilar alveolar infiltrates. However, consolidation or focal nodules are seen occasionally. Diagnosis can be confirmed from induced sputum in ~60–70% of HIV cases, but this procedure is less effective in non-HIV immunocompromised patients (as there are less organisms). Bronchoscopy with BAL and subsequent silver or immunofluorescent staining is diagnostic in >90% of cases. Occasionally, transbronchial biopsy or surgical lung biopsy may be required. If PCP is strongly suspected and the patient is unwell, treatment is started before confirmation, as pneumocysts are detectable for up to 2 weeks.

PCP is treated with:

- **High-dose co-trimoxazole** (120 mg/kg in four divided intravenous doses daily and then orally with improvement) for 2–3 weeks. Side effects, including rashes, vomiting and blood disorders occur in ~30% of cases. Pentamidine, atovaquone, and dapsone with trimethoprim are second-line alternatives.

- **High-dose steroids** (prednisolone 40–80 mg/day for 5 days, tapering over 2 weeks) are given if the patient has respiratory failure.

- **Supportive therapy** includes high-dose oxygen therapy, CPAP, and, when appropriate, mechanical ventilation. Liaise with infectious disease and HIV specialists early, and consider introduction of highly active antiretroviral therapy (HAART) in newly presenting HIV cases.

Mortality is <10% in HIV (60% in those requiring mechanical ventilation) and ~30% in cancer patients. Prophylaxis with co-trimoxazole (480 mg/day) is indicated if the CD4 count is <200 x 10^6/L in HIV patients, and after initial infection, as relapse is common (>50% in 12 months).

Other fungal pneumonias

- **Candida pneumonia.** *Candida* is part of the normal human flora. Invasive disease, usually candidaemia, occurs in the immunocompromised (e.g. transplant patients), following surgery, and in those with central lines (e.g. parenteral nutrition). Pulmonary involvement is rare, non-specific, and usually occurs in association with high fever and systemic infection (e.g. eyes, skin, liver, CNS). Confirmation of lung disease usually involves transbronchial or surgical lung biopsy. Patients with confirmed or treated *Candida* pneumonia require fundoscopy and review by an ophthalmologist. CXR may show nodules or infiltrates. Treatment is with fluconazole (400 mg daily) or intravenous amphotericin. Central lines should be removed. Candidaemia mortality is 30–40%.

- **Cryptococcal pneumonia.** *Cryptococcus neoformans* is found in bird droppings worldwide. After inhalation, it propagates asymptomatically in alveoli and then migrates to the CNS where it causes meningoencephalitis in patients with impaired cell-mediated immunity (e.g. AIDS, lymphoma, steroid use). Clinical lung disease is rare and usually associated with meningitis. Onset is acute or chronic, with fever, cough, and non-specific CXR changes. The diagnosis is established, using India ink stains or culture of CSF, BAL, sputum, blood, or urine, or the cryptococcal antigen test which is both sensitive and specific. Immunocompromised patients are treated with amphotericin and flucytosine for 2–3 weeks, followed by fluconazole. Observation alone is often adequate in immunocompetent patients, but some cases require fluconazole therapy.

- **Endemic mycoses.** Cause pulmonary disease in specific regions. Infection is usually asymptomatic, mild, and self-limiting within 2–4 weeks in the immunocompetent. However, patients with impaired T cell-mediated immunity (e.g. AIDS, steroid therapy, lymphoma) are at risk of severe, widespread disease. Sporadic cases or outbreaks can occur. Progressive disease and immunocompromised patients may need to be treated with long courses of oral itraconazole (3–24 months) or intravenous amphotericin in severe cases.

  - **Histoplasmosis.** *Histoplasma capsulatum* is found in soil contaminated by bat and bird droppings in southeast USA, Mexico, and South America. Following fungal inhalation, infective manifestations are very variable. They include asymptomatic cases with normal CXR or nodules (which calcify to form 'target lesions'); acute flu-like illnesses, following heavy fungal exposure (e.g. cavers); progression to respiratory failure, with widespread alveolar infiltrates on CXR; chronic progressive disease with cavitation; and widespread pulmonary and systemic dissemination in the immunocompromised. Rare features include mediastinal fibrosis with compression of airways, oesophagus, and superior vena cava, broncholithiasis, erythema nodosum, arthritis, and pericarditis. Serological or culture diagnosis can take several weeks.

- **Blastomycosis.** Infection with *Blastomyces dermatitis* follows inhalation of spores from infected soil (the fungus, which appears as a white cottony mould, lives in soil and rotten wood near lakes and rivers) in southeast USA, Africa, India, and the Middle East. It is less common than histoplasmosis. It may present with an acute flu-like illness, ARDS-like respiratory failure, and chronic or disseminated disease (with characteristic ulcerated, verrucous, dermal lesions in 60% of cases). Staining or culture of infected material is usually diagnostic. Treatment with itraconazole for at least 6 months is usually recommended.

- **Coccidioidomycosis** ('valley fever', 'California fever') is due to inhalation of *Coccidioides immitis* spores from infected soil (where it grows as a mycelium) in southwest USA and Mexico. It causes acute, chronic, or disseminated disease, including symptomatic CAP, but most are asymptomatic and self-limiting. Fluconazole is the treatment of choice.

- **Paracoccidioidomycosis** occurs in Mexico and Central or South America. Acute, disseminated infection occurs in the immunocompromised, with infected lymphadenopathy and mucosal lesions (e.g. lips, oral) but typically it causes a chronic pulmonary disease. Prolonged treatment with itraconazole is required.

Parasitic lung disease

Many parasites can infect the lungs, but clinical disease is rare in temperate climates. Pulmonary disease is due to:

- **Direct infection**, for example:
  - **Pulmonary hydatid disease** (see Chapter 6) is the commonest parasitic lung disease and occurs mainly in sheep-raising areas. It follows ingestion of parasitic eggs from adult worms found in sheep, dogs, horses, and camels. It usually occurs as cystic disease when *Echinococcus granulosus* larvae grow slowly in lungs. Most human infection is asymptomatic. Presentation is with cough, haemoptysis, chest discomfort, and rounded cysts, occasionally with calcified walls, in the lower lobes on CXR. Cyst rupture causes wheeze, eosinophilia, and spread (e.g. to pleura). Alveolar hydatid disease due to *E. multilocularis* is much less common but is fatal if untreated. Infection initially develops almost exclusively in the liver. It causes tissue invasion, and the associated CXR masses are less well delineated. Serology is highly sensitive and specific. Avoid aspiration of cysts which causes dissemination and hypersensitivity. Most cases require surgical resection. Albendazole is used in those unfit for surgery or with disseminated disease.
  - **Amoebic pulmonary disease** (see Chapter 6) is usually secondary to intestinal or liver infection. Pulmonary features include lung abscesses, empyema,

and occasionally hepatobronchial fistulae with large volumes of brown, 'anchovy sauce' sputum. Serology and identification of trophozoites in stool or sputum establish the diagnosis. Treatment is with metronidazole and iodoquinol or diloxanide.

- **Hypersensitivity reactions**, for example, eosinophilic lung disease or Loeffler's syndrome due to helminths like ascariasis, toxocara, and liver flukes.
  - **Pulmonary ascariasis** occurs during maturation of *Ascaris lumbricoides* (roundworm) and presents with hypersensitivity, including fever, cough, wheeze, peripheral eosinophilia, and CXR infiltrates. Detection of eggs in stool confirms the diagnosis. Symptoms resolve spontaneously within 2 weeks. Treat bowel infections with mebendazole 100 mg bd for 3 days.
  - **Toxocara canis** causes visceral larva migrans, with eye (e.g. blindness) and visceral (e.g. fever, hepatomegaly) involvement. It follows ingestion of eggs from contaminated soil. Dogs are the primary host. An immune response to migration of larvae through the lungs causes wheeze, cough, and eosinophilia. Larvae may be seen in the eyes. Serology is diagnostic. Treatment may not be required, but steroids can alleviate symptoms.
  - **Strongyloides stercoralis** (a parasitic roundworm/threadworm) occurs in the tropics and is transmitted when infectious larvae penetrate skin that comes in contact with infected soil. It causes cutaneous larva migrans (e.g. migrating urticaria) and Loeffler's syndrome, with wheeze, eosinophilia, and CXR infiltrates. Dissemination with 'hyperinfection' occurs in the immunocompromised. Treatment is with thiabendazole or albendazole.
  - **Tropical pulmonary eosinophilia** follows infection with *Wuchereria bancrofti* or *Brugia malayi* in the tropics. Pulmonary involvement is common with a hypersensitivity reaction, including cough, wheeze, raised IgE, and CXR infiltrates. Treatment is with diethylcarbamazine.
  - **Schistosomiasis**, the commonest fluke disease, is contracted due to freshwater snails following skin penetration. Migration through the lungs to the liver may be associated with cough, wheeze, and infiltrates on CXR. Ova may be detected in sputum, urine, or stool. Treatment is with praziquantel (see Chapter 6).
  - **Paragonimiasis** occurs in the tropics. After ingestion of raw crayfish or crabs, migration of flukes into the lungs and pleura causes hypersensitivity respiratory symptoms. Ova are detected in sputum, BAL, or pleural fluid. Treatment is with praziquantel.

Lung abscess

A lung abscess is a localized area of suppurative lung infection, causing necrosis and cavitation. They are uncommon in the developed world. Most are the result of aspiration pneumonia and are associated with impaired consciousness, alcohol, and post-anaesthetic aspiration, sinusitis and poor dentition. Some pneumonias are more likely to cavitate, including *Staphylococcus aureus*, *Klebsiella* spp., and anaerobic infections. Severe pharyngitis with associated jugular vein thrombophlebitis due to *Fusobacterium necrophorum* and septic embolization is associated with lung abscesses (Lemierre's syndrome or necrobacillosis). Diabetics and the immunocompromised are more susceptible. HIV-positive patients are at risk of cavitating abscesses due to PCP, cryptococcal, and fungal infection. Intravenous drug users with right-sided, often staphylococcal, endocarditis develop multiple lung abscesses.

Presentation is often insidious, with fever, night sweats, dyspnoea, and non-specific systemic features, including malaise, anaemia, clubbing, and weight loss. A cough productive of large quantities of foul sputum and haemoptysis is common. There may be focal chest signs, but often chest examination is normal. The diagnosis is made from the history and detection of a cavity with an air-fluid level on CXR. About 50% of abscesses are in the posterior segment of the right upper lobe or the apical segments of both lower lobes. CT scans may be useful to differentiate an abscess from a pleural collection or to detect obstructing endobronchial lesions due to malignancy or foreign bodies. Microbiological investigation includes culture of blood and sputum. Percutaneous needle aspiration usually detects a mixed bacterial infection, including anaerobes (e.g. *Bacteroides*) and aerobes (e.g. *Streptococcus milleri*, *Klebsiella*). Differentiation from a cavitating bronchial carcinoma, vasculitis, infarcts, tuberculosis, and aspergillomas can be difficult.

Prolonged antibiotic therapy, usually 2 weeks intravenously, followed by 2–4 weeks orally with broad-spectrum aerobic and anaerobic cover (e.g. co-amoxiclav) is recommended. Spontaneous bronchial drainage is common with the production of large quantities of foul, bloodstained sputum and is aided by postural drainage and physiotherapy. Percutaneous drainage may help those not responding to antibiotic therapy but risks pleural infection. Surgery is rarely necessary. The prognosis is usually good (90% cure rates), but mortality can be 20–30% in the elderly and those with underlying lung disease, large abscesses (>6 cm), immunodeficiency (e.g. HIV infection), and *S. aureus* infection.

Further reading

American Thoracic Society (2005). Guidelines for the management of adults with hospital-acquired, ventilator-associated, and health-care-associated pneumonia. *American Journal of Respiratory and Critical Care Medicine*, **171**, 388–416 (currently undergoing revision).

Best Health. Lungs and breathing. <http://besthealth.bmj.com/x/set/topic/condition-centre/15.html>.

Boyton RJ, Mitchell DM, Kon OM (2003). The pulmonary physician in critical care. HIV-associated pneumonia. *Thorax*, **58**, 721–5.

British Lung Foundation Breathe Easy Group. <http://www.lunguk.org>.

British Thoracic Society (2009). Guidelines for the management of community-acquired pneumonia in adults: update 2009. *Thorax*, **64**, S1–61.

Chest Heart & Stroke Scotland. <http://www.chss.org.uk/>.

Greenberg SB (2002). Respiratory viral infections in adults. *Current Opinion in Pulmonary Medicine*, **8**, 201–8.

Lung Foundation Australia. <http://www.lungfoundation.com.au/>.

Mandell LA, Wunderink RG, Anzueto A, *et al.* (2007). Infectious Disease Society of America/American Thoracic Society: Consensus guidelines on the management of community-acquired pneumonia in adults. *Clinical Infectious Diseases*, **44**, S1–46.

National Institute for Health and Clinical Excellence (2014). NICE clinical guideline 191: pneumonia: diagnosis and management of community- and hospital-acquired pneumonia in adults. <http://www.nice.org.uk/guidance/cg191/resources/guidance-pneumonia-pdf>.

Patient UK. <http://www.patient.co.uk/>.

Peiris JSM, Yuen KY, Osterhaus AD, Stöhr K (2003). The severe acute respiratory syndrome. *New England Journal of Medicine*, **349**, 2431–41.

Rotstein C, Evans G, Born A, *et al.* (2008). Clinical practice guidelines for hospital-acquired pneumonia and ventilator-associated pneumonia in adults. *Canadian Journal of Infectious Diseases & Medical Microbiology*, **19**, 19–53.

Mycobacterial infection

Mycobacterium tuberculosis (MTB)

Worldwide, MTB affects 10 million people and causes 2 million deaths a year despite being a curable disease. It is the second commonest cause of infectious mortality after AIDS. MTB incidence is highest in sub-Saharan Africa, but >50% of global cases occur in Asia (i.e. India, China) due to the high population density. MTB incidence is increasing in Eastern Europe and Russia due to economic decline and deteriorating health services, and about 10% are multidrug-resistant (MDR). The incidence of MTB in the UK in 2013 was about twice that in Western Europe at 12.3 per 100,000 population, with 73% occurring in people born outside the UK but only 15% of these were recent migrants (i.e. diagnosed within two years of entering the UK). Globally, 10% of MTB cases are co-infected with HIV. However, co-infection rates vary geographically, affecting 35–40% of sub-Saharan African cases, 2.7% of UK cases, and 1–2% in China.

Pathophysiology

MTB is spread in respiratory droplets that can remain airborne for hours after expectoration. Household contacts of a sputum-positive case have a 25% chance of being infected, and clinical disease develops in 5–10% of those infected. The risk is higher in contacts with HIV co-infection. Following inhalation, MTB is initially ingested by, and replicates within, alveolar macrophages in the subpleural, midzone terminal airspaces. It may be contained locally or spread via lymphatics to nearby lymph nodes and/or by the bloodstream to other organs where latent infection can persist for many years. Cell-mediated immunity leads to granuloma formation by activated T lymphocytes and macrophages, inhibits further replication and spread, and prevents development of active disease.

- **Primary MTB infection** usually occurs in childhood in endemic areas but often develops later in developed countries. Following inhalation and initial replication, the immune response usually limits pulmonary infection to a localized granulomatous lesion in the midzone termed the Ghon focus. If combined with infection and enlargement of local lymph nodes, it is referred to as the 'primary complex'. This initial infection lasts 3–8 weeks. It is associated with the development of an inflammatory reaction to injection of tubercular protein (tuberculin) into the skin, which is used as a diagnostic test (Mantoux). The primary infection is usually followed by healing, fibrosis and calcification, and immunity to further infection. However, in 5% of cases, especially children and immunocompromised adults, progressive active disease develops due to failure of the host's immune response to contain MTB replication. Although the lungs are most commonly involved, any organ may be affected due to haematogenous dissemination.
- **Post-primary MTB infection** accounts for most adult TB. It is due to reactivation of MTB which has lain dormant in a previous Ghon focus or site of primary haematogenous spread (e.g. meninges, kidneys), following an initial childhood infection.

Risk factors for active TB

Table 5.12 lists risk factors for TB. The lifetime risk of developing active clinical disease in a child infected with MTB is ~10%. Those who are elderly, malnourished, or immunosuppressed are more susceptible, and there may be a genetic predisposition in Asian, Chinese, and West Indian people.

TB tends to occur in younger age groups and has an equal sex distribution in the black and Asian groups. In contrast, older males are more commonly affected in the Caucasian population. Overcrowding, poverty, smoking, and vitamin D deficiency increase the risk of clinical TB.

Clinical features

Primary MTB infection is often asymptomatic. It may cause a mild febrile illness, erythema nodosum, and small pleural effusions. Very occasionally, bronchial compression by enlarged hilar lymph nodes causes wheeze and lobar collapse, followed by late bronchiectasis

Post-primary MTB infection is often pulmonary (~80%). The main features are productive cough and systemic symptoms, including weight loss, fever, night sweats, and loss of appetite. Breathlessness and chest pain occur occasionally. Small-volume haemoptysis affects a third of cases, especially those with cavitatory disease. Massive haemoptysis is rare. Examination is often normal and signs non-specific, including weight loss, lymphadenopathy, and crepitations or consolidation on chest auscultation. Pulmonary complications include;

- **Pleural TB** with cough, pleuritic pain, and unilateral pleural effusion. It is most common after primary MTB infection and is often self-limiting, although many develop active disease within 3 years. Pleural aspiration and biopsy confirm the diagnosis (see 'Pleural disease').
- **Pneumothorax** is rare (<1%) but predisposes to the formation of a bronchopleural fistula.
- **Right middle lobe syndrome** is due to hilar lymph node compression of the right middle lobe bronchus, with subsequent lobar collapse.

Table 5.12 Risk factors for TB, non-compliance with therapy, and resistant disease

a. Risk factors for tuberculosis
1. Ethnic origin, sex, and age
   - Caucasian; >50 y old; M > F
   - Asian/Chinese; <50 y old; M = F
   - Afro/Caribbean; <30 y old; M = F
2. Medical factors
   - Diabetes, renal and malignant disease
   - Immunosupression (chemotherapy, steroids)
   - Immunomodulatory drugs (infliximab)
   - Vitamin D deficiency
   - Smoking
3. Poverty, poor nutrition, homelessness
4. HIV/AIDS
5. Alcohol addiction

b. Risk factors for non-compliance
1. Alcohol addiction
2. Homelessness
3. Drug abuse
4. Mental illness

c. Factors associated with resistant MTB
1. Treatment failure, inadequate therapy
2. Contact with resistant disease
3. HIV infection
4. Immigration from area of high resistance

- *Aspergillosis and aspergilloma* may develop in secondarily infected apical cavities.
- *Bronchiectasis* follows inadequately treated disease, endobronchial infection, or airways obstruction.

Extrapulmonary TB occurs in 45% of patients and >50% of cases with coexisting HIV infection. It is often associated with a strong tuberculin reaction, as it usually represents reactivation, rather than primary MTB, but not if HIV-infected. Almost any organ may be affected:

- *Lymph node TB* presents with painless, enlarged, or matted nodes due to primary infection, reactivation, or spread. The cervical nodes are affected in 70% (scrofula) of cases, with systemic symptoms in 30–60%. The nodes may eventually break down to form discharging sinuses and chronic skin lesions.
- *Cerebral TB*, including meningitis and space-occupying tuberculomas, can cause permanent neurological damage without prompt treatment. Meningeal TB presents insidiously over 2–8 weeks with non-specific headache, neck stiffness, and fever, followed by reduced consciousness, epilepsy, and focal neurological signs, including cranial nerve palsies. Cerebrospinal fluid (CSF) contains lymphocytes, high protein, and low glucose levels. Culture of MTB confirms the diagnosis but is frequently negative.
- *Pericardial TB* may present with acute pericarditis, chronic pericardial effusion, with or without tamponade, or chronic constrictive pericarditis. Pericardial fluid and biopsy may not be diagnostic, but the tuberculin test is positive in 85% of cases. The CXR may show pericardial calcification in constrictive pericarditis. Echocardiography determines the need for drainage.
- *Bone or joint TB* (see Figure 5.18) can affect any bone or joint. Spinal involvement (Pott's disease) is commonest in the thoracic spine. Vertebral collapse can cause severe spinal angulation (gibbus). Surgery is required for spinal instability or cord compression. Paravertebral abscess may need drainage.
- *Renal and genitourinary TB* is rare. It causes a sterile pyuria. Prostatitis and epididymitis occur in men and infertility in women.
- *Miliary or disseminated TB* follows blood spread in chronic disease or following immunosuppresssion. Onset is often insidious with non-specific symptoms of fever, malaise, and weight loss. Pulmonary, cerebral, and liver involvement are most common. Choroidal tubercules may occur in up to 50% and are pathognomonic when

seen at fundoscopy. CXR typically, but not universally, reveals multiple miliary (millet seed), 1–2 mm, lung field nodules. Miliary disease has a higher mortality.

Investigation

Diagnosis is usually established from sputum smears or other infected material like pus, urine, or CSF (ideally three samples), culture, or by detecting caseating granulomas in tissue. Baseline full blood count, biochemistry, and liver function tests should precede chemotherapy.

- *Sputum examination* by Ziehl–Neelsen (ZN) or auramine staining or culture, is required to confirm the diagnosis and to assess drug sensitivity. Diagnosis from induced sputum samples is as effective as bronchoalveolar lavage (BAL), but caution is required in multidrug-resistant disease (MDR), as aerosolized particles may endanger health workers. Culture takes 6 weeks. Non-tuberculous mycobacteria occur in lower concentrations and are less likely to be seen on smear examinations, but grow rapidly and are detected earlier on culture.
- *CXR* usually reveals upper lobe infiltrates and cavitation (see Figure 5.19) and associated hilar or paratracheal adenopathy. HIV-infected patients are more likely to have atypical changes or even normal X-rays.
- *Tuberculin skin tests (TST)* are interpreted in relation to the patient's history, ethnic origin, BCG vaccination status, and TB exposure. In the Mantoux test, the reaction to intradermal injection of 10 tuberculin units (0.1 mL of 1,000 ppd solution) is assessed. An inflammatory response < 5mm in diameter is negative, 4–15 mm positive, and >15 mm strongly positive. Heaf testing is used less often at present due to concerns about cross-infection.
- *Interferon-gamma release assays (IGRA)* use more MTB-specific antigens than the TST (i.e. ESAT-6 and CFP10) to detect TB infection via blood samples. Consider interferon-gamma testing for people whose Mantoux testing shows positive results, or in people for whom Mantoux testing may be less reliable, for example BCG-vaccinated people.
- *Biopsy samples* from extrapulmonary nodes often confirm the diagnosis. In miliary TB, diagnostic yield from bone marrow and liver biopsies is high.
- *CT scan* is more sensitive than CXR. A 'tree in bud' appearance suggests active airways disease.

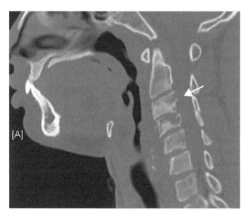

Figure 5.18 Tuberculosis of the cervical spine (arrow).

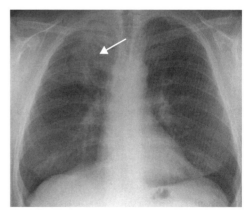

Figure 5.19 Right apical infiltration and early cavitation (arrow) in mycobacterial tuberculosis.

- **Bronchoscopy** may be required to obtain BAL samples in patients who are sputum-negative or cannot provide adequate samples. It occasionally reveals ulcerating endobronchial TB or discharging, perforated nodes.
- **Early-morning urine (EMU)** samples (ideally three) are required if renal disease is suspected and have good yield in miliary or disseminated disease.

Treatment

The aims of therapy are to cure TB, prevent transmission, and prevent relapse and drug resistance. Treatment is usually started after microbiological confirmation but before drug sensitivities are available. Most patients can be treated as outpatients. Following onset of therapy, smear-positive, non-MDR, HIV-negative cases usually become smear-negative within 2 weeks. They should be isolated in hospital or at home during this period. Patients admitted to hospital with suspected TB should be admitted to a negative-pressure side room and should be considered infectious, particularly to immunocompromised patients (e.g. HIV-positive). Whilst the patient is potentially infectious, staff should wear face masks when entering the side room. However, if a patient is found to have TB on an open ward, the risk to other patients is small, and only those in close proximity need contact tracing. The doctor making the diagnosis of TB, even if after death, has a legal responsibility to notify the disease which allows contact tracing and surveillance.

The standard TB treatment regime has two phases:

- An initial intensive period lasting 8 weeks which kills active mycobacteria using four drugs (rifampicin (R), isoniazid (I), pyrazinamide (P), ethambutol). This has superseded previous guidelines recommending three drug regimes because background isoniazid resistance has increased, especially in immigrants, ethnic minority groups, HIV-positive and previously treated patients.
- A follow-up phase of 16 weeks which eliminates residual bacteria using a two-drug regime, usually isoniazid and rifampicin.

Drug doses are calculated according to weight (see Table 5.13), and should be given as combination preparations (e.g. Rifater® contains I, R, and P and Rifinah® I and R). Baseline renal and liver function tests (LFT) should be checked, and, if normal, guidelines suggest that they need not be routinely rechecked. Pyridoxine (vitamin B6) 10 mg daily is given to patients with a poor diet (e.g. alcoholics), diabetes, renal failure, or HIV. First-line drugs include:

- **Rifampicin** is bactericidal and is given once daily. It can cause hepatitis, colitis, renal impairment, and thrombocytopenia. Hepatic metabolism of drugs via cytochrome P450 (including the oral contraceptive pill (OCP) and steroids) is increased. Before treatment, steroid doses

are doubled and women on the OCP given advice regarding alternative methods of contraception.
- **Isoniazid** is bactericidal, given once daily, and usually well tolerated. Hepatitis is the main side effect and is aggravated by alcohol. Associated peripheral neuropathy is prevented by supplemental pyridoxine.
- **Pyrazinamide** is bactericidal and given as a single daily dose. It can cause gastrointestinal upset, hepatic toxicity, and arthralgia. Renal excretion causes hyperuricaemia which may exacerbate gout.
- **Ethambutol** is mainly bacteriostatic, given once daily, and is usually well tolerated. Optic neuritis, with loss of visual acuity and/or colour vision, is the main, but uncommon side effect. Check visual acuity (Snellen chart) and/or colour vision (Ishihara charts) both before, and during treatment.

Second-line drugs include streptomycin, rifabutin, amikacin, ofloxacin, azithromycin, capreomycin, ciprofloxacin, clarithromycin, ethionamide, thiacetazone, and PAS. They are required in those with intolerance to first-line drugs or drug-resistant MTB. Drug intolerance requiring a change of therapy occurs in 5–10% of patients and is more common in HIV-positive cases, following previous therapy, after contact with drug-resistant disease and in those on non-standard TB drug regimes. Drug resistance is uncommon, affecting <5% of Caucasians in the UK, but levels are higher in HIV-positive patients and ethnic minority groups. In the UK, in 2013, 7.1% of isolates were resistant to isoniazid, 1.9% to rifampicin, and 1.6% were MDR. Monoresistant treatment regimes include three drugs to which the TB is sensitive. MDR-TB is discussed in the section on multiple drug resistance TB (MDR-TB).

Specific treatment advice. Cerebral TB, including meningitis, is treated for 12 months. Non-cerebral TB usually responds to 6 months' therapy. Steroid therapy should be considered in patients with meningitis (especially with cranial nerve involvement), cerebral TB, constrictive pericarditis, large pleural effusions, ureteric involvement, and to suppress hypersensitivity reactions to TB drugs.

Before starting therapy, advise patients about:
- Red urine and red contact lens (due to rifampicin).
- Nausea and abdominal pain. If vomiting or jaundice develop, stop the drugs, and contact the doctor.
- Reduced efficacy of the OCP.
- Common drug interactions. Rifampicin decreases levels of warfarin, phenytoin, digoxin, methadone, sulfonylureas, steroids, theophylline, ciclosporin, and antifungal agents. Isoniazid increases levels of phenytoin, carbamazepine, warfarin, and diazepam.
- Loss of visual acuity and colour vision with ethambutol. Stop therapy immediately, and contact the doctor.

Table 5.13 Standard anti-tuberculous drug doses

Drug	Daily dose	DOT (x3 weekly)
Isoniazid	300 mg	15 mg/kg x3 weekly
Rifampicin <50 kg	450 mg	600–900 mg x3 weekly
Rifampicin >50 kg	600 mg	600–900 mg x3 weekly
Pyrazinamide <50 kg	1.5 g	2.0 g x3 weekly
Pyrazinamide >50 kg	2.0 g	2.5 g x3 weekly
Ethambutol	15 mg/kg	30 mg/kg x3 weekly

Therapy in patients with comorbid conditions

- **Liver disease.** Liver function tests (LFTs) may be raised in alcoholics and new TB patients. Therapy should not be withheld, as liver function usually improves or remains stable with therapy. Viral hepatitis should be excluded. In chronic liver disease (CLD), baseline LFT should be followed by regular monitoring (i.e. weekly for 2 weeks, then every 2 weeks). If AST and ALT are >2 times normal, continue to monitor weekly. If >5 times normal or if bilirubin increases, stop therapy until LFTs recover. Reintroduce drugs individually at reduced doses whilst monitoring LFT and clinical condition. Exclude an offending drug if there is a recurrence. Treatment duration may, therefore, need to be extended or a second-line alternative considered. Patients with CLD should be managed by a TB expert, as drug-induced hepatitis can be fatal.
- **Renal disease.** Isoniazid, rifampicin, and pyrazinamide are given in normal doses in renal disease, as they have biliary excretion. Ethambutol accumulates, and the dose should be reduced to avoid optic neuropathy. Pyridoxine is required to prevent isoniazid-induced neuropathy. Drugs should be given after dialysis in end-stage renal failure.
- **HIV-positive patients** are treated with the standard four-drug regime. Rifampicin may significantly reduce levels of protease or non-nucleoside reverse transcriptase inhibitors used to treat HIV, and rifabutin may provide an alternative. Concurrent treatment for TB and HIV increases the frequency of paradoxical worsening of TB, and so physicians may choose to delay anti-HIV treatment where possible. Starting anti-HIV treatment in patients with subclinical or latent TB may 'unmask' the TB diagnosis.
- **Pregnancy** is not associated with an increased risk of TB. Presentation is identical, but diagnosis is often delayed, as initial non-specific symptoms are attributed to pregnancy and CXR is avoided. Tuberculin skin tests are not affected. However, a negative test should not be followed by BCG, as live vaccines are contraindicated in pregnancy. Diagnosis in the first trimester has a similar outcome to that in non-pregnant women. Diagnosis in the second or third trimester, particularly when associated with inadequate treatment, is associated with pre-eclampsia, small-for-date babies, spontaneous abortion, and increased preterm labour and obstetric mortality, particularly in Third World countries. Standard therapy is not teratogenic and is recommended for 6 months in non-CNS TB. Early pregnancy morning sickness may impair absorption, causing drug resistance. Second-line drugs have variable toxicity and should be used only after specialist advice (e.g. streptomycin causes fetal ototoxicity). Babies of sputum-positive mothers who have been treated for <2 weeks at delivery should be treated with isoniazid and skin-tested at 6 weeks. If the skin test is negative, the isoniazid is stopped and BCG given 1 week later (BCG is sensitive to isoniazid). Drug concentrations in breast milk are low, and breastfeeding is safe.

Treatment failure is often due to poor adherence, with alcoholics, the homeless, and drug abusers being at high risk. Drug resistance may develop in these cases. Dosette boxes aid adherence and may ensure correct treatment in those with poor understanding. If there is concern about adherence, consideration should be given to directly observed therapy (DOT), in which ingestion of medication is witnessed by a suitable individual. This may be achieved with daily or three times a week DOT, depending on individual circumstances.

Multiple drug resistance TB (MDR-TB)

MDR-TB is defined as resistance to two or more first-line agents, including isoniazid and rifampicin. Although infectivity is no different from normal TB, treatment is more complex, as second-line drugs are more toxic and less effective than first-line agents. Management must involve a specialist experienced in the treatment of MDR-TB, isolation in a negative-pressure room, close supervision, and monitoring for drug toxicity and compliance. Initial treatment is with ≥5 drugs to which the organism is sensitive until sputum cultures are negative, followed by therapy with three drugs to which the bacillus is sensitive for a total of 18–24 months. Contacts of MDR-TB may be treated with two drugs (depending on sensitivities in the index case) for 6 months, although there is no evidence to validate this treatment period. If the resistance is extensive in the index case, no chemoprophylactic regime may be suitable, and contacts require close follow-up. The BTS provide an expert advice panel to assist with the management of MDR-TB.

Latent TB

Latent TB, defined as a positive skin test or IGRA, with normal CXR and no symptoms, is due to small numbers of MTB. Treatment with chemoprophylaxis should be considered and is usually given in these cases (see 2011 NICE guidance). This prevents progression to active disease in 60–90% of cases. Daily rifampicin and isoniazid is given for 3 months, but isoniazid for 6 months has a lower side effect profile. In HIV-positive patients, tuberculin skin testing may be falsely negative due to anergy.

Contact tracing

Contact tracing identifies patients with active TB, latent TB, and those who require BCG vaccination. About 1% of contacts develop TB, and contact tracing detects about 10% of all TB. About 10% of close contacts develop TB and these contacts require symptom assessment, tuberculin testing, CXR, and enquiry about BCG vaccination status. Casual contacts (e.g. occupational) only require tracing if the index case was smear-positive or the contacts are at high risk. Smear-negative patients are less infective, but close contact tracing is still recommended.

BCG vaccination

In the UK and USA, routine BCG vaccination of children is no longer recommended. However, BCG vaccination is offered to patients at high risk, including children of infected mothers and immigrants.

Non-tuberculous mycobacteria (NTM)

NTM, also called atypical, environmental, or opportunistic mycobacteria, are ubiquitous and are found in water (i.e. tap water), soil, dust, birds, animals, and milk. To date, 125 different species have been identified. They are low-grade pathogens, and only a few cause significant human illness. In the USA, the commonest pulmonary pathogens are M. avium complex (MAC), M. kansasii, and M. abscessus. In the UK, M. kansasii is the most common pulmonary pathogen, but, in some areas, the incidence of M. malmoense and M. xenopi is similar.

Pulmonary infection is most common and affects older adults with pre-existing lung disease (e.g. bronchiectasis). Non-pulmonary infection is less common, usually occurs in the immunodeficient, and involves many sites:

- Lymphadenitis (e.g. MAC, *M. malmoense*) occurs in children (1–5 years old). It presents with non-tender, cervical lymphadenopathy and a normal CXR. Affected nodes should be surgically resected. Antituberculous drug therapy is reserved for post-operative recurrence or to shrink large nodes prior to resection.
- Widespread dissemination (e.g. MAC) occurs in the immunocompromised (e.g. HIV-positive).
- Skin and soft tissue lesions (e.g. *M. marinum*, *M. abscessus*, *M. chelonae*) follow local invasion (e.g. injection with a tap water contaminated needle).

Diagnosis requires >1 positive culture specimen because NTM is often isolated due to culture contamination. The decision to treat depends on the likelihood of infection determined from clinical, radiographic, and microbiological progression. BTS guidelines suggest that NTM lung disease is likely if the CXR (± symptoms) is consistent and ≥3 positive sputum samples are obtained >7 days apart; or if one positive culture is obtained from a sterile site (e.g. pleural fluid, biopsy); or two cultures from BAL on separate occasions.

Symptoms and signs are non-specific and frequently mimic those of TB. Most cases present with a subacute illness, productive cough, weight loss, fatigue, dyspnoea, fever, and occasional haemoptysis. Some may present with atypical progression of the underlying lung disease (e.g. COPD). Occasionally, a hypersensitivity type illness occurs. For example, in MAC-associated 'hot tub syndrome', symptoms usually resolve, following cessation of hot tub exposure, although steroids and antibiotics may be required.

Radiographic features in NTM lung disease are characterized by either fibrocavitatory changes (often indistinguishable from TB; see Figure 5.20) or clusters of small nodules (<5 mm) and multifocal bronchiectasis, typically located in the mid- and lower lung. A CXR may be sufficient for evaluation of fibrocavitary disease, but HRCT is often required to confirm nodular/bronchiectatic disease.

Mycobacterial culture of NTM is essential for the diagnosis of NTM lung disease. Presumptive diagnosis, based on clinical and radiographic features, is not adequate to initiate therapy. Three sputum samples should be collected on

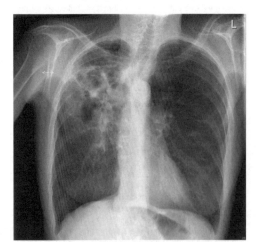

Figure 5.20 Non-mycobacterial tuberculosis with cavitation and fibrosis in right upper lobe.

three separate days to optimize the predictive value of sputum analysis. Correlation of MAC culture with new radiographic cavitation and infiltration demonstrated that >2 positive cultures (from three specimens) was associated with radiographic progression in >90% of cases, whereas a single positive culture was not.

Management depends on the organism, but antibiotic choice is best determined by clinical response, as improvement does not always correlate with documented sensitivities. Notification is not required in NTM infection, as the risk of cross-infection is low, and patients previously notified as having MTB can be 'denotified':

- *M. kansasii* is usually acquired from tap water. Lung disease occurs in geographic clusters in south-east England, Wales, and central USA. It mainly affects elderly white men with pre-existing lung disease, healed TB or emphysema (see Figure 5.19), alcoholism, or immunodeficiency. It progresses without therapy. Treatment is with rifampicin and ethambutol for at least 9 months or >2 years if immunocompromised. Isoniazid, clarithromycin, and ethionamide are also effective. Sputum conversion rates are 100%, cure rates >90%, and relapse rates <10% with rifampicin-containing treatment regimes.
- *M. avium complex (MAC)* is acquired from natural water sources, indoor pools, and hot tubs. Apical fibrocavitary lung disease occurs in middle-aged, male smokers who drink excessive alcohol. It progresses to severe lung destruction over 1–2 years if untreated. In contrast, 'Lady Windermere syndrome' progresses slowly and occurs in post-menopausal, non-smoking white females who are often thin with scoliosis and pectus excavatum. It affects mainly the right middle and lingular lobes and is characterized by HRCT scan findings of peripheral nodules and bronchiectasis. MAC is usually macrolide-sensitive, but resistance occurs with monotherapy. Therefore, most treatment regimes include rifampicin and ethambutol. Sputum clearance occurs in 70–90%. The primary goal is 12 months of negative sputum cultures whilst on therapy.
- *Other NTM* (e.g. *M. malmoense*, *M. xenopi*) show varying sensitivity to treatment, and specialist advice is required. Optimal treatment regimens include rifampicin, clarithromycin, ethambutol, and isoniazid (± ciprofloxacin, moxifloxacin) continued until sputum cultures have been negative for 12 months. Although sputum conversion occurs rapidly, relapse rates are high. *M. abscessus* requires resection of localized lung disease and multidrug therapy.

In HIV-positive patients, MAC is responsible for >90% of cases of NTM infection. Treatment should be considered lifelong, unless immune restoration is achieved with antiretroviral therapy. The risk of drug interactions between rifampicin, macrolides, protease inhibitors, and non-nucleoside reverse transcription inhibitors should be considered. MAC prophylaxis is achieved with azithromycin 1,200 mg weekly or clarithromycin 500 mg twice daily.

Further reading

American Thoracic Society, CDC, and Infectious Diseases Society of America (2003). Treatment of tuberculosis. *MMWR Recommendations and Reports*, **52** (RR11), 1–88. Currently undergoing revision.

British Thoracic Society (2000). Management of opportunistic mycobacterial infections: Joint Tuberculosis Committee Guidelines 1999. *Thorax*, **55**, 210–18. Revision guidelines due in Jan 2016.

Griffith DE, Aksamit T, Brown-Elliott BA, *et al.* (2007). An official ATS/IDSA statement: diagnosis, treatment, and prevention of non-tuberculous mycobacterial disease. *American Journal of Respiratory and Critical Care Medicine*, **175**, 367–416.

Joint Tuberculosis Committee of the British Thoracic Society (2000). Control and prevention of tuberculosis in the United Kingdom: code of practice 2000. *Thorax*, **55**, 887–901.

National Institute for Health and Clinical Excellence (2006). Tuberculosis: clinical diagnosis and management of tuberculosis and measures for its prevention and control. Clinical guideline 33. <http://www.nice.org.uk/cg033>.

National Institute for Health and Clinical Excellence (2011). Tuberculosis: clinical diagnosis and management of tuberculosis and measures for its prevention and control. Clinical guideline 117. <http://www.nice.org.uk/guidance/CG117>.

Public Health England (2014). Tuberculosis (TB) in the UK: annual report. <https://www.gov.uk/government/uploads/system/uploads/attachment_data/file/360335/TB_Annual_report__4_0_300914.pdf>.

Smego RA and Ahmed N (2003). A systematic review of the adjunctive use of systemic corticosteroids for pulmonary tuberculosis. *International Journal of Tuberculosis and Lung Disease*, **7**, 208–13.

Asthma

Definition

There is no universal definition of asthma. It is best described as a disorder due to chronic, often eosinophilic, bronchial inflammation, characterized by airway hyperreactivity to a variety of non-specific stimuli. The accompanying widespread, variable airways obstruction is usually reversible, either spontaneously or with treatment, and causes recurrent episodic wheeze, chest tightness, breathlessness, and cough, often at night or in the early morning

Epidemiology

Worldwide, asthma prevalence is increasing, especially in English-speaking countries, and, although the cause is unknown, it correlates with increased sensitization to common allergens. In the UK, asthma prevalence is ~10% and affects >5.4 million people, of whom 1.1 million are children. In 2014, the all party Parliamentary group (APPG) inquiry into respiratory deaths reported that there are ~65,000 asthma-related hospital admissions and 1,000–1,400 asthma deaths annually. It is estimated that 90% of these asthma-associated deaths could have been prevented.

The financial burden of asthma is considerable. Stable asthma costs ~£110–130/patient/year, with difficult asthma costing ~£350–450/patient/year. The direct cost to the UK health service is about £1 billion/year, with lost productivity costing a further £1.25 billion/annually.

Aetiology

Asthma is due to a combination of environmental and genetic factors.

- **Genetic factors.** There is a well-established hereditary basis for atopy and allergy, with linkage to chromosomes 5, 11, 13, 14, 16 and the high affinity IgE receptor and T helper 2 (Th2) cytokine genes.
- **Immunological mechanisms.** Atopic asthmatics react to an antigen challenge by causing B lymphocytes to produce IgE which forms IgE-antigen complexes and bind to mast cells, macrophages, and basophils. This causes these cells to release preformed mediators like histamine and eosinophilic chemotactic factor which precipitate bronchoconstriction and airways oedema. The inflammatory response also includes many other pathways (e.g. leukotrienes, kinins, and prostaglandins).
- **Hygiene theory.** Large epidemiological studies support the hypothesis that early-life exposure to allergens reduces allergen sensitivity in later life by deactivating Th2-mediated allergic responses like asthma and eczema.
- **Other environmental factors.** Obesity, westernized diet, affluence, immunization, inactivity, and reduced childhood respiratory infections have all been linked to the increased prevalence of asthma.

Pathophysiology

The commonest histopathological change in asthma is chronic, eosinophilic, bronchial inflammation affecting large and small airways, including infiltration of eosinophils, lymphocytes, Th2 cells, and mast cells, with associated cytokine production (e.g. IL-4, IL-5, leukotrienes). However, these findings are not specific, and some patients with reversible airways obstruction and bronchial hyperreactivity have no eosinophilic inflammation whilst others without asthma symptoms do. Subsequent airways obstruction occurs due to smooth muscle contraction, airway mucosal thickening, and increased viscid secretion production. This airways

obstruction may become irreversible over time due to airway remodelling with smooth muscle hyperplasia and hypertrophy, epithelial damage, collagen deposition, and basement membrane thickening.

Clinical features and diagnosis

Asthma is a clinical diagnosis. The characteristic triad of wheeze, breathlessness, and chest tightness occurs in 90% of patients, but these symptoms are non-specific and must be differentiated from other conditions, including chronic obstructive pulmonary disease (COPD) and heart disease (see Box 5.4). Attacks are typically episodic and variable, often occurring at night or in the early morning, and frequently precipitated by exposure to specific (e.g. pollen, house dust mite, animal dander) and non-specific (e.g. cold air, perfumes, chemicals) triggers of airways hyperreactivity. Cough (e.g. cough variant asthma) and exertional dyspnoea may be the only presenting features of asthma in up to 30% of cases. Asthma-associated cough is usually non-productive, frequently nocturnal, sometimes chronic, and precipitated by similar triggers to classical asthma. Although more common in children, cough may be the presenting feature in 10% of asthmatics over 50 years old.

Examination may reveal expiratory wheeze but is usually normal between attacks, except in those with severe, chronic asthma in whom the chest may be hyperinflated and deformed. Paradoxical chest wall movement and a silent chest with absence of wheeze on auscultation suggest a severe, life-threatening asthma attack.

Clinical assessment should include evaluation of:

- **Disease severity.** Lung function declines more rapidly than normal in asthmatics, especially smokers.
- **Potential triggers and exacerbating factors**, include aeroantigens (e.g. pollens), cold air, chemicals (e.g. bleach, perfumes), and occupational exposures. Allergy may be associated with hay fever, atopic dermatitis, eczema, nasal obstruction due to polyps, and post-nasal drip. Consider aspirin sensitivity (see 'Other asthma syndromes'), and assess family history. Food allergies, gastro-oesophageal reflux, stress and social factors may also aggravate asthma control.
- **Atypical presentations.** Consider asthma in patients with recurrent isolated or nocturnal cough or chest tightness despite the absence of wheeze, suspected hyperventilation syndrome, and exercise-induced cough or breathlessness.

Box 5.4 Asthma differential diagnosis

- COPD
- Bronchiolitis
- Heart failure
- Interstitial lung disease
- Upper airways obstruction (e.g. stridor, typical flow volume trace)
- Thromboembolic disease
- Allergic bronchopulmonary aspergillosis
- Eosinophilic lung diseases (e.g. Churg–Strauss syndrome)
- gastrooesophageal reflux disease
- Laryngospasm
- Hyperventilation syndrome
- Tumours (e.g. carcinoid may cause wheeze)

- **Morbidity assessment.** Ask if the patient has had their normal asthma symptoms during the day (e.g. wheeze, dyspnoea), difficulty sleeping because of asthma symptoms, or if asthma has interfered with normal activity (e.g. work) during the last week or month.

Investigation

Characteristically, airways obstruction reduces peak expiratory flow (PEF) and forced expiratory volume in 1 second (FEV_1). These measures are often normal between exacerbations. Asthma diagnosis should be based on objective evidence of variable airflow obstruction. Investigations might include:

- **Serial PEF and spirometry measurements** to assess variability in airways obstruction and response to treatment (see Figure 5.21). Diagnosis is confirmed if there is >20% diurnal variation on 3 days/week of diary card PEF measurement or if FEV_1 increases by >15% (and 200 mL) after a 2-week trial of oral steroid (e.g. prednisolone 30 mg daily) or if FEV_1 decreases by >15% after 6 min of exercise. Asthma is unlikely, and the diagnosis should be reconsidered if PEF or FEV_1 are normal and/or there is no variability.
- **Bronchodilator reversibility of airways obstruction.** An increase in FEV_1 >15% after bronchodilation with a short-acting beta-2-agonist (e.g. salbutamol 400 mcg by metered dose inhaler) is confirmatory.
- **Blood tests** include IgE to assess atopy and eosinophilia (e.g. to exclude Churg–Strauss syndrome). Allergic bronchopulmonary aspergillosis is detected with skin tests or RAST (Radioallergosorbent test) to aspergillus, as this is an IgE/eosinophil-driven condition. *Aspergillus* precipitins are sometimes positive but should be used as a test in aspergilloma, not ABPA (because up to 10% of normal asthma patients may be positive for precipitins).
- **Chest radiograph (CXR).** This is usually normal, apart from hyperinflation, but is performed to exclude other causes.
- **Skin prick testing** assesses atopy and potential asthma triggers.
- **Sputum analysis** may reveal eosinophilia, aiding asthma diagnosis.
- **ENT assessment** may detect nasal polyps, vocal cord dysfunction, and upper airway obstruction.
- **Methacholine (or histamine) provocation tests** measure bronchial hyperreactivity (BHR) as a PC20, the concentration of inhaled methacholine (or histamine) required to provoke a 20% fall in FEV_1. Normal subjects require >16 mg/mL. The lower the PC20, the more

likely asthma, and a PC20 <8 mg/mL would be suggestive. However, the level varies with the challenge method used.

- **Provocation tests** may confirm BHR to inhalation of a suspected trigger agent, usually in occupational asthma. Measurement of PEF at work, home, during weekends, and on holiday is usually more helpful.
- **Bronchoscopy/lung biopsy** are occasionally required to exclude other causes (e.g. bronchiolitis obliterans).

Clinical forms of asthma

The spectrum of clinical presentations of asthma is so wide that clinicians have found it useful to develop subcategories of asthma to aid management (e.g. acute, stable, difficult, and occupational). All share the common features of recurrent wheeze, dyspnoea, chest tightness, and/or cough with reversible airflow obstruction and BHR. The most common are discussed in this text, but the reader is referred to the *Oxford Desk Reference of Respiratory Medicine* for further details.

Acute severe asthma

This is the most frequent respiratory emergency in acute medicine. In the USA, it accounts for ~2 million emergency room visits each year, of which ~10% require admission. It is most commonly precipitated by acute respiratory tract infection, usually viral, but other precipitants include bacterial infection (e.g. *M. pneumoniae*), drugs (e.g. beta-blockers), non-compliance with medication, and emotional crises. Knowledge of the cause helps to predict the likely duration of an attack but has no implications for initial management.

Assessment and monitoring of acute asthma

Diagnosis rarely presents difficulty, but, as signs and symptoms correlate poorly with the severity of airflow obstruction, PEF or FEV_1 should be measured at presentation, repeated 15–30 minutes after starting treatment, and subsequently monitored to assess progress and response to therapy. Oximetry should be measured and oxygen saturation (SaO_2) maintained at 94–98% with oxygen therapy (see Chapter 1 and section 'Hypoxaemia, respiratory failure, and oxygen therapy' earlier in this chapter). Arterial blood gases (ABG) should be checked if the SaO_2 <92% or if respiratory failure is suspected. A typical ABG profile during an acute asthma attack shows mild hypoxaemia (PaO_2 9–11 kPa) and hypocapnia ($PaCO_2$ 3.5–4 kPa). Respiratory drive is invariably increased, and even a normal $PaCO_2$ indicates severe airflow obstruction and tiring of the respiratory muscles. A high $PaCO_2$ is a life-threatening emergency in acute asthma and requires immediate ICU assessment for ventilatory support. A CXR is usually not required, unless a pneumothorax or infection is suspected. Check heart rate, respiratory rate, glucose, and potassium levels.

Regardless of the cause, the first step is to assess the severity of the airflow obstruction and initiate treatment. Early discussion of potential ICU admissions is essential (see Box 5.5).

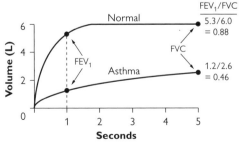

Figure 5.21 Spirometry in a normal subject and an asthmatic patient during an attack. FEV_1, forced expired volume in 1 s; FVC, forced vital capacity. Normal FEV_1/FVC is >0.8.

Box 5.5 Factors indicating the need for ICU admission

- Deteriorating PEF or FEV_1
- Hypercapnia
- Acidosis (respiratory or metabolic)
- Persistent or worsening hypoxia
- Exhaustion, poor respiratory effort
- Respiratory arrest
- Confusion, drowsiness, coma

- **Moderate asthma** describes increasing asthma symptoms, with a PEF >50–75% of predicted or the patient's best normal value. If, 1 h after emergency room treatment, PEF is >75% of best normal value, consider discharge home, following adjustment of asthma medication (e.g. oral steroids, bronchodilators). Consider admission for observation in pregnant patients, previous 'brittle' asthmatics, exacerbations that follow recent oral steroid therapy, and in those considered at risk (i.e. living alone, learning difficulty).
- **Severe asthma** is defined as any one of PEF 33–50% predicted or best normal value, respiratory rate >25/min, heart rate >110 beats/min, and difficulty completing sentences in one breath and accessory muscle use. Pulsus paradoxus occurs during severe asthma. However, measurement is discouraged, as it takes time to perform and adds nothing to the assessment.
- **Life-threatening asthma** describes severe asthma plus any of PEF <33% predicted or best normal value, cyanosis, poor respiratory effort, paradoxical thoracoabdominal excursions (outward abdominal and inward sternal movement during inspiration), silent chest, SaO_2 <92%, PaO_2 <8 kPa, normal $PaCO_2$ (4.5–6 kPa), exhaustion, confusion, coma, and bradycardia, hypotension, or arrhythmia.
- **Near-fatal asthma** is characterized by raised $PaCO_2$ and the need for mechanical ventilation with raised inflationary pressures. Fatal asthma is due to cardiac arrest due to hypoxia and acidosis and may be prevented with high-flow oxygen. Box 5.6 shows risk factors for near-fatal or fatal asthma. Most asthma deaths occur before hospital admission in patients with severe chronic asthma, behavioural difficulties, and psychosocial problems who are receiving inadequate therapy, often despite recent medical review for deteriorating symptoms.

Treatment

Treatment should be started as soon as possible, following baseline measurements and assessment of severity. Most asthma attacks respond well to pharmacological therapy and do not require hospital admission. Some hospitalized patients will need admission to ICU for monitoring, and a small proportion will require intubation and mechanical ventilation.

Box 5.6 Risk factors for near-fatal and fatal asthma

- **Previous life-threatening asthma**
  - Ventilation, ICU admission
  - Previous respiratory acidosis
  - Brittle asthma
- **Hospital/emergency room (ER) history**
  ≥3 ER visits within past year
  ≥2 hospitalizations within past year
  Hospital admission/ER visit in the last month
- **Medication history**
  - Treatment with ≥3 types of drug
  - >2 inhalers/month of SA beta-2-agonist
  - Recent use of oral steroids
- **Adverse behavioural/psychological factors**
- **Low socio-economic status**
- **Concurrent cardiorespiratory disease**
- **Illicit drug use**

SA= short acting, ICU=intensive care unit, ER=emergency room.

Pharmacotherapy

- **Intravenous fluid** replacement may be required, as patients are often dehydrated
- **High-dose oxygen** is given to maintain SaO_2 94–98%.
- **Inhaled bronchodilators.** All patients should be treated with a beta-2-agonist, given by nebulizer (e.g. salbutamol (albuterol) 2.5-5mg), driven by oxygen or a metered-dose inhaler (MDI). Repeated doses (every 30 min–4 h) or continuous nebulizer therapy is given in severe exacerbations and should be titrated to subsequent improvement in airflow obstruction. Anticholinergic therapy with ipratropium bromide, given by nebulizer (0.5 mg 6-hourly) or MDI, has additive bronchodilator effects when added to a beta-2-agonist in severe asthma. Be aware of the risk of hypokalaemia and lactic acidosis in patients on high-dose beta-2-agonists and steroids.
- **Intravenous bronchodilators** like beta-2-agonist (e.g. salbutamol) and methylxanthines (e.g. aminophylline) are no longer recommended in the routine management of acute asthma, unless inhaled therapy is impossible. Recent studies have shown no additional bronchodilator effect, compared to inhaled therapy alone, but adverse events (e.g. arrhythmias) increase (and may be fatal). Occasionally, intravenous aminophylline may be beneficial in severe or life-threatening asthma that fails to respond to initial therapy but should be used with caution. A loading dose of 5 mg/kg over 20 minutes (which is not needed if the patient is on oral therapy) is followed by a continuous infusion of 0.5 mg/kg/h, with levels monitored. Side effects include nausea, palpitations, and potentially life-threatening arrhythmias.
- **Early steroid therapy** improves outcome. Oral treatment is as effective as intravenous therapy. A prednisolone dose of 30–40 mg for 5–14 days, or until PEF is maintained for >5 days, is recommended,. This should be followed by ongoing inhaled steroid (ICS) therapy (started during oral therapy). Steroid therapy can be stopped abruptly, provided the patient has not been on long-term steroids or had repeated short steroid courses, in which case gradual weaning may be more appropriate.
- **Intravenous magnesium sulfate** (1.2 g infused over 20 min) has bronchodilator properties and may be beneficial in severe asthma responding poorly to initial therapy.
- **Antibiotics** are not indicated, unless there is good reason to suspect a bacterial infection. They are often overused, as viral infections are a common cause of exacerbations.

Ventilatory support

HDU/ICU admission (see Box 5.5) is required if severe asthma deteriorates during initial therapy, fails to improve after more than 6h treatment, or if complications (e.g. pneumothorax, arrhythmia) occur.

Mechanical ventilation is indicated in coma, cardiopulmonary arrest, and when respiratory failure with hypercapnia, exhaustion, or impending respiratory arrest occurs despite maximal pharmacological therapy. Initiation of mechanical ventilation may precipitate cardiovascular collapse (hypotension, reduced cardiac output), as venous return to the right atrium is impeded by increased airwaaessures and hyperinflation. In addition, inadequate alveolar ventilation may exacerbate hypercapnia.

Strategies to prevent hyperinflation, improve alveolar ventilation, and limit barotrauma have reduced ventilator-associated asthma mortality almost to zero. They include reducing respiratory rate (prolonging expiration), limiting peak inspiratory pressures, optimizing inspiratory/

expiratory patterns, and cautious use of positive end expiratory pressure (PEEP) to maximize expiratory volume and reduce work of breathing. In general, non-invasive ventilation is not recommended in acute severe asthma and may worsen outcome by delaying mechanical ventilation.

Discharge
Discharge is considered when patients have stopped nebulizer therapy and been stable on inhalers for over 24h and PEF is >75% predicted, with minimal diurnal variation. Before discharge, review the patient's self-management plan; check inhaler technique, and ensure appropriate follow-up.

Stable asthma
The aims of stable asthma management are: (a) to minimize symptoms and prevent exacerbations; (b) improve quality of life; (c) prevent the consequences of chronic airways inflammation which leads to airways remodelling and irreversible airways obstruction; and (d) to ensure patient education and development of patient self-management plans.

Ideally, on minimum treatment, there should be:
- No daytime or night-time symptoms, normal physical activity, and no exacerbations.
- Normal lung function and minimal diurnal variation.
- Ideally no, or minimal use (i.e. <3 short-acting beta-2-agonist inhaler actuations/week) of short-acting 'reliever' medication.

Ensure each patient has an action plan for exacerbations, and identify high-risk patients at risk of a poor outcome. The Royal College of Physicians (UK) suggests the following three questions to assess asthma control in the preceding week (or month):
- Have you had difficulty sleeping due to your asthma symptoms (e.g. cough)?
- Have you had your usual asthma symptoms during the day (e.g. wheeze, dyspnoea, chest tightness)?
- Has your asthma interfered with your normal activities (e.g. housework)?

Pharmacological management
The British Thoracic Society guidelines recommend a step-up, step-down approach to treatment, using five levels of therapy, depending on disease severity (see Figure 5.22). However, in 2014, the BTS and Scottish Intercollegiate Guidelines Network (SIGN) further developed this stepwise approach in the 'British guideline on the management of asthma; a national clinical guideline' and these changes, including the altered step headings, are included below. History, spirometry, and previous therapy determine the initial level of treatment. Referral to a respiratory specialist should be considered at step 4.
- **Step 1. Mild intermittent asthma.** Treat with 'as required' short-acting beta-2-agonist (SA beta-2A). Poor control is indicated by the use of more than ten inhalations of SA beta-2A/day or two canisters per month. Minimize or eliminate potential triggers. Consider spacer and dry powder devices if compliance or inhaler technique is poor.
- **Step 2. Regular Preventer Therapy**; BTS/SIGN (previously mild persistent asthma; BTS). Add regular 'preventer therapy' with inhaled corticosteroid therapy (ICS). Start at a dose of ICS appropriate to the severity of the asthma. Initially, beclometasone or budesonide 200 mcg twice daily is a typical starting dose in many patients. This is subsequently titrated to the lowest effective dose for symptom control.
- **Step 3. Initial add-on therapy**; BTS/SIGN (previously moderate persistent asthma; BTS). If symptoms persist,

Outcome: asthma control		Outcome: best possible control	

| Control therapy: None | Control therapy: Daily ICS | Control therapy: Daily ICS Daily inhaled long-acting (LA) beta-2-agonist | Control therapy: Daily ICS Daily inhaled LA beta-2-agonist (± if needed) -theophylline SR -leukotriene antagonist -oral LA beta-2-agonist -oral corticosteroid | Control therapy: Step 4 + continuous or frequent use of oral steroid at the lowest effective dose |

Reliever: Rapid-acting inhaled beta-2-agonist

STEP 1 Intermittent	STEP 2 Mild persistent	STEP 3 Moderate persistent	STEP 4 Severe persistent	STEP 5 Steroid therapy

Figure 5.22 British Thoracic Society guideline for the management of asthma. Reproduced with permission from BTS/SIGN British Guideline on the Management of Asthma, May 2008, Revised January 2012, Figure 4.

the first choice as add-on therapy to ICS is an inhaled long-acting beta-2-agonist (LA beta-2A), which should be considered before going above a dose of 400 micrograms beclometasone (BDP, or equivalent) per day (and certainly before going above 800 micrograms BDP). Following the addition of LA beta-2A assess the asthma control. If the asthma control remains suboptimal (after the addition of an inhaled LA beta-2A) then the dose of inhaled corticosteroids should be increased to 800 micrograms/day. If, as occasionally happens, there is no response to inhaled LA beta-2A, stop the LA beta-2A and increase the dose of ICS to 800 micrograms BDP/day. If control in these patients (without LA beta-2A) remains suboptimal consider adding a theophylline or a leukotriene antagonist. At ICS daily doses >800 mcg, side effects may include sore throat, dysphonia, oral Candida, and bone density effects. Consider use of a combined ICS and LA beta-2A inhaler (e.g. Symbicort®, Seretide®) to simplify the treatment regime and improve compliance. A SA beta-2A 'reliever' inhaler continues to be used to alleviate acute symptoms but addition of short-acting anticholinergics is generally of no value.

- **Step 4. Persistent poor control**; BTS/SIGN (previously severe persistent asthma; BTS). Consider increasing ICS to 2,000 micrograms BDP (or budesonide) daily or adding a fourth drug if control remains poor despite use of a combined ICS (800 mcg/day) and LA beta-2A. Theophyllines are effective bronchodilators but may precipitate cardiovascular side effects, including arrhythmias at high serum concentrations. They require therapeutic drug monitoring at doses >200 mg twice daily. Nausea and gastrointestinal side effects limit use in 30% of cases. A trial of leukotriene receptor antagonists may be beneficial in about 30% of cases, particularly atopic asthmatics and those with exercise-induced asthma. It should be withdrawn if unhelpful after 6–8 weeks. Slow-release oral beta-2-agonists may also be considered. Long-acting muscarinic antagonists also appear to be effective in fixed airways obstruction and may be superior to doubling the dose of ICS. There also appears to be benefit in adding tiotropium to ICS and LA beta-2A in patients who remain symptomatic despite these medications. However further evidence is required.

- **Step 5. Continuous or frequent use of oral steroids.** The lowest effective dose of steroid should be used. Warn patients about potential side effects. These usually occur after 3 months' continuous therapy or 3–4 courses of oral steroids each year. Side effects include hypertension, diabetes, peptic ulceration, osteoporosis, and cataracts. Consider treating patients at risk of, or with symptoms, of peptic ulceration with proton pump inhibitors. Monitor bone densitometry, and consider prophylactic therapy with calcium supplements or a bisphosphonate (e.g. alendronic acid 35–70 mg weekly).

- **Alternative pharmacotherapies**, including anti-IgE immunotherapy (e.g. omalizumab) and steroid-sparing therapies (e.g. methotrexate, gold, ciclosporin) may be helpful if initial management is ineffective. They should only be used by respiratory specialists and are discussed in the section on difficult asthma.

Non-pharmacological management
Despite the availability of effective pharmacotherapy, recent studies suggest that up to 75% of asthma patients are inadequately controlled. Non-compliance is the most important factor, as less than 50% of asthmatics are fully compliant with pharmacological therapy, although poor inhaler technique, inadequate education, and failure to recognize dete-

rioration are also factors. Consequently, simple maintenance regimes (i.e. twice daily), using the least number of inhaler devices (i.e. combination inhalers) and similar formulations (i.e. MDI or dry powder inhalers (DPI)), are recommended. Inhaler device and technique are vital for asthma control, as recent studies suggest that about 50% of patients are unable to use an MDI effectively. MDI spacer devices and DPI improve inhaler technique and lung drug deposition.

Patients require simple written self-management plans, education about their asthma, and a peak flow meter to detect asthma deterioration. Patients on low-dose ICS should be instructed to increase the dose at the onset of deterioration, whereas those on high-dose ICS may be provided with an emergency steroid course.

Other non-pharmacological strategies to improve asthma control include:

- **Smoking cessation.**
- **Weight reduction** is helpful in obese asthmatics.
- **Allergen avoidance**, including aggressive control of house dust mites (e.g. removal of carpets, hoovering beds) and pet removal, may be useful in atopic patients. However, evidence for benefit is relatively poor. Exclusion diets have not been helpful. However, fish oils may be beneficial.
- **Allergen-specific immunotherapy** for desensitization may be helpful in a few patients
- **Breathing techniques** reduce SA beta-2A and ICS use but do not alter lung function

Difficult (e.g. 'brittle', steroid-resistant) asthma

Asthma is refractory or difficult to treat in <5% of patients, and early referral to an asthma specialist is recommended. Labile disease, frequent exacerbations (± hospitalization), or severe chronic airflow obstruction, despite aggressive therapy, identify difficult asthma. In these patients, oral steroids often fail to completely reverse airways obstruction; beta-2-agonists responses are poor, and airflow obstruction, bronchial hyperresponsiveness, and diurnal PEF variation are more severe. The likely cause is ongoing airway inflammation, remodelling, and fibrosis, but steroid resistance, beta-2-receptor downregulation, and other disease process should be considered.

Initially, review the diagnosis of asthma, and confirm the reversibility of airflow limitation (e.g. steroid trial). Exclude other causes of cough, breathlessness, and wheeze, including COPD, bronchiectasis, vasculitis (e.g Churg–Strauss, eosinophilic syndromes), allergic bronchopulmonary aspergillosis (ABPA), sinus and upper airways disease, cardiac dysfunction, gastro-oesophageal reflux disease (GORD), hyperventilation syndrome, or psychiatric disease. Ensure compliance with therapy by checking pharmacy records, plasma steroid levels, and inhaler technique before labelling asthma-refractory.

Treatment includes standard high-dose ICS and LA beta-2A. The oral steroid dose is titrated to the lowest dose compatible with symptom control. If this remains >15 mg/day, with no obvious cause for increased steroid clearance (e.g. rifampicin therapy), steroid-sparing agents and alternative therapies should be considered. These are briefly reported below, but detailed data are available in the *Oxford Desk Reference of Respiratory Medicine*.

- **Adjustable ICS maintenance dosing (AMD)** regimes, in which the patient is taught to adjust the level of medication in response to symptom severity, has been demonstrated to improve asthma control.

- **The 'SMART' concept** of asthma management recommends the use of a combined ICS and LA beta-2A inhaler for both maintenance and reliever therapy. A low-dose background maintenance regime is supplemented by reliever doses of the combined inhaler when symptoms occur. There is no use of a SA beta-2A. This regime aims to tailor the intake of ICS to symptoms and has been demonstrated to improved asthma control with a reduction in the total ICS dose.
- **Steroid-sparing agents** include methotrexate, ciclosporin, gold, and macrolide antibiotics. Response is variable, but steroid dose reductions of up to 50% over 3–6 months have been reported. Unfortunately, there have been no confirmatory, randomized controlled trials. Haematological, renal, and liver function monitoring is required.
- **New steroids.** Research is ongoing into 'dissociated' steroid therapy in which the anti-inflammatory effects are dissociated from the side effects.
- **Anti-IgE allergen immunotherapy.** Omalizamub, a humanized anti-IgE antibody, is effective in moderate to severe asthma associated with atopy and high serum IgE levels. Targeting IgE blocks the allergic response, rather than specific allergens or triggers which are often unknown. Two controlled trials reported reduced exacerbation frequencies of 28% and 58%, respectively, and a reduction in ICS use. Although expensive, safety profiles were excellent.
- **Other drugs** currently under investigation include eosinophil inhibitors (e.g. anti-IL-5), cytokine modulators (e.g. anti-TNF-alpha), and phosphodiesterase-4 inhibitors (e.g. roflumilast).
  Specific difficult asthma syndromes include:
- **Steroid-resistant asthma** is rare. It tends to occur in middle-aged, obese women. Diagnoses other than asthma are likely. Treatment is supportive, avoiding high-dose steroids.

Occupational asthma

Asthma due to specific workplace sensitizers accounts for ~10% of adult asthma and is different from asthma exacerbated by 'workplace triggers'. Many agents (e.g. isocyanates, metals, disinfectants, amine dyes, wood dusts, biological enzymes, animal antigens) may cause occupational asthma. Referral to a specialist is recommended, as diagnosis can be difficult and may have significant economic consequences for the patient.

Time from first exposure to symptom onset is variable but can be prolonged. However, once sensitized, low doses can precipitate asthma. It can be difficult to diagnose, but, typically, asthma and serial PEF improve when the patient is away from work, at weekends, and when on holiday. Bronchial provocation tests and skin prick testing confirm the diagnosis and the likely sensitizer. Delayed diagnosis leads to progressive inflammatory airways obstruction. Early recognition and removal from the workplace improves outcome. The *Oxford Desk Reference of Respiratory Medicine* provides details of individual occupational asthma syndromes.

Asthma in pregnancy

One-third of pregnant asthmatic women improve; one-third deteriorate and one-third is unchanged. However, severe asthma is more likely to deteriorate than mild asthma in pregnancy. The course of asthma in successive pregnancies is usually similar. Suggested mechanisms include changes related to maternal hormones, beta-2-adrenoreceptor responsiveness, fetal sex, and altered immune function.

The risk of low birthweight babies increases twofold in mothers with asthma exacerbations during pregnancy (i.e. equivalent to smoking during pregnancy). Preterm delivery and pre-eclampsia were not significantly increased on meta-analysis. The main risk factors for acute exacerbations during pregnancy are severe asthma prior to pregnancy, inappropriate (i.e. patient-initiated) discontinuation of ICS, and increased susceptibility to viral infection. Exacerbations can occur at any time but predominantly late in the second trimester.

Pregnant women should be advised to continue their usual asthma medications. The maternal and fetal risks of poorly controlled asthma far outweigh the small risks from standard therapy. Mothers tend to underreport symptoms and clinicians often undertreat acute exacerbations which should be managed as normal, with additional fetal monitoring. Steroids and nebulized bronchodilators are used at normal doses and SaO_2 maintained >95%. Suggestions that oral steroids are associated with preterm labour and pre-eclampsia are unfounded. Leukotriene antagonists are not commenced during pregnancy due to limited safety data. However, they should be continued in those who have failed to achieve control with other agents in the past.

Acute asthma is unusual during labour. However, patients on more than 7.5 mg of oral steroid daily for longer than 2 weeks prior to delivery should be given intravenous hydrocortisone 100 mg 8-hourly during labour. Dinoprostone (prostaglandin E2) Prostaglandin E2 can be safely used to induce labour, but dinoprost (prostaglandin F2α) prostaglandin F2-alpha for post-partum haemorrhage may induce bronchospasm. Regional anaesthetic blockade (e.g. subdural anaesthesia) is preferable to general anaesthesia in asthmatic patients.

Breastfeeding reduces the incidence of atopy in the children of asthmatic mothers and should be strongly encouraged. Even when the mother is on high-dose prednisolone, which is secreted in breast milk, the infant is only exposed to small, and clinically irrelevant, doses.

Other asthma syndromes

See *Oxford Desk Reference of Respiratory Medicine* for detailed information.
- **Informal descriptive asthma categories** have developed to describe the extensive spectrum of clinical presentations of asthma, but few have formal diagnostic criteria.
  - **The extrinsic and intrinsic classification** arose from the perceived differences in the role of allergy in asthma. Extrinsic 'childhood or early-onset' asthma was associated with allergen sensitization, allergic rhinitis, positive skin prick tests, and raised IgE, whereas patients with intrinsic 'adult-onset' asthma lacked such features. The validity of this classification has been eroded by the finding that IgE levels are raised when corrected for age in intrinsic asthma and that pathological changes are identical in both types.
  - **Nocturnal asthma** describes night-time waking due to asthma symptoms and affects >90% of asthmatics monthly and >35% nightly. It is so common that it is considered a normal feature, rather than a subcategory, of asthma.
  - **Exercise-induced bronchospasm** affects most asthmatics and is thought to be due to evaporative water (± heat) loss during increased ventilation. Osmolality changes provoke mediator release from mast cells and afferent nerve endings, with subsequent bronchoconstriction.

This term is usually reserved for those who only develop bronchoconstriction during exercise. It is usually prevented by pre-exercise beta-2-agonist use.

- **Aspirin-induced asthma.** Asthma is precipitated by aspirin or other non-steroidal anti-inflammatory drugs in 1–20% of asthmatics. The likely mechanism is inhibition of the cyclo-oxygenase pathway, with excess leukotriene production by the lipo-oxygenase pathway. It tends to occur in 'late-onset' asthmatics, is more common in women, and is associated with rhinoconjunctivitis and nasal polyps. Treatment with anti-leukotrienes may help, but avoiding non-steroidal anti-inflammatory drugs is the definitive therapy.

- **Allergic bronchopulmonary aspergillosis** is a rare form of asthma due to hypersensitivity to fungus, usually *Aspergillus fumigatus*, colonizing the bronchial mucosa. It is characterized by eosinophilia, high IgE levels, serum *Aspergillus* antibodies, positive skin prick testing, and recurrent localized CXR infiltrates. Treatment is usually with oral steroids and may prevent bronchiectasis developing.

- **Oral allergy syndrome.** Patients with allergy to some pollens develop lip angioedema immediately after eating certain fresh fruits that share cross-reactivity. Birch pollen cross-reacts with potato, apple, and hazelnuts, whereas ragwort reacts with bananas and melon. Cooked fruit does not cause the same reaction, presumably due to protein denaturation.

Further reading

All Party Parliamentary Group (APPG) on Respiratory Health (June 2014). Report on Inquiry into Respiratory Deaths. <https://www.blf.org.uk/Page/Report-on-inquiry-into-respiratory-deaths>.

ASH. Stopping smoking. <http://www.ash.org.uk>.

Asthma UK. <http://www.asthma.org.uk>.

Asthma and Allergy UK. <http://www.allergyuk.org>.

Best Health. Lungs and breathing. <http://besthealth.bmj.com/x/set/topic/condition-centre/15.html>.

British Lung Foundation Breathe Easy Group. <http://www.lunguk.org>.

British Thoracic Society (2012). British Thoracic Society guidelines for the management of asthma. Thorax, **58**, S1–54.

British Thoracic Society and Scottish Intercollegiate Guidelines Network (2014). British guideline on the management of asthma. A national clinical guideline. <https://www.brit-thoracic.org.uk/document-library/clinical-information/asthma/btssign-asthma-guideline-2014/>.

Chest Heart & Stroke Scotland. <http://www.chss.org.uk/>.

Chung KF, Godard P, Adelroth E, *et al.* (1999). Difficult/therapy resistant asthma: the need for an integrated approach to define clinical phenotypes, evaluate risk factors, understand pathophysiology and find novel therapies. ERS Task Force on Difficult/Therapy Resistant Asthma. European Respiratory Society. *European Respiratory Journal*, **13**, 1198–208.

Chung KF, Wenzel SE, Brozek JL, *et al.* (2014). International ERS/ATS guidelines on definition, evaluation and treatment of severe asthma. *European Respiratory Journal*, **43**, 343–373.

Drazen JM and Silverman EK (1997). Genetics of asthma: conference summary. *American Journal of Respiratory and Critical Care Medicine*, **156**, S69–71.

Lanier BQ, Corren J, Lumry W, Liu J, Fowler-Taylor A, Gupta N (2003). Omalizumab is effective in the long-term control of severe allergic asthma. *Annals of Allergy, Asthma & Immunology*, **91**, 154–9.

Lung Foundation Australia. <http://www.lungfoundation.com.au/>.

Murphy VE, Clifton VL, Gibson PE (2006). Asthma exacerbations during pregnancy: incidence and association with adverse pregnancy outcomes. *Thorax*, **61**, 169–76.

Murphy VE, Gibson PG, Smith R, Clifton VL (2005). Asthma during pregnancy: mechanisms and treatment implications. *European Respiratory Journal*, **25**, 731–50.

NHS Choices. Asthma. <http://www.nhs.uk/conditions/Asthma/Pages/Introduction.aspx>.

NHS SmokeFree: Smoking—advice to help you stop smoking. <http://smokefree.nhs.uk/>.

No authors listed (1998). Worldwide variations in the prevalence of asthma, allergic rhinoconjunctivitis, and atopic eczema: ISAAC. The International Study of Asthma and Allergies in Childhood Steering Committee. *Lancet*, **351**, 1225–32.

O'Byrne PM, Barnes PJ, Rodriguez-Roisin R, *et al.* (2001). Low dose inhaled budesonide and formoterol in mild persistent asthma: the OPTIMA randomised trial. *American Journal of Respiratory and Critical Care Medicine*, **164**, 1392–7.

Partridge MR, van der Molen T, Myrseth S-E, Busse WW (2006). Attitudes and actions of asthma patients on regular maintenance therapy: the INSPIRE study. *BMC Pulmonary Medicine*, **6**, 13.

Pauwels RA, Löfdahl CG, Postma DS, *et al.* (1997). Effect of inhaled formoterol and budesonide on exacerbations of asthma. Formoterol and Corticosteroids Establishing Therapy (FACET) International Study Group. *New England Journal of Medicine*, **337**, 1405–11.

Reddel HK, Taylor DR, Bateman ED, *et al.* (2009) An Official American Thoracic Society/European Respiratory Society Statement: Asthma Control and Exacerbations. Standardizing Endpoints for Clinical Asthma Trials and Clinical Practice. *American Journal of Respiratory and Critical Care Medicine*, **180**, 59–99.

Sly RM (1999). Changing prevalence of allergic rhinitis and asthma. *Annals of Allergy, Asthma & Immunology*, **82**, 233–48.

Wiener C (1993). Ventilatory management of respiratory failure in asthma. *JAMA*, **269**, 2128–31.

Chronic obstructive pulmonary disease

Chronic obstructive pulmonary disease (COPD) is a common, slowly progressive disease that causes a gradual, irreversible decline in lung function, chronic respiratory symptoms (e.g. cough, wheeze, exertional dyspnoea), intermittent exacerbations, disability, respiratory failure, and eventually death. It is usually caused by cigarette smoke (>80%), but other noxious gases or particles can cause COPD. It is likely that all smokers develop some degree of airway inflammation, and there is evidence of genetic susceptibility. If they live long enough, up to 50% of smokers will develop pathophysiological and clinical features of COPD. These features include airflow obstruction that is partially reversible, destruction of the lung parenchyma (emphysema), secondary pulmonary vasculopathy, and important systemic consequences.

Although now slightly outdated, chronic bronchitis is defined by the MRC for epidemiological purposes as 'the presence of chronic cough and sputum production for at least three months in two consecutive years in the absence of other diseases recognised to cause sputum production'. It does not always signify the presence of airways obstruction or the diagnosis of COPD. However, it is airways obstruction, not mucus hypersecretion, that is the main cause of morbidity and mortality in COPD.

Several COPD guidelines have been published, which differ in detail. This chapter complies with the National Institute for Health and Clinical Excellence (NICE, UK) guidelines (2010), the ATS/ERS standards for the diagnosis and treatment of patients with COPD position paper (2004), the National Institute for Health (USA) Global Initiative for Chronic Obstructive Lung Disease (GOLD; 2015), the American Thoracic Society guidelines (2011), and the UK curriculum requirements for Acute and Internal Medicine (breathlessness and COPD; RCP; 2006).

Epidemiology

A diagnosis of COPD has been established in 0.9 million of the UK population (13% of people over 35 years of age have COPD), although the true prevalence is probably about 3.0 million (i.e. ~70% unidentified). Estimates suggest 24 million cases in the USA, and the BOLD study has shown the prevalence to be about 8% in many countries. Worldwide, COPD

Box 5.7 Risk factors for COPD
Smoking
Age >50 years old; prevalence ~5–10%
Male gender
Childhood chest infections
Airways hyperreactivity
• Asthma/atopy
Low socio-economic status
Alpha-1-antitrypsin deficiency
Heavy metal/dust exposure
• Cadmium, silica (pottery workers)
Atmospheric pollution

is the third leading cause of death and the only preventable cause that is increasing. In 2014, there were 26,267 deaths attributable to COPD in England and Wales (i.e. fifth commonest cause of death and responsible for about 5% of all deaths). However, it was a comorbid condition in many more deaths. Currently, COPD exacerbations account for ~12% of all emergency hospital admissions in the UK and is not more frequent in the winter months as is often believed. Yearly mortality is ~25% when FEV_1 is <0.8 L and is increased by coexisting cor pulmonale, hypercapnia, and weight loss.

Pathogenesis

COPD is a classic example of a disease arising from gene-environment interaction. The cumulative inhalation of particulates and fumes causes a dose-dependent airway inflammation that is influenced by genetic susceptibility. Smoking is the most obvious risk factor. Others are listed in Box 5.7. Figure 5.23 illustrates the traditional concept of an accelerated decline in FEV_1 over time that has been used to define disease progression in COPD. However, more recent evidence suggests early, rapid FEV_1 loss, and slowing of the rate of progression later. This is important as it emphasizes the importance of early diagnosis and the opportunity for prompt intervention.

Deficiency of alpha-1-proteinase inhibitor is associated with early-onset emphysema in 2% of COPD patients.

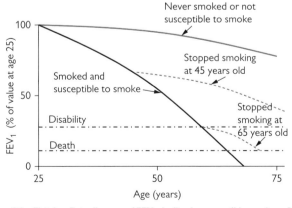

Figure 5.23 Modification of the Fletcher Peto diagram of FEV_1 decline in susceptible smokers. Reproduced from *British Medical Journal*, Fletcher C, Peto R, 'The natural history of chronic airflow obstruction', 1, 6077, pp. 1645–1648, copyright 1977, with permission from BMJ Publishing Group Ltd.

Alpha-1-antitrypsin is a protease inhibitor which prevents alveolar damage. Normal alpha-1-antitrypsin production requires two M genes (i.e. phenotype MM). Several genes, including S (partial deficiency), Z (severe deficiency), and null (complete deficiency), cause alpha-1-proteinase inhibitor deficiency. Homozygotes (e.g. SS, ZZ) have very low plasma alpha-1-proteinase inhibitor levels and develop emphysema in the third or fourth decade of life. Heterozygotes (e.g. MS, MZ) have reduced levels and are at greater risk of emphysema, particularly if smokers. The American Thoracic Society currently recommends screening all patients with airflow obstruction that is not obviously asthma for alpha-1-proteinase inhibitor phenotype.

Pathophysiology

The pathophysiological processes of emphysema, chronic bronchitis, and airflow obstruction usually coexist in COPD, and it is difficult to define the relative importance of each in an individual patient.

- **Emphysema** is associated with destruction of alveolar septa and capillaries due to protease and oxidant damage. Typically, tobacco smoke causes centrilobular or proximal emphysema, with predominantly upper lobe involvement, whereas alpha-1-proteinase inhibitor deficiency causes panacinar emphysema and usually affects the lower lobes. The type of emphysema has little clinical relevance, except when considering lung volume reduction surgery or endobronchial valve placement. Loss of lung tissue leads to the formation of bullae (large airspaces), reduces elastic recoil, and impairs diffusing capacity. It also contributes to airways obstruction as a result of the loss of 'elastic' radial traction that normally maintains airway patency.
- **Chronic bronchitis** causes airways obstruction as a result of chronic mucosal inflammation, fibrosis, mucus hypersecretion, and bronchospasm. Associated V/Q mismatch is due to early airways closure in expiration, redistribution of blood flow or alveolar collapse if the airway is completely obstructed.
- **Pulmonary hypertension.** Hypoxia leads to arteriolar remodelling and secondary pulmonary hypertension. In emphysema, extensive capillary loss may also contribute to PHT. Although the PHT may worsen over time, its severity is modest by comparison with primary pulmonary arterial hypertension (PAH), and its clinical relevance is uncertain.

COPD symptoms correlate poorly with the degree of airflow obstruction measured by spirometry, and hyperinflation is probably the major physiological mechanism leading to breathlessness. 'Static' hyperinflation describes air trapping present at rest as a result of loss of lung elastic recoil and gas trapping as a result of premature closure of the airways during exhalation. 'Dynamic' hyperinflation describes the additional air trapping that occurs when the breathing frequency increases during exercise, reducing the time available for exhalation. The 'horizontal' position of the ribs and flat diaphragms produced by hyperinflation place inspiratory muscles at a mechanical disadvantage, increasing the elastic work of breathing. The raised intrathoracic pressure due to hyperinflation can also reduce venous return to the right heart and decrease cardiac output, causing cardiovascular impairment.

- **Clinical features** of COPD include a morning cough productive of mucoid sputum, exertional dyspnoea, and sometimes wheezing. Weight loss, ankle oedema, nocturnal waking, and fatigue may occur. Haemoptysis and chest pain are unusual and raise the possibility of other diagnoses (e.g. lung cancer). Significant airways obstruction often precedes clinical features. The concept of emphysematous 'pink puffers' and bronchitic 'blue bloaters' is unreliable and outdated, and these terms should not now be used. Most patients have a mixture of airflow obstruction, emphysema, and chronic bronchitis, and the clinical features reflect all these pathologies. Patients with predominant emphysema are often more breathless, but less hypoxaemic, and have signs of hyperinflation and malnutrition, including thin body habitus, tachypnoea, barrel chest, purse-lipped breathing, and accessory muscle use. Chest auscultation reveals quiet breath and heart sounds, with prolonged expiratory time (>4 s) and wheeze.
- Patients with predominant chronic bronchitis are often less breathless despite being hypoxaemic. In extreme cases, impaired CO_2 clearance is associated with bounding pulse, confusion, headache, flapping tremor, vasodilation, and papilloedema.

Cor pulmonale, with characteristic hepatomegaly, ankle oedema, and raised JVP, is probably due to fluid retention, rather than right heart failure per se.

Pulmonary hypertension (PHT) is a late feature. It is partially reversed by oxygen therapy.

COPD is associated with low grade systemic inflammation and the intensity of this inflammation increases during exacerbations. The mechanism is not established but it is not simply linked to 'spill-over' pulmonary inflammation and appears to involve other factors including smoking, tissue hypoxia, and skeletal muscle dysfunction. Nevertheless this inflammation has been implicated in the pathogenesis of the majority of so-called 'systemic effects of COPD', including weight loss, skeletal muscle dysfunction, cardiovascular disease, depression, and osteoporosis. Available evidence suggests that the inflammation can be reduced by steroid therapy (both oral and inhaled). For example, a retrospective analysis suggested that the risk of acute myocardial infarction in patients with COPD was reduced by >30% in those receiving low dose ICS. However, the potential effects on clinically relevant outcomes in these patients (e.g. mortality, health status) remains to be demonstrated, and the opportunities for treatment require further study.

Defining the severity of COPD

This is a complex issue. Most guidelines use FEV_1 thresholds to define different degrees of airflow obstruction and use these to guide therapy. For example, the NICE guidelines define severe airflow obstruction as <30% of predicted FEV_1, moderate airflow obstruction as 30–49%, and mild airflow obstruction as 50–80%, but individual guidelines differ. Thus, in patients with an FEV_1/FVC <0.7, the GOLD (Global Strategy for the Diagnosis, Management, and Prevention of COPD) guidelines define very severe COPD as an FEV_1 <30% predicted, severe as <50% but >30% predicted, moderate as <80% but >50% predicted, and mild COPD as an FEV_1/FVC ratio <0.7 but with an FEV_1 >80% predicted. However, there is a poor correlation between the degree of airflow obstruction (FEV_1 on spirometry) and symptoms, disability, and quality of life. In this regard, a true assessment of the severity of COPD should be multidimensional and include factors such as exacerbation frequency, degree of breathlessness, symptom assessment, health related quality of life, body mass index (BMI), exercise capacity, and degree of hypoxia.

A simple measure of breathlessness is the modified Medical Research Council Questionnaire (mMRCQ) which grades breathlessness as follows: Grade 0 – only breathless with strenuous exercise; Grade 1 – short of breath when hurrying on the level or walking up a slight hill; Grade 2 – walking slower than people of the same age on the same level because of breathlessness or having to stop for breath when walking at the patient's own pace on the level; Grade 3 – the need to stop for breath after walking for about 100 metres or after a few minutes on the level; Grade 4 – too breathless to leave the house or breathless when dressing or undressing. (Reprinted from *Journal of the American College of Cardiology*, 54, 1, Simonneau G et al., 'Updated Clinical Classification of Pulmonary Hypertension', pp. S43-S54, Copyright 2009, with permission from Elsevier and American College of Cardiology.)

Symptomatic assessment of COPD using comprehensive disease-specific, health-related, quality of life questionnaires like the St George's Respiratory Questionnaire (SGRQ) is too cumbersome for routine clinical practice. However, the COPD Assessment Test (CAT), an eight-item unidimensional measure of health status impairment in COPD, is a comprehensive measure of symptoms including systemic effects. The score ranges from 0–40 and correlates closely with the SGRQ; a score of 10 or more indicates a high level of symptoms.

As COPD exacerbations are associated with an increase in lung function decline and risk of death, they can be regarded as an indicator of poor outcome. The best predictor of frequent exacerbations (i.e. two or more a year) is the previous history of COPD exacerbations. Admission to hospital with COPD exacerbations also correlates with a poor prognosis. Although not a precise measure in the individual patient, spirometric grading correlates with the increased risk of exacerbations, hospitalization, and death. In particular the risk of exacerbations increases significantly in GOLD spirometric grading levels 3 (severe) and 4 (very severe).

In order to understand the impact of COPD on an individual patient, and to provide a more meaningful classification of COPD, the 2015 GOLD guidelines have suggested combining:

(a) Symptoms; using symptomatic assessment of breathlessness (i.e. CAT or mMRCQ scores) to define patients with 'More' or 'Less' symptoms.

(b) Risk; by assessing spirometric classification, risk of exacerbations and hospital admissions to define patients as either 'High' or 'Low' risk.

This assessment of both risk and symptoms (e.g. 'Low risk', 'More symptoms') is thought to reflect the complexity of COPD better than an isolated measurement of airflow obstruction and, consequently, may help guide and improve subsequent treatment decisions.

Diagnosis

The diagnosis of COPD should be considered in patients with suspicious symptoms, such as exertional dyspnoea and productive cough, and/or a history of risk factors (e.g. smoking, air pollution, occupational dust, or chemical exposure). Early presentation is often masked because patients reduce their level of physical activity to avoid dyspnoea. The diagnosis is suspected on the basis of the history and confirmed on spirometry (see Figure 5.24) if post-bronchodilator FEV_1/FVC ratio is <0.7. The NICE criteria no longer include an FEV_1 <80% predicted as this may overlook early airflow limitation in patients where the FEV_1/FVC ratio is below the lower limit of normal and yet FEV_1 and FVC remain >80% predicted, and it may be important to identify these early cases. Further assessment should include routine blood tests, pulse oximetry, and a CXR to exclude other conditions (e.g. lung cancer). The clinical scenario determines the

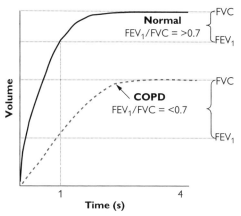

Figure 5.24 Spirometry. FEV_1 and FEV_1/FVC ratio are decreased in COPD.

need for further investigation (e.g. arterial blood gases (ABG), alpha-1-proteinase inhibitor levels, gas transfer, lung volumes, CT scan, sputum culture, ECG, etc.).

- **Chest radiography** may reveal hyperinflation (e.g. flat diaphragms, large retrosternal airspace, >7 posterior ribs visible, horizontal ribs), narrow mediastinum, hyperlucency, reduced peripheral vascular markings, and apical bullae which may be mistaken for pneumothoraces.
- **Lung function test** may show increased lung volumes (TLC, FRC, RV) and impaired diffusion (DLCO, KCO).

Management

Recent guidelines and healthcare priorities recommend:

1. **Early diagnosis of COPD**, based on smoking history and routine spirometry (± reversibility) measurements.
2. **Prevention of disease progression** by encouraging smoking cessation and reducing risk factors (e.g. occupational dust exposure, air pollution).
3. **Optimization of medical therapy in stable COPD** to improve the quality and length of life of patients and to prevent acute exacerbations and associated hospital admissions.
4. **Early discharge**, following hospital admission for acute exacerbations, and ongoing community support (e.g. outreach teams).

Stable COPD management

Optimal management of stable COPD requires both pharmacological and non-pharmacological interventions. The recommended stepwise increase in inhaler therapy as COPD deteriorates differs slightly between individual guidelines (e.g. GOLD, NICE). For some patients with mild intermittent symptoms, short-acting bronchodilators used as needed are sufficient, but, if symptoms persist, long-acting bronchodilators (beta-2-agonist or anticholinergic) should be prescribed alone or in combination. If symptoms remain uncontrolled, combined long-acting beta-2-agonist/inhaled steroid inhalers should be used in preference to long-acting beta-2-agonists alone, particularly if patients are experiencing frequent exacerbations. Table 5.14 provides a useful synthesis of the different management guidelines for stable COPD and remains a simple, practical guide to pharmacotherapy.

Table 5.14 Summary of current guidelines for pharmacological and non-pharmacological management of COPD: (↓) European guidelines (⋮) American guidelines

Clinical stage	Pharmacological therapy		Non-pharmacological therapy
At risk			Smoking cessation +++
Intermittent symptoms	Short acting bronchodilators (e.g. salbutamol and/or ipratropium bromide) initially 'as required'.		Vaccination, e.g. influenza
Persistent symptoms	Tiotropium Salbutamol	Long-acting beta-2-agonist Ipratropium, salbutamol	Pulmonary rehabilitation Nutrition Antidepressants
	Tiotropium Long-acting beta-2-agonist (± theophyllines, mucolytics)		
With frequent exacerbations	Tiotropium + long-acting beta-2-agonist Inhaled corticosteroid (± theophyllines, mucolytics, oral steroids)		Consider ambulatory oxygen therapy if exercise desaturation
Respiratory failure			Long-term oxygen therapy Non-invasive ventilation Lung reduction surgery

Adapted by permission from BMJ Publishing Group Limited. *British Medical Journal*, Cooper CB, Tashkin DP, 'Recent developments in inhaled therapy in stable chronic obstructive pulmonary disease', 330, pp. 640–644, copyright 2005.

Non pharmacological therapy

Smoking cessation is the most effective and cost-efficient intervention to reduce the risk of COPD and decrease the smoking-related decline in lung function (see Figure 5.23). Even a 3-min period of counselling, urging a smoker to 'quit', in a clear, strong, personalized manner can be effective, and, at the very least, this should be done for every smoker at each visit. Anti-smoking pharmacotherapies, including nicotine replacement therapy, bupropion, or varenicline (± behavioural support schemes) achieve quit rates of 20–40% at 12 weeks and 15–25% at 12 months. Even without pharmacotherapy, 'quit rates' of 15–20% at 12 weeks are reported with intensive behavioural support alone (e.g. ASH, NHS). Electronic cigarettes are battery powered vapourizers designed to simulate smoking and use heat to vaporize a liquid-based solution containing nicotine, glycerine, propylene glycol, and flavourings into an aerosol mist. They have been proposed as a way to help smokers quit. Their use is often termed 'vaping' and they are used by ~2 million people in the UK and ~8.5% of the population in the USA in 2013. Their role/value in smoking cessation or harm reduction has not been established but UK regulation is expected in 2016.

Pulmonary rehabilitation (PR) is a multidisciplinary programme that effectively increases exercise performance and muscle strength, enhances quality of life, increases physical and emotional involvement in everyday life, and reduces symptoms and hospital admissions. The mainstay of PR is graded exercise to prevent muscle wasting and deconditioning. However, interventions to address altered mood and social isolation, improve education (e.g. breathing techniques), and prevent weight loss are equally important.

Control of breathing exercises. 'Breathing retraining', using various techniques, works by slowing breathing frequency and thus reducing air trapping and hyperinflation. For example, during COPD exacerbations, air trapping can be reduced by slowing breathing frequency (i.e. longer expiration) and 'purse-lip' breathing (i.e. to 'splint' open small airways) which increases expiratory, and subsequent inspiratory, volumes and improves minute ventilation.

Nutrition. Body mass index (BMI) should be maintained in the range >20 to <30. When BMI is <20, improving nutritional status improves respiratory muscle strength and prognosis. Similarly, when BMI is >30, reducing weight improves functional status and reduces dyspnoea.

Pharmacological therapy

Inhaler and drug therapy aim to alleviate symptoms, prevent exacerbations and reduce long term risk. There is increasingly good evidence to suggest that smoking cessation, reduction of exacerbations, and maintenance of higher levels of physical activity (all of which can be achieved with inhaled pharmacotherapy) have a positive effect on survival.

Bronchodilators (see Table 5.14) are central to the symptomatic management of COPD, and use depends on the severity and persistence of symptoms at the time of diagnosis. Initially prescribed on an 'as required' basis, they are subsequently given regularly to prevent or relieve symptoms. When given by the preferred inhaled route, attention to inhaler technique is vital; many patients (~50%) use metered-dose inhalers (MDI) incorrectly. Spirometric improvements with inhaled bronchodilators are often small, but the associated reduction in functional residual capacity (FRC) and hyperinflation correlates well with improved functional status, dyspnoea index, and quality of life (QOL) measures. Side effects are mild, predictable, and dose-dependent. Patients with distressing breathlessness, despite maximal inhaler therapy, may be considered for supervised home nebulizer therapy, although the evidence for additional benefit is limited.

- **Inhaled short-acting beta-2-sympathomimetic agonists (SABA)** have a rapid onset of action (<5 min) and are often used as first-line therapy. They are initially prescribed as short-acting agents (e.g. salbutamol, albuterol).

- **Inhaled short-acting muscarinic antagonists** (SAMA e.g. ipratropium bromide) have a slower onset of action than SABAs (>20 min) but are equally effective bronchodilators in COPD when compared with SABAs. If patients require regular short-acting muscarinic antagonist therapy, they should be switched to a once-daily long-acting muscarinic antagonist (LAMA) therapy which is more effective.

- **Inhaled long-acting beta-2-sympathomimetic agonists** (LABA e.g. salmeterol, formoterol, arformoterol, indacaterol, vilanterol, olodaterol) are used if symptoms persist. Formoterol has a speed of onset of action similar to salbutamol, whereas salmeterol has a slower onset of action. LABAs improve health status and reduce exacerbation rates to a greater extent than short-acting drugs.
- **Inhaled long-acting muscarinic antagonists** (LAMA e.g. tiotropium) are given once daily. They improve health status, reduce hyperinflation, and reduce exacerbation rates. They also appear to reduce mortality and possibly slow the rate of decline in FEV_1. Combinations of a beta-2-sympathomimetic agonist and muscarinic antagonist agents are synergistic, with greater additive effects than either agent alone. Both tiotropium bromide and ipratropium bromide have an affinity for, and bind to, the muscarinic receptors M1, M2, and M3 (where M1 and M3 binding mediates bronchodilation, and M2 mediates bronchoconstriction). However, tiotropium dissociates very slowly from M1 and particularly M3 receptors compared with ipratropium and more rapidly from the M2 receptors. For tiotropium, this prolonged duration of action, higher affinity, and functional selectivity for M3 receptors produces greater improvement in airflow limitation when compared with ipratropium. Therefore, theoretically, tiotropium and ipratropium bromide should not be used at the same time.
- **Inhaled long-acting beta-2-sympathomimetic agonist/corticosteroid combinations** (e.g. salmeterol/fluticasone, formoterol/budesonide, vilanterol/fluticasone) are now generally indicated to reduce exacerbation frequency. Long-acting beta-2-sympathomimetic agonist/corticosteroid combinations improve health status and reduce exacerbation rates to a greater extent than LABAs alone, and they appear to reduce mortality and slow the rate of decline in FEV_1. However, inhaled corticosteroids (ICS) are associated with an increased risk of pneumonia but a recent Cochrane database review demonstrated that neither fluticasone or budesonide ICS significantly affected mortality compared with controls. Comparison of these two ICS drugs revealed no statistically significant difference in serious pneumonias, mortality, or adverse risk, although fluticasone was associated with higher risk of any pneumonia when compared with budesonide (i.e. less serious cases dealt with in the community).
- **Inhaled LAMA–LABA combinations** (e.g. umeclidinium and vilanterol) offer the combined effects of both long-acting bronchodilator classes and are just becoming available.
- **Methylxanthines** (e.g. theophylline, aminophylline) are usually prescribed as slow-release oral preparations and improve exercise tolerance and blood gases but have negligible effects on spirometry. In addition to bronchodilator effects, they may improve respiratory drive, diaphragmatic strength, and mucociliary clearance. Unfortunately, potential toxicity and the need for monitoring of plasma levels at higher doses limit usefulness.

Corticosteroids. Inhaled corticosteroids (ICS) should only be given in combination with LABAs. Combination therapy is indicated if symptoms persist or if patients have recurring exacerbations despite long-acting bronchodilator therapy (as previously described). However, as reported above, the use of the ICS fluticasone or budesonide in COPD is associated with an increased risk of serious pneumonia but not mortality. Long-term treatment with oral steroids is not recommended, as <25% of COPD patients benefit, and steroid-induced myopathy and systemic side effects contribute to muscle weakness and early respiratory failure. They also worsen osteoporosis.

Other pharmacological therapies include:
- **Vaccination** against influenza and pneumococcal infection is vital. Influenza vaccination reduces serious illness and death due to influenza by about 50% in COPD patients.
- **Azithromycin** maintenance treatment (250mg daily) has been shown to decrease the exacerbation rate (~17%) and improves quality of life in patients with COPD. It should be considered in patients who have the frequent exacerbator phenotype and are refractory to standard care. However, the potential cardiovascular risks of azithromycin (as with other macrolides) on QT interval and the prevalence of cardiovascular disease in patients with COPD can make 'selection' of patients a challenge. A cautious approach would exclude patients with known risks of cardiovascular disease or QTc prolongation on initial ECG and those on other medications known to prolong QTc.
- **Mucolytic agents** may assist some patients with excessive sputum production, but antitussive agents are not recommended.
- **Phosphodiesterase-4 (PDE4) inhibitors** are now available. In the 2015 GOLD guidelines the oral PDE4 inhibitor roflumilast is included as a potential 'add on' to bronchodilator therapy for maintenance treatment in severe COPD (GOLD spirometric grade 3–4: FEV_1 postbronchodilator <50% predicted) and those patients with a history of frequent exacerbations. In this patient population, roflumilast 500µg once-daily reduces exacerbation rate and marginally improves lung function.
- **Antidepressant and sedative pharmacotherapy.** Antidepressants should be considered in depressed patients. However, benzodiazepines and narcotics are respiratory depressants and may worsen hypercapnia. They are not recommended, except in end-stage palliative COPD when they may relieve dyspnoea.
- **Alpha-1-proteinase inhibitor augmentation** is expensive and of unproven value and is not recommended for routine use (NICE).
- **Other agents**, including antioxidants, respiratory stimulants, regular antibiotics, and immunoregulatory therapies, are not recommended in stable COPD.

Long-term oxygen therapy (LTOT)

Oxygen therapy used for >15 h/day improves survival in hypoxaemic patients. It also has beneficial effects on haemodynamics, polycythaemia, exercise capacity, and mental state. LTOT is indicated when PaO_2 is <7.3 kPa, with or without hypercapnia, in clinically stable COPD patients. When PaO_2 is >7.3 kPa but <8 kPa, LTOT may be appropriate if one of secondary polycythaemia, nocturnal hypoxaemia, peripheral oedema, or pulmonary hypertension is present. LTOT should only be prescribed after full assessment by a respiratory physician. Ideally, whenever LTOT is prescribed, there should be provision of a portable oxygen system to help patients remain physically active.

Endoscopic lung volume reduction and surgery
In advanced disease, lung volume reduction surgery (thoracoscopic or open) or lung transplantation may be indicated. Emphysema is a component of COPD characterized by hyperinflation resulting in reduced gas exchange and interference with breathing mechanics. Where emphysema is heterogeneous, the worst affected areas of lung expand disproportionately, restricting the ventilation of relatively more healthy areas. Lung volume reduction surgery (LVRS) to resect these emphysematous areas has been clearly shown to improve outcomes in selected patient groups. However, this surgical intervention is associated with significant morbidity and an early mortality rate of about 5%.

Endoscopic lung volume reduction (ELVR) uses one-way valves to induce atelectasis in pre-selected hyperinflated lobes and is less invasive than open or thoracoscopic lung volume reduction surgery. Selected patients have the potential for significant benefit in terms of lung function, exercise capacity, and possibly even survival. The evidence from clinical trials indicates that complete lobar occlusion in the absence of collateral ventilation or where there is an intact lobar fissure are the key predictors for clinical success. For example in unselected patients the overall benefits were relatively small (FEV$_1$ increase ~7%) but in carefully selected patients who developed sustained postprocedure atelectasis, clinically useful benefit was achieved (FEV$_1$ increase ~17%, improved exercise tolerance). The proportion of patients that respond to treatment improves from 20% in the unselected population to 75% with appropriate patient selection and assessment of collateral ventilation is fundamental to this patient selection. Other indicators for success are greater heterogeneity in disease distribution between upper and lower lobes. The main adverse events observed were an excess of pneumothoraces. All patients undergoing ELVR should be included in appropriate trials.

Bullectomy, surgical lung volume reduction, or transplantation may be indicated in carefully selected patients with advanced COPD. However, specialist advice should be sought.

Palliative care
As the disease progresses, a palliative care approach to symptom control should be considered. This may include the use of opiates and benzodiazepines for symptom control. Advance care planning is important, and patients should be encouraged to discuss issues, such as the use of mechanical ventilation and CPR.

Management of exacerbations
COPD exacerbations have been defined as a sustained worsening of the patient's usual stable state that is acute in onset and includes worsening breathlessness, cough, and an increase in discoloured sputum production. Exacerbations are common and, when severe, may require hospital admission (± critical care). They are often due to bacterial or viral infections. The differential diagnosis includes pulmonary embolism, pneumothorax, ischaemic heart disease, heart failure, and arrhythmias (e.g. atrial fibrillation due to medications, metabolic upset, or atrial enlargement). Frequent exacerbations probably accelerate the rate of decline in FEV$_1$. In the UK, the average length of hospital admission for an acute COPD exacerbation is 5 days and costs between £1,500 and £3,500. The readmission rate is >30% and mortality >10% within 3 months of the initial admission. Following ICU admission, 12-month mortality is ~40%.

General measures
Controlled oxygen therapy is vital in acute COPD exacerbations. In most patients, oxygen therapy (OT) leads to a small increase in PaCO$_2$ which is of no consequence, but, unfortunately, about 10% of COPD patients develop hypercapnic respiratory failure (HCRF), with a significant increase in PaCO$_2$ (primarily due to impaired CO$_2$ elimination (see section 'Hypoxaemia, respiratory failure, and oxygen therapy' earlier in this chapter)). Nevertheless, these patients still benefit from low-dose 'controlled' OT (24–28%) because even a small increase in PaO$_2$ on the steep part of the oxygen-haemoglobin dissociation curve significantly increases arterial oxygen content without causing significant CO$_2$ retention. In these patients, the response to an increase in oxygen concentration should be monitored with arterial blood gas (ABG) measurements to achieve a PaO$_2$ >8 kPa without a substantial rise in PaCO$_2$.

Patients with a previous history of HCRF should be given an oxygen alert card (± 24% Venturi mask) to give to healthcare personnel in the event of a further COPD exacerbation. In these patients, the target oxygen saturation (SaO$_2$) should be 88–92%, pending arterial blood gas (ABG) analysis. A higher SaO$_2$ has few advantages but may result in hypoventilation, hypercapnia, and respiratory acidosis. In the absence of an oximeter, selecting the appropriate dose of pre-hospital OT can be difficult. During short periods (<20 min) of pre-hospital transport and A+E department assessment, 28–35% O$_2$ therapy should be started. If drowsiness develops or if HCRF has occurred previously (i.e. patient has an oxygen alert card), give 'controlled' OT, using a fixed performance (24–28%) 'Venturi' mask.

If initial ABG measurements confirm HCRF, ongoing OT, administered through a Venturi mask, should be titrated to the lowest concentration required to achieve an SaO$_2$ 88–92% (PaO$_2$ ~8 kPa). ABG must be monitored regularly. If the PaCO$_2$ rises (>8 kPa) and pH falls (<7.35), or if the patient becomes drowsy or fatigued, non-invasive positive pressure ventilation (NIPPV) should be initiated (see section on ventilatory support). If despite NIPPV, hypercapnia and respiratory acidosis progress, but intubation and mechanical ventilation are considered inappropriate (i.e. end-stage disease), management should focus on optimizing ventilatory drive. FiO$_2$ may be reduced to stimulate hypoxic drive and spontaneous ventilation, thereby decreasing PaCO$_2$. SaO$_2$ will fall to <85%, but aim to maintain PaO$_2$ at >6.5 kPa (SaO$_2$ <80–85%).

In COPD patients at low risk of developing HCRF or if PaCO$_2$ is normal on the initial ABG measurement, OT should aim for the normal target SaO$_2$ range of 94–98% if aged <70 years and 92–98% if aged >70 years (i.e. wider normal range in the elderly). These higher ranges are on the plateau of the oxygen-haemoglobin dissociation curve where haemoglobin is fully saturated. Further increases in PaO$_2$ have no impact on oxygen delivery, as very little oxygen dissolves in plasma. In these patients, OT, delivered by nasal prongs, is more comfortable and allows normal communication, drinking, and eating. Oxygen conserving devices can also be very effective at improving oxygenation with lower oxygen flow requirements. ABG should be checked 30–60 minutes after a change in oxygen dose.

Other general measures include:
- **Physiotherapy** to assist secretion clearance (e.g. breathing and coughing techniques).
- **Fluid and electrolyte management** can be difficult in 'cor pulmonale' and requires careful monitoring and electrolyte correction (e.g. hypophosphataemia, hypokalaemia).

- **Nutritional support** (2,000 calorie intake daily) improves respiratory muscle strength and endurance. Although it is possible to generate excessive CO_2 production by overfeeding with carbohydrate, this is rarely a problem. Low-carbohydrate, high-lipid feeds (to reduce CO_2 generation) are rarely necessary.
- **Thromboembolic prophylaxis** is vital in immobile cases. Options include low-dose subcutaneous heparin, sequential compression devices, or graded elastic stockings where anticoagulants are contraindicated.

Pharmacological therapy

Bronchodilators. The first step in adjusting pharmacotherapy for a COPD exacerbation should be intensification of inhaled bronchodilator therapy. High-dose, aerosolized short-acting beta-2-sympathomimetic agonists (e.g. salbutamol 2.5–5 mg qds) and muscarinic antagonists (e.g. ipratropium bromide 0.5 mg qds) bronchodilators are initially delivered by nebulizer to relieve symptoms and improve gas exchange. Nebulizers should be driven with compressed air in hypercapnic patients. Handheld inhalers are used as soon as the acute exacerbation has stabilized.

Oral corticosteroids. In the absence of contraindications, oral corticosteroids should be used to improve lung function and hasten recovery in severe COPD exacerbations that do not immediately respond to intensification of bronchodilator therapy. Early treatment maximizes benefit. Current evidence suggests that in most cases prednisolone 30–40mg daily orally should be prescribed for 5–7 days. Current evidence suggests that treating COPD exacerbations with corticosteroids for ~5 days is no less effective than treating patients for 7–14 days or longer. A recent comparison of prednisolone 40mg daily for 5 versus 14 days showed no difference in outcomes, including time to death, exacerbation recovery times, relapse rates, death, or recovery of lung function. These findings are reflected in the recent GOLD guidelines (2015) which now recommend a shorter course of oral steroid therapy instead of the 7–14 days of treatment previously advised. Since systemic corticosteroids are considered undesirable in the maintenance therapy of COPD, they should be weaned off as soon as possible during recovery from an exacerbation. Osteoporosis prophylaxis should be considered in those requiring frequent courses of steroids.

Antibiotic therapy is recommended in COPD exacerbations if there is purulent sputum. Sputum culture is not routinely recommended, and antibiotic therapy is directed against the most likely organisms (e.g. *H. influenzae*, *S. pneumoniae*, *M. catarrhalis*) and adjusted, according to microbiological results. Initial empirical therapy should be with an aminopenicillin (amoxicillin 250 mg tds for 3–5days), a macrolide (e.g. clarithromycin 250 mg bd for 3–5 days), or a tetracycline (e.g. doxycycline 100 mg daily for 5 days).

Theophyllines can be used as an adjunct if the response to nebulized bronchodilators is inadequate. To prevent toxicity, plasma theophylline levels should be measured within 24 hours of starting therapy and interactions with other drugs reviewed. Be especially aware of the possibility of inducing toxicity in patients already taking a methylxanthine.

Respiratory stimulants are only appropriate when non-invasive ventilation is not available.

Ventilatory support

Non-invasive positive pressure ventilation (NIPPV)

This is effective in the management of hypercapnic ventilatory failure occurring during severe COPD exacerbations despite optimal medical therapy. It is best delivered by well-trained staff in an appropriate setting (e.g. high dependency area). Criteria for NIPPV include severe dyspnoea, moderate acidosis (pH 7.25–7.35), hypercapnia ($PaCO_2$ 6–8 kPa), and breathing frequency >25 breaths/min. Exclusion criteria include severe acidosis (pH <7.15), cardiovascular instability, impaired consciousness, respiratory arrest, lack of cooperation, risk of aspiration, facial surgery, or other factors preventing use of face masks.

NIPPV reduces endotracheal intubation rates and in-hospital mortality in hypercapnic COPD exacerbations with hypercapnic acidosis (pH 7.3–7.35). Rapid improvements in pH, $PaCO_2$, respiratory rate, and breathlessness were associated with a ~30% fall in endotracheal intubation rates, a 10% decrease in mortality, and a 4–6 day reduction in hospital stay. However, these studies included highly selected COPD cases with moderate respiratory failure (pH <7.35; $PaCO_2$ 6–8 kPa; breathing frequency >25 breaths/min) and also revealed failure rates of 20–30%, as judged by death or the need for intubation. Higher failure rates (35–49%) were reported in subsequent series of less carefully selected patients. Most investigators report that the response to the first 2 hours of NIPPV (as measured by the improvements in pH and $PaCO_2$) is predictive of success or failure.

Mechanical ventilation

In severe COPD exacerbations, mechanical ventilation may be lifesaving, but otherwise it should be avoided, whenever possible, because:

- Most COPD patients without advanced cor pulmonale tolerate hypoxaemia and acidosis well.
- Spontaneously breathing patients have an effective cough.
- COPD patients are at high risk of ventilator-associated complications (e.g. barotrauma, pneumothorax).
- Weaning can be difficult due to respiratory muscle weakness and the associated increase in work of breathing associated with hyperinflation.

Indications for mechanical ventilation include hypoxaemia (PaO_2 <5.3 kPa), tachypnoea >35 breaths/min, acidosis (pH <7.25), hypercapnia ($PaCO_2$ >8 kPa), respiratory arrest, NIPPV failure, confusion, poor cough, and haemodynamic instability.

Mortality in ventilated COPD patients is about 20% but, contrary to general opinion, is less than in ventilated non-COPD cases. It is higher in those requiring >72 h mechanical ventilation (37%) and after a failed extubation attempt (36%). Mean duration of mechanical ventilation is 5–9 days.

In end-stage COPD patients on palliative treatment, with limited exercise tolerance, resting breathlessness, and loss of independence, it may be appropriate to limit ventilatory support to NIPPV. The decision not to mechanically ventilate a patient should be based on health status, and an estimate of survival time based on previous functional status, body mass index, LTOT requirements, comorbidities, exacerbation rate, and previous ICU/hospital admissions. Neither age nor FEV_1 should be used in isolation when assessing suitability for mechanical ventilation. A clear statement of the patient's wishes, in the form of an advance directive or 'living will', always makes these difficult decisions easier.

- Weaning (discontinuation of mechanical ventilation) can be difficult in COPD patients but is undertaken as soon as possible. The best method is debated, but abrupt reductions in the level of ventilatory support that induce respiratory muscle fatigue must be avoided. Whether pressure support or a T-piece trial is used, weaning is shortened when a clinical protocol is adopted. Several recent trials indicate that NIPPV can facilitate and shorten the weaning process in COPD patients and may reduce ICU length of stay, decrease nosocomial pneumonia, and improve survival rates.

Before hospital discharge, the patient must be clinically stable and re-established on optimal inhaled bronchodilator therapy. Appropriate discharge support and follow-up should have been arranged (e.g. oxygen delivery, visiting nurse).

Further reading

Action on Smoking and Health. Stopping smoking. <http://www.ash.org.uk/>.

All Party Parliamentary Group (APPG) on Respiratory Health (June 2014). Report on Inquiry into Respiratory Deaths. <https://www.blf.org.uk/Page/Report-on-inquiry-into-respiratory-deaths>.

American Thoracic Society and European Respiratory Society (2004). Standards for the diagnosis and management of patients with COPD. <www.thoracic.org/clinical/copd-guidelines/resources/copddoc.pdf>.

Barnes PJ and Stockley RA (2005). COPD; current therapeutic interventions and future approaches. *European Respiratory Journal*, **25**, 1084–106.

Bateman NT and Leach RM (1998). Acute oxygen therapy. ABC of oxygen. *BMJ*, **317**, 798–801.

Best Health. Lungs and breathing. <http://besthealth.bmj.com/x/set/topic/condition-centre/15.html>.

British Lung Foundation Breathe Easy Group. <http://www.lunguk.org>.

Calfee CS and Matthay MA (2005). Recent advances in mechanical ventilation. *American Journal of Medicine*, **118**, 584–91.

Calverly PMA and Koulouris NG (2005). Flow limitation and dynamic hyperinflation: key concepts in modern respiratory physiology. *European Respiratory Journal*, **25**, 186–99.

Celli BR and MacNee W (ATS/ERS Task Force) (2004). Standards for the diagnosis and treatment of patients with COPD. *European Respiratory Journal*, **23**, 932–46.

Chest, Heart & Stroke Scotland. <http://www.chss.org.uk/>.

Cooper CB and Tashkin DP (2005). Recent developments in inhaled therapy in stable chronic obstructive pulmonary disease. *BMJ*, **330**, 640–4.

Emphysema Foundation. <http://www.emphysema.net/>.

Federation of Royal Colleges of Physicians (2006). The physician of tomorrow; Draft Medical competencies of curriculum for acute & internal medicine. Federation of Royal Colleges of Physicians. <www.jrcptb.org.uk/.../2007%20General%20Internal%20Medicine%20(Acute)%20Level%201>.

Kew KM, Seniukovich A (2014). Inhaled steroids and risk of pneumonia for chronic obstructive pulmonary disease. *Cochrane Database of Systematic Reviews*, 10;3:CD010115.<http://www.ncbi.nlm.nih.gov/pubmed/24615270>.

Leuppi JD, Schuetz P, Bingisser R, et al. (2013). Short-term vs conventional glucocorticoid therapy in acute exacerbations of chronic obstructive pulmonary disease: the REDUCE randomized clinical trial. *Journal of the American Medical Association*, **309**, 2223–2231.

Lung Foundation Australia. COPD information. <http://www.lung-foundation.com.au/lung-information/copd/>.

National Clinical Guidance Centre (2004). Chronic obstructive pulmonary disease. National clinical guideline on management of chronic obstructive pulmonary disease in adults in primary and secondary care. *Thorax*, **59** (Suppl 1), 1–232; <http://www.nice.org.uk/nicemedia/live/13029/49425/49425.pdf>.

National Institute for Health and Clinical Excellence (2010). Chronic obstructive pulmonary disease: Management of chronic obstructive pulmonary disease in adults in primary and secondary care (partial update). NICE clinical guideline 101. <https://www.nice.org.uk/guidance/cg101>.

National Institute for Health and Clinical Excellence (2013). Insertion of endobronchial valves for lung volume reduction in emphysema. NICE interventional procedure guidance 465. <http://www.nice.org.uk/guidance/ipg465/chapter/1-Recommendations>.

National Institutes of Health (2015). Global initiative for chronic obstructive lung disease. Global strategy for the diagnosis, management, and prevention of chronic obstructive pulmonary disease. <http://www.goldcopd.org/uploads/users/files/GOLD_Report_2015_Apr2.pdf>.

Nava S, Ambrosino N, Clini E, et al. (1998). Non-invasive mechanical ventilation in the weaning of patients with respiratory failure due to chronic obstructive pulmonary disease. A randomised controlled trial. *Annals of Internal Medicine*, **128**, 721–8.

NHS SmokeFree: Smoking—advice to help you stop smoking. <http://smokefree.nhs.uk/>.

O'Driscoll BR, Howard LS, Davison AG (2008). British Thoracic Society guideline for emergency oxygen use in adults. *Thorax*, **63** (Suppl 6), vi1–68.

Patient UK. Chronic obstructive pulmonary disease. <http://www.patient.co.uk/showdoc/23068705>.

Qaseem A, Wilt TJ, Weinberger SE, et al. (2011). Diagnosis and Management of Stable Chronic Obstructive Pulmonary Disease: A Clinical Practice Guideline Update from the American College of Physicians, American College of Chest Physicians, and European Respiratory Society. *Annals of Internal Medicine*, **155**, 179–191.

Ram F, Picot J, Lightowler J, Wedzicha J (2004). Non-invasive positive pressure ventilation for the treatment of respiratory failure due to exacerbations of chronic obstructive pulmonary disease. *Cochrane Database of Systematic Reviews*, **1**, CD004104.

Sciurba FC, Ernst A, Herth FJF, et al. (2010). A randomized study of endobronchial valves for advanced emphysema. *New England Journal of Medicine*, **363**, 1233–44.

Shah PL, Herth FJ (2014). Current status of bronchoscopic lung volume reduction with endobronchial valves. *Thorax*, **69**, 280–6.

Tantucci C, Modina D (2012). Lung function decline in COPD. *International Journal of Chronic Obstructive Pulmonary Disease*, **7**, 95–99.

Uzun S, Djamin RS, Kluytmans JA, et al. (2014). Azithromycin maintenance treatment in patients with frequent exacerbations of chronic obstructive pulmonary disease (COLUMBUS): a randomised, double-blind, placebo-controlled trial. *Lancet* **2**, 361–368.

Lung cancer

Lung cancer may present as unexpected CXR abnormalities, acute respiratory illnesses (e.g. pneumonia), paraneoplastic phenomena, and, occasionally, as respiratory emergencies like massive haemoptysis (see Box 5.8). The role of the acute physician is to recognize the possibility of lung cancer, initiate diagnostic investigations, and ensure timely referral to a respiratory specialist. This chapter will focus on the clinical presentations and initial diagnosis of lung cancer. A brief review of management and outcome is presented. The *Oxford Desk Reference of Respiratory Medicine* provides specialist details.

Epidemiology
Lung cancer is mainly due to cigarette smoking. In the USA and Europe, the incidence and mortality associated with lung cancer increased steadily from 1930 to 1995. Since 1995, it has decreased by 20–30% in men and is stable in women due to smoking cessation. However, it remains the commonest cause of cancer death in men and women in these countries.

In the UK, ~34,000 lung cancer deaths occur each year, and, after prostate cancer, it is the second commonest cancer in men, causing ~22,000 new cases/year. In women, it is the third commonest cancer after breast and bowel cancer, causing ~16,000 new cases/year. The incidence varies across Europe, with the highest rates in Hungary (>100/10⁵) and the lowest in Sweden (<25/10⁵).

Risk factors for lung cancer
- **Tobacco smoking** is responsible for 85–90% of lung cancer cases. Risk increases with earlier age of onset of smoking, number of cigarettes smoked daily, type of cigarette (i.e. unfiltered, high tar), and duration of smoking (i.e. one pack per day for 40 years is more hazardous than two packs per day for 20 years). The lifetime risk in heavy smokers (i.e. >20 pack years) is 10%, about 10–30 times greater than for lifetime non-smokers (<0.3%). Smoking cessation gradually reduces risk over 15 years, but it always remains raised. Periods (>3 months) of smoking cessation reduce cancer risk, compared to smokers with no non-smoking intervals.
- **Occupational exposure** to a variety of proven and suspected carcinogens increases the risk of lung cancer, particularly in workers who also smoke cigarettes (see Table 5.15). Asbestos exposure is associated with a 10-fold increase in the risk of developing lung cancer, and the risk in an individual with both smoking and asbestos exposure is greater than the sum of each individual risk.

Table 5.15 Proven and suspected carcinogens in lung cancer

Proven	Suspected
Arsenic	Heavy metals (e.g. beryllium, admium)
Asbestos	
Chromium	Vinyl chloride
Nickel	Silica
Polycyclic aromatic hydrocarbons, Bis(chloromethyl)ether	Iron ore
Ionizing radiation	Wood dust

- **Radon gas**, found naturally in rocks, soils, and ground water, increases lung cancer risk in some areas.
- **Genetic/familial predispositions.** Only 10–15% of heavy smokers develop lung cancer, suggesting that genetic susceptibility also plays an important role. Many polymorphisms in genes encoding enzymes that are important in DNA repair and the metabolism of tobacco smoke derived carcinogens, have been identified in patients with lung cancer, but sample sizes have been too small to demonstrate reproducibility at this stage.
- **Scar tissue.** An association between chronic lung disease (particularly idiopathic pulmonary fibrosis) and parenchymal scar tissue (e.g. following pulmonary tuberculosis) and lung cancer is recognized.

Classification
The WHO classification (1999) identifies seven histological types of lung cancer (see Box 5.9), but, for practical purposes, they are divided into two groups, which influence management, treatment, and prognosis:
1. **Non-small cell lung cancers (NSCLC)** account for 75–85% of lung cancer. There are three main histological types:
   - **Squamous cell cancer (SCC)** is most strongly associated with smoking and is still the commonest histological type in countries with a high percentage of smokers. These tumours develop in airway epithelium and, therefore, tend to be central.
   - **Adenocarcinoma** (and bronchoalveolar carcinoma) prevalence is increasing, particularly in women (~10–30%). It is the commonest histological type in non-smokers and, in countries with a low smoking

Box 5.8 Potential ways in which lung cancer can present to the acute physician

1. Incidental finding on chest X-ray
2. Acute respiratory illness (e.g. pneumonia, stridor, pleural effusion, haemoptysis)
3. Lung cancer complications (e.g. metastases to the brain or spine, paraneoplastic (e.g. hyponatraemia or hypercalcaemia), superior vena cava obstruction)
4. Treatment complications (e.g. neutropenic sepsis, radiation oesophagitis, and pneumonitis)
5. Disease progression requiring end of life care

Box 5.9 WHO classification of lung tumours (1999)

Squamous cell carcinoma
Small cell carcinoma
Adenocarcinoma
Large cell carcinoma
Adenosquamous carcinoma
Pleomorphic/sarcomatoid
Carcinoid tumour

incidence, is as common as SCC. Consequently, adenocarcinoma (33%) has overtaken SCC (30%) as the leading histological lung cancer type in the USA. Adenocarcinomas tend to arise peripherally and can arise on a background of interstitial fibrosis. Local invasion of the visceral pleura is common, with a resultant pleural effusion.

Bronchoalveolar carcinoma is rare and arises from type II pneumocytes that occur along alveolar septa. It is more common in women and non-smokers, rarely metastasizes, and may be associated with copious sputum production (bronchorrhoea). The CXR reveals diffuse infiltration which can be difficult to distinguish from lobar pneumonia.

- **Large cell carcinoma** (~10–15%) typically presents as a large peripheral mass, often with invasion of local structures. They are undifferentiated and lack the features of adenocarcinoma or SCC and are, therefore, a histological diagnosis of exclusion.

2. **Small cell lung cancers (SCLC)** cause 15–25% of lung cancers, arise from neuroendocrine cells in the bronchial mucosa, and typically present as a central mass with lymph node enlargement. They are aggressive tumours that invade blood vessels and lymphatics. Haematogenous spread often leads to widespread metastasis before diagnosis. Survival is <6 months from the time of diagnosis if untreated. Surgery is rarely appropriate, and, although the tumour is chemo- and radio-sensitive, survival time is usually only 12–14 months with therapy. The syndrome of inappropriate antidiuretic hormone secretion is common in SCLC.

Clinical presentations

The principal role of the acute physician in lung cancer management is recognition of the possible diagnosis, as diagnostic confirmation and therapy require early specialist involvement. Most patients are 50–70 year old smokers, with non-specific respiratory symptoms and signs, who are found to have an abnormality on CXR (see Figure 5.25). Less than 10% of cases are incidental findings in asymptomatic patients undergoing CXR for employment or immigration purposes or during assessment of other medical conditions.

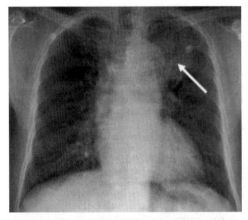

Figure 5.25 Chest radiograph showing a collapsed left upper lobe (→) due to non-small cell lung cancer.

Local tumour effects

- **Common symptoms** at presentation include new persistent cough or changed pattern of previous cough (70%), dyspnoea due to airway obstruction or pleural effusions (40%), chest pain due to chest wall involvement (30%), and minor haemoptysis with 'streaks' of blood or small clots in expectorated sputum (25%).

- **Less common symptoms** (<5%) include wheeze or stridor due to airways obstruction, hoarseness due to tumour invasion of the left recurrent laryngeal nerve, dysphagia due to oesophageal involvement, shoulder pain due to diaphragmatic invasion, pericardial effusions and diaphragmatic paralysis due to phrenic nerve damage.

- **Apical 'Pancoast' tumours** occasionally cause Horner's syndrome, with meiosis, ptosis, enophthalmos, and anhidrosis. Alternatively, it may cause brachial plexus compression, with direct wasting and weakness of small hand muscles.

- **Central versus peripheral lung tumours.** Central lesions usually present with cough, dyspnoea, haemoptysis, and wheeze. Peripheral lesions are asymptomatic for longer and may cause chest wall pain or dyspnoea due to tumour invasion or pleural effusions. Mediastinal involvement is not uncommon, with associated superior vena caval obstruction (SVCO), hoarseness, and dysphagia.

Superior vena caval obstruction (SVCO) may be due to: (1) external compression and/or invasion by local tumour (right:left lung ratio 4:1), lymph nodes, or other mediastinal structures, or (2) thrombosis within the vein.

Lung cancer and lymphoma account for >90% of SVCO. About 4% of lung cancer patients develop SVCO, and 10% of SCLC present with SVCO. Less common malignant causes include mediastinal tumours (e.g. thymoma) and metastases (e.g. breast). Benign causes may be iatrogenic (e.g. central lines, pacemaker wires), due to goitres or granulomatous diseases, and, rarely, infective (e.g. aspergillosis).

Onset may be rapid, over days or weeks, in malignant cases. Typical features include severe facial and upper body oedema, distension of neck veins, and a plethoric, cyanosed appearance due to congestion. Breathlessness, headache, hoarseness, confusion, and syncope also occur due to reduced venous return. Development of a collateral circulation produces distension of superficial chest wall veins. SVCO is not life-threatening, except when associated with stridor or laryngeal oedema, but patients are frequently extremely distressed by the symptoms.

Whilst establishing the diagnosis, sit the patient upright to reduce venous congestion, and provide high-flow oxygen. Arrange an urgent thoracic CT scan, and refer immediately to a respiratory specialist, who will arrange an appropriate means of biopsy. Steroids should not be given empirically, as there is no evidence for efficacy in lung cancer, and they may prevent an accurate histological diagnosis in lymphoma. Definitive oncological treatment (e.g. chemotherapy, radiotherapy, or both) results in resolution of SVCO symptoms in the majority of patients within 21 days. For patients with florid, distressing, or life-threatening symptoms, an urgent intravascular stent should be arranged which will relieve symptoms within 24–48 hours. Iatrogenic thrombosis (e.g. central lines) is treated with thrombolysis if the clot is less than 5 days old. Prophylactic anticoagulation in SVCO is controversial, but prevention of SVC thrombosis after treatment probably outweighs the small risk of intracerebral bleeding.

Metastatic tumour

Extrathoracic metastases are present in 30% at presentation, including liver, adrenals, bone, and brain. Most are asymptomatic. Bone metastases may be associated with bone pain, hypercalcaemia, and pathological fractures. Hypercalcaemia, due to bone metastases, occurs in at least 10% of cases (see further text). Brain metastases have a particularly poor prognosis, with a median survival of 2 months. Dysphagia may occur due to tumour invasion of the oesophagus or compression by enlarged mediastinal lymph nodes.

- **Lymphangitis carcinomatosis** is due to lymphatic spread of the primary tumour and occurs in advanced disease. Reticular and septal lines observed on CXR and CT thorax can be difficult to distinguish from pulmonary oedema. Management is focused on the palliation of dyspnoea.

- **Spinal cord compression** is usually due to spread from a vertebral metastasis but is occasionally due to direct spread from a primary tumour in the posterior mediastinum. Typically, back pain (due to vertebral collapse) is followed by constipation, urinary incontinence, lower limb weakness, and sensory loss, although pain is not universal. Urgent plain spinal X-rays and an MRI scan of the spine to confirm the diagnosis should be followed rapidly by consideration of neurosurgery and radiotherapy to maximize the chance of avoiding permanent neurological deficit. High-dose dexamethasone (16 mg IV, then 4 mg PO qds) may help to reduce oedema (and symptoms) around a confirmed spinal tumour.

Malignant pleural effusions are discussed in the section on 'Pleural disease' later in this chapter.

Paraneoplastic syndromes
Paraneoplastic syndromes are characteristic constellations of symptoms and signs, associated with lung and other cancers, but not directly related to the tumour or its metastases. They may precede clinical and radiographic tumour detection. Tumour hormone secretion or hormone-like substances, serum autoantibodies (e.g. anti-Hu), growth or other factors may be responsible. Paraneoplastic syndromes are often non-specific and include:

1. **Constitutional symptoms**, for example, fever, anorexia, cachexia, and wasting.

2. **Clubbing and hypertrophic pulmonary osteoarthropathy**, which occurs with all histological types of lung cancer, but most commonly SCC and adenocarcinoma (see Figure 5.26). There are many other causes of clubbing (e.g. cyanotic heart disease, chronic infection), but the pathogenesis has not been established. The prevailing theory suggests the release of humoral substances from malignant or hypoxic tissue, for example, platelet-derived growth factors which activate nail bed connective tissue cells. A striking feature is reversal when lung cancer is surgically removed.

3. **Cutaneous manifestations.** Acanthosis nigricans (hyperpigmentation in flexor areas (e.g. axilla)) is associated with malignancy in 60% of cases (often lung cancer). Similarly dermatomyositis/polymyositis and scleroderma are associated with lung and other malignancies in 5–15% of cases.

4. **Neurological syndromes**, which are common, rapidly progressive and often severe. They may be reversible with treatment of the causative cancer. About half are due to lung cancers. Type 1 antineuronal nuclear antibody (ANNA-1), also known as 'anti-Hu', is a marker of neurological autoimmunity and is strongly linked with SCLC (97%). Typical paraneoplastic neurological syndromes include:

- Peripheral neuropathy, mainly sensory.
- Cerebellar syndrome with progressive ataxia.
- Limbic encephalitis.
- Eaton–Lambert syndrome is a myasthenia-like syndrome caused by ANNA-1 or IgG autoantibodies. It may predate detectable cancer by 2–4 years. Typically, initial weakness and hyporeflexia improve in proximal limbs and the trunk with repeated muscle contractions. Autonomic involvement may also occur. It does not respond to edrophonium.

5. **Endocrine syndromes** include:

- **Ectopic adrenocorticotrophic hormone (ACTH).** This is the commonest paraendocrine disorder and is classically associated with SCLC. Due to its rapid development, patients do not develop classical Cushing's syndrome but present with hypokalaemia, alkalosis, and mild hypertension. Slow-growing and carcinoid tumours occasionally manifest as typical Cushing's syndrome.

- **Syndrome of inappropriate antidiuretic hormone (SIADH)** occurs in 15% of SCLC cases, 0.7% of NSCLC cases, and with many other tumours (e.g. head, neck). Non-malignant causes of SIADH include drugs (e.g. carbamazepine, fluoxetine), pneumonia,

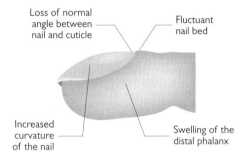

Loss of normal angle between nail and cuticle

Fluctuant nail bed

Increased curvature of the nail

Swelling of the distal phalanx

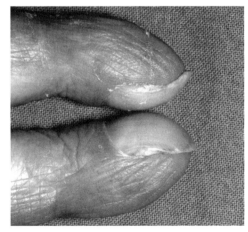

Figure 5.26 Clubbing. Reproduced from Longmore *et al.*, *Oxford Handbook of Clinical Medicine*, eighth edition, 2010, Figure 2, page 30, with permission from Oxford University Press

CNS disorders (e.g. strokes, infection), HIV disease, and post-surgery. Inappropriate antidiuretic hormone (ADH) production and activity promotes excessive water retention, with associated hyponatraemia (<135 mmol/L) and serum hypo-osmolality.

SIADH presents with lethargy and confusion when serum sodium falls below 120–130 mmol/L. Diagnosis is confirmed in hyponatraemic patients and distinguished from sodium depletion or water overload by a low serum osmolality (<280 mmol/L) in the presence of a high urine osmolality (>100 mOsm/L) and/or urinary sodium (>40 mmol/L) but normal acid-base balance and renal function. Patients are managed by restricting fluid intake (initially ~1 L/day). Demeclocycline (150–300 mg twice daily), a tetracycline derivative that blocks ADH action in distal renal tubules, is occasionally required. Hypertonic saline should only rarely be considered in severe hyponatraemia associated with seizures, as rapid increases in osmolality can cause irreversible central pontine demyelinolysis.

- **Hypercalcaemia** occurs during the course of the disease in 40% of patients with lung cancer. It is most commonly the result of bone metastases but may also be the result of ectopic parathyroid hormone-related peptide (PTHrP) production by NSCLC. Hypercalcaemic symptoms are most apparent at levels >3 mmol/L and include confusion, weakness, constipation, and nausea. Renal failure may occur, and the ECG QT interval may be short. Diagnosis is confirmed by measuring serum corrected calcium. Measurement of PTHrP does not alter management. Specific symptoms suggestive of bone metastases should be followed up with imaging.

Initial treatment should correct dehydration (3–4 L 0.9% normal saline (IV) over 24 hours). Intravenous bisphosphonates (e.g. disodium pamidronate; 30–60 mg infused over 2 hours) impede bone reabsorption and reduce hypercalcaemia within days. They are effective for several weeks and reduce metastatic bone pain and pathological fractures.

- **Melanocyte-stimulating hormone** may cause hyperpigmentation

6. **Thromboembolic events.** Deep vein thrombosis (including of the superior vena cava) and pulmonary embolus (PE) are common in patients with lung cancer. In particular, it is important to maintain a high index of suspicion for PE when a patient presents with breathlessness in the absence of obvious new chest X-ray changes. Anticoagulation with low molecular weight heparin is preferable to warfarin due to difficulty in maintaining a stable INR in patients with malignancy.

Pulmonary nodules

Pulmonary nodules (PN) are defined as focal lung opacities, measuring <3 cm in diameter, and most are benign (see Table 5.16). The Early Lung Cancer Action Project detected non-calcified PN in 7% of baseline CXR and 23% of CT scans in 1,000 symptom-free smokers (>10 pack years) over 60 years old. On subsequent biopsy, ~11% of the CT scan PN were malignant. In smokers with a normal CXR, about 1–2.5% of PN detected on CT scan were malignant. The ability to detect small PN improves with each new generation of CT scanners. Multidetector row CT scans can detect PNs as small as 1–2 mm in diameter, and recent screening studies report PNs in up to 51% of smokers, aged 50 years or older, on initial CT scans, with a new PN developing during a 1-year follow-up period in about 10%.

Table 5.16 Causes of pulmonary nodules

Benign	Malignant
Bronchial adenoma	Primary lung cancer
Benign carcinoid tumour	Metastases
Infectious granulomata (e.g. tuberculosis)	
Non-infectious granulomata (e.g. sarcoidosis)	
Benign hamartoma	

The probability of a PN being malignant increases with size. Less than 1% of PN <5 mm are malignant, even in smokers, whereas 10–20% of 8 mm PN will eventually show malignant change. Cigarette smoking, certain PN features (see following section), and increasing age (i.e. malignancy is rare in patients <35 years old) correlate with increasing likelihood of lung cancer.

- **Features of malignant PNs** include size >0.8 cm, an irregular or 'spiculated' margin (~20% of malignant PN have a smooth margin), cavitation with thick irregular walls, rapid growth, contrast enhancement (i.e. increased vascularity), and smoking, especially in older age groups. 'Solid', rather than ground glass, opacities are more likely to be malignant and have a more rapid growth rate.
- **Features of benign PNs** include size <0.5 cm, smooth and well-defined margin, calcification (e.g. diffuse, 'popcorn-like', laminated), stable or smaller with time, poor contrast enhancement, cavitation with thin, smooth walls, fat within the nodule (hamartoma), young age, and non-smokers.

A PN in a patient with an extrathoracic malignancy could be a metastasis, a new primary lung cancer, or a benign nodule. This partly depends on the histology of the extrathoracic malignancy and smoking history. A primary lung tumour is more likely if the extrathoracic tumour is in the stomach, prostate, bladder, oesophagus, or breast; a metastasis is more likely if the extrathoracic tumour is a melanoma, sarcoma, or testicular tumour.

Unfortunately, neither CT-guided biopsy nor positron emission tomography (PET) are reliable in lesions <7 mm in diameter, and, until recently, it was recommended that all PNs were scanned at regular intervals for at least 2 years to monitor change in size over time. If the PN increased in size or showed malignant features on repeat CT scans, a surgical biopsy or surgical resection was considered (see section on clinical assessment). However, this policy required large numbers of scans, with limited cost benefit and the associated radiation exposure.

Recent guidelines suggest a graded approach to investigation and repeat CT scanning, depending on PN size, clinical presentation, CT features, and the potential for malignant change (see Table 5.17).

1. **Very small PNs <4 mm** in a non-smoker do not require follow-up imaging. In high-risk patients with a PN <4 mm, a single CT at 12 months is required.
2. **Small PNs <8 mm** in low-risk patients are followed up with CT at 6–12 months and then at 24 months if no change is detected. In smokers, they are followed up at 3–6 months, then at 9–12 months, and finally 24 months if no change.
3. **Large PNs > 8 mm** are followed up with CT at 3, 9, and 24 months in either group. Patient choice is important. Smokers may choose an excision biopsy, rather than CT

Table 5.17 NSCLC stage, terminology, and treatment survival times from the 2009 IASLC clinical and pathological staging system

Stage	TNM	Terminology	5-year survival with clinical (c) or pathological staging (p)
1A	T1, N0, M0	T1—tumour size ≤2–3 cm	c 50% p 73%
1B	T2a, N0, M0	T2a—tumour size >3 cm –<5 cm	c 47% p 58%
IIA	T1, N1, M0	T2b—tumour size >5 cm–<7 cm	c 36% p 46%
IIB	T2a, N1, M0	N0—no regional nodes	c 26% p 36%
	T2b, N0, M0	N1—ipsilateral hilar nodes	
	T3, N0, M0	T3—> tumour size 7 cm or any tumour that invades local structures (e.g. chest wall) or a separate nodule in the same lobe	
IIIA	T1, N2, M0	N2—ipsilateral mediastinal nodes	c 19% p 24%
IIIB	T2, N2, M0	N3—contralateral hilar, mediastinal, or any supraclavicular lymph node	c 19% p 9%
	T3, N1–2, M0	T4—additional nodules in a different, ipsilateral lobe to the primary tumour or mediastinal invasion	
	T4, N0, M0		
	T4, N1, M0		
	T1–3, N3, M0		
	T4, N2, M0		
IV	Any T or N, M1	M1a—intrathoracic metastases (+ pleural effusion/involvement)	c 2% p 13%
		M1b—distant metastasis	

Reproduced from Rusch V, et al., 'The IASLC Lung Cancer Staging Project: A Proposal for a New International Lymph Node Map in the Forthcoming Seventh Edition of the TNM Classification for Lung Cancer', *Journal of Thoracic Oncology*, 4, 5, pp. 568– 577, copyright 2009, with permission from International Association for the Study of Cancer.

follow-up. PET-CT has a high false negative rate for PNs <1 cm, so cannot be used to avoid CT follow-up if negative, but is useful if positive.

Any increase in the size of a PN in a smoker should lead to excision biopsy if the patient is fit for this. PNs should be followed up by a specialist lung cancer multidisciplinary team (MDT).

When a diagnosis of PN malignancy has been established, treatment depends on the histological type (e.g. SCLC) and whether the nodule is a primary lung tumour or metastasis. Primary tumours are staged and treated, as described for individual histological types. Metastatic nodules should be discussed in a multidisciplinary meeting to establish the appropriate therapy.

Massive haemoptysis

Lung cancer may rarely present with life-threatening haemoptysis, the management of which is discussed in the section 'Haemoptysis' in 'Clinical presentations of respiratory disease' at the start of this chapter.

Clinical assessment

Smokers with new chest symptoms (i.e. haemoptysis, cough, chest/shoulder pain, weight loss, hoarse voice, or cervical lymphadenopathy) lasting more than 3 weeks, especially those greater than 50 years old, require a CXR. In the UK, patients with suspected lung cancer are seen urgently under the 2-week cancer wait scheme.

Initial investigations

- **Blood tests** include sodium, calcium, liver function, and a clotting profile if biopsies are planned.
- **Sputum cytology**, although inexpensive, has a high false negative rate and is only considered in patients unfit for bronchoscopy or biopsy.
- **Spirometry** should be undertaken before biopsy or surgery.

- **Aspirate pleural fluid**, if present, under ultrasound guidance, and send for cytology as well as standard biochemical tests and culture.
- **Staging CT thorax and upper abdomen.** It is vital to stage the tumour, plan the most appropriate means of obtaining a tissue diagnosis, and identify complications requiring urgent management (e.g. central airway tumours requiring stenting, vertebral metastases threatening the spinal cord). Lymphadenopathy seen on a CT scan can result from superimposed infection and requires further assessment if the tumour is otherwise resectable. Head CT scans are not performed routinely in asymptomatic patients at presentation.
- **Positron emission tomography (PET)** utilizes uptake of labelled 18-fluorodeoxyglucose (18FDG) by metabolically active tissue to identify malignant lesions. The use of integrated PET-CT scans has greater sensitivity (72–100%) and specificity (67–100%) than PET alone. False positives do occur in non-malignant tissue, usually associated with inflammation (e.g. pulmonary sarcoidosis, infective granulomata). False negatives occur in patients with hyperglycaemia, small nodules of <1 cm, and in bronchoalveolar cell carcinoma.

Integrated PET-CTs are requested, following review by the lung cancer MDT, for the evaluation of solitary pulmonary nodules of >1 cm and to fully stage all patients with confirmed NSCLC for whom radical therapy is planned.

Other imaging sometimes employed:

- **Bone scans** aid detection of bone metastases in those with hypercalcaemia, raised alkaline phosphatase or bone pain.
- **MRI scans** assess brachial plexus invasion by apical lung cancers but have no role in nodule evaluation.
- **Ultrasound scans** aid assessment and biopsy of cervical lymph nodes and liver metastases, and guide safe pleural aspiration.

Histological diagnosis

When feasible, the site of most advanced disease, as demonstrated by imaging, should be selected to achieve both histological diagnosis and full staging in a single procedure.

- **CT- or ultrasound-guided biopsy of metastatic lesion** (e.g. liver, adrenal).
- **Ultrasound-guided needle aspiration** of supraclavicular nodes (impalpable but >5 mm on ultrasound) yields positive results in 75% of cases and avoids more invasive tests in 42%.
- **Pleural aspiration/biopsy** (CT-guided pleural biopsy or local anaesthetic thoracoscopy to obtain pleural tissue).

Bronchoscopy

This allows visualization and biopsy of proximal endobronchial tumours. It is often important in assessing surgical resectability of localized tumours. Ideally, it is performed with the facility of endobronchial ultrasound (EBUS) and transbronchial needle biopsy (TBNA), so that enlarged subcarinal, hilar, and pretracheal lymph nodes can also be aspirated and staged.

- **CT-guided lung biopsy** has >85% sensitivity in peripheral lung lesions >2 cm. Before biopsy, clotting and spirometry must be checked. Haemoptysis occurs in ~5% and pneumothorax in ~20% (3% require a chest drain) after biopsy.
- **Mediastinoscopy or mediastinotomy**, with biopsy of enlarged mediastinal lymph nodes, can assist diagnosis (>90% sensitivity and specificity) and subsequent staging.
- **Surgical biopsy**, with frozen section, may be the most appropriate investigation in fit patients with radiologically localized disease, as the surgeon can proceed to complete resection if lung cancer is confirmed.

Staging

1. Small cell lung cancer (SCLC) is staged, on the basis of clinical evaluation, CT scans, and imaging of symptomatic areas as either:

- **Limited disease.** Defined as a tumour that can be encompassed within one radiotherapy field. It includes patients with tumour confined to one hemithorax (including pleural effusion) and involving bilateral hilar and/or supraclavicular lymphadenopathy. About 40% of cases are classified as 'limited' at diagnosis. Untreated, median survival is 4–6 months.
- **Extensive disease** (60% at presentation). Describes widespread disease beyond the definition of 'limited' disease and includes distant metastases (e.g. cerebral) and involvement of the contralateral lung. Untreated, median survival is 3 months.

2. Non-small cell lung cancer (NSCLC) staging aims to establish whether the cancer is surgically curable. If not curable, it determines prognosis and the most appropriate therapy (e.g. chemotherapy, radiotherapy, supportive care). It is based on the International Association for the Study of Lung Cancer (IASLC) classification which has been in routine use since 2009 (see Table 5.17).

Staging may be clinical (c), based on physical examination and radiology; or pathological (p) by examining tissue from lymph node biopsy, bronchoscopy, and/or mediastinoscopy. Surgical staging is required if accurate evaluation of the mediastinal nodes is necessary to determine therapy.

The 2009 classification identifies five sizes of tumour with significantly different survivals. Five-year survival rates for the five tumour size groups were: pT1a <2 cm, 77%; pT1b >2 but <3 cm, 71%; pT2a >3 but <5 cm, 58%; pT2b >5 but <7 cm, 49%; and pT3 >7 cm, 35%. The survival rates were similar when based on clinical staging. In this new classification, T1 tumours are subdivided into T1a <2 cm and T1b >2 but <3cm. T2 tumours are subdivided into T2a >3 but <5 cm and T2b >5 but <7 cm. T3 tumours are >7 cm or have additional nodules in the same lobe as the primary tumour, and T4 tumours include nodules in an ipsilateral lobe.

Nodal classification is unchanged: N0, no nodes; N1, ipsilateral hilar nodes; N2, ipsilateral mediastinal or subcarinal nodes; and N3, as contralateral, scalene, or supraclavicular nodes. Five-year survivals for pN0, pN1, pN2, and pN3 were 56%, 38%, 22%, and 6%, respectively.

Metastasis was reclassified as: M0, no distant metastases; M1a, intrathoracic metastases, including tumour nodules in the contralateral lung and pleural involvement; and M1b, distant metastases. Five-year survival for M1a and M1b metastases were ~4% and 1%, respectively .

At diagnosis, stages I and II account for 20%, stage III 35%, and stage IV 45% of cases.

Treatment of non-small cell lung cancer (NSCLC)

In the UK, patients suitable for therapy must be treated within 31 days of the decision to treat and within 62 days of referral. Following discussion at a local lung cancer multidisciplinary team meeting (MDM), NSCLC patients are usually classified into three groups, reflecting disease extent and treatment approach.

Surgical group

Stages I and II tumours are resectable by wedge resection, lobectomy, or pneumonectomy in patients of adequate performance status and FEV_1. Mean 5-year survival following surgery is 69% in stage IA, falling to 33% in IIB. Some stage IIIA patients are considered for surgery, but only 25% are completely resectable, and 75% of these will not be alive at 5 years. Adjuvant chemotherapy improves survival, compared to surgery alone, in patients with a macroscopically complete resection. The perioperative mortality rate for pneumonectomy is 6%, lobectomy 3%, and wedge resection 1%. Lymph node sampling for pathological staging should occur during all surgical resections. Endobronchial techniques (e.g. photodynamic therapy, Nd-Yag laser ablation, cryotherapy) are being evaluated for the treatment of *in situ* tumours and palliation.

Radiotherapy and chemotherapy group

- **Radiotherapy.** High-dose, 'curative', continuous hyperfractionated accelerated radiotherapy (CHART) is given to patients with resectable disease who have medical contraindications to, or do not want, surgery. CHART is given as small doses 3 times a day for 12 days (total 54 Gy). It improves 2-year survival (i.e. 29 vs 20%), compared with conventional high-dose radiotherapy.

  Palliative radiotherapy is very effective in the management of haemoptysis, SVCO, painful lymphadenopathy, pain from bony metastases, and airway obstruction.

- **Chemotherapy** improves symptoms and quality of life in advanced lung cancer (stages III, IV) in patients with good performance status (WHO 0–1), although survival gains are only 2–4 months, compared with best supportive care. First-line chemotherapy combines a platinum drug (e.g. cisplatin) with a third-generation drug (e.g. gemcitabine) which avoids alopecia. Repeat CT scans establish response. Second-line monotherapy (e.g. docetaxel, pemetrexed, pacitaxel) is used in relapse for locally

Table 5.18 Palliative symptom management

Symptoms	Management
Breathlessness	External beam radiotherapy Bronchoscopy procedures (e.g. debulking, stents) Pleural effusion drainage Talc pleurodesis
Cough, pain, haemoptysis	External beam radiotherapy
Superior vena cava obstruction	Chemo- and radiotherapy and occasionally stenting
Brain metastasis, spinal cord compression	Steroids and radiotherapy ± surgery for spinal cord compression
Bone metastases	Analgesia ± radiotherapy

advanced or metastatic disease but causes alopecia. The reader is referred to the *Oxford Desk Reference of Respiratory Medicine* for details of rescue chemotherapy and biological agents. Combined chemoradiotherapy improves quality of life and survival but is associated with more side effects.

Supportive care

The majority of patients with NSCLC have advanced disease at presentation, and, of these, only one-third are fit for palliative chemotherapy. Good symptom palliation, with effective management of dyspnoea, pain, and anxiety and depression (consider oxygen, opiates, anxiolytics), palliative radiotherapy, careful management of pleural effusions and coexistent pulmonary embolism and psychological support, is essential. Management within a specialist multidisciplinary team, working closely with the patient's general practitioner or family physician, is important, as patients need close follow-up to allow early recognition and management of symptoms (e.g. see Table 5.18).

Treatment of small cell lung cancer (SCLC)

Surgery

Most SCLCs are unsuitable for surgery as haematogenous spread will have occurred before diagnosis. However, if full staging, including sampling of mediastinal lymph nodes, indicates that full resection is possible with a lobectomy, this should be considered, as median survival is probably superior to chemotherapy alone in this group.

Chemotherapy

Chemotherapy is the mainstay of treatment, with a response rate of 80–90% in limited and 60–80% in extensive disease. Response is associated with quality of life benefits, even in patients of poor performance status. Unfortunately, relapse is usually rapid.

- **First-line chemotherapy** is usually with a platinum agent (e.g. cisplatin) and etoposide, given every 3 weeks for six cycles. Mean survival time with this regime is 14.5 months, 2-year survival 14%, and 5-year survival 5%. Although beneficial for poor prognosis groups, a less intense outpatient regime is often more appropriate in patients with a poor performance status.
- **Second-line chemotherapy** is considered for patients who made a response to first-line chemotherapy which was sustained for at least 3 months and have maintained a reasonable performance status.

Radiotherapy

SCLC is radiosensitive, and radiotherapy has an important role in treatment.

- **Thoracic radiotherapy** is indicated in patients with 'limited' disease, with a partial response, or better, from chemotherapy. The median survival benefit is about 1 month, with a 6% improvement in 2-year survival (i.e. chemotherapy alone 13% vs the addition of radiotherapy 19%). In extensive disease, thoracic radiotherapy is considered if there was a good response to chemotherapy at distant sites and a partial response in the chest.
  Palliative radiotherapy is effective for symptoms related to the primary tumour or metastases (e.g. airway compression, haemoptysis, SVCO).
- **Prophylactic cranial irradiation (PCI).** The brain is the primary site of extrathoracic recurrence, as cytotoxic drugs penetrate the blood–brain barrier poorly. Consequently, PCI is advised, on completion of chemotherapy, to eradicate occult cerebral micrometastases in patients with limited disease who have had a complete, or good partial, response to initial chemotherapy. Overall survival is improved by 5%.

Follow-up and supportive care

Palliative care is provided by multidisciplinary teams and specialist palliative care services. Management includes supportive measures for symptom control (e.g. weight loss, depression, pain) and specific interventions (e.g. see Table 5.18).

Prognosis

In NSCLC, 5-year survival rate is 14% in the USA but is closer to 8% in Europe, as ~75% of patients present with advanced disease. In stage IIIB disease, 5-year survival is <5%. In SCLC, prognosis is determined by disease extent (i.e. 'limited, extensive') and factors that indicate 'good' or 'poor' prognosis. The most significant factors indicating poor prognosis are impaired performance status, elevated lactate dehydrogenase level, age, and male sex. However, median survival, even in good prognostic groups, is only 12–14 months, with 2-year and 5-year survival rates of 20% and 10%, respectively.

Pulmonary carcinoid

These are rare neuroendocrine lung tumours that present equally in men and women at 40–50 years old. They account for 1–2% of lung tumours. Although typically slow-growing and benign, they can be malignant with metastases. Most are endobronchial lesions, presenting with wheeze, haemoptysis, and lobar collapse. Peripheral parenchymal carcinoids are often asymptomatic incidental CXR findings. Rare presentations include:

- Carcinoid syndrome (1%) with flushing, wheeze, tachycardia, and diarrhoea.
- Cushing's syndrome due to ectopic ACTH production.

CXR and CT scans reveal well-defined tumours or multiple 'tumourlets'. Endobronchial carcinoids appear as smooth cherry red lesions at bronchoscopy. Biopsy is often avoided, as it can cause profuse bleeding, but CT-guided biopsy may be helpful in peripheral lesions. Histologically, carcinoids must be differentiated from SCLC. They are classified as:

- **Typical carcinoids** with few mitoses. Local lymph nodes metastases occur in 10%, but distant spread is rare. Five- and ten-year survival rates are 100% and >85%, respectively.

- **Atypical carcinoids** have more mitotic activity. Local lymph node metastases occur in 50% and distant metastases in 20%. Five- and 10-year survival rates are ~70% and 50%, respectively.

Localized carcinoid tumours are surgically resected, with perioperative lymph node sampling, as tumour size does not relate to lymph node metastases. Carcinoid symptoms resolve following resection. Patients should be followed up with annual CXRs.

In the 1% with carcinoid syndrome, serotonin antagonists (e.g. octreotide) can be used for treatment. Arterial embolization may be considered in the treatment of isolated liver metastases. Chemotherapy is used for aggressive metastatic carcinoids.

Further reading

American National Cancer Institute. <http://www.cancer.org/treatment/.../nci-cancer-center-programs>.

Best Health. Lungs and breathing. <http://besthealth.bmj.com/x/set/topic/condition-centre/15.html>.

British Lung Foundation. <http://www.lunguk.org>. Tel: 0845 850 5020.

British Thoracic Society (2006). The burden of lung disease, 2nd edn. <https://www.brit-thoracic.org.uk/document-library/delivery-of-respiratory-care/burden-of-lung-disease/burden-of-lung-disease-2006/>.

Cancer Research UK. <http://www.cancerresearchuk.org>. Helpline tel: 0800 800 4040.

Colby TV, Corrin B, Shimosato Y, et al. (1999). Histological typing of lung and pleural tumours. In WD Travis and LH Sobin, eds. WHO international histological classification of tumors. 3rd edn. Springer Verlag, Berlin.

Doll R and Hill AB (1950). Smoking and carcinoma of the lung. BMJ, ii, 739–48.

Henschke, McCauley DI, Yankelevitz DF, et al. (1999). Early lung cancer action project: overall design and findings from baseline screening. Lancet, 354, 99–105.

Kumaran M, Benamore R E, Vaidhyanath R, et al. (2005). Ultrasound-guided cytological aspiration of supraclavicular lymph nodes in patients with suspected lung cancer. Thorax, 60, 229–33.

Lung Cancer Alliance.<http://www.lungcanceronline.org>.

MacMahon H, Austin JHM, Gamsu G, et al. (2005). Guidelines for management of small pulmonary nodules detected on CT scans: a statement from the Fleischner Society. Radiology, 237, 395–400.

Macmillan Cancer Support. <http://www.macmillan.org.uk>. Tel: 0808 808 0000.

Mountain CF (1997). Revisions in the International System for Staging Lung Cancer. Chest, 111, 1710–17.

National Institute for Health and Clinical Excellence (2011). NICE clinical guideline 121. Lung cancer: The diagnosis and treatment of lung cancer. <https://www.nice.org.uk/guidance/cg121>.

NHS SmokeFree: Smoking—advice to help you stop smoking. <http://smokefree.nhs.uk/>.

Office for National Statistics (2000). Mortality statistics by cause. Series DH2 no.26. The Stationery Office: London.

Rami-Porta R, et al. (2009). The revised TMN staging system for lung cancer. Annals of Thoracic and Cardiovascular Surgery, 15, 49.

Quint L, Park CH, Iannettoni MD (2000). Solitary pulmonary nodule with extra pulmonary neoplasms. Radiology, 217, 257–61.

Ries LAG, Melbert D, Krapcho M, et al., eds. (2005). SEER cancer statistics review, 1975–2005, National Cancer Institute, Bethesda. <http://seer.cancer.gov/csr/1975_2005/>.

Roy Castle Lung Cancer Foundation. <http://www.roycastle.org>. Tel: 0800 358 7200.

Samson DJ, Seidenfeld J, Simon GR, et al. (2007). Evidence for management of small cell lung cancer: ACCP evidence-based clinical practical guidelines (2nd edn). Chest, 132, 314S–23S.

Saunders M, Dische S, Barrett A, Harvey A, Gibson D, Parmar M (1997). CHART vs conventional radiotherapy. Lancet, 350, 161–5.

Schreiber G and McCrory DC (2003). Performance characteristics of different modalities for diagnosis of suspected lung cancer: summary of published evidence. Chest, 123 (1 Suppl), 115S–28S.

Stopping Smoking. <http://www.ash.org.uk/>.

Mediastinal lesions

The mediastinum is illustrated in Figure 5.27. Typical mediastinal symptoms include cough, chest pain, dyspnoea, and those due to compression of vital structures, including stridor, dysphagia, and superior vena caval obstruction. Many abnormalities are detected as asymptomatic CXR findings. Table 5.19 lists the causes of mediastinal masses.

Thymoma

Thymoma is a rare epithelial tumour arising in the thymus gland and often containing functional thymic tissue. Rare before 20 years old, they are equally common in men and women. Myasthenia gravis (MG) occurs in 35% of cases and may not resolve following thymectomy. They are usually benign, but those extending beyond the thymic capsule are malignant and invade local structures or metastasize. Dyspnoea, chest pain, and dysphagia are common. Treatment is by surgical excision of the thymus. Avoid needle aspiration or biopsy which may seed tumour outside the capsule. Consider post-operative radiotherapy for malignant tumours and those not fully resected. In MG, thymoma is detected in 20% of cases, usually men >50 years old, with acetylcholine receptor (AChR) autoantibodies. Consider thymectomy in all MG patients, even those without thymoma, as most improve symptomatically, although the young with severe, early disease and AChR antibodies do best.

Other thymic cysts and tumours

Thymic cysts are congenital or inflammatory. They are asymptomatic, unless large, and, although usually benign, are often excised, as diagnosis is difficult. Thymic carcinoids are aggressive, with local invasion and metastases. Cushing's syndrome may occur but not MG. Treatment involves surgical excision, chemotherapy, and octreotide therapy. Thymic carcinomas, hyperplasia, and lipomas also occur.

Germ cell tumours

Germ cell tumours arise from immature germ cells during development. They are usually midline.
- **Cystic teratomas** cause 80% of germ cell tumours. They are benign, occur in young adults, and are detected as well-defined masses, with flecks of calcification, on CXR.

Table 5.19 Mediastinal masses by anatomical site

Anterior mediastinal mass
Thymoma, lymphoma, germ cell tumours, pleuropericardial cysts, pericardial fat pad, anterior diaphragmatic hernia (Morgagni)

Posterior mediastinal mass
Neural tumours (neurofibroma), lymphoma + lymph node enlargement, aortic aneurysms, posterior diaphragmatic hernia (Bochdalek)

Superior mediastinal mass
Retrosternal thyroid, oesophageal + bronchogenic cysts

Although usually asymptomatic, they can cause pressure on surrounding structures. Treatment is by surgical excision.
- **Seminomas** are painful and malignant and occur in 20–40-year-old men. They usually arise from the thymus but are indistinguishable from testicular seminomas, so examine the testes. The CXR mass is not calcified, and diagnosis is confirmed by CT scan. Cisplatin-based chemotherapy is first-line therapy, as surgical excision is rarely complete. Subsequent radiotherapy is useful. Long-term survival is ~80%.
- **Non-seminomatous tumours** (e.g. choriocarcinoma) are malignant and symptomatic due to local invasion and occur in men 30–40 years old. Raised alpha-fetoprotein and alpha-HCG act as tumour markers, falling with tumour regression. Treatment is with cisplatin-based chemotherapy. Outcome is worse than with seminomas.

Retrosternal thyroid goitres

Retrosternal thyroid goitres usually occur in women. They are usually asymptomatic unless compressing the trachea and causing breathlessness, stridor, and a 'flattened' flow-volume loop. CXR detection is confirmed by CT or radioiodine scans. Tracheomalacia may follow surgical excision.

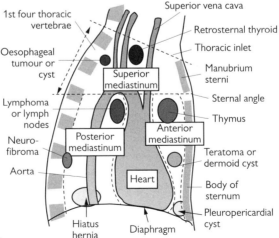

Figure 5.27 The mediastinum.

Neural tumours

Neural tumours are benign in 75% of cases. Nerve sheath tumours may be slow-growing and benign (e.g. schwannomas, neurofibromas) or malignant with local invasion and metastatic spread (e.g. neurosarcomas). Autonomic nervous system tumours include neuroblastomas and ganglioneuromas. Surgical excision is the treatment of choice, with chemotherapy and radiotherapy if malignant.

Enlarged lymph nodes

Enlarged lymph nodes may be due to infection (e.g. tuberculosis), lymphoma (e.g. Hodgkin's), or malignant metastases (e.g. oesophagus). Giant lymph node hyperplasia (Castleman's disease) is rare, occurring as:

- Localised, unicentric Castelman's Disease due to non-progressive angiofollicular lymph node hyperplasia causing mediastinal enlargement. Although often asymptomatic, it may cause fever, raised ESR, and cough and wheeze due to bronchial compression. It usually occurs in young adults and is curable by surgical resection of the involved lymph nodes.
- Generalised, multicentric Castleman's disease is a lymphoproliferative disease with systemic symptoms, adenopathy, hepatosplenomegaly, skin rash, and paraproteinaemia. It undergoes malignant transformation and is usually associated with HIV (and associated HHV-8, a gammaherpesvirus) infection. Treatment is with steroids, antivirals, rituximab, and chemotherapy, but prognosis is poor.

Cysts

Cysts include:

- **Pleuropericardial (or spring water) cysts** occur in the cardiophrenic angles and are usually asymptomatic. Management is usually conservative.
- **Foregut cysts** are related to the oesophagus or airway and lined by respiratory epithelium. Due to limited space for expansion, they cause dyspnoea, cough, and stridor and are often diagnosed in childhood on CXR or CT scan. Treatment is by excision.

Mediastinal inflammation

- **Mediastinitis** follows oesophageal perforation due to vomiting (Boerhaave's syndrome), malignancy, or gastroscopy. Patients are usually unwell with pain and fever. CXR shows mediastinal air, pleural fluid, and pneumothorax. Despite antibiotics, parenteral nutrition, and surgical repair, morbidity and mortality are often high.
- **Mediastinal fibrosis** is a rare idiopathic condition, occurring in middle age. It may be associated with autoimmune disease, retroperitoneal fibrosis, radiotherapy, drugs (e.g. methysergide), and infection (e.g. TB, histoplasmosis, *Nocardia*). Symptoms include breathlessness, wheeze, stridor, haemoptysis, dysphagia, SVCO, and pulmonary hypertension. Treatment is supportive, as steroids and surgery are ineffective. Prognosis depends on structures involved.

Further reading

Duwe BV, Sterman DH, Musani AI (2005). Tumors of the mediastinum. *Chest*, **128**, 2893–2909.

Pneumothorax

Pneumothorax is defined as a collection of air between the visceral and parietal pleura, causing a real, rather than potential, pleural space. Early recognition and drainage can be lifesaving. Pneumothorax is usually classified into the following categories.

Primary spontaneous pneumothorax

Primary spontaneous pneumothorax (PSP) is the commonest type of pneumothorax and occurs spontaneously in healthy lungs. Pathogenesis is poorly understood, but it may follow rupture of an apical subpleural air cyst ('bleb'). Small airways inflammation is often present and may contribute to air trapping and emphysema-like changes close to the visceral pleura. PSP usually affects tall, thin 20–40-year-old men. Prevalence is 8/100,000/year, rising to 20/100,000/year in subjects >1.9 m in height. It is less common in women (male:female ratio 5:1). PSP is rarely associated with significant physiological disturbance. Smoking is a major risk factor, and recurrence is more likely in tall men and those aged >60 years old. About 30% (range 16–54%) of first PSP recur, usually within the first 2 years. Probability of recurrence increases with further PSP to 40% after a second and >50% after a third PSP. Surgical pleurodesis is recommended after a second PSP to fuse the visceral and parietal pleura, remove blebs, and abrase subpleural cysts.

Secondary pneumothorax

Secondary pneumothorax (SP) is due to underlying lung diseases that damage lung architecture. It occurs most frequently in chronic obstructive pulmonary disease (COPD; ~60%), but also asthma, interstitial lung diseases (ILD), infection (e.g. *Pneumocystis carinii* pneumonia, necrotizing pneumonia), and rare or inherited disorders (e.g. Marfan's syndrome, cystic fibrosis, lymphangioleiomyomatosis (LAM)). The incidence of SP increases with age and the severity of the underlying lung disease. Other risk factors include ILD and emphysema. Hospital admission is usually required, as even a small SP may have serious implications if respiratory reserve is reduced. Mechanically ventilated patients with lung disease are at particular risk due to high pressures (i.e. barotrauma) and alveolar overdistension (i.e. volutrauma). Low-pressure, small-volume 'protective' ventilation strategies reduce this risk. In SP, mortality is 10%. Recurrence occurs in ~40% of cases but may be as high as 80% in patients with Langerhans' cell histiocytosis or LAM.

Traumatic pneumothorax

Traumatic pneumothorax (TP) may be due to blunt (e.g. road traffic accident) or penetrating (e.g. stab wounds) chest wounds, oesophageal rupture during gastroscopy, or mechanical ventilation (e.g. barotraumas, volutrauma).

Iatrogenic pneumothorax

Iatrogenic pneumothorax (IP) usually follows therapeutic procedures, including line insertion, transbronchial biopsy, pleural aspiration or biopsy, liver biopsy, cardiac massage, and chest surgery. Presentation may occur several hours, or even days, after the procedure.

Tension pneumothorax

Tension pneumothorax occurs when air enters the pleural space at each inspiration but is unable to escape on expiration. The resulting increase in intrathoracic pressure causes mediastinal shift, lung compression, and impaired venous return, with shock and reduced cardiac output. It is most common in TP and mechanically ventilated patients, but it may complicate PSP or SP. It is fatal if not rapidly relieved by drainage.

Clinical assessment

Classically, patients present with sudden pleuritic pain and/or breathlessness. Most PSP are small and cause few symptoms other than pain. Clinical signs can be surprisingly difficult to detect. A large pneumothorax limits expansion, reduces breath sounds, and causes hyperresonant percussion over one hemithorax. It may be associated with tachypnoea and cyanosis. Hamman's sign is unusual and refers to a 'click' on chest auscultation in time with the heart sounds. Rapid cardiorespiratory compromise can develop with a tension pneumothorax or during mechanical ventilation and indicates the need for immediate drainage. Subcutaneous emphysema may occur and is associated with a palpable crackling sensation around the root of the neck and upper chest.

Diagnosis is usually established at CXR (see Figure 5.28) which reveals a lung edge and absent peripheral lung markings. The width of the rim of air between the lung edge and the chest wall at the level of the hilum classifies pneumothoraces into large (>2 cm) and small (<2 cm). A pneumothorax with a 2 cm rim of air occupies 50% of the hemithorax. Lateral and lateral decubitus CXR are performed if clinical suspicion is high, but the posterior-anterior (PA) CXR is normal. They may aid detection of clinically important small SP. A lateral decubitus radiograph is as sensitive as a CT scan at detecting pneumothoraces. A CT scan is recommended to differentiate pneumothorax from complex bullous disease, particularly when aberrant tube placement is

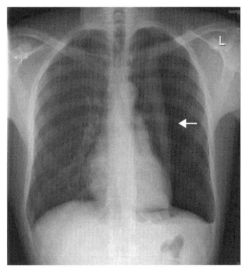

Figure 5.28 Large left-sided pneumothorax and collapsed left lung (→).

suspected or when surgical emphysema, following trauma, obscures the lung edge on CXR. Arterial blood gases often reveal hypoxia, and hypercapnia occurs in 15% of cases, usually those with SP.

Management

Figure 5.29 shows the current (2010) BTS recommended treatment algorithm for PSP and SP. Immediate supportive management includes analgesia for associated pain, treatment of the underlying cause in SP, and high-flow (10 L/min) oxygen, unless hypercapnia is a concern. By reducing nitrogen partial pressure in blood, high-concentration oxygen increases reabsorption of pleural air and encourages resolution of a pneumothorax. Management depends on breathlessness, haemodynamic compromise, the presence of associated lung disease, and the size of the pneumothorax.

Management of primary spontaneous pneumothorax

• **Observation.** Patients with minimal symptoms and a small (<2 cm rim) PSP do not require active intervention and can be observed and managed as outpatients. Patients discharged home should be asked to return if

breathlessness deteriorates. Typically, the pneumothorax is reabsorbed over 2–3 weeks, and resolution is confirmed on follow-up outpatient CXR. In managing PSP, the size of the pneumothorax is less important than the degree of clinical compromise.

• **Simple aspiration** (see Chapter 19) is recommended as first-line therapy in all PSP patients requiring intervention, including those with breathlessness and large pneumothoraces (>2 cm). Do not aspirate >2.5 L, as this suggests a persistent air leak, and stop if the procedure is painful or excessive cough occurs. Aspiration is successful in 60–80% of cases and confirmed by complete or near complete lung re-expansion on repeat CXR. Although the ideal time for a repeat CXR is unknown, it should be delayed for several hours in order to detect slow air leaks. Simple aspiration should not be repeated, unless there were technical difficulties. Compared to intercostal tube drainage, aspiration is associated with less recurrence and may avoid the need for hospital admission.

• Small bore (<14 Fr) intercostal chest drainage is occasionally required if aspiration fails or in large PSP with respiratory failure.

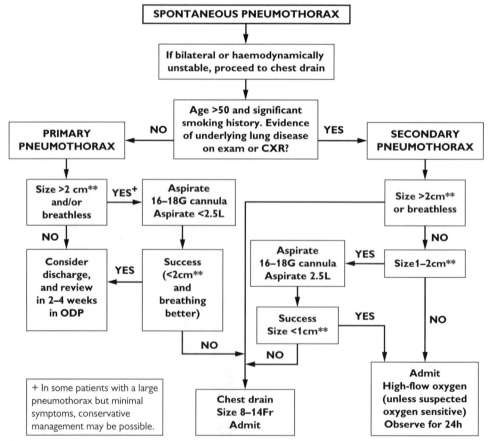

Figure 5.29 Management of spontaneous pneumothorax. (** is the distance from the lung edge to chest wall at the level of the hilum.) Reproduced from *Thorax*, 'Management of spontaneous pneumothorax: British Thoracic Society pleural disease guideline 2010', MacDuff A *et al.*, 65, Suppl 2, pp. ii18–ii31, Copyright 2010, with permission from BMJ Publishing Group Ltd.

Management of secondary pneumothorax

Secondary pneumothorax has a significant mortality and should be managed more aggressively.

- **Observation alone** is only recommended in patients with small (<1 cm) or apical SP. They should be hospitalized for observation.
- **Simple aspiration** achieves lung re-expansion in 35–65% of cases but is less successful than in PSP, particularly in patients with chronic lung disease, >50 years old, and with larger pneumothoraces. Aspiration is currently recommended as initial treatment in minimally breathless patients, <50 years old, with small SP. Successfully aspirated SP should be observed in hospital for at least 24 h before discharge.
- **Intercostal tube drainage** (see Chapter 19) is recommended in breathless patients, >50 years old, with large (>2 cm) SP. In most cases, a small drain (10–14 Fr) is adequate. Large drains (24–28 Fr) may be required in patients with large air leaks, during mechanical ventilation, and for subcutaneous emphysema. If the drain water level does not swing with respiration, check for blockages, incorrect tube positioning on CXR, or 'kinking' of the tubing. Chest drains can be safely removed when CXR confirms lung expansion, and there has been no air leakage (i.e. 'bubbling') through the drain for >24 h.

In general, drains should not be clamped before removal. Following adequate analgesia, the drain is pulled out at the end of a full inspiration and the drain site closed with previously inserted mattress sutures. However, some clinicians do clamp the drain for several hours before removal and repeat the CXR before removal to detect slow air leaks, thus avoiding inappropriate removal and the need for reinsertion. However, the benefit of this practice is controversial and should only be considered on specialist wards. A bubbling chest drain should never be clamped.

Chest drain insertion with both 'Seldinger' (insertion over a guide wire) and blunt dissection techniques is associated with significant morbidity and mortality. In complex pneumothoraces or if pleural fluid is present, ultrasound-guided insertion is advised in recent guidelines. Heimlich valves are an increasingly popular alternative to underwater bottle drainage, as they allow mobilization and, in some cases, outpatient management.

Management of traumatic pneumothorax

Traumatic pneumothorax and pneumothoraces during mechanical ventilation usually require chest drain insertion and intercostal drainage. High airways and positive end expiratory pressures (PEEP) encourage persistent leaks, and this can be minimized with 'protective' mechanical ventilation strategies, using small tidal volumes and the lowest airway pressures compatible with adequate gas exchange.

Management of iatrogenic pneumothoraces

Iatrogenic pneumothoraces (e.g. due to central line insertion) do not usually require intervention and resolve with observation alone, although aspiration is occasionally required. The exceptions are COPD and mechanically ventilated patients who often require intercostal tube drainage.

Management of tension pneumothorax

A tension pneumothorax is a medical emergency and must be drained immediately. Severity is not proportional to pneumothorax size. For example, patients with air trapping due to obstructive airways disease can develop significant tension with small pneumothoraces. Detection relies on a clinical examination. It should be considered in patients with acute respiratory distress, tracheal deviation away from the affected side and reduced air entry on the side of the pneumothorax, raised jugular venous pressure, hypotension, and, occasionally, cardiac arrest. Awaiting CXR confirmation may be life-threatening in severely compromised patients. Immediate drainage with a 14 G needle in the second intercostal space in the mid-clavicular line is essential. A characteristic 'hiss' of escaping air confirms the diagnosis. Further aspiration alleviates symptoms. The cannula is left *in situ* until an intercostal chest drain has been inserted.

Specific management problems

Chest drainage is associated with a number of potential practical and clinical problems.

- **Re-expansion pulmonary oedema** is suggested by breathlessness and cough, following lung re-expansion. It is associated with CXR features of pulmonary oedema and may affect both lungs. It is present radiologically in 14% of cases and is more common in patients who present late and those with large PSP. Although usually self-resolving, it can rarely be severe, requiring diuretics, nitrates, or mechanical ventilation, and is occasionally fatal.
- **Persistent drain leaks.** A persistent air leak is one that lasts >48 h after chest drain insertion and suggests the development of a bronchopleural fistula. After checking the chest drain for leaks and incorrect positioning, use high-flow wall suction, with pressures of −5 to −20 cmH₂O and a large-bore chest drain (24–28 Fr), to try and oppose visceral and parietal pleura, allowing spontaneous pleurodesis. Early surgical advice for consideration of operative intervention is essential (see section on surgical management).
- **Subcutaneous emphysema** occurs when parenchymal air dissects along perivascular sheaths into the mediastinum and then the neck. It may cause localized swelling (e.g. neck, chest) or grotesque facial and body distension. Palpation of the skin overlying the swelling produces a characteristic 'crackling' sensation. The voice may have a nasal quality, and auscultation over the precordium may reveal a 'crunch' with each heart beat (Hamman's sign). Management includes good drainage of associated pneumothoraces and 'protective' mechanical ventilation strategies. Failure of spontaneous resolution should prompt investigation (e.g. CT scan) to detect unrecognized bronchial air leaks and assessment of the drainage system to detect leaks.

Surgical management

Indications for referral of a patient with a pneumothorax to the thoracic surgical team for further investigation or pleurodesis include:

- Persistent air leaks (after >5 days of drainage).
- If the current episode is due to a second ipsilateral PSP.
- If the current episode is due to a contralateral PSP (i.e. after a previous pneumothorax in the other hemithorax).
- Bilateral PSP.
- Professions at risk after a first PSP (e.g. divers).

Surgical treatment aims to obliterate the 'pleural leak', close bronchopleural fistulae, and oppose and fuse the parietal and visceral pleural surfaces (pleurodesis). In young patients with PSP, video-assisted thoracoscopy (VATS) with pleural abrasion pleurodesis is preferred to open thoracotomy, as it is less invasive, with shorter recovery times, although recurrence rates are slightly higher than with open thoracotomy (i.e. 4% vs 1%). VATS is also as effective as thoracotomy at correcting bronchopleural fistula and causes less respiratory dysfunction.

Chemical pleurodesis performed by injecting a talc slurry through an intercostal drain is only recommended in frail patients and if surgery is not an option (e.g. COPD, malignant pleural effusions), as it is associated with 10–20% failure rate.

Specific pneumothorax and other air leaks

- **Catamenial pneumothorax** occurs with menstruation and is often recurrent. The cause is unknown, but it is usually associated with pleural endometriosis or diaphragmatic defects. Treatment options include suppression of the ovulatory cycle, chemical pleurodesis, or VATS pleurodesis with diaphragmatic repair.
- **Pneumothorax in HIV** is often associated with *Pneumocystis jirovecii* pneumonia and requires empirical treatment (see Chapters 6 and 13 and the 'Pneumonia' section in this chapter). Intercostal drainage is usually needed, and early surgical referral is recommended, as lung re-expansion may be difficult to achieve in this group of patients. Nebulized pentamidine increases the risk of pneumothorax.
- **Air leaks** follow ventilator-induced barotrauma or traumatic damage to the trachea (e.g. tracheostomy), bronchus, and oesophagus. A pneumomediastinum may

develop due to air in the mediastinal-pleural reflection and is detected as an air outline around the heart and great vessels on CXR. Occasionally, air may also collect in the pericardium, causing a pneumopericardium with associated tamponade.

Further reading

Barker A, Maratos EC, Edmonds L, *et al.* (2007). Recurrence rates of video-assisted thoracoscopic versus open surgery in the prevention of recurrent pneumothorax: a systemic review of randomised and non-randomised trials. *Lancet,* **370**, 329–35.

Davies RJO, Gleeson FV, Ali N, *et al.* (2010). BTS guidelines for the management of pleural disease. *Thorax,* **65** (Suppl 2), 1–40.

MacDuff A, Arnold A, Harvey J on behalf of the BTS Pleural Disease Guideline Group (2010). Management of spontaneous pneumothorax: British Thoracic Society pleural disease guideline. *Thorax,* **65**, ii18–ii31.

Millar AC and Harvey JE, on behalf of Standards of Care Committee, British Thoracic Society (1993). Guidelines for the management of spontaneous pneumothorax. *BMJ,* **307**, 114–16.

No authors listed (2000). Ventilation with lower tidal volumes as compared with traditional tidal volumes for acute lung injury and the acute respiratory distress syndrome. The Acute Respiratory Distress Syndrome Network. *New England Journal of Medicine,* **342**, 1301–8.

Vohra HA, Adamson L, Weeden DF (2008). Does video-assisted thoracoscopic pleurectomy result in better outcomes than open pleurectomy for primary spontaneous pneumothorax? *Interactive CardioVascular and Thoracic Surgery,* **7**, 673–7.

Pleural disease

Pleural effusion

A pleural effusion is an abnormal accumulation of fluid (>25 mL) in the pleural space. Normally, the pleural space contains about 0.26 mL/kg of fluid (~20 mL). Pleural fluid production and absorption is ~0.01 mL/kg/h or 15 mL/day, mainly by parietal pleura. Maximum fluid drainage is about 0.2 mL/kg/h or 300 mL/day. Normal pleural fluid contains similar concentrations of albumin to interstitial fluid, small numbers of macrophages (75%), lymphocytes (23%), mesothelial cells (1%), neutrophils (1%), and some larger molecular weight proteins such as lactate dehydrogenase (LDH). It has more bicarbonate, less sodium, and similar glucose levels, compared to plasma.

Clinical features

Pleural effusions are common and associated with a wide range of diseases, most commonly malignancy, heart failure, pneumonia, and pulmonary embolism. Small effusions may be asymptomatic. Larger effusions are associated with chest tightness, dyspnoea, and dry cough. Pleuritic chest pain is usually due to pleural inflammation and is often referred to the shoulder or abdomen. Examination reveals reduced chest expansion, quiet breath sounds, 'stony dull' percussion note, reduced tactile vocal fremitus, and a 'friction' rub when there is pleural inflammation, which disappears as the pleural effusion develops, separating the pleural surfaces. There may be bronchial breathing just above the fluid level. Radiological imaging confirms the presence of a pleural effusion and aids diagnosis. For example, bilateral effusions and cardiomegaly suggests heart failure, whereas massive unilateral effusions are usually malignant.

Chest radiography

Posterior-anterior (PA) CXRs detect pleural effusions >200 mL and lateral CXRs as little as 50 mL. Sequential blunting of the posterior, lateral, and anterior costophrenic angles occurs as effusions increase in size. A large effusion appears as a basal opacity, with concave upper border that obscures the hemidiaphagm (see Figure 5.30). Massive effusions show 'white-out' in the whole hemithorax, with mediastinal displacement away from the side of the effusion. Lack of displacement suggests collapse of underlying lung due to, for example, malignant bronchial occlusion or frozen mediastinum (commonly due to malignancy). Loculated 'interlobar' effusions produce well-defined round shadows. Diffuse opacification of a hemithorax on a supine film is characteristic of an effusion (e.g. in ICU).

Ultrasound scanning

Chest ultrasound scans (USS) differentiate fluid from pleural thickening and identify fibrinous septations and fluid loculations better than CT scans. Recent UK guidelines recommend that it should be used to guide aspiration of small collections and drainage of most pleural effusions.

Computer tomography scans

Chest computer tomography (CT) scans of pleural effusions should be performed with contrast to aid detection of pleural thickening and differentiation between benign and malignant disease. Nodular, irregular, circumferential, and mediastinal pleural thickening >1 cm suggest malignancy, with a specificity >90%. Detection of lymphadenopathy and

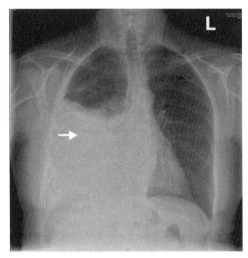

Figure 5.30 Right-sided pleural effusion (→).

parenchymal disease on CT scans aids diagnosis of many other diseases (e.g. tuberculosis).

Assessment of a pleural effusion

The initial aim is to establish the diagnosis and provide symptom relief until definitive treatment of the pleural effusion can be instituted. Assessment (see Figure 5.31) involves:

1. **Clinical assessment.**

   History, examination, and CXR can accurately determine the cause of most bilateral transudative effusions (e.g. left ventricular failure (LVF), hypoalbuminaemia, renal impairment, dialysis). These effusions do not need to be sampled, unless the appearance is atypical (e.g. unilateral effusion, fever, chest pain) or they fail to respond to treatment (e.g. diuresis improves heart failure effusions within 2–3 days).

2. **Pleural aspiration (thoracentesis).**

   Pleural aspiration (thoracentesis) is the primary means of evaluating a pleural effusion and is used to guide further investigation and management. It may be diagnostic or therapeutic (i.e. relieves breathlessness), depending on the volume of fluid removed. After the appearance of the fluid has been recorded, the sample is placed in sterile containers for protein and lactate dehydrogenase (LDH) and for microbiology including Gram stains and microscopy, culture, and acid-fast bacilli (AFB) stain and culture. A 20 mL fresh sample is sent to cytology to examine for malignant cells and differential cell counts. Use of a 3.8% sodium citrate tube may aid cell preservation in cytology samples. Blood culture bottle samples should also be sent for microbiology. A non-purulent, heparinized sample is processed in the arterial blood gas analyser for pH (without exposure to air or lidocaine). Measurement with pH litmus paper or pH meters is not reliable. Purulent

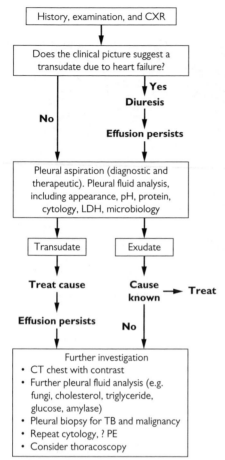

Figure 5.31 Diagnostic algorithm for the patient with a pleural effusion. Reproduced from *Thorax*, Davies HE, Davies RJO, and Davies CWH, 'Management of pleural infection British Thoracic Society pleural disease guidelines', 65, Suppl 2, pp. ii41–ii53, copyright 2003, with permission from BMJ Publishing Group Ltd.

Table 5.20 Causes of pleural effusions

Transudates	Exudates
Common causes	**Common causes**
Left ventricular failure	Parapneumonic effusions
Hypoalbuminaemia	Malignancy (>90%)
Cirrhosis (± ascites)	Pulmonary embolism (>80%)
Peritoneal dialysis	Rheumatoid arthritis
Nephrotic syndrome	Mesothelioma
Pulmonary embolism (<20%)	Tuberculous
Less common causes	**Less common causes**
Hypothyroidism	Autoimmune (e.g. SLE)
Constrictive pericarditis	Empyema
Mitral stenosis	Pancreatitis
Meig's syndrome	Post-cardiac injury
Malignancy (<10%)	Drugs
	Other infection (e.g. fungal)

samples should never be examined, as they may damage the analyser.

3. **Pleural fluid analysis.**

Pleural fluid analysis initially determines whether the effusion is a transudate or an exudate which aids diagnosis (see Table 5.20). A transudate is due to increased hydrostatic pressure (e.g. left ventricular failure) or reduced oncotic pressure (e.g. hypoalbuminaemia) in the microvascular circulation, resulting in increased serum but not albumin leakage. Light's criteria are used to determine if the fluid is a transudate or an exudate. The pleural fluid is an exudate if one of the following criteria is present: (a) pleural fluid protein/serum protein ratio is >0.5, (b) pleural fluid LDH/serum LDH ratio is >0.6, or (c) pleural fluid LDH is greater than two-thirds the upper limit of normal of serum LDH. These criteria are sensitive but may occasionally incorrectly identify a transudate as an exudate.

- **Appearance** may be bloody (e.g. trauma, malignancy, pulmonary infarction, infection, dissection), turbid

(e.g. empyema, chylothorax, pseudochylothorax; clear supernatant after centrifuging favours empyema), foul-smelling (e.g. anaerobic empyema), contain food particles (e.g. ruptured oesophagus), like 'anchovy sauce' (amoebic liver abscess rupture), or viscous (e.g. mesothelioma).

- **Differential cell counts** may indicate specific causes. Neutrophils occur in most acute effusions (e.g. parapneumonic, infarction). Lymphocytes are characteristic of tuberculosis (TB), especially if >80%, but also occur in rheumatoid, sarcoid, and malignant (including lymphoma) effusions. Pleural fluid eosinophilia, defined as >10% of eosinophils in the pleural fluid, is not very helpful in diagnosis; most are benign (e.g. TB, parapneumonic, drug-induced, infarction, parasitic, Churg–Strauss syndrome), but up to 25% are associated with malignancy, and, in many, no aetiology is ever established.

- **Pleural fluid glucose** of <3.3 mmol/L occurs in exudative effusions due to empyema (or paraneumonic), lupus, rheumatoid disease, TB, malignancy, and oesophageal rupture. The lowest glucose levels occur in rheumatoid pleurisy (<1.6 mmol/L in ~70% and <2.8 mmol/L in 80%) and empyema.

- **Pleural fluid pH** is normally ~7.6. A low pleural fluid pH is often associated with, and occurs in, the same diagnoses as a low pleural glucose but is mainly used to identify pleural infection. In parapneumonic effusions and empyema, a pleural fluid pH <7.2 indicates the need for pleural drainage, as infection is unlikely to resolve with antibiotics alone. In malignancy, a pH <7.3 is associated with positive cytology in 90% of cases, a poor outcome (median survival 2.1 months), and decreased success of pleurodesis (50%).

- **Pleural fluid cytology** is positive in 60% (study ranges 54–73%) of malignant effusions. The yield is increased by up to a further 25% by a second sample but not by a third or further samples.

- **Pleural amylase** is raised (> upper limit of serum amylase) in pleural malignancy, oesophageal rupture (both salivary amylase), and pancreatitis (pancreatic amylase).

- **Pleural lipids** are measured in turbid or milky pleural effusions. Chylothorax, following disruption of the thoracic duct (e.g. trauma, surgery, malignancy, especially lymphoma, lymphangioleiomyomatosis (LAM)), is associated with a pleural fluid triglyceride >110 mg/dL and chylomicrons. Pseudochylothorax occurs due to cholesterol crystal deposition in chronic effusions (e.g. TB, rheumatoid disease) and is associated with a raised pleural fluid cholesterol >200 mg/dL and cholesterol crystals on microscopy.

4. Further investigation.

Further investigations (± chest physician referral) should be considered if the diagnosis remains unclear. These include:

- Additional pleural fluid analysis, including cholesterol, triglyceride, glucose, amylase, fungal stains, haematocrit, and repeat pleural cytology.
- Consider pulmonary embolism, and arrange appropriate investigations.
- CT scan of the chest with contrast, preferably before complete fluid drainage, which aids assessment of the pleural surfaces and differentiation between benign and malignant pleural disease.
- Thoracoscopy is often diagnostic in difficult cases. Bronchoscopy is unhelpful, unless there is haemoptysis or the CXR/CT scan is abnormal, and is performed after drainage which decompresses the airways.
- Pleural tissue biopsy is essential for histology and TB culture. Image-guided (e.g. CT scan, ultrasound) 'closed' biopsies improve diagnostic yields in malignancy and reduce the risk of 'malignant seeding' in the biopsy tract. Unguided Abram's needle biopsies may occasionally be used if TB is suspected. Thoracoscopic biopsy is frequently the sampling technique of choice, has a sensitivity of 90% for malignancy, and allows simultaneous pleurodesis.

Management

Management of specific conditions is discussed in the following sections. However, most patients do not require a chest drain and can be managed as outpatients. Admission and chest drainage is considered in those with malignant effusions requiring pleurodesis, infected pleural effusions, and large symptomatic effusions.

Parapneumonic pleural effusion and empyema

Parapneumonic pleural effusions (PPE) occur in 40% of patients hospitalized with pneumonia, especially the paediatric and elderly populations, resulting in about 600,000 cases of PPE annually in the USA. These patients have a 3.4-fold increase in mortality. Iatrogenic and primary pleural infections also occur, and the incidence of pleural infection is increasing by 2.8% annually. A sterile initial exudate (simple PPE) may progress in some cases to a complicated PPE and then empyema. The classification and characteristics of PPE and empyema are summarized in Table 5.21.

'Simple parapneumonic pleural effusion'

The initial exudatative effusion contains raised cytokines and an LDH <300% of that in serum and has a pH >7.2 and a normal glucose. At this stage, observation and antibiotic therapy is recommended.

'Complicated parapneumonic pleural effusion'

Complicated PPE describes the early infective, fibrinopurulent stage when the effusion is not overtly purulent but has septa formation. Aspiration reveals inflammation and neutrophil phagocytosis, increased lactic acid production, and decreased pH. Increased metabolic activity reduces glucose levels, and LDH is elevated due to leucocyte cell death. Chest tube drainage is recommended for complicated PPE. Surgical drainage is required in ~15–40% of cases.

Empyema

Empyema describes the presence of frank pus. It has an estimated mortality of 15–20%. A poor outcome is associated with increased age, hypotension, low serum albumin, renal impairment, and hospital-acquired infection. Chest drainage is required, and outcome improves if loculated pus and thickened pleura are treated during video-assisted thoracoscopy (VATS).

Clinical features of parapneumonic pleural effusion

Are similar to those of pneumonia, with fever, dyspnoea, chest pain, and cough. The diagnosis should be considered in patients with 'slow to respond' pneumonia, pleural effusion with fever, or in high-risk patients with non-specific symptoms, including weight loss. It may occasionally follow oesophageal rupture (e.g. vomiting, gastroscopy) when it will be associated with a raised pleural fluid amylase. Anaerobic empyema often presents less acutely with

---

Table 5.21 Classification and characteristics of a parapneumonic pleural effusion (PPE) and empyema

Stages	Fluid	Pleural fluid characteristics	Management
Simple PPE	Clear	pH >7.2 LDH <1,000 IU/L Glucose >2.2 mmol/L No organisms on staining/culture	Usually clears spontaneously with antibiotic therapy alone. Chest tube drainage only for symptomatic relief
Complicated PPE	Clear or cloudy	pH <7.2 LDH >1,000 IU/L Glucose <2.2 mmol/L May be organisms on staining/culture	Requires chest tube drainage
Empyema	Frank pus	No additional biochemical tests needed May be organisms on staining/culture	Requires chest tube drainage ± surgery/VATS

general ill health, weight loss, and often without fever. It is usually associated with aspiration or poor dental hygiene.

Microbiology

Aerobic Gram-positive bacteria are the most frequently identified organisms, but pleural fluid cultures are negative in ~40% of infected PPE. Blood cultures are only positive in 13% of cases but are often the only positive microbiology.

- **Community-acquired infections** (CAI) include *Streptococcus milleri* (~30%), *Streptococcus pneumoniae* (~15%) and staphylococci (~10%), although many other organisms are implicated.
- **Hospital-acquired infections** (HAI) are often due to MRSA and other staphylococci (~50%). Gram-negative organisms, mainly *E. Coli*, *Enterobacter* spp., and *Pseudomonas*, are responsible for the majority of the remainder.
- **Mixed infections.** Gram-negative organisms (e.g. *E. coli*, *Pseudomonas*, *H. influenzae*, *Klebsiella*) are usually part of mixed infections with anaerobes and rarely occur in isolation. In both CAI and HAI, anaerobes occur in 12–34% but have been reported in up to 76% of cases.

Diagnosis

Diagnostic algorithms aid diagnosis and management of patients with suspected pleural infections, see Figure 5.32.

- **Diagnostic pleural aspiration** is essential if pleural infection is suspected. A pleural fluid pH <7.2 has highest accuracy for pleural infection, followed by glucose <2.2 mmol/L and LDH >300% upper normal limit for serum.

Detection of anaerobes is improved by inoculating blood culture bottles with pleural fluid. Frank pus does not need further pH or biochemical evaluation. Pleural fluid adenosine deaminase may be of value in countries where tuberculosis is prevalent (see section on tuberculous effusions).

- **Pleural biopsy** should be considered if a tuberculous effusion is suspected, as combined histology and culture increases diagnostic yield.
- **Ultrasound scans (USS)** improve visualization of septations and pleural thickening which occur in 86–100% of empyemas and ~50–60% of exudative PPEs. Recent guidelines recommend that all pleural fluid sampling should be performed under USS guidance, especially if effusions are small or loculated. The pH may vary between locules.
- **Contrast–enhanced chest CT scans** are performed in difficult cases to delineate the size and position of loculations and to guide drainage. Empyema is associated with attenuation of extrapleural subcostal fat and pleural enhancement, which may result in the 'split pleura sign' of enhanced, but separated, visceral and parietal pleura. CT scans also differentiate between parenchymal and pleural disease (e.g. lung abscess). Bronchoscopy is only indicated if a bronchial lesion is suspected.

Management

Small (i.e. maximal thickness <10 mm on USS) or simple PPE should be treated with antibiotics and observed, with pleural fluid sampling only if the effusion enlarges. Large,

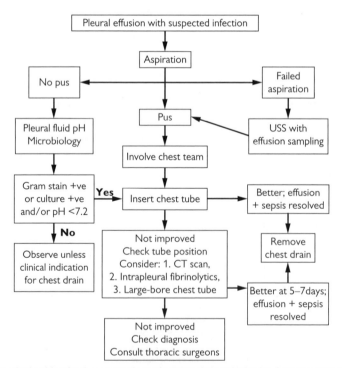

Figure 5.32 Diagnostic algorithm for the management of suspected pleural infection. Reproduced from *Thorax*, Davies HE, Davies RJO, and Davies CWH, 'Management of pleural infection British Thoracic Society pleural disease guidelines', 65, Suppl 2, pp. ii41–ii53, copyright 2003, with permission from BMJ Publishing Group Ltd.

infected effusions may require further intervention, including chest drainage.

Antibiotics
Antibiotics are required in all potentially infected PPE. Antibiotic therapy should be guided by local hospital guidelines and microbiological results. Empirical antibiotic treatment of:

• **Community-acquired infection** is with second-generation cephalosporins (e.g. cefuroxime) or penicillin ± beta-lactamase inhibitors (e.g. co-amoxiclav) which have good pleural space penetration and cover most expected organisms. Metronidazole is added for suspected anaerobic infection. Alternatively, clindamycin, with or without ciprofloxacin, may be used. Benzylpenicillin and a quinolone gives the same spectrum, with less risk of *C. difficile* diarrhoea. If microbiology is negative, antibiotics should initially cover community-acquired bacterial pathogens and anaerobic organisms.

• **Hospital-acquired infection** should cover Gram-positive, Gram-negative, and anaerobic organisms. Postoperative and trauma cases require staphylococcal cover. Recommended antibiotics include piperacillin with tazobactam, ticarcillin with clavulinic acid, carbapenems or third-generation cephalosporins. Aminoglycosides are avoided because they have poor pleural space penetration and are less active in acidic pleural fluid. MRSA infection is common and may require vancomycin cover.

There is no clear evidence regarding length of treatment, but, provided there is adequate pleural drainage, treatment for 3 weeks is probably adequate. Once the systemic symptoms and fever resolve, oral antibiotics may be used, and co-amoxiclav is a useful single agent that provides anaerobic cover.

Chest tube drainage
Chest drainage is required when pleural fluid is frankly purulent or cloudy/turbid, when microbiology is positive, and if pH <7.2, glucose <2.2 mmol/L, or LDH is >300% upper normal limit of serum. Consider early drainage in the elderly, those with comorbid conditions, and in loculated effusions, as these are associated with poor outcome. Small-bore (10–14 Fr) tubes are more comfortable and have been demonstrated to be as effective as large drains. Nevertheless, large-bore drains may be more appropriate for thick, viscid purulent fluid. The position of the drain is more important than the size, and tube insertion is best carried out under image guidance. Drains should be flushed 8-hourly with 30 mL of normal saline to prevent occlusion. Remove drains when clinical improvement occurs.

Surgical review
Surgical review is recommended if the patient does not improve or deteriorates despite antibiotics and tube drainage. Consider surgical referral in patients with ongoing weight loss and sepsis or if there is residual pleural fluid with loculations and pleural thickening after 7 days. Surgical options include:

• **Video-assisted thoracoscopic surgery** (VATS) to break down adhesions and drain residual collections. However, it may be unsuccessful in chronic empyema with substantially thickened visceral pleura.

• **Thoracotomy** for pleural decortication and removal of pleural debris. This is a major surgical procedure.

• **Rib resection and open drainage** which can be performed under local anaesthetic.

Other therapies
• **Pleural lavage and intrapleural antiseptics** have been reported to be beneficial in the treatment of pleural infection in several small studies. However, there are no randomized trial data, and this cannot be recommended as routine practice at present. The technique involves chest drain lavage with 750–1,000 mL/day of normal saline until the fluid from the chest clears.

• **Intrapleural fibrinolytics** have no benefit in terms of mortality, surgery, or hospital stay, and routine use is not recommended. However, they may be considered for use in large symptomatic loculated effusions in poor surgical candidates.

• **Nutritional support** is often required, as hypoalbuminaemia is associated with a poor outcome. Supplementary nasogastric feeding and parenteral nutrition should be considered from the time of diagnosis.

Management difficulties
Failure to improve, despite antibiotics and chest drainage, should initially lead to review of the microbiology and antibiotic adjustment. Check the chest drain tube for positioning and kinks, and ensure good drainage by flushing with saline. Consider a repeat CT scan to assess the extent of residual collection. Remove persistently blocked tubes, and insert image-guided new drains into loculated collections (recent evidence suggests large bore chest drains are better tolerated with less tube blockage). If surgical intervention is not an option, consider large-bore drains and lavage or rib resection under local anaesthetic with subsequent open drainage.

Complications
Residual pleural thickening occurs in 13.8% of empyema cases after 6 months but does not usually impair lung function. Surgical therapy is considered when there is significant impairment in lung function, with reduced TLC (<60% predicted) and >50% reduction of lung perfusion. Decortication is the definitive treatment, but general agreement is to wait for 6 months before considering surgery, as diffuse pleural thickening may resolve spontaneously over a few months.

Malignant pleural effusions
Malignancy is the commonest cause of exudative pleural effusion in patients >60 years of age and is responsible for about 40,000 cases a year in the UK. Most are metastatic, with lung and breast common primary sites (see Table 5.22). Median survival after diagnosis is 3–12 months, shortest in lung cancer and longest following ovarian cancer or mesothelioma. Effusions are often large, and breathlessness is the main symptom. Chest pain, cough, and weight loss are frequent. Occasionally, asymptomatic cases occur.

Table 5.22 The source (primary site) and frequency of malignant pleural effusions

Lung	~40%
Breast	~15%
Lymphoma	~10%
Mesothelioma	~10%
Genitourinary tract	~10%
Gastrointestinal tract	~5–7%
Unknown primary	~10%

Although rare, myeloma, leukaemia, sarcoma, melanoma can all cause pleural effusion. (Mesothelioma is discussed in Asbestos-related lung disease.)

Key diagnostic investigations

- **CT scan with pleural contrast** aids detection of pleural malignancy, as described previously.
- **Pleural fluid**. A pH <7.20 is associated with positive cytology, the possibility of failed pleurodesis, and a reduced median survival of 2.1 months (see 'Assessment of a pleural effusion'). However, it is not useful in predicting 3-month mortality.
- **Pleural fluid cytology** confirms the diagnosis in 60% of cases. A second sample, but not a third, increases the diagnostic yield. Cell immunostaining may suggest the primary site.
- **Serum tumour markers**, including CEA, CA-125, CA19-9, and PSA, may be useful when the primary tumour remains undetected. However, elevated tumour markers should be interpreted with caution (and supporting evidence) because they can be raised in up to 50% of benign effusions.
- **Pleural biopsy**, with CT or USS guidance, is more reliable than 'blind' Abram's pleural biopsy (sensitivity ~90% vs ~<60%, respectively) and should be considered in cytology-negative cases.
- **Thoracoscopy** is considered in patients with a good performance status when less invasive tests have failed to provide a diagnosis and allows direct visualization of the pleura. In less robust patients, the complications often outweigh the benefit. Diagnostic sensitivity is 95% for malignancy and it detects malignancy in ~65–70% of patients with previously negative cytology or closed pleural biopsy. Therapeutic talc pleurodesis is possible during thoracoscopy and is successful in >80% of cases.

Management

Management is determined by symptoms, performance status, disease stage, and the sensitivity of the primary tumour to chemotherapy. Some pleural effusions improve if the primary tumour responds to chemotherapy (e.g. lymphomas, breast, small cell cancer). In patients with unresponsive tumours, therapeutic and palliative aspiration of 1–2 L pleural fluid alleviates breathlessness. However, most effusions recur within a month, and repeated aspirations can be unpleasant. These patients should be considered for pleurodesis which aims to fuse the parietal and visceral pleura. Following intercostal tube drainage and full lung expansion, pleurodesis (see Chapter 19) is achieved by injecting a talc slurry (i.e. 5 g talc in 50 mL normal saline) or doxycycline 500 mg into the pleural space though the chest drain. Allow the sclerosant to dwell for 1–2 h before unclamping the drain. Success depends on apposition of the pleural surfaces and is prevented by incomplete expansion of the lung due to airway obstruction, air leaks, fibrotic processes (e.g. tuberculosis), and encasement of the visceral pleura by tumour with subsequent 'lung trapping'. Suction encourages lung expansion and may facilitate pleurodesis in patients with trapped lung and pneumo- or hydropneumothorax. An alternative approach is to insert an indwelling pleural catheter. With this, the patient drains their pleural effusion at home.

Treatment options in those with lungs that fail to expand include the insertion of an indwelling pleural catheter or pleuroperitoneal shunt. In patients with loculated pleural effusions, thoracoscopy or intrapleural fibrinolytics may be considered to disrupt loculations. However, neither thoracoscopy nor fibrinolytics are useful or used for trapped lung. Repeated pleural aspiration and long-term pleural drains may be required for some patients.

Other pleural effusions

- **Tuberculous pleural effusions** are a common feature of primary tuberculosis (TB) in children and may follow reactivation of TB or co-infection with HIV in adults. Clinical features are similar to those of pulmonary TB, with fever, night sweats, dyspnoea, and weight loss, although acute presentations with fever and pleuritic chest pain may mimic pneumonia. Effusions are usually small or moderate in size but can be massive. CXR shows associated pulmonary infiltrates in <33% of cases. Pleural fluid reveals a lymphocytosis, moderately reduced pH, and an elevated LDH. Acid-fast bacilli (AFB) are detected in 10–20%, with positive cultures in 25–50% at 6 weeks. Abram's pleural biopsy, combined with culture, detects 90% and thoracoscopic biopsies nearly 100% of cases. About 50% of patients with pleural TB have positive sputum culture. Pleural fluid adenosine deaminase, an enzyme released by macrophages after phagocytosis of mycobacteria, is sensitive for TB, but not specific, and is raised in empyema and occasionally malignancy. PCR for mycobacterial DNA has been disappointing and is not recommended.

  The majority of tuberculous effusions resolve spontaneously without treatment, but >65% of patients develop pulmonary TB within 5 years. Consequently, treatment (as for pulmonary TB) is recommended. Pleural fluid volumes may increase during treatment, requiring therapeutic aspiration and occasionally steroid therapy. Pleural thickening and calcification are long-term consequences.

- **Rheumatoid arthritis** (RA) associated effusions occur in 5% of cases. The effusions may be the first manifestation of RA, can be unilateral or bilateral, are more common in men, and often persist for months. Pleural fluid glucose is low (<1.6 mmol/L in ~70% and <2.8 mmol/L in 80%) and pH reduced (<7.3). Some cases respond to steroids.

- **Pulmonary embolism** (PE) associated effusions are usually small, unilateral, and bloodstained (~80%) and occur after 40% of PE. In the USA, PE is the fourth commonest cause of pleural effusion. Pleural fluid analysis is not diagnostic, although almost all are exudates. PE should be considered in patients with undiagnosed pleural effusion, particularly if there is a history of pleuritic chest pain or breathlessness or unexplained hypoxaemia.

- **Pleural effusions following asbestos exposure** are either benign asbestos pleural effusions or due to mesothelioma and are discussed in Asbestos related disease.

- **Pleural effusions in HIV infection** occur in 7–27% of hospitalized HIV patients. The commonest causes are Kaposi's sarcoma (30%), PPE (28%), TB (14%), PCP (10%), and lymphoma (7%).

- **Chylothorax** is usually due to malignancy (50%), trauma, or surgery (25%). Other causes include TB, sarcoidosis, LAM, amyloidosis, or cirrhosis. Pseudochylothorax is associated with TB, RA, and empyema.

- **Connective tissue disease**, including SLE.

- **Haemothorax** (defined as a pleural effusion with a haematocrit >50% of peripheral blood haematocrit) has a wide variety of causes, including trauma, malignancy, infarction, pneumonia, aortic rupture, and endometriosis.

Further reading

Anyunes G, Neville E, Duffy J, Ali N; Pleural Diseases Group, Standards of Care Committee, British Thoracic Society (2003). BTS guidelines for the management of malignant pleural effusions. *Thorax*, **58** (Suppl II), ii29–38.

Best Health. Lungs and breathing. <http://besthealth.bmj.com/x/set/topic/condition-centre/15.html>.

British Lung Foundation Breathe Easy Group. <http://www.lunguk.org>.

Cameron R and Davies HR (2008). Intra-pleural fibrinolytic therapy vs conservative management in the treatment of adult parapneumonic effusions and empyema. *Cochrane Database of Systematic Reviews*, **2**, CD002312.

Chest, Heart & Stroke Scotland. <http://www.chss.org.uk/>.

Davies CWH, Gleeson FV, Davies RJ; Pleural Diseases Group, Standards of Care Committee, British Thoracic Society (2003). BTS guidelines for the management of pleural infection. *Thorax*, **58** (Suppl II), 18–28.

Davies HE, Davies RJO, Davies CWH (2010). Management of pleural infection. British Thoracic Society pleural disease guidelines. *Thorax*, **65** (Suppl 2), ii41–53.

Davies RJO, Gleeson FV, Ali N, et al. (2003). BTS guidelines for the management of pleural disease. *Thorax*, **58** (Suppl II), ii1–59.

Hooper C, Lee YCG, Maskell N; BTS Pleural Guideline Group (2010). BTS guidelines for the investigation of a unilateral effusion in adults. British Thoracic Society pleural disease guidelines. *Thorax*, **65**, ii4–ii17.

Light RW (2001). Pleural effusion due to pulmonary emboli. *Current Opinion in Pulmonary Medicine*, **7**, 198–201.

Light RW (2002). Pleural effusion. *New England Journal of Medicine*, **346**, 1971–7.

Maskell NA and Butland RJA (2003). BTS guidelines for the investigation of a unilateral effusion in adults. *Thorax*, **58** (Suppl II), ii8–17.

Maskell NA, Gleeson FV, Davies RJO (2003). Standard pleural biopsy versus CT guided cutting needle biopsy for the diagnosis of pleural malignancy in pleural effusions: a randomised controlled trial. *Lancet*, **361**, 1326–31.

Maskell NA, Davies CW, Nunn AJ, et al. (2005). UK controlled trial of intrapleural streptokinase for pleural infection. *New England Journal of Medicine*, **352**, 865–74.

Roberts M, Neville E, Berrisford R, Antunes G, Ali N; BTS Pleural Disease Guideline Group (2010). BTS guidelines for the management of malignant pleural effusions. British Thoracic Society pleural disease guidelines. *Thorax*, **65**, ii32–ii40.

Asbestos-related lung disease

Asbestos, a naturally occurring hydrated silica fibre, occurs in two forms which differ in pathogenicity and lung clearance.

- **Curly serpentine fibres** include chrysotile (white asbestos), which is the only fibre still in commercial use. Severe restrictions limit its use in developed economies, and it is mainly employed in developing countries.
- **Straight, needle-like fibres** (amphiboles) include amosite (brown asbestos), crocidolite (blue asbestos), tremolite, and anthrophylite. They are more carcinogenic than chrysotile and clear slowly from the lung.

Asbestos causes benign and malignant disease. All types of asbestos are lung carcinogens, but the long latency periods, exposure to mixed fibre types, and confounding factors, such as smoking, make it difficult to quantify the carcinogenicity of each fibre type accurately.

Exposure is usually occupational and occurs during mining, construction (e.g. fireproofing, insulation), demolition work, or manufacturing (e.g. brake linings). However, domestic exposure is also well recognized due to 'carry home' fibres on clothing, geological exposure in some regions (e.g. Corsica), and during domestic refurbishment.

In the UK, peak industrial asbestos use occurred in the 1970s, and asbestos-related disease is likely to remain a significant problem for the next 20 years. The incidence of mesothelioma is expected to peak in about 2020. The coroner should be notified of any proven or suspected asbestos-related deaths.

If asbestos-related disease is suspected, a careful occupational history, including dates and type of exposure and the name of employer, is essential for future medico-legal purposes. In the UK, compensation can be claimed from:

- **The Government** through schemes administered by the Department for Work and Pensions (DWP), including the Industrial Injuries Disablement Benefit (IIDB) scheme. Industrial Injuries Disablement Benefit is available for a list of prescribed diseases, including a number or asbestos-related conditions. Benefit is available for diffuse pleural thickening (DPT), asbestosis, lung cancer, and mesothelioma (Form BI100PN). There are also three schemes that provide lump sum payments to those with asbestos-related diseases who are eligible. A DWP scheme set up under the 'Pneumoconiosis etc (Workers Compensation) Act' 1979 which provides a lump sum for patients suffering with certain asbestos-related conditions, where they are unable to claim damages because their employer has gone out of business. The 2008 'Diffuse Mesothelioma Payments' scheme which provides an immediate lump sum to a patient with mesothelioma whilst awaiting compensation from other sources, recognizing that most sufferers only survive for a few months. It also covers those not previously eligible for help (e.g. self-employed, domestic exposure) and operates alongside the scheme established by the 1979 Act for those unable to benefit from it. Payments in this scheme are subsequently recovered from successful civil compensation claims. From 2014 the new 'Diffuse Mesothelioma Payment Scheme' (DMPS) can make payments to those exposed to asbestos and diagnosed with mesothelioma after July 2012 who are unable to bring a claim against the previous employer or that employer's liability insurer. The 2014 scheme will operate alongside the 2008 scheme. The War Disablement Pension Scheme may provide compensation for disease resulting from asbestos exposure during employment in the armed forces (Form WPA1).
- **The courts** as common law compensation from a previous employer and their insurer, even if the employer is no longer in existence. Legal proceedings must start within 3 years of the diagnosis; otherwise, they become 'statute-barred' and cannot be pursued in the courts. Patients are not eligible for compensation if exposure occurred whilst they were self-employed.

Benign asbestos-related pleural disease

Asbestos exposure is associated with a number of benign pathologies, including:

- **Pleural plaques** (± calcification) occur in the parietal pleura of ~50% of asbestos-exposed workers, 20–30 years after exposure, but are not pre-malignant. They are often bilateral, mainly over the posterolateral chest wall and diaphragmatic dome. They are typically asymptomatic and best detected on high-resolution CT scan (HRCT). Compensation is not available for pleural plaques alone.
- **Benign asbestos-related pleural effusions** occur within 10 years of exposure and are usually small, unilateral, bloodstained exudates with a characteristic eosinophilic effusion in ~25%. Although often asymptomatic, they may be associated with pleurisy, fever, and dyspnoea. Benign pleural effusions may precede the development of diffuse pleural thickening, but there is no association with mesothelioma. Treatment is symptomatic with analgesics for pain and aspiration for breathlessness.
- **Diffuse pleural thickening** is due to fibrosis of the visceral pleura with parietal pleural adhesions and pleural symphisis which usually starts in the bases and gradually progresses to complete obliteration (see Figure 5.33). Unlike pleural plaques, its margins are ill-defined, and it should involve the costophrenic angle. It may also involve the apices and interlobar fissures.

On CXR, it appears as smooth pleural thickening, affecting more than 25% of the chest wall. Occasionally, contraction of visceral pleura ensnares underlying lung, resulting in a characteristic round, pleurally based mass, greater than 2.5 cm in diameter, with a 'comet tail' of vessels and bronchi

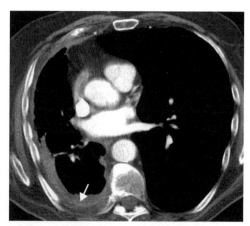

Figure 5.33 High-resolution CT scan of the chest demonstrating diffuse pleural thickening (→).

converging on the mass (it is also known as Blesovsky's syndrome or rounded atelectasis).

Exertional dyspnoea, chest pain, and, occasionally, respiratory failure are due to the associated restrictive defect. There is no association with mesothelioma.

DPT has characteristic radiological features (i.e. smooth outline, predominantly visceral involvement, subpleural fibrosis), and biopsy is seldom required. Indicators for biopsy include nodular invasion of the lung, mediastinal involvement, and >1 cm thickening of the parietal pleural.

Asbestosis

Asbestosis is due to asbestos inhalation, with a latency period of 20–40 years from first exposure. There is a clear dose-response relationship between the degree and length of asbestos exposure. Amphiboles are more fibrogenic, and the disease is accelerated by smoking.

Clinical onset is insidious with dyspnoea, dry cough, bilateral, late inspiratory basal crepitations, clubbing (~40%), and later respiratory failure. Pulmonary function testing usually demonstrates a restrictive defect with reduced gas transfer, although obstructive and mixed patterns occur which may reflect asbestos-induced small airways disease.

The CXR usually reveals bilateral reticulonodular shadowing, affecting mainly the lower lobes peripherally (± pleural plaques and diffuse pleural thickening). However, the CXR is normal in ~15% of proven cases. In these patients, HRCT is more sensitive and reveals ground glass shadowing in early disease and subpleural and/or interlobular fibrosis with later honeycombing and traction bronchiectasis.

Asbestos bodies may be demonstrated on histological examination, but diagnosis is usually based on history and clinical features. These patients are at increased risk of lung cancer. Treatment is supportive (e.g. supplemental oxygen, smoking cessation, influenza vaccination), as pharmacological therapy is ineffective.

Prognosis varies widely, and there is an increased risk of developing lung cancer. After removal from exposure, progression occurs in between 10 and 40% of cases over 10 years. Patients with greater exposure tend to progress more rapidly, but rapid progression (i.e. over 1–2 years) is unusual and more in keeping with usual interstitial pneumonitis (see section 'Diffuse parenchymal (interstitial) lung disease' later in this chapter). Prognosis is better in patients with fewer CXR opacities.

Mesothelioma

Mesothelioma, a malignant tumour of the pleura and peritoneum, is due to asbestos exposure in ~90% of cases. Other causes include exposure to non-asbestos fibres like erionite in certain geological areas (e.g. Turkey). Unlike asbestosis or lung cancer, there is no association with smoking or relationship with the level of asbestos exposure. Mean latency period from first exposure to death is ~40 years.

Clinical features include dull, aching (boring) chest pain, breathlessness, night sweats, pleural thickening or effusions, and chest wall invasion at chest drain or thoracoscopy biopsy sites. The CXR often reveals pleural thickening and/or a pleural effusion. Radiographic HRCT imaging (see Figure 5.34) detects pleural nodularity (± effusion) with contrast enhancement, local invasion (e.g. chest wall, peritoneum), and a 'constricted' small hemithorax.

Pleural fluid cytology is rarely diagnostic, although it may exclude other pathology (e.g. adenocarcinoma). Image-guided (e.g. ultrasound or CT scan) pleural biopsy is diagnostic in >90%. Thoracoscopy is now preferred by many

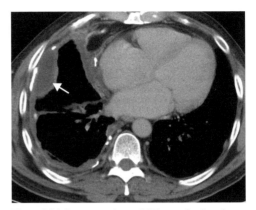

Figure 5.34 Contrast-enhanced CT scan of a pleural mesothelioma with pleural thickening, nodularity, and a pleural mass (→).

chest physicians, as it can be combined with talc pleurodesis, with a success rate of >90%. Blind biopsy is no longer recommended and should be discouraged. Thoracoscopy, chest drain, and biopsy sites should be marked for future prophylactic radiotherapy. Epithelioid histology (~50%) is associated with a better prognosis than sarcomatous or mixed cell types.

Median survival is poor (8–14 months). In many cases, treatment is symptomatic, including analgesia, nerve blocks, supplemental oxygen, and talc pleurodesis (preferably thoracoscopic), indwelling long-term drain, or repeated aspiration for pleural effusions. Early prophylactic radiotherapy (i.e. within 4 weeks) reduces chest wall invasion at thoracoscopy, chest drain, or biopsy sites from about 40% to 0%. Radiotherapy may also alleviate chest wall pain but is less effective in superior vena caval obstruction.

In specialized centres, radical surgery (± radiotherapy and chemotherapy) may be considered in selected cases for localized epithelioid tumours, although recent trials have shown only limited benefit. The role of chemotherapy alone has not been established. However, new chemotherapeutic regimes and immunotherapies (e.g. recombinant interferon-alpha) appear promising. For example, pemetrexed, an expensive NICE-approved chemotherapeutic agent (in combination with cisplatin), produces an objective response (>50% tumour shrinkage) in 41% of treated patients and prolongs survival by about 3 months when compared to cisplatin alone.

Lung cancer

There is a dose-response relationship between exposure to asbestos and lung cancer risk. Recent studies suggest a six-fold increase in the risk of lung cancer in the absence of a smoking history. Smoking increases the risk of dying of lung cancer in asbestos workers by 16-fold if they smoked more than 20 cigarettes/day and 9-fold if they smoked less than 20 cigarettes/day, compared to non-smokers.

Workers with asbestosis are at even greater risk of lung cancer, although it is unclear if this is because asbestosis is a marker for heavier asbestos exposure or if the inflammatory process is important per se in promoting carcinogenesis.

Further reading

British Thoracic Society Standards of Care Committee (2007). Statement on malignant mesothelioma in the United Kingdom. *Thorax*, **62**, ii1–ii9.

Camus M, Siemiatycki J, Meek B (1998). Non-occupational exposure to chrysotile asbestos and the risk of lung cancer. *New England Journal of Medicine*, **338**, 1565–71.

Davies RJO, Gleeson FV, Ali N, *et al.* (2003). BTS guidelines for the management of pleural disease. *Thorax*, **58** (Suppl II), ii1–59.

Department for Work and Pensions. Provides advice on benefits and application forms. A claim for Industrial Injuries Disablement Benefit requires Form BI100PN. The War Disablement Pensions Scheme may provide compensation for disease resulting from asbestos exposure in the armed forces and requires form WPA1.

GOV.UK. Industrial injuries disablement benefit scheme (for information on the Pneumoconiosis (Workers Compensation) Act 1979 with appropriate contacts and links). <https://www.gov.uk/industrial-injuries-disablement-benefit/further-information>.

Guidotti TL, Miller A, Christiani D, *et al.* (2004). Diagnosis and initial management of non-malignant diseases related to asbestos. *American Journal of Respiratory and Critical Care Medicine*, **170**, 691–715.

Mesothelioma Act 2014. <http://www.legislation.gov.uk/ukpga/2014/1/pdfs/ukpga_20140001_en.pdf>.

Mesothelioma UK. <http://www.mesothelioma.uk.com>.

Support and advice on compensation to patients, relatives and legal advisers. <http://www.patient.co.uk>.

Robinson BWS and Lake RA (2005). Advances in malignant mesothelioma. *New England Journal of Medicine*, **353**, 1591–603.

Sterman DH and Albeda SM (2005). Advances in the diagnosis, evaluation, and management of malignant pleural mesothelioma. *Respirology*, **10**, 266–83.

The Mesothelioma Center. <http://www.mesotheliomacenter.org>.

Diffuse parenchymal (interstitial) lung disease

The term diffuse parenchymal (interstitial) lung disease (DPLD/ILD) describes a group of disorders characterized by inflammation and/or fibrosis, primarily involving the pulmonary interstitium (i.e. the tissue between the alveolar epithelium and the capillary endothelium) and/or the bronchovascular and septal tissues comprising the lung's fibrous framework. However, the alveolar airspaces, distal airways, and vasculature are also frequently involved.

Clinical presentation and preliminary investigations

Typically, DPLD/ILD present with an insidious onset of dyspnoea, decreasing exercise tolerance, and cough. Examination may reveal finger clubbing, cyanosis, and fine (occasionally coarse) bilateral inspiratory crackles on chest auscultation. Exercise-induced desaturation may occur with disease progression; resting hypoxaemia and right heart failure may be evident in advanced disease. Initial investigations include:

- **Pulmonary function tests**. A restrictive spirometric defect is often evident, with a reduction in total lung capacity (TLC), functional residual capacity (FRC), and residual volume (RV) due to reduced lung compliance. Gas transfer (DLCO) is decreased due to impaired gas exchange at the alveolar-capillary interface.
- **Plain chest radiography** (CXR) is abnormal (>90%) with interstitial, alveolar, nodular, or mixed opacities.
- **Bronchoscopy and bronchoalveolar lavage** (BAL) help exclude other diseases (e.g. malignancy, infection). An increase in BAL inflammatory cells, indicating alveolitis, may correlate with ground glass opacification (GGO) on high-resolution computed tomography (HRCT); however, GGO may also represent fine fibrosis, rather than pure inflammation.
- **HRCT scans (± histology)** may be required for diagnosis and classification. Qualitative information from HRCT is crucial for determining the ILD 'phenotype' during investigational work-up.

DPLD/ILD classification and terminology

DPLD/ILD terminology and classification have been a source of confusion for many years. However, consensus has improved, following the American Thoracic and European Respiratory Societies (ATS/ERS) reclassification in 2001 (and further updated in 2013), which is now largely incorporated into the 2008 British Thoracic Society (BTS) DPLD/ILD guidelines and the 2013 NICE Idiopathic Pulmonary Fibrosis Guideline.

DPLD/ILD can be classified into four main categories, although there is considerable overlap.

Idiopathic interstitial pneumonias (IIPs)
- **Idiopathic Pulmonary Fibrosis (IPF)/Usual interstitial pneumonia** (UIP), the commonest IIP, previously known as cryptogenic fibrosing alveolitis (CFA).
- **Non-usual interstitial pneumonias** are less common, but distinct, disorders and include:
  - Idiopathic non-specific interstitial pneumonia (NSIP).
  - Cryptogenic organizing pneumonia (COP), previously known as bronchiolitis obliterans organizing pneumonia (BOOP).
  - Acute interstitial pneumonia (AIP), formerly known as Hamman–Rich syndrome.

- Respiratory bronchiolitis-associated interstitial lung disease (RB-ILD).
- Desquamative interstitial pneumonia/lung disease (DIP).
- Rare idiopathic lymphoid interstitial lung disease (LIP).
- Rare idiopathic pleuroparenchymal fibroelastosis.
- Unclassifiable idiopathic interstitial pneumonias.

ILDs due to specific causes or associations
- Medication (e.g. amiodarone, methotrexate).
- Hypersensitivity pneumonitis (HP, e.g. farmer's lung).
- Connective tissue disease (CTD, e.g. systemic sclerosis).
- Pneumoconioses (e.g. silicosis, asbestosis).
- Autoimmune (e.g. inflammatory bowel disease).

Granulomatous ILD
- Sarcoidosis (see 'Sarcoidosis').

Other rare causes of ILD
- Langerhans cell histiocytosis (LCH), previously histiocytosis X or pulmonary eosinophilic granuloma.
- Lymphangioleiomyomatosis (LAM).
- Infiltrative disorders (e.g. amyloidosis, Gaucher's disease, alveolar proteinosis).
- Malignancy (e.g. lymphangitis carcinomatosis).
- Post-inflammatory (e.g. ARDS, vasculitis, bronchiolitis).
- Infective and post-infective (e.g. HIV).
- Bone marrow transplantation.

Diagnosis

Tables 5.23 and 5.24 illustrate a diagnostic approach to DPLD/ILD, the main objective being to identify the most likely diagnosis in the fewest steps. Cases due to occupational exposure, drugs, CTD, and hypersensitivity pneumonitis are usually obvious, following a comprehensive consultation, including recreational and work history. Careful examination for features suggestive of a CTD, appropriate blood tests (e.g. rheumatoid factor, antinuclear antibodies), serology (e.g. avian precipitins), lung function testing, and radiological imaging is required. Similarly, the clinical, radiological, and histological features of sarcoidosis are characteristic (see 'Sarcoidosis').

Diagnosis of idiopathic interstitial pneumonia (IIP) is initially one of exclusion, having failed to detect an alternative cause (e.g. chronic HP). Subsequent IIP classification is difficult on clinical grounds alone. The ATS/ERS (2001, 2013) and BTS (2008) consensus panels and the updated guidelines for diagnosis and management of IPF published jointly by the ATS/ERS/JRS and ALAT (2011) emphasize an integrated clinical, radiological, and pathological approach to diagnosis and classification of IIP because accurate diagnosis of IPF/UIP has crucial therapeutic and prognostic implications.

Idiopathic pulmonary fibrosis (IPF) is the commonest IIP. It is a chronic, progressive fibrosing interstitial pneumonia of unknown cause, occurring primarily in older adults, limited to the lungs, and associated with the histopathologic and/or radiologic pattern of UIP (see next paragraph). The definition of IPF requires the exclusion of other forms of ILD, including other IIP and those associated with environmental exposure, medication, or systemic disease.

Table 5.23 Classification of diffuse parenchymal lung diseases (DPLD)

Types of DPLD	Examples
1. Idiopathic interstitial pneumonia (IIP)	• Idiopathic pulmonary fibrosis/Usual interstitial pneumonia (IPF/UIP)
	• Non-usual interstitial pneumonia (non-UIP e.g. NSIP, DIP)
2. DPLD due to specific causes	• Drug-induced
	• Hypersensitivity pneumonitis
	• Connective tissue disease
	• Occupational lung disease
3. Granulomatous DPLD	• Sarcoidosis
	• Granulomatous lung diseases
4. Unusual causes of DPLD	• Infiltrative (e.g. amyloidosis)
	• Malignant (e.g. lymphangitis carcinomatosis)
	• Infective or post-infective (e.g. HIV, mycoplasma)
	• Post-inflammatory (ARDS)
	• Langerhans cell histiocytosis (LCH)
	• Bone marrow transplant

Data from 'American Thoracic Society/European Respiratory Society International Multidisciplinary Consensus Classification of the Idiopathic Interstitial Pneumonias', *American Journal of Respiratory Critical Care Medicine*, 165, pp. 277–304, 2002.

IPF/UIP accounts for ~70% of IIP, is not steroid-sensitive, and has a poor prognosis (median survival <5 years). Non-UIP diseases account for ~30% of IIP, many of which are steroid-sensitive, with a good prognosis (median survival >10 years). However, some non-UIP diseases like AIP have a much worse prognosis than UIP (see further text).

High-resolution CT (HRCT) of the chest is integral to the evaluation of patients with DPLD/ILD. In IIP, its primary role is to help to distinguish confidently UIP from another disease (e.g. NSIP, DIP). Characteristic HRCT findings (see Table 5.25) include a bilateral, predominantly basal, and subpleural pattern of septal reticulation, with tractional air-way changes and honeycombing. Consolidation and nodules are rare. On these criteria, the accuracy of UIP diagnosis on HRCT scan has a reported sensitivity of 43–78% and specificity of ≥90% for biopsy-proven UIP. When expert radiologists were confident in the diagnosis of UIP, which occurred in ~50% of cases, the sensitivity was 87%, specificity 95%, and positive predictive value 96%.

On this basis, the presence of classical HRCT features of UIP (see Table 5.25), in the right clinical context, is considered diagnostic of IPF and obviates the need for surgical biopsy in >50% of cases. When the HRCT criteria for UIP are not fulfilled, surgical lung biopsy may be required. The previous

Table 5.24 Diagnostic process in diffuse parenchymal lung diseases (DPLD)

Diagnostic process	Outcomes
STEP 1. History, examination, CXR and lung function tests may suggest possible DPLD	a. Possible idiopathic interstitial pneumonia (IIP)
	b. Probably not IIP (e.g. drug-related, occupational, CTD, ARDS)
STEP 2. Arrange High Resolution CT if possible IIP	a. Characteristic CT (and clinical) features of usual interstitial pneumonia (UIP); surgical biopsy not required
	b. Confident diagnosis of another DPLD (e.g. sarcoidosis, LCH); surgical biopsy not required
	c. Atypical CT features for UIP or suspected other DPLD or non-UIP IIP (e.g. NSIP, AIP, DIP)
STEP 3. Obtain tissue/cell samples for histological examination (e.g. TBBx, surgical biopsy, BAL) if atypical CT scan features for UIP or suspected other DPLD (e.g. CTD, sarcoidosis) or non-UIP IIP (e.g. NSIP, AIP, DIP)	a. TBBx + BAL diagnostic in sarcoidosis in 60-90%
	b. Surgical biopsy to establish diagnosis:
	→ UIP
	→ Non-UIP idiopathic interstitial pneumonia e.g. NSIP, DIP, RB-ILD, COP, LIP, AIP
	→ Not IIP (e.g. CTD, sarcoidosis)

IIP = idiopathic interstitial pneumonia; TBBx = transbronchial biopsy; AIP = acute interstitial pneumonia; BAL = bronchioalveolar lavage; COP = organizing pneumonia; CTD = connective tissue disease; DIP = desquamative interstitial pneumonia; DPLD = diffuse parenchymal lung disease; HP = hypersensitivity pneumonitis; LIP = lymphoctic interstitial pneumonia; NSIP = non-specific interstitial pneumonia; RB-ILD = respiratory bronchiolitis-associated interstitial lung disease; UIP = usual interstitial pneumonia

Data from 'American Thoracic Society/European Respiratory Society International Multidisciplinary Consensus Classification of the Idiopathic Interstitial Pneumonias', *American Journal of Respiratory Critical Care Medicine*, 165, pp. 277–304, 2002.

Table 5.25 High-resolution computed tomography criteria for UIP pattern

UIP pattern (all four features)	Possible UIP pattern (all three features)	Inconsistent with UIP (any of the following)
• Subpleural, basal predominance • Reticular abnormality • Honeycombing, with or without traction bronchiectasis • Absence of features listed as inconsistent with UIP pattern	• Subpleural, basal predominance • Reticular abnormality • Absence of features listed as inconsistent with UIP pattern	• Upper or mid-lung predominance • Peribronchovascular predominance • Extensive ground glass abnormality (i.e. >reticular abnormality) • Profuse micronodules (bilateral, predominantly upper lobes) • Discrete cysts (multiple, bilateral, away from areas of honeycombing) • Diffuse mosaic attenuation/air trapping (bilateral in ≥3 lobes) • Consolidation in bronchopulmonary segments/lobe

Reproduced from *Thorax*, Wells AU and Hirani N, 'Interstitial lung disease guideline', 63, Suppl 5, pp. v1–v58, copyright 2008, with permission from BMJ Publishing Group Ltd and the British Thoracic Society.

major and minor criteria recommended in the 2002 ATS/ERS consensus statement for the non-surgical diagnosis of IPF/UIP have been superseded in the most recent 2011 guidelines and are no longer recommended for IPF/UIP diagnosis.

Transbronchial biopsies (TBBx) provide inadequate tissue for histological assessment in most non-UIP disorders, but CT imaging may identify conditions like sarcoidosis in which TBBx can be diagnostic.

Treatment
The optimal treatment of DPLD/ILD and IIP has not been established in the absence of robust data from randomized controlled trials. Non-disease-directed management includes nutritional supplementation, supplemental oxygen therapy, pulmonary rehabilitation, antireflux agents, withdrawal of ineffective medications, smoking cessation, and timely supportive/palliative care.

Steroids and immunosupressive therapies (e.g. azathioprine, colchicine, cyclophosphamide, penicillamine, ciclosporin) are often ineffective and have significant side effects. In practice, a treatment trial may be considered when there are severe or progressive symptoms, prominent ground glass opacification on HRCT, or in patients who request treatment, even if evidence for benefit is unclear, provided side effects have been discussed.

In potentially steroid-sensitive conditions (e.g. COP), high-dose steroids (e.g. prednisolone 0.5–1 mg/kg) may be tried. In IPF/UIP, in which steroids may exert serious side effects with little benefit, initial 'triple therapy' with low-dose prednisolone, azathioprine, and acetylcysteine has the only evidence of benefit (see further text). Early referral for lung transplantation may improve outcome in suitable candidates. The reader is referred to the *Oxford Desk Reference of Respiratory Medicine* for a further discussion.

Idiopathic interstitial pneumonias
For many years, the pathogenesis of IIP was thought to be the result of unspecified lung injury, promoting interstitial inflammation and subsequently parenchymal fibrosis. Aspects of this linear 'inflammatory' model may apply to some steroid-sensitive non-UIP interstitial lung diseases (e.g. NSIP, DIP, sarcoidosis, hypersensitivity pneumonitis) but may be relevant for only a few (if any) cases of UIP. The concept that UIP represents the final common pathway for all forms of lung injury remains unproven. Recent studies suggest that irreversible lung fibrosis is more likely to be due to abnormal parenchymal wound healing, following alveolar epithelial cell damage, a process involving aberrant epithelial-mesenchymal cell transformation.

Histological typing thus forms one aspect/basis for the current classification of IIP. In the absence of contraindications, surgical biopsy should be considered in most patients with suspected IIP, with the exception of patients with clinical and HRCT features highly suggestive of UIP. Differences in natural history, radiology, histopathological pattern, and prognostic outcome between individual IIPs suggest that they are separate clinicopathologic entities. These differences are summarized in Table 5.26.

Usual interstitial pneumonia (UIP)
This is the pathological correlate of the clinical picture of idiopathic pulmonary fibrosis (IPF). Its incidence is ~5–10/10^5 population. In recent clinical series, in well-defined UIP cases, median survival times were 2–3 years, with a 5-year survival range of 30–50%. Patients are usually >50 (median 70) years old, male, with dyspnoea of >6 months, digital clubbing (~25–40%), and fine 'velcro-like' inspiratory crepitations. Smoking is associated with a worse outcome.

IPF/UIP is a fatal lung disease, but the clinical history is variable and unpredictable. The usual clinical course is one of progressive deterioration over several years, often with periods of stability but also with episodes of acute decline. A minority of patients with mild to moderate UIP may remain stable for relatively long periods, whereas others experience accelerated phases, with rapid decline and subsequent death. These accelerated phases ('acute exacerbations') characterize the course of UIP and suggest a poor prognosis. They are associated with a histological pattern of acute lung injury (i.e. diffuse alveolar damage) on a background of UIP.

Bronchoalveolar lavage (BAL) may reveal an excess of neutrophils and eosinophils. Lymphocytosis is uncommon. BAL eosinophilia of >20% should prompt consideration of an eosinophilic lung disease. The HRCT scan shows peripheral reticular opacities, with traction bronchiectasis, associated volume loss, and characteristic, mainly basal, subpleural honeycombing (see Figure 5.35). Ground glass opacification (GGO) may occur as a minor component. Histological features include prominent fibroblastic foci and a distribution of fibrosis that is spatially heterogeneous (adjacent fibrotic and normal lung) but also temporally variable (areas of fibrosis of varying ages). Micro- and macrocystic honeycombing is expected. The histology of idiopathic UIP may bear similarities to UIP occurring in CTD, hypersensitivity pneumonitis, and asbestosis.

No anti-inflammatory therapy has thus far been shown to alter the course of IPF/UIP. The 2008 BTS guidelines suggest initial treatment of IPF/UIP with 'triple therapy', including low-dose prednisolone (0.5 mg/kg/day, tapering to

Table 5.26 Summary of the clinical features, age at onset, histologic pattern, and radiographic features of idiopathic interstitial pneumonias (IIPs)

Clinical name	Age, sex	Clinical features, relation to smoking, and response to treatment	Typical CT findings	CT distribution
IPF/UIP	50–80 y M >> F	Gradual onset, acute exacerbation, worse outcome in smokers. BAL shows neutrophils (± eosinophils). Poor/no response to immunosuppressive agents. Median survival 3–5 y from diagnosis.	Inter- and intralobular reticulation, honeycombing, traction bronchiectasis	Peripheral, basal + subpleural
NSIP	30–60 y F ≥ M	Gradual onset (over 6–30 months). Two-thirds non-smokers. Prognosis better than UIP, especially the cellular form. Most improve with steroids (± other immunosuppressives).	GGO, reticular opacities	Peripheral, subpleural
COP	~55 y M = F	Acute or subacute onset, fulminant form recognized. More common in non-smokers. Most respond to steroids but may be slow (>6 months).	Patchy consolidation and/or nodules	Patchy, basal, subpleural, peribronchial
RB-ILD	30–50 y M:F 2:1	Occurs in heavy active smokers. Typically pigmented intraluminal macrophages in bronchioles. Many improve with smoking cessation, but a short course of steroids may be required.	Bronchial wall thickening, patchy GGO, loose centrilobular nodules	Upper lobe predominant or diffuse
DIP	40–70 y M >> F	More extensive disease than RB-ILD. Strong smoking history. Pigment-laden alveolar macrophages. Fibrosis in <20%. Prognosis >10 y after smoking cessation (± steroids).	Coarse GGO, reticular opacities, coexisting emphysema	Lower zone, mainly peripheral
AIP	Any age M = F	Rapidly progressive disease with widespread GGO, consolidation, and fibrosis (similar to ARDS). No effective therapy. Mortality >50% within 4–8 weeks of onset. Recurrence or progressive fibrosis may occur in survivors.	Marked GGO, exudative changes, consolidation, architectural distortion	Diffuse
LIP	Any age F > M	Idiopathic LIP is rare; secondary LIP associated with CTD, lymphoproliferative disorders and HIV. BAL lymphocytosis common. Most respond to steroids; a minority develop fibrosis.	GGO, perivascular cysts, small nodules, reticular lines	Diffuse

IPF, idiopathic pulmonary fibrosis; UIP, usual interstitial pneumonia; NSIP, non-specific interstitial pneumonia; COP, cryptogenic organizing pneumonia; RB-ILD, respiratory bronchiolitis-associated interstitial lung disease; DIP, desquamative interstitial pneumonia; AIP, acute interstitial pneumonia; LIP, lymphocytic interstitial pneumonia; GGO, ground glass opacification; BAL, bronchoalveolar lavage; CTD, connective tissue disease.

10 mg daily over 3 months), azathioprine (50 mg daily, increasing to 2 mg/kg, maximum dose 150 mg), and acetyl-cysteine (600 mg three times daily), especially in patients

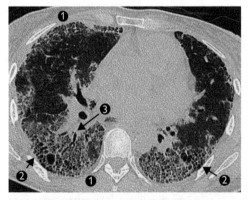

Figure 5.35 HRCT image of classical UIP, showing established subpleural fibrosis (1), honeycombing (2), and traction bronchiectasis (3).

with a potentially favourable outcome (i.e. early disease, GGO). Although usually well-tolerated, azathioprine must be monitored for hepatotoxicity, renal dysfunction, and bone marrow suppression, with regular blood tests at 2, then 6 weekly intervals.

The 2011 ATS/ERS/JRS/ALAT guidelines for diagnosis and management of IPF/UIP are less supportive of the use of 'triple therapy', as described previously, and recommend that the majority of patients should not be treated but that it may be a reasonable choice in a minority of patients with early disease and features suggestive of favourable out-come.

Initial high-dose steroid monotherapy is not recommend-ed in IPF/UIP, as neither survival nor disease course are improved and side effects are universal. When there is gen-uine doubt about the diagnosis, a steroid trial, with monitor-ing of benefit (i.e. VC, DLCO) and side effects, may be warranted. Pre-treatment tuberculin testing and osteopo-rosis prophylaxis are recommended.

The 2011 ATS/ERS/JRS/ALAT guidelines do not recom-mend the use of colchicine, ciclosporin, interferon gamma-1b (Iγ-1b), etanercept (a soluble human tumour necrosis factor receptor that binds to TNF and neutralizes its activity), bosentan (an endothelin receptor A and B antagonist), or combination corticosteroid and immunomodulator therapy (e.g. cyclophosphamide or azathioprine), as there are no convincing data to suggest benefit, and treatment toxicity is a major factor in many patients. Likewise, the 2013 NICE guidelines for the diagnosis and management of suspected IPF suggest there is no conclusive evidence to support the use of any drugs to increase the survival of people with IPF. Specifically, they do not recommend the use of azathioprine, ambrisentan, bosentan, mycophenolate mofetil, prednisolone, sildenafil, warfarin, or co-trimoxazole. Pirfenidone may be considered in some cases and patients taking acetylcysteine should be advised that the benefits are uncertain. NICE recommends that in those patients already taking prednisolone or azathioprine the potential risks and benefits of discontinuing, continuing, or altering therapy should be discussed with the patient.

Early lung transplant referral improves outcome in suitable candidates, reducing the risk of death by 75% following single lung transplantation, compared with patients on the transplant waiting list.

Non-specific interstitial pneumonia (NSIP)

This is a subgroup of IIP, with a better prognosis than UIP and is now recognized as a specific clinicopathological entity in the updated ATS/ERS guideline (2013). It comprises a heterogenous group of disorders and subsets of patients with varying clinical courses. Idiopathic NSIP is uncommon and has only recently been characterized. In the CTD setting, NSIP may precede the development of extrapulmonary manifestations by months to years. An NSIP-like radiological pattern may also be encountered following occupational exposures, drug toxicity, lung infections, immunosuppression, and hypersensitivity pneumonitis. Radiological NSIP may be predominantly 'cellular', 'fibrotic', or a combination of both. Although 'cellular' NSIP may precede fibrotic development, this is not a universally held notion. Unlike UIP, the fibrosis in NSIP is usually uniform (homogeneously distributed), rather than patchy, as in UIP. Fibroblastic foci and honeycombing are rare.

NSIP remains a problem for clinicians due to the lack of a distinctive clinical phenotype. Age of onset is earlier than in UIP at 40–50 years old, with no male predominance and no association with smoking. Onset is often insidious, with cough, dyspnoea, and inspiratory crackles, but a subacute course has been reported. BAL frequently shows lymphocytosis. HRCT imaging of fibrotic NSIP typically shows bilateral diffuse GGO, with irregular reticular opacities that might spare the immediate subpleural rim. Traction bronchiectasis indicates the presence of fibrosis (see Figure 5.36). Prognosis is better than in UIP, especially for those with a predominantly cellular pathology at presentation. Some patients experience almost complete recovery, with most stabilizing or improving with immunosuppressive therapy.

Respiratory bronchiolitis-associated interstitial lung disease (RB-ILD)

Respiratory bronchiolitis (RB) is common in heavy smokers and may be asymptomatic. RB-ILD is more diffuse and clinically significant than RB. It is denoted pathologically by the presence of intrabronchiolar pigmented macrophages. Most patients with RB-ILD are male (M:F, 2:1), between 30 and 50 years old, and active smokers (>25 pack years). Symptoms include progressive dyspnoea, cough, and occasional hypoxaemia. Heavy smokers (2–3 packs/day for >10 years) may present earlier. HRCT findings include centrilobular nodules, patchy GGO, and thickened central or peripheral bronchial walls. Its relationship with smoking means that it is often associated with emphysema. Although many patients improve with smoking cessation, steroid therapy may be required.

Desquamative interstitial pneumonia (DIP)

This is recognized as a more severe form of smoking-induced ILD than RB-ILD. A characteristic accumulation of pigment-laden macrophages diffusely filling alveolar spaces defines its pathological phenotype. DIP is almost invariably associated with smoking but may rarely occur with environmental exposures or passive smoke inhalation. It affects mainly middle-aged male smokers who insidiously develop dyspnoea and cough. Progression to respiratory failure may develop over months. Clubbing occurs in 50%, and lung physiology usually shows normal or mildly restrictive spirometry with a moderately decreased DLCO. BAL fluid analysis may show macrophages with intracellular granules of yellow or brown pigment. HRCT (see Figure 5.37) commonly shows quite coarse GGO, with a lower zone predilection and peripheral distribution. Mild, uniform reticular fibrosis may occur in many cases; progression to fibrosis occurs in a small number. True honeycombing is unusual, and coexisting emphysema may be mistaken for it. Prognosis is good after smoking cessation (± steroids), with resolution of GGO and a 70% 10-year survival rate.

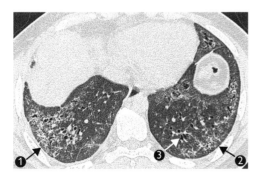

Figure 5.36 In fibrotic NSIP, HRCT findings include prominent ground glass and reticular opacities (1), areas of subpleural margin sparing (2), and traction bronchiectasis (3) signifying parenchymal fibrosis.

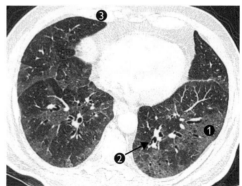

Figure 5.37 HRCT image showing areas of coarse ground glass opacification (1), thickened airways (2), and apparent background mosaicism, in a case of biopsy-proven DIP. Spared lung is also discernible (3).

Cryptogenic organizing pneumonia (COP)
Previously bronchiolitis obliterans organizing pneumonia (BOOP), this describes the histopathological pattern of organizing pneumonia within alveolar spaces, often with granulation material within adjacent bronchioles. It may be idiopathic or associated with CTD, drugs, or occur post-infection. Age at onset is 40–60 years old, and non-smokers outnumber smokers by 2:1. One typical presentation is with a short duration of cough, dyspnoea, and constitutional upset, following a suspected lower respiratory tract infection. Localized crepitations and hypoxaemia are common, but clubbing is absent. Inflammatory markers and neutrophils may be raised, and lung function tests confirm a mild to moderate restrictive pattern with reduced DLCO. HRCT shows bilateral patchy consolidation (90%), nodular opacities along the bronchovascular bundles (15–50%), and GGO (~60%), most frequently in the lower zones. Most patients recover with oral steroids, but some require prolonged therapy. An 'explosive' form of COP is recognized; at biopsy, diffuse alveolar damage (DAD) ± parenchymal fibrosis are characteristic findings.

Acute interstitial pneumonia (AIP)
This is a rapidly progressive, histologically distinct form of IIP, previously known as Hamman–Rich syndrome. The histopathological picture is that of DAD, indistinguishable from acute respiratory distress syndrome (ARDS). It affects all age groups (mean 50 years old), with no gender predominance or smoking association. Patients may recall an antecedent respiratory infection. They may have diffuse chest signs and invariably develop very high oxygen requirements. Radiological abnormalities may be dominated by extensive GGO, reticular opacities, exudative changes, and/or architectural distortion. There is no effective therapy, and mortality is very high. Recurrence or progressive fibrosis may occur in survivors.

Lymphoid interstitial pneumonia (LIP)
This is characterized by diffuse interstitial lymphocytic and plasma cell infiltration. Once considered pre-neoplastic and a precursor to pulmonary lymphoma, only a few cases undergo malignant transformation. Many cases, previously labelled as LIP, were probably non-Hodgkin's low-grade B cell (MALT) lymphomas. Idiopathic LIP is rare, and many cases have been reclassified as NSIP. LIP is often associated with an underlying autoimmune condition (e.g. rheumatoid arthritis, SLE, primary biliary cirrhosis) or HIV/AIDS which must be excluded. BAL reveals lymphocytosis without clonality. Some cases showing striking cyst formation on HRCT. The fibrogenic potential of LIP remains unknown, and, in general, most patients respond to steroid treatment.

Idiopathic Pleuroparenchymal Fibroelastosis
This is a rare condition that causes fibrosis involving the pleural and subpleural lung parenchyma, mainly in the upper lobes. It presents in adults with a median age of 57 years old,

affects both sexes equally, and a small proportion have familial ILD and non-specific auto-antibodies. Recurrent chest infections and pneumothorax are common. HRCT shows dense subpleural consolidation, traction bronchiectasis, and upper lobe volume loss. The disease is progressive in 60% and causes death in 40%.

DPLD/ILD due to specific causes
Drug-induced DPLD/ILD
Box 5.10 lists commonly implicated drugs. Four mechanisms of drug-induced injury are recognized but occur with considerable overlap:

- **Oxidant-mediated injury.** Nitrofurantoin produces DPLD by generating oxygen radicals within lung cells and overwhelming antioxidant defence mechanisms.
- **Direct cytotoxic effects** (e.g. DNA-scission) due to chemotherapeutic agents like bleomycin.
- **Phospholipid deposition** within alveolar macrophages and type II cells by amphophilic drugs (e.g. amiodarone).
- **Immune system-mediated injury** due to drug-induced systemic lupus erythematosus. Hydralazine, isoniazid, and penicillamine may induce this response.

Treatment requires drug withdrawal and occasionally systemic corticosteroids. Unfortunately, the DPLD/ILD may already be irreversible by the time of diagnosis.

Hypersensitivity pneumonitis (HP)
Also known as extrinsic allergic alveolitis, this describes a group of lung diseases caused by inhalation of mainly organic antigens but, occasionally, inorganic chemicals or drugs to which the individual has become sensitized. It is probably due to a type III or IV hypersensitivity reaction, with granuloma and antibody-antigen complex formation, respectively. It is not an atopic disease, and IgE and tissue eosinophils are not raised. Most affected individuals are non-smokers. Table 5.27 lists only a few common examples; certain forms of HP are rare in the UK (e.g. Japanese summer-type HP). About 5–10% of farmers and bird keepers may develop HP. Clinical HP syndromes are described as acute, subacute, or chronic:

Box 5.10 Drug-induced DPLD

Antibiotics (e.g. nitrofurantoin, sulfonamides)
Antiarrhythmics (e.g. amiodarone, procainamide)
Anti-inflammatories (e.g. gold salt, penicillamine)
Anticonvulsants (e.g. carbamazepine)
Antihypertensives (e.g. hydralazine)
Cytotoxics (e.g. bleomycin, mitomycin, methotrexate, busulfan)
Oxygen toxicity
Paraquat
Narcotics (inhaled or intravenous)
Thoracic irradiation

Table 5.27 Examples of hypersensitivity pneumonia

Antigen	Sources	Disease
Organisms		
Thermophilic actinomycetes	Mouldy hay, mushrooms, compost, sugarcane, contaminated water (e.g. humidifiers)	Farmer's lung, mushroom worker's lung, compost lung, bagassosis, humidifier lung
Aspergillus clavatus	Mouldy barley	Malt worker's lung
Animal protein		
Avian proteins	Bird feather bloom and droppings	Bird fancier's lung
Chemicals		
Toluene diisocyanate	Paint and resins	Isocyanate HP

- **Acute HP** presents 4–12 hours after short periods of heavy antigen exposure, with fever, myalgia, headache, cough, and dyspnoea, and has usually subsided by 48 hours. Diffuse small nodules and ground glass infiltrates are usually seen on CXR, occasionally sparing the apices and bases. HRCT shows diffuse or patchy GGO, 'loose' centrilobular nodules, and air trapping (visible as mosaic patterning on expiration).
- **Subacute and chronic HP** occur with ongoing lower-level antigen exposure. Dyspnoea, cough, weight loss, and fatigue develop insidiously, often without a history of acute symptoms. Chronic HP may cause a DPLD/ILD that must be distinguished from UIP, fibrotic NSIP, and DIP. Reticular or reticulonodular changes mainly affect the upper lobes on CXR. HRCT shows diffuse or zonal reticular opacities, mosaicism, air trapping, traction bronchiectasis with occasional cysts and/or honey-combing.

Inflammatory markers and serum precipitins to specific antigens may be detected in many cases (e.g. avian precipitins), but blood eosinophilia is not a feature of HP. Restrictive spirometry and a decreased DLCO are common. BAL typically shows lymphocytosis. Occasionally surgical biopsy may be required to establish the diagnosis, as TBBx usually provides inadequate tissue.

Avoidance of the causative antigen, when identified, is the most important aspect of treatment and can produce clinical resolution in acute and subacute HP. Face masks and air filters may help, but continued exposure risks progression to pulmonary fibrosis. Steroids hasten resolution of severe acute HP and may have a role in treating progressive disease.

Connective tissue diseases (CTD)
In this group, the highest frequency of DPLD/ILD occurs in rheumatoid arthritis (RA); however, only 5–10% may show changes on CXR. RA-associated ILD most commonly affects patients who are seropositive, male, smokers, have multisystem disease, associated vasculitis, rheumatoid nodules, and/or high ANA titres. DPLD/ILD occurs in >50% of patients with systemic sclerosis (SSc) (particularly if ANA or Scl-70 positive). Symptomatic disease (i.e. dyspnoea, cough) also occurs in 20–50% of polymyositis and dermatomyositis (PM/DM), SLE (5–10% with acute pneumonitis, 20% with abnormal HRCT), Sjögren's syndrome (15–20%, particularly the primary form), and ankylosing spondylitis (2%). In some cases, iatrogenic lung reactions may complicate the identification of CTD-ILD (e.g. due to methotrexate, gold salt, or penicillamine).

NSIP is the predominant DPLD/ILD subtype in CTD, although up to 50% of RA-ILD may have a UIP pattern. While imaging and pathological changes may not directly guide treatment choices, the finding of an organizing pneumonia (or DIP) pattern may indicate greater steroid responsiveness.

Treatment should be considered in progressive DPLD/ILD, severe physiological impairment, or a short duration of systemic disease, but side effects may be significant. Induction-maintenance therapy may vary substantially from 'rescue' treatment. With the exception of SSc, initial treatment of DPLD/ILD is with prednisolone (0.5–1 mg/kg/day, tapering to <10 mg/day) ± adjunct oral azathioprine (up to 2 mg/kg) or cyclophosphamide. SSc-associated DPLD/ILD is treated with low-dose oral prednisolone (10mg/day) and oral/IV cyclophosphamide, although azathioprine is also frequently used. In SSc, high-dose steroids may precipitate a renal crisis and should be used with extreme caution.

Table 5.28 Examples of occupational lung diseases

Dust and exposure	Disease
Coal dust during mining	Simple pneumoconiosis
	Progressive massive fibrosis
Silica during mining, stone masonry, pottery	Silicosis
Beryllium in engineering	Acute berylliosis
	Granulomatous berylliosis
Asbestos during mining, construction, and removal of insulation	Asbestosis
	Mesothelioma
	Lung cancer
Iron dust or fumes during mining or arc welding	Siderosis
Talc exposure	Talc pneumoconiosis
Tin oxide during mining	Stannosis
Aluminium	Bauxite worker's lung

Pneumoconioses (or occupational lung diseases)
These are caused by inhalation of mineral, occasionally organic, dusts (see Table 5.28). Particles <5 micron reach alveoli and terminal bronchioles where they cause inflammatory reactions. HP due to organic dusts is as discussed previously. Mineral dusts are non-fibrous (e.g. coal, silica, talc, clay), fibrous (e.g. asbestos), or metallic (e.g. iron, aluminium). Pneumoconioses are less common due to better protection (± reduced mining).

- **Coal worker's pneumoconiosis** (CWP) is either simple or complicated. In simple CWP, coal dust is engulfed by alveolar macrophages, causing inflammation, fibroblast activation, and bronchiolar dilation in the apices of upper and lower lobes. Small anthracotic macules/nodules and focal emphysema develop over time. This is a benign, asymptomatic condition. Apical nodular (1.5–10 mm) opacities are seen on CXR and HRCT, that are proportional to severity, and thus used to grade CWP.

For unclear reasons, some patients progress to complicated CWP, also known as progressive massive fibrosis (PMF), in which fibrotic nodules aggregate to form lesions 2–10 cm in diameter. Symptoms include productive cough and progressive dyspnoea (± cor pulmonale), with a normal chest examination. CXR and HRCT confirm the diagnosis if more than one opacity of >1 cm in diameter is detected. Lesions may cavitate or calcify, are usually located in lung apices, and progress, even after dust exposure ceases.

Prevention of CWP involves reducing dust exposure and regular CXR. No therapy will reverse the damage, but patients may be eligible for compensation. CWP is associated with increased rates of TB but not lung cancer. Caplan's syndrome occurs in miners with seropositive RA who develop large nodules that may cavitate but are usually asymptomatic and have no malignant potential.

- **Silicosis** is a nodular, fibrosing disease caused by inhalation of silica particles during stone mining or masonry, pottery, and brick-making. The pattern of disease depends on the level and duration of dust exposure. An acute, rapidly symptomatic form can occur during intense exposure to fine silica dust (e.g. sand-blasting), characterized pathologically by proteinaceous exudate-filled alveoli and adjacent fibrosis.

In subacute and chronic silicosis, a long time lag may occur between exposure and overt disease. An insidious dry cough and progressive dyspnoea are early symptoms. Upper and midzone nodules (3–5 mm diameter), with occasional fibrosis and 'eggshell' calcification of hilar lymph nodes, are detected on CXR and may progress, even after exposure ceases. Nodules may coalesce and calcify and progress to PMF. Patients with silicosis are prone to tuberculosis, and the risk of lung cancer is slightly increased. These patients may be eligible for compensation.

- **Beryllium**, a strong light metal, is used in fluorescent tubes, radiological equipment, and heat retardants. Berylliosis is now rare due to stringent regulation.

Acute berylliosis, a potentially fatal, but rare, alveolitis, follows high-dose inhalation of fumes containing beryllium salt. Steroids prevent progression and hasten recovery, but residual impairment may exist.

Chronic berylliosis is a hypersensitivity lung and skin disease that shares many features with sarcoidosis. The period between exposure and granuloma formation can be >10 years. Symptoms include cough, dyspnoea, fever, and dermatitis. Clubbing and crepitations occur with established lung fibrosis. CXR usually shows upper and midzonal reticulonodular changes with bihilar enlargement. On HRCT, peribronchovascular and fissural nodularity, GGO, bronchial wall thickening, and adenopathy are evident. Development of fibrosis produces traction bronchiectasis and basal honeycombing. Long-term steroids are required to retard such progressive changes.

Granulomatous DPLD/ILD

Excluding patients with radiographic stage I bihilar lympadenopathy (BHL) disease, sarcoidosis is the second most common DPLD/ILD. It has an incidence of about 3/100,000 population, assuming a mean disease duration of 2 years. Sarcoidosis and the other granulomatous ILDs are discussed in the next section.

Rare causes of DPLD/ILD

There are many other potential causes of DPLD/ILD; eosinophilic lung diseases, pulmonary vasculitis, ARDS, and infective causes are discussed elsewhere.

Langerhans cell histiocytosis (LCH)

This was previously known as pulmonary histiocytosis X or pulmonary eosinophilic granuloma. It is a rare granulomatous condition, affecting 20–40 year olds who are usually heavy smokers. It is characterized by pulmonary infiltration with histiocytes (Langerhans cells) and overlaps with other conditions with similar pathology, that affect single organs (e.g. eosinophilic granuloma of bone) or cause systemic disease (e.g. pituitary, skin, bone, cardiac and gastrointestinal tract; Hand–Schuller–Christian syndrome). It may also be associated with lymphoma. HRCT shows diffuse ill-defined nodules (± cavitation), reticulonodular opacities, and/or cystic lesions, with basal lung sparing. In some cases, smoking cessation promotes resolution. There is little evidence to support the routine use of steroids. A few patients deteriorate rapidly with respiratory failure, but, for most, median survival is 10–15 years.

Lymphangioleiomyomatosis (LAM)

This is a rare hormone-dependent disorder of smooth muscle proliferation, involving airways, lymphatic and blood vessels. Cyst formation, pneumothorax, chylothorax, and occasional pulmonary haemorrhage are features of a disease that affects women of childbearing age. HRCT shows multiple small (<1 cm) thin-walled cysts and occasional pleural effusions. Excess oestrogen states may accelerate disease progression. Treatment is largely symptomatic, and lung transplantation remains the only option to extend survival. Trials of hormone manipulation have been unsuccessful.

Amyloidosis

This arises from the extracellular deposition of insoluble low molecular weight proteins that bear a beta-pleated structure (see 'Rare pulmomary diseases'). It may be hereditary, primary due to plasma cell dyscrasias, or secondary to chronic disease. Any organ may be involved, including the lung where it may manifest as localized or diffuse reticulonodular abnormalities, often with adenopathy and pleural effusion.

Further reading

American Thoracic Society. <http://www.thoracic.org>.

American Thoracic Society and European Respiratory Society (2002). Joint statement of the American Thoracic Society (ATS) and the European Respiratory Society (ERS). International multidisciplinary consensus classification of the idiopathic interstitial pneumonias. International Consensus Statement 1999. *American Journal of Respiratory and Critical Care Medicine*, **165**, 277–304.

British Thoracic Society. <http://www.brit-thoracic.org.uk>.

Centre for Occupational and Environmental Health (COEH). Surveillance of work-related and occupational respiratory disease scheme (SWORD). <http://www.population-health.manchester.ac.uk/epidemiology/COEH/research/thor/schemes/sword/>.

Coal Health Claims. <http://webarchive.nationalarchives.gov.uk/+/http://www.dti.gov.uk/coalhealth/>.

du Bois R and King TE Jr (2007). Challenges in pulmonary fibrosis x5: the NSIP/UIP debate. *Thorax*, **62**, 1008–12.

Hirschmann JV, Pipavath SNJ, Godwin JD (2009). Hypersensitivity pneumonitis: a historical, clinical and radiologic review. *RadioGraphics*, **29**, 1921–38.

IPFnet. <http://www.ipfnet.org>.

King TE Jr (2005). Clinical advances in the diagnosis and therapy of the interstitial lung diseases. *American Journal of Respiratory and Critical Care Medicine*, **172**, 268–79.

LAM Action. <http://www.lamaction.org>.

Morgenthau AS and Padilla ML (2009). Spectrum of fibrosing diffuse parenchymal lung disease. *Mount Sinai Journal of Medicine*, **76**, 2–23.

Mueller-Mang C, Grosse C, Schmid K, Stiebellehner L, Bankier AA (2007). What every radiologist should know about the idiopathic interstitial pneumonias. *RadioGraphics*, **27**, 595–615.

National Institute for Health and Clinical Excellence (2013). Idiopathic pulmonary fibrosis: The diagnosis and management of suspected idiopathic pulmonary fibrosis. NICE clinical guideline 163. <https://www.nice.org.uk/guidance/cg163/resources/guidance-idiopathic-pulmonary-fibrosis-pdf>.

Noth I and Martinez FJ (2007). Recent advances in idiopathic pulmonary fibrosis. *Chest*, **132**, 637–50.

Raghu G, Collard HR, Egan JJ, et al. (2011). An official ATS/ERS/JRS/ALAT statement. Idiopathic pulmonary fibrosis: evidence-based guidelines for diagnosis and management. *American Journal of Respiratory and Critical Care Medicine*, **183**, 788–824.

Richeldi L, Davies HR, Ferrara G, Franco F (2003). Corticosteroids for idiopathic pulmonary fibrosis. *Cochrane Database of Systematic Reviews*, **3**, CD002880.

Travis WD, Costabel U, Hansell DM, et al. (2013). An official American Thoracic Society/European Respiratory Society Statement: Update of the International Multidisciplinary Classification of the Idiopathic Interstitial Pneumonias. *American Journal of Respiratory and Critical Care Medicine*, **188**, 733–748.

Travis WD, Hunninghake G, King TE Jr., et al. (2008). Idiopathic non-specific interstitial pneumonia. Report of an ATS project. *American Journal of Respiratory and Critical Care Medicine*, **177**, 1338–447.

Wells AU, Desai SR, Rubens MB, et al. (2003). Idiopathic pulmonary fibrosis: a composite physiologic index derived from disease extent observed by computed tomography. *American Journal of Respiratory and Critical Care Medicine*, **167**, 962–9.

Wells AU, Hirani N, on behalf of the British Thoracic Society Interstitial Lung Disease Guideline Group (2008). Interstitial lung disease guideline: BTS in collaboration with TSANZ and ITS. *Thorax*, **63** (Suppl V), v1–58.

Willis BC and Borok Z (2007). TGF-beta-induced EMT: mechanisms and implications for fibrotic lung disease. *American Journal of Physiology, Lung Cellular and Molecular Physiology*, **293**, L525–34.

Sarcoidosis

Sarcoidosis is a benign multisystem inflammatory disorder of unknown cause that can affect most organs, but most commonly the respiratory system. Spontaneous resolution occurs in >50% of cases over 1–5 years, but chronic progressive disease may occur. Sarcoidosis typically occurs in 20–40 years olds; it is unusual in children. African Americans, Scandinavians, and the Irish are most commonly affected as are those with first- or second-degree relatives with sarcoidosis. Black populations are susceptible to an aggressive systemic form of the disease. Geographically, incidence varies from $5–100/10^5$ population, and is $\sim10/10^5$ population in the UK.

Aetiology
The cause of sarcoidosis is unknown, but current evidence suggests that it occurs when a genetically susceptible individual is exposed to an antigenic trigger. Both ethnic and familial susceptibilities indicate a genetic predisposition. A link has been identified with chromosome 6, and certain alleles appear to confer susceptibility to the disease (e.g. HLA-DR11, 12, 14, 15, 17), whilst others provide protection (e.g. HLA-DR1, DR4). Potential antigenic triggers include infectious agents (e.g. mycobacteria, propionibacteria, viral), geographical (e.g. pine pollen) and occupational irritants (e.g. beryllium, talc, aluminium), or occupation-associated (e.g. firefighters). There is no firm evidence that sarcoidosis is an autoimmune disease at present.

Pathophysiology
Histologically, sarcoidosis is characterized by non-caseating, well-formed granulomata. Box 5.11 illustrates other causes of lung granulomata. Briefly, an antigenic stimulus triggers an abnormal CD4 (helper) Th-1-biased T cell response, with interferon gamma (IFN-γ) and IL-2 production. T cell activity stimulates B cells, with immunoglobulin and immune complex formation. Macrophages are activated, releasing serum angiotensin-converting enzyme, and IFN-γ enhanced granuloma formation stimulates tissue fibroblasts, which can lead to fibrosis in some cases. Sarcoid-like reactions occur with malignancy and, rarely, with antiretroviral therapy in HIV. Delayed hypersensitivity responses (e.g. to tuberculin) are depressed due to migration of T cells to involved tissue.

Clinical features
Although sarcoidosis can affect any system (e.g. eyes, skin), >90% have pulmonary involvement.

Pulmonary sarcoidosis may be asymptomatic (~30%) or cause non-productive cough, dyspnoea, and chest dis-

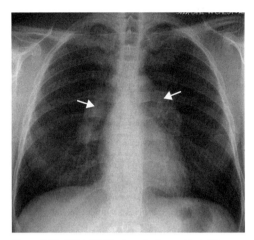

Figure 5.38 CXR of bihilar lymphadenopathy (→) in sarcoidosis.

comfort (30–50%). Constitutional symptoms, including fever, malaise, and weight loss, occur in 30% and fatigue in 70% of cases. In contrast to idiopathic pulmonary fibrosis, physical findings are unusual. Clubbing is infrequent, and crepitations occur in <20% of patients (despite extensive radiographic infiltrates).

Pulmonary sarcoidosis has two distinct clinical courses:
- **Mild, acute, non-progressive disease** (Löfgren's syndrome) which presents mainly in Caucasians with fever, erythema nodosum, arthralgia, and bihilar lymphadenopathy (BHL; see Figure 5.38). However, many cases are asymptomatic, and lymphadenopathy is detected incidentally on CXR. Other causes of BHL (see Box 5.12) should be excluded which may require a high-resolution CT scan (HRCT) and node biopsy. The course is usually benign, with symptoms and BHL resolving spontaneously in >80% of cases within 0.5–2 years. Non-steroidal anti-inflammatory drugs alleviate symptoms; steroids are rarely required. About 10% develop progressive lung disease.
- **Progressive, infiltrative lung disease** is often asymptomatic. However, it may present with dyspnoea, dry cough, chest pain and constitutional symptoms. It may also be associated with systemic disease. Pulmonary infiltrates are often present on CXR (see Figure 5.39), and, in some cases, there may be BHL. Infiltrates may resolve or progress to fibrosis and respiratory failure. Lung function tests typically reveal a restrictive defect with reduced gas transfer, but obstructive spirometry is not unusual. In the

---

Box 5.11 Causes of lung granuloma

Idiopathic: sarcoidosis
Infective: tuberculosis, leprosy, brucellosis, fungal, schistosomiasis, cat-scratch fever, syphilis, brucellosis
Malignant: lymphoma
Allergic: extrinsic allergic alveolitis
Vasculitic: Wegener's granulomatosis, giant cell arteritis, polyarteritis nodosa, Takayasu's arteritis
Gastrointestinal: Crohn's disease, primary biliary cirrhosis
Occupational: berylliosis, silicosis
Others: thyroiditis, Langerhans cell histiocytosis, hypogammaglobulinaemia, orchitis

---

Box 5.12 Causes of CXR bihilar lymphadenopathy

Sarcoidosis
Tuberculosis
Lymphoma, leukaemia
Hypogammaglobulinaemia (+ recurrent infection)
Fungal infections (e.g. histoplasmosis)
Berylliosis

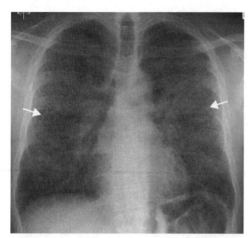

Figure 5.39 CXR of pulmonary infiltrates (→) in sarcoidosis.

Histological confirmation is important if the clinical presentation is unusual. However, detection of granulomatous disease in a single organ does not necessarily confirm the diagnosis, as granulomata occur in other diseases. It is the combination of the clinical picture and histological findings that is important. The initial evaluation of sarcoidosis is illustrated in Box 5.13 and aims to assess the extent, activity, and likely response to therapy.

Disease progression is best monitored by serial evaluation of clinical features, pulmonary function tests (spirometry ± DLCO), and CXR; as well as biochemical screening of U&E, liver function, sACE, and calcium levels. No single investigation is reliable.

Serum angiotensin-converting enzyme (sACE) is raised in 80% of patients with acute sarcoidosis but is not specific (e.g. it is often raised in tuberculosis). It is suppressed by steroids and may increase when steroids are stopped, independent of sarcoid activity. Nevertheless, it can be useful to monitor the clinical course.

High-resolution CT scan (HRCT) is superior to CXR in delineating mediastinal, parenchymal, and hilar structures but is not necessary for routine evaluation of pulmonary sarcoidosis. It is helpful in about 30% of cases when the CXR is normal, but sarcoidosis is suspected, to discriminate between active inflammation and fibrosis in stage II or III disease, and to detect specific complications (e.g. bronchiectasis, infection). Characteristic features include micronodules, nodules, and ground glass opacities in a subpleural, bronchovascular, and fissural distribution (see Figure 5.40).

USA, 87% of sarcoidosis-related deaths are due to pulmonary involvement; in Japan, cardiac complications account for 77% of deaths.

Radiographic classification

Table 5.29 shows the radiographic staging system for pulmonary sarcoidosis, introduced 40 years ago. The CXR is abnormal in >90% of patients, but ~30% are asymptomatic with incidental CXR findings. BHL (± right paratracheal lymph nodes) occurs in 50–85%, whereas unilateral hilar lymphadenopathy is rare (<10%). Pulmonary parenchymal infiltrates, usually central or in the upper lobes, with or without BHL, occur in 25–50% of cases.

Prognosis is best with stage I and poorest in stage IV radiographic classifications. Spontaneous remission is associated with a low relapse rate and occurs in 60–90% of stage I, 40–60% of stage II, and 10–20% of stage III radiographic disease. However, considerable variability occurs within different ethnic and geographical regions. Spontaneous remission usually occurs within 2–3 years, and failure to remit during this time predicts a chronic, persistent course (10–30%), with death in 2–5% of cases.

Diagnosis and monitoring

Diagnosis of sarcoidosis is established by demonstrating:
- A compatible clinical and radiological picture.
- Histological confirmation of non-caseating granulomata.
- Exclusion of other diseases with similar clinical or histological profile.

Table 5.29 Radiographic staging in sarcoidosis

Stage	Finding
0	Normal chest radiograph
I	Bilateral hilar lymphadenopathy (BHL)
II	BHL plus pulmonary infiltrates
III	Pulmonary infiltrates (without BHL)
IV	Pulmonary fibrosis (± bullae)

Reproduced from *British Medical Journal*, Scadding JG, 'Prognosis of intrathoracic sarcoidosis in England', 2, pp. 1165–1172, copyright 1961, with permission from BMJ Publishing Group Ltd.

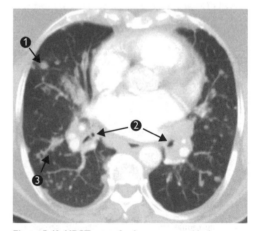

Figure 5.40 HRCT scan of pulmonary sarcoidosis showing parenchymal nodules (1→), bihilar adenopathy (2→), and peribronchovascular nodularity (3→).

Mediastinal and hilar adenopathy and irregular septal and non-septal thickening are common. Endobronchial disease occurs in >50%, with air trapping due to small airways obstruction by bronchiolar granulomata. Only in progressive fibrotic sarcoidosis is there development of traction bronchiectasis, fibrous bands, cystic/bullous changes, and hilar retraction. Positron emission tomography and gallium scans may also detect disease activity but are non-specific.

Histological confirmation is not needed in asymptomatic patients with symmetrical BHL and/or a typical acute presentation (as previously described). However, histological confirmation is strongly recommended in symptomatic patients with asymmetrical or massive BHL or large paratracheal lymph nodes, as a significant proportion (~11%) will have malignancy.

- Flexible fibreoptic bronchoscopy with transbronchial lung biopsy (TBBx) provides histological confirmation in 60–90% of cases, even in patients with stage I disease without parenchymal involvement on CXR. Bronchial mucosal biopsies detect non-caseating granulomata in 40–60%, even if the mucosa appears normal, and 90% if there is mucosal nodularity, oedema, or hypervascularity.
- A bronchoalveolar lavage (BAL) CD4:CD8 ratio of >3.5 is specific for sarcoidosis, with a sensitivity of ~60% and a specificity 95%, and provides reliable confirmation of the diagnosis. A BAL lymphocytosis >2 x 10^5 cells/mL supports the diagnosis, especially if peripheral lymphopenia is also present.
- Endobronchial ultrasound (EBUS) guided transbronchial lymph node biopsy is a reliable and less invasive technique than mediastinoscopy, parasternal mini-thoracotomy, or surgical lung biopsy which may occasionally be required to obtain biopsies from central or paratracheal lymph nodes and/or lung tissue.
- Other potentially diagnostic procedures include easily accessible skin or salivary/parotid gland biopsies. Liver biopsy is not specific. The Kveim test, an assessment of the granulomatous reaction to injection of homogenized splenic tissue from a sarcoid patient, is no longer used due to risk of transmissible disease. A positive Mantoux test makes sarcoidosis unlikely (as previously described).

Pulmonary function tests (PFT) are abnormal in 20% of cases with stage I and 40–70% of stages II–IV disease. Although CXR correlation is only moderate, PFT provide a baseline for monitoring disease progression and should be performed at presentation in every patient. The most sensitive tests are DLCO and the vital capacity. Even with a normal CXR, FVC and DLCO are reduced in 15–25% and 25–50% of patients, respectively. The typical finding is a restrictive pattern, but obstructive defects (i.e. reduced FEV$_1$/FVC) occur in ~30–50% of patients, particularly in those with parenchymal involvement.

Management

Most patients with pulmonary sarcoidosis do not require treatment. Asymptomatic BHL or pulmonary infiltration on CXR (stages II, III) is usually monitored. Indications for steroid therapy in sarcoidosis are summarized in Box 5.14. Avoid futile steroid therapy in end-stage disease (e.g. honeycomb lung), as there is little benefit and the side effects may be harmful.

Steroid therapy
Steroid dose and duration of therapy is determined by disease location (e.g. pulmonary, neurological) and therapeutic response. However, the optimal doses and duration of treatment are unknown.

> **Box 5.14** ATS/ERS criteria for steroid therapy in sarcoidosis
>
> Progressive symptomatic pulmonary disease
> Asymptomatic pulmonary disease with persistent or progressive loss of lung function
> Cardiac disease
> Neurological disease
> Eye disease not responding to topical therapy
> Symptomatic hypercalcaemia
> Other symptomatic/progressive extrapulmonary disease
>
> ATS, American Thoracic Society; ERS, European Respiratory Society.
> Data from American Thoracic Society, 'Statement on Sarcoidosis', American Journal of Respiratory and Critical Care Medicine, 160, 2, (1999), pp. 736–755, doi: 10.1164/ajrccm.160.2.ats4-99.

Initial high-dose prednisolone 0.5 mg/kg/day (20–40 mg/day) aims to control active pulmonary or systemic disease. Lower initial doses (e.g. 20 mg/daily) may control symptomatic disease (e.g. fever, arthralgia). The response is evaluated after 1–2 months. In steroid responders, the dose is reduced to 10–15 mg/daily for ~3 months, then tapered and continued at 5–7.5 mg/daily for 6–24 months before a trial of withdrawal.

Patients should be monitored for relapse during and after dosage reduction or steroid withdrawal. For example, in stage III radiographic disease, steroid therapy usually results in radiographic and histological improvement, but longitudinal studies report that more than 33% of patients relapse within 2 years of stopping treatment. Recurrent relapses occur in some patients and may require long-term low-dose therapy. Patients who do not respond to steroids within 3 months are unlikely to respond to further therapy, and other causes for failure should be sought (e.g. non-compliance, fibrotic change or steroid resistance, or wrong diagnosis). Bisphosphonates should be considered during steroid therapy to prevent osteoporosis. Prophylactic agents to prevent gastric ulceration may be required in those at risk.

Inhaled corticosteroid therapy
The concept of inhaled steroids (ICS) is attractive because of their steroid-sparing effects, and, because pulmonary pathological processes are distributed around bronchovascular bundles and bronchial infiltration, hyperresponsiveness and cough are common. Unfortunately, controlled trials of ICS for both initial and/or maintenance therapy did not show significant benefit. However, ICS may be considered for symptom control (e.g. cough) in some patients.

Immunosuppresive/immunomodulatory therapies
Immunosuppressive therapy can be used in the treatment of pulmonary sarcoidosis. It should be considered in patients with steroid-insensitive disease and significant steroid side effects, or as a steroid-sparing agent in patients requiring >15 mg prednisolone daily for disease control.

- **Methotrexate** is beneficial in 40–60% of patients with chronic pulmonary, systemic, and skin sarcoid. A dose of 10–25 mg/week has significant steroid-sparing effects after 6 months. It should be avoided in liver or renal disease. Side effects include myelosuppresion, hepatotoxicity (± hepatic fibrosis with prolonged use), interstitial pneumonitis, peripheral eosinophilia (50%), hilar lymphadenopathy (15%), low-level oncogenic potential, and pleural effusion (10%). Monitor blood tests 4–8-weekly for myelosuppression and hepatotoxicity.

- **Azathioprine** is often used in steroid-resistant stages II and III pulmonary sarcoidosis and neurosarcoid. It is usually used in combination with low-dose oral steroids (e.g. prednisolone 5–10 mg daily). The initial dose of azathioprine is 50 mg/day for 2 weeks, increasing by 25 mg/day every 2 weeks until the recommended dose of 2 mg/kg is achieved (usually 100–150 mg/day: maximum dose 200 mg/day). Response rate varies from 20 to 80%, but benefit may not occur for 3–6 months. The enzyme thiopurine methyltransferase (TPMT) metabolizes azathioprine and must be measured before treatment, as myelosuppression is greater in patients with low TPMT enzyme activity. Routine blood tests to monitor for myelosuppression are essential at 4-weekly intervals for 3 months and then every 8 weeks. Nausea, diarrhoea, fever, rash, and abnormal LFT are the other main side effects. There is associated teratogenic and low oncogenic potential.
- **Others cytotoxic agents**, including cyclophosphamide, chlorambucil, and ciclosporin, are limited by their toxicity profiles (see *Oxford Desk Reference of Respiratory Medicine*).

Immunomodulatory therapies
Immunomodulatory therapies inhibit macrophage TNF-alpha production which is implicated in granuloma formation. The antimalarial drugs chloroquine and hydroxycholoroquine are effective in hypercalcaemia, skin, or neurosarcoid and reduce disease activity in pulmonary disease. They are also steroid-sparing and can be combined with other immunosuppressant drugs in severe sarcoidosis. Hydroxychloroquine (200 mg od/bd) is preferred, as it is less oculotoxic and can be used for longer periods than chloroquine (i.e. >6 months). Other unproven immunomodulatory drugs include thalidomide, pentoxifylline, and infliximab (see *Oxford Desk Reference of Respiratory Medicine*).

Lung transplant
Lung transplant may be considered in end-stage, rapidly progressive, oxygen-dependent patients with sarcoid lung disease. Granuloma recur in transplanted lung but do not cause higher rates of graft failure.

Prognosis
Acute inflammatory manifestations, including erythema nodosum, polyarthritis, and fever, indicate a good prognosis, with spontaneous remission rates of >85%. Factors associated with a poor prognosis and a chronic relapsing course include age >40 years old at onset, hypercalcaemia, ethnic origin (e.g. black race), extrathoracic disease, splenomegaly, lupus pernio, chronic uveitis, bone, CNS and cardiac involvement. Lower family income is also associated with a worse outcome.

Prognosis can also be determined by CXR appearance and is best with stage I and poorest in stage IV disease (see Table 5.30). Spontaneous remission occurs in 60–90% of stage I, 40–60% of stage II, and 10–20% of stage III. Spontaneous remission usually occurs within 2–3 years, and failure to remit during this time predicts chronic or persistent disease. At the onset, pulmonary function tests have little prognostic value, but serial measurements of FVC and DLCO detect progressive pulmonary fibrosis which has a poor outcome.

Extrathoracic disease
Extrathoracic involvement varies, according to ethnic origin and sex. Systemic symptoms are most common with fever, weight loss, malaise, and arthralgia of the ankles, feet, elbows, and wrists.

- **Skin involvement** occurs in 25% of cases. Women are more frequently involved. Erythema nodosum (EN) describes raised, shiny, tender, indurated, and occasionally bruised plaques or nodules, usually over the shins. Sarcoid induration also occurs in tattoos and scars. Lupus pernio produces indurated skin lesions with a bluish tingle over the nose, cheeks, and ears, usually in chronic disease. Treatment of EN is initially with topical therapy. Lupus pernio requires systemic steroids. Hydroxychloroquine and methotrexate are often effective.
- **Eye involvement**, including uveitis, scleritis, conjunctivitis, glaucoma, retinal disease affects more than 25% of cases, especially women and Afro-Caribbeans. It may be asymptomatic or cause a painful red eye with photophobia and visual impairment without treatment. Lacrimal gland enlargement is associated with dry, painful red eyes. Ophthalmology assessment is essential. Systemic steroids may be required if there is no response to steroid eye drops.
- **Cardiac involvement** occurs in 5% of patients with pulmonary disease. In Japan, it accounts for >70% of deaths and <5% in the USA. Typical features include chest pain, arrhythmias, heart block, valvular dysfunction, and cardiac failure due to fibrosis. Treatment is with high-dose steroids and appropriate specific therapies (e.g. antiarrhythmics, pacemakers).
- **CNS involvement** affects 5–15% of patients. Lower motor neurone lesions of the facial and optic nerves are most common. Mononeuritis multiplex, cerebral lesions, and hypothalamic involvement with diabetes insipidus and hypersomnolence also occur. It is always treated with systemic steroids but can be resistant to therapy, requiring additional immunosuppressants.
- **Hypercalcaemia** is due to the conversion of vitamin D to 1,25-dihydroxycholecalciferol which increases intestinal calcium absorption. Hypercalcaemia may have systemic effects and is associated with renal damage and hypercalciuria. It is more common in men and Caucasians. Steroid therapy is effective, often at low dose when the hypercalcaemia is controlled.
- **Other organs** are frequently involved. Parotid and salivary gland swelling are associated with dry mouth. Liver biopsy demonstrates hepatic granulomata in 60% of cases. Splenomegaly, anaemia, and thrombocytopenia all occur. A degree of renal impairment occurs in 35% of cases. Bone cysts can develop in the terminal phalanges.

Further reading
American Thoracic Society (1999). Statement on sarcoidosis. *American Journal of Respiratory and Critical Care Medicine*, **160**, 736–55.

Baughman RP and Lower EE (1997). Alternatives to corticosteroids in the treatment of sarcoidosis. *Sarcoidosis*, **14**, 121–30.

Baughman RP, Lower EE, du Bois RM (2003). Sarcoidosis. *Lancet*, **361**, 1111–18.

British Thoracic Society Guideline Group (2008). Interstitial lung disease guideline. *Thorax*, **63** (Suppl V), v1–56.

Drent M and Costabel U, eds. (2005). *European respiratory monograph. Sarcoidosis*, volume 10. European Respiratory Society Journals Ltd, Wakefield.

Gibson GJ, Prescott RJ, Muers MF, et al. (1996). British Thoracic Society Sarcoidosis Study; effects of long term corticosteroid treatment. *Thorax*, **51**, 238–47.

Grutters JC and van den Bosch JMM (2006). Corticosteroid treatment in sarcoidosis. *European Respiratory Journal*, **28**, 627–36.

Paramothyayan NS, Lasserson TJ, Jones PW (2005). Corticosteroids for pulmonary sarcoidosis. *Cochrane Database of Systematic Reviews*, **18**, CD001114.

Sarcoid Networking Association. <http://www.sarcoidosisnetwork.org>.

Sarcoidosis Online Sites. <http://www.sarcoidosisonlinesites.com>.

Sarcoidosis Support. <http://www.sarcoidlife.org>.

Scadding J (1961). Prognosis of intrathoracic sarcoidosis in England: a review of 136 cases after five years observation. *BMJ*, **2**, 1165–72.

UK Sarcoidosis Information and Support Group. <http://www.sarcoidosissupport.ning.com>.

World Association of Sarcoidosis and Other Granulomatous Disorders. <http://www.wasog.org/>.

Pulmonary hypertension

Definitions

Pulmonary hypertension (PHT) is defined (Dana Point Consensus Conference 2009) as a mean pulmonary artery pressure (PAP) ≥25 mmHg at rest, as assessed by right heart catheterization (RHC). Normal mean PAP is 14 ± 3 mmHg, with an upper limit of normal of ~20 mmHg. The definition of PHT on exercise as a mean PAP >30 mmHg, as assessed by RHC, is not supported by published data.

In precapillary PHT, the pulmonary capillary wedge pressure (PCWP) is ≤15 mmHg, whereas, in post-capillary PHT, PCWP is ≥15 mmHg. Cardiac output is normal or reduced in both pre- and post-capillary PHT. Pulmonary vascular resistance grading is not specified as a requirement in the most recent definition but was >240 dynes/s/cm^2 (>3 mmHg/L/min (Wood units)) in previous classifications.

Pulmonary arterial hypertension (PAH) is a clinical condition characterized by the presence of precapillary PHT in the absence of other causes of precapillary PHT, including lung, thromboembolic, or other rare diseases (Table 5.30). Increased PAP may be due to increased pulmonary vascular resistance (e.g. hypoxia, pulmonary embolism), an increase in pulmonary blood flow (e.g. atrial septal defect), or a rise in pulmonary venous pressure (e.g. left heart failure).

Classification and epidemiology

The 2009 'Dana Point' classification has replaced the earlier 'Venice' (2003) and 'Evian' (1998) PHT classifications (Table 5.30). The 2003 and 2009 classifications have abandoned the term primary pulmonary hypertension, replacing it with 'pulmonary arterial hypertension' (PAH). The risk

Table 5.30. Dana Point clinical classification of PHT 2009

1. Pulmonary arterial hypertension (PAH)
  1.1. Idiopathic (IPAH)
  1.2. Heritable (HPAH); BMPR2, ALK-1, endoglin
  1.3. Drug and toxin induced
  1.4. Associated with (APAH) CTD, HIV infection, portal hypertension (cirrhosis), CHD, schistosomiasis, chronic haemolytic anaemia
  1.5. Persistent PHT in the newborn (PPHN)
2. Pulmonary veno-occlusive disease and/or pulmonary capillary haemangiomatosis
3. PHT due to left heart disease including systolic or diastolic dysfunction, or valvular disease.
4. PHT due to lung diseases (±hypoxia) including COPD, ILD, sleep-disordered breathing, alveolar hypoventilation, chronic high altitude exposure, and developmental abnormalities
5. PHT due to chronic thromboembolism
6. PHT with unclear (±multifactorial) mechanisms including haematological disorders, systemic disorders (e.g. sarcoidosis, Langerhans cell histiocytosis, lymphangiomatosis), metabolic disorders (e.g. thyroid, GSD), and other causes (e.g. tumour obstruction, dialysis) PHT, pulmonary hypertension; GSD, glycogen storage disease; COPD, chronic obstructive pulmonary disease; CTD, connective tissue disease; ILD, interstitial lung disease; CHD, congenital heart disease.

Reprinted from *Journal of the American College of Cardiology*, 54, 1, Simonneau G et al., 'Updated Clinical Classification of Pulmonary Hypertension', pp. S43–S54, Copyright 2009, with permission from Elsevier and American College of Cardiology.

Table 5.31 Risk factors and associated conditions in the development of PAH

1. Drugs and toxins
  1.1. Definite: anorexigens (e.g. fenfluramine), toxic rapeseed oil
  1.2. Very likely: amphetamines, L-tryptophan
  1.3. Possible: cocaine, chemotherapeutic agents
  1.4. Unlikely: OCP, antidepressants, cigarette smoking
2. Demographic and medical conditions
  2.1. Definite: gender (females > males)
  2.2. Possible: pregnancy, systemic hypertension
  2.3. Unlikely: obesity
3. Diseases
  3.1. Definite: HIV infection
  3.2. Likely: portal hypertension, liver disease, CTD, cardiac shunts
  3.3. Possible: thyroid disorders, haematological (e.g. splenectomy, SCD, thalassaemia, chronic myeloproliferative disorders), rare genetic/metabolic disorders (e.g. GSD, Gaucher's disease, HHT)

PAH, pulmonary arterial hypertension; OC, oral contraceptives; CTD, connective tissue disease; SCD, sickle cell disease; GSD, glycogen storage disease; HHT, hereditary haemorrhagic telangiectasia.

Reproduced from Galiè N, et al., 'Guidelines on diagnosis and treatment of pulmonary arterial hypertension: The Task Force on Diagnosis and Treatment of Pulmonary Arterial Hypertension of the European Society of Cardiology', *European Heart Journal*, 2004, 25, 24, pp. 2243–2278, by permission of Oxford University Press.

factors (e.g. anorexigenic drugs) and associated conditions in PAH are reported in Table 5.31. Functional status of PHT patients is based on the New York Health Association (NYHA)/WHO functional class (WHO-FC). In Europe and the USA, PAH prevalence is in the range of 15–30/10^6 population, with ~40% due to idiopathic PAH (IPAH) and 4% heritable PAH (HPAH). The female to male ratio is 2:1, with a mean age at diagnosis of 36 years old. Although rare, diagnosis is important, as it affects a young age group and has a poor prognosis without treatment.

Pathophysiology

Characteristic luminal occlusion due to vascular remodelling and microthrombosis in peripheral 'resistance' vessels is thought to be due to endothelial injury, impaired vasodilation, potassium channel dysfunction, and proliferative stimuli, although the exact mechanisms are unknown. Resting pulmonary hypertension suggests that >70% of the vascular bed has been lost. Mutations of the bone morphogenetic protein receptor 2 (BMPR2), a member of the transforming growth factor (TGF-beta) superfamily, are present in most HPAH. These patients should be offered genetic counselling. However, <20% of subjects with the BMPR2 mutation develop PAH, suggesting other gene mutations and environmental factors are involved. For example, mutations of ALK-1 and endoglin genes are associated with PHT in patients with hereditary haemorrhagic telangiectasia (HHT).

Clinical features

Symptoms and signs are those of PHT, with the features of associated underlying disease if present (e.g. connective tissue disease, heart disease, and hypoxic lung disease).

Symptoms of PHT are often non-specific and a feature of advanced disease. A history of slowly progressive dyspnoea and non-specific cardiac features, including chest discomfort, syncope, and tiredness, should raise clinical suspicion, particularly when overt signs of pulmonary or cardiac disease are absent and spirometry is normal. Examination may reveal cyanosis, right ventricular heave, tricuspid regurgitation, a loud pulmonary component of the second heart sound, jugular distension, and features of right heart failure. In 90% of patients with IPAH, the CXR is abnormal at the time of diagnosis. Cardiac enlargement with pulmonary artery prominence and peripheral blood vessel 'pruning' should raise the possibility of PHT.

Diagnosis

An ECG and transthoracic Doppler echocardiography (TTE) should be performed since these are abnormal in 80–90% of suspected cases of PHT. The ECG demonstrates right ventricular hypertrophy in 87% and right axis deviation in 79% of patients with IPAH. However, the ECG is a poor screening tool for PH, with low sensitivity (55%) and specificity (70%). TTE shows right heart chamber enlargement, abnormal motion of the interventricular septum, and tricuspid insufficiency.

The pulmonary artery systolic pressure (PASP) can be estimated, using Doppler techniques, and is <40 mmHg in 95% of normal subjects. It is equivalent to the right ventricular systolic pressure (RVSP) in the absence of pulmonary outflow obstruction. The RVSP is determined from the systolic regurgitant tricuspid flow velocity (v) and an estimate of the right atrial pressure (RAP), applied to the formula $RVSP = 4v^2 + RAP$, where RAP is estimated from the inferior vena cava characteristics or jugular venous distension. Tricuspid regurgitant jets can be assessed in 74% of patients with PHT. PASP estimated with TTE correlates well with measurements using right heart catheterization. In studies of healthy controls, normal RVSP is reported to be 28 ± 5 mmHg.

Investigations

Guidelines recommend a stepwise approach to diagnosis.
1. Symptoms (± signs) raise the clinical suspicion of PHT.
2. Detection or confirmation with ECG, CXR, and TTE.
3. Classification requires pulmonary function tests, arterial blood gases, ventilation/perfusion (V/Q) scan, contrast-enhanced or high-resolution spiral CT scans (HRCT), or pulmonary angiography. Consider referral to a specialist centre if investigation suggests PHT is not due to a cardiac or respiratory cause.
4. Evaluation includes blood tests, immunology, HIV test, abdominal ultrasound scan, and 6-min walking tests. Cardiopulmonary exercise testing (CPET) measures exercise tolerance and peak VO$_2$. RHC and vasoreactivity testing assess haemodynamics.

Spirometry excludes chronic lung disease as a cause, but gas transfer (TLCO) is often slightly reduced in PAH (40–80% predicted). V/Q scans detect chronic thromboembolic pulmonary hypertension (CTEPH), which causes segmental perfusion defects and distinguishes between IPAH and CTEPH, with a sensitivity of 90–100% and specificity of 94–100%. Some cases of PAH may show small peripheral non-segmental perfusion defects.

A high-resolution CT scan excludes obstructive airways and interstitial lung disease. Pulmonary venous occlusive disease is associated with diffuse central ground glass opacification. The presence of small, centrilobular, poorly circumscribed nodular opacities suggests pulmonary capillary haemangiomatosis. Contrast-enhanced CT scans may also exclude pulmonary emboli, but pulmonary angiography identifies distal obstruction better and is still required to help to identify those patients with small distal emboli and those requiring endarterectomy.

Routine blood tests should include a thrombophilia screen (e.g. antiphospholipid antibodies), autoantibodies (e.g. antinuclear antibody) to exclude connective tissue disease, and HIV serology. Abdominal ultrasound scan excludes liver cirrhosis and portal hypertension as a potential cause. The 6-min walk (6MW) is a simple and inexpensive test to evaluate disease severity and response to treatment. It is predictive of survival in IPAH and inversely correlated with functional status. A 10% fall in saturation during 6MW is associated with a 2.9 increase in mortality over 26 months.

RHC is required to confirm the diagnosis of PAH and to test the vasoreactivity of the pulmonary circulation. It is best performed at a specialist centre. Early referral is recommended to avoid the need for repeat testing in late referrals. RHC is recommended in symptomatic patients (NYHA classes 2, 3, 4, see section on 'Heart Failure' Chapter 4) detected by Doppler TTE. It has prognostic significance with raised right atrial pressure (RAP) and PAP and reduced cardiac output and central venous saturation, identifying IPAH patients with the worst prognosis. PCWP distinguishes between arterial and venous hypertension in left heart disease.

Acute vasodilator testing with short-acting pulmonary vasodilators like intravenous adenosine and prostacyclin or inhaled nitric oxide identifies patients who may benefit from long-term calcium channel blocker (CCB) therapy. A positive response, with a reduction in PAP of >10 mmHg to a mean of <40 mmHg, is detected in about 15% of IPAH patients. Long-term CCB can only safely be used in positive responders to vasodilator testing and is beneficial in about 50% of these responders in the long term.

Treatment

Only patients in group 1 of the Dana Point classification (i.e. IPAH, HPAH, and APAH) should receive specific treatment for PHT. However, where an underlying cause for PHT is established, this must be treated. Figure 5.41 summarizes the treatment of PAH (group 1). The last two decades have witnessed major advances in PAH treatment, with at least four licensed medical therapies targeting specific pathogenic pathways. Several new treatments and combination therapies are currently being assessed. Patients with PAH and CTEPH and those where the diagnosis is unclear or PHT is unusually severe (PASP >60 mmHg) should be managed in specialist centres.

Supportive management

- **Treat the cause** (e.g. COPD, sarcoidosis), and ensure appropriate immunizations and exercise.
- **Pregnancy** is associated with a high maternal mortality (>30%), and counselling with clear contraceptive advice is essential. Early termination of pregnancy should be offered.
- **Supplemental oxygen** is used to maintain SaO2 >90%, as hypoxia is a pulmonary vasoconstrictor.
- **Anticoagulation** with warfarin (INR 1.5–2.5) is recommended in IPAH and CTEPH. Prevention of microscopic thrombosis has been demonstrated to improve survival in IPAH, FPAH, and PAH due to anorexigens. In PAH due

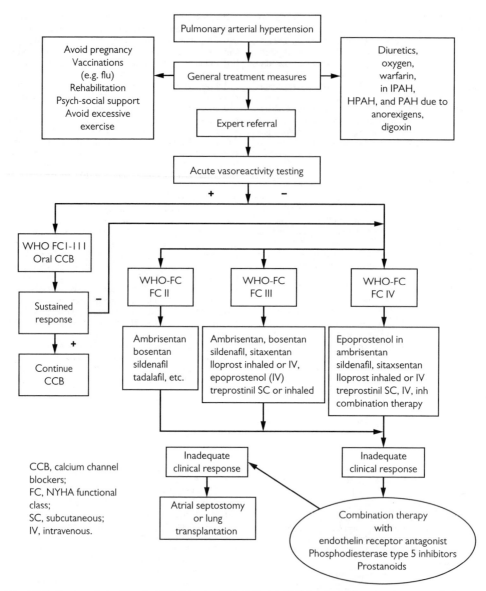

Figure 5.41 Treatment algorithm for PAH. Reproduced from Galiè et al., 'Guidelines for the diagnosis and treatment of pulmonary hypertension: The Task Force for the Diagnosis and Treatment of Pulmonary Hypertension of the European Society of Cardiology (ESC) and the European Respiratory Society (ERS), endorsed by the International Society of Heart and Lung Transplantation (ISHLT)', *European Heart Journal*, 2009, 30, 20, pp. 2493–2537, by permission of European Society of Cardiology and Oxford University Press.

to other aetiologies (e.g. scleroderma), anticoagulation is controversial. However, during therapy with intravenous epoprostenol, anticoagulation is recommended to reduce the risk associated with catheter-induced thrombosis.

- **Diuretics** may be required in right ventricular failure (RVF) but risks systemic hypotension due to hypovolaemia, renal insufficiency, and electrolyte abnormalities.
- **Digoxin** is occasionally used in refractory RVF and for rate control of the atrial dysrhythmias that occasionally

complicate severe PAH with RVF. Atrial arrhythmias are often fatal in PAH.

Pharmacological management

- **Calcium channel blockers (CCB).** Of the 10% of IPAH patients who respond to acute vasodilators (e.g. adenosine), only about 50% have sustained vasodilation, with improved long-term survival using high-dose CCB. Nifedipine 120–240 mg/day is used in patients with relative bradycardia, and diltiazem 240–720 mg/day in patients with relative tachycardia. Treatment is started at low dose, with careful monitoring for systemic hypotension and peripheral oedema. CCB therapy in those patients without an acute vasodilator response (and untested patients) is potentially dangerous and is not recommended. CCB should never be used in a patient who has not been vasoreactivity-tested or in those with a negative study because of the potentially severe side effects (e.g. hypotension and RHF).

- **Phosphodiesterase-5 inhibitors.** Sildenafil (20–80 mg tds) is an orally active, potent inhibitor of cGMP-phosphodiesterase type 5 which increases cGMP, augmenting relaxation and reducing proliferation in lung vascular smooth muscle. In large randomized controlled trials, it improved exercise capacity, functional class, and haemodynamics in PAH patients (WHO-FC II and III). Tadalafil is a once-daily alternative.
- **Endothelin receptor antagonists.** Endothelin-1 (ET-1), a potent vasoconstrictor and smooth muscle mitogen, is increased in PAH and correlates with severity. Bosentan, a dual ETA and ETB receptor antagonist, improves exercise tolerance, symptoms, haemodynamics, and functional class. It is licensed for WHO-FC II and III PAH. Start therapy with 62.5 mg twice daily for 4 weeks, increasing to 125 mg twice daily thereafter. Monitor liver function tests due to the risk of hepatic toxicity. Bosentan also causes anaemia, oedema, testicular atrophy, male infertility, and teratogenicity. Two selective ETA receptor antagonists, sitaxsentan (100 mg daily) and ambrisentan (5–10 mg daily) have also been demonstrated to be effective in WHO-FC II and III patients with IPAH and APAH.
- **Prostanoids.** Prostacyclin is a metabolite of arachidonic acid produced in vascular endothelium. It is a potent pulmonary (and systemic) vasodilator, has antiplatelet effects, and is relatively deficient in PAH.
  - **Epoprostenol** by continuous intravenous infusions improves exercise capacity, haemodynamics, and survival, compared to conventional therapy (e.g. anticoagulants, diuretics), in both IPAH and the scleroderma spectrum of diseases. Benefit is maintained for many years. Therapeutic difficulties are due to the short half-life, the need for continuous central venous infusion (e.g. infection, thrombosis), and rebound hypertension during therapeutic interruptions. Side effects include headache, nausea, jaw pain, diarrhoea, rash, musculoskeletal pain, and hypotension. It is licensed for WHO-FC III–IV PAH but is reserved for disease refractory to oral therapies.
  - **Treprostinil** has a longer half-life (3 h), and subcutaneous infusion is associated with modest improvements in 6MW and haemodynamic parameters when compared to placebo. It is licensed for subcutaneous and intravenous use in WHO-FC II–IV PAH.
  - **Iloprost** has a half-life of 20 minutes, and inhalation 6–9 times daily improves 6MW, haemodynamics, and functional class. Cough, flushing, and headache are the principal side effects. It is licensed for NYHA class III PAH and may be a useful adjunct to oral therapy.
- **Combination therapy** has become the standard of care in many centres and may be associated with improved

outcomes, although long-term safety and efficacy have not been adequately established.

Interventional/surgical therapies

Atrial septostomy creates a right-to-left shunt and decompresses the failing right heart. It is a palliative procedure or bridge to lung transplantation. Patient selection, timing, and septostomy size are vital. Lung transplantation is reserved for failed medical therapy. One-year survival is ~65–75%.

Prognosis

In IPAH, the mean survival without treatment is 2 years. Survival with therapy is variable and depends on PAP, haemodynamic variable, response to vasodilators, and NYHA stage, with a mean of 3–4 years. These patients are at risk of progressive RHF and sudden death. In COPD, PHT is also associated with a much worse prognosis; 5-year survival in those with a PAP >45 mmHg is <10%, compared with >90% for those with a PAP <25 mmHg.

Further reading

Galiè N, Corris PA, Frost A, et al. (2013). Updated Treatment Algorithm of Pulmonary Arterial Hypertension. *Journal of the American College of Cardiology*, **62**, 25–S.

Galiè N, Hoeper MM, Humbert M, et al. (2009). ESC/ERS guidelines for the diagnosis and treatment of pulmonary hypertension. *European Respiratory Journal*, **34**, 1219–63.

Galiè N, Hoeper MM, Humbert M, et al. (2009). Guidelines for the diagnosis and treatment of pulmonary hypertension: The Task Force for the Diagnosis and Treatment of Pulmonary Hypertension of the European Society of Cardiology (ESC) and the European Respiratory Society (ERS), endorsed by the International Society of Heart and Lung Transplantation (ISHLT). *European Heart Journal*, **30**, 2493–2537.

Galiè N, Seeger W, Naeije, et al. (2004). Comparative analysis of clinical trials and evidence-based treatment algorithm in pulmonary arterial hypertension. *Journal of the American College of Cardiology*, **43**, 81S–8S.

Galiè N, Torbicki A, Barst R, et al. (2004). Guidelines on the diagnosis and treatment of pulmonary arterial hypertension. *European Heart Journal*, **25**, 2243–78.

National Pulmonary Hypertension Centres of the UK and Ireland (2008). Consensus statement on the management of pulmonary hypertension in clinical practice in the UK and Ireland. *Thorax*, **63** (Suppl II), ii1–ii41; *Heart*, **94** (Suppl 1), i1–41.

National Pulmonary Hypertension Service. <http://www.imperial.nhs.uk/services/cardiology/pulmonaryhypertension/index.htm>. Tel: 020 3313 2330.

Pulmonary Hypertension Association UK. <http://www.phassociation.uk.com/>.

Rubin LJ (2006). Pulmonary arterial hypertension. *Proceedings of the American Thoracic Society*, **3**, 111–15.

Simonneau G, Robbins I, Beghetti M, et al. (2009). Updated clinical classification of pulmonary hypertension. *Journal of the American College of Cardiology*, **54**, 43S–54S.

Scottish Pulmonary Vascular Unit. <http://www.spvu.co.uk>. Tel: 0141 211 6327.

Taichman DB, Ornelas J, Chung L, et al. (2014). Pharmacologic Therapy for Pulmonary Arterial Hypertension in Adults: Chest Guideline and Expert Panel Report. *Chest*, **146**, 449–475.

(There are nine designated pulmonary hypertension centres in the UK and Ireland—Clydebank, Newcastle-upon-Tyne, Sheffield, Cambridge, London (Hammersmith, Royal Brompton, Royal Free, and Great Ormond Street Hospitals), and Dublin.)

Acute respiratory distress syndrome

Pathophysiology
Acute respiratory distress syndrome (ARDS) is best described as 'leaky lung syndrome' or 'low pressure, non-cardiogenic pulmonary oedema'. It is an acute inflammatory lung injury, often in previously healthy lungs, mediated by a uniform pulmonary pathological process in response to a variety of direct (i.e. inhaled) or indirect (i.e. blood-borne) insults (see Table 5.32).

The pathophysiological response occurs in two stages:
- **An initial acute inflammatory phase** (days 3–10) in which cytokine-activated neutrophils and monocytes adhere to the alveolar epithelium and capillary endothelium and release pro-inflammatory mediators. These damage the integrity of the alveolar capillary membrane, increase permeability, and cause alveolar oedema. A reduction in surfactant causes alveolar collapse, hyaline membrane formation, and reduced lung compliance. Subsequent severe V/Q mismatch and shunting cause progressive hypoxaemia, respiratory failure, and pulmonary hypertension. Hyperventilation of remaining functional alveoli is usually sufficient to prevent significant hypercapnia.
- **A later healing, fibroproliferative phase** (>10 days) is initially associated with resolution of pulmonary infiltrates, increased type 2 pneumocytes (i.e. surfactant production), myofibroblasts, and early collagen formation. Ongoing pulmonary fibrosis distorts lung architecture, reduces compliance (stiff lungs), and is associated with pulmonary hypertension.

Definition and diagnosis
The recent internationally agreed criteria for the diagnosis of ARDS (Berlin Definition 2012) include:
- **Acute onset** within 1 week of the causative insult.
- **Bilateral diffuse opacities on CXR** (see Figure 5.42).
- **Non-cardiac origin for pulmonary oedema** (nor fluid overload).

Oxygenation (degree of hypoxaemia) defines the severity of the ARDS; mild ARDS equates to a PaO_2/FiO_2 (P/F) of 200–300 mmHg; moderate 100–200 mmHg; severe <100 mmHg (all with PEEP/CPAP ≤5cm H_2O). P/F is calculated as follows; if PaO_2 is 80 mmHg on 80% inspired oxygen; $PaO_2/FiO_2 = 80/0.8 = 100$ mmHg.

Mild ARDS equates to the previous definition of acute lung injury.

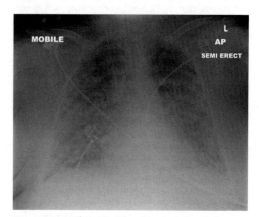

Figure 5.42 ARDS with diffuse alveolar infiltration, following gastric acid aspiration post-operatively.

Epidemiology and prognosis
The incidence of moderate and severe ARDS is ~2–8 cases/10^5/year, but its precursor mild ARDS is more common and often unrecognized. Improvements in survival over the last 20 years are due to better supportive care, rather than modification of the inflammatory process. Mortality is ~27% in mild, ~32% in moderate, and ~45% in severe ARDS. It is worse with pulmonary causes (trauma <35%, sepsis ~50%, aspiration pneumonia ~80% mortality) and increases with age (>60 years) and sepsis.

Early deaths are usually due to the precipitating condition and later deaths to multiorgan failure (MOF) and complications, with <20% dying from hypoxaemia alone. Residual lung damage, including restrictive defects and reduced gas transfer occurs in 50% of survivors but is often mild, reflecting the lungs' regenerative capacity.

Clinical features
ARDS usually presents 1–2 days after the onset of the precipitating cause (e.g. pancreatitis, trauma). Typical features include increasing dyspnoea, dry cough, tachypnoea, cyanosis, increased work of breathing due to reduced compliance, confusion, and rapidly progressive hypoxaemia. Rapidly increasing concentrations of supplemental oxygen are required. Chest examination reveals coarse crepitations on auscultation, and the CXR shows diffuse alveolar infiltration (see Figure 5.42).

Early CT scans often demonstrate dependent consolidation and later scans pneumothoraces, pneumatoceles, and fibrosis (see Figure 5.43). These features are not diagnostic and must be differentiated from heart failure, diffuse alveolar haemorrhage, vasculitis, infection, and infiltrative disorders like lymphangitis carcinomatosis.

During the healing, fibroproliferative phase pneumothoraces are common. Secondary nosocomial infections affect 50% of cases and require constant surveillance (e.g. bronchoalveolar lavage).

Other complications include venous thromboembolism, gastrointestinal haemorrhage, and myopathy associated with steroids, paralysing agents, and poor glycaemic control.

Table 5.32 Common causes of ARDS

Direct pulmonary	Indirect pulmonary injury
Infective (e.g. pneumonia, TB)	Sepsis
Pulmonary trauma	Non-thoracic trauma
Near drowning	Haemorrhage/large transfusions
Toxic gas inhalation	
• Smoke	Post-arrest
• NO_2, NH_3, Cl_2	Burns
• Phosgene	Bowel infarction, pancreatitis
Oxygen toxicity (FiO_2 0.8)	Drugs (e.g. salicylates)
Inhalation of gastric contents	Uraemia, eclampsia, toxins
	Anaphylaxis

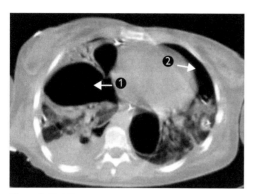

Figure 5.43 CT scan showing pneumatoceles (→) and a pneumothorax (→) due to barotrauma in ARDS.

Management

Initially, the precipitating cause must be identified and treated. In mild ARDS, supportive therapy with supplemental oxygen, diuretics to minimize alveolar oedema, and physiotherapy aimed at optimizing gas exchange and V/Q matching will maintain gas exchange whilst awaiting recovery.

In some cases, non-invasive, mask-delivered respiratory support with continuous positive airways pressure (CPAP) to correct hypoxaemia or bilevel positive airways pressure (BIPAP), which also aids ventilation by reducing work of breathing, may avoid the need for mechanical ventilation (MV).

In severe ARDS, intubation and mechanical ventilation are usually indicated. High peak inspiratory pressures (PIP) are required to achieve normal tidal volumes (Tv) due to reduced lung compliance. These high pressures cause alveolar damage termed 'barotrauma' (e.g. pneumothorax). The reduced compliance of diseased or consolidated alveoli also results in the available Tv causing overdistension and damage to otherwise healthy alveoli, an effect termed 'volutrauma'.

- **Mechanical ventilation** aims to limit pressure-induced lung damage and volutrauma, prevent oxygen toxicity (i.e. FiO_2 <80%), optimize alveolar recruitment and oxygenation, and avoid circulatory compromise due to high intrathoracic pressures. A 'protective' lung ventilation strategy of low Tv (6 mL/kg) and low PIP (<30 cmH_2O) prevent lung damage, whilst high positive end expiratory pressures (PEEP; >10 cmH_2O) and long inspiratory to expiratory (I:E) times (i.e. 2:1 instead of the normal 1:2) recruit collapsed alveoli. No ventilatory mode is proven to be superior, although pressure-controlled modes which tend to improve alveolar recruitment are generally favoured. The resulting CO_2 retention, termed 'permissive hypercapnia', resulting from this low Tv strategy, is usually tolerated with adequate sedation.
- **Conservative fluid management** reduces alveolar oedema caused by increased alveolar permeability. The aim is to maintain organ perfusion whilst reducing the pulmonary capillary hydrostatic pressure which generates alveolar oedema, often by using inotropes or vasoactive drugs, rather than with excessive fluid administration. In the acute phase, diuretics reduce pulmonary oedema and may improve oxygenation.

- **General measures** include good nursing care, physiotherapy, nutrition, sedation, and infection control. Bronchoscopy improves ventilation and V/Q matching by removing sputum plugs and secretions. Minimize metabolic demand and associated oxygen consumption (VO_2) by preventing fever (VO_2 increases by >10% for every degree rise above 37°C) and shivering (can double or triple VO_2) and controlling agitation with sedatives.
- **Pharmacotherapy.** No drug therapy, including steroids, anti-inflammatory agents, or surfactant, has been consistently effective in clinical ARDS trials. The role of corticosteroids in late-stage ARDS remains controversial and generally cautious. One consensus group has supported a 'weak' recommendation for use of low-to-moderate doses in ARDS of <14 days duration. If corticosteroids are used, strict infection surveillance, avoidance of neuromuscular blockers, and gradual weaning are recommended.
- **Future developments** include inhaled nitric oxide to increase perfusion of ventilated alveoli by vasodilating surrounding vessels, improving V/Q matching, and reducing overall shunt fraction. Unfortunately, the initial PaO_2 improvement is not sustained, and there is no survival benefit. As consolidation is usually dependent and blood flow is greatest in the dependent areas, prone positioning aims to improve V/Q match by turning the patient so that non-consolidated ventilated lung is dependent. Although oxygenation is improved, there is no survival benefit. Extracorporeal membrane oxygenation (ECMO), techniques to oxygenate blood or remove CO_2 are effective in children and increasing recent evidence suggests significant benefit in adults.

Further reading

American Thoracic Society (1999). International consensus conference in Intensive Care Medicine: ventilator-associated lung injury in ARDS. *American Journal of Respiratory and Critical Care Medicine*, **160**, 2118–24.

ARDS Definition Task Force, Ranieri VM, Rubenfeld GD, Thompson BT, *et al.* (2012). Acute respiratory distress syndrome: the Berlin Definition. *Journal of the American Medical Association*, **307**, 2526–33.

ARDS Support Center. <http://www.ards.org>.

Artigas A, Bernard GR, Carlet J, *et al.* (1998). The American-European consensus conference on ARDS Part 2: Ventilatory, pharmacologic, supportive therapy, study design strategies and issues related to recovery and remodelling. *American Journal of Respiratory and Critical Care Medicine*, **157**, 1332–47.

Calfee CS and Matthay MA (2007). Nonventilatory treatments for acute lung injury and ARDS. *Chest*, **131**, 913–20.

Girard TD and Bernard GR (2007). Mechanical ventilation in ARDS: a state-of-the-art review. *Chest*, **131**, 921–9.

Hong Kong Society of Critical Care Medicine. Murray score calculator. <http://www.hksccm.org/index.php?option=com_content&view=article&id=1596:2010-mar-20-murray-score-calculator&catid=197&Itemid=87&lang=en>.

No authors listed (1998). Round table conference. Acute lung injury. *American Journal of Respiratory and Critical Care Medicine*, **158**, 675–9.

Sessler CN, Gay PC (2010). Are corticosteroids useful in late-stage acute respiratory distress syndrome? *Respiratory Care*, **55**, 43–55.

Ware LB and Matthay MA (2000). The acute respiratory distress syndrome. *New England Journal of Medicine*, **342**, 1334–49.

Wheeler AP and Bernard GR (2007). Acute lung injury and the acute respiratory distress syndrome. A clinical review. *Lancet*, **369**, 1553–64.

Bronchiectasis and cystic fibrosis

Bronchiectasis

A disease characterized by irreversible, abnormal dilation of one or more bronchi, often with chronic airways obstruction and inflammation and chronic sputum production. Secretion retention and secondary infection with bacteria that tend to reduce sputum clearance like *Pseudomonas aeruginosa* results in a cycle of inflammation, progressive damage, and bronchial dilation. Prevalence is about 1/1,000 but is falling due to vaccinations and better treatment of childhood chest infections (e.g. whooping cough, tuberculosis (TB)).

Aetiology

Aetiology is related to distribution:

- **Localized disease** follows severe chest infection and occurs distal to obstruction (e.g. foreign body) or extrabronchial compression (e.g. hilar TB nodes in Brock's syndrome).
- **Generalized disease** has many causes but is usually due to cystic fibrosis (CF), immune deficiency, or infection:
  - **Genetic** (e.g. cystic fibrosis, pulmonary sequestration).
  - **Post-infective** (e.g. TB, atypical mycobacteria (ATM), whooping cough, measles, pneumonia, allergic bronchopulmonary aspergillosis (ABPA)).
  - **Mucociliary clearance defects** (e.g. primary ciliary dyskinesia, Kartagener's syndrome (a gene mutation causing ciliary dyskinesia with associated sinusitis, situs inversus, and male infertility), Young's syndrome (due to viscid mucus with sinusitis and obstructive azoospermia)).
  - **Immune deficiency**, both primary (e.g. IgA or IgM hypogammaglobulinaemia) and secondary (e.g. HIV, CLL).
  - **Toxic insults** (e.g. aspiration, inhaled gases).
  - **Associated with systemic disease** (e.g. rheumatoid arthritis (RA), SLE, Sjögren's syndrome, traction in interstitial lung disease, ulcerative colitis, Crohn's disease) and rare causes (e.g. Marfan's syndrome, alpha-1-antitrypsin deficiency, yellow nail syndrome).

Clinical features

Some patients are asymptomatic, but classical symptoms include chronic cough productive of large volumes of mucopurulent, often foul-smelling, sputum, breathlessness, lethargy, minor haemoptysis (~50%), and infective pleurisy. Signs include anaemia, cyanosis, finger clubbing, coarse crepitations, and airways obstruction with wheeze. Features of systemic disease (e.g. RA, ABPA) or those associated with the underlying condition (e.g. sinusitis, situs inversus) may be present. Frequent complications include respiratory failure (RF), pneumonia, major haemoptysis, pleural effusions, cerebral abscesses, and amyloidosis.

Investigation

CXR usually shows ring (cystic) shadows, with thickened (tramline) bronchial walls, but is normal in ~10%. High-resolution CT scans confirm the diagnosis and assess the extent of the disease. The cause should be determined, and tests should include serum immunoglobulins, CF sweat tests, *Aspergillus* precipitins, IgE, and bronchoscopy to exclude a proximal obstruction. Spirometry detects airways obstruction and reversibility. Assess the time for nasal saccharin to reach the taste buds or perform electron microscopy to detect ciliary dyskinesia. Sputum culture detects bacterial

pathogens, including *Haemophilus* spp. and *Pseudomonas* spp., and excludes atypical organisms (e.g. *Aspergillus*, ATM).

Management

This includes:

- **General therapy**, including annual influenza vaccination, oxygen therapy in RF, and twice-daily postural drainage or supervised physiotherapy during exacerbations. Treat reversible airways obstruction with beta-2-agonists and anticholinergic bronchodilators and inhaled steroids. Mucolytic acetylcysteine and regular nebulized 0.9% normal or 7% hypertonic saline, may aid expectoration (although potential bronchoconstricton associated with hypertonic saline may require pre-treatment bronchodilator therapy).
- **Specific therapy**, includes high-dose antibiotic therapy, prescribed according to bacterial sensitivities in infective exacerbations. *Pseudomonas* infections may require two antibiotics for prolonged periods (>14 days). Frequent exacerbations may necessitate continuous, rotating prophylactic antibiotic therapy (e.g. azithromycin 250mg three times weekly, which may also have anti-inflammatory, as well as antimicrobial, effects). Immunoglobulin replacement in hypogammaglobulinaemia reduces infections. Surgery may be indicated for local disease or severe haemoptysis.

Cystic fibrosis

The commonest autosomal recessive genetic disorder in Caucasians, with a carrier frequency of ~1 in 25 and an incidence of 1 in 2,500 live births. It is caused by mutation of the CF transmembrane conductance regulator (CFTR) gene on chromosome 7 (>800 identified), a cellular chloride (Cl^-) channel that controls movement of salt and water across membranes. The associated changes in surface airways fluid predispose the lung to recurrent infection and bronchiectasis. The $\Delta F508$ mutation causes 70% of European CF and is associated with severe disease and pancreatic insufficiency.

Clinical features

CF may present with failure to thrive, meconium ileus, or rectal prolapse in neonates. Lungs are normal at birth, but recurrent childhood chest infections cause early upper lobe bronchiectasis, progressive airway obstruction, pneumothorax (10%), hyperinflation, and dyspnoea. Viscid intestinal secretions cause pancreatic insufficiency with malabsorption (>85%), diabetes mellitus (DM; ~30% by late teens) and steatorrhoea, distal intestinal obstruction, gallstones, and cirrhosis. Additional features include male infertility (95%), sinusitis, nasal polyps, immune complex-mediated arthropathy, osteoporosis, and vasculitis. Clinical signs include cyanosis, clubbing, and bilateral lung crepitations.

Diagnosis

This is based on compatible clinical findings with biochemical and genetic confirmation. Although most CF is diagnosed in childhood, acute physicians must be alert to the possibility, as even relatively mild bronchiectasis presenting in middle age can be due to CF and has important management implications. Consider the possibility in upper lobe disease or with malnutrition, DM, or *H. influenzae* or Pseudomonas infection. Routine diagnostic sweat chloride test reveals a sodium (Na^+) and Cl^- >60 mmol/L ($Cl^- > Na^+$), but some CF mutations have normal sweat Cl^- levels. Genetic screening for common mutations identifies 90% of cases.

Management

Early diagnosis, improved nutrition, effective treatment of respiratory infections, and early referral to, and management by, specialist multidisciplinary teams have improved median survival to >30 years. Lung disease is managed as for bronchiectasis (see 'Bronchiectasis'). Monitor bacteriology; resistant organisms may need prolonged therapy with >2 high-dose antibiotics. Prophylactic and nebulized (tobramycin) antibiotics are often given. Recombinant DNase is a useful mucolytic in 30–50% of cases. Pancreatic enzyme replacement, fat-soluble vitamin supplements, and screening for DM, osteoporosis, and cirrhosis are required. Treat arthritis, sinusitis, and vasculitis, and provide genetic and fertility counselling. Transplantation should be considered in end-stage disease. Although currently ineffective, it is hoped gene therapy may be useful in the future.

Further reading

Colombo C, Littlewood J (2011). The implementation of standards of care in Europe: State of the art. *Journal of Cystic Fibrosis*, **10**, S7–S15.

Cystic Fibrosis Foundation (USA). <http://www.cff.org/>.

Cystic Fibrosis Trust. <https://www.cysticfibrosis.org.uk/>.

Mogayzel PJ, Naureckas ET, Robinson KA, *et al.* (2013). Cystic Fibrosis Pulmonary Guidelines Chronic Medications for Maintenance of Lung Health. *American Journal of Respiratory and Critical Care Medicine*, **187**, 680–89.

Pasteur MC, Bilton D, Hill AT (2010). British Thoracic Society guideline for non-CF bronchiectasis. *Thorax*, **65**, i1–58.

Smyth AR, Bell SC, Bojcin S, *et al.* (2014). European Cystic Fibrosis Society Standards of Care: Best Practice guidelines. *Journal of Cystic Fibrosis*, **13**, S23–42.

Team Cystic Fibrosis. <http://www.teamcysticfibrosis.co.uk/>.

Bronchiolitis

Bronchioles are small airways (<2 mm diameter) with no cartilage in their walls. Bronchiolitis describes non-specific epithelial inflammation in bronchioles and may occur alone or in combination with more diffuse lung disease (e.g. cryptogenic organizing pneumonia (COP), respiratory bronchiolitis interstitial lung disease, Langerhans cell histiocytosis). There are two main pathological patterns of bronchiolitis.

1. **Proliferative bronchiolitis** (cryptogenic organizing pneumonia), the more common of the two, is a non-specific response to bronchiolar injury which results in organizing intraluminal exudates and proliferation of fibrotic buds (Masson bodies) in the bronchioles and alveoli, with associated alveolar wall inflammation and foamy macrophages in alveolar spaces. The pathology is similar to COP. Causes are shown in Table 5.33. Complete or partial resolution may occur, and it often responds to steroids.

2. **Constrictive bronchiolitis** is rare. It causes patchy circumferential bronchial narrowing due to cellular wall infiltration and smooth muscle hyperplasia, with potential occlusion, peribronchiolar inflammation, distortion, and scarring. The causes are shown in Table 5.34. It is a progressive condition that is unresponsive to steroids and eventually results in respiratory failure and death.

Clinical features

Bronchiolitis presents with a gradual onset of cough and breathlessness over weeks or months. It is most common after viral chest infections, especially respiratory syncitial virus (RSV) in children, in association with connective tissue and interstitial lung diseases, and following lung or bone marrow transplants. There may be a history of drug exposure or dust inhalation.

Diagnosis

- Pulmonary function tests (PFT) often show an obstructive picture with no bronchodilator reversibility.
- Chest radiography may be normal. Diffuse migratory infiltrates occur in proliferative bronchiolitis and hyperinflation in constrictive bronchiolitis.
- High-resolution CT (HRCT) scans performed prone (to minimize gravity-dependent effects) and in full expiration shows air trapping with a mosaic pattern and areas of atelectasis. The inflamed, dilated walls of bronchioles may cause a 'tree in bud' appearance.
- Open lung biopsy histologically confirms bronchiolitis, but transbronchial biopsies are usually inadequate.

Table 5.33 Causes of proliferative bronchiolitis (± organizing pneumonia)

Common causes
COP, acute organizing infection (e.g. mycoplasma, PCP, influenza, cytomegalovirus), connective tissue diseases (e.g. rheumatoid arthritis, dermatomyositis), chronic pulmonary eosinophilia, hypersensitivity pneumonitis, post-transplant (e.g. lung, bone marrow)

Rare causes
Drug-induced (e.g. busulfan), vasculitis (e.g. Wegener's), ARDS, ulcerative colitis, radiation pneumonitis

Table 5.34 Causes of constrictive bronchiolitis

Common causes
Infection (e.g. adenovirus, influenza, respiratory syncytial virus), connective tissue disease (e.g. rheumatoid arthritis), drug-induced (e.g. penicillamine), post-transplant chronic rejection (i.e bronchiolitis obliterans syndrome)

Rare causes
Dust inhalation (e.g. talc, iron, asbestos, silica, coal, sulphur dioxide, chlorine, ammonia), Japanese panbronchiolitis, ulcerative colitis, hypersensitivity reactions, idiopathic (which occurs mainly in females >40 years old)

Management

The underlying condition must be treated. In proliferative bronchiolitis, the associated cryptogenic organizing pneumonia is reduced by high-dose steroids which may also be useful in the early and late stages of inhalational injury. Steroids are less effective in constrictive bronchiolitis but are often the mainstay of therapy. Long-term, low-dose macrolide antibiotics like erythromycin (200–400 mg daily) may improve symptoms and PFT and reduce mortality in those with diffuse panbronchiolitis or cryptogenic bronchiolitis. Early experience with TNF-alpha inhibitors (e.g. infliximab) as a second-line therapy for bronchiolitis following bone marrow transplantation has reported some success but like other immunomodulatory therapies (e.g. rituximab) requires further assessment.

Specific conditions

Bronchiolitis obliterans syndrome (BOS)
This is a fibroplastic process affecting small airways and is a manifestation of chronic rejection syndrome, following lung, heart, and bone marrow transplants. Although uncommon in the first 6 months, it affects two-thirds of transplant patients by 5 years. It presents with insidious cough and breathlessness and is manifest as expiratory air trapping and peripheral bronchiectasis on HRCT scan and a sustained fall in FEV_1 to <80% of the best post-transplant value. CXR is unhelpful. Bronchial infection with *P. aeruginosa* is common. Treatment with increased immunosuppression slows progression. Mortality is 40% within 2 years of diagnosis. For unknown reasons, patients taking statins post-transplant are less affected.

Acute (post-infectious) bronchiolitis obliterans
This usually occurs in infants and follows infection with adenovirus or RSV, but also influenza, and mycoplasma. It presents with tachypnoea, wheeze, and breathlessness. Treatment is supportive with oxygen, bronchodilators, and steroid therapy. Outcomes in children tend to be better than in adults.

Diffuse panbronchiolitis (Japanese panbronchiolitis)
This is common in Japan and rare outside south-east Asia. Fifty-year-old men are most commonly affected, and there is a familial predisposition associated with HLA Bw54 in Japan. It is thought to be post-infective, but no specific organism has been found. It tends to occur in non-smokers, and there may be a preceding history of chronic sinusitis.

Patients have a productive cough, with purulent sputum production, wheeze, and exertional dyspnoea. Examination reveals weight loss and respiratory failure, with crepitations and wheeze on auscultation. Sputum cultures are often positive (e.g. *H. influenzae*, *S. pneumoniae*), and infection should be treated. PFT usually detect an obstructive or mixed pattern, with little reversibility and reduced gas transfer (DLCO). CXR and HRCT scans show ill-defined nodules, bronchiectasis, and air trapping. Open lung biopsy is diagnostic, with bronchiolar histology showing transmural infiltrates of lymphocytes, plasma cells, foamy macrophages, and organizing intraluminal exudates/plugs.

The relatively recent (~1985) introduction of longterm treatment with low-dose erythromycin (200–600 mg/day) or other macrolides (e.g. clarithromycin, roxithromycin) and better symptomatic and infection control has substantially improved survival in diffuse panbronchiolitis (10-year survival rate ~90%, previously ~33%). The value of macrolide therapy appears to be due to its anti-inflammatory, rather than antibacterial, effects. In comparison, corticosteroid and immunosuppressant (e.g. azathioprine) therapy are of limited value. Without treatment, there is a 50% 5-year mortality.

Further reading
Barker AF, Bergeron A, Rom WN, Hertz MI (2014). Obliterative Bronchiolitis. *New England Journal of Medicine*, **370**, 1820–1828

Meyer KC, Raghu G, Verleden GM, *et al.* (2014). An international ISHLT/ATS/ERS clinical practice guideline: diagnosis and management of bronchiolitis obliterans syndrome. *European Respiratory Journal*, **44**, 1479–1503.

Ryu JH, Myers JL, Swensen SJ (2003). Bronchiolar disorders. *American Journal of Respiratory and Critical Care Medicine*, **168**, 1277–92.

Eosinophilic lung disease

Pulmonary eosinophilia describes a group of diseases characterized by lung infiltration with eosinophils, with or without blood eosinophilia, and associated with diffuse CXR shadowing. Eosinophils are phagocytes that circulate in the blood for ~8–12 h after release from the bone marrow, with tightly regulated counts <0.4 x 10^9/L (1–4% of white cells), before accumulating in the gastrointestinal tract. In allergic diseases, parasitic infections, and cancer, blood eosinophils can migrate to other tissues if attracted by mast cell activation or other chemoattractants. In these areas persistently high eosinophil levels cause damage due to their proinflammatory effects. Eosinophil counts >0.4 x 10^9/L are seen in asthma and pulmonary eosinophilia, but levels >1 x 10^9/L suggest the possibility of hypereosinophilia or Churg–Strauss syndromes. Clinical features of individual diseases are summarized in the following sections.

Specific eosinophilic lung diseases (i.e. cause known)

Asthma and allergic bronchopulmonary aspergillosis (ABPA)
In these patients, type 1 and 2 hypersensitivity to *Aspergillus fumigatus* causes fever and worsening asthma, with blood eosinophilia, raised IgE levels, increased serum *Aspergillus precipitins*, a positive *Aspergillus* skin prick test, and fleeting CXR shadows (see 'Asthma' section in this chapter). Treatment with steroid therapy and antifungal agents (e.g. itraconazole) may be required.

Drug-induced pulmonary eosinophilia
This is due to an allergic reaction in the wall of pulmonary vessels that develops within hours or days of starting a new drug. It resolves on stopping the drug and recurs on re-exposure. The severity of the associated illness varies from mild to severe, with fever, cough, breathlessness, and hypoxia. Skin reactions may occasionally occur. Despite tissue eosinophilia, blood eosinophilia does not always occur. Treatment with steroid therapy is occasionally required. There are many potentially causative drugs (e.g. penicillins, tetracyclines, aspirin, diclofenac, phenytoin).

Simple pulmonary eosinophilia (Loeffler's syndrome)
This is due to parasitic infection with *Ascaris lumbricoides* (or *Strongyloides*) and occurs worldwide (see Chapter 6). Parasitic eggs found in soil are ingested, and, ~10–14 days later, larvae migrate via the lymph and blood to the liver and then lung. In the lung, they cause an allergic reaction which may be asymptomatic or cause a low-grade fever, cough, wheeze, dyspnoea, and constitutional symptoms, including anorexia, malaise, sweats, and transient bilateral perihilar shadows, which last about 2 weeks. Low-level blood and sputum eosinophilia occur. The larvae subsequently pass along the bronchial tree, are swallowed, develop into roundworms in the gastrointestinal tract and are detected in the stool 8–12 weeks later. The roundworms are treated with mebendazole for 3 days or levamisole as a single dose. Steroids are required for severe respiratory symptoms.

Tropical pulmonary eosinophilia
This is due to hypersensitivity to the migrating larvae of the filarial worms *Wuchereria bancrofti* (or *Brugia malayi*) found in India, South East Asia, and the south Pacific (see Chapter 6). Symptoms, which include cough, wheeze, dyspnoea, chest pain and associated fever, malaise, and weight loss, may last for many months, with remissions and relapses. Blood and sputum eosinophil counts and IgE are raised.

Filarial complement tests are positive. CXR shows bilateral mottling of the middle and lower zones. Histology confirms eosinophilic bronchopneumonia. Treatment with diethylcarbamazine rapidly relieves symptoms.

Idiopathic eosinophilic lung disease (cause unknown)

Acute eosinophilic pneumonia
This is an acute febrile illness lasting <5 days that occurs at any age without an obvious cause (e.g. ABPA, parasites, drugs). Presentation is with fever, cough, breathlessness, myalgia, and interstitial or alveolar CXR infiltrates (see Figures 5.44 and 5.45). It may cause hypoxic respiratory failure, requiring ventilatory support. Bronchoalveolar lavage (BAL) reveals a high eosinophil count (>25%), but there is no blood eosinophilia. Rapid improvement follows high-

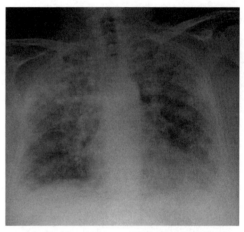

Figure 5.44 Alveolar infiltrates on the chest radiograph of a patient with acute eosinophilic pneumonia, presenting with fever, cough, breathlessness, and respiratory failure, before steroid therapy.

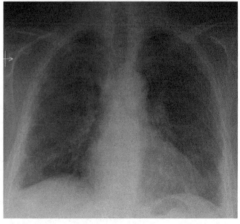

Figure 5.45 Chest radiograph showing rapid resolution of the alveolar infiltrates due to acute eosinophilic pneumonia seen in Figure 5.44 with steroid therapy.

dose steroids (prednisolone 40 mg daily) which are given until the respiratory failure resolves and then tapered over the next 2–4 weeks. Relapse does not occur.

Chronic eosinophilic pneumonia

This has an insidious onset over weeks to months, with cough, dyspnoea, recent-onset asthma, occasional haemoptysis, and constitutional features of high fever, night sweats, raised ESR, and weight loss. It must be differentiated from tuberculosis. It is more common in middle-aged women. CXR shows characteristic dense peripheral opacities. The BAL eosinophil count is high, but blood counts may be normal. Response to high-dose steroid therapy is rapid, with resolution of CXR opacities in 3–14 days. Low-dose steroids are continued for 6 months, but relapse is common, requiring further steroid therapy.

Hypereosinophilic syndrome

This is a rare disease of unknown cause that is most common in men aged 30–40 years old. It is often associated with systemic symptoms and involves other organs. Presentation is with fever, night sweats, weight loss, cough, and pruritus for weeks to months. Blood eosinophilia is marked ($>1.5 \times 10^9$/L, 70% WCC), and IgE levels are raised. Histology confirms eosinophilic tissue infiltration. CXR shows interstitial infiltrates ($\pm$ pleural effusions). Systemic involvement may be cardiovascular (e.g. myocarditis, restrictive cardiomyopathy, mural thrombus), dermatalogical (e.g. urticaria, angioedema), neurological (e.g. encephalopathy, peripheral neuropathy), or gastrointestinal (e.g. hepatosplenomegaly, nausea, alcohol intolerance). Eosinophilic infiltration can involve the joints, kidneys, and muscles. About half of cases improve with high-dose steroids (prednisolone 30–60 mg daily), but additional therapy with immunosuppressants (e.g. azathioprine, cyclophosphamide) may be required. Treatment should be gradually tapered, according to eosinophil and organ response, but many require long-term treatment.

Vasculitic eosinophilic lung diseases

Churg–Strauss syndrome

This is a small or medium-sized vessel vasculitis (see 'Vasculitis' section later in this chapter) associated with late-onset, severe asthma, blood eosinophilia, and CXR infiltrates. Antineutrophil cytoplasmic antibody (ANCA) is positive in 60–70% of cases. Treatment is with high-dose steroid and immunosuppressants.

Others

For example, polyarteritis nodosa, Hodgkin's lymphoma.

Further reading

Allen JD and Davis WB (1994). Eosinophilic lung disease. *American Journal of Respiratory and Critical Care Medicine*, **150**, 1423–38.

Burden of Obstructive Lung Disease Initiative. <http://www.boldstudy.org/>.

Kauffman HF, Tomee JFC, van der Werf TS, *et al.* (1995). Review of fungus-induced asthmatic reactions. *American Journal of Respiratory and Critical Care Medicine*, **151**, 2109–16.

Klion AD, Bochner BS, Gleich GJ, *et al.* (2006). Approaches to the treatment of hypereosinophilic syndromes: a workshop summary report. *Journal of Allergy and Clinical Immunology*, **117**, 1292–302.

Orphanet. <http://www.orpha.net>.

Philit P and Cordier J-F (2006). Idiopathic acute eosinophilic pneumonia. *Orphanet Journal of Rare Diseases*, 1, 11. <http://www.ojrd.com/content/1/1/11>.

Rare Disease. <http://raredisease.org>.

Airways obstruction, aspiration syndromes, and near-drowning

Acute upper airways obstruction

Partially masticated food is the most commonly aspirated solid particulate matter (the 'café coronary' syndrome), but coins, teeth, or confectionery may also be inhaled. Upper airways may also be blocked by vomit, sputum plugs, blood clots, laryngospasm, or airway stenosis. Inflammatory oedema due to inhaled toxic gases, burns, trauma, anaphylaxis, or laryngeal angio-oedema also occludes airways. Occasionally, childhood infections, including epiglottitis or diphtheria, can cause acute laryngeal obstruction. Pharyngeal occlusion by the tongue should be excluded and is usually due to loss of pharyngeal muscle tone caused by drugs, alcohol, unconsciousness, or neurological events.

Upper airways obstruction is either:

• **Complete** with inability to speak, distress, rapid-onset cyanosis, marked respiratory effort, paradoxical abdominal and chest wall movement (classically described as see-saw breathing), and use of accessory muscles of respiration. If not rapidly corrected, it causes coma, collapse, cardiovascular instability, and finally cardiac arrest. Look for chest wall and abdominal movement, and listen and feel for airflow at the nose and mouth.

• **Partial upper airways obstruction** causes noisy breathing, with stridor, snoring, wheeze, and cough.

Management

If there is a witnessed episode of choking, consider a sharp blow to the back of the chest to dislodge the obstructing particle. If this fails, attempt the Heimlich manoeuvre by standing behind the patient, with arms around the costal margin and the hands clenched below the xiphoid process. Pull the hands backwards sharply, compressing the upper abdomen. The increase in thoracic pressure may dislodge the obstructing particle, which is exhaled by the patient.

If these manoeuvres fail and the patient loses consciousness, call for help and then:

• **Inspect the oral cavity** for obstructions, and remove with a finger sweep. Suction out secretions. Leave well-fitting dentures in place.

• **Open the airway** with backwards head tilt, chin lift, and jaw thrust (see Chapters 1 and 18). In trauma, use jaw thrust only to avoid further potential injury to the cervical spine.

• **Insert an oropharyngeal (or nasopharyngeal) airway** if the patient is breathing. Maintain oxygenation with supplemental oxygen (10–15 L/min) therapy. If there is no spontaneous respiratory effort, attempt mask ventilation with a self-inflating bag. If this fails, consider a laryngeal mask or endotracheal intubation (ETI).

• **Emergency cricothyroidectomy** is attempted if the patient is not breathing and cannot be ventilated. It will only be successful if the obstruction is at the level of the larynx. A large-bore needle or sharp knife is inserted through the cricothyroid membrane, which is palpable just below the thyroid cartilage. If using a knife, insert the blade horizontally through the cricothyroid membrane and then turn it gently to the vertical position which will create an opening and allows insertion of a tube (largest available, e.g. biro casing) to aid ventilation. Feed oxygen down the needle or tube, if available.

• **Urgent bronchoscopy or thoracic surgery** is performed to remove the obstruction. A history of recurrent pneumonia with radiological changes following an episode of aspiration suggests the need for exploration to recover an obstructing foreign body (e.g. peanut).

• **Heliox**, a mixture of helium and oxygen, is a temporary measure to improve ventilation past an airways obstruction, as helium has a lower density than nitrogen.

• **Nebulized epinephrine/adrenaline** temporarily reduces airways obstruction due to laryngeal or airways oedema whilst awaiting the effects of definitive treatment.

Laryngospasm

Irritation of the upper airways by blood, pharyngeal secretions, toxic inhaled gases, burns, aspirated food or vomit, and extubation can cause laryngeal spasm, oedema, stridor, and respiratory distress. Immediate intubation is required, if severe. In less critical situations, intubation may be avoided by using nebulized adrenaline (2–3 mL 1:1,000 adrenaline), salbutamol, and intravenous hydrocortisone (100–200 mg initial dose) to reduce laryngeal oedema and airways spasm. Heliox may be considered as a temporary measure.

Anaphylaxis and angioedema

Sensitized humans may develop life-threatening anaphylactic reactions within minutes of exposure to a specific antigen. It usually presents with respiratory distress and cardiovascular collapse. Laryngeal oedema and bronchial obstruction cause hoarseness, stridor, chest tightness, and wheeze. Cutaneous manifestations include pruritus, urticaria, and angioedema. The urticarial eruptions are intensely pruritic and may coalesce to form giant hives. They seldom persist for >48 hours. Angioedema is a deeper cutaneous oedematous process that can cause severe airways obstruction in the larynx, epiglottis, or upper trachea. Rhinitis, abdominal pain, vomiting, diarrhoea, and preceding apprehension may also occur. Typical precipitating allergens include foods (e.g. peanuts, fish), bee stings, drugs (e.g. anaesthetic agents), latex, pollen, contrast media, and enzymes. Anaphylaxis is an IgE-mediated type I hypersensitivity reaction in which histamine release causes the clinical syndrome. Histamine and levels of IgE are raised. Urticaria and angioedema may be associated with a variety of autoimmune or vasculitic diseases. Rarely, it is a hereditary condition due to an autosomal dominant deficiency of C1 inhibitor, and it may also be acquired in certain lymphoproliferative disorders.

Management

Initially, call for help, as this is a potentially life-threatening emergency. Remove potential allergens; start supplemental oxygen therapy, and ensure a patent airway. Immediately treat cardiorespiratory emergencies with intravenous epinephrine/adrenaline (0.5–1 mg), hydrocortisone (200 mg), and chlorphenamine (10 mg). Start fluid resuscitation in hypotensive shock, and treat bronchospasm with nebulized salbutamol (± intravenous aminophylline). Consider early ETI in cases with severe upper airways obstruction. Nebulized epinephrine/adrenaline reduces laryngeal oedema and may avoid the need for ETI in less critical cases. If intubation is not possible due to laryngeal obstruction (e.g. oedema), an emergency cricothyroidotomy must be performed. Before discharge, provide an auto-injector (e.g. intramuscular self-administered adrenaline); give advice about future episodes, and provide a medic alert bracelet. Consider referral to an allergy clinic, especially if the allergen is unknown. Allergen desensitization may be beneficial when allergen exposure cannot be avoided (e.g. pollen).

Trauma, toxic inhalational injury, and burns

Trauma, hot inspired gases in burns victims, inhaled toxins (e.g. sulphur dioxide), and aspirated chemicals (e.g. bleach, hydrocarbons) can cause injury, oedema, and obstruction to upper airways. These are discussed in Chapter 18 and may all require ETI or tracheostomy.

Upper respiratory tract infections (URTI)

Acute upper respiratory tract infections include sinusitis, pharyngitis, tonsillitis, and epiglottitis.

- **Acute bacterial sinusitis** complicates 0.5% of viral URTI. *S. pneumoniae* and *H. influenzae* are the commonest organisms, although mixed anaerobic infection occurs in 10%. *Pseudomonas* may occur in cystic fibrosis. It presents with fever, headache, and sinus pain (worse leaning forward). Post-nasal drip can cause cough. Sinusitis lasting for >3 months is defined as chronic. In these cases anaerobic, and fungal infections are more common, particularly in atopic, diabetic, and immunocompromised patients. Sinus radiographs may reveal fluid levels and thickened mucosa, but CT scans are more sensitive. Treatment with analgesics, topical decongestants (e.g. nasal steroid sprays), and antibiotics are usually effective. Surgery to correct anatomical abnormalities may be warranted for recurrent infections.
- **Acute epiglottitis** is potentially life-threatening. It is usually due to infection with *H. influenzae*, streptococci, or staphylococci. It is commoner in children. Sore throat, dysphagia, stridor, airways obstruction, and CXR infiltrates (due to high negative intrathoracic pressures) are characteristic. Initially, treat with a third-generation cephalosporin to cover beta-lactam producing *H. influenzae*. ETI or tracheostomy may be required for airways obstruction.
- **Acute pharyngitis and tonsillitis** (see Chapter 6) are due to viral (e.g. adenovirus) URTI in >80% of cases, although secondary bacterial infections (e.g. *H. influenzae*, *S. pneumoniae*, group B streptococci) are common. Most cases present with sore throat that is often self-limiting, fever, malaise, headache, and lymphadenopathy. Treatment is largely supportive, but anti-streptococcal antibiotics (e.g. penicillin; macrolides in penicillin allergy) may be appropriate in severe infections.
  - Infectious mononucleosis (glandular fever), due to Epstein–Barr virus infection, is associated with pharyngitis. Diagnosis is confirmed by Paul Bunnell testing and detection of atypical mononuclear cells in blood samples. Amoxicillin can cause a rash in these cases.
  - Herpes simplex and Coxsackie A virus infections cause ulcerating vesicles on the tonsils and pharynx.
  - Cytomegalovirus (CMV) and infectious mononucleosis pharyngitis are associated with splenomegaly and lymphadenopathy.

  Rare, but severe, causes of pharyngitis include:
- **Corynebacterium diphtheriae** in unvaccinated patients. A pharyngeal membrane forms and obstructs the upper airways. It is associated with marked cervical, 'bull neck' lymphadenopathy, low-grade fever, tachycardia, and systemic symptoms. Treat urgently with diphtheria antitoxin.
- **Lemierre's syndrome** (necrobacilliosis), due to the anaerobe *Fusobacterium necrophorum*, causes severe pharyngitis, jugular vein suppurative thrombophlebitis (± thrombosis), and lung (± systemic) abscesses.

- **Vincent's angina** is caused by Gram-negative *Borrelia vincentia* and other anaerobic organisms in those with poor mouth hygiene. Treat with penicillin.
- **Group A Streptococcus** may cause severe systemic upset and dysphagia due to pharyngeal oedema.

  The main complication of pharyngitis is peritonsillar ('quinsy'), retropharyngeal, or cervical abscess formation, requiring antibiotics and occasional surgical drainage.
- **Laryngitis** causes hoarse voice and aphonia and is due to *M. catarrhalis* infection in 50% of cases. It may be due to laryngeal or lung cancer (recurrent laryngeal nerve paralysis), inhaled steroid, acid reflux, and other rare infections (e.g. fungal, CMV).
- **Tracheobronchitis** usually follows viral URTI and has increased winter prevalence. Secondary bacterial infection with *S. pneumoniae* or *H. influenzae* is common. Symptoms include fever, cough, blood-streaked sputum and retrosternal chest pain with tracheitis. Treatment is usually symptomatic, with antibiotics if secondary infection is suspected.

Fluid aspiration syndromes

A high index of suspicion is required to detect pulmonary aspiration, as it is not often witnessed. The volume and type of fluid aspirated determines the clinical scenario. For example, ARDS follows aspiration of large volumes of gastric fluid, whereas repeated microaspiration of nasopharyngeal secretions causes pneumonia. High-risk groups include perioperative, ICU, and emergency room patients and those with reduced consciousness (e.g. overdose, epilepsy) or laryngeal incompetence (e.g. bulbar syndromes, Guillain–Barré). Other risk factors include nasogastric feeding, gastrointestinal haemorrhage, supine posture, gastric lavage, tracheo-oesophageal fistulae (e.g. trauma, malignancy), and leakage past the endotracheal tube cuff during mechanical ventilation. During non-invasive ventilation, tight-fitting face masks impede airway clearance and swallowed gas may promote vomiting, both of which increase the risk of aspiration.

Aspiration of gastric contents

Aspiration of gastric contents (pH <2.5) causes tachypnoea, wheeze, cyanosis, hypotension, and hypoxaemia. The right lower lobe is most commonly affected (~60%), as the right main bronchus is the most direct path for aspirated material. Associated ARDS has a high mortality (>80%) and as treatment is relatively ineffective, prevention is essential. Tracheal suctioning or bronchoscopy remove excess fluid and debris but do not prevent acid-induced lung injury. Respiratory support includes high-dose oxygen, bronchodilator, and antibiotic therapy. Continuous positive airways pressure mask ventilation may improve oxygenation. Early steroid therapy is ineffective.

Recurrent microaspiration

Recurrent microaspiration (e.g. following bulbar palsy or during mechanical ventilation) causes nosocomial (hospital acquired) pneumonia. Onset is slower and symptoms more subtle, but morbidity and mortality may be significant. Microaspiration is confirmed by observing dye introduced into the mouth or food in tracheobronchial secretions or by detecting glucose in these secretions with glucose oxidase reagent strips. Strategies to reduce microaspiration include semi-recumbent nursing (30% head up) and thickened feed. Early enteral feeding and sucralfate prevent gastric microbial overgrowth due to stress ulcer prophylaxis.

Near-drowning and water aspiration

Near-drowning and water aspiration are a common cause of accidental death and are often associated with alcohol consumption. Although more frequent in areas near natural water sources, deaths may occur in small volumes of water (e.g. a shallow bath) in any home. Primary medical events (e.g. myocardial infarction), whilst swimming, often precipitate near-drowning. The amount and type of water aspirated determines the severity of the pulmonary damage, although 10% of patients do not aspirate due to laryngospasm and breath-holding.

- **Freshwater aspiration** impairs lung surfactant, causing atelectasis, shunt, and hypoxaemia. Initial hypervolaemia follows rapid absorption of the aspirated water into the pulmonary circulation. Plasma hypotonicity occurs if sufficient water is absorbed, causing intravascular haemolysis, hyperkalaemia, and renal impairment due to free haemoglobin. Hypovolaemia rapidly follows due to pulmonary oedema.

- **Hypertonic seawater aspiration** pulls plasma water into alveoli, causing shunt and hypovolaemia.

Respiratory features, including tachypnoea, wheeze, cyanosis, and pulmonary oedema, depend on the amount of water aspirated, the level of contamination, and the risk of infection. Intrapulmonary shunt can increase to 25–75% (PaO_2 <8 kPa) within 3 minutes of aspiration of 2.5 mL/kg of water, and 85% of survivors aspirate <22 mL/kg. Pulmonary oedema can be delayed for over 12 hours, and asymptomatic cases should be admitted for observation. Mortality is similar in freshwater and seawater drowning.

Cold (<10°C) water immersion causes uncontrollable hyperventilation and reduces breath-hold time to <10 seconds, increasing aspiration risk in turbulent water or when escaping from a submerged vehicle. Body temperatures <28°C impair neuromuscular performance, making swimming difficult, and reduce cardiac conduction, increasing the risk of arrhythmia, particularly during rough handling. Profound hypothermia (<30°C) slows cerebral metabolism and may reduce neurological damage during prolonged (<30 min) asphyxia, particularly in children.

The primary aims during the initial treatment of near-drowning are to reverse hypoxaemia, restore cardiovascular stability, prevent further heat loss, correct acidosis and electrolyte imbalance, and prevent hypoxaemic brain injury. At the scene, the patient must be retrieved from the water and cardiopulmonary resuscitation (CPR) initiated. Abdominal thrust (Heimlich) manoeuvres do not aid drainage of lung fluid and may precipitate arrhythmias, which are difficult to reverse in the hypothermic patient, or may cause vomiting (± aspiration) due to the gastric dilation associated with near-drowning. Gravitational drainage is equally effective.

Hypothermia is associated with resistant arrhythmias, and, if initial defibrillation is unsuccessful, it should be discontinued until the core body temperature is >29°C. Rewarm patients before terminating CPR because recovery after prolonged cold submersion is reported. Stable patients are rewarmed at 1°C/h, using warmed inspired gas, intravenous fluids, and blankets. Rapid rewarming, with peritoneal dialysis, bladder irrigation, gastric or pleural lavage, is considered if core temperature is <28°C because of the risk of ventricular arrhythmias. Extracorporeal rewarming with haemofiltration or cardiopulmonary bypass rapidly restores normothermia (~10°C/h) and removes fluid in pulmonary oedema.

Fluid resuscitation is essential, and electrolyte imbalance, although infrequent, must be corrected. Oxygen therapy is given until hypoxaemia resolves. The chest radiograph is normal in 20% of cases at hospital admission, although most show infiltrates or pulmonary oedema. In seawater aspiration, non-invasive mask ventilation with CPAP usually corrects hypoxaemia, whereas mechanical ventilation is often required following freshwater aspiration due to the associated alterations in pulmonary surfactant. Antibiotics are withheld, unless there is evidence of infection or the aspirated water was contaminated.

The degree of hypoxic brain injury often determines outcome. Survival is not improved by intracranial pressure monitoring, steroid therapy, deliberate hypothermia, or barbiturate-induced coma. Prolonged submersion, delayed resuscitation, severe acidosis (pH <7.1), fixed and dilated pupils, and a low Glasgow coma score (<5) are usually associated with increased mortality and brain injury, although none of these predictors are infallible.

Hydrocarbon aspiration

Hydrocarbon aspiration (e.g. petrol, furniture polish) accounts for ~15% of accidental childhood poisoning. Pulmonary toxicity follows inhalation during ingestion or subsequent vomiting. The odour of hydrocarbon is readily detected, and an oropharyngeal burning sensation is reported. Central nervous system irritability with lethargy, dizziness, twitching, and, less commonly, convulsions may occur. Progressive respiratory failure with pulmonary oedema and hypoxaemia develops over 24 hours. Small aspirations usually recover over 2–5 days. Gastric lavage is not recommended, as pulmonary aspiration, rather than gastrointestinal absorption, is the life-threatening event.

Blood aspiration

Blood aspiration occurs during haematemesis, intrapulmonary haemorrhage, and upper airways surgery. It mimics the acute phase of gastric acid inhalation, but these symptoms usually settle rapidly, with few long-term sequelae. Laryngeal blood may precipitate severe laryngospasm, a serious complication during and after upper airways surgery.

Tracheo-oesophageal fistula (TOF)

TOF due to tumour, trauma, or mediastinal sepsis may cause recurrent occult aspiration. Diagnosis is difficult and requires bronchoscopy, oesophagoscopy, gastrograffin imaging, and CT scan. Management is determined by the underlying cause.

Further reading

Best Health. Lungs and breathing. <http://besthealth.bmj.com/x/set/topic/condition-centre/15.html>.

British Lung Foundation Breathe Easy Group. <http://www.lunguk.org>.

Calderwood HW, Modell JH, Ruiz BC (1975). The ineffectiveness of steroid therapy in treatment of fresh-water near-drowning. *Anaesthesiology*, **43**, 642–50.

Chest Heart and Stroke Scotland. <http://www.chss.org.uk/>.

Giammona ST and Modell JH (1967). Drowning by total immersion: effects on pulmonary surfactant of distilled water, isotonic saline and seawater. *American Journal of Diseases of Children*, **114**, 612–16.

Golden F, Tipton MJ, Scott RC (1997). Immersion, near drowning and drowning. *British Journal of Anaesthesia*, **79**, 214–225.

Lomotan JR, George SS, Brandstetter RD (1997). Aspiration pneumonia. Strategies for early recognition and prevention. *Postgraduate Medicine*, **102**, 229–231.

Lung Foundation Australia. <http://www.lungnet.com.au/>.

Modell HH (1993). Drowning. *New England Journal of Medicine*, **328**, 253–6.

Soar J, Perkins GD, Abbas G, *et al.* (2010). European Resuscitation Council Guidelines for Resuscitation 2010. Section 8. Cardiac arrest in special circumstances: Electrolyte abnormalities, poisoning, drowning, accidental hypothermia, hyperthermia, asthma, anaphylaxis, cardiac surgery, trauma, pregnancy, electrocution. *Resuscitation*, **81**, 1219–1276.

Vanden Hoek TL, Morrison LJ, Shuster M, *et al.* (2010). Guidelines for Cardiopulmonary Resuscitation and Emergency Cardiovascular Care. Part 12: Cardiac Arrest in Special Situations: 2010 American Heart Association. *Circulation*, **122**, S829–S861.

Your Lung Health. <http://www.yourlunghealth.org/>.

Pulmonary vasculitis

The vasculitides are rare conditions with a high untreated mortality. They are non-specific and mimic other conditions, including infection and cancer. Typical systemic features include low-grade fever, weight loss, haematuria, proteinuria, renal impairment, raised ESR, and autoantibodies. Pulmonary involvement usually occurs as part of a systemic vasculitis. Typical respiratory features include dyspnoea, wheeze, haemoptysis, sinus and nasal disease, exercise desaturation, hypoxaemia, CXR infiltrates, and abnormal gas transfer (KCO).

Primary pathology

Inflammation and necrosis of blood vessels. The classification of vasculitis adopted by the 2012 International Chapel Hill Consensus Conference on the 'Nomenclature of Vasculitides' is illustrated in Table 5.35. Small vessel vasculitides most commonly affect the lung interstitium. Neutrophil infiltration and fibrinoid necrosis cause damage to vessel walls. Capillary rupture releases red cells into the alveolus, causing alveolar haemorrhage.

Antineutrophil cytoplasmic antibodies (ANCA)

ANCA are markers of pulmonary vasculitis and may have a role in pathogenesis. Indirect immunofluorescence detects the reaction of ANCA with cytoplasmic granule enzymes in neutrophils. The resulting staining pattern is either diffusely cytoplasmic (c-ANCA) or perinuclear (p-ANCA). Modern ELISA (enzyme-linked immunosorbant assay) testing identifies ANCA as specific antibodies that target proteinase 3 (anti-PR3 antibodies) and myeloperoxidase (anti-MPO antibodies).

- **c-ANCA pattern** is associated with anti-PR3 antibodies and occurs in ~75% of Wegener's granulomatosis (granulomatosis with polyangiitis) and ~45% of microscopic polyangiitis. c-ANCA levels are most useful diagnostically. They are of limited value in assessing disease activity, but rising titres may precede a clinical relapse.

- **p-ANCA pattern** occurs with anti-MPO antibodies. It is associated with many diseases, including other vasculitides, autoimmune disease, pulmonary fibrosis, HIV, lung cancer, and pulmonary emboli.

Wegener's granulomatosis (granulomatosis with polyangiitis)

Wegener's granulomatosis (WG) is a rare necrotizing systemic, 'granuloma-forming' vasculitis. It affects $3/10^5$ of the population, mainly Caucasian people (>80%) of all ages but usually 40–55 years old. Sex distribution is equal. It involves mainly small and medium-sized vessels. At presentation, WG is often 'generalized' and includes the classical triad of sinusitis (90%), lower respiratory tract disease (>85%), and renal impairment (80%). However, non-specific upper airway disease, arthralgia, and eye features, including conjunctivitis, scleritis, visual loss, proptosis, and eye pain, may precede the diagnosis by several months. The heart, skin (~45%), and central nervous system (CNS) may also be involved. About 25% of cases, typically young women, present with 'limited' disease, affecting the upper and lower airways, although 80% eventually develop renal (± general) involvement. Acute cases may present with respiratory distress, alveolar haemorrhage, acute renal failure, and overwhelming systemic vasculitis. Some manifestations, such as subglottic tracheal stenosis, present insidiously when other aspects of the disease appear to be in remission.

Investigations

Typical findings include normocytic, normochromic anaemia, raised ESR, leucocytosis, and thrombocytosis. Renal impairment, proteinuria, haematuria, and urinary casts suggest glomerular disease.

Table 5.35 Vasculitis Classification

Large vessel vasculitis (LVV)	Takayasu arteritis (TAK), Giant cell arteritis (GCA)
Medium vessel vasculitis (MVV)	Polyarteritis nodosa (PAN), Kawasaki disease (KD)
Small vessel vasculitis (SVV)	Antineutrophil cytoplasmic antibody (ANCA)-associated vasculitis (AAV), Microscopic polyangiitis (MPA), Granulomatosis with polyangiitis (Wegener's) (GPA), Eosinophilic granulomatosis with polyangiitis (Churg-Strauss) (EGPA), Immune complex SVV, Anti-glomerular basement membrane (anti-GBM) disease, Cryoglobulinemic vasculitis (CV), IgA vasculitis (Henoch-Schönlein) (IgAV), Hypocomplementemic urticarial vasculitis (HUV) (anti-C1q vasculitis)
Variable vessel vasculitis (VVV)	Behçet's disease (BD), Cogan's syndrome (CS)
Single-organ vasculitis (SOV)	Cutaneous leukocytoclastic angiitis, Cutaneous arteritis, Primary central nervous system vasculitis, Isolated aortitis, Others
Vasculitis associated with systemic disease	Lupus vasculitis, Rheumatoid vasculitis, Sarcoid vasculitis, Others
Vasculitis associated with probable etiology	Hepatitis C virus-associated cryoglobulinemic vasculitis, Hepatitis B virus-associated vasculitis, Syphilis-associated aortitis, Drug-associated immune complex vasculitis, Drug-associated ANCA-associated vasculitis, Cancer-associated vasculitis, Others

Reproduced from Jennette JC et al., '2012 Revised International Chapel Hill Consensus Conference Nomenclature of Vasculitides', *Arthritis and Rheumatism*, 65, 1, Table 2, pp. 1–11, Wiley, Copyright © 2013 by the American College of Rheumatology.

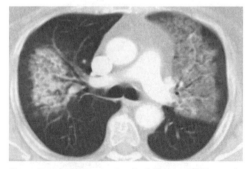

Figure 5.46 HRCT scan: alveolar infiltrates in Wegener's granulomatosis.

HRCT lung scans (see Figure 5.46) reveal alveolar infiltrates, haemorrhage, and 0.5–10 cm subpleural nodules, with cavitation in 20–50% of those >2 cm. Pleural lesions may mimic infarcts.

- **ANCA** (75–90% anti-PR3) are detected in ~90% of active generalized WG. Dual ANCA positivity can occur but suggests disorders like systemic lupus erythematosus (SLE). WG limited to the kidneys is associated with p-ANCA (75–80%). About 40% of 'limited' disease is ANCA-negative, and biopsy is required for diagnosis. A positive c-ANCA differentiates alveolar haemorrhage due to WG from other causes like Goodpasture's syndrome and SLE.
- **Biopsy confirmation** is usually required before immunosuppressant (± cytotoxic) therapy, but gravely ill patients may require immediate therapy. Upper airway and skin biopsies are simple and non-invasive. Transbronchial biopsy yield is low (<10%), even with HRCT guidance, and open lung biopsy may be indicated for local disease. Renal biopsy risks haemorrhage and may not differentiate histologically between microscopic polyangiitis and WG, although this is not important clinically.

Management
Management requires a multidisciplinary approach, involving chest, renal, and specialist teams. Early therapy aims to prevent end-organ damage.

- The standard regime to induce remission in progressive pulmonary, renal, or CNS disease combines oral prednisolone (1 mg/kg/day for 1 month, tapered over 6–12 months) with cyclophosphamide (2 mg/kg/day; maximum 200 mg daily for 3–6 months). About 90% respond within 6 months, although recovery may take up to a year. The regime is repeated in relapse which occurs in 50% of patients. Low-dose methotrexate is used in mild disease if cyclophosphamide is not tolerated. Maintenance therapy with either methotrexate or azathioprine, and low-dose steroid is given for a minimum of 2 years to reduce relapse. PCP prophylaxis and bone protection are also required. Control sinusitus with antibiotics and nasal steroids; long-term co-trimoxazole reduces the risk of relapse.
- Severely ill patients with rapidly progressive renal failure or alveolar haemorrhage are treated with pulsed methylprednisolone (0.5–1 g/day for 3 days) and intravenous cyclophosphamide (600 mg/m^2). Remission can be achieved faster with plasma exchange/plasmapheresis and then consolidated with standard therapy.

Prognosis
Without treatment, 80–90% of severe WG cases die within 2 years. With therapy, survival is 72–80% at 5 years and 65% at 10 years. Prolonged cyclophosphamide therapy is associated with lymphoma and bladder and skin cancer.

Microscopic polyangiitis

Microscopic polyangiitis (MPA) is as common as, but difficult to distinguish from, WG. This is unimportant, as clinical management is the same. MPA occurs mainly in Caucasians, aged ~50 years old, with an equal sex distribution. It mainly affects the kidneys, causing a small-vessel necrotizing vasculitis and is associated with proteinuria and haematuria. Renal biopsy reveals focal segmental glomerulonephritis. Pulmonary involvement occurs in ~40%, with associated asthma, pleurisy, alveolar haemorrhage, and haemoptysis. It is p- and c-ANCA-positive. Treatment is as for WG, with steroids and cyclophosphamide, followed by azathioprine or methotrexate if renal function is impaired.

Churg–Strauss syndrome (eosinophilic granulomatosis with polyangiitis)

Churg–Strauss syndrome (CSS) is a rare necrotizing vasculitis of unknown cause in small and medium-sized arteries. It affects about 2.4/10^6 of the population, usually in middle age, with a male to female ratio of 2:1. It is characterized by late onset, difficult-to-control asthma, with associated nasal polyps, sinus disease, pulmonary infiltrates, vasculitic neuropathy (± mononeuritis multiplex), blood eosinophilia (>10%), and extravascular eosinophils on biopsy, including eosinophilic granulomatous inflammation of the respiratory tract. Other features include fever, arthralgia, myositis, cardiomyopathy, alveolar haemorrhage, focal segmental glomerulonephritis (although renal failure is rare), purpura, and skin nodules. It usually presents with asthma, followed by eosinophilia and then systemic vasculitis, often many years later.

Investigation
The CXR reveals flitting peripheral infiltrates with multifocal consolidation. HRCT scans show ground glass shadowing, peripheral nodules, and alveolar haemorrhage. Blood and bronchoalveolar lavage reveal eosinophilia. Two-thirds of cases are p-ANCA-positive. Histological evidence of eosinophilic granulomata, and ideally necrotizing vasculitis, from biopsy samples confirms the diagnosis.

Treatment
Treatment depends on disease severity. Isolated pulmonary involvement is treated with high-dose prednisolone (60 mg/day for 1 month or until the disease is controlled; taper over 1 year, with increases for relapses). In severe disease, pulsed methylprednisolone for 3 days is followed by high-dose steroids. Cyclophosphamide is used in severe disease with cardiac, neurological, or gastrointestinal involvement. Remission is usually maintained with steroids and azathioprine. Untreated survival is 25% at 5 years. Response to steroid treatment is good in isolated pulmonary disease. Renal impairment, cardiac, neurological, and gastrointestinal involvement are associated with a poor prognosis.

Goodpasture's syndrome (anti-glomerular basement membrane (anti-GBM) disease)

Goodpasture's syndrome (GPS) is due to linear IgG deposition on the basement membranes of alveoli and glomeruli. This damages collagen and causes blood leakage in the lungs. The cause is unknown, but it is associated with HLA DR2 (65%), and it often follows a viral infection. It is rare, affecting 0.5–1/10^6 of the population, occurs most frequently in the third decade of life and mainly in men (M:F = 4:1). It presents with dyspnoea, cough, renal impairment, and inspiratory crackles on examination. Haemoptysis occurs in 80–90% of cases. Proteinuria, haematuria, and casts are detected in urine. CXR and CT scan shows bilateral patchy airspace shadowing. Pulmonary function tests demonstrate a restrictive defect, with raised gas transfer (KCO) due to pulmonary haemorrhage. Diagnosis is confirmed by renal biopsy which shows crescentic glomerulonephritis. Lung biopsy reveals alveolar haemorrhage, with haemosiderin-laden macrophages. Treatment is with high-dose steroids, cyclophosphamide, and, occasionally, plasma exchange. Dialysis may be required. Recurrence is uncommon once controlled, but renal and pulmonary function may not recover.

Giant cell arteritis (GCA)

GCA is the commonest systemic vasculitis, involving mainly large arteries. It affects 24/10^5 of the population, mainly elderly females. It presents with fever, weight loss, headache, and scalp tenderness. Optic neuritis may cause amaurosis fugax and visual symptoms. In particular, vasculitic occlusion of the ophthalmic artery, a branch of the internal carotid artery, is a medical emergency which can cause irreversible ischaemia and blindness if not treated promptly with corticosteroids. Aortitis is being diagnosed more commonly, using PET-CT imaging. Mild pulmonary involvement (<25%) causes cough and sore throat. The ESR is high. Temporal artery biopsy showing arteritis and giant cells confirms the diagnosis. Response to steroids is good. They should be continued for 1–2 years.

Takayasu's arteritis

Involves the aorta, its major branches, and large pulmonary vessels. It affects young Asian women. Clinical features include fever, weight loss, absent peripheral pulses, arterial bruits, and, occasionally, pulmonary artery stenosis. Angiography confirms the diagnosis, and PET-CT is useful in documenting the extent of large vessel involvement. Angioplasty treats complications. Steroids reduce symptoms but not mortality. Spontaneous remissions may occur.

Polyarteritis nodosa

Polyarteritis nodosa is similar to MPA, affecting middle-sized vessels, but lung involvement is unusual. It may overlap with CSS and WG. Occasionally, it is associated with hepatitis B (and rarely C).

Further reading

Best Health. Lungs and breathing. <http://besthealth.bmj.com/x/set/topic/condition-centre/15.html>.

Booth AD, Pusey CD, Jayne DR (2004). Renal vasculitis—an update in 2004. *Nephrology Dialysis Transplantation*, **19**, 1964.

British Lung Foundation Breathe Easy Group. <http://www.lunguk.org>.

Jennette JC, Falk RJ, Bacon PA, *et al.* (2013). 2012 revised International Chapel Hill Consensus Conference Nomenclature of Vasculitides. *Arthritis & Rheumatology*, **65**, 1–11.

Lane SE, Watts RA, Shepstone L, Scott DG (2005). Primary systemic vasculitis: clinical features and mortality. *QJM*, **98**, 97–111.

Langford C and Hoffman G (1999). Wegener's granulomatosis. Rare diseases 3. *Thorax*, **54**, 629–63.

Ntatsaki E, Carruthers D, Chakravarty K, D'Cruz D, *et al.* (2013). BSR and BHPR guideline for the management of adults with ANCA-associated vasculitis. <http://www.rheumatology.org.uk/includes/documents/cm_docs/2014/2/2014vasculitisfull_guidelines_new.pdf>.

Noth I, *et al.* (2003). Churg–Strauss syndrome. *Lancet*, **361**, 587–94.

Schwarz M and Brown K (2000). Small vessel vasculitis. Rare diseases 10. *Thorax*, **55**, 502–10.

Vasculitis Foundation. <http://www.VasculitisFoundation.org>.

VOICE4VASCULITIS. <https://sites.google.com/site/voice4vasculitis/>.

The immunocompromised host

Respiratory disease is a frequent cause of morbidity and mortality in the immunocompromised host. It is most common following chemotherapy or in those infected with human immunodeficiency virus (HIV). Other causes include malignancy (e.g. lymphoma, leukaemia), immunosuppression (e.g. steroids, azathioprine), and after renal or bone marrow transplant. The non-specific clinical presentation, with fever, dyspnoea, hypoxia, dry cough, chest discomfort, and inconclusive investigations often makes diagnosis difficult. However, rate of onset (e.g. rapid with bacterial infection, slow with malignancy), recent drug therapy (e.g. methotrexate), and associated extrapulmonary features (e.g. shingles, Kaposi's sarcoma) are helpful.

Investigation

Investigation should include blood and pleural fluid microscopy, culture, and serology. Sputum may detect *Aspergillus* and mycobacteria, and induced sputum *Pneumocystis jirovecii* pneumonia (PCP). Arterial blood gases determine the degree of hypoxaemia. Initial CXR findings (e.g. diffuse infiltration, nodules, consolidation) are non-specific, but serial changes indicate treatment response. Chest CT scans may be diagnostic (e.g. lymphangitis carcinomatosis, aspergillosis (e.g. halo sign), pulmonary embolism), reveal the extent and location of pulmonary disease, and aid invasive sampling. Bronchoscopy with bronchoalveolar lavage (BAL) and appropriate microbiology (e.g. bacterial pneumonia), stains (e.g. *Aspergillus*, mycobacteria, malignancy), immunofluorescence (e.g. PCP), and serology (e.g. CMV, *Cryptococcus*) are diagnostic in 50–60% of cases and should be considered early in management. Transbronchial, percutaneous fine needle, and formal lung biopsies all have potential risks but aid diagnosis.

Cause

This is infectious in >75% and non-infectious in <25% of immunocompromised patients with lung disease.

• **Infection** depends on the immunological defect (see Table 5.36) and previous use of prophylactic therapy (e.g. PCP). However, there is considerable overlap.

• **Non-infectious disease** presents with similar clinical (e.g. fever) and radiological features to infection. Causes include: pulmonary oedema (e.g. post-transplant); acute respiratory distress syndrome (ARDS) secondary to sepsis or drugs, underlying disease (e.g. lymphoma, leukaemia, connective tissue disease); diffuse alveolar haemorrhage; pulmonary embolism; drug-induced disease (e.g. bleomycin, azathioprine, busulfan, methotrexate, cyclophosphamide); bone marrow transplant-associated idiopathic pneumonia; radiation-induced pneumonitis; pulmonary alveolar proteinosis;

and chronic graft-versus-host disease. More than one cause is often present (~30%).

Treatment

Treatment with antimicrobial agents may be required before the diagnosis has been established in neutropenic patients with fever and/or pulmonary infiltrates because these cases are at risk of life-threatening sepsis. Blood cultures should always precede antibiotic therapy. Subsequent invasive diagnostic procedures are reserved for those who fail to improve after 2–3 days' therapy. It is often possible to withhold antibiotics in non-neutropenic patients until the appropriate investigations are completed.

• **Antibiotic** choice is determined by the condition and local antibiotic policy, but neutropenic patients are usually treated with broad-spectrum antibiotics (e.g. piperacillin, gentamicin, ± vancomycin, ± antifungal agents). PCP and CMV therapy have major toxic side effects and are best started after definitive diagnosis. Nevertheless, if suspicion of PCP is high, treatment is started empirically, as it can be detected for up to 2 weeks after onset of therapy. Treatment of mycobacterial infection is only ever started after definitive diagnosis.

• **Steroid therapy** is recommended in PCP, radiation- or drug-induced lung disease, alveolar haemorrhage, and the idiopathic pneumonia of bone marrow transplantation.

• **Supportive therapies** include diuretics for pulmonary oedema, supplemental oxygen, and non-invasive or mechanical ventilation. Occasionally, surgical resection is needed in invasive aspergillosis. Respiratory failure has a poor outcome in the immunocompromised host.

The HIV-positive, immunocompromised patient

Respiratory disease in HIV-positive patients should be managed in association with an HIV specialist. Factors influencing infection are compliance with highly active antiretroviral therapy (HAART) and prophylactic antibiotics, source of infection (i.e. TB is more common in intravenous drug users), and geography (e.g. histoplasmosis and coccidioidomycosis are more common in the USA). Extrapulmonary features may suggest the cause of pulmonary disease (e.g. Kaposi's sarcoma). Investigation and treatment are similar to those in non-HIV immunocompromised cases.

1. **Infectious causes** of chest disease in HIV infection are:
   • **Bacterial** (e.g. S. pneumoniae, S. aureus, Nocardia).
   • **Pneumocystis jiroveci pneumonia** (PCP).
   • **Viral** (e.g. adenovirus, influenza, herpes simplex, CMV).

Table 5.36 Infectious causes of respiratory disease in immunocompromised patients

Immunological defect	Clinical conditions	Types of infection
Neutropenia	Chemotherapy, aplastic anaemia, leukaemia	Bacterial (e.g. *E. coli*), fungal (e.g. *Aspergillus*)
Impaired T cell function	Transplantation, HIV, lymphoma, steroids, chemotherapy	Bacteria (e.g. *Mycobacterium tuberculosis*), fungi (e.g. PCP), viruses (e.g. CMV)
Impaired B cell function	Lymphoma, leukaemia, myeloma, hypogammaglobulinaemia	*Streptococcus pneumoniae, Haemophilus influenzae*
Impaired complement	Genetic causes, mannose-lectin deficiency	*Streptococcus pneumoniae*

- **Fungal** (e.g. *Aspergillus*, *Cryptococcus*).
- **Mycobacterial** (e.g. *Mycobacterium avian intracellulare*, *Mycobacterium tuberculosis*, *Mycobacterium kansasii*).
- **Parasites** (e.g. *Strongyloides stercoralis*).

2. **Non-infectious causes** include lymphoma, Kaposi's sarcoma, lymphocytic and non-specific interstitial pneumonitis, drug-induced lung disease, and heart failure.

Further reading

National AIDS Trust. <http://www.nat.org.uk>.

Rosen MJ (2008). Pulmonary complications of HIV infection. *Respirology*, **13**,181–90.

St Peters House Project. <http://www.stpetershouse.org.uk>.

Terrence Higgins Trust. <http://www.tht.org.uk>.

Vento S, Cainelli F, Temesgen Z (2008) Lung infections after cancer chemotherapy. *Lancet Oncology*, **9**, 982–92.

Sleep apnoea

Sleep apnoea may be due to upper airways obstruction, described as obstructive sleep apnoea (OSA), or disturbances of control of breathing collectively termed central sleep apnoea (CSA). If severe, OSA causes significant daytime symptoms, especially sleepiness, impairs quality of life (QOL), reduces performance, and increases the risk of serious accidents and other cardiovascular and systemic diseases (e.g. hypertension, angina).

Obstructive sleep apnoea (OSA)/hypopnoea (OSAH)

OSA is defined as upper airways narrowing, provoked by sleep, causing sufficient sleep fragmentation to result in daytime symptoms, mainly sleepiness, and called OSAH syndrome. It is a common disorder, but prevalence depends on the thresholds used to define significant symptoms or abnormal sleep studies. However, 0.5–1% of men and 0.1–0.2% of women are candidates for treatment with nasal continuous positive airways pressure (CPAP) to splint open the upper airway during sleep. Prevalence increases with obesity and is determined by fat distribution, with causative truncal body and neck obesity more common in men.

Mechanism

Upper airways patency decreases during sleep due to loss of dilator muscle activity in the pharynx. This muscle relaxation is increased by neuromuscular diseases (e.g. stroke, dystrophies), age, and muscle relaxants (e.g. sedatives, alcohol). The pharyngeal airway is further narrowed by obesity, myxoedema, tonsillar enlargement, craniofacial factors (e.g. micrognathia), and specific syndromes (e.g. Marfan's, acromegaly). In severe OSA, repetitive upper airways collapse (± hypoxaemia), and subsequent arousal, to reactivate pharyngeal dilator muscles, may occur every minute throughout the night. Recurrent arousal fragments sleep, causes daytime sleepiness, and is associated with increases in cardiovascular risk factors like hypertension.

Clinical features

These include unrefreshing sleep, excessive sleepiness, poor concentration, and nocturia. Risk of road traffic and work-associated accidents is increased. Sleepiness can be difficult to assess due to concerns over driving, licensing, and employment. The Epworth scale scores the tendency to fall asleep; >10 is considered abnormally sleepy. Partners are often concerned by loud snoring, choking episodes, and apnoeic periods. Reduced libido, oesophageal reflux, and nocturnal sweating may also occur. Most patients are male and tend to have upper body obesity (neck size >17 in) and a small or set-back mandible.

Investigation

This requires routine blood tests, including glucose, thyroid, and appropriate endocrine function tests and lipid profiles, as these patients have a high risk cardiovascular profile. Overnight oximetry alone (see Figure 5.47) identifies most OSA cases, if its limitations are recognized, and allows onward referral for CPAP. In COPD or other patients with a low baseline SaO_2, some caution is required when diagnosing OSA on the basis of oximetry alone. False negatives studies occur in younger, thinner patients, in whom it is the compensatory reflex increases in inspiratory effort that arouse the patient, rather than hypoxaemia, which is less likely due to the larger oxygen stores in the lungs of less obese patients. Limited sleep studies, in which oximetry is combined with monitoring of snoring, chest/abdominal movement, heart rate, and oronasal airflow, are the routine investigation in most sleep units. Full polysomnography (PSG), including EEG, EMG, and eye movements is used to stage sleep electrophysiologically.

Management

Factors determining the need to treat include the impact of symptoms on quality of life (QOL), impact on livelihood (e.g. HGV driving), the presence of associated obesity or COPD, and motivation to undergo treatment. There is no evidence

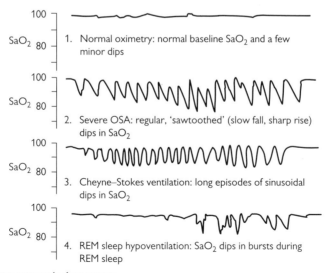

1. Normal oximetry: normal baseline SaO_2 and a few minor dips

2. Severe OSA: regular, 'sawtoothed' (slow fall, sharp rise) dips in SaO_2

3. Cheyne–Stokes ventilation: long episodes of sinusoidal dips in SaO_2

4. REM sleep hypoventilation: SaO_2 dips in bursts during REM sleep

Figure 5.47 Oximetry patterns in sleep apnoea.

that hypertension, heart failure, or angina should influence the decision, but may reduce the threshold, to treat.

Simple therapeutic measures include weight loss and reduced consumption of alcohol in the evening. Patients should be encouraged to avoid sleeping supine. Some snorers with good dentition may benefit from mandibular advancement devices. In significant OSA, nasal CPAP can improve daytime symptoms and QOL dramatically. Tonsillectomy or mandibular surgery can be beneficial occasionally, but outcome from pharyngeal surgery is usually poor. Bariatric surgery (e.g. gastroplasty) may be considered in severe obesity. Patients with raised $PaCO_2$ (± acidosis) may require a period of non-invasive positive pressure ventilation (NIPPV) prior to CPAP.

Central sleep apnoea

Central sleep apnoea (CSA) is much less common than OSA and is defined by short repetitive central apnoeas or more prolonged periods of hypoventilation. CSA is usually used to describe actual apnoeas and is termed Cheyne–Stokes breathing when there is regular symmetrical waxing and waning of ventilation, as in heart failure. Periodic breathing describes regular fluctuations in breathing (± apnoeas).

The causes of CSA include 'lung failure, brain failure, and heart failure'.

- **Failure of mechanical ability to ventilate**, due to inspiratory muscle impairment in many neuromuscular diseases (e.g. motor neurone disease, muscular dystrophies or post-polio syndrome (in which recurrence of inspiratory muscle weakness occurs decades after the initial illness)) and obstructive (e.g. COPD) or restrictive (e.g. kyphoscoliosis) disorders, results in the use of accessory muscles to maintain ventilation. However, during non-REM sleep, recruitment of accessory muscles is attenuated, causing hypoventilation, and, during REM sleep, physiological paralysis of all postural muscles (i.e. REM atonia) results in isolated diaphragmatic breathing, with profound hypoventilation and apnoea.
- **Impaired ventilatory drive** may be congenital or due to brainstem involvement in strokes, trauma, malignancy, or syringobulbia. These patients have no obvious respiratory or neuromuscular cause for hypoventilation. They maintain adequate daytime ventilation, as there is a non-metabolic 'awake' ventilatory drive equivalent to ~5 L/min. During non-REM sleep, the 'awake' drive is lost, and ventilation is dependent on blood gas stimulation (i.e. hypoxaemia, hypercapnia), although 'awake-like' drive may return during REM sleep.
- **Cheyne–Stokes breathing** occurs in heart failure or at high altitude. In left heart failure, J receptor stimulation (i.e. due to raised left atrial pressure) and hypoxaemia increase ventilatory drive, causing respiratory alkalosis. At sleep onset, the $PaCO_2$ threshold increases by 1 kPa and, with the loss of 'awake' ventilatory drive, causes hypoventilation and/or apnoea. Eventually, increasing $PaCO_2$ (± hypoxia) causes arousal with associated hyperventilation and hypocapnia again, and the cycle repeats. Similarly, at high altitude, hypoxia causes respiratory stimulation with hypocapnia, and, at sleep onset, the loss of 'awake' ventilatory drive allows hypoventilation (± apnoeas).

Investigation

This includes simple spirometry to characterize respiratory muscle weakness and airways obstruction. Supine vital capacity may reveal diaphragmatic weakness masked during erect testing. Arterial blood gases detect respiratory failure.

Sleep studies are required to confirm CSA:

- Oximetry alone is variable and may show persistent oscillations (due to repeated arousals) or isolated REM sleep-related SaO_2 dips (see Figure 5.47). In OSA, the fall in SaO_2 is gradual, as oxygen stores are utilized, followed by a rapid recovery with the first deep breath after apnoea giving a 'sawtoothed' pattern. During Cheyne–Stokes breathing, the SaO_2 oscillations are sinusoidal as the breathing pattern tends to wax and wane. However, it may mimic OSA if sudden arousals follow apnoea. In COPD, the findings are related to baseline SaO_2, with dramatic dips occurring during REM sleep. The combination of hypoxic COPD and OSA can produce particularly dramatic oximetry traces and requires fuller sleep study evidence of OSA.
- Limited respiratory sleep studies confirm SaO_2 falls with hypoventilation but detects no evidence of obstruction or snoring.
- Full PSG may be required in some cases and identifies the relationship to sleep stage.

Management depends on symptoms. Improved treatment of the underlying condition (e.g. heart failure, COPD) or raising inspired oxygen concentration (FiO_2) in hypoxaemic patients may be helpful. If this fails to alleviate Cheyne–Stokes ventilation and sleep continues to be fragmented with associated daytime respiratory failure, consider trials of acetazolamide, benzodiazepines, or CPAP, although evidence of benefit is limited.

In patients with hypercapnia, raising FiO_2 may be detrimental. In these patients, overnight nasal or full face mask NIPPV may be beneficial. Likewise, in patients with sleep disturbance or respiratory failure due to slowly progressive neuromuscular disorders or chest wall restrictions (e.g. kyphoscoliosis), the response to NIPPV can be dramatic. However, increasing dependence on NIPPV, which is not designed to be life-sustaining, can raise difficult issues with progressive respiratory failure.

Further reading

CPAPMAN. <http://www.cpapman.com>.

Greenstone M and Hack M (2014). Obstructive sleep apnoea (clinical review). *BMJ*, **348**: g3745. <www.bmj.com>.

Lanfranchi PA and Somers VK (2003). Sleep disordered breathing in heart failure: characteristics and implications. *Respiratory Physiology & Neurobiology*, **136**, 153–65.

Malhotra A and White DP (2002). Obstructive sleep apnoea. *Lancet*, **360**, 237–45.

MedlinePlus. Sleep disorders. <http://www.nlm.nih.gov/medlineplus/tutorials/sleepdisorders/htm/_no_50_no_0.htm>.

National Institute for Health and Care Excellence (2008). Continuous positive airway pressure for the treatment of obstructive sleep apnoea/hypopnoea syndrome. NICE technology appraisal 139. <http://www.nice.org.uk/guidance/TA139>.

National Institute for Health and Care Excellence (2015). Obstructive sleep apnoea syndrome. Clinical knowledge summaries. <http://cks.nice.org.uk/obstructive-sleep-apnoea-syndrome>.

No authors listed (2014). British Thoracic Society Position statement on driving and obstructive sleep apnoea (OSA)/obstructive sleep apnoea syndrome (OSAS). <https://www.brit-thoracic.org.uk/document-library/about-bts/documents/bts-position-statement-on-driving-and-obstructive-sleep-apnoea/>.

Parati G, Lombardi C, Hedner J, et al. (2013). Recommendations for the management of patients with obstructive sleep apnoea and hypertension. *European Respiratory Journal*, **41**, 523–538.

Scottish Intercollegiate Guidelines Network/British Thoracic Society Guidelines (2003). <http://www.sign.ac.uk/guidelines/fulltext/73/index.html>.

Sleep Apnoea Trust Association. <http://www.sleep-apnoea-trust.org>.

Sleep Home Pages. <http://www.sleephomepages.org>.

Rare pulmonary diseases

These rare conditions are only discussed briefly. Comprehensive texts can be found in *Oxford Desk Reference of Respiratory Medicine*.

Pulmonary arteriovenous malformations

Pulmonary arteriovenous malformations (PAVM; see Figure 5.48) are abnormal shunt vessels between the arterial and venous circulations. They vary in size from telangiectasia to large aneurysmal lesions and enlarge throughout life, particularly during puberty. PAVM affect <1 in 15,000 people. About 80% of cases have hereditary haemorrhagic telangiectasia (HHT), with the associated risk of acute stroke and focal neurological signs. Most are associated with low pulmonary vascular resistance, haemorrhage, vascular remodelling, high cardiac output, and, occasionally, embolic strokes.

Characteristic clinical features include dyspnoea, haemoptysis (10%), chest pain (10%), cyanosis, clubbing, orthodeoxia (desaturation on standing up), telangiectasia, and vascular bruits, but 50% are asymptomatic. Most cases present with hypoxaemia or a CXR finding of a round, smooth mass with feeding and drainage vessels. CT confirms the diagnosis and assesses suitability for embolization. Shunt can be quantified at angiography, echocardiography, or with 100% oxygen rebreathing studies.

Embolization with coils is effective in most cases, although a small shunt often persists, requiring antibiotic prophylaxis during dental/surgical procedures to reduce the risk of abscess formation. Surgical resection is required in some cases. Family members must always be screened for HHT. Advise young women to delay pregnancy until after PAVM treatment to avoid the risk of further enlargement.

Pulmonary alveolar proteinosis

Pulmonary alveolar proteinosis is a rare alveolar filling defect, affecting 2–3/10^6 of the population; mainly middle-aged, male smokers. It is due to the presence of antibodies to granulocyte macrophage-stimulating factor (GM-CSF). This inhibits alveolar macrophage clearance of surfactant

and results in the accumulation of a PAS-positive, proteinaceous phospholipid deposit. Other causes include congenital surfactant gene mutations, dust exposure, amphiphilic drugs (e.g. amiodarone), lymphoma, and leukaemia. Most cases present with breathlessness, non-productive cough, hypoxaemia, secondary chest infections (e.g. mycobacteria, fungi, *Nocardia*), clubbing (30%), and crepitations on chest auscultation. Lung function is restrictive and gas transfer reduced. CXR shows bilateral, often perihilar, airspace consolidation. CT scans reveal a characteristic 'crazy paving' pattern of alternating airspace consolidation and normal lung (which also occurs in alveolar cell carcinoma). Endoscopic whole lung lavage (i.e. 40 L washouts) is the most effective therapy. Prognosis varies; a third resolves spontaneously; a third remain stable, and a third progress to respiratory failure.

Amyloidosis

Amyloidosis is due to extracellular deposition of insoluble, low molecular weight protein fibrils. Clinically significant respiratory disease is usually due to primary amyloid, in which the fibrils are derived from monoclonal immunoglobulin light chain fragments in plasma cell dyscrasias (e.g. myeloma). Fibril deposition may be systemic, affecting many organs, and includes parenchymal amyloid with diffuse alveolar deposition or multiple peripheral pulmonary nodules; or localized to specific organs or areas (e.g. laryngeal or tracheobronchial nodules or infiltration). Secondary amyloid is a rare complication of chronic inflammation (e.g. rheumatoid). The fibrils are fragments of acute phase proteins, and respiratory involvement is rare. Other inherited, dialysis-related, and organ-specific (e.g. Alzheimer's) types of amyloid rarely affect the lung.

Idiopathic pulmonary haemosiderosis

Idiopathic pulmonary haemosiderosis is a rare disease that presents in childhood (85%). It is characterized by recurrent alveolar haemorrhage and haemoptysis, progressive dyspnoea, chronic iron deficiency anaemia, lymphadenopathy, hepatosplenomegaly, and clubbing (25%). Although the cause is unknown, an autoimmune mechanism is suspected, as it is associated with other autoimmune diseases (e.g. rheumatoid, thyrotoxicosis). Steroids and immunosuppressive drugs are beneficial in acute bleeds but do not affect long-term outcome.

Primary ciliary dyskinesia

Primary ciliary dyskinesia (PCD) is a rare genetic (autosomal recessive) cause of ciliary dysfunction that affects the lungs, brain ventricles, and Fallopian tubes. It often presents in childhood, with rhinitis, cough, 'glue' ear, and situs invertus. Adult bronchiectasis, chronic respiratory disease, and infertility (e.g. Kartagener's syndrome) occur later. The saccharin test and ciliary biopsy establish the diagnosis. Treatment is as for bronchiectasis.

Alveolar microlithiasis

Alveolar microlithiasis is a rare interstitial lung disease of unknown cause, characterized by the accumulation of calcified lesions in the alveolar spaces. It has a familial tendency and is more common in women. Presentation occurs at 30–40 years old, with breathlessness and micronodular lung calcification on CXR and CT scan. It progresses to respiratory failure and death. No medical therapy is available, but

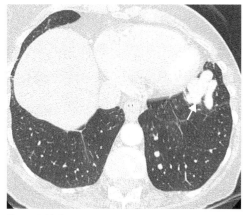

Figure 5.48 Pulmonary arteriovenous malformation (arrow) on a CT scan pulmonary angiogram in a 65-year-old woman with progressive dyspnoea, hypoxaemia, and orthodeoxia.

lung transplantation has been successful. Lungs are often 'rock-hard' at post-mortem.

Recurrent respiratory papillomatosis

Recurrent respiratory papillomatosis are warts of the upper respiratory tract caused by human papilloma virus. They are often confined to the larynx, but bronchial involvement occurs in 25% of cases. It causes voice loss and airways obstruction. Treatment with interferon-alpha achieves complete (30%) or partial (30%) remission, but relapse is common. Aciclovir, cidofovir, and ribavirin have also been used. Microdebridement, photodynamic and laser therapy are used to maintain airway patency.

Further reading

Association of Cancer Online Resources. Amyloid online support. <http://listserv.acor.org/SCRIPTS/WA-ACOR.EXE?A0= amyloid>.

British Orphan Lung Disease (BOLD) project. <http://www.BTS. org>.

Gillmore JD and Hawkins PN (1999). Amyloidosis and the respiratory tract. *Thorax*, **54**, 444–51.

HHT groups. <http://www.hht.org> and <http://www.telangiectasia.co.uk>.

Primary Ciliary Dyskinesia Family Support Group. <http://www. pcdsupport.org.uk/>.

Seymour JF and Presneill JJ (2002). Pulmonary alveolar proteinosis: progress in the first 44 years. *American Journal of Respiratory and Critical Care Medicine*, **166**, 215–35.

Shovlin CL and Letarte M (1999). Hereditary haemorrhagic telangiectasia and pulmonary arteriovenous malformation. *Thorax*, **54**, 714–29.

Infectious diseases and emergencies

Clinical features, history, and examination

The clinical history

The traditional emphasis on the pre-eminence of the clinical history and physical examination is not better exemplified than in the approach to the patient with a suspected infectious disease.

'Fever' is a cardinal clinical feature of infection, but, strictly speaking, this is a clinical sign and not a symptom. Some patients take their own temperature, but, in most instances, the presence of fever is surmised from symptoms, such as feeling 'hot', cold 'chills', and excessive sweatiness. It is useful to elicit the presence of 'drenching' night sweats (i.e. patients need to change night clothes or shower), which can occur, for example, in tuberculosis or lymphoproliferative disorders. True rigors are a frequent accompaniment of bacteraemia.

Focal symptoms usually direct the clinician to the source of infection. However, not infrequently, these are absent or indeterminant and localizing the source can be difficult. It is important to ascertain the duration, as, with the exception of recurrent or secondary infectious complications, relatively few infectious diseases cause febrile illnesses that last several weeks. Where the diagnosis or source is elusive, the most likely causes and approach to management are outlined in a later section in this chapter 'Fever of unknown origin (FUO)'.

Every history should also include a detailed enquiry into foreign travel (see 'Fever in the returning traveller'). Animal contact, particularly scratches and bites from pets, may be significant, and infections involving contact with farm or wild animals may involve occupational and recreational risks (see Table 6.1). In particular, tick bites and visits to woodland or heathland inhabited by ticks are risk factors for Lyme disease.

The past medical history may indicate relapse of a previous condition (e.g. acute cholecystitis), and a history of recurrent, severe, or unusual infections should raise the possibility of an underlying immunodeficiency state. The presence of implanted prosthetic materials (e.g. heart valves, vascular grafts, and joints) that provide a potential site for bacterial adherence should also be noted. Recent hospitalization and, in particular, instrumentation (e.g. vascular catheterization) may point towards a hospital-acquired infection. Immunization makes some conditions less likely, but patients may not recall childhood vaccinations, and some are not highly effective in adulthood (e.g. BCG). It is important to take a drug history since immunosuppressive therapy predisposes to opportunistic infections and drug reactions can manifest as a febrile illness.

The social history can be important, as transmission of some infections is increased amongst closed or overcrowded populations, such as student halls of residence and military camps (e.g. meningococcal infection). Louse-borne infections are diseases of poverty, famine, and overcrowding (e.g. 'trench fever' in the homeless and epidemic typhus

Table 6.1 Some specific exposure risks for infections

Risk	Endemic conditions	Non-endemic conditions
Water contact (f, fresh; s, sea)	*Aeromonas hydrophila* (f), Leptospirosis (f), *Mycobacterium marinum* (s and f), *Naegleria fowleri* (f)	Acute schistosomiasis (f), *Vibrio vulnificans* (s), meliodosis (f)
Animal contact	Capnocytophagia (dogs > cats) Cat scratch fever (cats) Leptospirosis (rodents) Pasteurellosis (cats > dogs) *Mycobacterium marinum* (tropical fish) Psittacosis (birds) Q fever (cattle, sheep, goats) Rat bite fever (rodents)	Anthrax (herbivores, e.g. cattle, goats) Avian influenza (birds) Brucellosis (cattle, camels, goats, sheep) Hantavirus (rodents) Histoplasmosis (bats, poultry) Plague (wild rodents) Rabies (dogs, cats, wild carnivores, e.g. bats, foxes) Tularaemia (small mammals, e.g. rabbits) VHF (see **Table 6.7**)
Tick bite	Lyme disease	Babesiosis, CCHF (see **Table 6.7**), tick typhus, RMSF, relapsing fever, tularaemia
Occupational and recreational	Anthrax (handling imported skins and furs, e.g. tanners) Leptospirosis (farm and sewer workers, water sports) Lyme (hiking, camping)	Brucellosis (farm, abattoir, and laboratory workers) Histoplasmosis (agricultural and construction workers, poultry farmers, spelunkers) Plague (hunters, farmers) Q fever (farm and abattoir workers, meatpackers) Rabies (biologists, hunters) Tick typhus (camping safari) Tularaemia (trappers, hunters)
Human contacts	Viral exanthems, meningococcal infections, group A *Streptococcus*	VHF
Sexual	HIV, HAV, HBV, HSV, gonorrhoea	
Injecting drug use	Group A *Streptococcus*, *Staphylococcus aureus*, botulism, tetanus, HIV, HBV, HCV	

CCHF, Congo-Crimean haemorrhagic fever; HIV, human immunodeficiency virus; HAV, hepatitis A virus; HBV, hepatitis B virus; HCV, hepatitis C virus; HSV, herpes simplex virus; RMSF, Rocky Mountain spotted fever; VHF, viral haemorrhagic fever.

in refugee camps). Enquiry after recent contacts with similar symptoms may be useful for a limited number of conditions (e.g. norovirus). It is often unrewarding, or even misleading, to enquire about what has recently been consumed. However, a cluster of simultaneous cases arising after a shared meal suggests food poisoning (e.g. *Campylobacter* after a barbecue). A sexual history, which includes assessment of HIV risk, should be routine. Family history, in the sense of inherited conditions, is only really relevant if one of the rare periodic febrile syndromes, such as familial Mediterranean fever, is suspected (see 'Fever of unknown origin').

Physical examination

A comprehensive examination of all systems is essential. The temperature pattern is generally unhelpful, except for a high 'swinging' fever that is often seen in pyogenic abscesses. Careful inspection of the oral cavity may show tonsillar enlargement and pharyngitis. Vesicles and ulcers suggest viral infections (e.g. herpes simplex, varicella-zoster, and enteroviruses); 'snail track' mouth ulcers occur in secondary syphilis; HIV infection is associated with thrush and hairy leucoplakia of the tongue, and Koplik's spots on the buccal mucosa are pathognomonic of measles. Poor dentition is associated with dental abscesses, endocarditis, and microaspiration. The presence of vascular and urinary catheters should be noted, and, in particular, IV cannulae sites should be inspected closely for evidence of infection or phlebitis after removal. Splinter haemorrhages may be microembolic manifestations of endovascular infection.

A skin rash accompanies many infectious illnesses but is not always obvious, and a thorough search over the body should be made in good light. In particular, recognition of the non-blanching petechial rash of meningococcaemia demands urgent treatment. Important causes of specific types of rash are shown in Table 6.2 and include some non-infectious conditions that are often associated with fever. These can be the result of micro-organisms multiplying in the skin, toxin-mediated effects, inflammatory reactions, or mechanisms that cause vascular leak.

Lymphadenopathy (a practical guide is any node ≥1cm) should be sought at all sites (the axillae are frequently omitted). Table 6.3 shows some important causes of lymphadenopathy depending on the duration and site. Regional lymphadenopathy often occurs at sites proximal to inflamed or infected skin and soft tissue. Lymphoma and malignancy are always in the list of differential diagnoses, whether regional or generalized. Supraclavicular nodes are more frequently malignant. Regional lymph nodes with suppuration include pyogenic infections (e.g. group A *Streptococcus* or *Staphylococcus aureus*), scrofula, meliodosis, plague, and tularaemia. Splenomegaly may be found in association with the causes of generalized lymphadenopathy, but, when present in isolation, it is associated with a diverse range of conditions (e.g. infective endocarditis, malaria, visceral leishmaniasis).

Basic blood tests

Routine haematology and biochemistry can provide a helpful initial pointer to the aetiology of a suspected infection in the emergency setting. Many bacterial infections are characteristically associated with a neutrophil leucocytosis, sometimes with a 'left shift' caused by the release of immature leucocytes. However, careful interpretation is needed, since there is sometimes failure to mount a normal immune response (e.g. especially in the elderly), and leucopenia can also be a feature of overwhelming bacterial sepsis. The total white cell count is not characteristically elevated in most viral infections. Although lymphopenia commonly occurs in glandular fever and primary cytomegalovirus infections, lymphocytosis is characteristic and 'atypical' lymphocytes may be seen on a blood film. Pancytopenia occurs in parvo-

Table 6.2 Causes of a febrile illness associated with skin manifestations

	Maculopapular/ macular	Petechial/ purpuric	Vesicular/pustular	Nodular	Miscellaneous rashes/lesions
ENDEMIC	Drug reaction Enteroviruses EBV (esp. with amoxicillin) HIV HHV-6 Measles Parvovirus B19 Rat bite fever Rubella Still's disease Syphilis Trench fever (Bartonellosis)	DIC (severe sepsis) Endocarditis Leptospirosis Meningococcaemia Henoch–Schönlein purpura Vasculitis	HSV VZV *Staphylococcus aureus,* e.g. impetigo Group A *Streptococcus* N. *gonorrhoeae* Hand-foot-and-mouth disease Stevens–Johnson syndrome Toxic epidermal necrolysis Pemphigus Pemphigoid	Erythema nodosum Cryptococcosis* Ecthyma gangrenosum* Mycobacteria	Anthrax (eschar) Erythema marginatum (rheumatic fever) Erythema migrans (Lyme disease) Kawasaki disease Toxic shock syndrome Scarlet fever
NON-ENDEMIC	African trypanosomiasis Rickettsial infections Typhoid Dengue fever	Relapsing fever Rickettsial infections VHF	Orthopoxviruses	Histoplasmosis* Coccidioidomycosis* Blastomycosis Paracoccidioidomycosis* Leprosy	Acute schistosomiasis (urticaria) African trypanosomiasis (chancre) Strongyloidiasis (Larva currens, urticaria)

DIC, disseminated intravascular coagulation; EBV, Epstein–Barr virus; HHV-6, human herpes-6 virus; VZV, herpes varicella zoster virus.

*Typically in immunocompromised hosts.

Table 6.3 Selected infections causing lymphadenopathy and non-infectious differential diagnoses

	Generalized	Regional		
		Cervical	Inguinal	Mediastinal
ACUTE	Brucellosis	Cat scratch	Chancroid	
	EBV	Group A *Streptococcus*	HSV	
	CMV	Viral pharyngitis	Lower limb cellulitis	
	HIV	Still's disease	LGV	
	Still's disease		Plague	Tuberculosis
	Syphilis		Syphilis	Sarcoidosis
	Toxoplasmosis			Histoplasmosis
				Coccidioidomycosis
CHRONIC	Castleman's disease	TB	Lymphatic filariasis	Sarcoidosis
	Coccidioidomycosis	Toxoplasmosis		Castleman's disease
	Histoplasmosis	Kikuchi's disease		
	HIV			
	Syphilis			
	TB			

LGV, lymphogranuloma venerum.

virus B19 infection (failure of red cell production is associated with reduced reticulocyte numbers).

Inflammatory indices, such as the C-reactive protein (CRP) or erythrocyte sedimentation rate (ESR), are significantly more elevated in bacterial than viral infections, although these are not always dependable markers.

Thrombocytopenia with a normal white cell count should prompt review of the travel history in case malaria has been overlooked. Varying degrees of renal and liver impairment can be features of some specific, fulminant infections (e.g. leptospirosis) but may also reflect multiorgan failure in any patient with septic shock.

The febrile patient with skin lesions or rash

There are many ways that the febrile patient with skin lesions or rash can be classified (e.g. mechanism or causative agent), but the most helpful way is to work backwards from the appearance of the rash.

Generalized macular and maculopapular rashes

Viruses

These account for the majority of cases and are covered in the sections on Classic viral exanthems and mumps, and 'Mononucleosis' syndromes.

Syphilis

The clinical features of secondary syphilis start 2–8 weeks after the primary chancre (this may be still present). The manifestations are protean but include: low-grade fever, pharyngitis, arthralgia, generalized lymphadenopathy (epitrochlear lymph node enlargement, detected just above the elbow on the inner arm, is a unique finding), and a skin rash (90% of cases).

Macular skin lesions initially appear on the upper trunk, limb flexures, soles, and palms. After 3 months, the lesions become papular and follow skin creases. Lesions in hairy areas cause small, discrete areas of alopecia of the scalp, beard, and eyebrows. By 6 months, moist, flat-topped papules (condylomata lata) develop in the intertrigenous areas (beneath the breasts, anus, axillae, and around the genitalia). Snail track ulcers may also be visible in the mucous membrane of the oral cavity by this stage.

The differential diagnosis of the rash can be broad and includes HIV seroconversion (see 'Mononucleosis' syndromes), pityriasis rosea (also follows skin cleavage lines), and guttate psoriasis. Definitive diagnosis includes identification of *Treponema pallidum* in fluid from a chancre by dark field microscopy or using serological tests. Treatment is with intramuscular (IM) benzathine benzylpenicillin, 2.4 million units, once only. Second-line treatment is doxycycline 100 mg PO twice daily for 14 days.

Rat bite fever

Rat bite fever ('Haverhill' fever) is a rare systemic illness transmitted by rodent bites. The causative organisms are *Streptobacillus moniliformis* or *Spirillum minor*. Fever, rash, and polyarthritis are the main clinical features. Penicillin or tetracycline (e.g. if allergic to penicillin) are effective.

Trench fever

Bartonella quintana, found in the excreta of the human body louse (*Pediculus humanus*), is the cause of trench fever and enters the circulation through broken skin. It is a disease that affects the homeless in western society. Patients complain of fever, myalgia, musculoskeletal pains, and a transient rash. The illness can last several weeks and may be the result of sustained or recurrent bacteraemia. Endocarditis can be a complication. The diagnosis is most easily confirmed serologically, but cross-reactivity between *B. quintana* and *B. henselae* (the cause of cat scratch disease) make definitive species identification difficult. Treatment is with azithromycin or doxycycline for 4 weeks. Patients with endocarditis may need longer courses or valve replacement.

Non-endemic infections

These are important causes of fever and maculopapular rash in the returning traveller from tropical and subtropical regions (see 'Fever in the returning traveller'). The rash of dengue fever may resemble 'sunburn', which blanches on pressure. The 'rose spots' of typhoid fever are most commonly seen on the trunk of fair-skinned individuals during the second week of illness. A careful search for a tick eschar (black scab) should be made in African tick typhus. This may be hidden in an obscure site where the tick has crawled, such as the axillae, groin, natal cleft, perineum, etc.

Non-infective causes

Drug reactions are a common cause of fever and rash. The cutaneous manifestations cross all categories, but the simple maculopapular type is most common. Frequently implicated drugs include penicillins, sulfonamides, phenytoin, and non-steroidal anti-inflammatory agents. Photosensitivity is caused by some drugs, e.g. tetracyclines, amiodarone, and thiazides. When examining a list of drugs likely to cause a reaction, drugs added within the last month are the most likely culprits. Amoxicillin-induced rashes appear 5–14 days after treatment is initiated and thus are often seen after a course of treatment has been finished. Amoxicillin frequently precipitates a rash in patients with glandular fever. The evanescent rash of Still's disease is described below (see 'Fever of unknown origin').

Widespread petechial and purpuric rashes

This group of rashes encompasses the most severe and life-threatening of infectious condition and always requires immediate attention.

Meningococcaemia

Acute meningococcaemia can occur in the absence of meningitis and presents as a severe sepsis syndrome with high fever. The non-blanching purpuric rash of meningococcaemia usually occurs on the extremities and evolves over hours. Petechiae coalesce to form ecchymoses, and the extent of the rash corresponds to the degree of thrombocytopenia resulting from disseminated intravascular coagulation (DIC).

Blood cultures are positive in ~50%, and Gram stains of skin lesions are positive in ~70%. Throat swabs to detect carriage are also useful in this setting. However, collection of specimens should never delay treatment, and a lumbar puncture does not need to be performed if a typical rash is present. Chronic meningococcaemia is much less common than the other syndromes and presents with fever, joint pain, and rash over days to weeks (skin lesions are most commonly maculopapular but may be petechial or pustular). The management of meningococcal sepsis is described in detail in Meningococcal disease later in this chapter.

Endocarditis

Petechiae can also be seen in patients with new regurgitant cardiac murmurs due to infective endocarditis. A search for other peripheral stigmata (e.g. Osler's nodes, Janeway lesions, and Roth spots) should be undertaken, although these will be absent in the vast majority. Microscopic haematuria may be detected on urine dipstick, and at least three sets of blood cultures should be obtained before starting antibiotic treatment.

Leptospirosis

If there is an appropriate history of exposure, leptospirosis should be considered, particularly if there is evidence of renal and liver failure (see 'Fever in the returning traveller'). The rash is a product of coagulopathy and immune-mediated vascular leak.

Non-endemic infections

These are covered in the following sections and include the viral haemorrhagic fevers, which characteristically have a high mortality. If a viral haemorrhagic fever is suspected, the case should be discussed immediately with a local infectious diseases expert. In addition, to prevent person-to-person transmission, there are specific infection control measures that should be instituted immediately and strictly adhered to.

The rash of rickettsial infections is the result of a cutaneous vasculitis, which may also become haemorrhagic or petechial. This is especially the case for Rocky Mountain spotted fever, which is frequently more severe than other rickettsial infections.

Vasculitides

These include Henoch–Schönlein purpura, polyarteritis nodosa, and Churg–Strauss syndrome. Henoch–Schönlein purpura is characterized by palpable purpura on the extensor surfaces of the limbs, especially ankles, buttocks, and elbows. There is associated glomerulonephritis (IgA nephropathy), polyarthritis involving large joints (knees and ankles), and abdominal pain.

Generalized vesicular and pustular rashes

Disseminated gonococcal infection

Less than 2% of gonococcal infections become disseminated. A characteristic syndrome of polyarthritis and dermatitis are the most predominant manifestations. The classic skin lesions are one or more crops of macules or papules, which subsequently become pustular. *Neisseria gonorrhoeae* is a relatively common cause of septic arthritis in young adults, particularly involving knees, elbows, wrists, and more distal joints. Often, ≥2 joints are involved, and the arthritis may be migratory. Gonococcal endocarditis was common in the pre-antibiotic era.

N. gonorrhoeae can be cultured directly from skin lesions or from blood (30%). Treatment of patients with the arthritis-dermatitis syndrome should be started with intravenous ceftriaxone 1 g daily. Immune complex deposition is partly responsible for arthritis, and, therefore, joint washout may not be required if there is a definite clinical improvement at 48 hours. At this point, therapy can be switched to oral ciprofloxacin 500 mg twice daily (alternatively, penicillins or tetracyclines, if sensitive) for a total of 7–10 days.

Impetigo and scalded skin syndrome (or Lyell's syndrome)

Impetigo is a very superficial skin infection on exposed skin areas (e.g. face and legs) and is characterized by the formation of large vesicopustules and secondary rupture with crusting. Impetigo is at the mild end of a spectrum of blistering skin diseases caused by an exfoliative toxin produced by *S. aureus*. The other extreme is represented by widespread painful blistering of the skin and superficial denudation (the staphylococcal scalded skin syndrome). Both are diseases of infants <5 years old.

Herpesviruses and poxviruses

These are examples of skin rashes that directly involve the virus itself. The vesiculopustular rash of herpes simplex is characteristically localized (e.g. genital herpes or herpetic whitlow). However, a severe and disseminated form can develop in patients with eczema (i.e. eczema herpeticum). Varicella is described in detail in the section Classic viral exanthems and mumps below.

Smallpox, monkeypox, and cowpox are all orthopoxviruses. Smallpox (variola virus) was eradicated from humans in 1977, but there is the fear that stocks of illegally held virus may be released as a biological weapon. Smallpox transmission is by contact with respiratory secretions and skin lesions. Papules first appear, which then develop into umbilicated vesicles, then pustules, and finally crusts. The rash is distinguished from chickenpox by the more peripheral distribution of lesions, including on the soles and palms. The lesions are also less superficial than in chickenpox and have a more uniform appearance since they do not arise in crops, leading to lesions at different stages of development. Mortality is ≤40%.

Cowpox is rare in the UK and transmitted by direct introduction of the virus from an animal source. Person-to-person transmission does not occur, and, despite the name, contact with the domestic cat is responsible for most infections. Monkeypox is confined to the tropical rainforests in western and central Africa.

Specific skin reactions and disorders

Erythema multiforme is regarded as a cutaneous reaction to a variety of agents, including drugs (e.g. phenytoin, sulphonamides, penicillins) and infections, most commonly herpes simplex and *Mycoplasma pneumoniae*.

The characteristic rash is symmetrically distributed on the extremities, with erythematous, coin-shaped 'target' lesions, which may blister and recur. No cause is found in 50%. Mucous membranes (eyes, mouth, and genitalia) may also become involved. Stevens–Johnson syndrome is the term used when the blistering and mucosal lesions are severe.

Toxic epidermal necrolysis is a more severe condition, characterized by widespread blistering and separation of the epidermis, resembling staphylococcal 'scalded skin syndrome' (as previously described).

Other dermatological syndromes that may have systemic features include pemphigus and pemphigoid.

Widespread macronodular skin lesions

Fungal infections

Skin lesions directly due to fungi are manifestations of disseminated infection and occur mainly in the immunocompromised host. Nodular, veruccous, or ulcerating skin lesions are caused by the non-endemic, dimorphic fungi (i.e. histoplasmosis, coccidiodomycosis, and blastomycosis) and are seen in patients with impaired cell-mediated immunity (see 'Fungal infections').

There is a wide range of skin manifestations (e.g. papules, pustules, ulcerations, and plaques) associated with disseminated cryptococcosis (see 'Fungal infections'). In particular, patients with HIV (CD4 <200 mm^3) may develop umbilicated lesions resembling molluscum contagiosum.

Fusarium is most common in the immunocompromised, with neutropenia being the strongest risk factor. The characteristic feature is erythematous, nodular, and ulcerated skin lesions.

Treatment includes voriconazole and amphotericin (there is intrinsic resistance to fluconazole, itraconazole, and echinocandins).

Erythema nodosum

Erythema nodosum is a focal panniculitis in the deep dermis and subcutaneous tissue. There are many precipitants, but these include reactions to: infection (e.g. *Streptococcus pyogenes* and *Mycobacterium tuberculosis*), sarcoidosis, inflammatory bowel disease, lymphoproliferative disorders, pregnancy, and various drugs (e.g. oral contraceptives, sulfonamides, etc.). Tender, raised lesions most frequently appear on the surface of the shins but, occasionally, the thighs and arms. Erythema nodosum is often accompanied by fever, malaise, and arthralgia but commonly resolves with bruising over 3 weeks.

Erythrodermic and miscellaneous rashes and skin lesions

Scarlet fever

Scarlet fever is mainly a disease of children and caused by infection with a specific pyrogenic exotoxin producing strains of *Streptococcus pyogenes* or group A *Streptococcus*. In some sense, it can be regarded as an abortive form of toxic shock syndrome, described below in Toxic shock syndrome. After an incubation period of 2–5 days, there is sore throat with fever. On the second day, a punctate erythematous rash develops, usually on the upper trunk first, which then becomes generalized over the next few hours to days. A characteristic sign is transverse red streaks at the site of skinfolds, which are due to capillary damage (Pastia's lines). Although the skin of the face is erythematous, there is circumoral pallor. Exudative tonsillitis is present, and a white coating appears on the tongue surface, through which red papillae protrude ('strawberry tongue'). A week later, there is desquamation on the hands and feet.

Therapy is aimed towards prevention of rheumatic fever and suppurative complications. Oral phenoxymethylpenicillin for 10 days is the treatment of first choice. Erythromycin is an alternative in penicillin-allergic patients.

Toxic shock syndrome

Toxic shock syndrome starts abruptly, and prominent initial symptoms include myalgia, fever, vomiting, and diarrhoea. Severe hypotension follows, and a deep red, erythematous ('sunburn') rash develops within a few hours and is accompanied by conjunctival injection. Multiorgan involvement is essential for diagnosis, including renal failure, hepatitis, thrombocytopenia, ARDS, and confusion without focal neurological signs. There is subsequent desquamation, especially on the palms and soles.

Toxic shock syndrome is caused by either *Staphylococcus aureus* (subdivided into menstrual and non-menstrual disease, also called 'staphylococcal scarlet fever') or *Streptococcus pyogenes* (associated with deep soft tissue infection, e.g. necrotizing fasciitis). Toxic shock syndrome toxin-1 (TSST-1) or enterotoxins produced by *Staphylococcus aureus* and pyrogenic exotoxins (scarlatina toxins, erythrotoxins) produced by *Streptococcus pyogenes* are responsible for the pathogenesis. Toxic shock syndrome is described in detail in the Toxic shock syndrome section later in this chapter.

Rheumatic fever

Rheumatic fever is an immunologically driven disease occurring after a group A streptococcal infection. Nowadays, the condition is rare in the UK, but erythema marginatum is a specific (but rare) feature. It consists of distinctive rings or arcs of erythema, which make discrete or enlarged polycyclic patterns. The rings fade over hours or days and then reappear at different sites of the body, over many weeks (hence the classic 'serpiginous' description of the rash).

Lyme disease

Ticks usually feed on blood from wild mammals and birds but may occasionally bite humans who visit woodland, heathland, or deer parks. *B. burgdorferi* is present in the tick (*Ixodes*) salivary gland, and bites that transmit infection are typically painless. Patients may, therefore, not recall a bite, but there should be a history of likely tick exposure (e.g. visiting the New Forest, South Downs, Lake District,

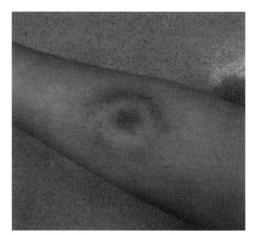

Figure 6.1 Rash of erythema migrans. The patient was bitten by a tick walking through a forest in Poland.

Exmoor, or the Scottish Highlands). Peak times of the year for tick bites are late spring and early summer.

There are two stages to infection. Three to 30 days after the tick bite, a characteristic rash of erythema migrans develops at the site of inoculation (patients may have removed ticks from the same place on their skin). The classic appearance is a large, flat, well-demarcated, erythematous lesion with central clearing (see Figure 6.1). Single lesions represent localized infection, but multiple lesions can result from haematogenous spread to other areas of skin. Systemic symptoms may be present, including malaise, fever, chills, arthralgia, myalgia, and headache. These features usually represent dissemination of infection around the body. Cardiac conduction defects, meningitis, and cranial nerve palsies may also occur at this time. There is usually spontaneous resolution after several weeks or months, but 'late' Lyme disease develops months after the initial bite and is the result of persistent infection. Features include chronic or recurrent arthritis and neurological syndromes of encephalopathy and polyneuropathy. Chronic skin changes called acrodermatitis chronicum atrophicans may also develop in the late phase.

The diagnosis of 'early' Lyme disease can be made clinically on the basis of a characteristic erythema migrans rash with a history of likely exposure. Interpretation of *Borrelia* serology can be difficult. However, serology is useful where a rash has recently faded or when 'late' Lyme disease is suspected. Oral doxycycline 100 mg twice daily or amoxicillin 500 mg three times daily for 14 days is effective treatment for patients with erythema migrans. Patients with 'late' Lyme disease require longer treatment courses (3–4 weeks). Except for isolated facial nerve palsy, which can be treated with an oral regimen, central or peripheral nervous system involvement is treated with parenteral antibiotics (e.g. intravenous ceftriaxone 2 g daily). A single prophylactic dose of doxycycline 200 mg taken ≤72 hours after a tick bite from a known endemic area is effective in preventing the development of Lyme disease.

Leprosy

Leprosy now only occurs in developing countries with a warm climate (e.g. Asia, Africa, and South America). *Mycobacterium leprae* is the causative organism, and transmission is by the respiratory route from aerosols produced by patients with nasal discharge. Bacilli cannot pass through intact skin.

Clinical disease ranges from tuberculoid to lepromatous leprosy. The pattern of illness is principally determined by the strength of the cell-mediated immune response, but subclinical disease is far more common than overt infection.

- **Tuberculoid leprosy**. There are well-demarcated, hypopigmented skin patches located anywhere on the body. Sensation of pain and temperature is lost over these lesions, and thickened peripheral nerves are palpable, e.g. ulnar, radial, lateral popliteal, posterior tibial, and great auricular nerves.
- **Lepromatous leprosy**. There are widespread nodular, macular, and plaque-like skin lesions, which appear erythematous and inflamed. Diffuse sensory loss may occur. Patients can be systemically unwell with fever and nasal congestion. Blindness may also occur from direct bacillary invasion or hypersensitivity (most commonly an iridocyclitis).
- **Borderline leprosy** is a mixed form, but the disease is unstable and may shift either way along the spectrum. In addition, inflammatory skin reactions can develop spontaneously, which may be localized ('reversal' reactions) or generalized (e.g. erythema nodosum leprosum).

Antimicrobial treatment depends on the clinical subtype and may involve rifampicin, clofazimine, and dapsone, given for months to years. Steroids are given for intense inflammatory reactions or eye involvement.

Tuberculosis

Skin involvement can be the result of direct skin invasion from an underlying infected structure, e.g. lymph nodes (called scrofula) or bone, and appears as a purple nodule. More rarely, it develops as multiple papular lesions, following haematogenous spread in miliary TB.

The tuberculides are a group of cutaneous inflammatory reactions to distant mycobacterial antigen. These include erythema nodosum (as described previously), Bazin's disease or erythema induratum (i.e. nodular and ulcerated lesions on the calves), papulonecrotic tuberculid (i.e. widespread necrotic papules with crusting), and lichen scrofulosum (i.e. minute lichenoid papules on the limbs, rather than trunk).

Cutaneous ulcerations

Cutaneous anthrax is caused by entry of *Bacillus anthracis* spores through breaks in the skin, particularly after contact with infected herbivores (e.g. goats, sheep, cattle, horses, swine, and deer) or their hair, wool, and skin. Sporadic cases are very rare in the UK and sometimes associated with occupational exposure (e.g. working with imported animal hides). An outbreak in intravenous drug users was reported in the UK in 2010, caused by sharing contaminated heroin. A painless, black eschar develops at the site of bacterial entry, with an incubation period of 1–7 days. Prominent surrounding oedema is a characteristic finding.

Gram stain, microscopy (i.e. spore-forming Grampositive rods), and culture of skin lesion samples are diagnostic. Cutaneous anthrax has a mortality rate of up to 20%, and treatment success depends on early recognition. Penicillin, doxycycline, or ciprofloxacin are effective in cutaneous infections.

Other ulcerations associated with an acute systemic illness include tularaemia and ecthyma gangrenosum. Tularaemia is distributed throughout much of North America (especially the south central and western states) and Eurasia. *Francisella tularensis* is the causative bacterium and is transmitted to humans by handling infected rodents or from a tick bite. Ecthyma gangrenosum occurs in neutropenic patients with *Pseudomonas aeruginosa* bacteraemia.

Chronic ulcerations without systemic symptoms include cutaneous leishmaniasis and Buruli ulcer (*Mycobacterium ulcerans*). Cutaneous leishmaniasis is geographically distributed in Central and South America, parts of Africa, India, and the Middle East. Buruli ulcer is endemic in tropical climates, particularly Africa.

Cellulitis associated with specific exposure risks

- Cellulitis associated with dog, cat, and human bites contain a variety of anaerobic organisms, e.g. *Pasteurella multocida* (associated with cat and, less commonly, dog bites) and *Capnocytophaga canimorsus* (dog bites). *Pasteurella multocida* is resistant to flucloxacillin but sensitive to other beta-lactams; in addition, it is sensitive to tetracyclines, macrolides, and quinolones. Co-amoxiclav is a good choice for human or animal bites.
- *Aeromonas hydrophila* can cause an aggressive form of cellulitis, following skin injuries and lacerations occurring in freshwater lakes and streams. It is sensitive to quinolones, co-trimoxazole, aminoglycosides, and third-generation cephalosporins.
- *Mycobacterium marinum* can contaminate water fleas (*Daphnia*) in fish food and cause cellulitis or granulomas, following cuts and abrasions on the skin surfaces exposed to water in aquariums or following injuries in swimming pools. Systemic features of infection are frequently absent. Rifampicin plus ethambutol are effective, but there are many suggested regimens and no comparative trials of efficacy.
- *Vibrio vulnificus* is part of the normal marine flora in temperate climates and can cause severe cellulitis if wounds are exposed to sea or brackish water. Treatment is surgical debridement and abscess drainage, combined with doxycycline or cefotaxime therapy.
- *Pseudomonas aeruginosa* causes cellulitis in burn wounds. Treatment depends on the antimicrobial sensitivity pattern and includes the use of quinolones, ceftazidime, carbapenems, and aminoglycoside antibiotics.

Kawasaki disease

Kawasaki disease is an acute febrile condition, usually affecting children <5 years, and is characterized by a polymorphic rash (e.g. morbilliform, scarlatiniform, urticariform, or erythema multiforme-like), painful cervical lymphadenopathy, conjunctival injection, and mucocutaneous changes causing red lips. Although most common in Japan, it has been reported all over the world. Many infectious agents have been implicated (e.g. viruses, *Rickettsia*, streptococci, staphylococci, etc.), but, in most cases, none is found. The fever lasts for more than 5 days, and, when it settles, there is desquamation of the skin, and the child may develop arthralgia. Cardiac complications also occur.

Further reading

Mygland A, Ljostad U, Fingerle V, Rupprecht T, Schmutzhard E, Steiner I; European Federation of Neurological Societies (2010). EFNS guidelines on the diagnosis and management of European Lyme neuroborreliosis. *European Journal of Neurology*, **17**, 8–16.

Wormser GP, Dattwyler RJ, Shapiro ED, *et al.* (2006). The clinical assessment, treatment, and prevention of Lyme disease, human granulocytic anaplasmosis and babesiosis: clinical practice guidelines by the Infectious Diseases Society of America. *Clinical Infectious Diseases*, **43**, 1089–134.

Hospital-acquired (nosocomial) infections

Hospital-acquired infections (HAI) are an increasingly important cause of morbidity and mortality on medical and surgical wards, high dependency units, and in nursing homes. The prevalence (3–12%) varies between settings and institutions (i.e. higher on intensive care units and in teaching hospitals). Hospital-acquired pneumonia, wound infection, and bacteraemia increase average hospital length of stay by ~12–14 days.

Causative organisms (see Table 6.4) are often virulent, antibiotic-resistant, and spore-forming, features which impede environmental eradication and encourage recurrent infection. Frequent causes are meticillin resistant *Staphylococcus aureus* (MRSA), *Clostridium difficile*, and multidrug-resistant (MDR) Gram-negative bacilli (e.g. *Pseudomonas*).

Commonest sites of infection are:

- Urinary tract (~40%).
- Surgical wounds (~15–20%).
- Respiratory tract (~15–20%).
- Line-related bacteraemia (~10%).
- Colitis (<10%).

Risk factors are listed in Table 6.5 and include host, environmental, and pathogen-related factors. Prevention of HAI requires identification and isolation of carriers of causative organisms, elimination of reservoirs, prevention of transmission, and appropriate antibiotic usage.

In order to limit the emergence and spread of resistant organisms, antibiotics must be used rationally and sparingly:

- They should only be prescribed when clearly indicated.
- Use narrow-spectrum agents whenever possible.

Table 6.5 Risk factors for nosocomial infection

Patient factors
- Underlying disease (e.g. SLE, diabetes)
- Nutritional status, immunosuppression (e.g. steroids)
- Multiple or prolonged antibiotic use (i.e. resistance)
- Integrity of natural defences (e.g. lines, wounds, burns)

Environmental factors
- Inadequate infection control (e.g. hand washing, isolation)
- Inadequate or inexperienced staff
- Iatrogenic infection (i.e. line insertions)
- Transmission (e.g. overcrowding, prolonged stay)

Organism factors
- Prevalence, resilience (e.g. spore formation), colonization
- Antibiotic resistance and selection
- Pathogenicity

- Treat for short periods (e.g. 5 days).
- Avoid unnecessary treatment of colonization.
- Use of prophylactic antibiotics must be carefully controlled.

Line-related sepsis

Line-related sepsis is a common and preventable cause of HAI and is discussed in the Vascular access device-associated infection section below. Five days after insertion of central venous catheters (CVC), about 10–20% are colonized and 2–5% develop bacteraemia. The average bacteraemia rate for CVC is ~5 per 1,000 CVC days but varies

Table 6.4 Organisms responsible for most HAI infections

• Meticillin-resistant *Staphylococcus aureus* (MRSA)	Rising prevalence. Colonizes and infects. Easily treated, but glycopeptide resistance is increasing
• Coagulase-negative *Staphylococcus* (CNS)	Frequent skin colonization. Low virulence organisms. Increasing cause of nosocomial infections
• *Enterococcus faecalis* (vancomycin-resistant *Enterococcus* (VRE))	Emerge with third-generation cephalosporin use. Often sensitive to ampicillin but resistance to aminoglycosides, ampicillin, and vancomycin increasing (e.g. VRE)
• *Pseudomonas aeruginosa*	Broad spectrum of antibiotic resistance. Common in ICU and chronic lung disease
• *Stenotrophomonas maltophilia*	Environmental organism. Increasingly common. Broad spectrum of antibiotic resistance
• *Acinetobacter baumanii*	Increasingly common. Resistant to antibiotics but may be sensitive to carbapenems
• *Klebsiella* spp.	Extended beta-lactam resistance ± multi-resistant to antibiotics
• *Enterobacter* spp.	Occur in normal intestinal flora and develop extended beta-lactam resistance
• *E. coli*	Variable resistance seems to correspond with use of quinolones
• *Proteus* spp., *Serratia marcescens*	Broad spectrums of antibiotic resistance
• *Clostridium difficile*	Spore-forming, antibiotic-resistant bacillus that colonizes the intestine in hospital patients
• *Candida* spp.	Overgrowth due to antibiotic pressures. Diagnosis suggested by growth in >2 sites

between patients (e.g. burns, surgical), severity of illness, CVC type (e.g. urgent, tunnelled, insertion site, antibiotic/silver impregnation), and the environment (e.g. medical ward, critical care units). Long, antecubital peripheral venous catheters (PVC; >12 cm) are associated with bacteraemia on 0.8 per 1,000 catheter days, and short PVC (i.e. <12 cm) are even less, although local phlebitis is common. Peripheral intra-arterial lines (e.g. radial) are less frequently colonized (~4–5% 5 days after insertion), and bacteraemia occurs on 2.9 per 1,000 catheter days. The commonest organisms associated with line-related infections are *S. epidermidis* (~35%), *S. aureus* (~15%), and Gram-negative bacilli (e.g. *E. coli*; ~15%).

Risk factors for line infection are listed in Box 6.1. Factors that prevent line infection include strict aseptic insertion technique (i.e. handwashing, mask, sterile gown, gloves, drapes), appropriate assistance during line insertion (i.e. to maintain sterility), good skin antisepsis (i.e. 2% aqueous chlorhexidine to clean skin and allow to dry), the type of cannulae (i.e antimicrobial or antiseptic-impregnated CVC (e.g. silver) catheters), insertion site (as above), a firmly secured cannula (i.e. movement risks infection), use of transparent dressings to allow regular line inspection (i.e. for signs of local infection), and good line management with use of closed systems, cleansing of access ports with 70% alcohol, and avoidance of 3-way tap contamination. Total parenteral nutrition must always be given through a dedicated CVC lumen, and administration sets should be replaced at ≥72 h, unless used to administer lipid, blood, or blood products when they should be changed at 24 h.

Timing of line replacements

Peripheral venous catheters should be changed at 72–96 hours. Regular scheduled CVC and arterial line replacements do not reduce line-related bacteraemia and are not required for normally functioning catheters with no evidence of local or systemic complications. Lines must be inspected daily for signs of insertion site infection and replaced if infection is suspected. All intravenous lines should be removed promptly when no longer needed. Line replacement, particularly CVC lines, is associated with a surprising number of complications (e.g. pneumothorax, haemorrhage), and the risk to benefit ratio must always be considered.

Management

If line-related infection is suspected (i.e. sepsis ± positive blood cultures), remove the line, and send the tip for culture. If needed, new lines should be inserted at different sites (i.e. placement of a new line over a guidewire at a previous insertion site risks reinfection). Empiric antibiotic therapy is usually started whilst awaiting microbiology results. However, fever and symptoms often resolve spontaneously after line removal.

Meticillin-resistant *Staphylococcus aureus*

Meticillin-resistant *Staphylococcus aureus* (MRSA) infection has rapidly increased over the last 5–10 years. Although largely associated with hospital and residential homes, it is increasingly common in community settings. Community MRSA is partly due to 'silent' healthcare acquisition during the previous year. Once MRSA is established within healthcare environments, it is difficult to eradicate.

Prevention

Prevention depends on identification and isolation of carriers of MRSA, elimination of potential reservoirs, prevention of transmission, and protocol-driven antibiotic usage to prevent development. Unrecognized MRSA carriage (e.g. asymptomatic skin colonization) is present in about 3% of hospital patients and about 30% of ICU admissions and constitutes the main reservoir and source of hospital transmission. Antibiotic restriction policies and protocols, combined with reduced usage and avoidance of some antibiotics (e.g. quinolones, cephalosporins), decreases MRSA infection rates.

Detection

Detection requires active surveillance, especially in high-risk patients. These include patients over 75 years old, those treated with antibiotics within the last 6 months, patients hospitalized within the last year, those with a urinary catheter at admission, and especially patients on critical care units. Early diagnosis, using rapid molecular screening techniques, and prompt patient isolation reduce MRSA acquisitions.

Decolonization

Decolonization aims to reduce MRSA carriage, an important risk factor for subsequent infection and transmission. Although intranasal mupirocin and chlorhexidine-based skin cleaning are commonly used, evidence for benefit is limited. However, environmental cleaning and disinfection may be effective.

Antibiotic therapy

MRSA may be resistant to fluoroquinolones (~80%), macrolides (~70%), trimethoprim (~35%), gentamicin (12%), and mupirocin (12%).

Most MRSA isolates are susceptible to tetracycline, fusidic acid, and rifampicin. Treatment with vancomycin, teicoplanin, and linezolid should be reserved for patients with severe line-related or neutropenic sepsis, burns, serious soft tissue infections, and prosthetic valve infections.

A minimum treatment period of 14 days is required for bacteraemia and longer in endocarditis. Vancomycin and teicoplanin levels must be monitored to ensure therapeutic levels and avoid toxicity. Tetracyclines, trimethoprim, and combinations of rifampicin and fusidic acid are effective in cellulitis, urinary and respiratory tract infections, and as part of eradication therapy. Inadequate therapy may contribute to excess mortality in critically ill patients.

Clostridium difficile

C. difficile is a ubiquitous, Gram-positive, anaerobic, motile, spore-forming bacillus that colonizes the intestines of nursing home or long-stay hospital patients. Acquisition is estimated to occur in ~13% of patients with a hospital stay of up to 2 weeks, and in ~50% of those with hospital stays longer than 4 weeks. It is resistant to most antibiotics and forms heat and disinfectant resistant spores. Consequently, *C. difficile* survives for long periods in hospital environments. Fortunately, bleach-containing disinfectants destroy the organism.

C. difficile induced diarrhoea has been linked to the use of certain broad-spectrum antibiotics, including cephalosporins, clindamycin, and especially quinolones (e.g. ciprofloxacin).

Clinical features

Spores are transmitted by the faecal-oral route. Following ingestion, they pass through the stomach because they are acid-resistant, and then change to their active form and multiply in the colon. In small numbers, *C. difficile* does not cause significant disease, but, after disruption of normal intestinal flora by broad-spectrum antibiotic therapy (especially quinolones, cephalosporins), overgrowth may cause a spectrum of symptoms. These range from asymptomatic colonization to severe, life-threatening diarrhoea with pseudomembranous colitis and, occasionally, bowel perforation. Pathogenic *C. difficile* produces toxins responsible for the diarrhoea and inflammation. The best characterized of these are enterotoxins (toxin A) and cytotoxin (toxin B).

Diagnosis

Diagnosis is based on clinical features (e.g. odorous diarrhoea, antibiotic exposure), detection of toxins A + B, and characteristic CT scan features (e.g. colonic wall thickening >4 mm, pericolonic stranding, ascites, and colon wall nodularity). Toxin assessment is by enzyme-linked immunoabsorbent assay (ELISA). It is important to test for both toxins, as some hospital strains only express toxin B. Delayed diagnosis risks bowel perforation and increases mortality.

Treatment

In symptomatic patients, the initial choice of drugs to eliminate *C. difficile* is oral metronidazole (500 mg three times daily). Oral vancomycin (125 mg four times daily) is second-line therapy and can be used in severe disease, if metronidazole is ineffective or the organism is resistant to metronidazole, and in pregnant patients. There is a theoretical risk of converting intestinal flora into vancomycin-resistant organisms. Linezolid may also be used. In relapse, the addition of rifampicin to vancomycin may be effective. Asymptomatic patients may not require antibiotic therapy.

Antidiarrhoeal drugs (e.g. loperamide) are contraindicated, as they prolong toxin-induced colonic damage. Probiotics (i.e. 'good' intestinal flora) may be beneficial and help prevent relapse. Colestyramine (4 g daily) binds toxin and slows bowel motility, which may reduce dehydration. Intravenous immunoglobulin is a last resort treatment in immunocompromised patients. Colectomy may be required in patients who develop systemic symptoms of *C. difficile*.

Prevention

Prevention includes avoiding inappropriate antibiotic therapy (especially in the elderly), the use of gloves, and appropriate infection control measures to reduce transmission. The value of prophylactic probiotics has not been established.

Prognosis

Normally, only 1–5% of affected patients develop severe disease leading to colectomy, intensive care, or death. The elderly and immunocompromised are most at risk. However, there have been a number of recent hospital outbreaks, with particularly virulent strains (e.g. Quebec strain), which cause increased morbidity and mortality (~5–10%).

Urinary tract infections

Urinary tract infections (UTI) account for about 40% of all nosocomial infections, but mortality rates are generally low. UTI can follow introduction of perineal organisms into the bladder during catheterization. Although mortality rates are low, aseptic catheterization, closed unobstructed drainage, and a well-secured catheter to prevent movement and patient discomfort reduce infection risk.

Wound infection

Wound infections account for about 15–20% of all nosocomial infections and are usually caused by autogenous infection at the time of surgery. Risk factors include:

- **Type of surgery.** In clean elective surgery, the incidence of infection should be less than 10%. In prolonged or 'dirty' procedures (e.g. bowel surgery), the incidence is ~15%. In contaminated (e.g. bowel perforation) or 'already infected' surgery, wound infection may occur in 20–40%.
- **Surgical ability.** Rates are higher for junior surgeons.
- **Host factors.** Wound infection is more common in the elderly and poorly nourished and those with diabetes, renal failure, or receiving steroids.
- **Prophylactic antibiotic use** is controversial, but there is some evidence for reduction of secondary or wound infections in 'dirty' or potentially contaminated procedures.

Infection is heralded by fever, pain, redness, or cellulitis around the wound site and purulent discharge. Commonly implicated organisms include *S. aureus*, streptococci, *E. coli*, enterococci, *P. aeruginosa*, and *Enterobacter* spp.

Norovirus

Norovirus, also known as the Norwalk agent/virus, winter vomiting disease, stomach flu, viral gastroenteritis, and snow mountain virus, is an RNA virus of the Calicividae virus family. It is a small, round structured virus (SRSV), 35 nm in diameter, found in 'used' water and concentrated in shellfish, oysters, and plankton.

Norovirus was first identified as the cause of epidemic gastroenteritis in 1972 by immune electron microscopy of stored stool samples from an outbreak at Bronson elementary school in Norwalk, Ohio in 1968. There are five genogroups, of which GI, GII, and GIV infect humans, but GII, genotype 4 (GII.4), causes the majority of epidemic outbreaks in adults. Susceptibility is linked to human blood type, and individuals with blood type O are more often infected than those with blood types B and AB which confer some protection against symptomatic infection.

Norovirus accounts for about 90% of worldwide epidemic non-bacterial outbreaks of gastroenteritis, and it is responsible for about 50% of food-borne outbreaks of gastroenteritis in the USA. Annually, there are ~250 million cases worldwide and 0.6–1 million cases in the UK. Outbreaks often occur in closed communities, including hospitals, nursing homes, prisons, cruise ships, and military camps where infection spreads rapidly from person to person (~80%) or through contaminated food (~20%). In 2004, there were 148 outbreaks in England and Wales, of which 110 were in hospitals or residential homes.

The norovirus is highly contagious, with as few as ten virus particles being able to cause infection. Transmission is mainly by the faecal-oral route but may be airborne due to aerosolization of vomit, with infection occurring after eating food prepared near to a site of vomiting (even if carefully cleaned up). Many outbreaks have been traced to food that was handled by a single infected person. The source of water-borne outbreaks includes wells, lakes, swimming pools, municipal water supplies, and ice-making machines. Shellfish and salad ingredients (i.e. washed in infected water) are the most common food sources. The viruses continue to be shed for many weeks after symptoms have subsided.

Handwashing is an effective method to reduce the spread of norovirus pathogens. They are also rapidly killed by heat and chlorine-based disinfectants but are less susceptible to alcohols and detergents, as they do not have lipid capsules.

Following infection, rapid multiplication of norovirus occurs in the small intestine. Acute gastroenteritis develops 1–2 days after infection. Associated symptoms include nausea, vomiting (often projectile), watery diarrhoea (without blood), abdominal cramps, and, occasionally, loss of taste lasting for 12–60 hours, although the diarrhoea may last a little longer. General weakness, lethargy, muscle aches, headache, low-grade fever, and, very occasionally, seizures may occur. Severe illness is rare, and most patients do not need admission to hospital. However, 300 deaths occur annually in the USA and 80 in England and Wales, usually in the elderly, very young, or immunosuppressed, especially if dehydration is inadequately managed. Unfortunately, immunity is short-lived (~14 weeks), and reinfection can occur at any age, although multiple infections do confer some protection against future episodes.

Diagnosis of norovirus infection is routinely made by polymerase chain reaction (PCR) or real-time PCR assays on stool samples, which give a result within hours. These assays are very sensitive and can detect concentrations as low as 10–15 virus particles. Commercially available enzyme-linked immunosorbent assay (ELISA) tests lack specificity and sensitivity.

Treatment, other than oral fluids, is usually unnecessary. Intravenous fluids and electrolyte replacement may be required in the elderly or very young. Antiemetics and anti-diarrhoeals are rarely necessary. Hand hygiene is vital, and infected patients should not prepare food for others for at least 3 days. Environmental cleaning with bleach, especially in bathrooms and kitchens, is important to prevent spread. Hospital outbreaks are shortened when wards are closed to new admissions within 4 days of the beginning of an outbreak and strict hygiene measures (e.g. barrier nursing) are implemented.

Vancomycin-resistant *Enterococcus*

Enterococci (e.g. *Enterococcus faecalis*, *Enterococcus faecium*) are Gram-positive coccoid-shaped bacteria, usually found in the digestive and urinary tracts of most humans, which occasionally cause infection (e.g. urinary tract, wound). They are amongst the most antibiotic-resistant bacteria isolated from humans, and, in 1986, the first vancomycin-resistant enterococci (VRE) was described. The genetic material that confers this resistance was probably acquired from other bacteria that do not cause human disease. Currently, there are six types of VRE, of which three types occur in clinical practice. Van-A is resistant to vanco-

mycin and teicoplanin; Van-B is resistant to vancomycin, but sensitive to teicoplanin, and Van-C is partly resistant to vancomycin and sensitive to teicoplanin.

Enterococci cause one in eight hospital infections, of which about 30% are due to VRE. Transmission is usually by the oro-faecal route and can be reduced by isolation, barrier nursing, and good hand and environmental hygiene.

VRE can be carried by healthy people who have come into contact with the bacteria, particularly in hospital. Intensively farmed chickens and farm animals also frequently carry VRE, and humans may acquire asymptomatic intestinal colonization after eating meat from these animals. Following admission to hospital, antibiotic pressure can cause VRE overgrowth, infection, and spread (e.g. bacteraemia). Restricting antibiotic use (including in veterinary practice) may also decrease the risk of VRE development.

VRE cause the same range of infections (e.g. urinary tract, bacteraemia, wound infection) as vancomycin-sensitive enterococci and are no more likely to cause infection. They are common in patients who have been in hospital for long periods and who have been treated with certain antibiotics, including cephalosporins, vancomycin, and teicoplanin, or fed via nasogastric tubes.

In normal healthy people, illness due to VRE is rare despite colonization. However, the risk of symptomatic infection is increased in the immunocompromised, following major surgery and in those treated with prolonged antibiotic courses or with long-term urinary catheters or central venous lines. Outbreaks of VRE infection have been reported from transplant, haematology, renal dialysis, and intensive care departments.

The range of antibiotics available for treating VRE infections is limited, and effective treatment may be delayed whilst awaiting laboratory antibiotic sensitivities. Potentially effective antibiotics include penicillins (e.g. ampicillin) and linezolid. New antibiotics effective against VRE are currently being developed. Asymptomatic colonization does not usually require treatment, and many cases will spontaneously clear over a period of time. *Lactobacillus rhamnosus* GG (LGG) is a Gram-positive facultative anaerobic bacterium that is able to survive stomach acid and intestinal bile, and when used as a probiotic, was reported to successfully treat gastrointestinal carriage of VRE in renal patients in 2005.

Further reading

Cooper BS, Stone SP, Kibbler C, *et al.* (2004). Isolation measures in the hospital management of methicilin resistant *Staphylococcus aureus* (MRSA): systemic review of the literature. *BMJ*, **329**, 533–41.

Edgeworth JD, Treacher DF, Eykyn SJ (1999). A 25-year study of nosocomial bacteraemia in an adult intensive care unit. *Critical Care Medicine*, **27**, 1421–8.

Loo VG, Poirier L, Miller MA, *et al.* (2005). A predominantly clonal multi-institutional outbreak of *Clostridium difficile*-associated diarrhea with high morbidity and mortality. *New England Journal of Medicine*, **353**, 2442–9.

Lorente L, Henry C, Martin MM, *et al.* (2005). Central venous catheter-related infection in a prospective and observational study of 2,595 catheters. *Critical Care*, **9**, 631–5.

Manley KJ, Fraenkel MB, Mayall BC, *et al*, (2007). Probiotic treatment of vancomycin-resistant enterococci: a randomized controlled trial. *Medical Journal of Australia*, **186**, 454–57.

Mascini EM, Troelstra A, Beitsma M, *et al.* (2006). Genotyping and preemptive isolation to control an outbreak of vancomycin-resistant Enterococcus faecium. *Clinical Infectious Diseases*, **42**, 739–46.

Nelson R (2007). Antibiotic treatment for *Clostridium difficile*-associated diarrhea in adults. *Cochrane Database of Systematic Reviews*, **3**, CD004610.

Newsom SWB (2004). MRSA - Past present and future. *Journal of the Royal Society of Medicine*, **97**, 509–10.

Public Health England. Norovirus Working Party; an equal partnership of professional organisations (Health Protection Agency; British Infection Association; Healthcare Infection Society; Infection Prevention Society; National Concern for Healthcare Infections; NHS Confederation) (2012). Guidelines for the management of norovirus outbreaks in acute and community health and social care settings. <https://www.gov.uk/government/publications/norovirus-managing-outbreaks-in-acute-and-community-health-and-social-care-settings>.

Public Health England (2014). Norovirus: guidance, data and analysis. <https://www.gov.uk/government/collections/norovirus-guidance-data-and-analysis>.

Siebenga JJ, Vennema H, Zheng DP, *et al.* (2009). Norovirus illness is a global problem: Emergence and spread of Norovirus GII.4 variants, 2001–2007. *Journal of Infectious Diseases*, **200**, 802–12.

Traore O, Liotier J, Souweina B, *et al.* (2005). Prospective study of arterial and central venous catheter colonization and of arterial and central venous catheter-related bacteremia in intensive care units. *Critical Care Medicine*, **33**, 1276–80.

Vincent JL, Bihari DJ, Suter PM, *et al.* (1995). The prevalence of nosocomial infection in intensive care units in Europe. Results of the European Prevalence of Infection in Intensive Care (EPIC) study. EPIC International Advisory Committee. *JAMA*, **274**, 639–44.

Zar FA, Bakkanagari SR, Moorthi KM, *et al.* (2007). A comparison of vancomycin and metranidazole for the treatment of *Clostridium difficile* associated diarrhea, stratified by disease severity. *Clinical Infectious Diseases*, **45**, 302–7.

Classic viral exanthems and mumps

Measles (first disease)

Epidemiology

- Measles is caused by a morbillivirus (RNA virus), which belongs to the paramyxovirus family. Measles is one of the most infectious conditions known, and respiratory droplets are the main mechanism of transmission.
- Vaccination against MMR (measles, mumps, and rubella) was introduced in 1988 for children less than 5 years and has dramatically reduced the incidence of these viruses in the UK. However, measles, mumps, and rubella are increasingly seen in a susceptible cohort of young adults who were either not vaccinated (as they were too old when mass vaccination was introduced) or who received only one of the three doses needed for full protective immunity.

Clinical features

Incubation period is 8–12 days.
- The typical prodromal phase, lasting 3–4 days, starts with fever, cough, coryza, conjunctivitis, and pharyngitis. In the mouth, tiny white plaques that are pathognomonic of measles may be visible on the buccal mucosa (Koplik's spots).
- Around day 4, a maculopapular rash appears on the forehead. This spreads to involve the rest of the face and progresses down from head to feet over a period of 2–3 days. Large areas of the rash become confluent and then begin to fade away. Desquamation is sometimes seen afterwards.

Acute complications include those of secondary bacterial infection (e.g. pneumonia, otitis media) and meningoencephalitis (1 per 1,000 cases). Complications are more frequent and serious in adults. Hepatitis may be a prominent feature in adults. Infection may be more severe during pregnancy and is sometimes associated with fetal loss after 25 weeks' gestation.

Investigations

- The diagnosis is made clinically but confirmed serologically. Measles IgM appears at the same time as the rash.
- A PCR-based assay exists for diagnosis from saliva and urine.

Management

- Most cases require supportive care only, and the illness is self-limiting. Vitamin A supplementation is sometimes given, especially in the developing world where malnourishment is associated with more severe disease. Adult infection is generally more severe, and hepatitis can be a significant feature.
- Immune globulin (human normal immunoglobulin) is given to susceptible contacts, such as non-immune pregnant women, infants, and immunocompromised individuals. Measles has a suppressive effect on the cellular immune system for many months after acute infection. For example, this may mean that a tuberculin skin test is unreactive.
- Subacute sclerosing panencephalitis (SSPE) is a rare late complication, occurring after 1/100,000 episodes of measles and 1/1,000,000 vaccinations. SSPE is caused by chronic infection with the virus and develops several years after the initial attack.

Rubella (German measles, third disease)

Epidemiology

- Rubella is caused by a togavirus (RNA virus). Airborne transmission by respiratory droplets is responsible for the spread of rubella. After an attack, immunity is lifelong.
- Vaccination is highly effective, and rubella is rare in countries where vaccination is widespread.

Clinical features

Incubation period is 16–18 days, and subclinical infections are common. There is rarely any prodrome in children, but adults may have pharyngitis, fever, headache, eye pain, cough, and myalgia. Following this, a fine, rose-pink maculopapular rash that starts on the face and spreads to the distal extremities within 24 hours is classic. Patients may not feel or look particularly unwell. Post-auricular and suboccipital lymphadenopathy is often palpable. The rash fades after 3 days, but, during this time, polyarthralgia is often present and may last for several weeks.

Of note, there is a high risk of congenital rubella syndrome in non-immune pregnant women exposed to rubella. Features include cataract, microcephaly, deafness, congenital heart defects, mental retardation, and diabetes. The risk to the fetus is greatest during the first 12 weeks of gestation. Rubella is infectious 5 days before, and 5 days after, the rash develops.

Investigations

- Serology should be performed on a suspected case, and all women are routinely screened for rubella during early pregnancy.
- Rubella may also be cultured from nasopharyngeal secretions and other body fluids.

Management

- Rubella is usually a very mild illness, and recovery is the rule. There is no specific treatment.
- If active infection is identified in non-immune pregnant women before 16 weeks' gestation, termination of pregnancy may be discussed.
- Post-infectious encephalitis and immune thrombocytopenia are rare complications.

Parvovirus B19 (erythema infectiosum, fifth disease)

Epidemiology

- Parvovirus B19 is a DNA virus belonging to the parvoviridae family. Transmission is by droplet inhalation or direct contact with respiratory secretions.
- Children aged 6–10 years are particularly affected, and most infections occur before middle age. Immunity is lifelong.
- It is more common in winter or spring months.

Clinical features

Incubation period is 13–18 days. Parvovirus B19 is commonly asymptomatic in children. Symptomatic infection begins with a characteristic erythematous rash on the child's cheeks that looks as if they have been slapped, hence 'slapped cheek syndrome'. Fever is unusual. The rash then spreads to involve the rest of the body over the next 1–2 weeks and then fades away, with a particular lacy or reticular appearance on the legs as it fades.

In adults, the rash may be absent, but symmetrical arthralgia involving the hands, wrists, and ankles may develop. The rash and arthralgia are immunologically mediated and develop at the same time as specific IgM appears. Patients are no longer infectious when the rash develops.

In patients with chronic haemolytic anaemia, particularly sickle cell disease, an 'aplastic crisis' can result, lasting 1–2 weeks. This is associated with fever, chills, myalgia, malaise, arthralgia, and a maculopapular rash. Red cell production is temporarily halted, and the patient can become severely anaemic.

Chronic infection can develop in immunocompromised patients (including those infected with HIV). This is characterized by chronic persistent or recurrent episodes of anaemia, and the rash is usually absent.

Fetal death may result if pregnant women become infected. Congenital abnormalities do not occur.

Investigations
- Anaemia with a transient reduction in reticulocytes is characteristic of aplastic crises.
- Specific IgM may be absent in immunocompromised hosts, but viral DNA can be detected in blood by PCR.
- 'Giant' pronormoblasts may be seen in the bone marrow.

Management
- No specific treatment is available.
- Chronic B19 infection can persist for years in immunocompromised patients. Chronic anaemia may be treated with intravenous immunoglobulin.

Human herpesvirus-6 (sixth disease, roseola infantum)
Human herpesvirus-6 is the cause of exanthema subitum (or roseola infantum) in young children.

Characteristic features are fever, a mild respiratory illness, lymphadenopathy, and a fine, generalized maculopapular rash. It is a frequent cause of febrile convulsions in infants. The illness is short-lived, and full recovery is usual.

In adolescents and adults, primary infection can produce a self-limiting glandular fever-type syndrome.

Varicella-zoster (chickenpox, shingles)
Epidemiology
- Varicella-zoster virus (VZV) is transmitted by the respiratory route or contact with vesicle fluid from patients with chickenpox or shingles.
- VZV is responsible for two distinct clinical diseases: chickenpox (varicella), following primary infection, and shingles (zoster), resulting from reactivation of latent infection within dorsal root ganglia.
- 90% of UK adults have had chickenpox, the vast majority in childhood. VZV is highly contagious, and the attack rate within a household is 90%.
- After primary infection, up to 20% develop shingles at some point subsequently, usually in later life. Shingles occurs in ~10% of patients with HIV.

Clinical features of chickenpox (varicella)
- Incubation period is 10–21 days, and patients are infectious for 48 hours prior to the rash developing and afterwards, until every skin lesion has scabbed over (~5 days).
- Chickenpox is primarily a mild febrile illness of healthy children and characterized by the appearance of pruritic, erythematous maculopapules that initially appear on the face and trunk and progress through vesicular, pustular,

and crusting stages over a period of 3–4 days. New 'crops' appear, but rarely on the palms and soles, and skin lesions are typically at different stages of evolution. Ulcerating vesicles may also be seen on the oropharyngeal mucosa.

- In adults, varicella may be much more serious. Life-threatening pneumonitis (~1 in 400 cases) may develop, especially in smokers and pregnant women.
- Encephalitis (0.1–0.2%) is a life-threatening complication in adults (mortality up to 20%). Post-infectious cerebellar encephalitis may develop in children ≤15 years old (1/4,000 cases). Ataxia is the most frequent presentation and can appear as late as 21 days after the onset of rash. Complete recovery is usual.
- Immunocompromised patients develop disseminated infection with pneumonitis (most commonly), encephalitis, and hepatitis. The rash may become haemorrhagic, and healing of cutaneous lesions is delayed. Patients with lymphoproliferative malignancies and persons undergoing bone marrow transplantation are most at risk (mortality 15%).
- Chickenpox in early pregnancy may result in congenital malformations and fatal infection in the newborn if acquired 7 days before or after delivery.

Clinical features of shingles (zoster)
- The first symptom is usually pain or itching in the area of nerve where the virus is reactivating. An identical rash to that seen in chickenpox subsequently appears (commonly on the chest wall) but restricted to the distribution of a dermatome. Less commonly, more than one dermatome can be involved, but the painful rash never crosses the midline and is usually present for about a week.
- Depending on the branches affected, fifth (Vth; trigeminal) cranial nerve involvement may produce a sight-threatening keratitis (zoster ophthalmicus), in association with lesions on the eyelids and tip of the nose (1st and 2nd branches); or on the palate, tonsillar fossa, floor of mouth, and tongue (2nd and 3rd branches). Involvement of the geniculate ganglion of the seventh (VIIth; facial) cranial nerve (Ramsay Hunt syndrome) produces lesions in the external auditory meatus, ipsilateral facial palsy, and loss of taste to the anterior two-thirds of the tongue.
- Motor paralysis (anterior horn cell involvement) can cause paralysis akin to polio and is characteristically associated with severe neuropathic pain.
- Extracutaneous sites of reactivation include the CNS, resulting in encephalitis and meningoencephalitis. A rare manifestation is granulomatous cerebral angiitis, which usually follows zoster ophthalmicus.
- Cutaneous and visceral dissemination can occur in immunocompromised patients, but this is rarely fatal, unlike primary infection.
- If covered by clothing, shingles does not represent a significant infection control risk, and isolation is not needed.
- Post-herpetic neuralgia develops in 25–50% of patients >50 years old.

Investigations
- The diagnosis of chickenpox (or shingles) can usually be made clinically. However, scrapings from the base of vesicular lesions may enable a rapid identification of VZV by immunofluorescence or electron microscopy.

- The chest X-ray in chickenpox pneumonia shows small discrete opacities throughout both lungs and lesions, which may calcify after recovery.
- PCR analysis of CSF is useful in suspected VZV encephalitis.

Management

- In children, no treatment is required for varicella, apart from symptom relief.
- In adults with chickenpox, oral aciclovir 800 mg PO five times/day for 7 days, commenced ≤24 hours after onset of the rash, shortens the illness.
- All immunocompromised patients or chickenpox pneumonia should be treated with either intravenous aciclovir 10 mg/kg three times daily or oral valaciclovir 1 g three times daily for 7–10 days. Patients with encephalitis may need extended treatment.
- Zoster immunoglobulin is also given to immunocompromised patients and women without protective serum anti-VZV antibodies, who become exposed during pregnancy.
- Either aciclovir 800 mg five times daily orally for 7 days or valaciclovir 1 g three times daily orally for 7 days is given for shingles. The sooner treatment is started, the better, but there is little value in doing this after 72 hours of the rash onset. There is evidence that antiviral treatment may reduce the incidence of post-herpetic neuralgia.
- Urgent ophthalmological input should be sought if there is suspected involvement of the eye.

Enteroviruses

- Enteroviruses belong to the picornavirus group ('pico-' small RNA viruses). They include echoviruses and Coxsackie viruses, which are sometimes associated with exanthems. Spread is by the faecal oral route, and humans are the only natural reservoir.
- Most infections occur in children or young people (<20 years old). Infections are more common in summer and autumn. The incubation period for enterovirus infections is usually 2–10 days.
- Hand, foot, and mouth disease (Coxsackie A16) mainly affects young children. There are vesicles on the hands and feet, and ulcers in the mouth identical to herpangina (small red spots at the back of the mouth, progress to vesicles and then small (2-4 mm diameter), painful ulcers).
- Fever with maculopapular rash (i.e. rubelliform, morbilliform, and roseoliform) can occur in children. Occasionally, the rash may appear purpuric.

There is no specific antiviral therapy, and treatment is supportive.

Mumps

Epidemiology

- Mumps is an RNA virus belonging to the paramyxovirus family which causes mumps. Respiratory droplets and direct contact with infected saliva are the modes of transmission.
- Mumps is as contagious as influenza and rubella but not as infectious as chickenpox or measles.
- Mumps usually affects children and adolescents and was the commonest cause of viral meningitis in children before the introduction of MMR. In the last decade, there has been a 10-fold increase in mumps, 90% in those aged >15 years old due to inadequate vaccination (see section on measles).

Clinical features

- The incubation period is 17–19 days.
- Many infections are subclinical.
- Fever, headache, sore throat, myalgia, and, in two-thirds of cases, tender enlargement of the parotid glands develop. The fever and swelling resolve over 1–2 weeks.
- Some cases, especially in adolescents, may present with epididymo-orchitis (usually unilateral) or meningitis, without parotid swelling. Pancreatitis, oophoritis, deafness, and arthritis may also occur.

Investigations

- The diagnosis is made clinically and confirmed serologically.
- The virus can also be cultured in CSF, saliva, or urine.

Management

- A full recovery is usual. The treatment is entirely for symptoms, especially analgesia for orchitis, which may require opiate analgesics and cool compresses.
- Meningitis is self-limiting. Encephalitis is rare but can be fatal.
- Sterility following epididymo-orchitis is very uncommon.

Further reading

Gnann JW (2002). Varicella-Zoster virus; atypical presentations and unusual complications. *Journal of Infectious Diseases*, **186**, S91–8.

Tunbridge AJ, Breuer J, Jeffrey KJ, *et al.*, British Infection Society (2008). Chickenpox in adults—clinical management. *Journal of Infection*, **57**, 95–102.

'Mononucleosis' syndromes

Epstein–Barr virus (glandular fever, infectious mononucleosis)

Epidemiology

- Epstein–Barr virus (EBV) is a herpesvirus and the cause of glandular fever. Infection is by contact with the virus in infected saliva. Transmission is, therefore, direct, such as by kissing, or indirectly via contaminated hands.
- In western countries, 50% of children are infected by the age of 5 years old, but children in developing nations acquire the EBV earlier. Symptomatic infections occur most commonly in adolescents, and 90% of human beings have evidence of infection by adulthood.

Clinical features

Incubation period is 2–6 weeks. Infection in children is usually asymptomatic.

Primary infection presents with a prodrome of fever, tiredness, and malaise, followed by sore throat, fever, and lymphadenopathy. An exudative tonsillitis is seen, and petechiae may be visible on the palate. There is generalized lymphadenopathy and splenomegaly.

A skin rash develops in <10%, but, if patients are mistakenly given amoxicillin or ampicillin, a maculopapular rash develops in ≥90%. The illness usually resolves in 1–2 weeks, but, occasionally, the fever and fatigue may persist for longer.

Complications are exceptionally rare but include haemolytic anaemia, severe hepatitis, splenic rupture, myocarditis, Guillain–Barré syndrome, and meningoencephalitis.

Investigations

- Characteristic findings in the peripheral blood are a lymphocytosis and lymphocytes with an atypical appearance. Liver function tests often show a slight increase in serum transaminases.
- Heterophile antibodies may be detected rapidly (e.g. Paul Bunnell or Monospot test), but these tests are not specific, and, in 10–15%, heterophile antibodies do not develop.
- Specific EBV antibodies confirm acute infection.

Management

- There is no specific treatment other than symptomatic relief.
- Steroids are not recommended for uncomplicated illness but have been recommended in patients with impending airway obstruction, severe thrombocytopenia, or haemolytic anaemia.

Cytomegalovirus

Clinical features

Cytomegalovirus (CMV) is a herpes virus transmitted in body fluids (blood, semen, cervical fluids, urine, and saliva) by intimate or sexual contact. It is found worldwide, and approximately 50% of adults have antibodies in their blood, indicating previous infection. The vast majority of cytomegalovirus (CMV) infections are completely unnoticed.

- Symptomatic primary infection produces a febrile illness very similar to glandular fever ('CMV-mononucleosis'), but rash is not typical. Atypical lymphocytes on the blood film and lymphocytosis are also commonly seen. A mild hepatitis may also occur at the same time but can sometimes be the presenting feature. The fever may persist for a couple of weeks, but CMV-mononucleosis usually resolves spontaneously without any long-term sequelae. Diagnosis is confirmed by specific serology.
- Congenital infection occurs when mothers experience primary infection during pregnancy.
- Primary CMV or reactivation of latent infection can cause life-threatening diseases in the immunosuppressed host:
  - Pneumonitis, gastrointestinal disease, hepatitis, and retinitis usually develop ≤3 months post-transplantation. IV ganciclovir is the drug of choice. Valganciclovir is an oral alternative.
  - CMV can cause colitis, sight-threatening retinitis, and encephalitis in patients with advanced HIV infection. CMV retinitis should be managed in conjunction with an ophthalmologist, and an intravitreal ganciclovir implant may be given.

Other differential diagnoses

HIV seroconversion

- Incubation is 1–6 weeks after exposure, with a peak at 3 weeks.
- Presentation may be with pharyngitis, fever, widespread lymphadenopathy, splenomegaly, and, in two-thirds, a generalized macular skin rash. It may be indistinguishable from glandular fever in young adults, but lymphopenia (not lymphocytosis) is typical.
- Aseptic meningitis and diarrhoea can also be presenting features.

Primary toxoplasmosis

- Only 10–20% of primary infections are symptomatic.
- Patients present with enlarged lymph nodes, usually in the cervical region, but any or all lymph nodes may be involved. Often, there are no other symptoms, but malaise, sore throat, sweats, and a low-grade fever may be reported. There is no rash. Symptoms and lymphadenopathy may sometimes persist for many months.
- Serologic tests are the primary method of diagnosis in most cases. Toxoplasmosis may also be demonstrated in tissue samples obtained by biopsy.
- Congenital toxoplasmosis is acquired *in utero* when pregnant women become infected. Infection may be asymptomatic or produce signs present at birth, which include hydrocephalus, mental retardation, and chorioretinitis. The risk of severe disease is increased if infection occurs in the first trimester. Spiramycin should be given as soon as possible after the diagnosis is made.

Fungal infections

Fungi are ubiquitous in the environment, but few cause human infection. Fungal infection can be divided into two broad groups: 'opportunistic' fungi that cause infection in immunocompromised patients and 'pathogenic' fungi which cause systemic infection in immunocompetent hosts and more serious disseminated infections in the immunocompromised. Many pathogenic fungi have specific geographical distributions. They cause systemic 'granulomatous' infections.

'Opportunistic' fungal infections
Candidiasis
Candida is ubiquitous in the soil and a normal commensal of the mouth, gastrointestinal tract, and vagina. The vast majority of infections are local (e.g. oral or vaginal candidiasis) and are caused by *Candida albicans*. Disseminated candidiasis occurs in the immunocompromised host and may also involve other species derived from the patient's endogenous flora, e.g. *C. tropicalis, C. parapsilosis, C. krusei*, and *C. lusitaniae*.

Risk factors are neutropenia (especially acute leukaemia), organ transplantation (especially liver), burns, indwelling central venous catheters, intravenous drug use, gastrointestinal surgery, parenteral nutrition, and broad-spectrum antibiotic exposure. Candidaemia can be asymptomatic or present as septic shock with fever. Multiple microabscesses may be found in affected organs, such as the liver, spleen, kidneys, and brain. Visual disturbance should be taken very seriously, and every patient with candidaemia should be examined by an ophthalmologist to exclude endophthalmitis (~10%).

The diagnosis of disseminated candidiasis is usually made by positive blood cultures. Disseminated candidiasis is treated with azoles (e.g. fluconazole), echinocandins (e.g. caspofungin), or amphotericin. Fluconazole resistance may be encountered, especially in bone marrow transplantation units where fluconazole prophylaxis is used. Infected intravenous lines, which are frequently the portal of entry, should be removed.

Aspergillosis
Aspergillus species are found worldwide and grow in soil and moist decaying vegetation, such as compost piles or stored hay. Human disease is acquired by inhalation, and most infections are caused by *Aspergillus fumigatus*. The clinical feature of aspergillosis result from either an allergic response to fungal colonization (e.g. allergic bronchopulmonary aspergillosis) or various degrees of 'invasive' infection, discussed further in this section.

- Acute invasive pulmonary aspergillosis (see Figure 6.2a) occurs in patients with profound neutropenia (especially acute leukaemia), prolonged neutropenia (≥12 days), high-dose steroid therapy, advanced AIDS, and organ transplantation. Cough, haemoptysis, chest pain, and fever are the most common features. Nodular infiltrates are the most frequent finding on the chest X-ray (see Figure 6.2b). Pulmonary infarction is commonly followed by secondary cavitation. CT imaging (see Figure 6.2c), may show nodular infiltrates, cavitation, and an area of ground glass opacification around a pulmonary nodule (the 'halo sign'), which is highly suggestive of 'angioinvasive' aspergillosis. Culture of sputum or bronchoalveolar lavage samples only has a yield of ≤40%, and lung biopsy

may be required for definitive proof of infection (see Figure 6.2a). However, if suspected, treatment is started promptly since invasive aspergillosis may be rapidly progressive and fatal (mortality ≥20%). Detection of circulating antigen (e.g. galactomannan), specific antibody, or molecular assays have been incorporated into some diagnostic criteria, but these have variable performance and may not be readily available.

- Haematogenous dissemination may follow acute invasive pulmonary aspergillosis, especially to the brain, which can manifest as a single 'granuloma' or multiple abscesses. Other sites include skin, liver, kidneys, and spleen.
- Invasive sino-orbital aspergillosis is also observed in acute leukaemia and bone marrow transplantion and is the result of extension from infected sinuses. Features include fever, periorbital swelling, retro-orbital pain, and headache. Surgical debridement is often required, in addition to antifungal agents.
- Chronic necrotizing pulmonary aspergillosis is a semi-invasive form of infection, which occurs in patients with 'mild' immune suppression (e.g. diabetes mellitus, steroid therapy, alcoholism) and chronic lung disease (e.g. COPD). These conditions are slowly progressive and result in cavitation and aspergilloma formation within cavities. Patients present with fever, weight loss, cough, and haemoptysis. Surgical resection is required, in addition to antifungal agents.
- Intravenous (IV) amphotericin and voriconazole are the drugs of choice for invasive aspergillosis. Echinocandins can also be used.
- Aspergilloma result from heavy *Aspergillus* colonization of a pre-existing lung cavity produced, for example, by 'old' tuberculosis. Imaging may show the fungal ball within the cavity, producing an 'air crescent' sign. Erosion into the wall of the cavity can result in bleeding; consequently, haemoptysis is a common symptom. Haemoptysis is mostly minor and self-limiting, and patients are simply observed. Occasionally, massive haemoptysis is life-threatening. Antifungals have no proven role, and definitive treatment is surgical resection.

Cryptococcosis
Cryptococcus neoformans causes cryptococcosis. It is widely present in soil and pigeon droppings. Transmission is by inhalation, and risk factors for infection include HIV infection, steroid therapy, organ transplantation, leukaemia, and lymphoma. *C. neoformans* is the commonest cause of meningitis in patients with advanced HIV infection (CD4 count <100 cells/mm^3). More rarely, disseminated infection may involve other organs, such as the lungs and skin. The diagnosis is made by direct visualization of cryptococci in CSF stained with India ink and by culture. In patients with meningitis, cryptococcal antigen can be detected in serum (80–95%) and CSF (99%).

Initial treatment of cryptococcal meningitis in AIDS is with intravenous amphotericin 0.7 mg/kg plus flucytosine 25 mg/kg orally four times daily for 2 weeks. This is followed by long-term maintenance therapy with oral fluconazole 200–400 mg daily. Very elevated intracranial pressure causes coma and blindness and should be treated by repeated CSF removal to keep the CSF opening pressure ≤20 cmH$_2$O.

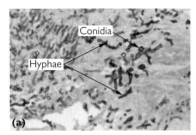

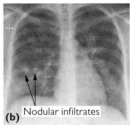

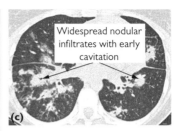

Figure 6.2a Bronchial biopsy histology showing invasive *Aspergillus* hyphae and conidia (*Aspergillus* spores) in an immunocompromised patient (cyclophosphamide therapy) with invasive aspergillosis.

Figure 6.2b Chest radiograph showing nodular infiltrates in pulmonary aspergillosis.

Figure 6.2c Chest CT scan showing nodular infiltrates with early cavitation in pulmonary aspergillosis.

Pneumocystis jirovecii

Pneumocystis jirovecii (formerly *Pneumocystis carinii*) almost never causes illness in healthy individuals but can cause a potentially fatal pneumonia in individuals with impaired cell-mediated immunity. In particular, until the widespread use of effective chemoprophylaxis, it occurred in up to 85% of patients with HIV infection (CD4 <200 mm^3). It is also a complication of haematological malignancies, organ transplantation, and immunosuppressive or cytotoxic therapy.

Characteristic clinical features include dry cough, breathlessness, and fever over a 1–2 week period. The classic radiological picture is bilateral infiltrates, extending outwards from the perihilar regions (see Figure 6.3). However, plain films can appear normal in early presentations and focal or lobar consolidation may be the presenting abnormality in a few cases. Exercise-induced oxygen desaturation at the bedside can demonstrate the presence of an interstitial barrier to gas diffusion produced by *Pneumocystis jirovecii*.

Examination of bronchoalveolar lavage or induced sputum samples with histochemical stains (typically silver stains, such as Grocott–Gomori methenamine silver stain) or immunofluorescent stains is highly sensitive for identifying *Pneumocystis jirovecii* in the setting of HIV (≥90%) and remains positive for 2–3 days after initiation of specific ther-

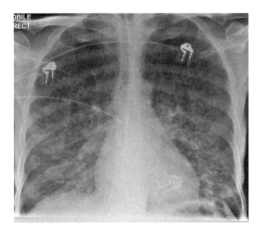

Figure 6.3 Diffuse alveolar infiltration on chest radiography in a HIV-positive patient presenting with *Pneumocystis jirovecii* pneumonia.

apy. In some centres, induced sputum sampling techniques approach the same sensitivity as bronchoalveolar lavage and are less invasive.

First-line therapy is with co-trimoxazole. Dosing for moderate to severe infection is 120 mg/kg/day for the first 3 days and 90 mg/kg/day for a further 18 days (the total daily dose may be divided into three or four times daily). Individuals with a PaO$_2$ <9.3 kPa (<70 mmHg) or O$_2$ saturation on room air <92% should initially receive oral prednisolone 40 mg twice daily, which is weaned down after day 5 (intravenous methylprednisolone is recommended if the patient is unable to take oral treatment). Adjunctive steroids are of greatest benefit when they are commenced within 72 hours of starting specific anti-*P. jirovecii* therapy. For mild to moderate infections, oral co-trimoxazole 1,920 mg tds for 21 days may be used.

There is little to choose from between the various second-line treatment regimens. For moderate to severe PCP, either intravenous clindamycin (600–900 mg tds or qds) or oral clindamycin (300–450 mg tds or qds) can be given, in addition to oral primaquine (15–30 mg daily), for a total of 21 days. Intravenous pentamidine (4 mg/kg daily) is an alternative, but many favour clindamycin-based therapy because of the toxicity associated with pentamidine.

In mild to moderate disease, other oral options include trimethoprim (20 mg/kg/day) and dapsone (100 mg daily) for 21 days. Atovaquone liquid suspension (750 mg twice daily) for 21 days is another alternative. It should be noted that G6PDH levels should be checked prior to co-trimoxazole, dapsone, or primaquine use, but, if co-trimoxazole therapy needs to be started immediately, levels should be determined as soon as possible.

Mucormycosis

Mucormycosis refers to a spectrum of conditions caused by filamentous fungi belonging to the order *Mucorales*. The most common agents are *Rhizopus*, *Rhizomucor*, *Absidia*, and *Cunninghamella*. Risk factors include poorly controlled diabetes (especially after diabetic ketoacidosis), acute leukaemia with prolonged neutropenia, organ transplantation, iron overload states and therapy with desferrioxamine or steroids. Rhinocerebral mucormycosis occurs following inhalation of spores. A rapidly progressive, invasive sinusitis proceeds to involve the orbits and skull base. Nasal congestion and facial pain are early symptoms. A black eschar on the hard palate is the classic sign of mucormycosis. Other signs are proptosis, orbital cellulitis, double vision, and serial cranial nerve palsies, especially Vth and

VIIth. Brain invasion may result in cavernous sinus or carotid artery thrombosis and cerebral abscess formation. Extensive surgical debridement is required, in addition to amphotericin. Other syndromes include fulminant pulmonary infection with angioinvasion and infarction (especially in patients with prolonged neutropenia and antecedent broad-spectrum antibiotics) and disseminated infection.

Pathogenic fungi

Histoplasmosis

Histoplasmosis is caused by *Histoplasma capsulatum*, a dimorphic soil-based fungus. It is the most common systemic mycosis in the USA. There is a strong association between decaying faeces from birds or bats and contaminated soil. The classic endemic region is the Ohio and Mississippi River valleys where large flocks of starlings congregate. In South America, histoplasmosis is associated with chicken coops and bat caves. Disruption of the soil, particularly by construction or excavation, releases infectious particles into the air that are inhaled. Spelunkers (cave explorers) are, therefore, also at specific risk. There are also discrete foci in Africa and Asia.

The vast majority of infections (>90%) are asymptomatic or very mild lower respiratory tract illnesses. Chronic pulmonary histoplasmosis occurs in individuals with underlying emphysema. Patients have a low-grade fever, productive cough, and weight loss. Disseminated histoplasmosis occurs in patients with impaired cell-mediated immunity, and, in particular, reactivation of latent infection occurs in patients who are HIV co-infected. Fever, weight loss, generalized lymphadenopathy, and hepatosplenomegaly are often found. Nodular skin lesions, ulceration of the gastrointestinal tract, and meningitis can also develop. The clinical course may be chronic or rapidly progressive and fatal.

Serological tests can identify both specific antibodies in blood and *H. capsulatum* antigens in blood or urine. Demonstrating yeast cells in clinical samples, e.g. sputum, liver, bone marrow, and skin, is also diagnostic (cultures may take several weeks to grow). Hilar lymphadenopathy and patchy lung infiltrates are seen in acute primary infections on the chest X-ray. Upper lobe cavities are seen in chronic pulmonary infection and a widespread nodular pattern in disseminated disease.

Most cases require no treatment, but itraconazole may be given to immunocompetent patients with symptomatic infections. Severe infections that occur in the immunocompromised patient should be treated with amphotericin.

Coccidioidomycosis

Coccidioides immitis is transmitted by inhalation of contaminated dust in dry desert climates. It is most common in the south-western United States and primarily causes a pneumonic illness. Most infections are self-limiting. Disseminated infections can also cause meningitis.

Blastomycosis

Blastomyces dermatitidis has a similar distribution to histoplasmosis in the USA, but there are also foci in Africa, India, and the Middle East. It is associated with dust exposure and can cause acute or chronic infection of the lungs, skin, or bone.

Paracoccidioidomycosis

Infections caused by *Paracoccidioides brasiliensis* occur sporadically throughout Central and South America, particularly in agricultural workers. An acute form in children and young adults presents with fever, lymphadenopathy, and weight loss. Chronic disease in older individuals presents with pulmonary disease and oral mucocutaneous lesions.

Further reading

Nelson M, Dockrell D, Edwards S (2010). British HIV association guidelines for the treatment of opportunistic infection in HIV-positive individuals 2010. <http://www.liv.ac.uk/hiv/2010_BHIVA_OI-GuidelineConsultationVersion.pdf>.

Pappas PJ, Kauffman CA, Andes D, *et al.* (2000). Clinical practice guidelines for the management of candidiasis: 2009 update by the Infectious Diseases Society of America. *Clinical Infectious Diseases*, **48,** 503–35.

Perfect JR, Dismukes WE, Dromer F, *et al.* Clinical practice guidelines for the management of cryptococcocal disease: 2010 update by the Infectious Diseases Society of America. *Clinical Infectious Diseases*, **50,** 291–322.

Walsh TJ, Anaissie EJ, Denning DW, *et al.* (2008). Treatment of aspergillosis: clinical practice guidelines of the Infectious Diseases Society of America. *Clinical Infectious Diseases*, **30,** 327–60.

Fever in the returning traveller

A travel history should accurately document where a patient has been and for how long. Dates of entry and exit from countries should be obtained, since the onset of illness can be compared with the incubation periods of specific infections. This is one of the most valuable pieces of information, since some conditions can immediately be ruled out if the returning patient became symptomatic after the incubation period has elapsed (see Table 6.6). Depending on what is suspected, it is sometimes necessary to obtain details of the exact places visited or the nature of the region, e.g. transmission of Lassa fever is associated with travel to specific rural areas in West Africa.

The general approach to the febrile patient is similar to that outlined previously, but there are some direct exposure risk questions that need to be asked. In particular, **water contact** is an important risk for leptospirosis (e.g. white water rafting), and swimming in the African lakes may result in Katayama fever (acute schistosomiasis). In general, it is unhelpful to ask about bites from mosquitoes or flies, but **tick bites** are an exception. Visits to African game parks, camping safaris, and walking or riding in the bush, heathland, or forests are exposure risks for ticks. Tick bites are painless and, therefore, often go unnoticed, but a patient may recall removing ticks from their skin. It is useful to know that vaccination against hepatitis A, typhoid, and yellow fever are effective, but anti-malaria chemoprophylaxis is not fail-safe and is frequently not taken with full compliance.

The peripheral blood white cell and platelet count is particularly helpful in the assessment of 'tropical' fevers (see Table 6.6). Typical clinical features and findings on investigation are covered in more detail for the most important of these infections in this section.

Protozoa
Malaria
Malaria is discussed in detail in a later section.

Amoebiasis
Epidemiology
- Amoebiasis has a worldwide distribution (it is only 'tropical' in the sense that it is found in areas of the world where sanitation is poor).
- Infection is through ingestion of food or water contaminated with *Entamoeba histolytica* in the form of 'cysts'.
- Asymptomatic human carriage is extremely common, and, following excretion in stool, cysts are resistant to dehydration in the environment.
- Transmission in the UK can occur without travel, very rarely, e.g. sexual transmission between an asymptomatic immigrant male carrier and another male.

Clinical features
- The incubation period is difficult to define but often weeks or even months.
- Amoebic dysentery is the commonest symptomatic state. There is gradual-onset diarrhoea, and the stool often contains blood and/or mucus. The patient can remain ambulant, and the presence of fever is variable. Occasionally, a fulminant colitis may develop that is mistaken for inflammatory bowel disease.

Table 6.6 Incubation periods, laboratory indicators, and diagnosis of imported infections

Incubation	Infection	White cells	Platelets	Definite diagnosis
≤1 week	Dengue fever	$\rightarrow \downarrow$	$\downarrow$	S
	Relapsing fever	$\uparrow$neutrophils		S, BF
	Plague*			C
	CCHF*	$\downarrow \rightarrow \uparrow$	$\downarrow$	S
1–3 weeks	Malaria	$\rightarrow$	$\downarrow$	BF
	Typhoid	$\rightarrow$		C
	Tick typhus	$\rightarrow$		S
	Brucellosis*	$\rightarrow$		C, S
	Leptospirosis	$\rightarrow \uparrow$neutrophils		S, urine microscopy
	VHF*	$\downarrow \rightarrow \uparrow$	$\downarrow$	PCR on blood, S
	African trypanosomiasis (*T. brucei rhodesiense*)			S, BF
>3 weeks	Malaria	$\rightarrow$	$\downarrow$	BF
	Viral hepatitis	$\rightarrow$		S
	Amoebic liver abscess	$\uparrow$ neutrophils		S
	Acute schistosomiasis	$\uparrow$ eosinophils		S, urine microscopy
	Brucellosis*	$\rightarrow$		C, S
	HIV	$\rightarrow \downarrow$	$\rightarrow \downarrow$	S
	African trypanosomiasis (*T. brucei gambiense*)	$\rightarrow \downarrow$	$\downarrow$	S, BF
	Visceral leishmaniasis	$\uparrow$ eosinophils		S, histology, C
	Filariasis			BF, S

* Samples require special handling; if suspected, discuss with laboratory before sending.

C, culture; S, serology; BF, blood film; CCHF, Crimean-Congo haemorrhagic fever; VHF, viral haemorrhagic fever.

- An amoebic liver abscess may develop directly as a result of an attack of amoebic dysentery or many years after leaving an endemic area, with no history of a preceding dysenteric illness. Pain over the liver and fever are typical. The liver is often tender and enlarged, but clinical jaundice is rare. Sometimes, the patient may have a dry cough, and there may be reduced breath sounds or crackles at the right lung base. Spontaneous rupture into local structures can lead to pericarditis, empyema, and peritonitis. A sinus may develop if there is rupture through the overlying skin.
- Rarely, a chronic inflammatory mass may develop in the abdomen that results from thickening of the bowel wall ('amoeboma'). The ileocaecal region is most commonly affected and may be mistaken for a carcinoma.
- Blood-borne metastatic infection to the lung or brain is extremely rare.

Investigations
- A neutrophil leucocytosis in the peripheral blood and significantly raised inflammatory indices are universal. Liver function derangement is common in amoebic liver abscess, but jaundice is very atypical.

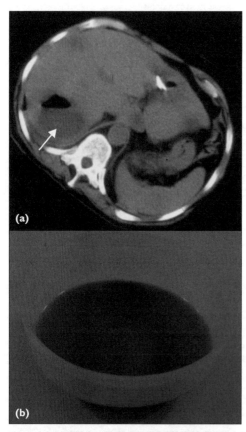

Figure 6.4 (a) CT scan showing an amoebic liver abscess in the right lobe of the liver (arrow) and (b) non-offensive smelling amoebic pus following drainage.

- The presence of *E. histolytica* cysts in stool does not mean that the patient has invasive amoebiasis, since asymptomatic cyst excretion is common.
- Dysentery: microscopy performed on a fresh stool sample, showing red cell ingestion by amoebic trophozoites, is diagnostic. Sigmoidoscopy may show shallow ulcers or colitis in severe cases.
- Liver abscess: ultrasound shows one or more focal lesions, most commonly in the right lobe. Pus aspirated from these (resembles 'anchovy sauce') is non-offensive smelling, in contrast to that from a pyogenic abscess (see Figure 6.4). Amoebae may be seen in aspirates by microscopy, and very few neutrophils are present.
- Rapid serological tests are both highly sensitive and specific for invasive amoebiasis.

Management
- Most forms of amoebiasis respond to treatment, but life-threatening complications may develop if untreated, e.g. liver abscess rupture, colonic perforation, or haematogenous spread.
- Drainage is usually performed if liver abscesses are very large or in order to prevent imminent spontaneous rupture.
- Metronidazole (400–800 mg three times daily for 5–10 days) is the drug treatment of choice for all forms of amoebiasis, but this has no activity against amoebic cysts. Diloxanide furoate (500 mg three times daily) is, therefore, given for 10 days afterwards to eradicate cyst carriage and to prevent future relapse.

Visceral leishmaniasis (kala-azar)
Epidemiology
- Visceral leishmaniasis is found in India and East Africa (*Leishmania donovani*), Latin America (*L. chagasi*), and the Mediterranean basin (*L. infantum*). It mainly affects children in Southern Europe and occurs in epidemics in the Indian subcontinent, especially in malnourished individuals.
- Infection is transmitted by small, biting female sandflies. (Sandflies have a short flight range and, therefore, seldom bite people sleeping on the first floor of a building.)
- The reservoirs of infection are animals, such as wild dogs, rodents, and man. In the Mediterranean, domesticated dogs are the major reservoir.
- Intracellular parasites may persist in the body in a dormant state for many years until the host immunity deteriorates. Visceral leishmaniasis is an opportunistic infection in HIV-positive individuals (CD4 count <200 cells/mm^3). This combination is relatively more common in Southern Europe.

Clinical features
Incubation period is 3–18 months. Asymptomatic infections are relatively common. Fever and sweating often occur, but patients remain relatively well until the disease is well advanced. The fever may relapse and remit, and the course is typically prolonged. Lymphadenopathy is variable, but hepatosplenomegaly is common. The spleen can be enormous.

In the later stages of infection, patients become increasingly weak and emaciated and usually die from intercurrent infections.

Investigations
- Pancytopenia, low albumin, and a normal or raised total protein are characteristic. This is due to marrow infiltration and a polyclonal increase in immunoglobulins.

- Specific serology is sensitive but is reduced in HIV co-infection.
- Direct microscopic diagnosis involves identifying amastigotes (protist cells that do not have visible external flagella or cilia; a phase in the life-cycle of trypanosome protozoans) in bone marrow aspirates or liver biopsy tissue. An aspirate obtained by splenic puncture has an excellent yield but is rarely performed nowadays due to the risk of haemorrhage.
- Amastigotes and non-caseating granuloma may be seen on liver biopsy tissue.
- Culture of blood may occasionally be positive, using special medium, but is rarely performed.

Management
- Intravenous amphotericin (1–3 mg/kg/day for 10–21 days) is effective and the standard therapy, but miltefosine is the first effective oral drug.
- Relapses are common, necessitating careful post-treatment follow-up.
- Sometimes, after apparently successful treatment, a nodular skin eruption, called post-kala-azar dermal leishmaniasis, develops on the face and is caused by the persistence of large numbers of amastigotes in the skin.

Trypanosomiasis
African trypanosomiasis
- African trypanosomiasis is caused by two *Trypanosoma* species: *T. brucei rhodesiense* occurs in East Africa (wild buck and cattle are the reservoir), and *T. brucei gambiense* in West and Central Africa (humans from rural communities are the main reservoir).
- Transmission is from a tsetse fly bite (typically painful). It is extremely rare in returning travellers but may be acquired on visits to safari game parks.
- The clinical course has two phases: (1) a painful chancre initially develops at the bite site, with regional lymphadenopathy; an influenza-like illness then follows, with a relapsing and remitting pattern, lasting weeks to months; (2) a dementia-like illness subsequently evolves with behavioural changes; patients become increasingly somnolent (hence, 'sleeping sickness') and slip into coma. *T. brucei rhodesiense* is more rapidly progressive and frequently fatal than *T. brucei gambiense*.
- Diagnosis is made by direct visualization of trypanosomes in a thick blood film or stained aspirates from the chancre, lymph nodes, bone marrow, or CSF. Serology is available.
- Suramin is used in early infections, but only melarsoprol, an arsenic compound, is effective in patients with established meningoencephalitis. However, melarsoprol itself may induce fatal encephalopathy.

South American trypanosomiasis (Chagas' disease)
Caused by *Trypanosoma cruzi*, South American trypanosomiasis is confined to the Southern USA and Argentina. Most infections occur in children living in poor, rural areas, and imported UK cases are exceptionally rare. Human transmission is by the infected faeces of reduviid bugs, which are rubbed into bite wounds or mucous membranes. Transmission from blood transfusion also occurs.

In the acute phase, there is cutaneous oedema at the initial entry site (or unilateral orbital oedema, if inoculation is via the conjunctiva), and the patient is systemically unwell. A quarter of infections become chronic, and complications resulting from subsequent tissue fibrosis include dilated cardiomyopathy, cardiac conduction defects, megaoesophagus, and megacolon. Diagnosis is by visualization of trypanosomes in peripheral blood and serology. Reduviid bugs are used for xenodiagnosis in Latin America.

Treatment of acute infections is with nifurtimox. There is no specific treatment for chronic infections, apart from managing the complications, e.g. pacemaker insertion or surgery.

Bacterial infections
Typhoid and paratyphoid fevers (enteric fevers)
Epidemiology
- The causative organisms of typhoid and paratyphoid fevers are *Salmonella typhi* and *S. paratyphi*, respectively. Both are Gram-negative bacilli from the *Enterobacteriaceae* group.
- Transmission is by the faecal-oral route via contaminated food or water. The most important reservoirs of infection are asymptomatic human carriers, in whom infection persists in either the gall bladder or urinary tract.
- The enteric fevers have a worldwide distribution but are commonest in parts of the world where standards of personal and environmental hygiene are particularly poor. Typhoid is only an imported infection in the UK.

Clinical features
Incubation is usually about 14 days but can be 1–3 weeks.

Fever, headache, and abdominal discomfort are the commonest symptoms during the first week of illness. Constipation and dry cough are also relatively frequent.

In the second week of illness, physical signs become more apparent. A 'relative bradycardia' and splenomegaly may be present. 'Rose spots' (scanty pink macules that fade with pressure) may appear on the trunk of fair-skinned patients.

In the third week, complications may develop. The most common complications are gastrointestinal haemorrhage and perforated bowel, caused by ischaemia and necrosis of lymph follicles in the terminal ileum (Peyer's patches). Other complications affect every organ system and include hepatitis, cholecystitis, pneumonia, meningitis, transverse myelitis, myocarditis, and focal abscess formation.

Investigations
- The total peripheral white cell count is usually normal, and a considerably elevated C-reactive protein may help to distinguish enteric fever from a viral illness in the early phase of infection.
- Blood culture is the most useful of all, but stool and urine may yield positive cultures also. The highest yield is from bone marrow culture, which may be diagnostic, even after antibiotic treatment has been commenced.
- Serological diagnosis (Widal test) is not recommended because it is non-specific and difficult to interpret.

Management
- If untreated, enteric fever may be fatal, but, if diagnosed and treated early enough, the outcome is good.
- Ceftriaxone is the empiric agent of choice until drug sensitivities become available. Oral antibiotics can be used when the patient is stable (e.g. ciprofloxacin), but antibiotic resistance is a problem. A 10-day course of antibiotics is required.
- About 10% relapse after treatment. Relapses occur about 2 weeks after recovery. The illness is milder, and the antibiotic sensitivity pattern is usually identical to the first illness.

- The persistent carrier state must be excluded after recovery to prevent others from being infected. Food handlers who are also chronic carriers present a significant public health risk and should be cleared of infection before returning to work.

Leptospirosis
Epidemiology

- Leptospirosis has a worldwide distribution, including the UK. It is more common in temperate and tropical climates, especially after heavy rain. There are approximately 60 cases of leptospirosis in the UK each year.
- *Leptospira* are excreted in the urine of a large number of animals, including rodents, dogs, cats, wild mammals, fish, birds, and reptiles. Leptospirosis is caused by *Leptospira interrogans*, but the species contains hundreds of serovars. *L. icterohaemorrhagiae* is commonly pathogenic in humans and is the cause of the most severe manifestation, Weil's disease.
- Organisms may remain viable in water or soil for weeks to months, and human transmission occurs when bacteria enter through broken skin or mucous membranes. It is associated with farmers, sewer workers, veterinarians, and recreational activities involving water.

Clinical features
The incubation period is 7–14 days.

- The first phase is a flu-like syndrome that lasts up to a week (the so-called 'septicaemic phase'). There is sudden-onset high fever, rigors, conjunctival suffusion, headache, and myalgia. In many cases, there is no progression, and full recovery is made.
- The second phase may last 2–3 weeks ('immune phase', which corresponds to the development of specific IgM). After a 48-hour remission, there is a recurrence of fever, with severe muscle pain, headache, pneumonitis, and a maculopapular or haemorrhagic skin rash. Aseptic meningitis (with or without meningeal irritation) may also develop.
- In some cases, renal failure, deep jaundice, and haemorrhage also develop in the second phase (Weil's disease). This typically runs a fulminant course, with disseminated intravascular coagulation (DIC) and multiorgan failure.

Investigations

- A neutrophil leucocytosis in the blood is typical but not universal. Inflammatory indices are very elevated, and the platelet count may be low. Renal and liver function tests are abnormal in Weil's disease. Creatine phosphokinase is very elevated, indicating dissemination to muscle, and may help to differentiate leptopirosis from other causes of hepatitis.
- The diagnosis can be made by directly visualizing the organism in centrifuged urine or fresh blood by dark ground microscopy. However, serological tests and PCR-based assays in blood are more commonly used.

Management

- All cases should receive treatment. Mild cases may be given oral doxycycline or amoxicillin. Severe cases should be treated with IV benzylpenicillin or amoxicillin. Dialysis and blood products may be required in Weil's disease.
- As with any spirochaete infection, penicillin treatment can trigger a Jarisch–Herxheimer reaction (a reaction to endotoxin-like products released by the death of harmful microorganisms associated with fever, rigors, hypotension, headache, myalgia, tachycardia, hyperventilation, and vasodilation with flushing).

- Most cases recover fully. However, in jaundiced patients, the clinical cause can be fulminant, with multiorgan failure and massive haemorrhage, causing death in up to 10%.

Relapsing fever
Relapsing fever is caused by two species of *Borrelia* (spirochaetal organisms): *Borrelia recurrentis* (louse-borne relapsing fever) and *B. duttoni* (tick-borne relapsing fever).

- Tick-borne relapsing fever occurs in East Africa and is transmitted by bites from infected soft ticks (the reservoirs are rodents and the ticks themselves).
- The reservoir of infection in louse-borne relapsing fever is man, and infected fluids from the body louse (*Pediculus humanus*) are responsible for transmission. Louse-borne relapsing fever is found in any part of the world where there is poverty, overcrowding, and poor standards of hygiene.
- A relapsing pattern of fever, headache, and myalgia, lasting for several days, followed by spontaneous remission for a similar duration, is typical. The number of relapses can vary, e.g. two to 12 (tick-borne relapsing fever has more relapses but is less often fatal than louse-borne). Dry cough, hepatomegaly, splenomegaly, and lymphadenopathy may be present. Multiorgan involvement (e.g. jaundice, myocarditis, encephalitis), accompanied by DIC and a haemorrhagic skin rash, occurs in severe cases.
- There is typically a neutrophilia in the peripheral blood, and direct visualization of organisms on a stained thick blood film is diagnostic. Serological tests are available.
- Tetracycline is the agent of choice, but treatment may be complicated by a Jarisch–Herxheimer reaction.

Rickettsial infections
Epidemiology

Rickettsiae are intracellular Gram-negative bacteria with mammalian resevoirs (e.g. rodents) and are distributed in geographically distinct areas. Human transmission involves an arthropod vector, e.g. lice, ticks, and mites.

- Tick typhus from Africa and Boutonneuse fever from the Mediterranean (both *R. conori*) will be most often encountered in emergency departments in the UK. Tick bites also transmit Rocky Mountain spotted fever (*R. rickettsii*) in North and South America.
- Scrub typhus (*R. tsutsugamushi*) is transmitted by the trombiculid mite, which lives in well-demarcated 'islands' of secondary vegetation that regrows after felling of jungle forests in the Asiatic-Pacific region.
- Louse-borne ('epidemic') typhus (*R. prowazekii*) is transmitted by body lice and is a disease of human overcrowding, large-scale human catastrophe, and squalor. As such, it is found in populations throughout the world stricken by war, poverty, and famine.
- Murine ('endemic') typhus (*R. typhi*) is found most commonly in warm coastal ports of the Southern USA, Mediterranean, Middle East, Indian subcontinent, and South East Asia. Rats are the principal reservoir, and infected faeces from rat fleas that enter broken human skin (and sometimes flea bites) cause transmission.

Clinical features

- The incubation period is 1–3 weeks, and many patients will not recall the bite from the vector. However, enquiry should be made about outdoor activities and walking through long grass where transmission occurs (e.g. camping safaris, hiking through scrub, etc.).

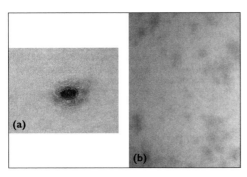

Figure 6.5 (a) **A typical tick bite 'eschar' in a traveller returning from safari in Zimbabwe;** (b) **A close-up of a generalized maculopapular skin rash in a patient with African tick typhus.**

- An 'eschar' (black scab), with secondary lymphadenitis, develops at the site of the bite, especially in African tick and scrub typhus (see Figure 6.5a). Several days later, fever, cough, conjunctivitis, lymphadenopathy, spleno-megaly, and a generalized rash develop. The rash is usu-ally maculopapular in type but may occasionally be petechial or even gangrenous (see Figure 6.5b).
- Different rickettsial species cause diseases of varying severity. Many are mild and self-limiting, but others can lead to DIC and multiorgan failure, especially involving the skin, brain, heart, lungs, and kidneys.

Investigations
- The white cell count is typically normal, and thrombocy-topenia is common.
- Specific serological tests are commonly used to confirm the diagnosis.
- *Rickettsiae* may also be identified by immunohistochemis-try or PCR in biopsy samples from the eschar or rash in the acute stages.

Management
- African tick typhus and Boutonneuse fever are often self-limiting infections and resolve without treatment.
- If required, the antibiotics of choice include doxycycline, ciprofloxacin, and chloramphenicol.
- Rocky Mountain spotted fever and epidemic typhus are the most severe rickettsial conditions. Rocky Mountain spotted fever causes encephalitis and non-cardiogenic pulmonary oedema and has a mortality rate of up to 10%. However, if treatment is started before complica-tions develop, the outlook is usually good.
- Epidemic typhus may recur after treatment (Brill–Zinsser disease).

Brucellosis
Epidemiology
- Brucellosis has a worldwide distribution and is transmit-ted to man from infected animals, such as sheep, goats, and cattle. Relatively few countries are brucellosis-free; these include the UK, Canada, New Zealand, and Japan.
- Brucellosis is caused by an intracellular Gram-negative bacterium. Four species of *Brucellae* are human patho-gens: *Brucella melitensis* (from goats, sheep, and camels), *B. abortus* (cattle), *B. suis* (swine), and *B. canis* (dogs).

- Transmission occurs through consumption of infected animal milk products, direct contact with contaminated animal parts (e.g. placenta), and inhalation of infected aerosols. Consumption of unpasteurized dairy produce is the most common mode of transmission, especially milk, soft cheese, butter, and ice cream.
- Brucellosis is also an occupational disease for those work-ing in abattoirs, farms, or microbiology laboratories. Without travel outside the UK, it may be useful to ask patients about food consumption from delicatessen shops, which import unpasteurized dairy produce.

Clinical features
- The incubation period is usually 2–4 weeks.
- Brucellosis has a myriad of clinical presentations: acute, chronic progressive, and relapsing and remitting.
- Non-specific, generalized symptoms, such as sweats and malaise, are usually present. Patients may have general-ized lymphadenopathy or hepatosplenomegaly. Additional symptoms and signs depend on which sites in the body are specifically affected.
- Brucellosis can involve nearly every organ system but most commonly affects the large joints (knees, hips, ankles, and wrists). Sacroiliitis and lumbar spondylitis may also occur.
- Epididymo-orchitis, meningoencephalitis, and brain abscess are rare complications. Brucella endocarditis is very rare.

Investigations
- The peripheral blood count shows a normal white cell count or slight leukopenia. A mild hepatitis is also com-mon, with raised transaminases.
- Blood cultures and bone marrow cultures may be posi-tive. In contrast to traditional teaching, modern tech-niques mean that prolonged culture is unnecessary. The diagnosis can also be made serologically.
- Granulomatous inflammation may be seen on biopsy tis-sue (e.g. liver).

Management
- In general, brucellosis responds well to antibiotic treat-ment. Combinations of antibiotics that penetrate well into cells are required. WHO guidelines recommend doxycycline with either rifampicin or streptomycin. Quinolones, aminoglycosides, and co-trimoxazole have also been used with success. Antibiotics are usually given for several weeks or months.
- The relapse rate is around 10%, but these usually result from initial inadequate treatment and most frequently occur in the first year.
- Endocarditis is the principal cause of death and usually requires valve replacement.

Viral infections
Dengue fever
Epidemiology
- Dengue fever is caused by a flavivirus (four serotypes: 1–4), which is transmitted by bites from infected mosqui-toes (*Aedes aegypti*). *A. aegypti* breeds in urban areas, for example, in domestic water tanks or abandoned car tyres filled with rain water.
- Transmission takes place in almost all tropical areas, with the highest burden in South East Asia. The incidence is

increasing in South America and the Caribbean. It causes up to 100 million infections each year worldwide.

- Dengue fever (unlike other arboviruses) is only transmitted between humans and has no significant animal reservoir. Most cases of dengue haemorrhagic fever are in young native-born children, and it is rare in travellers.

Clinical features

The incubation period is usually ≤7 days.

- Sudden onset of headache, musculoskeletal pains, and fever are typical. The headache is commonly retro-orbital and worse on eye movement. Musculoskeletal pains are frequently severe ('break-bone' fever).
- The fever is sometimes described as having a 'saddleback' pattern, since it may subside after 2–3 days and then recur. In this second phase, a generalized, blanching erythematous rash develops. The fever goes away, and a full recovery starts a few days after the rash appears.
- A very small proportion of patients suddenly develop 'dengue haemorrhagic fever' (DHF) 2–7 days into the illness. This manifestation of vascular endothelial leak results in the appearance of skin petechiae and, in more extreme cases, bleeding from multiple sites, e.g. melaena, haematemesis, haematuria, and epistaxis. The most severely ill develop circulatory collapse ('dengue shock syndrome').
- Encephalitis is an extremely rare complication.

Investigations

- Leucopenia and thrombocytopenia are characteristic.
- Raised haematocrit (>20% baseline) is an indicator of DHF.
- The diagnosis is confirmed retrospectively when serological results become available.

Management

- There is no specific treatment for dengue fever. Management is entirely supportive.
- In DHF, IV fluids and plasma expanders are given for hypotension, and blood products for bleeding and clotting abnormalities.
- The vascular leak typically resolves in 24–48 hours, and, with careful supportive management, mortality is <5%.

Yellow fever
Epidemiology

- Yellow fever is found in Africa, Central and South America, but not Asia. The WHO estimates that there are 200,000 cases per year, with 30,000 deaths.
- Yellow fever is a flavivirus transmitted by *Aedes aegyptes* from monkey to monkey in the forest canopies. Mosquitoes transmit infection to humans entering the forest.
- Spread from person to person occurs when infected humans enter a populated area, possibly a city, where the mosquito vector is also present. Direct person-to-person transmission, without the vector, has not been reported.
- A live attenuated vaccine is protective for 10 years. Many countries do not permit visitors to enter without certified proof of vaccination.

Clinical features

The incubation period is ≤7 days.

- Most infections are subclinical or cause a mild febrile illness.
- In severe infections, fever, headache, and vomiting are followed by renal and liver failure (jaundice gives the condi-

tion its name), severe vomiting, gastrointestinal haemorrhage, and shock.

Investigations

- Diagnosis requires a specialized laboratory to look for specific antibody.
- A liver biopsy (usually post-mortem) characteristically shows mid-zone necrosis and 'Councilman bodies' (an eosinophilic globule that indicates a hepatocyte that is undergoing apoptosis).

Management

- There is no specific treatment, and care is purely supportive.
- Florid infections are often fatal (especially if there is jaundice), but, if the patient survives, recovery is full.

Chikungunya

- Caused by a mosquito-borne alphavirus, with a wide geographical range that includes sub-Saharan Africa, India, and South East Asia. Sudden and dramatic outbreaks can occur.
- Incubation period is ≤7days. Features include fever, headache, and prominent arthralgia and myalgia. A truncal rash may also be seen, which may occasionally appear petechial or haemorrhagic.
- Diagnosis (usually retrospective) is by serology.
- There is no specific treatment, and recovery in 5–7 days is usual.

Viral haemorrhagic fevers

- Viral haemorrhagic fevers (VHF) are a miscellaneous group of acute viral infections that may result in uncontrolled haemorrhage from multiple sites and hypovolaemic shock. Either insect vectors or close contact with the animal reservoir is involved in transmission, and mortality from these conditions is characteristically high.
- Although extremely rare in the UK, four of these (Lassa, Ebola, Marburg, and Congo-Crimean haemorrhagic fever) are of particular concern in the UK due to the potential for person-to-person transmission through direct contact with infected body fluids, e.g. blood, sweat, urine, and semen. In clinical practice, Lassa fever is the most likely to be encountered, and most recently Ebola following the recent epidemic in West Africa (see Table 6.7).
- Although yellow fever and dengue haemorrhagic fever are classified as VHFs, they are not transmitted from person to person.
- Transmissible VHF should be suspected if the patient has a febrile illness and a history of travel to an endemic area (especially rural Africa and most recently Sierra Leone, Liberia and, Guinea in West Africa) within the last 21 days. The possibility of VHF is significantly increased if the individual:
  - Stayed in a house for >4 hours where there were ill or feverish persons, known or suspected to have VHF.
  - Took part in nursing or caring for ill or feverish persons, known or strongly suspected to have VHF, or had contact with body fluids, tissue, or the dead body of such a patient.
  - Works as a laboratory, healthcare, or other worker, likely to have come into contact with body fluids, tissue, or the dead body of a human or animal, known or strongly suspected to have VHF.
  - Has none of the above risks but develops an illness with multiorgan failure (± haemorrhage), and there is no alternative explanation, apart from a VHF.

- In addition, a patient should also be considered high risk if, during the 3 weeks before illness, they travelled to countries adjacent to endemic regions and have developed clinical evidence of VHF, with no alternative diagnosis.
- Following the 2013–16 Ebola epidemic in West Africa, patients with fever, headache, myalgia, weakness, fatigue, diarrhoea, vomiting, abdominal pain, or unexplained haemorrhage within 21 days of returning from this region should be immediately notified to the communicable disease authorities. They should be isolated and barrier nursed wearing appropriate personal protective equipment (PPE) by trained specialist infection control personnel.
- In the initial assessment, ONLY a malaria film should be performed, since, in the vast majority of instances, the diagnosis will turn out to be malaria. Further clinical samples for laboratory analysis should not be taken if this is negative, and the case should be urgently discussed with the local infectious diseases physician or consultant in communicable diseases control. Diagnosis requires a specialized laboratory to identify specific antibody, antigen, or culture the virus.
- Strongly suspected or confirmed cases are cared for in a specialized high-security infectious diseases unit, and there are strict guidelines about the taking and handling of clinical specimens and safe disposal of body waste.

Lassa fever
- Lassa fever is caused by an arenavirus, first identified in Lassa, Nigeria. Transmission is reported in rural areas of Sierra Leone, Mali, and 'middle belt' Nigeria.
- Lassa fever causes several thousand deaths each year, but many people from endemic areas have serological evidence of previous infection.
- The natural reservoir is the multimammate rat, and human infection may follow direct contact with infected rat urine.
- Ribavirin may be useful, but treatment is mainly supportive. Mortality is up to 50%.

Marburg and Ebola
- Marburg and Ebola viruses belong to the filovirus family. The natural reservoirs of both diseases are unknown but are suspected to be monkeys.
- Marburg virus was first identified in 1967 in German laboratory workers who had been exposed to blood or tissues from Ugandan, African green monkeys. A large Marburg virus outbreak occurred in 2005 in Angola. The mortality in infected individuals is up to 90%.
- Ebola virus disease was first described in 1976 in two simultaneous outbreaks in sub-Saharan Africa, and subsequent cases have been reported in Zaire, Congo, Gabon, and Sudan. The most widespread epidemic of Ebola occurred from 2013 16 in three West African countries. The outbreak began in Guinea in December 2013 and then spread to Liberia and Sierra Leone. Dysfunctional healthcare systems, extreme poverty, the local burial custom of washing the body after death, distrust of government officials, armed conflict, and delay in responding to the outbreak for several months all contributed to the initial failure to control the epidemic. It has caused significant mortality, with reported case fatality rates of up to 70% and about 55% in hospitalized patients. As of June 2015 the World Health Organization (WHO) and respective governments had reported a total of ~27,000 cases and ~11,500 deaths. However, the WHO believes that this substantially understates the magnitude of the outbreak. Many healthcare workers were also infected and died due to inadequate infection control and PPE. Recent reports (2016) suggest that the number of new cases has decreased substantially and the outbreak appears to have been controlled.

Congo-Crimean haemorrhagic fever
- Congo-Crimean haemorrhagic fever is endemic in many countries in Eastern Europe, the Middle East, Africa, and Asia. Outbreaks have been reported in Russia, Turkey, Iran, Kazakhstan, Albania, Pakistan Serbia, and South Africa in recent years.

Table 6.7 Viral haemorrhagic fevers

Family	Agent	Mode of transmission
Arenaviruses	Argentine HF (Junin)* Bolivian HF (Machupo)* Brazilian HF (Sabia)* **Lassa** Venezuelan HF (Guanarito)*	Aerosols of rodent excreta or other close contact
Bunyaviruses	**Congo-Crimean HF** Hantaan (HF with renal syndrome)* Rift Valley fever	Tick bite; contact with slaughtered cattle or sheep Aerosols of rodent excreta or other close contact Mosquito bite; contact with blood of domestic animals
Filoviruses	**Ebola*** Marburg	Close contact with body fluids of humans and non-human primates
Flaviviruses	Dengue Yellow fever Omsk HF Kyanasur forest disease	Mosquito Mosquito Tick Tick

HF, haemorrhagic fever.

Bold denotes agents of particular concern for the UK. * Indicates person-to-person transmission reported.

- Human transmission results from contact with blood or other infected tissues from livestock or infected Ixodid tick bites. Most cases have occurred in those involved with the livestock industry (e.g. farm or slaughterhouse workers and veterinarians).

Helminths

Schistosomiasis

Epidemiology

- There are three major species of blood flukes that infect man with different geographic distributions: *Schistosoma haematobium* (Africa and the Middle East), *S. mansoni* (Africa, Middle East, South America, and the Caribbean), and *S. japonicum* (China, Japan, Philippines and the Far East).
- Human transmission requires contact with a freshwater source, which is the natural habitat of the snail host (e.g. *Bulinus*), which is essential in the flukes' life cycle. In the returning traveller, this is often swimming in the great African freshwater lakes (e.g. Lake Malawi, Lake Kariba).

Clinical features

- Local dermatitis (or 'swimmer's itch') may occur 1–3 days after free-swimming larvae (cercariae) penetrate intact human skin.
- Six weeks later, an acute systemic hypersensitivity reaction to the release of eggs by mature flukes can occur ('Katayama fever' or acute schistosomiasis). Typical features include fever, cough, wheeze, diarrhoea, urticarial skin rash, and hepatosplenomegaly. This may be very severe but usually resolves spontaneously after a week or so.
- Features of chronic infection are the result of granulomatous inflammation and the subsequent fibrosis that develops in response to eggs deposited in the bladder (*S. haematobium*), bowel (*S. mansoni* and *S. japonicum*), and liver (all three species). Months to years later, haematuria is the commonest presenting feature of *S. haematobium* infection. In *S. mansoni* and *S. japonicum* infections, papilloma-type outgrowths develop on the colonic mucosa, which may ulcerate and bleed and cause intermittent bloody diarrhoea. Large numbers of eggs reaching the periportal regions of the liver lead to hepatomegaly and occlusion of the portal veins. Portal hypertension produces secondary splenomegaly, oesophageal varices and ascites, which in some patients can cause significant abdominal enlargement.
- Occasionally, ectopic worms or their eggs find their way into other organs, such as the brain or spinal cord, where they cause space-occupying lesions and focal neurological signs.

Investigations

- Blood eosinophilia is common.
- Urine microscopy may identify red cells and eggs. Eggs may also be seen in bladder and rectal biopsy specimens.
- Serology is very useful but remains positive for many years after successful treatment.
- Imaging may reveal irreversible obstructive uropathy due to fibrous stricture formation (e.g. hydroureter and hydronephrosis) or reduced bladder capacity due to thickening and rigidity of the bladder wall. There is an increased risk of bladder cancer in chronic infection, and all patients with microscopic haematuria should be referred for cystoscopy.

Management

- Praziquantel 40 mg/kg daily (single dose or split twice daily) for 3 days is the drug of choice for all species.
- Most infections that are treated, before obstructive renal disease or portal hypertension develops, respond well.

Lymphatic filariasis

Epidemiology

- Caused by the nematode filarial worms *Wuchereria bancrofti* and, less commonly, *Brugia malayi*. *W. bancrofti* is found in Africa, the Indian subcontinent, South East Asia, and Central and South America. Most infections occur in Asia.
- Infective larvae are transmitted to humans by bites from culicine and anopheline mosquitoes. They subsequently migrate to the lymphatic system and develop into adults.
- Adult worms (4–10 cm long) may survive for ≥10 years in humans.

Clinical features

Most patients are asymptomatic.

- The main features are recurrent episodes of fever and chills, associated with lymphangitis and lymphadenitis. Attacks last a week or two and then spontaneously resolve.
- Recurrent lymphangitis eventually leads to chronic lymphatic obstruction, gross lymphoedema, and massive overgrowth of the skin and subcutaneous tissues ('elephantiasis'). The legs and scrotum are most commonly affected.

Investigations

- Eosinophilia is very common, and serological tests may be positive.
- Microfilaria (produced by female adult worms after mating) may be seen on a blood film. Blood should be taken from the patient in the middle of the night because this is when microfilaria are taken up in the blood meal of biting mosquitos to complete the filarial life cycle.

Management

- Treatment is with diethylcarbamazine (DEC) over 2–3 weeks. This is usually well tolerated, but acute inflammatory reactions, provoked by dead and dying worms, are common.
- Surgical treatment of hydrocele is effective. Surgery and drugs have no effect on established limb elephantiasis.

Other important imported infections

Rabies

Epidemiology

- 'Classic' rabies (RNA virus) is a lyssa virus. There are several other closely related viruses found in bats, which belong to the same genus and produce an indistinguishable disease in humans.
- Rabies still poses a significant public health problem in Asia and Africa where 95% of human deaths occur. In India alone, there are 30–50,000 deaths/year. Many European countries (including the UK), Australia, New Zealand, and Japan are free of classic rabies.
- The few UK cases that have been recorded are mostly from dog bites acquired abroad, but, in 2002, a death resulted from a bat lyssa virus contracted in Scotland. In the USA, there are approximately two cases per year.
- Apart from bats, other wild mammals, such as wolves, foxes, racoons, and skunks, are also responsible for transmission in a minority of cases.

Clinical features

Human infection is usually transmitted by the bite of a rabid animal, but infected saliva on broken skin or mucous membranes from licks and scratches can also cause infection. Most cases are through infected dogs, cats, and wild carnivores, e.g. foxes, wolves, racoons, skunks, and bats. Herbivores, e.g. cattle, deer, horses, have the potential to transmit rabies, but this rarely occurs. Unprovoked animal bites are unusual and increase the suspicion of rabies.

- The incubation period can range from a few days to many years but is usually 20–90 days. The first sign is paraesthesiae, commonly itching or pain at the inoculation site. Fever may also be present. After a few days, either 'furious' or 'paralytic' rabies develops.
- Hydrophobia is a cardinal symptom of 'furious' rabies. Other key features are spasmodic contractions involving the muscles of the throat, diaphragm, and respiration. More generalized muscle spasms cause opisthotonus, and, during attacks, the patient appears filled with terror. The spasms can be precipitated by attempts to swallow fluids and blowing air onto the face ('aerophobia'). Other features include hypersalivation ('frothing at the mouth'), seizures, confusion, and extreme agitation, but there may be interspersed lucid intervals. Death usually occurs within a week, often at the end of a hydrophobic spasm from a cardiac or respiratory arrest.
- In 'paralytic' (or 'dumb') rabies, there is ascending, symmetric, or asymmetric flaccid paralysis, usually beginning in the bitten limb. Like furious rabies, coma develops, and death is inevitable.

Investigations

- Virus may be identified in body fluids (e.g. saliva, CSF, and tears) and tissue (brain and skin) by a number of techniques. These include detecting antigen by immunofluorescence, antibody (in unvaccinated individuals), and PCR-based assays.
- Since rabid dogs and cats usually succumb within 10 days of biting, the diagnosis can be excluded if the animal can be safely captured, observed in quarantine, and remains healthy for a 15-day period. Alternatively, examining its brain can make the diagnosis. The classic histopathological feature is dark staining aggregates of viral protein within the cytoplasm of neurones ('Negri bodies').

Management

- There is no effective treatment for rabies when clinical features develop.
- Following a bite, the wound should be cleaned vigorously with soap and water. Human tetanus immunoglobulin and antibiotics for secondary infection should be considered.
- The aim of post-exposure treatment (PET) using rabies vaccine with or without rabies immunoglobulin (HRIG) is to stop the virus reaching the central nervous system by producing or giving protective antibody. Given within days, it is 100% effective at preventing progression to fatal encephalitis.
- Treatment, including the decision as to whether or not to give post-exposure vaccination alone, or with HRIG, is based on assessment of risk i.e. country of exposure, category of exposure, and immune status of the individual. (see Public Health England website; Rabies: risk assessment, post-exposure treatment, management (2015), for further guidance).
- The UK schedule for 'at risk' and unimmunized individuals is to give live vaccine (± rabies immune globulin) at intervals of 0, 3, 7, 14, 28–30 days into the deltoid muscle by IM injection. Sequential doses should be given in alternate arms.
- Although the mainstay of rabies PET is rabies vaccine, HRIG may provide short term immunity in the 'high risk' individual during the first 7-10 day period after initiation of treatment before vaccine-induced immunity develops. HRIG 20 IU/kg should be infiltrated around the wound, if possible. If this is difficult or if the wound has healed, then HRIG should be given into the anterolateral thigh (vaccine and HRIG should never be given in the same anatomical site).
- Licks, scratches, and minor bites (to covered areas of limbs and trunk), without the skin being broken, are regarded as a lower risk. Major bites (multiple or on the face, head, finger, or neck) and transdermal bites, licks, or scratches on broken skin are regarded as high risk. Contamination of mucous membranes with mammal saliva (i.e. licks) or bat droppings and urine constitutes a major risk.
- Bat exposure risk is assessed differently to terrestrial animals. Bat bites do not cause an obvious break in the skin, and 50% of cases in the USA have resulted from unrecognized bat bites. Significant bat exposure may, therefore, occur without direct physical contact being appreciated, e.g. the discovery of a bat in the room of a sleeping individual or in the water supply.
- Two post-exposure vaccines are given to fully immunized individuals, but, if there is doubt, the patient should be treated as non-immune/not fully immunized.
- Treatment can be stopped if the captured dog/mammal remains healthy after 15 days or if examination of its brain proves negative for rabies as mentioned above. (This does not include bats, since they can carry rabies without signs of infection.)
- When rabies becomes clinically apparent, it is always fatal, and treatment is, therefore, palliative.

Hydatid disease
Epidemiology

- *Echinococcus* species are canine tapeworms, normally found in domestic dogs, wolves, and foxes. Transmission to humans is by ingestion of eggs, excreted in dog faeces, which hatch into larvae in the intestine.
- Cystic hydatid disease (*Echinococcus granulosus*) is most commonly encountered throughout the world, especially in rural, sheep-farming areas. Alveolar hydatid disease (*E. multilocularis*) occurs mainly in the Northern hemisphere. *E. vogeli* (very rare) is found in Central and South America.

Clinical features

- Almost any organ in the body can be involved, but most infections are asymptomatic.
- The liver is most often involved (50–70%). Abdominal discomfort and hepatomegaly related to pressure from the enlarging cysts may be present (~1 cm/year), but fever is not a typical feature.
- The lungs are the next most common organ involved (20–30%) and may present when there is cyst rupture into an airway and its contents are expectorate.
- Cyst rupture is the most serious complication, which can cause life-threatening anaphylaxis. Cholangitis can occur when there is rupture into the biliary tree. Cysts may also become secondarily infected, resulting in a pyogenic abscess.

- Alveolar hydatid disease is more invasive and likely to disseminate (e.g. to brain, bone, lungs, eyes). As a result it is sometimes mistaken for malignancy.

Diagnosis
- Most diagnoses are made by characteristic radiographic appearances, e.g. liver cyst, with characteristic multiple 'daughter' cysts on a CT or ultrasound scan.
- There is specific serology to support the diagnosis. Eosinophilia is not usually present until there is cyst rupture.
- Suspected cysts should not be routinely aspirated for diagnostic purposes because of the risk of rupture and disseminating infection. However, if inadvertently performed, protoscolex hooks may be seen on microscopy, using an appropriate stain.

Treatment
- Most liver cysts are amenable to percutaneous-aspiration-injection-re-aspiration (PAIR). A suitable scolicidal agent to inject is either hypertonic saline or 95% ethanol. Cure rates are >95%, but PAIR should only be performed at experienced centres.
- Albendazole is most effective in combination with PAIR or surgery for cystic hydatid disease. Some recommend albendazole 400 mg bd in three to six 4-week cycles, with a 14-day break between each cycle. Praziquantel may be used in combination if there is rupture
- If PAIR is not possible, consider surgical removal, particularly if there is the risk of imminent rupture or the cyst is causing significant pressure effects. An experienced surgeon in a specialist centre should perform this.

Cysticercosis
Cysticercosis can develop if pork tapeworm (*Taenia solium*) eggs are ingested with food or water contaminated with pig faeces. In the human intestine, larvae hatch from the eggs and invade host tissue. The CNS, muscle, skin, and eye are most affected, where larvae reside within cysts. Symptoms relate to viable and dying parasites and the long-term inflammatory reaction to degenerating cysts, e.g. calcification and fibrosis. It is widespread throughout the world, especially Africa, Asia, and South America.

Neurocysticercosis is the commonest cause of epilepsy worldwide. The number and distribution of cysts in the CNS varies considerably, and less common manifestations include behavioural change, hydrocephalus, meningitis, and focal neurological lesions. Small, firm cysts may be palpated under the skin and calcified cysts seen in muscle on X-ray. Ocular cysts may present with visual disturbance and progress to blindness.

Diagnosis is made by appearances on CT or MRI of the brain and serology. Lesions can be easily confused with tuberculoma radiologically. Treatment is with albendazole, but this needs to be considered carefully, as dying larvae can precipitate a host inflammatory response. Oral dexamethasone is, therefore, also given initially to reduce this potentially harmful effect. Surgery is reserved for cysts causing hydrocephalus or cord compression. Ocular cysts should not be treated with drugs and may need surgical intervention.

Strongyloidiasis
Epidemiology
- Strongyloidiasis (caused by the nematode worm *Strongyloides stercoralis*) is found widely throughout the tropics. Worms are able to live as free-living forms in soil or as parasitic forms in humans.

- Transmission occurs when larvae in the soil penetrate intact skin. Adult worms (<3 mm long) live in the small intestine, and females produces eggs that are passed with faeces into the soil.
- Some larvae hatch from eggs in the gut before being excreted. These invade the bowel wall and migrate back to the small intestine via the liver and lungs. This 'autoinfection' cycle means that infection can persist for decades in humans.

Clinical features
- Most infections are asymptomatic, but abdominal discomfort and chronic diarrhoea may occur. Fever is unusual. Migrating larvae sometimes produce a transient skin rash (larva currens on the trunk or generalized urticaria).
- In the immunocompromised host (e.g. HIV, HTLV-1, corticosteroids), the autoinfection cycle can produce a 'hyperinfection' syndrome, which may be fatal in ~80%. Features include diarrhoea, malabsorption, cough, and wheeze (Loeffler-like syndrome). Fever in this context is most likely to be related to Gram-negative bacteraemia from bowel wall invasion or the underlying immunodeficiency, e.g. lymphoma.

Diagnosis
- Eosinophilia is not invariably present.
- Diagnosis is by serology or demonstration of larvae in small intestinal aspirates/biopsies and stool.
- In hyperinfection, pulmonary infiltrates are visible on the X-ray, and larvae may be seen in the sputum by microscopy.
- A search should be made for the underlying immunodeficiency state in hyperinfection syndrome.

Management
- Standard treatment is with ivermectin 200 mcg/kg/day orally for 1–2 days. Albendazole is a significantly inferior alternative.
- Treatment may need to be repeated or prolonged in the hyperinfection syndrome. Patients with fever should receive intravenous antibiotics to cover Gram-negative bacteraemia.

Further reading
Brown K, Kirkbride H (2015). Public Health England guidelines on rabies post exposure treatment. <https://www.gov.uk/government/uploads/system/uploads/attachment_data/file/438926/PHE_clinical_rabies_service_Jun_2015.pdf>.

Department of Health Advisory Committee on Dangerous Pathogens (1996). Management and control of viral haemorrhagic fevers. The Stationery Office, London. <http://www.hpa.org.uk>.

Johnston V, Stockley JM, Dockrell D, *et al.* on behalf of the British Infection Society and the Hospital for Tropical Diseases (2009). Fever in returned travellers presenting in the United Kingdom; recommendations for investigation and initial management. *Journal of Infection*, **59**, 1–18.

Public Health England (2013). Rabies: The Green Book, Chapter 27. <https://www.gov.uk/government/publications/rabies-the-green-book-chapter-27>.

Public Health England (2015). Rabies: risk assessment, post-exposure treatment, management. <https://www.gov.uk/government/collections/rabies-risk-assessment-post-exposure-treatment-management>.

Fever of unknown origin (FUO)

Definition
In 1961, Petersdorf and Beeson defined FUO as a fever that is ≥38.3°C on several occasions, over a period of at least 3 weeks, the cause of which is not discovered after 1 week of inpatient investigation. However, with modern diagnostics and increased pressure to shorten the length of hospital stay, this definition has been updated to something more practical. FUO is, therefore, now strictly defined as a temperature of ≥38.3°C on several occasions for ≥3 weeks in duration, the cause of which is not identified after ≥3 days of inpatient investigation or ≥2 outpatient visits.

This definition helpfully excludes over 95% of the infections that are either treated effectively or self-limiting (e.g. viral infections). Strictly speaking, therefore, FUO is usually not an entity that can be diagnosed in a one-off emergency department encounter (a better term, in this context where there is no obvious source or aetiology, is 'unexplained' or 'undifferentiated' fever). The attending physician needs to be aware of the clinical approach with maximum diagnostic yield and whether and what to treat, especially if the patient's condition is deteriorating.

Epidemiology
The underlying cause falls into one of four classic categories: 'infection' (36%), 'neoplasia' (15%), 'autoimmune/inflammatory' (35%), and 'miscellaneous' (20%) (see Tables 6.8 and 6.9). The relative proportions in each group vary, depending upon the age of the patient, nationality, ethnic background, immune status, etc.

Tuberculosis is one of the most common causes of FUO and most frequently occurs in individuals from high-incidence countries or immigrant communities. Often there is no previous known contact with tuberculosis. In contrast, in individuals from low-risk ethnic backgrounds, a history of significant exposure should be sought (e.g. healthcare worker).

FUO in HIV-infected patients is often infective. Neoplastic causes, especially lymphoma, are also more common in this group. In neutropenic patients, fungal and bacterial infections predominate, but the underlying disease itself (e.g. a lymphoproliferative disorder) may sometimes be the culprit.

In the elderly, malignancy, temporal arteritis, chronic prostatitis, pulmonary emboli, drug fever, and tuberculosis are relatively more common. In young adults, SLE, Still's disease, and factitious fevers occur more frequently.

Clinical approach
The single most important diagnostic tool is a detailed clinical history and thorough examination. Where the patient volunteers no localizing symptoms, it is important to run through the review of systems in order not to overlook significant clues to the diagnosis. It is extremely useful to try and establish the duration and pattern of the illness. For example, relapsing and remitting fevers, with periods of normality between febrile episodes, may point to attacks of benign malaria or filariasis, flares of an autoimmune/vasculitic disorder, or a hereditary periodic condition (e.g. familial Mediterranean fever). Continuous febrile conditions with ≥1-year duration are unlikely to be infectious.

The history should be structured, as outlined in the previous paragraph, incorporating the relevant direct questions if there has been foreign travel. If no cause is found, a full history and examination should be repeated since important facts are sometimes remembered and physical signs evolve over time. It may be helpful to ask a colleague to see the patient since a 'fresh pair of eyes' can often be very helpful.

Pathology
Infections
Bacterial infections often take the form of occult intra-abdominal or pelvic collections, e.g. subdiaphragmatic, peri-

Table 6.8 Important infections causing FUO

Bacteria	Viral	Fungal	Protozoal and parasitic
Abscess (especially intra-abdominal)	EBV	*Pneumocystis jirovecii**	Toxocariasis
Bacterial endocarditis	CMV	Cryptococcosis*	Toxoplasmosis
Deep-seated focus (e.g. osteomyelitis)	HIV		
Leptospirosis	Parvovirus B19		
Lyme disease			
Opportunistic mycobacteria*			
Q fever			
Rat bite fever			
Syphilis			
Trench fever (Bartonellosis)			
Tuberculosis			
Brucellosis		Histoplasmosis*	Amoebiasis
Relapsing fever			Lymphatic filariasis
Rickettsial infections			Visceral leishmaniasis*
Typhoid			Malaria
Whipple's disease			Trichinosis
Yersiniosis			Trypanosomiasis

Bold indicates relatively more common cause.

* Especially in HIV-infected patients.

Table 6.9 Selected non-infectious causes of FUO

Neoplastic*	Connective tissue and rheumatological	Miscellaneous
Lymphoma	**Adult Still's disease**	Atrial myxoma
Leukaemia	Ankylosing spondylitis	Autoimmune haemolytic anaemia
Hepatoma	Behçet's disease	Castleman's disease
Hypernephroma	Cryoglobulinaemia	**Crohn's disease**
Intra-abdominal carcinoma	Giant cell arteritis	Cyclic neutropenia
Metastatic carcinoma	Gout and pseudogout	**Drug fever**
	Mixed connective tissue disease	Extrinsic allergic alveolitis
		Factitious fever
	Polyarteritis nodosa	Familial Mediterranean fever
	Polymyositis	Haematoma
	Relapsing polychondritis	Kawasaki's syndrome
	Rheumatic fever	Kikuchi's disease
	Rheumatoid disease	Metal fume fever
	Sjögren's syndrome	Pulmonary emboli
	SLE	Sarcoidosis
	Takayasu's aortitis	Seizures
	Wegener's granulomatosis	Thyroiditis

* Reported in all common malignancies.

Bold indicates relatively more common cause.

colic, and hepatic abscesses. Blood cultures in patients with endocarditis may initially be negative if one of the slow-growing Gram-negative organisms is involved (belonging to the HACEK group) or if the patient has received prior anti-biotics. The culture-negative causes of endocarditis should also be considered in patients with a heart murmur, such as Q fever, bartonellosis, brucellosis, *Chlamydia*, and legionel-losis. Occasionally, EBV and CMV may cause a prolonged febrile illness. As previously noted, tuberculosis is a major cause and usually takes the form of disseminated infection without miliary features on the chest X-ray or extrapulmo-nary disease without clear localizing features.

Whipple's disease (caused by *Tropheryma whipplei*) is rare, occurring most frequently in white, middle-aged males from mid-Europe. It presents mainly with weight loss, diar-rhoea (watery or steatorrhoea), and a chronic, migratory arthropathy affecting peripheral joints (one-third also have sacroiliac involvement). Fever is present in ~50%, and involvement of almost all organs has also been described, e.g. generalized lymphadenopathy, skin hyperpigmentation, and cardiac murmurs. Duodenal or jejunal lesions can be seen on endoscopy, and PAS-positive material is seen in macrophages from biopsy specimens. Culture is only per-formed in research laboratories. PCR on peripheral blood or tissue is helpful diagnostically. Untreated, Whipple's dis-ease can be fatal. Currently recommended treatment is with co-trimoxazole for 1 year, preceded by a 2-week course of IV ceftriaxone if the patient is severely ill or if there is evidence of CNS involvement.

Multisystem inflammatory diseases
Adult Still's disease (see Chapter 16) is the commonest rheumatologic cause of FUO and should be considered in young adults with a classic triad of high fever (>39°C), a transient ('evanescent') rash, and arthralgia, especially if sore throat is also present. Enlarged cervical lymph nodes, pericarditis, and splenomegaly may also feature. Anaemia, neutrophil leucocytosis, and a raised ESR are typical, although the acute phase protein, serum ferritin, may be disproportionately elevated into the 1,000s (not just 100s).

However, there is no definitive laboratory test, and other conditions with a similar clinical presentation need to be excluded before the diagnosis can be made.

In patients over 50 years old the potential diagnosis of temporal arteritis should be excluded. The classic physical signs of headache, jaw claudication, palpable temporal artery, and visual loss may be absent, but the inflammatory indices are usually very elevated (ESR >100 mm/h). Some have suggested that, in an elderly patient with FUO, a tem-poral artery biopsy should be performed routinely.

Neoplasia
Lymphoma is the commonest individual cause of an FUO. Constitutional or B symptoms (weight loss, night sweats, and fevers) are present in a minority of patients with lym-phoma. The classic 'Pel-Ebstein fever', characterized by intermittent febrile episodes lasting for days, followed by afebrile periods of days to weeks, is extremely rare. Whilst almost all tumours can cause FUO, fever appears to be more common in necrotic malignancies, those involving liver metastases, renal cell carcinoma, and adenocarcino-mas. A cardiac murmur may be absent in atrial myxoma, but a 'tumour plop' may be heard during diastole, and other features resembling endocarditis may be evident, e.g. arthralgia, rash, weight loss, anaemia, and raised inflamma-tory indices

Miscellaneous
This encompasses a large number of unrelated conditions, some obscure. Crohn's disease is a major cause and may present with weight loss, fever, and anaemia, without pro-nounced gastrointestinal symptoms. A haematoma may cause unexplained fever, especially if there has been a retro-peritoneal bleed. Drug fever develops 1–3 weeks after a new drug (e.g. phenytoin, sulfonamides, and beta-lactams). Factitious fever often occurs in well-looking young adults, and fraudulent behaviour is occasionally responsible for a genuine fever (e.g. deliberately contaminating IV lines, resulting in polymicrobial bacteraemias). Cyclic neutropenia

is notable for causing recurrent febrile episodes at fixed intervals of approximately 21 days.

Castleman's disease (or angiofollicular lymph node hyperplasia) may present with focal mediastinal or generalized lymphadenopathy. The localized type occurs in young adults and is curable by surgery. The generalized form affects older patients and may undergo malignant transformation. Kikuchi disease (also Kikuchi-Fujimoto disease) is an uncommon, idiopathic necrotizing lymphadenitis. It occurs mainly in young adults, with a slight female preponderance. Infectious and autoimmune aetiologies have been proposed, and it can be mistaken for SLE or lymphoma. The disease generally runs a benign and self-limiting course, but, in a small number of cases, it is recurrent. Lymphadenopathy most often resolves over several weeks to 6 months.

Sweet's syndrome is an acute-onset neutrophilic dermatosis. It is characterized by the sudden onset of fever, leucocytosis, tender and erythematous papules and plaques, which show dense neutrophilic infiltrates. Lesions most frequently appear on the upper body, including the face, but can appear anywhere. Although mostly idiopathic, Sweet's syndrome can be associated with haematological malignancies and inflammatory disorders, e.g. rheumatoid arthritis, inflammatory bowel disease, etc. Arthralgia is common. Treatment with systemic corticosteroids is usually effective.

Familial Mediterranean fever is a hereditary autosomal recessive condition that occurs in patients with Jewish, Turkish, Armenian, or Arab ancestry. It is characterized by recurrent attacks of fever, with polyserositis (peritonitis, arthritis, and pleuritis). Attacks only last for a few hours to days, and, between episodes, the patient is well. Ninety per cent of patients have their first attack before the age of 20 years, and, appendicectomy, following a misdiagnosed attack of abdominal pain, is almost the norm. The diagnosis can now be confirmed by identifying the defective gene (*MEFV*—the pyrin gene). The main complication is renal failure caused by amyloid deposition, which may be prevented with colchicine treatment.

Other rare hereditary periodic fevers include hyper-IgD syndrome and TNF-alpha receptor-associated periodic syndrome (TRAPS). Hyper-IgD syndrome is an autosomal recessive disease that starts before the first year of life in children of French and Dutch ancestry. Recurrent attacks continue throughout life and are characterized by fever, cervical lymphadenopathy, and abdominal pain, with diarrhoea or vomiting. Very high IgD levels are continuously found in

serum. TRAPS (originally called familial Hibernian fever) has autosomal dominant inheritance and begins in patients <20 years with Scottish and Irish ancestry. Uncontrolled inflammation, resulting from the inability to 'switch off' TNF-alpha signalling, is thought to be responsible for recurrent attacks of fever, myalgia, abdominal pain, and erythematous skin lesions.

Investigations

A list of routine tests and more specialized investigations is shown in Table 6.10. The peripheral white blood cell differential may give a useful clue to the diagnosis, as mentioned previously. Very high eosinophil counts (>3 × 10^9/L) are more suggestive of malignancy, drug reactions, and Churg–Strauss syndrome than parasitic infections. Raised inflammatory indices make factitious fever less likely, and very high inflammatory markers (ESR >100 mm/h) are frequently seen in Still's disease, drug fever, endocarditis, giant cell arteritis, myeloma, and other malignancies. Mild liver function test abnormalities occur in many causes, including, tuberculosis, viral infections, brucellosis, Q fever, Still's disease, and drug fever. Elevated alkaline phosphatase with no alternative explanation can indicate disseminated tuberculosis, and, in patients with advanced HIV infection, it may point to cryptosporidiosis or *Mycobacterium avium intracellulare* infection. Serum angiotensin-converting enzyme may be elevated in sarcoidosis or, more rarely, granulomatous infections.

Abnormal findings on urinalysis may point towards a renal tract source, but microscopic haematuria also occurs in endocarditis and other causes of renal vasculitis. Three blood culture sets should be performed to increase the chance of isolating a pathogen. Serum should be 'saved' early in the illness, so a specific antibody response to a suspected pathogen may be demonstrated in paired samples after a suitable interval. A Paul Bunnell test gives a rapid result, compared to specific EBV or CMV serology, but false negatives are not uncommon. Knowing the patient's HIV status at an early stage frequently assists the clinician to assess the likelihood of an opportunistic infection being involved. In general, most serological tests for infection and 'blind' autoantibody 'screens' have a low diagnostic yield in the setting of an FUO.

A positive Mantoux skin test (or immunoassay) does not allow differentiation between latent and active tuberculosis. However, extremely vigorous or blistering skin reactions

Table 6.10 Investigations for patients with an FUO

Routine	Specialized
FBC	Monospot or Paul Bunnell test
Blood film	Autoantibodies, e.g. rheumatoid factor, ANA, ANCA
Thick and thin malaria film if travel	Serum angiotensin-converting enzyme
U&E and liver function tests	Syphilis serology
C-reactive protein	HIV test
Urine dipstick	Serological tests, e.g. EBV, etc.
MSU	Serum save
Blood cultures (≥2 sets)	Tuberculin skin test
Chest X-ray	Early morning urine (if suspected renal or miliary TB)
	Urine microscopy, e.g. for red cell casts if suspected vasculitis
	Imaging, e.g. abdominal USS or CT chest, abdomen, and pelvis
	Echocardiogram
	Biopsy, e.g. liver, bone marrow, temporal artery, etc.
	Radionucleotide scan?

are more often seen in active infection. Early morning urine samples are not helpful, unless renal tract or miliary tuberculosis is possible.

Chest CT scans may reveal intrathoracic lymphadenopathy or miliary shadowing invisible on a plain chest film. Ultrasound or CT scans of the abdomen may reveal an occult collection, lymphadenopathy, or malignancy. Of note, some intra-abdominal structures may not be as easily visualized by ultrasound, especially if they are obscured by bowel gas or if the patient is grossly obese. Abdominal tuberculosis can be a particularly difficult diagnosis, and peritoneal 'thickening' or 'stranding' on a CT scan should alert the physician to this possibility. In such a situation, laparoscopic peritoneal biopsy should be considered, especially if intra-abdominal lymphadenopathy is present.

As a rule, it is helpful to biopsy tissue where possible, in particular, excision of lymph nodes (≥1 cm in diameter) or skin lesions. In sarcoidosis, non-caseating granulomas in tissue biopsies are characteristic. Liver biopsy demonstrates granulomas in 80–90% of cases of miliary tuberculosis. The presence of granulomas on biopsy samples may also point towards Q fever, brucellosis, sarcoidosis, and lymphoma, amongst other possibilities. Bone marrow biopsy is likely to show tuberculous granuloma in ~50% of miliary tuberculosis, but the yield is >80% when there are abnormalities in the peripheral blood (e.g. leucopenia or anaemia are present). Although a rapid visual result is not available, in advanced HIV infection, mycobacterial blood cultures have a similar culture yield for tuberculosis as bone marrow samples. Bone marrow examination may also be revealing in other disseminated infections (e.g. leishmaniasis, typhoid, histoplasmosis) and infiltrative malignancies.

An echocardiogram to look for vegetations on heart valves should be performed if there is a murmur or other stigmata of infective endocarditis. Radionucleotide scans have a controversial role in the investigation of FUO, as they often reveal little more than a CT scan of chest, abdomen, and pelvis.

Management

Empiric courses of treatment with antimicrobials are generally ill advised, unless the patient is unwell or severely immunocompromised. However, if empiric therapy is felt absolutely necessary, a full course of treatment should be given and only after material for culture has been obtained. In particular, once empiric anti-tuberculous therapy has been commenced, it is not recommended to stop prematurely, unless an alternative diagnosis is confirmed or if there are significant adverse drug effects. It is essential to exclude infection and lymphoma as far as possible if empiric steroids are thought necessary for a presumed autoimmune inflammatory disorder. If the patient remains relatively well and no cause is found, it is reasonable to monitor their progress at regular intervals as an outpatient. It is sometimes worth asking patients to purchase a digital thermometer and to monitor their own temperature between visits. Twenty per cent of patients remain undiagnosed; however, the prognosis for the majority is good, and the fever usually resolves within a few weeks.

Further reading

Arnow PM and Flaherty JP (1997). Fever of unknown origin. *Lancet*, **350**, 575–80.

British HIV Association. <http://www.bhiva.org>.

British Infection Society. <http://www.britishinfection.org>.

British Thoracic Society (excellent guidelines on all aspects of the management of tuberculosis). <http://www.brit-thoracic.org.uk>.

Centers for Disease Control and Prevention (USA). <http://www.cdc.gov>.

Drenth JPH and Van der Meer JVM (2001). Hereditary periodic fever. *New England Journal of Medicine*, **345**, 1748–57.

Infectious Diseases Society of America. <http://www.idsociety.org>.

Knockaert DC, Vannestse LJ, Bobbaers HJ (1993). Recurrent or episodic fever of unknown origin. *Medicine*, **72**, 184–96.

Larson EB (1984). Adult Still's disease. *Medicine*, **63**, 82–91.

Petersforf RG and Beeson PB (1961). Fever of unexplained origin: report on 100 cases. *Medicine*, **40**, 1–30.

Public Health England. <https://www.gov.uk/government/organisations/public-health-england>.

UK Department of Health Immunization against Infectious Diseases. <https://www.gov.uk/government/organisations/public-health-england/series/immunisation-against-infectious-disease-the-green-book>.

World Health Organization. <http://www.who.int/en>.

Principles and practice of antibiotic use

Since their discovery in the 1930s, antibiotics have generally been viewed as agents only capable of doing good to patients. Indeed, over the past six decades, their use has cured countless individuals of infections they would have died from in the pre-antibiotic era. However, it has become apparent in recent years that bacteria are quite capable of outwitting human endeavour in developing new antimicrobials to combat increasing antibiotic resistance. Although there have been several recently developed antibiotics active against Gram-positive bacteria, the pipeline for the development of agents active against Gram-negative bacteria looks decidedly unpromising.

Bacteria develop resistance to antibiotics by a process akin to Darwinian selection—the greater the antibiotic 'pressure', the higher the probability that resistant subpopulations will expand. Thus, many countries are now putting resources into controlling the use of antimicrobials in an effort to preserve their benefit. In addition, large outbreaks of highly transmissible, and apparently hypervirulent, strains of Clostridium difficile infection have been described in developed countries over recent years. This infection has a direct link to the prior use of antibiotics, particularly those with a broad-spectrum of activity.

How to choose the right antibiotic

Several decisions need to be made before the correct antibiotic can be prescribed:

- Attempt to make an accurate microbial diagnosis.
- Choose an antibiotic active against the relevant bacteria.
- Choose the right dose (and route of administration).
- Prescribe for the correct duration.

There is often significant uncertainty at all of these stages. The science behind choosing the correct duration, a parameter closely linked to both the generation of antimicrobial resistance and C. difficile infection, has a particularly weak evidence base.

The prescribing physician should also try to answer the question '**Is this infection community-acquired or hospital-acquired?**' because the former usually involves bacteria that are much more susceptible to antimicrobials than the latter. For example, Pseudomonas aeruginosa, an organism intrinsically resistant to many antibiotics, rarely causes infection in patients in the community. Therefore, empirical treatment of community-acquired infections rarely needs to cover this microbe. Hospital-acquired infections are usually defined as infections occurring more than two days into hospital admission. Similar 'hospital-type' organisms may be implicated in infections occurring in patients recently discharged from hospital or patients resident in long-term care facilities.

Making an accurate microbial diagnosis

As microbiological information is rarely available at the point of care, this usually relies on knowledge of the likely organisms that may cause the diagnosed infection. However, relevant specimens should be taken for culture (with or without initial Gram stain) prior to starting antibiotics. Some rapid tests are now available to identify specific microbes (e.g. group A streptococcal antigen tests for pharyngitis) and urinary Legionella and pneumococcal antigen tests (for pneumonia). For some specimens, discussion with the microbiology laboratory to request an urgent Gram stain will be appropriate, for example, aspirates of normally sterile sites or debrided tissue where necrotizing fasciitis is suspected.

Choosing an effective antibiotic

The prescriber needs to have a working knowledge of the antibacterial spectra of the antibiotics on his or her formulary. A knowledge of local antibiotic resistance patterns is also important, particularly for common pathogens, such as Streptococcus pneumoniae. Decreased susceptibility to penicillin for this organism ranges from around 5% to 40%, depending on the geographic location. Hospital-associated infections are generally caused by pathogens with a much broader array of resistance mechanisms. Consequently, empirical antibiotics for these infections are usually different from those aimed at community-associated infection.

Clinicians must actively pursue microbiological results in order to rationalize antibiotics. This may mean broadening cover where unexpected resistance is detected or narrowing the spectrum of the antibiotic, for example, switching to benzylpenicillin when a penicillin-susceptible Pneumococcus is detected in blood cultures. In general, an agent with the narrowest spectrum should be chosen. This will often limit the side effect profile, minimize the risk of Clostridium difficile infection, and have the least ecological impact on antimicrobial resistance in the environment. (Tables 6.11 and 6.12 provide a guide to the antibacterial activity of commonly prescribed agents.)

Choosing the right dose and route

Due attention should be given to the age of the patient and renal/liver function when prescribing an antibiotic. The minimum dose required to treat the infection should be prescribed. This will minimize both the cost of the antibiotic course and the risk of side effects. The oral route will be appropriate for the vast majority of infections. Parenteral antibiotics are preferred, at least initially, for the following situations:

- Endocarditis.
- Septic arthritis or osteomyelitis.
- Meningitis.
- Severe sepsis/septic shock.
- Vomiting or abnormal gastrointestinal absorption.
- Necrotizing soft tissue infections.
- Staphylococcus aureus bacteraemia.

Choosing the right duration

For many infections, there are few published data to help decide on an appropriate antibiotic duration. This statement is particularly true for hospital-acquired infections, such as ventilator-associated pneumonia where some authorities would recommend 21 days of antimicrobial therapy, whereas others would advocate just 5 days. Many virulent and antibiotic-susceptible bacteria (e.g. Neisseria meningitidis and penicillin-susceptible pneumococci) will be non-viable within hours of starting antibiotics: physicians must resist the temptation to give long antibiotic courses in these patients, however complicated their clinical course. (Table 6.13 lists suggested durations of therapy for selected infections.)

For certain life-threatening infections, there is evidence that the time taken to administer the first antibiotic dose is critical. In severe sepsis and septic shock, there are data to

Table 6.11 Relative activity of selected beta-lactam antibiotics against common pathogens

Bacteria	Antibiotic								
	Amoxicillin	Co-amoxiclav	Cefalexin/ cefadroxil	Cefuroxime	Cefoxitin	Ceftriaxone/ cefotaxime	Ceftazidime	Piperacillin-tazobactam	Meropenem
Streptococci	+++	+++	++	++	++	++	+	+++	+++
S. aureus (meticillin-susceptible)	+/–	+++	+	++	++	++	+	+++	+++
MRSA	–	–	–	–	–	–	–	–	–
Coagulase-negative staphylococci	+/–	+/–	–	+/–	+/–	+/–	–	+/–	+/–
Enterococcus faecalis	+++	+++	–	–	–	–	–	++	–
Enterococcus faecium	–	–	–	–	–	–	–	–	–
H. influenzae	+	+++	+	++	++	+++	+++	+++	+++
M. catarrhalis	-	+++	+	++	++	+++	+++	+++	+++
N. meningitidis	++	++	+	++	++	+++	+++	+++	+++
N. gonorrhoeae	+	++	+	++	++	+++	+++	+++	+++
E. coli	+	++	+	++	++	++	++	++	+++
Klebsiella spp.	–	++	+	++	++	++	++	++	+++
Serratia, Enterobacter, and Morganella species	–	–	–	–	–	+	+	+	+++
Pseudomonas aeruginosa	–	–	–	–	–	–	+++	+++	+++
Anaerobes	+	+++	–	–	++	–	–	+++	+++

MRSA, meticillin-resistant *S. Aureus*

show that, for each hour's delay in administering an effective antibiotic, the mortality increases by around 8%.

Combination therapy

There has been much debate over the years regarding the merits of antibiotic combinations. There are several potential reasons for adopting this approach, as detailed in the following paragraphs:

Prevention of resistance

Theoretical and animal data underpin the argument for using combination therapy to prevent the emergence of resistance. Indeed, there is sound clinical evidence for this approach in the management of some infections, notably tuberculosis and HIV infection. There is, however, no convincing evidence for this approach for the treatment of bacterial infections in general.

Synergistic action

The use of combination therapy for the initial treatment of neutropenic sepsis is widely practised. However, a recent meta-analysis did not suggest a benefit of two active agents

over one in the treatment of Gram-negative bacteraemia. The only possible exception to this is in *Pseudomonas aeruginosa* bacteraemia. This study did suggest some benefit in patients receiving two active agents, rather than one. The main rationale, therefore, for use of combination therapy in these patients is to ensure that at least one antibiotic is active against the infecting bacteria, rather than to achieve a synergistic action. The only infection for which there is evidence for clinical benefit of two synergistic antibiotics is endocarditis caused by the viridans group streptococci and *Enterococcus faecalis*. In both these settings, the combination of a penicillin and an aminoglycoside, a synergistic pairing *in vitro*, achieves higher, or more rapid, clinical cure rates. The main benefit of this approach in viridans streptococcal endocarditis is to allow the use of short 2-week antibiotic courses in uncomplicated cases. Its use in enterococcal endocarditis leads to higher cure rates than penicillin monotherapy.

Table 6.12 Relative activity of selected non-beta-lactam antibiotics against common pathogens

Bacteria	Antibiotic								
	Ciprofloxacin	Moxifloxacin	Clarithromycin	Gentamicin	Amikacin	Tigecycline	Daptomycin	Vancomycin/teicoplanin	Linezolid
Streptococci	+/-	++	++	–	–	+++	+++	+++	+++
S. aureus (meticillin-susceptible)	+	++	++	++	++	+++	+++	+++	+++
MRSA	–	–	+/-	+	+	+++	+++	+++	+++
Coagulase-negative staphylococci	+	+	+/-	+/-	+/-	+++	+++	+++	+++
Enterococcus faecalis	–	–	–	–	–	++	+++	++	+++
Enterococcus faecium	–	–	–	–	–	++	+++	++	+++
H. influenzae	+++	+++	+++	+	+	++	–	–	–
M. catarrhalis	+++	+++	+++	+	+	++	–	–	–
N. meningitidis	+++	+++	++	+	+	++	–	–	+
N. gonorrhoeae	+	+	++	+	+	++	–	–	+
E. coli	++	++	–	+++	+++	+++	–	–	–
Klebsiella spp.	++	++	–	+++	+++	+++	–	–	–
Serratia, Enterobacter, and Morganella species	++	++	–	+++	+++	+++ (except Morganella)	–	–	–
Pseudomonas aeruginosa	++	–	–	+++	+++	–	–	–	–
Anaerobes	–	–	+/-	–	+/-	+++	+/-	+	+

MRSA, meticillin-resistant S. Aureus

Table 6.13 Suggested durations of antimicrobial therapy for selected infections

Condition	Duration of treatment (days)	Comments
Uncomplicated urinary tract infection	3	7–14 days for men
Pyelonephritis	10–14	
Epididymo-orchitis	14	
Community-acquired pneumonia	7	14–21 days for *Legionella* infection
Empyema	14–42	Duration depends on adequacy of surgical drainage. 14 days appropriate for susceptible pathogens (e.g. penicillin-susceptible *S. pneumoniae*)
Acute exacerbation of COPD	7	
Acute otitis media or sinusitis	7	
Acute pharyngitis	10	If Penicillin V used
Cellulitis	7–10	
Diabetic foot infection (no osteomyelitis)	7–14	
Diabetic foot infection (osteomyelitis)	42–56	
Cholecystitis, peritonitis, cholangitis	7	
Spontaneous bacterial peritonitis	7	
Septic arthritis (native joint)	28–42	
Osteomyelitis	28–42	Longer courses may be necessary for vertebral osteomyelitis. Duration in chronic osteomyelitis depends on nature of surgical intervention
Meningitis (*N. meningitidis*)	5	
Meningitis (*S. pneumoniae*)	7–10	Longer courses may be required for organisms with intermediate or high level penicillin resistance
Meningitis (*H. influenzae*)	7–10	
Meningitis (*Listeria monocytogenes*)	21	
Infective endocarditis	14–42	Duration depends on organism and its susceptibility to prescribed antibiotic, whether native or prosthetic valve and whether patient undergoes surgery
Hospital-acquired pneumonia and ventilator-associated pneumonia	7	Longer courses may be necessary, especially if there is radiological evidence of cavitation
Aspiration pneumonitis	3	This short course is appropriate where antibiotics are started shortly after aspiration event (especially in the hospital setting)
Clostridium difficile infection	10–14	

Broad-spectrum activity

Many infections, particularly in surgical wards, are polymicrobial. In this setting, the use of more than one antibiotic is often appropriate to achieve activity against all relevant bacteria. Cefuroxime and metronidazole is a favoured combination in the UK for community-associated intra-abdominal sepsis: the former agent treats streptococci and coliforms, and the latter treats anaerobes.

Penicillin allergy

Hypersensitivity to penicillins affects around 2% of the general population. It may manifest as follows:
- Pruritic maculopapular rash.
- Hypotension (anaphylactic).
- Wheezing.
- Stridor (due to upper airway oedema).
- Facial swelling (angio-oedema).

Unfortunately, both patients and physicians overdiagnose the condition. In most series, only 10–20% of patients reporting penicillin allergy have true hypersensitivity on skin testing. Approximately 5–10% of patients with a penicillin allergy will also be allergic to cephalosporins. In addition, the cross-reactivity appears to be appreciably higher with first-generation cephalosporins than with second- or third-generation cephalosporins. In a recent meta-analysis in patients with penicillin allergy, the odds ratio for an allergic reaction to a cephalosporin was 4.79 (CI 3.71–6.17) for a first-generation, 1.13 (CI 0.61–2.12) for a second-generation, and 0.45 (CI 0.18–1.13) for a third-generation cephalosporin respectively.

As beta-lactam agents are the mainstay of treatment for so many infections, some of which are life-threatening, establishing the true allergy status of patients is extremely important. The first step is to ascertain the nature of the allergic reaction. In many cases, the symptoms reported clearly represent mere intolerance (e.g. diarrhoea). In patients reporting a reaction consistent with an allergy, the second step is to consider skin testing. This can often be arranged as an outpatient, particularly in those patients with chronic medical conditions that render them susceptible to infection. In an important minority of inpatients, urgent penicillin skin testing should be arranged, if available. This group mainly includes patients with serious infections requiring prolonged parenteral antibiotics, e.g. infective endocarditis, osteomyelitis, or S. aureus bacteraemia.

For obvious patient safety reasons, individuals with penicillin allergy should never be given antibiotics containing a penicillin, and all agents containing the beta-lactam ring should be avoided. Beta-lactam ring-based agents are listed as follows:
- Penicillins (e.g. benzylpenicillin, phenoxymethylpenicillin, flucloxacillin, amoxicillin).
- Penicillin/beta-lactamase inhibitor combinations (e.g. co-amoxiclav, piperacillin-tazobactam).
- Cephalosporins (e.g. cefalexin, cefuroxime, ceftazidime).
- Carbapenems (e.g. meropenem, imipenem).
- Monobactams (e.g. aztreonam).

In clinical practice, however, physicians are often faced with a reportedly penicillin-allergic patient with a life-threatening infection for which a beta-lactam agent is the optimal treatment. In such situations, a second- or third-generation cephalosporin or a carbapenem **may** be given but with resuscitation facilities nearby.

Prescription of antibiotics and antibiotic stewardship

In the current era of increasing antibiotic resistance and hypervirulent C. difficile strains, there is much interest in controlling antibiotic use both in the community and in healthcare environments. In addition, there is good evidence that such programmes are cost-effective and may enhance patient care. In the UK, antimicrobial stewardship programmes are now mandatory for all NHS Trusts. The main aims of these programmes are as follows:
1. To promote rational choice of antimicrobials through publication of antibiotic policies.
2. To promote a switch from intravenous to oral antibiotics as soon as clinically appropriate.

3. To promote rationalization of antibiotics when microbiological data are available.
4. To encourage accurate prescription of antibiotics, with documentation of indication for use and duration of prescription on drug charts.

Stewardship programmes should include specialist pharmacists, infectious disease physicians, microbiologists, and epidemiologists or information technology specialists. Control of antibiotic prescribing may be achieved using a range of different strategies, including:
- Antimicrobial ward rounds.
- Ward-based pharmacists questioning inappropriate prescriptions.
- Pharmacist-driven automatic stop dates for antibiotics after defined duration (e.g. 7 days).
- Regular audits of antibiotic use with feedback to prescribers.
- Designated controlled antibiotics that require authorization from an infection specialist (e.g. pharmacist, microbiologist, or infectious diseases physician) before they can be dispensed.
- Electronic prescribing (with appropriate automatic controls of antibiotic prescribing).

Further reading

Bliziotis IA, Samonis G, Vardakas KZ, Chrysanthopoulou S, Falagas ME (2005). Effect of aminoglycoside and beta-lactam combination therapy versus beta-lactam monotherapy on the emergence of antimicrobial resistance: a meta-analysis of randomized, controlled trials. *Clinical Infectious Diseases*, **41**, 149–58.

Dellit TH, Owens RC, McGowan JE, et al. (2007). Infectious Diseases Society of America and the Society for Healthcare Epidemiology of America guidelines for developing an institutional program to enhance antimicrobial stewardship. *Clinical Infectious Diseases*, **44**, 159–77.

Kumar A, Roberts D, Wood KE, et al. (2006). Duration of hypotension before initiation of effective antimicrobial therapy is the critical determinant of survival in human septic shock. *Critical Care Medicine*, **34**, 1589–96.

National Institute for Health and Clinical Excellence (NICE) QS61 (2014). Infection prevention and control. Quality statement 1: Antimicrobial stewardship. <https://www.nice.org.uk/guidance/qs61/chapter/quality-statement-1-antimicrobial-stewardship>.

Pichichero ME and Casey JR (2007). Safe use of selected cephalosporins in penicillin allergic patients: a meta-analysis. *Otolaryngology—Head and Neck Surgery*, **136**, 340–7.

Public Health England (2015). Antimicrobial stewardship: start smart, then focus. Toolkit for hospitals. <https://www.gov.uk/government/publications/antimicrobial-stewardship-start-smart-then-focus>.

Safdar N, Handelsman J, Maki DG (2004). Does combination antimicrobial therapy reduce mortality in Gram-negative bacteraemia? A meta-analysis. *Lancet Infectious Diseases*, **4**, 519–27.

Public health aspects of infectious disease

Introduction

The practice of clinical medicine and the focus of medical textbooks are predicated on the principle of curing individual patients by establishing the diagnosis and instituting appropriate therapy. By contrast, public health practitioners set their focus at the level of populations. Epidemiology provides the scientific basis for the analysis of threats to public health, whether they be infectious in origin or not. However, infectious diseases have the unique feature, when compared to other human diseases, that they are transmissible from person to person. Understanding the epidemiology of infectious diseases also requires an appreciation of the biology of infectious agents and the host-parasite interaction.

Public health officials are generally concerned with prevention of infectious diseases. This occurs at different levels. Within the hospital environment, the infection control department, usually led by a medical doctor with specialist training, is charged with identifying and dealing with the threat of infectious disease transmission. Public health services generally deal with local communities and national threats. Lastly, international infectious threats are addressed by bodies, such as the World Health Organization, working with national and supranational organizations, such as the European Centre for Disease Control. In England, for example, public health tasks are carried out by Public Health England (PHE), which is part of the Department of Health. This agency operates at a local level through Health Protection Teams (HPTs) that cover sections of the population; London, for example, has four such units. The HPTs have two main functions:

- **Proactive:** prevention of infectious diseases through promotion of immunization, support for hospitals in prevention of healthcare-associated infection, and provision of advice for prevention of travel-associated infection.
- **Reactive:** to prevent further cases once an incident has occurred. This includes surveillance to identify outbreaks, contact tracing, and epidemiological investigations of outbreaks.

Notification of infectious diseases

Most countries have a system for passive collection of epidemiological data on selected infectious diseases. This information is then used to monitor the incidence of infectious diseases, detect outbreaks, and plan interventions. As individual physicians will often only manage single cases, even large countrywide outbreaks may not be detected without effective reporting mechanisms.

Notification may be enshrined in law, as in the UK, where, since the 19th century, medical practitioners have been required to inform public health authorities when they diagnose or suspect certain infectious diseases (see Table 6.14). Importantly, microbiological confirmation of the aetiology of these infections is generally not required. Compliance with such legislation, however, can be poor. For example, in the UK, national statistics on the incidence of food poisoning are notoriously unreliable, partly because most cases are not severe enough to bring the patient to medical attention and partly because notification by doctors is unreliable. By contrast, notification of some infectious diseases, such as tuberculosis, is very good, as specific resources are available for the control of this infection.

Table 6.14 List of notifiable diseases under the Health Protection Legislation (England) 2010

Infectious disease or syndrome

- Acute encephalitis
- Acute infectious hepatitis
- Acute meningitis
- Acute poliomyelitis
- Anthrax
- Botulism
- Brucellosis
- Cholera
- Diphtheria
- Enteric fever (typhoid or paratyphoid fever)
- Food poisoning
- Haemolytic uraemic syndrome (HUS)
- Infectious bloody diarrhoea
- Invasive group A streptococcal disease
- Legionnaires' disease
- Leprosy
- Malaria
- Measles
- Meningococcal septicaemia
- Mumps
- Plague
- Rabies
- Rubella
- SARS
- Scarlet fever
- Smallpox
- Tetanus
- Tuberculosis
- Typhus
- Viral haemorrhagic fever (VHF)
- Whooping cough
- Yellow fever

<https://www.gov.uk/government/organisations/public-health-england>

In the UK, surveillance data for other infections are collected outside of the legal framework previously described. Some of this data collection is continuous, and some is finite in response to perceived public health threats. Examples of infections in these categories include listeriosis, *Legionella* infection, and invasive group A streptococcal infections.

Systems for recording epidemiological trends vary from country to country. In the USA, medical doctors are required by law to notify infectious diseases. In addition, Centers for Disease Control and Prevention coordinate a range of active surveillance schemes. For example, the Active Bacterial Core Surveillance Scheme actively records both laboratory and population-based data on selected bacterial infections from selected states in the USA. This more active surveillance, with its associated microbiological data, yields detailed national data essential for the consideration of novel interventions, such as group A streptococcal vaccination.

Public health aspects of selected infectious diseases

Public health professionals require notification of statutory notifiable diseases, because for some infections, specific and sometimes urgent interventions are necessary to prevent further transmission. A full discussion of all these approaches is beyond the remit of this chapter, but a few examples described in the following paragraphs illustrate many of the principles.

Measles

Measles is a highly transmissible viral infection: secondary attack rates in non-immune household contacts approach 90%. It also has a significant case fatality rate, even in the developed world. As there are several highly effective measles vaccines available, immunization is the key public health weapon in the fight against this disease. Measles vaccination in the UK started in the 1960s, and, in 1988, a combined measles-mumps-rubella (MMR) vaccine was introduced. Unfortunately, due to adverse publicity, vaccination rates have fallen in recent years, and measles incidence has subsequently risen. Suspected measles must be promptly notified, as the following interventions are required:

- Laboratory support may be necessary for confirmation (e.g. salivary IgM antibody testing in reference laboratories).
- Affected individuals should be kept away from childcare settings for 4 days after the onset of the rash.
- Non-immune pregnant women exposed to measles may require immunoprophylaxis with human normal immunoglobulin (HNIG) if presentation is within 6 days of exposure.
- Consideration should be given to the administration of HNIG to immunocompromised individuals and infants under 1 year of age.
- Non-immune exposed individuals should be offered MMR, ideally within 3 days of exposure.

Anthrax

Anthrax is a severe bacterial infection caused by *Bacillus anthracis*. The infection is very rare in developed countries: there were just six reported cases in the UK from 1999 to 2008. However, as infection may be acquired from infected imported animal products (whole animals for slaughter, hides, wool), it has public health importance. In addition, anthrax spores have potential for use as a bioterrorism vehicle. Public health officials must be notified of any suspected cases in order to carry out an investigation into the likely source of the infection. The main goal of such an investigation is to ensure other people are not put at risk. Of interest, a large outbreak of cutaneous anthrax in injecting drug users occurred in Scotland in 2010, with 119 cases and 14 deaths. Public health interventions in this outbreak included:

- Publicizing the epidemiological and clinical features amongst healthcare professionals.
- Providing information for drug users to facilitate early recognition of the symptoms.
- Working with police to identify the source of the anthrax spores (thought to be contaminated heroin).

Whooping cough

Whooping cough or pertussis, is cause by *Bordetella pertussis*. Although childhood immunization strategies have reduced the incidence of the disease in many countries, circulation of the infection may still occur in adolescents and young adults. Although significant morbidity may occur in adults with pertussis, the greatest mortality burden rests with infants less than 6 months of age. A resurgence of the disease has been documented in several developed countries. As a consequence, some countries have introduced adolescent or adult vaccination campaigns. Once a case of pertussis is identified, consideration should be given to the following:

- Chemoprophylaxis: erythromycin (or another macrolide) is recommended for non-immunized, or partially immunized, vulnerable contacts (particularly infants).
- Partially immunized contacts should complete their vaccination schedules.
- In the healthcare setting, particularly neonatal units, widespread chemoprophylaxis for both infants and exposed healthcare workers may be necessary.
- Affected individuals should be excluded from childcare facilities until 21 days after the onset of symptoms or 5 days after commencing effective antibiotics.

Malaria

Malaria is a relatively common imported tropical infection in the UK, with around 1,500 cases per year. Detailed epidemiological information on cases is collated by the Malaria Reference Laboratory (part of PHE). Trends are analysed on a regular basis. This informs public health drives to reduce imported malaria in the UK. The main focus for this is promotion of the three methods of malaria prevention in travellers: personal insect repellents, bed nets, and chemoprophylaxis. The main risk group at which this health message is aimed is travellers leaving the UK to visit friends and relatives in their country of origin. Malaria is not transmissible in the UK, although it was endemic in the South East of England in the 19th century. Thus, historically, notification data were used to identify foci of local malaria transmission. Small clusters of autochthonous malaria transmission still occasionally occur in southern parts of the USA.

Hepatitis A

Hepatitis A virus causes an acute hepatitis and is transmitted via the faeco-oral route. Natural infection leads to lifelong immunity, and available active vaccines are highly effective. In the UK, most infections occur after travel to tropical regions of the world or in high-risk groups (men who have sex with men and injecting drug users). Prompt telephone notification of acute hepatitis A (based on a positive IgM test) is essential to facilitate preventative interventions described in recent PHE publications:

- The index case should be excluded from childcare facilities or the work place until 7 days after the onset of jaundice.
- Single-dose monovalent hepatitis A vaccine is recommended for household and sexual contacts of the index case where vaccine can be administered within 7 days of onset of jaundice. HNIG is recommended if the onset of jaundice was 7–14 days earlier and may be used after 14 days, particularly in the elderly.
- For contacts with chronic liver disease, HNIG plus hepatitis A vaccine is recommended where duration of exposure is between 14 and 28 days.

- If the index case is a food handler, consideration should be given to vaccinating co-workers or recipients of high-risk food prepared by the index case.
- Where there are large numbers of cases (e.g. in injecting drug users), large-scale vaccination of the at-risk population may be warranted.

Further reading

Chorba TL, Berkelman RL, Safford SK, Gibbs NP, Hull HF (1989). Mandatory reporting of infectious diseases by clinicians. *JAMA*, **262**, 3018–26.

Dodhia H, Crowcroft NS, Bramley JC, Miller E (2002). UK guidelines for the use of erythromycin prophylaxis in persons exposed to pertussis. *Journal of Public Health Medicine*, **24**, 200–6.

Maki DG (2009). Coming to grips with foodborne infection: Peanut butter, peppers and nationwide Salmonella outbreaks. *New England Journal of Medicine*, **360**, 949–53.

Smith AD, Bradley DJ, Smith V, *et al.* (2008). Imported malaria and high risk groups: observational study using UK surveillance data 1987–2006. *BMJ*, **337**, a120.

Thomas L and the Hepatitis A Guidelines Group (2009). Guidance for the prevention and control of hepatitis A infection. <https://www.gov.uk/government/uploads/system/uploads/attachment_data/file/363023/Guidance_for_the_Prevention_and_Control_of_Hepatitis_A_Infection.pdf>.

Malaria

Epidemiology

Malaria is a parasitic infection caused by five species of *Plasmodium* (*P. falciparum, P. vivax, P. ovale, P. malariae,* and *P. knowlesi*), the last species only recently being described as a human pathogen. It is a major killer on the world stage, with around a million deaths per year, mainly affecting children in sub-Saharan Africa.

Although it is endemic in most parts of the tropical world, the intensity of transmission varies widely with Africa and, in particular, West Africa suffering the greatest parasite burden. As repeated infection leads to clinical immunity, the burden of malaria falls predominantly on children in areas of intense transmission but affects all age groups in areas with less intense, more seasonal malaria. Only one species, *Plasmodium falciparum,* is frequently lethal. The other species rarely kill, but *P. vivax* causes substantial morbidity on a global scale.

Imported malaria is a significant problem in many non-endemic countries. In the UK, 1,500–2,000 cases of malaria are reported every year, with around ten deaths. Although the majority of UK infections occur in immigrant populations visiting their country of origin, most deaths occur in non-immune Caucasian travellers. The case fatality rate for falciparum malaria in the UK is less than 1%.

Clinical features

If the diagnosis of malaria is not to be missed, a detailed travel history must be taken in patients with a febrile illness. Falciparum malaria usually causes symptoms within 1 month of return from endemic areas, but the other species may not manifest for several months.

Although a fever, or history of a fever, is almost invariable in patients with malaria, the hallmark of this disease is the **absence** of specific features. Chills, sweats, and rigors are common, but false localizing symptoms, such as cough or diarrhoea, may mislead the unwary clinician.

Physical signs, apart from fever, are few in uncomplicated infection, although jaundice, splenomegaly, and hepatomegaly occur in a significant minority.

Laboratory findings are helpful, with thrombocytopenia in around 60% of patients. A mild normocytic anaemia or a raised bilirubin are also common, whereas the white cell count is almost invariably normal or low.

Severe malaria

Severe malaria, almost always caused by *P. falciparum,* usually manifests as cerebral malaria, severe anaemia, acute respiratory distress syndrome (ARDS), acute renal failure, or shock. Table 6.15 lists the WHO defining features of severe malaria. Although jaundice is associated with severe malaria, its sole presence is not a good predictor of poor outcome.

The following groups are at higher risk of severe malaria and death: pregnant women, non-immune Caucasians, patients with asplenia or sickle cell disease, patients more than 60 years old, and cases with parasitaemia >2%.

- **Cerebral malaria** presents as drowsiness or confusion but may rapidly progress to unrousable coma. Focal neurological signs, such as decerebrate posturing and disconjugate eye movements, may develop in the later stages.
- **Severe anaemia** is mainly a disease of children presenting with respiratory distress secondary to cardiac failure, often with associated metabolic acidosis.

Table 6.15 Defining criteria for severe malaria

WHO criterion	Definition
Cerebral malaria	Unrousable coma or inability to sit up
Severe anaemia	Haemoglobin <5 g/dL
Acute renal failure	Serum creatinine >265 micromoles/L or renal output <0.4 mL/kg per hour
Acidosis	Arterial pH <7.3
Shock	Systolic blood pressure <90 mmHg
Hypoglycaemia	Blood glucose <2.2 mmol/L
Spontaneous bleeding ± DIC	Standard criteria
Pulmonary oedema or ARDS	Standard criteria

Data from World Health Organization. Severe Falciparum Malaria. *Transactions of the Royal Society of Tropical Medicine and Hygiene.*2000;94 (Suppl 1).

- **ARDS/pulmonary oedema** in malaria is indistinguishable from the syndrome caused by bacterial sepsis. It may develop 1 or 2 days into treatment and is associated with a mortality of up to 50%.
- **Acute renal failure** in malaria is secondary to acute tubular necrosis. The mortality associated with this condition is low in regions where renal replacement therapy is available, and renal function usually returns to normal after several weeks.
- **Shock** is uncommon in severe malaria and may reflect concomitant bacteraemia (a well-known complication of the condition).
- **Hypoglycaemia** is less common in adults than children with severe malaria. It is, however a common side effect of parenteral quinine treatment.

Pregnant women are particularly at risk from malaria, especially in the third trimester. They have increased susceptibility to severe malaria and have a particular predisposition to ARDS and hypoglycaemia.

Diagnosis

Once the diagnosis of malaria is suspected, an EDTA blood specimen for analysis should be collected without delay. Although thick and thin blood films stained using Giemsa remain the mainstay of parasitological diagnosis of malaria, many laboratories in the developed world use immunochromatographic tests (ICT). PCR-based methods are usually restricted to research or reference laboratories.

In general, ICT tests have very good diagnostic accuracy for *P. falciparum* but perform less well for the other species. In laboratories experienced in the diagnosis of malaria, thick films, QBC tests (a fluorescence-based microscopic screening test), and ICT kits have a very good negative predictive value for falciparum malaria.

Where the clinical suspicion is high, particularly in patients who may have self-treated or who have been taking chemoprophylaxis, up to three films may be necessary to exclude the diagnosis. Empirical treatment of patients for malaria is rarely appropriate in view of the high sensitivity of available diagnostic tests.

Management

Severe falciparum malaria

The first question to answer in patients with falciparum malaria is 'Does this patient have severe disease?' This involves a detailed clinical examination, paying attention to the cardinal features of severe malaria, plus, where facilities exist, a full blood count, renal and liver profile. The parasitaemia provides some prognostic value, although the relevance of a particular level will vary, depending on the immune status of the individual.

Current UK guidelines recommend treating all patients with a parasitaemia more than 2% as severe malaria, with parenteral quinine. However, a threshold level of 5% for parenteral treatment has been suggested by other authorities. Most recently two large randomized trials, one in adults in South East Asia and the other in children in Africa, have clearly shown that, compared with quinine, artesunate significantly reduces the mortality from severe malaria. Thus artesunate is now the drug of choice for this condition. A coagulation screen, arterial blood gases, blood cultures, chest radiograph, and baseline ECG should also be obtained in ill patients. Severe malaria should be managed in a high dependency or critical care environment where possible. Exchange transfusion is generally not recommended, especially when patients are treated with artesunate, a rapidly acting antimalarial.

- **Fluid resuscitation.** Although some degree of fluid depletion is common in patients with malaria, haemodynamic compromise is uncommon. Thus, unlike the management of bacterial sepsis, these patients should receive relatively cautious fluid resuscitation.
- **Intravenous artesunate.** 2.4 mg/kg on admission, then at 12 h and 24 h, then once daily until the blood film is clear of parasites. The course should be completed with an agent, such as artemether–lumefantrine (Riamet®) or atovaquone-proguanil eg Malarone®).
- **If artesunate is unavailable**, give intravenous quinine, with a loading dose of 20 mg/kg (maximum 1.4 g) intravenous quinine dihydrochloride in 500 mL 5% glucose (or 0.9% sodium chloride), infused over 4 hours, followed 8 hours later with a maintenance dose of 10 mg/kg (maximum 700 mg) in 500 mL 5% glucose (or 0.9% sodium chloride) infused over 4 hours every 8 hours. A loading dose should NOT be given if the patient has recently taken mefloquine or quinine. Patients need ECG monitoring (as quinine prolongs the QTc interval) and frequent blood glucose measurements (as quinine causes hypoglycaemia). Once able to swallow, patients should be converted to oral quinine 600 mg tds to complete 7 days. This should then be followed by doxycycline 200 mg od or clindamycin 450 mg three times daily for a further week.

- **Consider antibiotics** if there are signs of shock (e.g. ceftriaxone 2 g daily intravenously).

Uncomplicated falciparum malaria

Although UK guidance recommends inpatient management for all cases of falciparum malaria, there is accumulating evidence that ambulatory treatment is safe in selected cases. Decisions to manage these patients without hospital admission, however, should only be taken in consultation with infection specialists.

Uncomplicated infection is effectively treated with a 7-day course of oral quinine plus doxycycline 200 mg daily or clindamycin 450 mg three times daily. The second drug is given because compliance with 7 days of quinine is poor due to side effects. Pregnant women should be treated with the quinine/clindamycin combination, as doxycycline is contraindicated. Outside of pregnancy, however, better compliance is likely with the following preferred regimens:

- Atovaquone-proguanil (e.g Malarone®) four tablets daily for 3 days, or
- Artemether-lumefantrine (Riamet®) four tablets, then four tablets at 8, 24, 36, 48, and 60 hours.

Non-falciparum malaria

Patients with non-falciparum (benign) malaria can usually be managed as outpatients. For all parasites, chloroquine remains the treatment of choice, given as follows:

- 600 mg stat, followed by 300 mg at 6, 18, and 42 hours.

Two species P. ovale and P. vivax have a stage called the hypnozoite that develops in the liver. This form of the parasite is resistant to chloroquine therapy and leads to the phenomenon of relapses, if not specifically treated. Primaquine treatment is, therefore, necessary to achieve radical cure, given as 15 mg daily for P. ovale and 30 mg daily for P. vivax for a total of 2 weeks.

Primaquine frequently causes haemolysis in patients with glucose-6-phosphate dehydrogenase (G6PD) deficiency. Consequently, the G6PD level must be checked before primaquine is prescribed; if the level is low, seek expert advice.

P. malariae and P. knowlesi are reliably cured with chloroquine alone. The latter, however, frequently causes severe disease, for which intravenous artesunate is probably the drug of choice, as for P. falciparum.

Further reading

Bottieau E, Clerinx J, Colebunders R, et al. (2006). Selective ambulatory management of imported falciparum malaria: a 5-year prospective study. European Journal of Clinical Microiology & Infectious Diseases, **26**, 181–8.

Dondorp A, Nosten F, Stepniewska K, Day N, White N; South East Asian Quinine Artesunate Malaria Trial (SEAQUAMAT) group (2005). Artesunate versus quinine for the treatment of severe falciparum malaria; a randomized trial. Lancet, **366**, 717–25.

Lalloo DG, Shingadia D, Pasvol G, et al. (2007). UK malaria treatment guidelines. Journal of Infection, **54**, 111–21.

World Health Organization (2000). Severe falciparum malaria. Transactions of the Royal Society of Tropical Medicine and Hygiene. **94** (Suppl 1).

Meningococcal disease

Epidemiology

The aetiological agent *Neisseria meningitidis* is a Gram-negative coccus. It grows rapidly in conventional solid and liquid media in the laboratory and is easily identified, using a small number of biochemical characteristics. The bacterium has a polysaccharide capsule that acts as an important virulence determinant. Although there are 13 serologically defined polysaccharide types, most disease worldwide is caused by serogroups A, B, C, Y, and W135.

Epidemic meningococcal meningitis has been recognized as a clinical entity since the early 1800s, but it was not until 1887 when Weichselbaum established the aetiology of the infection by isolating the organism from the CSF of a patient with meningitis.

The epidemiology of the infection is characterized by both large epidemics and sporadic endemic disease. Predominant circulating serogroups vary markedly from country to country and over time. In the UK, for example, the predominant serogroup in the early 20th century was A, whereas now the disease is mainly caused by group B. Transmission of the organism generally requires close contact with infected or colonized individuals. Attack rates in household contacts may be over 500 times the background rate.

In the developed world, the highest incidence rates of the infection are in children less than 5 years of age, with a second peak in the late teenage years; infection in individuals older than 30 years of age is very uncommon. By contrast, in the 'meningitis belt' of Africa, stretching across the Sahel region from Sudan to Senegal, the infection affects all age groups and is characterized by large seasonal epidemics that follow the dry season. Case fatality rates in this setting may be substantial due to poor access to effective antimicrobials.

Highly effective conjugate vaccines have been developed for serogroup C infection, and, more recently, a tetravalent conjugate vaccine covering serogroups A, C, Y, and W135 has been licensed. Although a new serogroup B vaccine (Bexsero®) has recently been licensed in Europe, its role in prevention of meningococcal disease is currently uncertain.

Clinical features

About two-thirds of meningococcal infections manifest as meningitis, with most of the remainder presenting as a septicaemic illness marked by profound shock. The overall mortality rate in developed countries is 5–10%, with septicaemia carrying a higher mortality than meningitis alone.

Septicaemia

The septicaemic presentation is characterized by a short illness, often developing over hours, with fever, malaise and prostration. In most cases, there is a petechial or purpuric rash that may progress rapidly to affect large areas of the skin, sometimes with widespread necrosis, especially affecting the peripheries. It is important to recognize, however, that the rash may also be maculopapular and inconspicuous or indeed not present at all.

Cool peripheries and limb pain have recently been identified as useful predictors of this infection in young children. Diagnosis of early meningococcal infection in this age group is extremely difficult in the absence of the characteristic rash.

Patients usually have frank shock, with hypotension and organ hypoperfusion at, or soon after, presentation. Pathological bleeding from venepuncture sites, gums, or the gastrointestinal tract may result from disseminated intravascular coagulation.

Typical laboratory findings include leucocytosis, thrombocytopenia, prolonged prothrombin time, decreased fibrinogen, and elevated creatinine. The creatinine kinase may also be markedly elevated in children, reflecting muscle involvement.

Meningitis

The presentation of meningococcal meningitis is similar to other bacterial meningitides. The illness usually has a rapid onset with one or more of fever, neck stiffness, headache, photophobia, and altered mental status.

In a recent cohort study, however, the classic triad of fever, neck stiffness, and altered mental state was present in only 27% of culture-proven cases. In a minority of cases, there is a septicaemic element to the infection when the presence of rash is a useful clue to the aetiology.

Other presentations

Meningococcal infection has a number of rare manifestations, including:

- **Community-acquired pneumonia**. This condition mainly affects older adults.
- **Septic arthritis**.
- **Chronic meningococcaemia**. A relatively benign condition, manifesting as fever over several weeks with demonstrable meningococcaemia.
- **Urethritis.**

Diagnosis

The mainstay of diagnosis of meningococcal infection is the isolation of the organism from a normally sterile site. As the organism is rather fastidious, diagnostic samples should be incubated appropriately as soon as possible after collection. Blood cultures are the most important bacteriological investigation and are positive (within a day of incubation) in most septicaemic cases and the majority of meningitis cases. As the organism is exquisitely susceptible to antibiotics, blood **must** be drawn for culture prior to antibiotic administration wherever possible.

Cerebrospinal fluid findings in patients with meningitis are nearly always abnormal, with raised white cell counts (predominantly neutrophils), a low glucose, and high protein. Microscopy will demonstrate Gram-negative cocci in most patients where CSF is drawn prior to antibiotic administration. The yield of CSF Gram stain and culture decreases rapidly (within hours) after administration of effective antibiotics.

Culture of a throat swab for meningococci may be diagnostically useful, especially in young children in whom asymptomatic colonization rates are low. The laboratory must be informed of the clinical context so the swab can be incubated using the appropriate selective plates. Gram stain and culture of petechial lesions may also yield diagnostic information.

Diagnostic assays, based upon the polymerase chain reaction (PCR), have helped enormously in making a microbial diagnosis of meningococcal infection. Both CSF and blood (collected in an EDTA tube) may be examined for meningococcal DNA using PCR and are particularly useful when samples have been collected after antibiotic administration. The diagnostic yield of such samples remains high for up to 48 hours into antibiotic treatment.

In the UK, around a third of all cases of meningococcal disease are confirmed using PCR alone. In addition, as the technique can determine the serogroup involved, it contributes significantly to the surveillance of the disease from a public health perspective.

Management

Initial management of patients with meningococcal infection involves careful assessment of the degree of shock and appropriately aggressive fluid resuscitation. Where meningitis is suspected, in the absence of shock, decreased Glasgow coma scale, or evidence of a space-occupying lesion in the brain (papilloedema or focal neurological signs), a CSF sample should be collected without delay. Drug management is as follows:

- *Ceftriaxone* 4 g intravenously, followed by 2 g intravenously daily for 4 days. Benzylpenicillin 1.2 g intravenously 4-hourly is an alternative.
- *Consider dexamethasone in meningitis.* In adults, there is evidence that dexamethasone 10 mg four times daily intravenously (administered before, or with, the first dose of antibiotic) for 4 days improves outcome in bacterial meningitis. The benefit of this drug, however, appears to be greater in pneumococcal meningitis.

In patients with anaphylactic reaction to penicillin, give *chloramphenicol* 1 g four times daily intravenously. In patients with an uncertain, or a mild, allergy (rash alone) to penicillin, administration of ceftriaxone is justified. In the developing world, chloramphenicol remains the mainstay therapy for bacterial meningitis. Studies using single doses of an oily, long-acting preparation of chloramphenicol or ceftriaxone intramuscularly have yielded excellent results in the context of epidemic serogroup A meningitis in Africa.

Several adjunctive therapies (including hyperimmune serum and recombinant bactericidal permeability-increasing protein) have been trialled in meningococcal disease without conclusive benefits. The initial promise shown by the use of recombinant activated protein C in septic shock and meningococcal infection was not supported by further randomized controlled trial evidence, which showed no benefit. The drug was removed from the market in 2011.

In many countries, notification of suspected or confirmed meningococcal infection is required by law. This allows public health authorities to instigate measures to prevent further cases. Most authorities recommend chemoprophylaxis for household contacts and for healthcare workers with close contact with respiratory secretions (e.g. endotracheal intubation). Vaccination is appropriate in selected cases. Preferred agents are given in Table 6.16.

Table 6.16 Chemoprophylaxis and vaccination for contacts of meningococcal disease

Patient group	Antibiotic regimen
Household or healthcare worker contacts	**Rifampicin**—2-day course PO: 600 mg bd (adults) 10 mg/kg bd (1–12 years) 5 mg/kg bd (<1 year) or **Ciprofloxacin**—single dose PO: 500 mg (adult) 250 mg (5–12 years) 30 mg/kg – maximum 125 mg (>5 years)
Pregnant contacts	**Ceftriaxone** 250 mg IM stat **Azithromycin** 500 mg stat **Ciprofloxacin** (as above)
Vaccination (where serogroup known)	Recommended for non-immunized contacts where effective vaccine available (e.g. meningococcal C conjugate vaccine)

Data from Public Health England (2014). Guidance for public health management of meningococcal disease in the UK and <https://www.gov.uk/government/organisations/public-health-england>.

If cases of meningococcal disease are treated with penicillin, they must be given one of the chemoprophylactic agents listed in Table 6.16 to ensure eradication from the nasopharynx.

Further reading

Andrews SM, Pollard AJ (2014). A vaccine against serogroup B Neisseria meningitidis: dealing with uncertainty. *Lancet Infectious Diseases*, **14**, 426–34.

Greenwood B (1999). Manson Lecture. Meningococcal meningitis in Africa. *Transactions of the Royal Society of Tropical Medicine and Hygiene*, **93**, 341–53.

Heckenberg SG, de Gans J, Brouwer MC, *et al.* (2008). Clinical features, outcome and meningococcal genotype in 258 adults with meningococcal meningitis: a prospective cohort study. *Medicine (Baltimore)*, **87**, 185–92.

Nathan N, Borel T, Djibo A, *et al.* (2005). Ceftriaxone as effective as long-acting chloramphenicol in short-course of meningococcal meningitis during epidemics: a randomized non-inferiority study. *Lancet*, **366**, 308–13.

Public Health England (2014). Guidance for public health management of meningococcal disease in the UK. <https://www.gov.uk/government/uploads/system/uploads/attachment_data/file/322008/Guidance_for_management_of_meningococcal_disease_pdf.pdf>.

Public Health England. <https://www.gov.uk/government/organisations/public-health-england>.

Thompson MJ, Ninis N, Perera R, *et al.* (2006). Clinical recognition of meningococcal disease in children and adolescents. *Lancet*, **367**, 397–403.

Infections in pregnancy

Pregnancy is one of the most hazardous times of a woman's life. As the fetus grows, the woman becomes increasingly 'immunotolerant' in order not to reject the fetus. Specifically, the immunological profile of the mother shifts towards a Th2 phenotype, with suppression of interferon-γ and IL-12. As a result, particularly as she enters the third trimester, the woman becomes increasingly susceptible to a range of infections. This susceptibility manifests as clinical infections that would not have occurred in the absence of pregnancy (e.g. listeriosis) or, more commonly, a severe manifestation of the infection (e.g. chickenpox). A list of infections for which there is evidence for a higher incidence or increased severity in pregnancy is given in Table 6.17.

There are a few infections that, although they frequently only cause minor illness, in pregnant women, may have devastating effects on the fetus. The most important infections in this category are described in the following paragraphs, with an outline of their management.

Listeriosis

Listeria monocytogenes, a Gram-positive rod, is widely distributed in nature. It is prevalent in soil, water, vegetation, and the gastrointestinal tract of animals. The organism is easy to cultivate in the laboratory and, unusually, replicates at 4°C (refrigerator temperature). It is extremely prevalent in foodstuffs such that ingestion of the organism probably occurs on a daily basis. It is a classic opportunistic pathogen: clinical infection is extremely rare outside of risk groups, one of which is pregnant women, particularly those in the third trimester. Infection manifests as an acute, rather non-specific, febrile illness, often with myalgia and backache. Although the illness is usually self-limiting in the mother, infection of the fetus may be devastating. Overall, about a quarter of maternal infections lead to stillbirth or neonatal

Table 6.17 Infections that are more common or more severe in pregnancy

Infection	Effect of pregnancy
Listeriosis	Increased susceptibility to infection; neonatal infection
Chickenpox	Increased severity of infection; congenital varicella syndrome (rare)
Falciparum malaria	Increased susceptibility to, and severity of, infection; intrauterine growth retardation, stillbirth, premature labour
Hepatitis E	Increased severity of infection; mortality up to 25% described in developing world
Influenza (including 2009 pandemic H1N1)	Increased severity of infection
Hepatitis B virus	Higher blood viral loads; hepatitic flare in puerperium
Urinary tract infection	Increased susceptibility to urinary tract infection, including pyelonephritis
Group B streptococcal infection	Peripartum bacteraemia; chorioamnionitis leading to neonatal infection

death. Approximately two-thirds of live births that follow maternal *Listeria* infection are affected.

The diagnosis of listeriosis in pregnancy is usually made by isolating the organism from blood cultures. In cases of stillbirth or early-onset neonatal infection, the organism may first be recovered from fetal swabs or culture of amniotic fluid. Serological assays have been developed, but they have proven unhelpful in diagnosis.

Affected patients should be treated with high doses of amoxicillin (e.g. 2 g tds IV, switching to oral therapy following defervescence) for a total of 2 weeks. Antibiotic therapy in patients with penicillin allergy is problematic. Co-trimoxazole would be the preferred agent in the third trimester (when the risk of adverse fetal affects is minimal). Routine CSF analysis is not required in this disease, as meningitis, as a manifestation of listeriosis, in pregnancy is vanishingly rare. Treated mothers will require close monitoring of the fetus in view of the substantial risk of poor neonatal outcomes.

Toxoplasmosis

Toxoplasma gondii is a protozoan parasite, with a worldwide distribution. The natural lifecycle involves cats and a large array of other animals. Humans acquire infection by ingesting undercooked meat or food and water contaminated with *T. gondii* oocysts. As in immunocompetent individuals, most infections in pregnant women are asymptomatic. If symptoms are present, they are usually subtle and include fever and cervical lymphadenopathy.

The principal clinical importance of toxoplasmosis in pregnancy relates to the risk to the fetus. In immunocompetent women, transmission to the fetus only occurs as a result of acute primary infection during gestation. Although the risk of mother-to-child transmission is highest later in pregnancy, the risk of fetal infection, manifesting as symptomatic disease, is higher when transmission occurs in the first trimester. Thus, whenever infection is acquired during gestation, the chances of delivering an affected infant is 5–10%.

The diagnosis of toxoplasmosis in pregnancy is primarily serological, and some authorities recommend routine screening in early pregnancy. Initial IgG and IgM testing often requires specialist confirmatory tests, as it is critical to attempt to accurately date the time of acquisition. In addition, amniocentesis for molecular detection of *T. gondii* using PCR may be necessary. Pregnant women with confirmed acute toxoplasmosis may be offered antimicrobial treatment. There are, however, no randomized controlled trials to unequivocally support this intervention. The commonly advised agents are spiramycin before 18 weeks' gestation and sulfadiazine, pyrimethamine, and folinic acid after this period.

Rubella

In view of the potentially catastrophic effects on the fetus, the diagnosis of rubella must be considered in every pregnant woman with a rash. The infection is highly infectious and usually manifests as a relatively mild febrile illness, with a widespread maculopapular rash that starts on the face. Cervical lymphadenopathy in the posterior triangle may also be present. Infection in the first half of pregnancy carries a high risk of malformation in the fetus; the risk of adverse fetal outcomes is around 90% for mothers infected in the first 11 weeks of pregnancy, falling to 20% from 11 to

16 weeks. The diagnosis is usually easily confirmed with an IgM assay. There is no treatment for this infection, and termination may be recommended for severely affected cases.

Cytomegalovirus

Cytomegalovirus (CMV) is a very common herpesvirus infection. Infections are acquired throughout life, and seropositivity in women of childbearing age is around 50% in most settings. Although infection in pregnant women is nearly always asymptomatic, primary infections may lead to congenital infection. Rarely, symptomatic CMV infection in pregnancy presents as a non-specific febrile illness. In addition, it has been shown that seropositive mothers reinfected with a different strain may also give birth to congenitally infected babies.

First trimester infections are more likely to lead to the delivery of symptomatic infants. Most congenitally infected infants are asymptomatic at birth, but longitudinal studies in such children have shown significant neurological and audiological sequelae. Primary infection is diagnosed with a positive IgM assay or demonstration of seroconversion. Although treatment of pregnant women with primary infections is not routinely recommended, a recent uncontrolled study showed potential benefit with hyperimmune immunoglobulin therapy.

Parvovirus B19

Parvovirus B19 is a small DNA virus that was only discovered in 1974. Infection is frequently asymptomatic in all age groups. Symptomatic infection manifests as a non-specific febrile illness, with coryza and often gastrointestinal upset. Some patients develop a transient or recurrent maculopapular rash, affecting the trunk and limbs. Female patients, in particular, may also develop quite persistent arthralgia.

It is important to consider the infection in pregnant women with a rash, as infection in the first 20 weeks is an important cause of hydrops fetalis. The affected fetus develops a severe anaemia that causes heart failure; fetal loss ensues in about 10% of cases. The diagnosis of parvovirus B19 infection is usually easily made, using a commercial IgM assay. Although there is no antimicrobial therapy available for this virus, intrauterine transfusion may be beneficial in hydrops fetalis.

Syphilis

Most countries advocate screening pregnant women for syphilis in early pregnancy in order to prevent congenital infection. Although the fetus may be affected by maternal syphilis at all stages, the risk is highest with the spirochetaemia associated with primary and secondary syphilis. Maternal infection may cause stillbirth, late abortion, or an affected live birth.

The diagnosis of syphilis in pregnancy is largely serological, although dark-ground microscopy of lesions may confirm the diagnosis in symptomatic primary or secondary syphilis. The mother should be treated, in conjunction with genitourinary medicine physicians, along similar lines to non-pregnant adults with penicillin-based regimens. Alternative antimicrobials are of unproven efficacy in treating the affected fetus, so penicillin-allergic mothers should be considered for desensitization. Treatment of infected sexual partners is important both at a population level and in order to prevent reinfection of the mother.

Miscellaneous infections

Sepsis is an important cause of death in pregnant women. The commonest organism is *Streptococcus pyogenes*, with infections usually occurring in the third trimester or puerperium; recent delivery was cited as a risk factor in 4% of cases of invasive *S. pyogenes* infection in a recent surveillance study in the UK. Pregnant women are also predisposed to urinary tract infections due to the physiological ureteric dilatation that occurs during pregnancy.

Asymptomatic bacteriuria is a well-recognized risk factor for the subsequent development of pyelonephritis. As screening and treatment of asymptomatic bacteriuria have been shown to prevent pyelonephritis, this approach is widely recommended. Cephalosporins, such as cefalexin and cefadroxil, are the preferred agents for short-course (3-day) treatment of uncomplicated urinary tract infection or bacteriuria.

There is substantial circumstantial evidence that infections, such as tuberculosis, cryptococcosis, and coccidioidomycosis, may preferentially become manifest during the third trimester or early post-partum period of pregnancy. This is thought to reflect an immune reconstitution syndrome, with clinical symptoms coinciding with a restoration of the normal immune balance.

Further reading

Kingston M, French P, Goh B, *et al.* (2008). UK guidelines on management of syphilis. *International Journal of STD & AIDS*, **19**, 729–40.

Montoya JG and Remington JS (2008). Management of *Toxoplasma gondii* infection during pregnancy. *Clinical Infectious Diseases*, **47**, 554–66.

Mylonakis E, Paliou M, Hohmann EL, Calderwood SB, Wing EJ (2002). Listeriosis during pregnancy: a case series and review of 222 cases. *Medicine (Baltimore)*, **81**, 260–9.

Nigro G, Adler SP, La Torre R, Best AM; Congenital Cytomegalovirus Collaborating Group (2005). Passive immunization during pregnancy for congenital cytomegalovirus infection. *New England Journal of Medicine*, **353**, 1350–62.

Singh N and Perfect JR (2007). Immune reconstitution syndrome and exacerbation of infections after pregnancy. *Clinical Infectious Diseases*, **45**, 1192–9.

Vascular access device-associated infection

Epidemiology

Vascular access devices (VAD) are increasingly used in the modern healthcare setting. Devices range from peripheral venous cannulae, designed for short-term use, to tunnelled implanted central venous catheters (CVC), typically used over a period of months. The risk of infection related to these devices is highest for short-term peripheral and central catheters, and lowest for tunnelled catheters (e.g. Hickman lines and Port-o-Caths). Infections range in severity from local phlebitis, that resolves with catheter removal alone, to septic thrombophlebitis and bloodstream infections with associated sepsis. The highest risk site for bloodstream infections is for VAD in the femoral vein, followed by the internal jugular vein, then the subclavian vein. Rates of bloodstream infection for central lines range from 2 to 10 per 1,000 catheter days, and VAD-related infection may cause a significant proportion of bacteraemias in the hospital setting (see Table 6.18).

Microorganisms gain entry into the bloodstream via VADs in three ways:

- **Extraluminal** infection is caused by bacteria gaining access to the VAD via the exit site through the skin; this is the commonest mechanism for peripheral and non-tunnelled lines.
- **Endoluminal** infection occurs when organisms gain access to the inside of the catheter via the hub; this is the commonest mechanism for tunnelled central lines.
- **Infusate-related** infection is also endoluminal but is caused by infection of the infusate itself; Gram-negative organisms predominate, especially *Pseudomonas*, *Enterobacter*, and *Serratia* species. The most commonly implicated fluids are heparin solutions, blood products, and total parenteral nutrition.

In some instances, there is an infected thrombus at the site of the catheter, leading to the syndrome of septic thrombophlebitis. Arterial catheters may also lead to bloodstream infection, but the incidence rate is lower than that for venous devices.

A number of strategies reduce the risk of central line-related bloodstream infections:

- Education of staff involved in insertion and care of central lines.

- Use maximal sterile precautions at insertion (cap, mask, sterile gown, and gloves).
- Use all-inclusive catheter kit.
- Good hand hygiene at the time of insertion and before manipulations.
- Skin cleansing with chlorhexidine.
- Avoid using femoral vein site.
- Insertion sites should be inspected every shift (peripheral); daily (central).
- Use a sterile transparent semipermeable membrane dressing to cover the vascular access device insertion site.
- Flush and lock lumens with 0.9% normal saline solution.
- Change administration sets for blood every 12 hours; total parenteral nutrition every 24 hours.
- Change dressings, and clean the VAD site with chlorhexidine regularly.
- Disinfect hubs and ports with chlorhexidine before accessing the catheter.

There is also substantial evidence that antiseptic or antibiotic-coated central lines may also help to reduce the risk of infection. Use of these devices should be considered if the incidence of central line-associated infections is not controlled by the above measures. Routine replacement of central lines has not been shown to reduce the risk of infection and is, therefore, not recommended.

The evidence base for routinely changing peripheral access devices is not clear, although the CDC (Centers for Disease Control and Prevention) recommends changing these devices every 72–96 hours. As VADs inserted under emergency conditions are at greater risk for becoming infected, it may be sensible to replace these catheters at the earliest opportunity. Although antibiotic lock solutions should not be used routinely to prevent catheter-related bloodstream infections (NICE 2012), there is good evidence that routine use of antimicrobial lock solutions reduces the incidence on bloodstream infections in haemodialysis patients. However, there is still uncertainty about which is the optimal antimicrobial solution, including non-antibiotic agents, such as alcohol or taurolidine. In addition, studies have not adequately addressed the risk of infections caused by resistant organisms.

Clinical features

Local infection related to VADs manifests as pain and erythema at the insertion site, sometimes with pus or evidence of induration of the associated vein. Differentiating non-infectious from infectious phlebitis may be difficult, but the presence of pus, spreading cellulitis, or systemic upset strongly suggests an infectious cause.

VAD-related bloodstream infections present with fever, often with evidence of sepsis syndrome. If a peripheral VAD is the cause, there is usually evidence of local infection. However, evidence of line site inflammation is less common with central lines, especially those that are tunnelled. It follows that the suspicion of VAD-related sepsis should be high in hospital-acquired sepsis (or community-acquired sepsis in patients with tunnelled lines) where there is no other identifiable focus. Clinical suspicion of VAD-related infection should be further heightened in those receiving total parenteral nutrition (TPN).

Septic thrombophlebitis may follow the use of VADs and is usually associated with bloodstream infection. This is

Table 6.18 Relative frequency of implicated organisms in VAD-related bloodstream infections

VAD type	Organisms			
	S. aureus	Gram-negative rods	CNS	Yeasts
Peripheral	+++	+/−	+/−	+/−
Central (non-tunnelled)	++	+++	++	++
Central (tunnelled)	++	++	+++	+
Infusate-related infections	+/−	+++	+/−	+

CNS, coagulase-negative staphylococci.

commoner with large central catheters but can also occur with peripheral cannulae. It may be difficult to differentiate this from simple VAD-related bloodstream infection, as signs of thrombosis are usually absent. The main clinical clues to the presence of this condition are:

- Slow clinical response despite VAD removal and effective antimicrobial therapy.
- Persistently positive blood cultures.
- Development of features suggestive of septic pulmonary emboli (chest pain and dyspnoea, with multiple pulmonary opacities that may cavitate).

Diagnosis

Making a diagnosis of VAD-associated bloodstream infection starts with maintaining a high index of suspicion in septic hospitalized patients with no apparent focus of infection. As most infections secondary to peripheral VADs are associated with local inflammation, the diagnosis is usually readily established by isolating the same organism, typically S. aureus, from the exit site and/or the catheter tip.

Establishing a central catheter as the source of bloodstream infection is more problematic. The most commonly used technique is to culture the catheter tip by rolling it across an agar plate; culturing >15 colony-forming units of the same organism recovered from a peripherally drawn blood culture supports the diagnosis of VAD-related bloodstream infection. Quantitative cultures of blood drawn from long-term tunnelled catheters may also be useful but are not routinely available in most laboratories.

A diagnosis of septic thrombophlebitis of a peripheral vein can be made on clinical grounds and may be pathologically confirmed if the organism can be isolated from pus aspirated from the vein or from a surgically excised vein segment. Confirmation of septic thrombophlebitis of central veins is less straightforward, but, in the appropriate clinical context, radiological demonstration of thrombosis at the catheter site (usually by ultrasound) will support the diagnosis.

Management

The most important part of the management of VAD-associated infection is to promptly remove the device (and send it for microbiological analysis). Empirical treatment of exit site infections should be directed towards S. aureus. Penicillins, such as flucloxacillin, are appropriate where the risk of MRSA is low or a glycopeptide, such as vancomycin, if MRSA is more prevalent if the patient is colonized with this organism.

With documented bloodstream infection in the intensive care setting, several VADs may need to be removed. As arterial lines are less common sources of bacteraemia, they need not be routinely removed. However, they should be replaced if they are the only VAD in place, if blood cultures are persistently positive, or if the patient deteriorates clinically on appropriate therapy. Fluid and vasopressor use for VAD-associated sepsis should be utilized along similar lines to sepsis from other causes (see above and Chapter 2).

The empirical antibiotic management of VAD-associated bloodstream infection depends on:

1. Whether the affected VAD is peripheral or central.
2. Epidemiological setting (i.e. the risk of resistant organisms).
3. Whether there is sepsis or septic shock.

For example, in our intensive care unit, the policy is to use gentamicin alone for VAD-related sepsis, but to add in vancomycin if there is shock or the patient is MRSA-colonized.

Suggested antibiotic durations for VAD-related bloodstream infections with different organisms (assuming the VAD has been removed) are:

- **S. aureus.** Due to the risk of metastatic infection, a minimum of 2 weeks of therapy is recommended. A longer course is necessary (4–6 weeks) if there is evidence of suppurative thrombophlebitis, endocarditis, or bone and joint infection. Patients need to be assessed regularly for features of metastatic infection (especially a new regurgitant murmur or new back pain). Although some authorities recommend echocardiogram in all cases, this may be unnecessary if the clinical course is uncomplicated (i.e. rapid clinical resolution, negative follow-up blood cultures 2–3 days after VAD removal, and no clinical evidence of metastatic infection).

- **Gram-negative rods (including Pseudomonas species).** 3–5 days of an active antibiotic is adequate if clinical recovery is prompt. Clinical resolution may even occur spontaneously if VADs are removed promptly.

- **Coagulase-negative staphylococci.** Provided the offending VADs have been removed, antibiotics can be safely discontinued within 1–2 days in most cases.

- **Candida species.** 2 weeks' therapy after the last positive blood culture is recommended. Ophthalmological assessment within the first week is essential to diagnose endophthalmitis (occurs in 5–10% of candidaemias). Consider an echocardiogram in valvular heart disease. Similarly renal imaging may be necessary in neonates, as they are at risk of developing fungal masses in the kidneys. In general, fluconazole is the preferred therapeutic agent where the organism is known or likely to be susceptible. Echinocandins, such as caspofungin, or amphotericin preparations have an important role where a broader spectrum of activity is desirable, for example:

  - A known fluconazole-resistant isolate, usually C. glabrata or C. krusei, is present.
  - In an unstable patient with a high risk of a fluconazole-resistant isolate (e.g. recent exposure to fluconazole), especially if neutropenic.

Achieving successful clearance of bloodstream infection in the absence of catheter removal is always problematic. Where central catheters cannot be removed, antibiotic lock therapy may be tried. This technique involves instilling high concentrations of an antibiotic into the catheter lumen for a period of hours, the process being repeated on a regular basis. Cure rates with this technique are generally poor with virulent organisms, such as S. aureus or coliforms, but may approach 80% for coagulase-negative staphylococci.

Further reading

Marschall J, Mermel LA, Classen D, et al. (2008). Strategies to prevent central line-associated bloodstream infections in acute care hospitals. Infection Control and Hospital Epidemiology, **29**, S22–30.

National Institute for Health and Clinical Excellence (NICE) (2012). Clinical Guideline 139. Infection: Prevention and control of healthcare-associated infections in primary and community care. <https://www.nice.org.uk/guidance/cg139>.

National Institute for Health and Clinical Excellence (NICE) (2014). QS61. Infection prevention and control. Quality statement 5: Vascular Access Devices. <http://publications.nice.org.uk/infection-prevention-and-control-qs61/quality-statement-5-vascular-access-devices>.

O'Grady NP, Alexander M, Dellinger EP, et al. (2002). Guidelines for the prevention of intravascular catheter-related infections. Infection Control and Hospital Epidemiology, **23**, 759–69.

Pappas PG, Kauffman CA, Andes D, *et al.* (2009). Clinical practice guidelines for the management of candidiasis: a 2009 update by the Infectious Diseases Society of America. *Clinical Infectious Diseases*, **48**, 503–35.

Siegman-Igra Y, Anglim AM, Shapiro DE, Adal KA, Strain BA, Farr BM (1997). Diagnosis of vascular catheter-related bloodstream infection: a meta-analysis. *Journal of Clinical Microbiology*, **35**, 928–36.

Thwaites GE, Edgeworth JD, Gkrania-Klotsas E *et al.* (2011). Clinical Management of Staphylococcus aureus bacteraemia. *Lancet Infectious Diseases*, **11**, 208-22.

Yahav D, Rozen-Zvi B, Gafter-Gvili A, Leibovici L, Gafter U, Paul M (2008). Antimicrobial lock solutions for the prevention of infections associated with intravascular catheters in patients undergoing hemodialysis: systematic review and meta-analysis of randomized, controlled trials. *Clinical Infectious Diseases*, **47**, 83–93.

Toxic shock syndrome

Epidemiology

Toxic shock syndrome (TSS) is a term applied to two infectious causes of shock attributable to bacterial exotoxins. Both *Staphylococcus aureus* and *Streptococcus pyogenes* (group A streptococci) can cause the syndrome.

Staphylococcal TSS, although described in the early 20th century, became prominent in the 1980s when it was associated with the use of hyperabsorbable tampons. Around this time, the incidence of the disease, derived from active surveillance, reached 12 cases per 100,000 per year in the USA. The disease is caused by staphylococcal strains that produce toxins that have superantigen properties. This group of toxins has the ability to cross-link the V-beta domain of T cell receptors directly to MHC (major histocompatibility complex) class II receptors in a non-specific fashion. This has the effect of stimulating up to 20% of the T cell population, leading to a pro-inflammatory state that resembles Gram- negative endotoxic shock.

The most important of a range of staphylococcal superantigens, and the toxin most closely associated with menses-related TSS, is toxic shock syndrome toxin-1 (TSST-1). The most commonly implicated streptococcal superantigens are pyrogenic exotoxins, such as SPeA and SPeC.

Whereas staphylococcal TSS predominantly affects children, streptococcal TSS is more common in adults, particularly those with underlying chronic diseases. Certain serotypes, defined by the M protein on the surface of *S. pyogenes*, are particularly associated with TSS, particularly M1 and M3. Although estimates of mortality from this syndrome vary widely in the published literature, it is clear that staphylococcal infections have a much better outcome than streptococcal cases. Mortality from staphylococcal TSS ranges from 0 to 10%, whereas death in streptococcal TSS occurs in 20–50% of cases.

Clinical features

Staphylococcal TSS

Staphylococcal TSS is characterized by fever, hypotension, and a diffuse erythematous rash that usually desquamates 1–2 weeks after onset. Criteria for its diagnosis (alongside those for streptococcal TSS) are given in Table 6.19. Diarrhoea and vomiting are frequent early features and often lead to the syndrome initially being diagnosed as food poisoning.

As this disease is related to toxin production, and not invasive staphylococcal infection, the site of bacterial infection may be inconspicuous. In menses-related disease, the girl is usually menstruating at the time of onset of symptoms, and the tampon may still be present. Although there may be vaginal erythema on examination, the patient does not normally complain of vaginal symptoms.

Non-menstrual TSS may result from colonization of any body site and is often nosocomial in origin. Affected body sites include wounds (surgical or traumatic), other skin lesions, and the upper or lower respiratory tract. Similar to menstrual-related disease, there may be minimal, or no, inflammation at the site of staphylococcal colonization. In contrast to streptococcal TSS, bacteraemia is very uncommon. The main clue to the diagnosis is, therefore, the diffuse rash, in association with shock, particularly in a menstruating female.

Table 6.19 Diagnostic criteria for staphylococcal and streptococcal toxic shock syndrome

Staphylococcal TSS	Streptococcal TSS
Fever	Hypotension
Hypotension	Isolation of group A streptococci from: • Sterile site (definite case) • Non-sterile site (probable case)
Diffuse macular rash	Two or more of the following: • Renal dysfunction • Liver dysfunction • Acute respiratory distress syndrome • Soft tissue necrosis • Coagulopathy • Erythematous macular rash

Involvement of three or more of the following:
• Liver
• Blood
• Renal
• Gastrointestinal
• Central nervous system
• Muscular

Exclusion of other diagnoses

Supported by:
• Isolation of *S. aureus*
• Superantigen production by isolate

Data from: 'Defining the group A streptococcal toxic shock syndrome. Rational and Consensus Definition.' The Working Group on Severe Streptococcal Infections. *JAMA* 1993;269:390-391, and Wharton M *et al*. 'Case definitions for public health surveillance'. MMWR Recomm Rep 1990;39 (RR-13):1-43.

Streptococcal TSS

Streptococcal TSS is characterized by an abrupt onset of hypotension and organ dysfunction, similar to the staphylococcal form. Unlike the latter, however, there may be no rash. Another important distinction is the fact that streptococcal TSS is usually associated with isolation of the organism from a sterile site (e.g. blood, joint fluid, or pleural fluid), and therefore, there is invasive streptococcal infection as well as the toxin-related shock. In addition, streptococcal TSS is frequently associated with an overt, and often necrotizing, soft tissue infection. In children, there is a well-described association between this syndrome and varicella infection.

Diagnosis

The diagnosis of TSS is predominantly clinical; accepted diagnostic criteria are shown in Table 6.19. The presence of the diffuse rash is key to making the diagnosis of staphylococcal TSS as patients with streptococcal TSS often do not have a rash. The diagnosis in streptococcal TSS may be more difficult, although the presence of necrotizing soft tissue infection, or indeed microbiological evidence (streptococci in blood culture or Gram-positive cocci from fluid or tissue), should suggest the diagnosis in the presence of shock. Attempting to distinguish staphylococcal from streptococcal TSS is important. To this end, collecting appropriate samples for culture at presentation is key. Aside from blood cultures and cultures of other clinically directed sterile sites, samples for culture should be collected from:

• Nose.
• Throat.
• Wounds or other skin lesions (however minor).
• Vagina.

If any of the samples yield *S. aureus*, the isolate should be tested for production of superantigens (especially TSST-1).

Management

Patients should be promptly, and aggressively, fluid-resuscitated, as for other causes of septic shock. In addition, the focus of the infection must be sought carefully. In TSS in females, a vaginal examination should be performed to ensure there are no retained tampons. In streptococcal TSS, the main drive must be to identify, and surgically debride, any focus of necrotizing soft tissue infection. An antibiotic regimen should be chosen to provide adequate cover against staphylococci and streptococci. Penicillin-based therapy is key for the latter, but epidemiological factors should be assessed before deciding on antistaphylococcal therapy. In the USA, for example, where community-associated MRSA is highly prevalent, an antibiotic active against MRSA may be appropriate. There are good data from animal studies, and some clinical data, to support using antibiotics which directly affect protein synthesis in order to 'switch off' toxin production. To this end, most authorities recommend adding clindamycin to penicillin-based regimens. Recommended antibiotics are given in Table 6.20.

As TSS is thought to be driven by bacterial superantigens circulating in the bloodstream, there has been much interest in the potential benefit of pooled intravenous immunoglobulin (IVIG) as a therapeutic intervention. Several studies have shown that commercial preparations of IVIG are capable of neutralizing the superantigen properties of bacterial toxins *in vitro*, particularly for *Streptococcus pyogenes*. Although still controversial, several clinical studies, including a single underpowered randomized trial, have suggested that the addition of IVIG to standard therapy may provide significant clinical benefit in streptococcal TSS. We would,

Table 6.20 Antibiotic regimens in toxic shock syndrome

Infection syndrome	Antibiotic regimen (doses for adults)
Toxic shock syndrome (MRSA likely)	Vancomycin 1 g bd IV **plus** Clindamycin 600 mg 8-hourly IV **Or** Linezolid 600 mg bd IV
Toxic shock syndrome (MRSA unlikely)	Benzylpenicillin 1.2 g 4-hourly IV **plus** Flucloxacillin 2 g 6-hourly IV **plus** Clindamycin 600 mg 8-hourly IV **Use MRSA regimen if penicillin allergy**

therefore, recommend that, in cases where the diagnosis of streptococcal TSS is strongly suspected, IVIG should be administered without delay.

A suggested dose regimen would be 1 g/kg on day 1, followed by 0.5 g/kg on days 2 and 3. On current evidence, IVIG should not be routinely administered in staphylococcal TSS but may be considered (in higher doses than for streptococcal disease) in cases with severe refractory shock.

Recurrent episodes of staphylococcal TSS are well described and probably result from the poor humoral response to TSST-1. For this reason, it is worth considering administering a course of topical antiseptics to attempt decolonization in staphylococcal cases.

Further reading

Darenberg J, Ihendyane N, Sjölin J, *et al*. (2003). Intravenous immunoglobulin G therapy in streptococcal toxic shock syndrome: a European randomised, double-blind, placebo-controlled trial. *Clinical Infectious Diseases*, **37**, 333–40.

Hajjeh RA, Reingold A, Weil A, Shutt K, Schuchat A, Perkins BA (1999). Toxic shock syndrome in the United States, surveillance update 1979-1996. *Emerging Infectious Diseases*, **5**, 807–10.

Luca-Harari B, Darenberg J, Neal S, *et al*. (2009). Clinical and microbiological characteristics of severe *Streptococcus pyogenes* disease in Europe. *Journal of Clinical Microbiology*, **47**, 1155–65.

The Working Group on Severe Streptococcal Infections (1993). Defining the group A streptococcal toxic shock syndrome. Rational and consensus definition. *JAMA*, **269**, 390–1.

Wharton M, Chorba TL, Vogt RL, Morse DL, Buehler JW (1990). Case definitions for public health surveillance. *MMWR Recommendations and Reports*, **39** (RR–13), 1–43.

Chapter 7

Neurological diseases and emergencies

Headache

Although most primary headaches (migraine, tension-type headache, cluster and other miscellaneous headaches) are benign, they are a cause of considerable morbidity. Secondary headaches are heterogeneous, and classification is based on the underlying cause.

Migraine

Migraine is a paroxysmal syndrome characterized by recurrent attacks of headache, separated by symptom-free intervals. The headaches are usually associated with nausea and vomiting and preceded by an aura, but the aura may occur without any ensuing headache. Most patients experience visual auras (i.e. visual hallucinations and scotoma, arising from the occipital cortex), teichopsia (i.e. fortification spectra), and photopsia (i.e unformed flashes of light)).

Others experience sensory, motor, or speech disturbances, which may include temporal lobe phenomena. Migraine aura without headache may mimic partial epilepsy or transient ischaemic attacks.

Other forms of migraine include:

- **Vertebrobasilar migraine** in which symptoms arise from the brainstem, including dysarthria, vertigo, tinnitus, decreased hearing, diplopia, ataxia, impaired coordination, bilateral paraesthesiae, and episodes of transient loss of consciousness.
- **Retinal migraine** is due to constriction of the retinal arterioles, which impair vision in one eye, with or without photopsia. Usually, there is preceding headache or a dull ache behind the affected eye.
- **Familial hemiplegic migraine** causes transient weakness and associated headache but usually resolves without infarction.
- **Migrainous infarction** is defined as a neurological deficit that has occurred during a migraine attack that is typical of previous migrainous headaches.

Management

- **Avoidance of trigger factors** (e.g. red wine, chocolate).
- **General lifestyle measures**, including ensuring adequate sleep and regular diet. Limiting tea and coffee may be valuable.
- **Simple analgesia and antiemetic therapy.** Acute migraine headache may respond to simple analgesics alone or the combination of an analgesic (e.g. naproxen 500–750 mg orally at onset (max. daily dose 1,250 mg), ibuprofen 400–800 mg orally at onset (max. daily dose 2,400 mg)) and antiemetic (which may be given rectally to aid absorption) (domperidone 10 mg, metoclopramide 10 mg). Fixed-drug combinations are less satisfactory.
- **Specific anti-migraine therapy.** Triptans are the most effective agents in interrupting an attack; however, they are expensive, and the response is variable (e.g sumatriptan 50–100 mg; zolmitriptan 1.25–2.5 mg; naratriptan 1–2.5 mg; rizatriptan 5–10 mg (rizatriptan should not be used in vertebrobasilar or hemiplegic migraine)). They can be administered in different formulations (e.g. tablet, nasal spray, subcutaneous injection, sublingually, or as a suppository) and the time between, and frequency of, subsequent safe doses varies for individual preparations.
- **Prophylactic medications** include beta-blockers (e.g. propranolol 10–40 mg qds), sodium valproate (400–600 mg twice daily), serotonin antagonists, such as methysergide or pizotifen (0.5–2 mg daily), and calcium channel blockers, especially verapamil.

- **Tricyclic antidepressants** may be useful as an adjunct therapy (e.g. amitriptyline 25–75 mg nocte).

Tension-type headache

Tension headaches are highly variable but characterized by headache of mild to moderate intensity, which is bilateral and either pressing or tight. They may occur at least 10 times and last for between 30 minutes and 7 days. There is no associated photophobia, aurophobia, nausea, or vomiting, and usually no exertional worsening.

Tension headache may develop into chronic daily headache, particularly as a consequence of transformed migraine or analgesic overuse.

Management

- **General.** A psychological, physiological, and pharmacological approach to management is often effective.
- **Sympathetic attention** to the history and examination. Providing reassurance that the patient does not have a cerebral tumour or another serious intracranial neurological disorder is important.
- **Imaging** rarely identifies an underlying lesion, but, in practice, CT or MRI brain scan is undertaken either because the physician suspects an underlying lesion or to reassure the patient and their relatives.
- **Acute treatment** may be difficult. Most patients prefer to use non-steroidal anti-inflammatory drugs (NSAID), such as ibuprofen, rather than simple analgesia with aspirin or paracetamol. Others find caffeine, sedatives, or tranquillizers to be valuable. If analgesics are taken daily, they may lead to rebound headache, as their effect wears off, predisposing to chronic daily headache.
- **Prophylaxis.** Tricyclics are the drug of choice for prophylaxis, but their role is difficult to evaluate. Amitriptyline is the most widely used, and its effects seem to be independent of its antidepressant activity. Dothiepin is also widely used in low dose.
- **Anticonvulsants.** If tension-type headache persists, anticonvulsants may be indicated. Valuable drugs include valproate, gabapentin, and topiramate, but each has significant toxicity.
- **Complementary therapies.** Many patients derive considerable benefit from complementary techniques, including relaxation, biofeedback, cognitive behavioural therapy, and physical treatments, including transcutaneous nerve stimulation (TENS).

Short-lasting headaches

Cluster headaches

These are severe unilateral headaches associated with prominent autonomic features and a striking periodicity. The attacks consist of a unilateral excruciating pain in the orbital or temporal region, lasting between 45 and 90 minutes (although the pain can be present for up to 3 hours).

The onset and cessation are abrupt; the headache may be associated with a range of autonomic features, including lacrimation, nasal congestion, rhinorrhoea, facial sweating, miosis, ptosis, eyelid oedema, conjunctival injection, and a sense of restlessness.

Episodic cluster headaches recur in periods, lasting from 7 days to 1 year and separated by pain-free periods, with remission from 3 months to 3 years.

Management

- **Oxygen.** Acute attacks may be aborted by the provision of inhaled 100% oxygen by a face mask.
- **Corticosteroids and NSAIDs.** Corticosteroids, often together with a non-steroidal anti-inflammatory drug (NSAID), are effective in aborting bouts of episodic cluster headache when taken in short courses of 3–4 weeks.
- **Subcutaneous sumatriptan** (6 mg) causes rapid headache relief in most patients without the development of tachyphylaxis. In some patients, clusters occur regularly without remission.
- **Prophylactic treatment** may be necessary, using methysergide, ergotamine, lithium, or verapamil (starting dose 40–80 mg twice daily and maintenance doses up to 960 mg/day).

Paroxysmal hemicranias

These headaches occur with a higher frequency than cluster headaches, and the duration of individual attacks is shorter. They respond dramatically well to indomethacin.

SUNCT (short-lasting, unilateral, neuralgiform, orbital pain attacks, with conjunctival injection, tearing, sweating, and rhinorrhoea) is a rare syndrome. It usually occurs in males. The headaches are poorly responsive to treatment, but lamotrigine and gabapentin have been used.

Post-traumatic headache

Acute post-traumatic headache may follow significant head trauma, associated with loss of consciousness, post-traumatic amnesia, or abnormal neurological signs. It appears within 14 days and has resolved by 8 weeks after the trauma or regaining consciousness. It is often severe and throbbing in quality, associated with nausea, vomiting, photophobia, phonophobia, memory impairment, irritability, drowsiness, or vertigo. It is treated as part of the overall management of the head trauma, with supportive and symptomatic care, including simple analgesics and anti-inflammatory medications.

Chronic post-traumatic headache is a much more common clinical problem. This describes headaches that have continued for more than 8 weeks after regaining consciousness or the initial trauma. Most patients develop a muscle contraction (tension-type) headache, which persists for many months but may respond to conventional treatments. Anxiety, depression, other psychological factors, and the litigation process may exacerbate the headache.

Thunderclap headache

This is defined as a severe headache that takes seconds to minutes to reach maximum intensity. Most importantly, it occurs in vascular disorders including subarachnoid haemorrhage, cerebral venous sinus thrombosis, cerebral vascular aneurysms, and cervical artery dissection (see 'Vascular disorders' below). It may occasionally be indicative of other medical problems including hypertensive crises, pituitary apoplexy, reversible cerebral vasoconstriction syndrome, meningitis, cerebral haematoma, spontaneous intracranial hypotension, and stroke. In some cases, there are no other abnormalities, but the various causes may be associated with a wide variety of neurological features.

Vascular disorders

Vascular disorders may be associated with headache. For example:

- **Subarachnoid haemorrhage** is characterized by the sudden onset of severe and incapacitating headache ('thunderclap headache'), which is often occipital and associated with meningism and low back pain. Approximately 25% of patients with an intracranial aneurysm may present with a 'sentinel headache', suggesting intermittent leaking of the aneurysm.
- **Intracerebral haemorrhage** is often followed by headache, but this depends on the onset, size, and location of the haemorrhage.
- **Extradural haemorrhage** is characterized by the development of acute headache following head trauma
- **Subdural haematoma** may be associated with a fluctuating paroxysmal headache which occurs before the development of focal neurological signs.
- **Carotid or vertebral dissection** often gives rise to ipsilateral headache or cervical pain and may precede the development of neurological symptoms.

Giant cell arteritis

Giant cell arteritis is characterized by the presence of headache, a swollen and tender temporal artery, elevated ESR, and the typical inflammatory pathological features on temporal artery biopsy. The condition occurs in the elderly and responds rapidly to steroids. Headache is the presenting feature in 50% and may be unilateral or generalized. Sudden painless loss of vision is the presenting feature in 15%, but visual loss may occur in 7–60% of patients. Urgent treatment with steroids (e.g. prednisolone 60–80 mg daily) is indicated as soon as possible after the diagnosis.

Raised intracranial pressure

It is unusual for intracranial neoplasms to present with headache. The headache of raised intracranial pressure is characteristically bilateral, moderate to severe, and often worse during the night or on waking. It is classically associated with vomiting and diplopia.

Benign intracranial hypertension presents with generalized headache, associated with visual obscurations and intracranial noises. On examination, there is papilloedema and variable visual field defect.

Temporomandibular disorders

These are characterized by tenderness and pain in the temporomandibular joint and the associated muscles of mastication, trismus, limited or jerky jaw movements, and evidence of bruxism (teeth grinding). The pain may be felt as temporal headache and is often precipitated by movement and clenching teeth.

The condition should be treated conservatively with antidepressant medication, occlusal appliances, and rehabilitation; it usually resolves slowly.

Further reading

Afridi S, Giffin NJ, Kaube H, et al. (2005). A PET study in spontaneous migraine. Archives of Neurology, **62**, 1270–5.

Goadsby PJ, Lipton RB, Ferrari MD (2002). Migraine—current understanding and treatment. New England Journal of Medicine, **346**, 257–70.

Headache Classification Committee of the International Headache Society (2004). The international classification of headache disorders (2nd edition). Cephalalgia, **24**, 1–160.

Lipton RB and Bigal M (2006). Migraine and other headache disorders. Marcel Dekker, Taylor & Francis Books, Inc, New York.

National Institute for Health and Care Excellence (2012). Headaches: Diagnosis and management of headaches in young people and adults. NICE clinical guideline 150. <https://www.nice.org.uk/guidance/cg150>.

Olesen J, Tfelt-Hansen P, Ramadan N, et al. (2005). The headaches. Lippincott, Williams & Wilkins, Philadelphia.

Scottish Intercollegiate Guidelines Network (2008). Diagnosis and management of headache in adults. SIGN guideline 107. <http://www.sign.ac.uk/pdf/sign107.pdf>.

Silberstein SD, Lipton RB, Solomon S, et al. (2001). *Wolff's headache and other head pain*. Oxford University Press, Oxford.

Silberstein SD, Lipton RB, Goadsby PJ, et al. (2002). *Headache in clinical practice*. Martin Dunitz, London.

Silberstein SD, Holland S, Freitag F, et al. (2012). Evidence-based guideline update: pharmacologic treatment for episodic migraine prevention in adults: report of the Quality Standards Subcommittee of the American Academy of Neurology and the American Headache Society. *Neurology*, **78**, 1337–45.

Transient loss of consciousness

Transient loss of consciousness (TLC) is a brief clinical episode, characterized by rapid loss of normal responsiveness, loss or reduction of muscle tone or stiffness, and amnesia for the event. Recovery is spontaneous and complete without focal neurological deficits.

The causes include:

1. Syncope.
- **Reflex (neurally mediated) syncope** is associated with pain, fear, coughing, sneezing, micturition, swallowing, defecation, carotid sinus syncope.
- Orthostatic hypotension—associated with primary/ secondary (i.e. diabetes) autonomic failure.
- Cardiac syncope:
  - Arrhythmias (brady- and tachycardias).
  - Structural causes (valvular/ischaemic).

2. Epilepsy.
- Tonic and atonic seizures.

3. Non-organic.

4. Other.
- Vertebrobasilar or anterior cerebral artery transient ischaemic attacks (TIAs) and stroke.
- Subclavian steal syndrome.
- Cataplexy ± excessive daytime sleepiness.
- Central mechanical causes (i.e. third ventricular colloid cysts and posterior fossa tumours).
- Basilar artery migraine.
- Drop attacks.
- Ménière's disease.

Syncope

This is the commonest cause of TLC and is due to cerebral hypoperfusion.

- **Neurally mediated** (vasovagal, neurocardiogenic, or reflex) occurs in <40% of the general population and has a strong familial incidence. It is usually preceded (and followed) by autonomic activation of variable duration that includes nausea, pallor, and sweating. Vasovagal syncope is potentiated by hypovolaemia or peripheral vasodilation (e.g. vomiting, diarrhoea, blood loss, heat, fever, alcohol) and also by anxiety.

Following the initial phase of autonomic overflow, there is a brief loss of postural tone, followed, a few seconds later, by tonic and myoclonic jerks. Urinary incontinence occurs in a quarter of patients, but tongue biting is infrequent. Unconsciousness lasts <20s, but some patients lie still for longer after they have regained awareness. Typically, there is no post-ictal confusion.

- **Orthostatic syncope** can be caused by central autonomic failure (e.g. Parkinson's disease and multiple system atrophy), autonomic peripheral neuropathy (e.g. diabetes mellitus and amyloidosis), or can be precipitated by vasodilating or hypovolaemic agents.
- **Cardiogenic syncope** may be precipitated by exercise, particularly when due to structural heart disease, and arrhythmia; the latter is suspected in patients with repeated episodes without recognizable triggers or when lying down.

Sudden death in young relatives may be suggestive of cardiogenic syncope. Other important clues are ECG abnormalities, a previous history of cardiac disease, and palpitations before the syncope in older patients. Rarely, focal epileptic seizures may trigger cardiac asystole and anoxic seizures.

Epilepsy

Epileptic seizures are the second major cause of TLC, mainly tonic and atonic seizures. These occur mostly in children with severe epileptic encephalopathies and in adults with a long history of bilateral focal seizures. Differentiation between vasovagal syncope and epilepsy may be difficult. Prolonged syncope (as, for example, when patients are erroneously kept upright) results in cerebral hypoxia and reflex anoxic seizures, in which there are primitive motor behaviours, in particular, irregular myoclonus, spasms, or tonic extensions.

Occasionally, a true epileptic seizure follows syncope, with bilateral synchronous, usually clonic, convulsions (post-syncopal anoxic-epileptic seizure). Therefore, syncope of any cause can mimic a generalized convulsive seizure (of early or late onset) or an atonic seizure, but not complex partial seizures or absences, in which patients may become unresponsive and lose some tone but usually remains upright.

Patients with myoclonic seizures may fall either as a result of a violent generalized myoclonus or because of a negative component of collapse of muscle tone (i.e. epileptic negative myoclonus) but usually retain consciousness. The epilepsies will be treated separately in the next chapter.

Non-organic

Psychogenic syncope is suggested by the history when it occurs in a context of prior psychological problems or history of physical or sexual abuse. Repeated episodes that may occur when the patient is lying down, have no clear triggers, and are long-lasting, with the patient reporting that they are unable to move, are good indicators of psychogenic syncope-like episodes.

Differentiation is complicated by the fact that psychogenic syncope commonly occurs at the time vasovagal syncope is most likely to manifest (i.e. in the early teens).

Other causes

Although sleep disorders are not associated with loss of consciousness, episodes of cataplexy (i.e. either in the context of narcolepsy or in isolation) may be misdiagnosed as syncope, atonic seizure, or psychogenic attacks. Atonia may be partial and usually spreads gradually; there should be no 'ictal' unresponsiveness or 'post-ictal' clouding of consciousness, and tendon reflexes are temporary depressed or absent. Daytime naps of sudden onset in narcoleptic patients may also mimic syncope.

Other non-syncopal, non-epileptic drop attacks include:

- **Sudden otolithic dysfunction (e.g. Ménière's disease).**
- **Recurrent vertebrobasilar attacks** (e.g. due to vertebrobasilar stenosis, subclavian steal).
- **Anterior cerebral artery TIAs.**
- **Third ventricular colloid cysts and posterior fossa tumours.**
- **Basilar artery migraine.**

Further reading

Crompton DE and Berkovic SF (2009). The borderland of epilepsy: clinical and molecular features of phenomena that mimic epileptic seizures. *Lancet Neurology*, **8**, 370–81.

Lempert T (1996). Recognizing syncope: pitfalls and surprises. *Journal of the Royal Society of Medicine*, **89**, 372–5.

Lempert T, Bauer M, Schmidt D, *et al*. (1994). Syncope: a videometric analysis of 56 episodes of transient cerebral hypoxia. *Annals of Neurology*, **36**, 233–7.

National Institute for Health and Care Excellence (2012).Transient loss of consciousness ('blackouts') management in adults and young people. NICE clinical guideline 109. <https://www.nice.org.uk/guidance/cg109>.

National Institute for Health and Care Excellence (2014). Transient loss of consciousness. NICE quality standard 71. <https://www.nice.org.uk/guidance/qs71>.

Stephenson JBP (1990). *Fits and faints*. MacKeith Press, London.

States of impaired consciousness

Different patterns of arousal and awareness are difficult to assess, but characteristic clinical features allow recognition of a spectrum of states of conscious level.

Coma

Coma is a state from which patients cannot be roused. They lie with their eyes closed and show no evidence of consciousness. There is no spontaneous eye opening, response to voice, localization to painful stimuli, or verbal output.

Acute confusional state

Patients are drowsy, bewildered, disorientated in time, with poor short-term memory and comprehension. They have difficulty undertaking complex tasks and show day-night reversal.

Delirium

Delirium is a floridly abnormal mental state which develops acutely. Hypoactive periods, with drowsiness, disorientation, and reduced responsiveness, alternate with severe motor restlessness, anxiety, fear, irritability, misperception of sensory stimuli, and visual hallucinations.

Vegetative state

Patients appear to be awake with their eyes open but show no awareness of themselves or the environment. They are unable to interact with others and have no purposeful or voluntary behavioural responses to visual, auditory, tactile, or noxious stimuli. There is no evidence of language comprehension or expression. Patients breathe spontaneously and exhibit inconsistent non-purposive movements. Sleep-wake cycles, cranial nerve, brainstem, spinal and primitive reflexes are present. There is bladder and bowel incontinence.

The vegetative state develops after a variable period of coma. It may be partially or totally reversible or may progress to a permanent vegetative state or death.

Minimally conscious state

Patients show low-level behavioural responses, consistent with severe neurological impairment and disability. These include limited awareness, yes/no responses, intelligible speech, and purposeful behaviour. These patients may remain in minimally responsive states or recover some ability to communicate reliably or use objects functionally.

Locked-in syndrome

The locked-in syndrome is characterized by preservation of consciousness, with dissociation between automatic and volitional control of lower cranial nerve and limb function.

Although volitional control of respiratory, facial, bulbar, and limb function is lost, there is preserved awareness of the environment and self, and patients can usually communicate through vertical eye movements which are often slow and incomplete. There is usually a horizontal gaze palsy, anarthria (loss of the motor power to articulate speech), and tetraplegia. The most frequent causes of locked-in syndrome are occlusion of the vertebrobasilar system or pontine haemorrhage.

Management

Initial management of coma includes cardiopulmonary resuscitation, oxygenation, and airway protection (± tracheal intubation and mechanical ventilation). Intravenous access and maintenance of arterial blood pressure with fluids and/or inotropic drugs may be required. Obtain a full blood count, and determine blood levels of glucose, electrolytes, renal and hepatic function urgently.

In cases where the cause of coma is not immediately apparent, consider giving 50 mL of 20% glucose intravenously to exclude hypoglycaemia. If alcoholism or malnutrition are suspected, thiamine should also be administered to prevent the development of Wernicke's encephalopathy. Naloxone or flumazenil should be administered if narcotic or benzodiazepine overdose is suspected. Further acute management of the unconscious patient includes treatment of seizures, correction of electrolyte and acid-base disturbances, and supportive treatment, including adequate nutrition, nursing, and physiotherapy.

Medical assessment of coma

Initial assessment must include a detailed history obtained from as many sources as possible, particularly witnesses, family, and the attending paramedical staff. This will include details of the predisposing event (e.g. previous trauma, pyrexia), the prodromal symptoms (e.g. headache, neck stiffness, ataxia, epilepsy), previous similar episodes, a list of medications, and a psychiatric history.

Examination should include an assessment of the patient's breath for alcohol, ketones, hepatic or renal fetor, mucous membranes for cyanosis, anaemia, jaundice or carbon monoxide intoxication, and nails for splinter haemorrhages suggestive of endocarditis. The skin must be examined to detect purpuric or petechial rashes, coagulation disorders, and maculopapular lesions suggestive of viral meningoencephalitis or fungal infection. Bullous lesions may indicate barbiturate intoxication.

Systemic examination may detect pyrexia, abnormalities of cardiac rate, rhythm, and blood pressure, respiratory irregularities, meningism, retinopathy, papilloedema, and/or subhyaloid haemorrhage. Otoscopic examination may reveal otorrhoea or haemotympanum due to a basal skull fracture, and CSF rhinorrhoea can be confirmed by the presence of glucose in a watery nasal discharge.

Level of consciousness

Level of consciousness is determined from the ability to respond to stimuli of varying intensity and by speech, eye opening, and motor movements. The eyelids should be held open and the patient asked to move their eyes in a horizontal and vertical plane to detect locked-in syndrome. Visual, auditory, and painful stimuli of increasing intensity are then systematically presented bilaterally in cranial nerve and limb territories.

The Glasgow coma score (GCS)

GCS is the most widely used (and reproducible) scale for the assessment of the level of consciousness (see Table 1.2). It was designed as a simple, objective, reproducible scale to assess varying levels of consciousness in patients with head trauma. It facilitates early recognition of deteriorating consciousness due to raised intracranial pressure or herniation. It is most effective when regular serial observations are used. In practice, it has been demonstrated to be a valuable and durable tool because it is easily used by medical, nursing, and paramedical staff.

However, there are several limitations to the use of the GCS.

- The scale excludes assessment of many important neurological functions.
- It requires regular and consecutive observations to be effective.
- It is limited to the best response in a single limb (i.e. it cannot represent asymmetry).
- It has very poor diagnostic value.
- Interrater reliability in non-experienced observers is poor, not least because it is difficult to standardize the intensity of maximal auditory, visual, and painful stimuli.
- Full assessment cannot be undertaken in intubated patients or when soft tissue swelling prevents eye opening.
- The scale represents the addition of ordinal values which are neither equal nor independent of each other.
- It is relatively insensitive to changes in the level of consciousness at higher levels.

Although the GCS score is helpful, particularly in the context of traumatic brain injury, when assessing change in the level of consciousness, GCS cannot replace a detailed and careful neurological examination of the pattern of responsiveness.

Assessment of neurological function
Assessment should include the following.

Eyelids
In coma, opening of the eyelids by an examiner is followed by slow, spontaneous re-closure.

Pupillary responses
Pupillary responses indicate the functional state of the afferent (II; second (optic) cranial nerve) and efferent (III; third (oculomotor) nerve) pathways and the midbrain tegmentum.
- Equal, light-reactive pupils in a comatose patient indicate a metabolic, rather than structural, cause of coma.
- Bilateral pinpoint and mid-position pupils are associated with pontine lesions or opiates.
- In progressive compressive third nerve lesions, the initial sign is a sluggish pupillary response, followed by the development of fixed dilatation.
- Irregular oval, unequal pupils follow brainstem transtentorial herniation and midbrain infarction.

Ocular motor disorders
The preservation of normal eye movements demonstrates that the brainstem and cerebellar connections are intact.
- A complete third nerve palsy is manifest as pupillary dilatation, ptosis, and deviation of the eye downward and laterally.
- Oculomotor nerve palsies occur in midbrain lesions due to direct trauma or transtentorial herniation but have many other causes.
- A sixth nerve palsy causes inward deviation and failure of abduction by the lateral rectus muscle; it may be due to trauma or raised intracranial pressure but is a poor guide to localization.

Conjugate ocular deviation
Tonic horizontal conjugate ocular deviation is common in coma.
- The eyes usually deviate towards the side of a destructive hemispheric lesion and away from the hemiparesis (e.g. infarction, haemorrhage, or tumour).

- The eyes may deviate away from an irritative, epileptic focus or from a thalamic lesion.
- In a pontine gaze palsy, the eyes deviate away from the side of the lesion and look towards the hemiparesis.
- Tonic upward or downward deviation of the eyes is associated with metabolic coma and hypoxic-ischaemic damage.

Eye movements
Horizontal nystagmus, occurring in comatose patients, suggests an irritative or a supratentorial aversive epileptic focus, usually associated with other motor manifestations of seizures. The presence of spontaneous eye movements implies integrity of the brainstem oculomotor pathways and that coma is relatively light.

Repetitive rapid downbeat saccades, followed by slow movement back to the midline (ocular bobbing), is associated with intrinsic pontine or cerebellar lesions and metabolic or toxic coma.

Vestibulo-ocular reflexes (VOR) are the involuntary ocular movements which occur after stimulation of the vestibular apparatus and can be tested either by mechanical rotation of the head (oculocephalic) or caloric irrigation (oculovestibular). If supranuclear influences are absent, the eyes will normally remain fixed in space (i.e. continue to look forward). Reduced or absent oculovestibular reflexes indicate severe intrinsic brainstem impairment.

Other cranial nerves
The corneal reflex has a higher threshold in comatose patients but may be totally lost with deep sedation. Pontine lesions produce ipsilateral complete facial weakness, whilst supranuclear lesions produce contralateral facial weakness, sparing the forehead and orbicularis oculi.

Assessment of bulbar function in coma is difficult and unreliable. Several characteristic patterns of respiratory irregularity occur, but lesions are rarely localized, and coexisting pulmonary, cardiovascular, or autonomic influences may complicate the clinical picture.

Motor responses
Motor responses include assessment of the resting posture of the limbs and head, involuntary movements, spontaneous movements (purposeful or non-purposeful), and response to external stimuli.

The motor response to deep, painful stimuli is particularly valuable in assessing diagnosis and prognosis of coma. A predominantly extensor response in the upper extremities carries a poor prognosis. The pattern and asymmetry of muscle tone may be helpful in localizing focal structural lesions and in differentiating metabolic from structural coma.

Tonic-clonic or other stereotyped movements suggest generalized or focal seizures or epilepsia partialis continuans. Myoclonic jerks are seen with hypoxic-ischaemic encephalopathy, metabolic coma (e.g. hepatic encephalopathy), or following pontine infarction.

Distinction of toxic and metabolic coma from structural coma
Preceding medical history may suggest a metabolic abnormality. The onset is more likely to be acute in the presence of a structural lesion. Metabolic or toxic lesions usually result in coma, without lateralizing or brainstem signs, whilst structural lesions are suggested by asymmetrical motor signs.

Metabolic encephalopathy is favoured by the presence of involuntary limb movements (tremor, myoclonus, and asterixis) and a fluctuating level of consciousness.

Psychogenic unresponsiveness

Psychogenic unresponsiveness may be distinguished by history, examination, and, if necessary, investigations. Examination reveals inconsistent volitional responses, particularly on eyelid opening. Spontaneous saccadic eye movements are present, and pupillary constriction will occur on eye opening. Oculovestibular stimulation with cold stimulus shows preservation of the fast phase away from the stimulated side, and EEG has responsive alpha rhythms.

Causes of coma

Coma can be due to a large number of neurological and general medical disorders. In clinical practice, it is useful to classify the causes, using a simple scheme. The most effective of these is to identify the following in the initial assessment of the patient:

1. The presence of lateralizing signs.
2. The presence of meningism.
3. The pattern of brainstem reflexes.

These features can be used to categorize causes of coma and to aid diagnosis.

- Causes of coma with intact brainstem function, without meningism and without lateralizing signs include:
  - *Toxins* (e.g. carbon monoxide, methanol, lead, cyanide, thallium, others).
  - *Alcohol.*
  - *Drugs* (e.g. all sedatives, anaesthetics, and many other drugs, e.g. barbiturates, tranquillizers, opioids, psychotropics, salicylates, amphetamine).
  - *Extrapyramidal* (e.g. acute movement disorders (*status dystonicus*), neuroleptic malignant syndrome, serotonin syndrome).
  - *Seizures, epilepsy* (e.g. convulsive/non-convulsive status epilepticus, post-ictal, drug-induced, non-epileptic status).
  - *Psychiatric* (e.g. catatonia, conversion reactions, malingering).
  - *Anoxic-ischaemic encephalopathy.*
  - *Respiratory* (e.g. hypoxaemia, hypercarbia).
  - *Electrolyte disturbance* (e.g. hypo-/hypernatraemia; hypocalcaemia, hypercalcaemia; hypermagnesaemia).
  - *Diabetes mellitus* (e.g. hypoglycaemia, ketoacidosis, lactic acidosis, hyperosmolar non-ketotic diabetic coma).
  - *Uraemia/dialysis.*
  - *Hepatic encephalopathy.*
  - *Endocrine* (e.g. hypopituitarism, hypo-/hyperthyroidism, hypoadrenalism, Hashimoto's encephalopathy).
  - *Core temperature change* (e.g. hypothermia, hyperpyrexia).
  - *Nutritional* (e.g. Wernicke's encephalopathy).
  - *Inborn errors of metabolism* (e.g. hyperammoniacal states, aminoacidurias, organic acidurias).
  - *Others* (e.g. porphyria, Reye's syndrome (hepatic), idiopathic recurrent stupor, mitochondrial disease, hypothalamic lesions, septic encephalopathy, malaria).

- Causes of coma with meningism include:
  - *Infection* (e.g. meningitis, encephalitis, malaria, HIV-related).
  - *Vascular* (e.g. subarachnoid haemorrhage (spontaneous or traumatic)).
- Causes of coma with intact brainstem function and asymmetrical lateralizing signs include:
  - *Vascular* (infarction, e.g. ischaemia, embolic, hypoperfusion/hypotension; haemorrhage, e.g. extradural, subdural, subarachnoid, intracerebral (e.g. primary or secondary)).
  - *Vasculitis.*
  - *Venous thrombosis.*
  - *Mitochondrial disease.*
  - *Hypertensive encephalopathy.*
  - *Eclampsia.*
  - *Endocarditis.*
  - *Traumatic brain injury.*
  - *Infection.*
  - *Brain neoplasms.*
  - *White matter diseases* (multiple sclerosis, acute disseminated encephalomyelitis).
- Causes of coma with intact brainstem function and symmetrical lateralizing signs include:
  - *Diffuse axonal (traumatic) brain injury.*
  - *Bilateral subdural haematoma/empyema.*
  - *Vascular* (e.g. multiple infarcts, vasculitis).
- Causes of coma with signs of focal brainstem dysfunction include:
  - *Herniation syndromes.*
  - *Intrinsic brainstem disease.*
  - *Advanced metabolic/toxic encephalopathy.*
  - *Vascular.*
  - *Mass lesions.*
  - *Traumatic brain injury.*

Further reading

Bernat JL (2006). Chronic disorders of consciousness. *Lancet*, **367**, 1181.

Bleck TP (2006). Prognostication and management of patients who are comatose after cardiac arrest. *Neurology*, **67**, 556–7.

Howard RS, Kullmann DM, Hirsch NP, *et al.* (2003). Admission to neurological intensive care: who, when and why? *Journal of Neurology, Neurosurgery & Psychiatry*, **74** (Suppl 3), 2–9.

Howard RS, Radcliffe J, Hirsch NP, *et al.* (2003). General medical care on the neuromedical intensive care unit. *Journal of Neurology, Neurosurgery & Psychiatry*, **74** (Suppl 3), 10–16.

Laureys S, Owen, AM, Schiff, ND, *et al.* (2004). Brain function in coma, vegetative state, and related disorders. *Lancet Neurology*, **3**, 537.

Royal College of Physicians. Report of a working party. (2013). Prolonged disorders of consciousness: National clinical guidelines. RCP, London. <https://www.rcplondon.ac.uk/guidelines-policy/prolonged-disorders-consciousness-national-clinical-guidelines>.

Wijdicks EF (1995). Determining brain death in adults. *Neurology*, **45**, 1003–11.

Wijdicks EFM, Hijdra A, Young GB, *et al.* (2006). Practice parameter: prediction of outcome in comatose survivors after cardiopulmonary resuscitation (an evidence-based review): report of the Quality Standards Subcommittee of the American Academy of Neurology. *Neurology*, **67**, 203–10.

The dementias

Dementia may present acutely and have a non-progressive course, such as after a head injury or a hypoxaemic cerebral insult. Alternatively, they may have an insidious onset and progression, as in Alzheimer's disease. In approximately 10% of cases, there is a reversible or treatable cause, such as myxoedema or hydrocephalus.

Dementia describes a syndrome in which there is an acquired decline in cognitive function in an alert individual. The term cognitive impairment is used to include 'mild cognitive impairment' (insufficient to affect independence), dementia, and the acute confusional state (also termed delirium).

Acute confusional states are usually reversible global disorders of thinking and perception and may be secondary to medication, sepsis, or a toxic/metabolic disturbance; they need to be correctly diagnosed and treated. Similarly, expressive dysphasia, as seen in acute stroke, deafness, and the pseudodementia of depression should not be misdiagnosed as delirium or dementia. Cognitive impairment may also be seen in sleep apnoea, temporal lobe epilepsy, and transient global amnesia.

The social and economic costs of dementia are projected to increase greatly as the population of western economies ages. Dementia is estimated to affect 1% of 60–65 year olds and 10–35% of the over 85 year olds.

Cognitive function

- **Attention and concentration:** assessed by taking sevens away from 100, spelling 'world' backwards.
- **Language:** (e.g. aphasia) verbal fluency, naming, comprehension (verbal and written), reading, writing, repetition; listen for phonemic (shed for bed) and semantic errors (door for window).
- **Memory:** (e.g. amnesia) divided into implicit and explicit, and into short-term (online working memory, less than a minute) and long-term (minutes, hours, days to years).
  - **Short-term:** digit span—repeating numbers forwards (less than 6 abnormal in younger patients) and backwards (less than 4); immediate repetition of three word items.
  - **Long-term:** episodic (what did you do yesterday?) and semantic (what is the capital of France?).
- **Literacy and numeracy.**
- **Visuospatial perception.**
  - **Drawing:** clock face, interlocking pentagons, copy complex figure.
  - **Hemineglect:** bisecting a line.
- **Praxis** (c.f. apraxia): the ability to carry out a learned or imitated movement with normal sensory, motor, and cerebellar function.
- **Executive function:** ordering, planning, abstract reasoning.

Causes of dementia

- **Primary degenerative:**
  - Alzheimer's disease.
  - Frontotemporal dementias.
  - Dementia with Lewy bodies (DLB).
- **Other degenerative diseases in which dementia is a feature:**

- Parkinson's disease (PD), progressive supra-nuclear gaze palsy (PSP), Huntington's disease, multiple sclerosis, Wilson's disease, corticobasal degeneration (CBD).
- **Vascular:**
  - Multi-infarct disease.
  - Binswanger's disease.
  - Cerebral amyloid angiopathy.
  - CADASIL (cerebral autosomal dominant arteriopathy with subcortical infarcts and leukoencephalopathy).
- **Infective:**
  - Neurosyphilis, tuberculous, cryptococcal, and fungal meningitis.
  - Human immunodeficiency virus (HIV).
  - Progressive multifocal leukoencephalopathy (JC virus).
  - Encephalitic— herpes simplex virus (HSV), subacute sclerosing panencephalitis (SSPE; following measles).
  - Encephalitis lethargica.
  - Lyme disease and Whipple's disease.
- **Prion disease:**
  - CJD and variant CJD.
- **Metabolic endocrine:**
  - Uraemia, hepatic encephalopathy, hypothyroidism, hypopituitarism, hypoglycaemia, hypo- and hypercalcaemia, hypoadrenalism.
- **Nutritional deficiencies:**
  - Thiamine (Wernicke–Korsakoff), vitamin B_{12}, nicotinic acid (beriberi), multiple vitamin deficiency state.
- **Trauma, hypoxia, ischaemia:**
  - Head injury, dementia pugilistica.
  - Subdural haematoma.
  - Cerebral hypoxia, cerebral hypoxaemia.
- **Neoplastic:**
  - Glioma, meningioma, CNS lymphoma, cerebral metastases.
  - Carcinomatous meningitis.
  - Post-radiotherapy.
- **Obstructive hydrocephalus.**
- **Normal pressure hydrocephalus:**
  - Triad of incontinence, gait apraxia, and cognitive impairment.
- **Inflammatory/autoimmune:**
  - Limbic encephalitis—antineuronal antibodies and anti-voltage-gated potassium channel and NMDAR antibodies.
  - Behçet's; neurosarcoidosis.
  - Cerebral vasculitis.
- **Toxins and drugs:**
  - Alcohol, barbiturates, organic solvents, heavy metals, carbon monoxide.

There are three main cognitive syndromes in dementia

- Temporoparietal (e.g. Alzheimer's disease); early loss of recall and recognition memory and word-finding difficulties.

- Frontal, frontotemporal, or 'anterior cortical' (e.g. frontotemporal dementias); early change in personality and behaviour, loss of empathy, disinhibition.
- Subcortical (e.g. Huntington's disease); slowing of mental processing, loss of motivation, deficits in planning and attention.

Alzheimer's disease

Alzheimer's disease is the most common cause of dementia in all age groups; its incidence increases markedly with age. Pathology shows neuronal loss with tau-positive neurofibrillary tangles and extracellular amyloid plaque formation. Imaging characteristically shows loss of mesial temporal lobe volume and, specifically, hippocampal atrophy.

The classical clinical picture is early loss of recall and recognition, with disorientation in space, and deficits in language and calculation. About 5–10% have a family history and a number of genetic mutations have been identified including amyloid precursor protein, presenilin-1 (PS-1), and presenilin-2 (PS-2). In addition, individuals who are e4 homozygotes for the apolipoprotein polymorphism have a sixfold increased incidence of Alzheimer's disease when compared with the general population.

Dementia with Lewy bodies

In dementia with Lewy bodies (DLB), as in Parkinson's disease, there are widespread Lewy bodies in cortical and subcortical neurones. A proportion of patients with Parkinson's disease develop a dementia which is indistinguishable from DLB, but, for the diagnosis of DLB, there must be no evidence of clinical Parkinsonism until at least a year after the onset of dementia.

Classical features include fluctuating attention and cognition, excess daytime sleepiness, visual hallucinations (60–70%) often of people and animals, and REM sleep behaviour disorder. Parkinsonism and dysautonomia are common.

About 30–50% show neuroleptic (dopamine antagonist) supersensitivity, characterized by severe reversible Parkinsonism, impaired consciousness, and, in extreme cases, the neuroleptic malignant syndrome. Patients with DLB must not be prescribed these drugs (e.g. haloperidol, olanzapine).

Frontotemporal lobar degeneration

Frontotemporal lobar degeneration (FTD) includes a number of different syndromes which, histopathologically, divide into two groups, with either tau-positive or ubiquitin-positive inclusions; 7% have a motor neurone disease component to their clinical picture. About 20–30% are familial. FTD accounts for more than 10% of dementias presenting before the age of 65.

Three distinct syndromes are identified:

- Frontotemporal dementia with disinhibition, distractibility, apathy, loss of empathy, and perseveration, but with memory relatively preserved.
- Progressive non-fluent aphasia with loss of expressive language, word retrieval, phonemic and semantic errors, progressing to mutism; in contrast, reading and writing may be preserved late into the course of the disease.
- Semantic dementia: impairment of comprehension and naming in the context of fluent, effortless speech output; visual agnosia (impaired recognition of visually presented objects) but with relatively preserved repetition and ability to read out loud.

Vascular dementia

Vascular dementia accounts for approximately 20% of dementias across all age groups. The pathology is heterogeneous:

- **Small-vessel ischaemia** has a progressive course and a subcortical presentation, often with associated gait disturbance.
- **Lacunar infarcts** present with a classically stepwise decline in function.
- **Single or multiple salient hemispheric strokes**, result in focal cognitive deficits (e.g. memory: temporal lobe stroke; visuospatial and hemineglect: parietal lobe stroke).
- **CADASIL**, affects young adults without vascular risk factors and is associated with migraine and multiple white matter abnormalities on diagnostic imaging. It is caused by a mutation in the Notch 3 gene.

Prion disease

The most common of the transmissible spongiform encephalopathies, also known as prion diseases, is sporadic Creutzfeld–Jakob disease (CJD) with an incidence of 1–2 per million per year. The prion diseases are caused by accumulation of an insoluble isoform of the host-encoded prion protein. About 5–15% of cases are familial. Behaviour and mood changes, myoclonus, extrapyramidal and pyramidal signs (e.g. unsteady gait, lack of coordination) may develop through the course of the illness which, in sporadic CJD, usually results in death within a year of diagnosis. Variant CJD emerged in the 1990s and affects young adults; it is the human equivalent of bovine spongiform encephalopathy, and the majority of cases have been caused by ingestion of infected beef.

Management of patients with dementia

Prion disease, cerebral vasculitis, paraneoplastic, and autoimmune (e.g. voltage-gated potassium and NMDAR receptor antibody) disease should be included in the differential diagnosis of a rapidly progressive dementia. A specific diagnosis should be made in order to exclude a treatable cause of dementia. The history should detail activities of daily living, including driving, any change in personality or mood, as well as a detailed drug, medication, family, and social history.

The initial examination should include an assessment of the patient's alertness (as previously described) and a cognitive assessment. The mini-mental state examination (MMSE) gives a score out of 30 and is routinely used at the bedside and in clinic. It is sensitive for Alzheimer's disease but insensitive for the early detection of frontal and subcortical dementias, and, to detect these conditions, the inclusion of additional tests of abstract thinking, motor sequencing (Luria), and verbal fluency is useful. More detailed bedside tests include the CAMCOG (Cambridge Cognition Examination; a standardized test to measure the extent of dementia and cognitive impairment). Younger patients and patients with an unusual clinical picture should be referred for formal neuropsychometry.

The baseline investigations in all age groups should include a dementia blood screen, including vitamin B_{12}, thyroid function, and brain imaging with CT or MRI to exclude treatable causes. Further investigations, depending on clinical picture and course, may include electroencephalography (EEG), cerebrospinal fluid (CSF) analysis, and, in some cases a brain biopsy.

Patients and their families and carers need to be advised and counselled on the prognosis and progression, on social issues, such as working, benefits, and care provision, and on legal issues around driving. During the earlier stages of dementia, patients should be advised on setting up a power of attorney and asked about end-of-life wishes.

Pharmacological and behavioural interventions are available and may be useful for the management of depression and behavioural problems in patients with dementia. Therapies aimed at enhancing cognitive function include the cholinesterase inhibitors (e.g. donepezil 5–10 mg daily, rivastigmine 1.5–3 mg bd, galantamine initially 4 mg twice daily, increasing at 4-weekly intervals to 8–12 mg twice daily) and NMDA antagonists (e.g. memantine 5 mg od, maximum dose 10 mg twice daily).

NICE guidelines recommend the prescription of cholinesterase inhibitors as options in the management of moderate Alzheimer's disease where the MMSE is between 20 and 30. Memantine, an NMDA antagonist, has been approved in the USA and in some countries in Europe for the symptomatic management of moderate to severe Alzheimer's disease.

The search for disease-modifying therapies remains active and urgent.

Further reading

Alzheimer's Society. <http://alzheimers.org.uk/>.

Cambridge Cognition. <http://www.camcog.com/>.

Kester MI and Scheltens P (2009). Dementia. *Practical Neurology*, **9**, 241–51.

National Institute for Health and Clinical Excellence (2006). NICE guideline. Dementia. Supporting people with dementia and their carers in health and social care. <http://guidance.nice.org.uk/CG42/Guidance>.

National Institute for Health and Clinical Excellence (2010). Delirium: diagnosis, prevention and management. NICE clinical guideline 103. <http://www.nice.org.uk/guidance/cg103>.

National Institute of Neurological Disorders and Stroke. <http://www.ninds.nih.gov/>.

National Mental Health Development Unit (2009). The commissioning friend for mental health services. A guide for health and social care commissioners. <http://themhs.files.wordpress.com/2011/12/the-commissioning-friend-for-mental-health-services1.pdf>.

Psychological Assessment Resources. Mini-mental® state examination (MMSE®). (The mini-mental state examination (MMSE) was originally distributed free, but the current copyright holders are Psychological Assessment Resources (PAR).) <http://www4.parinc.com/products/product.aspx?Productid=MMSE>.

Rossor M, Collinge J, Fox N, *et al.* (2009). Cognitive impairment and dementia. In C Clarke, R Howard, M Rossor, S Shorvon, eds. *Neurology—A Queen Square textbook*, pp. 245–88. Wiley-Blackwell, Oxford.

Gait and disturbances of speech

Gait

Difficulty in walking is one of the commonest presenting symptoms in neurology. It is important to exclude joint disease, including painful arthritis and Charcot joint as a cause.

Several patterns can be recognized on inspection. These include:

- **Hemiparetic.** A narrow-based, stiff-legged gait with circumduction of the affected leg and scuffing of the toes or outer foot on the hemiparetic side that often causes the patient to trip.
- **Spastic paraparesis.** Bilateral spasticity causes a scissoring gait (tight hip adduction that causes the legs to cross the midline) in which both legs circumduct, with scuffing of the toes of both feet.
- **Extrapyramidal.** Slow shuffling, festinant (hurrying) gait, with poor arm swing. In idiopathic Parkinson's disease, this is often asymmetrical or even unilateral.
- **Involuntary movements.** Including chorea, myoclonus, and dystonia—may become obvious on walking.
- **Ataxic.** Broad-based, unsteady, and uncertain gait which may be caused by sensory loss, cerebellar disease, or weakness.

In sensory ataxia, the gait is often high-stepping, with the feet wide apart and lifted high off the ground. This is much worse in the dark.

In cerebellar ataxia, the patient often sways from side to side.

- **Apraxic.** Difficulty initiating gait, with a tendency to fall backwards, leading to severe imbalance. The patients remain able to move legs quickly and normally on the bed. The cause is usually diffuse cerebrovascular disease, but normal pressure hydrocephalus may be responsible.
- **Myopathy.** Gait is characterized by proximal weakness, causing a waddling gait because of failure to stabilize the pelvis on the femur when the opposite leg is lifted. Patients have difficulty getting out of a low chair, rising from a crouched position or climbing stairs.
- **Neuropathic.** Foot drop causes a tendency to trip and a high-stepping gait in which the foot slaps down as it hits the floor.
- **Non-organic.** A variety of bizarre patterns of gait may be seen, and these are usually variably inconsistent and non-reproducible. However, many disorders, initially labelled as non-organic or even malingering, turn out to be due to a movement or neuromuscular disorder.

Disturbances of speech

The contents and articulation of speech become apparent early in the process of history-taking.

Disturbances of speech include:

- **Dysphonia.** Voice production is impaired by mechanical abnormalities of the vocal cords or larynx. The content and articulation are preserved.
- **Dysarthria.** Disordered oral speech production (articulation), with intact language content, may be due to any abnormality in the motor pathway of speech production. Spastic dysarthria occurs in pseudobulbar palsy and is characterized by monotonous, stiff, slurred speech. Cerebellar dysarthria causes a more irregular explosive staccato pattern.
- **Dysphasia.** Disturbance in spontaneous speech (fluent and non-fluent), the content of speech, repetition, comprehension, writing, and reading. These occur as a result of lesions in the dominant cerebral hemisphere, and several patterns are recognized.
- **Global aphasia.** Impairment of all language functions (i.e. speech, naming, comprehension, reading, writing, and repetition). This is associated with extensive lesions of the dominant hemisphere.
- **Non-fluent (Broca's) aphasia.** The most common form of aphasia—often follows stroke. There is slow, incomplete production of language which is telegraphic, with impaired grammatical output and an inability to repeat phrases. Comprehension is preserved, but perseveration is common, and writing can be affected. The lesion is in the posterior frontal region.
- **Fluent (Wernicke's) aphasia.** Production of fluent speech with language that lacks meaning and content. Comprehension, writing, and reading are all severely impaired. The lesion lies in the posterior part of the superior temporal gyrus.
- **Conduction aphasia.** Characterized by an inability to repeat spoken words or phrases but with fluent speech and preserved comprehension. Associated with lesions of the arcuate fasciculus connecting speech areas.
- **Transcortical aphasia.** Fluent or non-fluent aphasia, with preserved ability to repeat spoken words or phrases. The lesion is subcortical and affects input to Broca's or Wernicke's speech areas.

Further reading

Clarke C, Howard R, Rossor M, et al. (2009). *Neurology—A Queen Square textbook*. Wiley-Blackwell, Oxford.

Stroke

Stroke is a clinical syndrome characterized by the rapid onset of a focal cerebral deficit, lasting at least 24 hours, and for which there is no cause other than a vascular one. Transient ischaemic attack (TIA) is now defined as a 'brief episode of neurological dysfunction caused by a focal disturbance of brain or retinal ischaemia, with clinical symptoms typically lasting less than 1 hour, and without evidence of infarction'. TIAs are an important determinant of stroke, with the greatest stroke risk apparent in the first week.

Burden of stroke
In the UK, the overall prevalence of stroke is estimated to be 47/10,000 population and, as such, is the most common cause of adult physical disability. Cognitive impairment (~33%), problems with lower limbs (~30%), and speech difficulties (~27%) are the most common residual impairments.

Presentation of transient ischaemic attack
Transient ischaemic attack is characterized by symptoms and signs that are focal, negative, of sudden onset, and maximal at onset, rather than progressive.
- **Non-focal symptoms**, such as faintness, dizziness, lightheadedness, confusion, mental disorientation, incontinence, and syncope are all very unlikely to be due to TIA.
- **Positive motor or sensory phenomena**, such as abnormal movements, are more likely to be due to epilepsy.
- **Migraine** often produces focal neurological symptoms but they are usually positive symptoms that develop over minutes, rather than the sudden onset typical of TIA.
- **If the patient is likely to have had a TIA**, it is important that he/she is seen and investigated urgently. Their risk of subsequent stroke can be estimated, using a validated scoring system, such as ABCD2.

ABCD2 algorithm[1]
The ABCD2 algorithm aims to identify patients at high risk of stroke following a TIA:
It is calculated from:
- **A—age** (≥60 years, 1 point).
- **B—blood pressure at presentation** (≥140/90 mmHg, 1 point).
- **C—clinical features** (unilateral weakness, 2 points; speech disturbance without weakness, 1 point).
- **D—duration of symptoms** (≥60 minutes, 2 points; 10–59 minutes, 1 point).
- **Plus diabetes.** Calculation of ABCD2 also includes the presence of diabetes (1 point).
  Total scores range from 0 (low risk) to 7 (high risk).

TIA at high risk of stroke
People who have had a suspected TIA who are at high risk of stroke (that is, with an ABCD2 score of 4 or above) should have:
- Aspirin (300 mg daily) started immediately.
- Specialist assessment and investigation within 24 hours of onset of symptoms.

- Measures for secondary prevention (see below) introduced as soon as the diagnosis is confirmed, including discussion of individual risk factors.

TIA at low risk of stroke
People who have had a suspected TIA who are at lower risk of stroke (that is, an ABCD2 score of 3 or below) should have:
- Aspirin (300 mg daily) started immediately.
- Specialist assessment and investigation as soon as possible, but definitely within 1 week of onset of symptoms.
- Measures for secondary prevention introduced as soon as the diagnosis is confirmed, including discussion of individual risk factors

Presentation of stroke
Stroke usually occurs without warning, and neurological symptoms most often develop suddenly although they can develop in a stuttering fashion over several hours. Classically, haemorrhage is associated with headache, vomiting, and sometimes clouding of consciousness.

Differential diagnosis
Many conditions can mimic stroke.
- **Space-occupying lesions**, such as cerebral neoplasm or abscess, may have presented with a more gradual onset, although tumours may remain silent until they haemorrhage, thus presenting in an identical way to stroke.
- **Subdural haematoma** more commonly presents with fluctuating clouding of consciousness or confusion and only minor focal signs. A history of head injury is only obtained in about 50% of cases of subdural haematoma.
- **Epilepsy** can leave a patient with residual focal neurological symptoms and signs for some days after a fit. There may be a history of previous events to provide a clue.
- **Migraine** is itself a cause of stroke, particularly in younger patients. Stroke should be suspected when the focal features persist.
- **Hypoglycaemia** must be excluded.

Acute stroke care
The appropriate management and good outcome depend on rapid access to acute stroke care. This requires:
- **Early recognition** of stroke signs and symptoms.
- **Prompt transport** and pre-hospital notification.
- **Immediate triage** and clinical examination.
- **Prompt laboratory studies and CT imaging.**
- **Diagnosis and decision** about appropriate therapy.
- **Administration of appropriate drugs** or other interventions.

Acute management
Acute management of patients with suspected stroke involves:
- Resuscitation (airway, breathing, and circulation).
- Cardiac monitoring.
- Establishing and maintaining intravenous access.
- Oxygen (as required, oxygen saturation (SaO_2) >92%).
- Assess for hypoglycaemia.
- Keep nil by mouth.

---

[1]Reprinted from *The Lancet*, 369, 9558, S Claiborne Johnston et al., 'Validation and refinement of scores to predict very early stroke risk after transient ischaemic attack', pp. 283–292, Copyright 2007, with permission from Elsevier.

- Alert receiving emergency department.
- Rapid transport to closest appropriate facility capable of treating acute stroke (hyperacute stroke unit (HASU)).
  Avoid the following in the acute situation:
- Dextrose-containing fluids in non-hypoglycaemic patients.
- Hypotension/excessive blood pressure reduction.
- Excessive intravenous fluids.

History
On admission, the history must include details of the onset of symptoms, recent events (e.g. stroke, myocardial infarction, trauma, surgery, bleeding, comorbid diseases, hypertension, diabetes mellitus), and medications (e.g. anticoagulants, insulin, and antihypertensives).

Time window
The intravenous thrombolytic tissue-type plasminogen activator (alteplase: 0.9 mg/kg, maximum dose 90 mg) is recommended for selected patients with acute ischaemic stroke who may be treated within 3 hours of onset. Infuse 0.9 mg/kg (maximum dose 90 mg) over 60 minutes, with 10% of the dose given as a bolus over 1 minute. The age criteria are for persons aged 18–80 years old.

Immediate diagnostic studies
Evaluation of a patient with suspected acute ischaemic stroke should include:

- **A non-contrast CT brain scan** for all patients. This accurately identifies most cases of intracranial haemorrhage and helps to discriminate non-vascular causes of neurological symptoms (e.g. brain tumour).
  CT can identify subtle early signs of ischaemic brain injury, including arterial occlusion (hyperdense vessel sign), loss of the grey-white differentiation in the cortical ribbon (particularly at the lateral margins of the insula) or the lentiform nucleus, and sulcal effacement. These changes can often be detected within 6 hours in up to 82% of patients with large-vessel anterior circulation occlusions and are associated with poorer outcomes.
  Multimodal CT include non-contrast CT, perfusion CT, and CT angiography studies.
  Baseline CT findings, including the presence of ischaemic changes involving more than one-third of a hemisphere, do not predict response to treatment with rtPA when the agent is administered within the 3-hour treatment window.
- **Further investigations** should include blood glucose, full blood count (FBC), serum electrolytes/renal function tests, ECG, markers of cardiac ischaemia, clotting screen, and SaO$_2$. In selected patients, hepatic function tests, toxicology screening, blood alcohol levels, pregnancy test, arterial blood gas tests (i.e. if hypoxia is suspected), chest radiography (if lung disease is suspected), lumbar puncture (i.e. if subarachnoid haemorrhage is suspected and CT scan is negative for blood), and electroencephalogram (i.e. if seizures are suspected) may be required.
- **Clotting studies.** Although it is desirable to know the results of the clotting screen before giving rtPA, thrombolytic therapy should not be delayed while awaiting the results, unless:
1. There is clinical suspicion of a bleeding abnormality or thrombocytopenia.
2. The patient has received heparin or warfarin.
3. The concurrent use of anticoagulants is not known.

Approach to arterial hypertension in acute ischaemic stroke
If the patient is eligible for treatment with intravenous rtPA or other acute reperfusion intervention, hypertension must be treated so that the systolic BP is <185 mmHg and diastolic BP is <110 mmHg.

- Labetalol 10–20 mg intravenously (IV) is given over 1–2 minutes and may be repeated once, but, if blood pressure does not decline and remains >185/110 mmHg, do not administer rtPA.

Management of blood pressure during and after treatment with rtPA or other acute reperfusion intervention
- Monitor blood pressure every 15 minutes during treatment and then for another 2 hours, then every 30 minutes for 6 hours, and then every hour for 16 hours.
- If systolic pressure is 180–230 mmHg or diastolic pressure 105–120 mmHg, give labetalol 10 mg IV over 1 to 2 minutes which may be repeated every 10–20 minutes, maximum dose of 300 mg; or labetalol 10 mg IV, followed by an infusion at 2–8 mg/min.
- If systolic pressure is >230 mmHg or diastolic 121–140 mmHg, give labetalol 10 mg IV over 1 to 2 minutes which may be repeated every 10–20 minutes to a maximum dose of 300 mg; or labetalol 10 mg IV, followed by an infusion at 2–8 mg/min. Alternatively, use a nicardipine infusion at 5 mg/h, and titrate up to the desired effect by increasing by 2.5 mg/h every 5 minutes to a maximum of 15 mg/h.
- If blood pressure remains uncontrolled, consider sodium nitroprusside.

Hypertension in the immediate post-stroke period
Arterial hypertension is a recognized risk factor for stroke and recurrent stroke. Patients with markedly elevated blood pressure may have their blood pressure lowered by about 15% during the first 24 hours after the onset of a stroke. The level of blood pressure that would mandate such treatment is not known, but consensus exists that medications should be withheld, unless the systolic pressure is >220 mmHg or the mean blood pressure is >120 mmHg.
Treatment should be with angiotensin receptor antagonists or angiotensin-converting enzyme (ACE) inhibitors.

Hyperglycaemia after acute stroke
Persistent hyperglycaemia (>7.8 mmol/L) during the first 24 hours after a stroke is associated with poor outcomes. Thus, it is generally agreed that hyperglycaemia should be treated aggressively, following acute ischaemic stroke. Raised serum glucose concentrations (~7.8–10.2 mmol/L) should probably trigger administration of insulin.

Heparin and oral anticoagulation
There is no indication for heparin or a LMW heparin following acute ischaemic stroke, and these medications increase the risk of symptomatic haemorrhagic transformation of ischaemic strokes, especially among persons with severe events, and are associated with a risk of serious systemic bleeding.
In patients with atrial fibrillation who have suffered an ischaemic stroke, anticoagulation should be commenced 7–10 days after the stroke. If there is a documented intracardiac clot and the stroke is small to moderate in size, then anticoagulation may be considered earlier (i.e. 24–48 hours after the incidence event).

Antiplatelet agents

The oral administration of aspirin (initial dose: 300 mg) within 24 to 48 hours after stroke onset is recommended in most patients. Clopidogrel alone, or in combination with aspirin, is not recommended for the treatment of acute ischaemic stroke.

Stroke units

Comprehensive stroke units lessen the rates of mortality and morbidity after stroke. The positive effects can persist for years. In addition, stroke unit care can be given to a broad number of patients, regardless of the interval from stroke or the severity of the neurological impairments, including patients who cannot be treated with thrombolytic therapy.

Secondary prevention strategies

Antiplatelet medication

The combination of aspirin and an extended-release dipyridamole after a first event, is recommended over aspirin alone, following evidence of benefit in recently published trials. Clopidogrel appears superior to aspirin alone in direct comparison trials. Addition of aspirin to clopidogrel increases the risk of haemorrhage and is not routinely recommended for ischaemic stroke or TIA patients. For patients allergic to aspirin, clopidogrel is a reasonable alternative. For patients who have had an ischaemic cerebrovascular event while taking aspirin, there is no evidence that increasing the dose of aspirin provides additional benefit. Current recommendations after an acute ischaemic stroke are to use aspirin 300 mg daily for 2 weeks, then change to a combination of aspirin 75 mg and an extended-release dipyridamole for 2 years. Subsequently, aspirin 75 mg daily (i.e. alone) should be prescribed.

Hypertension

There is a direct association between both systolic and diastolic blood pressures and the risk of ischaemic stroke. Meta-analyses of randomized controlled trials confirm an approximate 30–40% reduction in stroke risk with BP lowering. Antihypertensive treatment is recommended for both prevention of recurrent stroke and prevention of other vascular events in persons who have had an ischaemic stroke or TIA and are beyond the hyperacute period.

An absolute target blood pressure level and reduction are uncertain and should be individualized. However, benefit has been associated with an average systolic/diastolic reduction of 10/5 mmHg, and normal blood pressure levels have been defined as <120/80 mmHg. The optimal drug regimen remains uncertain; but, the available data support the use of diuretics or the combination of a diuretic and an ACE inhibitor.

Diabetes

More rigorous control of blood pressure and lipids should be considered in patients with diabetes. Although all major classes of antihypertensives are suitable for the control of blood pressure, most patients will require more than one agent. Glucose control is recommended to near-normoglycaemic levels among diabetics with ischaemic stroke or TIA to reduce microvascular complications. The goal for HbA1c should be <7%.

Smoking

Smoking increases the risk of stroke by around 50%. All ischaemic stroke or TIA patients who have smoked in the past year should be strongly encouraged to stop smoking and to avoid environmental smoke. Counselling, nicotine products, and oral smoking cessation medications have been found to be effective for smokers (see Chapter 3).

Cholesterol reduction

All patients with total cholesterol over 3.5 mmol/L should be treated with a statin and given dietary advice.

Carotid endarterectomy (CEA)

For patients with recent TIA or ischaemic stroke and ipsilateral severe (i.e. 70–99%) carotid artery stenosis, CEA is recommended by a surgeon, with a perioperative morbidity and mortality of <6%. When CEA is indicated, surgery should be undertaken within 2 weeks, rather than delayed.

In patients with symptomatic severe stenosis (>70%), in whom the stenosis is difficult to access surgically, or with comorbid medical conditions that greatly increase the risk for surgery, or when other specific circumstances exist, such as radiation-induced stenosis or restenosis after CEA, carotid artery stenting may be considered.

In asymptomatic carotid stenosis of >70%, there is a 2-year delayed benefit in outcome, suggesting that men aged 40–75 years old with a >70% stenosis without significant complicating comorbidities may be offered surgery, although there remains very mixed opinion. Control of vascular risk factors is more important. There is no conclusive benefit in women.

Stroke in young patients

The cause of stroke in young patients remains unknown in at least 40%.

- *Cardiac embolization* remains the commonest cause of stroke in young patients. The optimal therapy for prevention of recurrent stroke or transient ischaemic attack in patients with cryptogenic stroke and patent foramen ovale has not been defined. Treatment choices include medical therapy with antiplatelet agents or vitamin K antagonists, and percutaneous device closure, or open surgical repair of a patent foramen ovale.
- *Arterial dissection* accounts for 5–20% of strokes in individuals younger than 45 years. The most frequent presenting complaints in patients with cervicocephalic dissections are ischaemic symptoms that include transient ischaemic attack (TIA) or stroke. Symptoms include ipsilateral neck, scalp, or head pain, occurring in both carotid and vertebral artery dissections. Neurologic deficits reflect the ultimate site of ischaemia in the ipsilateral anterior or posterior circulations and may include an ipsilateral partial Horner's syndrome, ipsilateral cranial nerve palsies, particularly cranial nerves IX, X, XI, and XII. Examination may detect an audible bruit (e.g. carotid bruit).

Rehabilitation

Rehabilitation after stroke needs to begin immediately and should not wait until the patient is deemed to be medically 'stable'. The key components are:

- Involvement of the appropriate specialist staff, who may include physiotherapy, occupational therapy, speech and language therapy, psychology, dietitians, nurses, social workers, physicians, and psychiatrists.
- Using evidence-based guidelines to inform the decision-making process.
- Using a clear framework and assessment measures to structure the therapy process.
- Regular (at least weekly) team meetings to coordinate treatment and set achievable objectives for the patient.

- Involvement of the patient and carer in the rehabilitation process.
- Regular audit of the effectiveness of treatment being provided by the service.

Discharge from hospital

The hospital stroke service should maintain close working relationships with the primary care teams to ensure seamless care between hospital and home. The components of successful discharge will include:

- Detailed and rapid information exchange between hospital and primary care.
- Prior assessment of the home environment, with all necessary aids and adaptations having been made prior to discharge.
- Identification of the key individuals and clear routes of access to them, for support and treatment after discharge.
- Education and training given to the patient and their carers about living with the consequences of their stroke.
- A secondary prevention strategy.
- Recognition of the burden stroke places on the carers both psychologically and physically with a plan in place to support them.

Longer-term management

Recovery of neurological impairment after stroke can continue for many months after the acute event. Language, sensory, and higher cognitive deficits are often slower to recover than motor deficits. Specific issues that the primary care physician may need to consider will be:

- Driving.
- Work.
- Leisure.
- Post-stroke pain. Shoulder pain and central post-stroke pain are the two most frequent causes of pain.
- Epilepsy. Approximately 5% of stroke patients develop epilepsy following stroke. Referral to a neurologist for investigation and treatment is appropriate. Carbamazepine and phenytoin remain the most widely used drugs and, in most cases, are successful.

Primary intracerebral and subarachnoid haemorrhage

Spontaneous primary intracerebral haemorrhage (PICH) accounts for about 10% of all strokes. The incidence is higher in some ethnic groups. About 50% of patients die within the first month. The major risk factor for PICH is arterial hypertension. Other risk factors include excess alcohol consumption, male sex, increasing age, and smoking. These risk factors lead to small-vessel vascular disease and aneurysm formation which eventually may lead to PICH.

Detailed investigations in selected patients have shown an underlying arteriovenous malformation in about 20% and an aneurysm in about 13%. About 1 in 2,000 people are estimated to have an unruptured AVM, which if left alone, carries an annual risk of bleeding of ~1%, of which ~10% are fatal.

Causes

- Small-vessel disease (seen as leukoaraiosis on MRI).
- Amyloid angiopathy (e.g. lobar intracerebral haemorrhage without other underlying causes).
- Brain arteriovenous malformations (AVM) should be suspected if there is extension of blood into other compartments or calcified or enhancing vessels are detected on imaging.

- Cavernous malformations (clusters of abnormal, tiny blood vessels, and larger, thin-walled blood vessels filled with blood, usually in the brain) should be suspected if there is a personal or family history of PICH. Typically, there are small bleeds without extension of blood into other compartments.
- Cerebral venous thrombosis with haemorrhagic venous infarction is suspected if there is a history of raised intracranial pressure, headache, papilloedema, or venous thrombosis risk.
- Intracranial arterial aneurysm should be suspected if there is extension of blood into other compartments or the bleed is located near the sylvian or interhemispheric fissure.
- Dural arteriovenous (AV) fistula. These cases may have a history of pulsatile tinnitus.
- Clotting factor deficiency.
- Cerebral neoplasms may present with a bleed into the tumour.
- Vasculitis
- Infective endocarditis.

Investigations

Following radiological diagnosis on a brain CT scan, the following routine investigations are essential: FBC, coagulation screen, biochemistry, liver function tests, glucose, C-reactive protein, ESR, toxicology screen, ECG, chest radiograph, and a pregnancy test, if indicated. Early CT angiography is a quick and widely available first-line investigation for underlying aneurysm and AVM when these diagnoses are suspected. MRI is useful for cerebral venous thrombosis to detect venous infarction. CT venography may be superior at looking at the cerebral veins. Catheter angiography is the best investigation to detect intracranial arterial aneurysms.

Outcomes

The main predictors of death within 1 month are:

- Low GCS on admission.
- Increasing intracerebral haemorrhage volume.
- Infratentorial location.
- Intraventricular extension.
- Older age.

Treatment

Patients should be managed on a stroke unit or in an intensive care facility if they need ventilation or intracranial pressure monitoring. Although the risk of epileptic seizures is higher with lobar, rather than deep, intracerebral haemorrhages (14 vs 4%), the routine use of prophylactic anti-epileptic medication is not recommended.

Limited data are available to guide the decision on acute blood pressure lowering after PICH. For now, the use of antihypertensive agents seems necessary if there is end-organ damage, though the desirable parameters are uncertain.

Haemostatic drugs (recombinant factor VIIa) have not been shown to be of value in improving outcome despite the prevention of haematoma expansion when given under 3 hours.

Neurosurgical haematoma evacuation should be undertaken in some situations. In infratentorial haemorrhage, cerebellar haemorrhage that is causing deterioration in consciousness, brainstem compression, or hydrocephalus due to obstruction of CSF flow, then immediate neurosurgical intervention should be considered. Ventricular drainage may be enough to relieve the hydrocephalus, but, if further deterioration occurs, evacuation of the haematoma is required. The role of surgery for supratentorial haemorrhage has not been proven. The STITCH 2 trial is ongoing for haematoma <1 cm from cortical surface.

Aneurysm and arteriovenous malformations

- The International Subarachnoid Aneurysm Trial (IZAT) of coiling versus clipping for ruptured arterial aneurysms has shown that coiling is less likely to result in death at 5 years despite a higher risk of rebleeding after coiling.
- A recent primary prevention trial, the ARUBA study, for unruptured arteriovenous malformations (AVM) compared intervention with conservative therapy. It was stopped in 2014 because of a higher than expected event rate in the intervention group. Consequently there is currently no evidence for the treatment of unruptured AVMs, although this remains controversial.
- Ruptured AVMs with unfavourable angioarchitecture may be treated surgically by catheter embolization or stereotactic radiosurgery.

Cerebral venous thrombosis (CVT)

- The presentation is usually with raised intracranial pressure-type headaches and seizures secondary to venous infarction.
- Risk factors are the combined oral contraceptive pill and venous thrombophilia.
- Investigation is with CT or MR venography.
- Expert opinion and data from two randomized trials support the use of therapeutic anticoagulation for CVT. This does not seem to precipitate or worsen clinically important haemorrhage.
- Seizures are treated with conventional anti-epileptic medication.
- Treatment is usually for 6 months, with repeat imaging when anticoagulation is stopped.

Further reading

Adams RJ, Albers G, Alberts MJ, et al. (2008). Update to the AHA/ASA recommendations for the prevention of stroke in patients with stroke and transient ischaemic attack. Stroke, 39, 1647–52.

Albers GW, Caplan LR, Easton JD, et al., for the TIA Working Group (2002). Transient ischaemic attack: proposal for a new definition. New England Journal of Medicine, 347, 1713–16.

Bederson JB, Connolly ES Jr, Batjer HH, et al. (2009). Guidelines for the management of aneurysmal subarachnoid hemorrhage: a statement for healthcare professionals from a special writing group of the Stroke Council, American Heart Association (published correction appears in Stroke (2009), 40, e518); Stroke, 40, 994–1025.

Department of Health (2001). The National Service Framework for Older People. Department of Health, London.

Fairhead JF, Mehta Z, Rothwell PM (2005). Population-based study of delays in carotid imaging and surgery and the risk of recurrent stroke. Neurology, 65, 371–5.

Giles MF and Rothwell PM (2006). Prediction and prevention of stroke after transient ischaemic attack in the short and long term. Expert Review of Neurotherapeutics, 6, 381–95.

Hankey GJ and Warlow CP (1999). Treatment and secondary prevention of stroke: evidence, costs, and effects on individuals and populations. Lancet, 354, 1457–63.

Intercollegiate Stroke Working Party (2012). Royal College of Physicians National clinical guideline for stroke, fourth edition. Incorporating the recommendations from Stroke: national clinical guideline for diagnosis and initial management of acute stroke and transient ischaemic attack (TIA) by the National Institute for Health and Clinical Excellence <http://www.nice.org.uk/nicemedia/pdf/cg68niceguideline.pdf>. <http://www.rcplondon.ac.uk/sites/default/files/national-clinical-guidelines-for-stroke-fourth-edition.pdf>.

Mohr JP, Parides MK, Stapf C, et al. (2014). Medical management with or without interventional therapy for unruptured brain arteriovenous malformations (ARUBA): a multicentre, non-blinded, randomised trial. Lancet, 383, 614–21.

National Stroke Strategy (2009). <http://webarchive.nationalarchives.gov.uk/20130107105354/http://www.dh.gov.uk/en/Healthcare/Longtermconditions/Vascular/Stroke/DH_099065>.

National Institute for Health and Clinical Excellence (2008). Stroke: Diagnosis and initial management of acute stroke and transient ischaemic attack (TIA). NICE clinical guideline 68. <https://www.nice.org.uk/guidance/cg68>.

National Institute for Health and Clinical Excellence (2013). Stroke rehabilitation: Long-term rehabilitation after stroke. NICE clinical guideline 162. <https://www.nice.org.uk/guidance/cg162>.

Rothwell PM and Warlow CP (2005). Timing of TIAs preceding stroke: time window for prevention is very short. Neurology, 64, 817–20.

Russin J, Spetzler R (2014). Commentary: The ARUBA Trial. Neurosurgery, 75, E96–E97.

Scottish Intercollegiate Guidelines Network. Management of patients with stroke or TIA: assessment, investigation, immediate management and secondary prevention. A national clinical guideline 108. <http://www.sign.ac.uk/pdf/sign108.pdf>.

Stroke Unit Trialists' Collaboration (2007). Organized inpatient (stroke unit) care for stroke. Cochrane Database of Systematic Reviews, 4, CD000197.

The ARUBA Trial. <http://www.arubastudy.org>.

The National Institute of Neurological Disorders and Stroke rt-PA Stroke Study Group (1995). Tissue plasminogen activator for acute ischaemic stroke. New England Journal of Medicine, 333, 1581–7.

Wade D (1994). Stroke (acute cerebrovascular disease). In A Stevens, J Raftery, eds. Health care needs assessments, vol 1, pp. 111–255. Radcliffe Medical Press, Oxford.

Wahlgren N, Ahmed N, Davalos A, et al.; SITS-MOST investigators (2007). Thrombolysis with alteplase for acute ischaemic stroke in the Safe Implementation of Thrombolysis in Stroke-Monitoring Study (SITS-MOST): an observational study. Lancet, 369, 275–82.

Wardlaw JM, Seymour J, Cairns J, et al. (2004). Immediate computed tomography scanning of acute stroke is cost-effective and improves quality of life. Stroke, 35, 2477–83.

Warlow CP, Dennis MS, van Gijn J, et al. (2003). Stroke: a practical guide to management (2nd edn). Blackwell Science Ltd, Oxford.

Neuro-ophthalmology

A significant number of patients presenting with visual disturbances have primary neurological disorders and require neurological assessment.

Visual failure

Unilateral visual loss

- **Sudden onset of painless and fixed visual loss** is generally vascular (e.g. central or branch retinal artery occlusion, anterior ischaemic optic neuropathy, or vein occlusion).
- **Subacute loss over days with pain** is usually due to an inflammatory cause (e.g. optic neuritis).
- **Gradually progressive loss of vision** is more likely to be due to a compressive lesion (e.g. anterior communicating artery aneurysm, infections or mucocele of the paranasal sinuses).
- **Unilateral visual field defects** may also be due to focal retinal pathology, congenital optic nerve defects, glaucoma, or optic disc drusen (globules of mucoprotein/mucopolysaccharide that gradually calcify in the optic disc).
- **Transient unilateral visual loss** lasting several minutes is usually due to migraine or retinal emboli (i.e. amaurosis fugax), but ischaemia, venous occlusion, retinal hypoperfusion, or primary ocular disorders (e.g. glaucoma, retinal detachment) may cause a similar pattern. Obscurations due to raised intracranial pressure usually last for seconds.

Bilateral visual loss

- **Ocular disease** (e.g. refractive errors, cataracts, uveitis, macular degeneration, bilateral retinal disease) may cause bilateral visual loss.
- **Bilateral optic nerve disease**, causing slowly progressive visual failure, may be due to hereditary optic atrophy, atrophy secondary to chronic papilloedema, or optic nerve damage secondary to toxins, drugs, and radiation.
- **Compression of the optic chiasm** by mass lesions (e.g. pituitary adenoma, craniopharyngioma, meningioma) causes a bitemporal field loss.
- **Post-chiasmal disorders** affect the optic tract (continuation of the optic nerve from the optic chiasm to the lateral geniculate nucleus (LGN), pretectal nuclei, and superior colliculus), the optic radiation (from the LGN to the primary visual cortex) or the visual cortex and its association areas.

Optic nerve disease

- Optic nerve lesions generally lead to monocular visual loss, and pain is common. The most important causes are inflammatory (e.g. demyelination, infection, sarcoidosis, vasculitis), ischaemic, compressive (e.g. optic pathway tumours, thyroid ophthalmopathy), infiltrative (e.g. metastases, lymphoma), toxic (e.g. toxins, nutritional deficiencies, including B_1, B_{12} and folate, tobacco, alcohol, radiation), or degenerative.

Diplopia

Orbital disease

The principal causes of restricted ocular movement due to orbital disease include dysthyroid eye disease, orbital pseudotumour (myositis), primary or metastatic orbital tumours (e.g. lymphoma), intracranial masses extending into the orbit (e.g. mucocele or tumour), or caroticocavernous fistula.

Cavernous sinus thrombosis

A number of conditions may lead to thrombosis within the cavernous sinus. Infectious causes may spread from local structures either directly or via vascular pathways. Underlying medical conditions may predispose to thrombosis, including thrombophilia, diabetes mellitus, malignancy, and some collagen vascular diseases. There is periorbital pain, proptosis, chemosis, ptosis, and ophthalmoplegia, with early involvement of the VI nerve occurring before total ophthalmoplegia develops.

Cranial nerve palsies

Cranial nerve palsies include:

- **Oculomotor nerve (III nerve palsy).** The third nerve supplies the medial rectus, inferior oblique, inferior rectus and superior rectus muscles, the lid levator, and the parasympathetic innervation of the pupillary sphincter and ciliary body. With a complete lesion, there is ptosis; the eye is deviated 'downward and outward', with residual function only in abduction, and there may be a fixed, dilated pupil.

  Lesions may lie anywhere in the course of the nerve from the nucleus to the orbit. The commonest causes are vascular lesions in the nucleus or fascicle; microvascular damage to the nerve associated with diabetes mellitus and hypertension (the pupil is usually unaffected); and compressive lesions in the subarachnoid space and cavernous sinus due to aneurysmal compression, leading to partial or complete third nerve palsy with pupil involvement.

- **Abducens nerve (VI nerve palsy).** Abducens nerve palsy causes binocular horizontal diplopia due to ipsilateral rectus paresis, with a primary position esotropia (a 'squint' in which the eye turns inward). Nuclear lesions are commonly vascular, and several characteristic syndromes of pontine infarction occur (see *Oxford Desk Reference of Neurology*). Within the subarachnoid space, the abducens nerve may be involved by meningeal inflammation, infiltration, and raised intracranial pressure. Acute onset of a painful sixth nerve palsy is often due to microvascular ischaemia. Bilateral sixth nerve palsies are associated with raised intracranial pressure, subarachnoid haemorrhage, meningitis, Wernicke's encephalopathy, and tumours.

- **Trochlear nerve (IV nerve palsy).** Fourth nerve palsy causes binocular vertical diplopia, with tilting of objects (torsional diplopia), and is worse on looking down (and inwards) and is due to ipsilateral superior oblique weakness. There is elevation of the affected eye, with vertical diplopia and head tilt away from the side of the lesion. The commonest cause of trochlear palsy is trauma, but it may be due to microvascular ischaemic disease.

Painful and combined ophthalmoplegia

Multiple ocular motor palsies are usually unilateral and result from lesions in the cavernous sinus or superior orbital fissure. The principal causes include tumours (e.g. pituitary adenoma, nasopharyngeal carcinoma, meningioma, and metastases from breast, lung, and prostate), carotid aneurysm or occlusions, cavernous sinus thrombosis, and caroticocavernous fistula.

Bilateral lesions suggest a diffuse disorder of muscle, a neuromuscular abnormality (e.g. myasthenia gravis) or a neurogenic cause (e.g. Guillain–Barré syndrome, Miller–Fisher syndrome), diffuse infiltrative brainstem lesions, infection or neoplastic disease affecting the meninges.

Abnormalities of the visual pathway
Bitemporal and homonymous hemianopias

- **Bitemporal hemianopia** (loss of vision in the outer half of both right and left visual fields) is the characteristic clinical sign of chiasmal disease due to compression.
- **Homonymous hemianopia** (visual field loss on the same side in both eyes, either to the left or right of the vertical midline) is caused by unilateral lesions of the visual pathway posterior to the optic chiasm, i.e. optic tract, lateral geniculate body, optic radiation, and cerebral cortex.

  Clinically, these are often disabling, causing difficulty with reading and visual scanning. Patients may fail to notice relevant objects or obstacles on the affected side, causing collisions with approaching people or cars.

Specific patterns of acquired field defect
Specific patterns of acquired field defect occur with various lesions of the primary visual cortex. Occipital lobe lesions are the commonest cause of homonymous hemianopia and are usually due to infarction in the distribution of the posterior cerebral artery; other aetiologies include venous infarction, haemorrhagic arteriovenous malformations and fistulas, tumours, abscess, and trauma. Superior and inferior homonymous visual field defects, respecting the vertical and sometimes the horizontal meridians, occur with lesions of the occipital cortex.

Bilateral homonymous hemianopia
Bilateral homonymous hemianopia may occur with bilateral lesions of the occipital cortex, either simultaneously or consecutively. A variety of bilateral homonymous lesions may occur, ranging from complete bilateral homonymous hemianopia (e.g. cortical blindness) to bilateral macular sparing hemianopia (e.g. ring scotoma), quadrantanopias, or scotomatous and altitudinal defects. Patients with cortical blindness may appear to be unaware of their visual loss, deny any difficulty, and confabulate about what they are able to see, often being able to direct their gaze to auditory stimuli.

Abnormalities of the pupil
Pupillary changes rarely cause prominent symptoms, but they may indicate serious underlying neurological disease.

Complete afferent pupillary defect
When there is complete blindness due to a lesion in the anterior visual pathway or the eye, the pupil will show no reaction to direct light reflex, and there will be no response in the opposite eye. However, the pupil of the blind eye will respond to light shone into the opposite unaffected eye. A preserved light reflex, in the presence of apparent total blindness in the eye, indicates either that the blindness is feigned or that it arises from the posterior visual pathways.

Relative afferent pupillary defect
When light is directed into the affected eye, this will cause mild constriction of both pupils, and, when directed to the unaffected eye, it will cause a normal constriction of both pupils. When the light is rapidly alternated between the two eyes, the normal reaction in the good eye will override the poorer reaction in the affected eye so that the pupils in the affected eye react less well to the direct light source, and, in a severe case, the pupil in the affected eye actually dilates when the light is swung onto that eye. The presence of a relative afferent pupillary defect indicates that there is an abnormality in the optic pathway due to unilateral (or at least asymmetrical) optic nerve or retinal disease.

Argyll Robertson syndrome
The pupils are small and irregular and do not react to light but do react to accommodation (light-near dissociation). It occurs in tertiary syphilis but may be associated with diabetes, multiple sclerosis, or myotonic dystrophy.

Parinaud's syndrome
Parinaud's syndrome describes the combination of signs due to damage in the dorsal midbrain. It is seen with pineal tumours (usually pinealoma), other tumours in the same region, multiple sclerosis, acute hydrocephalus, and ischaemic or haemorrhagic stroke. The signs include dilated (or mid-dilated) pupils which do not react to light but which do react to accommodation; paralysis of voluntary upgaze, with preservation of downward gaze; convergence retraction nystagmus on attempted upgaze and eyelid retraction (Collier's sign).

Holmes–Adie syndrome
Holmes–Adie syndrome is characterized by a tonic (dilated) pupil, in which there is limited reaction to light and the response to accommodation is present but abnormally prolonged. The syndrome is associated with the absence of deep tendon reflexes (sometimes complete absence or sometimes with preservation of some reflexes) and impaired autonomic functions (e.g. anhidrosis).

Horner's syndrome
Horner's syndrome is associated with ptosis and miosis (i.e. constricted pupil). Other signs include upside-down ptosis (i.e. slight elevation of the lower lid), enophthalmos, conjunctival injection, and anhidrosis (i.e. decreased sweating). Thus, the ptosis caused by Horner's syndrome occurs with a constricted pupil whilst that caused by a third palsy is usually more severe and associated with a dilated pupil.

Horner's syndrome can be congenital but is usually acquired. The causes are almost all unilateral and can be due to involvement of the sympathetic nervous supply at any point in its long anatomical course. Preganglionic lesions in the hypothalamus, brainstem, or spinal cord are usually vascular (e.g. lateral medullary syndrome), inflammatory (e.g. multiple sclerosis), or structural (e.g. tumour, syrinx). Dissection of the carotid artery may present with a Horner's syndrome and ipsilateral neck or face pain. Pancoast tumours (i.e. carcinoma at the apex of the lung) may also present with a Horner's syndrome. Cluster headaches cause a transient Horner's syndrome.

Further reading
Acheson J and Riordan-Eva P (1999). *Fundamentals of clinical ophthalmology: neuro-ophthalmology*. BMJ Books, London.

Belcer LJ (2006). Clinical practice: optic neuritis. *New England Journal of Medicine*, **354**, 1273–80.

Bhatti MT (2007). Orbital syndromes. *Seminars in Neurology*, **27**, 269–87.

Brazis PW, Stewart M, Lee AG, *et al.* (2004). The uveo-meningeal syndromes. *The Neurologist*, **10**, 171–85.

Caplan LR (1980). 'Top of the basilar' syndrome. *Neurology*, **30**, 72–9.

Keane JR (2005). Bilateral involvement of a single cranial nerve: analysis of 578 cases. *Neurology*, **65**, 950–2.

Leigh RJ and Zee DS (2006). *The neurology of eye movements*, 4th edn. Oxford University Press, Oxford.

Miller NR and Newman NJ (2004). The eye in neurological disease. *Lancet*, **364**, 2045–54.

Spalton DJ, Hitchings RA, Hunter P, eds. (2004). *Atlas of clinical ophthalmology*, 3rd edn. Elsevier, London.

Epilepsies and epileptic states

The generic term 'epilepsy' is of limited clinical value. Well-defined epileptic syndromes are now recognized, with different clinical patterns, natural history, prognosis, and management.

Early treatment can reduce the risk of seizure recurrence, and its efficacy depends on the appropriate drug choice in relation to the particular clinical syndrome. Therefore, identification of the particular form or syndrome is the basis of management and often requires specialist neurological input.

Classification of epileptic seizures and epilepsy syndromes

Epilepsies are classified as **generalized** and **localized** (or partial/focal), and in terms of their aetiology as **idiopathic** (i.e. genetically determined, unrelated to structural brain pathology, and associated with normal neurological and neuropsychological status) and **symptomatic** (i.e. due to cerebral pathology).

- **Idiopathic generalized epilepsies (IGE)** manifest with generalized seizures (e.g. tonic-clonic, bilateral myoclonic, and typical absences). The different syndromes are characterized by clinical (i.e. seizure type(s) and combinations and the age at onset) and specific electroencephalogram (EEG) features. Prognosis is largely dependent on the particular subsyndrome and seizures are typically facilitated by sleep deprivation, alcohol and early awakening, and importantly by some anti-epileptic drugs (see further text).
- **Focal epilepsies** manifest with focal (i.e. simple and complex partial) seizures, with or without aura, and are traditionally classified according to the lobe (i.e. frontal,

temporal, occipital, and parietal) or the anatomical area (e.g. mesial or lateral temporal) from which seizures arise. They may become secondarily generalized. In contrast to IGEs, focal epilepsies may be amenable to surgical resection.

The main syndromes within each type and the relevant anti-epileptic drugs (AED) of choice are listed in Table 7.1.

Diagnosis

The diagnosis of epilepsy is primarily clinical and relies on obtaining an adequate history from the patient and witnesses of the seizures.

Seizure and syndrome diagnosis

Recognizing 'minor' seizures is the foundation for the diagnosis of the epilepsy type (IGE vs focal) and syndrome; for instance, **juvenile myoclonic epilepsy** (JME) is recognized by the myoclonic seizures (typically early morning clumsiness), while **temporal lobe epilepsy** (TLE) by the often conspicuous episodes of epigastric sensation or déjà vu.

- **Absences** are the commonest seizure type of IGE. They are brief blank spells without warning or post-ictal symptoms, frequently associated with manual or oral automatisms and sometimes with mild symmetrical twitching of the eyelids or mouth.
- **Myoclonic jerks** are the defining seizure type of JME. They are sudden, brief, bilateral, symmetrical, or asymmetrical clonic movements of distal, regional, or axial muscles that usually occur in clear consciousness while awake, mainly in the morning.
- **Simple partial seizures (SPS)** are focal epileptic seizures that manifest with a variety of symptoms (e.g.

Table 7.1 Main epilepsy types and syndromes and recommended/contraindicated# anti-epileptic drugs (AED)

Generalized		Recommended AED
Idiopathic	Benign myoclonic epilepsy in infancy	VPA
	Childhood absence epilepsy	VPA, ESX, LTG
	Juvenile absence epilepsy	VPA, LTG, LEV
	Juvenile myoclonic epilepsy	VPA, LEV, ZSM, LTG
	Epilepsy with GTCS only	VPA, LEV, TPM, LTG
	Mixed phenotypes*	
Symptomatic/cryptogenic	Myoclonic astatic epilepsy**	VPA, LEV, ESX, CLZ
	Epilepsy with myoclonic absences**	VPA, ESX, LTG, LEV, CLZ
	Infantile spasms (West syndrome)**	VPA, VGB, steroids
	Lennox Gastaut syndrome**	VPA, LTG, LEV
Focal/multifocal		
Idiopathic	Benign rolandic epilepsy***	
	Panayiotopoulos syndrome***	
	Benign occipital epilepsy***	
Symptomatic/cryptogenic	Lobar (frontal, temporal, parietal, occipital), including specific syndromes such as:	CBZ, OXC, LEV, TPM, LTG, TGB, VPA, CLB, PHT
	Rasmussen's encephalitis	
	Mesial temporal lobe epilepsy	

#, anti-epileptic drugs (AED) that are contraindicated for generalized epilepsies include CBZ, OXC, VGB, TGB, GBP, PHT; *, patients with phenotypes between JAE and JME (prominent myoclonic and absence components); **, idiopathic forms of these syndromes also exist; ***, often, no AED treatment is necessary; if yes, AED for symptomatic focal can be used; VPA, valproate; ESX, ethosuximide; LTG, lamotrigine; LEV, levetiracetam; TPM, topiramate; ZSM, zonisamide; CLZ, clonazepam; VGB, vigabatrine; CBZ, carbamazepine; OXC, oxcarbazepine; TGB, tiagabine; CLB, clobazam; PHT, phenytoin; GBP, gabapentin; GTCS, generalised tonic-clonic seizures; JAE, juvenile absence epilepsy; JME, juvenile myoclonic epilepsy.

auras) in apparently unaffected consciousness. Most auras have localizing value (i.e. indicate the area of brain primarily involved). For example:

- Olfactory, gustatory, epigastric, mnemonic, and psychic-experiential (i.e. déjà vu) suggest primary involvement of the mesial temporal area of the brain.
- Auditory, dysphasic, vestibular, and/or complex visual aura suggest lateral or posterior temporal brain activation.
- Visual hallucinations and amaurosis suggest occipital onset.
- Contralateral somatosensory and distortion of spatial perception point to parietal lobe.
- Focal motor, eye deviation, dysphasia, explosive peculiar automatisms, and forced thinking indicate frontal involvement.
- Autonomic symptoms (e.g. cardiac: tachycardia, bradycardia, or asystole; respiratory, gastrointestinal, genital sensations, pupillary changes, pallor, or flushing, etc.) indicate frontotemporal involvement, including the cingulate gyrus and the insula.

- **Complex partial seizures** (CPS) are focal seizures that manifest with unresponsiveness, automatisms, or asymmetric motor phenomena, such as unilateral dystonic posture which is usually contralateral to the site of seizure onset. They may, or may not, be preceded by a simple partial seizure; as a rule, they last longer than absences and are usually followed by post-ictal confusion. Such ictal clouding of consciousness indicates bilateral brain involvement in the seizure process.

Investigations
The interictal video EEG supports the clinical diagnosis by demonstrating epileptiform activity and contributing to the identification of the particular epilepsy type or syndrome. The interictal EEG alone cannot be used for establishing or excluding the diagnosis of epilepsy. The first interictal EEG can be normal in up to 50% of patients with seizures. Brain MRI may show a lesion in symptomatic epilepsies and guide management, but its nature and topography must be consistent with the clinical ictal symptoms. The use of interictal positron emission tomography (FDG-PET) is mainly limited to epilepsy surgery candidates.

Differential diagnosis
Paroxysmal events that alter, or appear to alter, neurological function to produce motor signs or sensory, autonomic, or psychic symptoms that, at least, superficially resemble those occurring during epileptic seizures are called non-epileptic seizures (NES). These can be either physiological (PhNES) or psychogenic (PsNES) in origin. More than 30% of patients referred to epilepsy centres have NES. PsNES and syncope are more frequent in adolescence, but both may start much earlier.

Physiological non-epileptic seizures
Physiological non-epileptic seizures (PhNES) present with:
- Abnormal paroxysmal motor phenomena.
  - In neonates and infants, these include jitteriness, startle, and benign myoclonus. Older children present with breath-holding attacks, tics, paroxysmal dyskinesias, and sleep-related motor disorders, including hypnic jerks, confusional arousals, and sleep terrors and/or walking.
  - Movement disorders may present during childhood, adolescence, or in adulthood and be either familial or

symptomatic. They include choreoathetosis, dystonia, paroxysmal dyskinesia, and myoclonus.
- Abnormal paroxysmal non-motor symptoms.
  - These may mimic simple partial seizures. Symptoms, including fear, as part of panic attacks, déjà vu, or smells and tastes, are of similar or identical quality to their epileptic counterparts and may be experienced by people without epileptic seizures. A long duration and high frequency over the years, with lack of a strict temporal relationship with other symptoms and signs that are unequivocally epileptic or lack of coexistent independent seizures, argue for a non-epileptic nature.
  - A particular flavour of a symptom may also be indicative. Fear or a panic sensation as symptom of an epileptic seizure for example, lasts for few seconds and commonly evolves into a complex partial seizure with unmistakable clinical features. It is also stereotypical, moderate in intensity, and not in context with situation; in contrast, a panic attack is typically longer, and the fear is intense and relevant to reality.

Sleep disorders
The diagnosis of sleep disorders and differentiation from seizure disorders is based on history, video EEG, and polysomnography (PSG), coupled with multiple sleep latency test (MSLT), and also on home videos. The following sleep-related disorders may cause diagnostic confusion:
- **Hypnic jerks** ('sleep starts') occur in about 60% of the population, mainly in adults at sleep onset or in light stages of sleep, and differ from myoclonic seizures, as the latter occur usually on awakening and are always associated with spike wave activity on the EEG.

  Diagnostic problems may arise when they are repetitive, frequent or violent, asymmetric, or associated with a sense of falling, brief formed images, noises, or a floating sensation.
- **Arousal parasomnias** (i.e. incomplete arousals from deep slow sleep, which is abundant during the first half of the sleep period). Patients with 'confusional arousals' look confused and may become agitated or aggressive if restrained. This can progress into sleep walking (somnambulism) or more complex acts, such as driving a car. Patients may become violent, either at the start of the sleepwalking period or when an attempt is made to arouse them. Somniloquy (i.e. random, slurred, non-sensical speech), somnambulistic eating, and abnormal sexual behaviours may occur, and adults may report fragments of dream recall during the ambulation period.

  Sleep terrors are associated with intense autonomic arousal and a typical non-epileptiform EEG response. The patient may scream and sit up in bed, with palpitations, mydriasis, being flushed, and sweating.
- **REM parasomnias** are behavioural disorders (REM-BD), arising mostly during the latter part of the night when REM sleep is more prevalent. Particularly unpleasant dreams are acted out because of the lack of atonia that usually characterizes the REM state. They are associated with underlying neurological conditions, such as Parkinson's disease and narcolepsy. PSG may show muscle tone during REM sleep, and, in contrast to focal epilepsies, patients do not report daytime events.
- **Cataplexy** may be misdiagnosed as atonic seizure, particularly when associated with some staring and possible

facial jerking. Excessive daytime sleepiness may account for reported episodes of 'losing a period of time' or 'not knowing how patients found themselves in bed' that could not be interpreted as of epileptic origin.

Non-epileptic amnesic and confusional paroxysmal episodes
These occur in the context of cerebrovascular dysfunction, such as transient global amnesia (TGA), transient ischaemic attack (TIA), and confusional migraine, in the course of encephalopathy (e.g. metabolic, infectious, or toxic), and in dementia (e.g. 'sundowning').

Psychogenic non-epileptic seizures (PsNES)
Psychogenic non-epileptic seizures (PsNES) form the majority of NES. They are associated with psychiatric disorders, including conversion, the most common cause, anxiety (i.e. panic, post-traumatic stress, and acute stress disorders), dissociative (i.e. mainly fugue and depersonalization) and factitious disorders. Malingering is also included here.

PsNES coexist in up to 20% of people with epilepsies, and confirmation of the diagnosis of PsNES, as in all other non-epileptic paroxysmal events, requires 'ictal' video EEG.

Clinical features suggestive of NES include multiple seizure types, frequently changing ictal symptoms with inconsistent temporal sequence and poor description, high seizure frequency and even 'status' despite adequate AED treatment, and an inconsistent response to AED.

Further reading

Engel J Jr (2006). ILAE classification of epilepsy syndromes. *Epilepsy Research*, **70S**, S5–10.

First Seizure Trial Group (FIRST Group) (1993). Randomized clinical trial on the efficacy of antiepileptic drugs in reducing the risk of relapse after a first unprovoked tonic-clonic seizure. *Neurology*, **43**, 478–83.

International League Against Epilepsy (2010). Report of the Commission on classification and terminology. <http://www.ilae.org/Visitors/Centre/ctf/ctfoverview.cfm>.

Krumholz A, Wiebe S, Gronseth GS, et al. (2015) Evidence-based guideline: Management of an unprovoked first seizure in adults. Report of the Guideline Development Subcommittee of the American Academy of Neurology and the American Epilepsy Society. *Neurology*, **84**, 1705–1713.

National Institute for Health and Clinical Excellence (2012). The epilepsies: the diagnosis and management of the epilepsies in adults and children in primary and secondary care. NICE clinical guideline 137. <https://www.nice.org.uk/guidance/cg137>.

Status epilepticus in adults

Generalized convulsive status epilepticus

Generalized convulsive status epilepticus (GCSE) is a medical emergency and is associated with an overall mortality of up to 8% in children and 30% in adults. An additional 5 to 10% of people have permanent sequelae, including vegetative state or cognitive difficulties. The longer the duration of the GCSE, the higher the risk for neuronal damage and serious systemic complications.

The aim of anticonvulsive medication is rapid and sustainable therapeutic effect, achieved without severe depressive, neurological, cardiovascular, or respiratory side effects.

Definition of GCSE

A continuous seizure lasting at least 5 minutes, or two or more seizures without complete recovery of consciousness between them. Serial seizures are defined as three or more seizures in an hour.

Clinical evolution

GCSE is customarily distinguished into early, established, and refractory stages.

- **Early status epilepticus** is associated with physiological mechanisms that compensate for the greatly enhanced metabolic activity.
- **Established status epilepticus** is defined as the stage beyond 30 minutes where the status continues despite early stage treatment. It is during this phase that the early physiological compensation mechanisms begin to fail.
- **Refractory status epilepticus (RSE)** is reached when seizures continue despite prompt therapy with two antiepileptic drugs (AED), a benzodiazepine and a longer-acting drug, in adequate doses. RSE is reached by 30-40% of patients with GCSE and the associated prognosis is poor.

Aetiology

Aetiology includes non-compliance with, or accidental withdrawal of, AED which is the commonest, and most probable, mechanism in patients already on AED treatment, traumatic brain injury, systemic infections, metabolic or electrolyte derangements, and alcoholic or toxic effects. Stroke, brain tumours, and central nervous system (CNS) infections have the poorest outcome.

Other factors that adversely affect outcome are duration greater than 1 hour, marked impairment of consciousness at presentation, and old age. About 10% of adults with a new diagnosis of epilepsy present in GCSE.

Management of GCSE

Treatment strategies depend on the stage of the status epilepticus (see Table 7.2 and Figure 7.1). The preferred anticonvulsant must: (i) afford good immediate, but also lasting, anti-epileptic effect and (ii) be free of serious effects on cardiorespiratory function and the level of consciousness.

Table 7.2 Treatment of convulsive status epilepticus

Prodromal phase	(If the patient is seen early, i.e. if brought with clustering of GTCS over the few preceding hours) **Buccal midazolam** 10 mg (if not available, use rectal diazepam 10–20 mg rectally)
Early status	(i.e. three or more seizures in an hour without full recovery in between or >5 min of generalized convulsions) **Lorazepam** (IV) 0.1 mg/kg (usually a 4 mg bolus, repeated once after 10–20 minutes; rate not critical) Give usual AED medication if already on treatment Prepare for IV **valproate acid** (in case seizures continue)
Established status	(Immediately after failure of lorazepam is appreciated—no need to wait for >30 minutes!) **Valproate acid** IV (12–15 mg/kg, targeting a concentration of 75 mg/L, or 25 mg/kg, targeting 100–150 mg/L, at 10 mg/kg/min) **Or** **Levetiracetam** (LEV) infused in 100 ml 0.9% sterile saline (100 mg/ml); well tolerated at high doses and fast infusion rates (2,000 mg in 5 min or 4,000 in 15 min) **Or** **Phenobarbital** bolus (10–15 mg/kg at 100 mg/min) **Or** **Phenytoin** infusion (15–18 mg/kg at 50 mg/min) or fosphenytoin infusion (15–20 mg phenytoin equivalents (PE)/kg at 50–100 mg PE/min); if continuous ECG monitoring is not available, dilute 250 mg in 100 mL of normal saline
Refractory status	(Seizures >60–90 minutes) Definitive treatment in ICU with: **Propofol:** IV bolus 2 mg/kg, repeated as necessary, followed by continuous infusion of 5–10 mg/kg/h, reducing to maintain EEG burst suppression (usually 1–3 mg/kg/h) **Or** **Thiopental:** IV 100–250 mg, given over 20 s, with further 50 mg boluses every 2–3 minutes until seizures are controlled. Then continuous infusion to maintain EEG burst suppression (usually 3–5 mg/kg/h) **Or** **Midazolam:** IV bolus 0.1–0.3 mg/kg at a rate not exceeding 4 mg/min initially, followed by continuous infusion at a dose sufficient to maintain EEG burst suppression (usually 0.05–0.4 mg/kg/h)

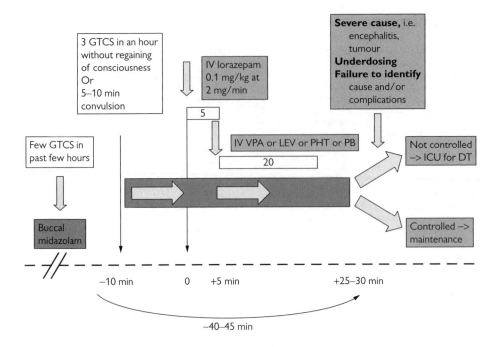

Figure 7.1 Management of GCSE over time. Progression to GCSE can be aborted using buccal midazolam if a 'prodromal phase' can be identified (left part of figure). Time '0' defines the diagnosis of the 'early phase' of GCSE when treatment with IV lorazepam should start (continuous infusion at 0.1 mg/kg may prevent underdosing in obese patients, compared to bolus). The two boxes 5 and 20 in the middle of the figure represent the approximate times allowed to appreciate the effects of lorazepam and the second-line AED (around 5 and 20 minutes, respectively). Lack of response to the second-line AED should prompt definitive treatment (DT) in the ICU setting, as it can only be positively appreciated a full 40–45 minutes from GCSE onset, at the very earliest, and assuming that the patient is closely monitored from the first convulsion (–10 min). Given that mortality increases exponentially after the first hour of status, there is no time to try a second second-line AED. The main reasons of treatment failure during the established phase appear in the grey box (top right). PHT, phenytoin; VPA, valproate acid; PB, phenobarbital; LEV, levetiracetam; ICU, intensive care unit.

- **The prodromal phase.** In some patients, there is a 'prodromal phase' of increasingly frequent seizures when prompt treatment can prevent evolution into status. Buccal midazolam is very useful in the 'out of hospital' environment, but overzealous use of any benzodiazepine should be discouraged because of the risk of cardiorespiratory depression.
- **Early status epilepticus.** The preferred AED in early status epilepticus (i.e. after more than 5 minutes of generalized convulsions, or three or more seizures in an hour without full recovery in between) is lorazepam plus the usual AED medication if the patient is already on treatment. The cause must be established from the history, examination, bloods, imaging, and other investigations (e.g. CSF examination) and the underlying cause treated accordingly.
- **Established status epilepticus.** If seizures continue, despite treatment with lorazepam (i.e. established status), prevent transition to refractory state by adding a longer-acting AED. The choice should be based on the patient's history and seizure type (primary vs secondary generalized). As the commonest cause of GCSE is failure to comply with the prescribed AED(s), it is logical to use the one that has already proven, or is expected to be,

effective. For example, in patients with idiopathic generalized epilepsies, sodium valproate (valproic acid; VPA) is the first choice. In those with known history of, or with suspected, focal seizure onset, as in post-traumatic GCSE, any of the options in Table 7.2, including VPA, can be considered. At this stage, it is important to identify and treat medical complications and prepare for potential admission to ICU for definitive treatment. Time is precious, as GCSE for >1 hour is associated with a mortality of 32% but only with 3% when <1 hour.

- **Refractory status epilepticus** occurs in up to 40% of patients with GCSE and carries high morbidity and mortality. The optimal duration of definitive treatment in the ICU is uncertain. Continuous AED infusions can be maintained for 24–48 hours, following which AED can be weaned gradually and the EEG re-examined for seizure activity. Maintenance treatment with VPA should be initiated at this stage.

Non-convulsive status epilepticus

Non-convulsive status epilepticus (NCSE) is classified into:

- **Complex partial status epilepticus** (CPSE) status with clinical features that may relate to localization.

- **Absence status epilepticus (ASE)** that occurs in idiopathic generalized epilepsy (IGE) and is essentially a long absence.

NCSE may last from 30 minutes to several days. Clinical presentation varies widely, but both states are essentially characterized by fluctuating confusion with 'focal' symptoms, such as dysmnesia (impaired memory) or dysphasia being more pronounced in CPSE. Distinct lobar epileptic states may manifest with more 'focal' symptoms:

- **Transient epileptic amnesia**, a type of temporal lobe seizure—status that may be mistaken for transient global amnesia, Korsakoff's psychosis, limbic encephalitis, or psychogenic amnesia.
- **Prolonged ictal dysphasic states** that involve the lateral temporal neocortex.
- **Occipital status** with visual hallucinations that may occur in association with posterior cortex lesions.

In clinical practice, the diagnosis of NCSE and the identification of its type (i.e. complex partial or absence status epilepticus) rely on the electroencephalogram (EEG).

Differential diagnosis

Non-epileptic states from which NCSE must be differentiated, depending on clinical presentation, include:

- **Localized brain lesions**, as in akinetic mutism (patient does not move or speak but appears aware), where imaging may reveal bilateral mesial frontal pathology in the absence of an ictal EEG.
- **Catatonic states** associated with depression, schizophrenia, limbic encephalitides, or orbitofrontal lesions.
- **Psychiatric states**, including conversion, interictal, post-ictal, or recurrent psychoses.
- **Prolonged post-ictal states.**
- **Malingering.**

Management

The management of complex partial status epilepticus differs between patients with known focal epilepsies and those with acute precipitated focal epileptic states. The former usually respond to oral benzodiazepines or buccal midazolam, but the latter, which occur in conditions associated with significantly increased mortality and morbidity, may need intravenous lorazepam or VPA.

Absence status may also respond to oral benzodiazepines but may need intravenous VPA. In these patients, phenytoin is strictly contraindicated as it may worsen absence seizures (as may carbamazepine, vigabatrin, tiagabine, oxcarbazepine, phenobarbital, and gabapentin). Overtreating patients with NCSE and known focal and IGE epilepsies should be avoided.

Further reading

Clarke C, Howard R, Rossor M, Shorvon S (2009). *Neurology—A Queen Square textbook*. Wiley-Blackwell, Oxford.

Kanner AM (2008). Intravenous valproate for status epilepticus. An effective, yet still merely empirical alternative! *Epilepsy Currents*, **8**, 66–7.

Koutroumanidis M (2009). Absence status epilepticus. In PW Kaplan, FW Drislane, eds. *Non-convulsive status epilepticus*, pp. 145–66. Demos Medical Publishing, New York.

National Institute for Health and Care Excellence (2012). The epilepsies: the diagnosis and management of the epilepsies in adults and children in primary and secondary care. NICE clinical guideline 137. <https://www.nice.org.uk/guidance/cg137>.

National Institute for Health and Clinical Excellence (2004). Appendix C Guidelines for treating status epilepticus in adults and children. <http://www.nice.org.uk/nicemedia/pdf/cg020full-guideline.pdf>.

Prasad K, Al-Roomi K, Krishnan PR, Sequeira R (2005). Anticonvulsant therapy for status epilepticus. *Cochrane Database of Systematic Reviews*, **4**, CD003723.

Shorvon S (1993). Tonic-clonic status epilepticus. *Journal of Neurology, Neurosurgery & Psychiatry*, **56,** 125–34.

Treiman DM, Meyers PD, Walton NY, *et al.* (1998). A comparison of four treatments for generalized convulsive status epilepticus: Veterans Affairs Status Epilepticus Cooperative Study Group. *New England Journal of Medicine*, **17**, 792–8.

Working Group (1993). Treatment of convulsive status epilepticus. Recommendations of the Epilepsy Foundation of America's Working Group on Status Epilepticus. *JAMA*, **270**, 854–9.

Infections of the nervous system

Bacterial meningitis

Bacterial meningitis (see also Chapter 6) is due to a primary infection within the subarachnoid space which causes acute inflammation of the meninges (pia and arachnoid mater).

Clinical presentation

Meningitis may evolve as a fulminating illness over a few hours, particularly in children, but it can present as a progressive subacute infection, evolving over several days.

Meningitis is characterized by fever, headache and meningism (i.e. neck stiffness on passive flexion), Kernig's sign (i.e. neck and back pain felt when the patient is in a supine position with the hip and knee flexed and subsequent extension of the knee is painful), and Brudzinski's sign (i.e. flexion of the neck results in spontaneous flexion of the hips and knees when the patient is in a supine position). There is nausea, vomiting, photophobia, progressive lethargy, stupor, or coma. Epileptic activity may develop, with seizures occurring in 40% which may be focal or generalized.

Complications are caused by the development of antibiotic resistance, cerebral oedema, subdural effusion or empyema, superior sagittal sinus thrombosis, hydrocephalus due to impaired cerebrospinal fluid (CSF) absorption and obstruction. Vasculitis, leading to vascular occlusion and infarction of the brain or spinal cord, may cause progressive cranial nerve lesions (particularly hearing loss) and systemic complications, including organ failure, pericardial effusion, polyarteritis, and limb infarction.

The commonest causes of bacterial meningitis, by age and risk factors, are:

- **Neonates** (<3 months): *E. coli*, group B *Streptococcus* and *Listeria monocytogenes*.
- **Infant and child** (>3 months): *Streptococcus pneumoniae* (i.e. pneumococcus), *Neisseria meningitides* (i.e meningococcus), and *Haemophilus influenzae*.
- **Adults** (healthy and immunocompetent): *Streptococcus pneumoniae*, *Neisseria meningitides*, and *Listeria monocytogenes* (usually in patients >50 years or pregnant women).

- **Associated with CSF leaks** (e.g. skull fracture, post-neurosurgery, shunts): *Staphylococcus epidermidis/aureus*, Gram-negatives (i.e. *Klebsiella, Proteus, Pseudomonas, E. coli, Serratia, Acinetobacter*), group A and group D streptococci, *Streptococcus pneumoniae*, and *H. influenzae*.
- **Immunosuppressed** (e.g. malignancy, alcohol, diabetes mellitus, septicaemia, UTI): *Listeria monocytogenes*, Gram-negatives, *Streptococcus pneumoniae*, group B *Streptococcus*, *Staphylococcus aureus*, and *Cryptococcus*.

Investigations

Imaging should be undertaken urgently to exclude mass lesions, hydrocephalus, or cerebral oedema which are contraindications to lumbar puncture. However, CSF examination should be undertaken whenever possible. In the absence of imaging, lumbar puncture should be avoided if there is impaired consciousness, focal neurological deficits, signs of shock or bleeding diathesis, purpuric or petechial rash, prolonged focal seizures, or signs of raised intracranial pressure or incipient herniation.

The CSF findings in different forms of meningitis are summarized in Table 7.3. Gram staining of the CSF is positive for meningococcus in <50% of patients with acute meningococcal meningitis. Blood cultures may be helpful but are unreliable. CSF tests may directly identify an organism and its nucleic acid or surface constituents by staining, culture, or capsular antigen detection. Polymerase chain reaction (PCR) is sensitive for *S. pneumoniae* and *N. meningitidis*.

Management

In severe meningitis, the first priority is to begin empirical antibiotic treatment, ideally after sending a blood culture. Benzylpenicillin should be commenced in any child suspected of having meningococcal meningitis before transfer to hospital. Otherwise, empirical therapy depends on the age and immune status of the patient and any other risk factors.

In the healthy, immunocompetent adult, treatment should be initiated with a third-generation cephalosporin, with the addition of ampicillin if *Listeria* infection is a possibility. If nosocomial infection is suspected (e.g. following surgery, trauma, or in the presence of a shunt), ceftazidine is

Table 7.3 Comparison of CSF findings in different forms of meningitis

	Normal	Acute bacterial	Viral meningitis	TB meningitis	Fungal meningitis
Appearance	Clear colourless	Turbid	Clear/opalescent	Clear/opalescent	Clear
Pressure	Normal	Increased	Normal or increased	Increased	Normal or increased
Cells	0–5/mm³	100–60,000/mm³	5–1,000/mm³	5–1,000/mm³	20–500/mm³
Polymorphs	None	>80%	< 50%	<50%	<50%
Glucose	>3.5 mmol/L (75% blood glucose)	Low (<40% blood glucose)	Normal	Low (<40% blood concentration)	Low (<80% blood concentration)
Protein	<0.4 g/L	>0.9 g/L (1–5 g/L)	0.4–0.9 g/L	>1 g/L (1–5 g/L)	>0.4 g/L (0.5–5 g/L)
Others		Gram stain positive <90% Culture positive <80% Blood culture positive <60%	Culture positive <50% PCR	ZN stain positive <10–80% Culture positive 50–80%	Gram stain negative Culture positive 25–50%

preferred. Vancomycin is also added to cover resistant *Staphylococcus*. If there is penicillin or cephalosporin allergy, chloramphenicol should be given with vancomycin.

Neisseria meningitidis (meningococcal meningitis)

Meningococcal meningitis is the most common cause of meningitis in children and young adults, with a mortality of approximately 10%. Isolated meningococcal meningitis (40%) carries a better prognosis than meningococcal septicaemia (10%) or a mixed picture (50%). Meningococcal septicaemia is associated with progressive vasomotor disturbance, culminating in profound hypotension, tachycardia, and a rising respiratory rate, indicating pulmonary oedema or raised intracranial pressure due to cerebral oedema. In Waterhouse–Friedrichsen syndrome, septicaemia is complicated by the development of bilateral haemorrhage into the adrenal glands. Disseminated intravascular coagulation (DIC) may also occur with a characteristic petechial rash that does not fade under pressure.

Management
- Immediate treatment with intravenous benzylpenicillin (2.4 g) should be commenced.
- Ceftriaxone (2 g IV 12-hourly for 14 days), cefotaxime (2 g IV 4–6-hourly for 14 days), or chloramphenicol (50 mg/kg IV 6-hourly) are alternatives if there is penicillin allergy.
- Septicaemic shock should be treated with appropriate volume replacement and, if necessary, elective intubation and mechanical ventilation.
- Patients may require inotropic support and correction of metabolic abnormalities.
- Coagulopathy and anaemia should also be appropriately treated.
- Meningococcal meningitis is a notifiable disease in the UK, and there is a high risk of family members developing the disease. All household close contacts should, therefore, be treated to eradicate nasopharyngeal carriage with rifampicin 600 mg bd or ciprofloxacin 750 mg once daily (see Chapter 6).

Streptococcus pneumoniae (pneumococcal meningitis)

Pneumococcal meningitis is the most common cause of meningitis in adults over the age of 18 years old, with a case fatality rate of about 20%. It is commonly due to local extension from otitis media, a paranasal source of infection, following a skull base fracture or sinus injury with dural tear.

Treatment is with benzylpenicillin (<2.4 g IV 4-hourly for 10–14 days, ceftriaxone or cefotaxime). If a penicillin-resistant pneumococcal infection is suspected, vancomycin (1 g IV 12-hourly for 14 days, with monitored blood levels) should be added. Adjuvant dexamethasone (10 mg 6-hourly intravenously for 4 days) improves the outcome and should be commenced before, or with, the first dose of antibiotics. Residual neurological sequelae are common and occur in >35% of patients (e.g. hydrocephalus, vasculitis, venous thrombosis, labyrinthitis, spinal cord involvement).

Listeria monocytogenes

Listeria monocytogenes is associated with contaminated food (e.g. soft cheese, unpasteurized milk, and occasionally raw meat). Predisposing factors include pregnancy, advanced age, or immunosuppression (e.g. malignancy, renal failure, organ transplantation, or steroid treatment). *Listeria* may cause meningitis, meningoencephalitis and seizures, or a brainstem encephalitis with cranial neuropathy, pyramidal and sensory signs.

Treatment is with ampicillin or penicillin for 3–4 weeks, although gentamicin (3–5 mg/kg/day in divided doses 8-hourly) is often added to enhance bactericidal activity.

Botulism

Botulism is caused by a highly potent neurotoxin, elaborated by *Clostridium botulinum*. The toxin is absorbed from the gastrointestinal tract and haematogenously disseminated before it binds irreversibly to the presynaptic membrane of peripheral neuromuscular and autonomic nerve junctions to inhibit acetylcholine release. Cure depends on the sprouting of new nerve terminals.

Characteristic features of botulism
Food-borne botulism has a mean incubation period of 2 days. Onset is with acute non-specific gastrointestinal symptoms (e.g. nausea, vomiting, anorexia, and abdominal pain).

There may be a descending flaccid paralysis. Cranial nerve deficits develop early, including blurred vision, diplopia, ptosis, and external ophthalmoplegia with mydriasis due to accommodation paresis. Facial weakness, dysarthria, dysphagia, and dysphonia also occur.

There is autonomic disturbance (e.g. dry mouth, unreactive pupils, paralytic ileus, gastric dilatation, bladder distension, orthostatic hypotension, and constipation), and ventilatory failure may develop.

Wound botulism has a longer incubation period, but the symptoms and signs are similar to food-borne botulism. This condition most commonly occurs as a result of subcutaneous injection (skin popping) of black tar heroin that has become contaminated with *Clostridium botulinum*, whilst being cut or diluted, prior to street sale.

C. botulinum may be isolated from the wound site, stool, or food, and the toxin is detected in serum, stool, and food by bioassay using mice. Nerve conduction studies are normal, but repetitive stimulation shows a decremental response at low rates and an incremental response at high rates. Needle EMG confirms small polyphasic motor units, and single-fibre studies show jitter and block.

Management
The following may be beneficial in botulism.
- Supportive care with admission to ITU, close bulbar and respiratory monitoring, and intubation and mechanical ventilation, if necessary.
- Attempt to remove unabsorbed food-borne botulinum toxin by inducing catharsis or enemas in the absence of ileus and if ingestion is recent.
- Antitoxin is helpful (particularly in type E) to eliminate circulating toxin but does not remove botulinum toxin that has entered the neuromuscular junctions. It should be administered as soon as possible, but there is a risk of allergic reactions with equine antitoxins, including urticaria and serum sickness.
- Wound treatment with debridement and antibiotic therapy, including penicillin, tetracyclines, metronidazole, or chloramphenicol.

Tetanus

Tetanus is caused by the neurotoxin tetanospasmin, elaborated by the anaerobic Gram-positive rod *Clostridium tetani*. The incubation period varies from a few days to several weeks. There is localized spasm and rigidity in the region of the wound, spreading to involve masseter muscles leading to trismus (i.e. lock jaw) and facial muscles (i.e. risus sardonicus). In addition:

- Localized stiffness develops near to the injury, with subsequent sustained rigidity of the axial muscles and involvement of the neck, back, and abdomen, and, in severe cases, reflex spasms and opisthotonus (hyperextension of the neck and spine).
- Paroxysmal muscle contractions occur in response to slight stimuli and, in severe cases, can be severe enough to cause limb fractures, tendon avulsion, and rhabdomyolysis. Respiratory muscle spasm may cause asphyxia, vocal cord obstruction, and aspiration due to the associated increase in bronchial secretions, hypersalivation, and dysphagia.
- Autonomic manifestations are common in severe tetanus, with profuse sweating, hypersalivation, and extreme hyperpyrexia. Fluctuations of blood pressure and heart rate are cardinal features, and these may be followed by arrhythmias and circulatory failure. There may be transient glycosuria. Excessive bronchial secretion, gastric stasis, diarrhoea, acute renal failure, and volume depletion also occur.
- The diagnosis is made on the basis of history of the spasms and examination. *Clostridium tetani* in a wound guides the diagnosis.

Treatment

Management in the ICU has resulted in a marked improvement in prognosis for patients with tetanus, but the mortality is still about 10%. Severe muscular rigidity may last for several weeks, with assisted ventilation being required for up to 3–4 weeks. Complete recovery is typical, although mild painful spasms can persist for months. Management involves:

- Eradication of the causative bacterium by debridement of the wound and antibiotics (e.g. metronidazole 500 mg 6-hourly for 7–10 days).
- Neutralization of any unbound toxin using equine or human antitoxin.
- Post-injury wound care.
- Supportive therapy during the acute phase includes nursing in a calm and quiet environment, cardiorespiratory monitoring, and management of fluid balance and nutrition. Muscle spasms are controlled with diazepam and midazolam, and neuromuscular blockade with vecuronium in mechanically ventilated patients.
- Prevention is achieved with vaccination, including primary childhood immunization programmes and boosters every 10 years.

Viral meningitis

Viruses cause an isolated aseptic meningitis, characterized by symptoms and signs of meningeal irritation with a CSF pleocytosis in the absence of bacterial, fungal, or parasitic infection.

Non-polio enteroviruses are, by far, the most common cause of viral meningitis and include Coxsackie and echovirus strains. Other agents are mumps, measles, herpes simplex virus 2, varicella-zoster virus, Epstein–Barr virus (EBV), cytomegalovirus (CMV), HHV6, arboviruses, and adenovirus.

Presentation is with a flu-like prodrome with pyrexia, sudden onset of intense headache, fever, and neck stiffness with photophobia, malaise, myalgia, and severe nausea and vomiting. A pruritic rash, pleurodynia (severe localised, pleuritic-type chest pain), or myocarditis may also be present.

The peripheral white cell count may be increased or decreased, and liver function may be abnormal. The CSF is clear and colourless, with normal to moderately elevated pressure, and the cell count may be <1,000 cells/mm^3 (usually <300) with mononuclear lymphocytes predominating, although polymorpholeucocytes may be present. Viral isolation is undertaken from the throat, urine, or stool, and viral antibody studies are possible in serum or CSF. Detection of viral RNA or DNA in the serum or CSF is undertaken using PCR.

Supportive care is usually adequate. Herpes virus meningitis can be treated with antiviral agents, including aciclovir, famciclovir, valaciclovir, ganciclovir, and foscarnet. Enterovirus meningitis includes the use of immune serum globulin, but the new antipicorna viral agent pleconaril may have an important role.

The prognosis in viral meningitis is good, with spontaneous recovery usually occurring within 1–2 weeks. However, there may be prolonged residual deficits in up to 5%, including malaise, fatigue, mild intellectual and language difficulties, seizures, isolated cranial nerve lesions, and optic neuritis.

Encephalitis

Encephalitis is acute infection of the parenchyma of the brain, usually caused by a virus, which results in a diffuse inflammatory process, often also involving the meninges.

Clinical features include fever (90%), seizures (common at presentation or early in the course), headache, pyrexia, behavioural and speech disturbances. Meningism suggests leptomeningeal irritation, and focal signs indicate parenchymal involvement (i.e. seizures and alteration of consciousness, progressing to stupor and coma). Abnormal movements are associated with lesions in the basal ganglia, and hypothermia follows involvement of the hypothalamus and pituitary.

The commonest causes of severe infectious encephalitis are herpes simplex virus I and II (HSV), varicella-zoster virus (VZV), Epstein–Barr virus (EBV), cytomegalovirus (CMV), human herpes viruses 6 and 7, enteroviruses (Coxsackie, echovirus, enterovirus 70 and 71, poliovirus), measles, mumps, rubella, parvovirus, adenovirus, influenza virus A and B, arbovirus, *Mycoplasma pneumoniae*, and HIV seroconversion.

Herpes simplex encephalitis is due to HSV1 in 90% of cases. Magnetic resonance imaging (MRI; T2W scans) shows high signal areas of unilateral focal oedema in the medial and inferior temporal lobes. The electroencephalogram (EEG) is characterized by periodic stereotyped, lateralized sharp and slow wave complexes. The CSF is clear and colourless, with a mild to moderate elevation in the protein (0.6–6 g/L), normal or mildly decreased glucose, and mononuclear pleocytosis (5–500/mm^3). PCR examination of the CSF is sensitive and specific for the detection of HSV DNA. It should be positive after about 5 days of infection but clears again after 14 days of illness. Brain biopsy is now rarely undertaken but may be considered if diagnostic uncertainty remains.

High-dose intravenous aciclovir (10–15 mg/kg body weight three times a day) reduces the mortality of herpes simplex encephalitis from 70% to 20%. It is also appropriate treatment for VZV-related CNS disease. Treatment is for 14–21 day or at least until the PCR has become negative. Occasionally, HSV may be resistant to aciclovir, and foscarnet is indicated. Seizures require specific treatment, and corticosteroids may be used if cerebral oedema develops. Intracranial pressure monitoring and surgical decompression may be necessary.

There is still significant morbidity, including severe memory impairment (up to 69%), personality/behavioural changes, dysphasia, and epilepsy. Early treatment is essential, particularly before the development of impairment of consciousness.

Late deterioration is usually the result of severe cerebral oedema, with diencephalic herniation or systemic complications, including generalized sepsis and aspiration. Progressive worsening of focal seizures may lead to status epilepticus. Aggressive treatment, including tracheal intubation and mechanical ventilation with appropriate sedation, should be instituted and seizures treated. Prolonged sedation or general anaesthesia may be necessary, and decompressive craniotomy has been undertaken to manage rapid brain swelling.

Other causes of infective encephalitis

- **Varicella-zoster (VZV).** Secondary reactivation leads to dermatomal shingles or disseminated herpes zoster. Neurological complications include a severe encephalitis, meningitis, myelitis, and cerebellar ataxia, occurring particularly in the immunosuppressed. Herpes zoster can be complicated by a vasculopathy affecting both small and large vessels which may cause infarction.
- **Cytomegalovirus (CMV)** is usually transient and asymptomatic, but it may cause encephalitis in the immunocompromised adult, particularly following organ transplant or in AIDS.
- **Epstein–Barr virus (EBV)** causes <5% of viral encephalitis and is associated with impaired level of consciousness, seizures, and focal deficits. Although recovery is usual, permanent deficit may occur, with residual chorea and cognitive impairment.

Cerebral malaria

Malaria (see also section on 'Malaria' in Chapter 6) is the most important parasitic disease of man, and it is estimated that >5% of the world population has been infected. Malaria is due to four parasitic protozoa of the genus *Plasmodium*, but only *falciparum* can cause severe generalized disease and, in particular, cerebral malaria.

The diagnosis is established by thick blood films with light microscopy, ensuring that large amounts of blood are available and a minimum of 100 fields are observed. A thin film assessment allows species recognition. Newer antigen tests are now available, based on recognition of the HRP-2 antigen of *falciparum*, and PCR techniques are specific and sensitive to *Plasmodium* but do not give an estimate of the parasite load.

Coma, occurring in patients with cerebral malaria, carries a mortality rate of up to 20% when appropriately treated and is invariably fatal if untreated. Complications include cerebral or dural venous thrombosis and cortical infarction.

Acute management of cerebral malaria involves supportive care, with appropriate attention to ventilation, fluid balance, renal and cardiac function, and seizures. *Plasmodium*

malariae, *ovale*, and *vivax* should be treated with a standard course of chloroquine over 48 hours. In severe cases, it may be necessary to treat with an intravenous infusion of chloroquine. Primaquine may be added to eradicate the exoerythrocytic forms and prevent relapses. Because chloroquine-resistant falciparum is widespread, treatment of mild infections is with oral quinine sulfate, followed by doxycycline or clindamycin to eradicate remaining asexual forms. Alternatives include mefloquine or co-artemether. Severe falciparum should be treated in intensive care with intravenous quinine sulfate or artesunate (see section on 'Malaria' in Chapter 6). Alternative treatments for falciparum or cerebral malaria include quinidine, and artemether.

Further reading

Britton WJ and Lockwood DN (2004). Leprosy. *Lancet*, **363**, 1209–19.

Centers for Disease Control and Prevention (2013). Treatment Guidelines. Treatment of Malaria (Guidelines For Clinicians). <http://www.cdc.gov/malaria/resources/pdf/clinicalguidance.pdf>.

Cherington M (1998). Clinical spectrum of botulism. *Muscle nerve*, **21**, 701–10.

Davies NWS, Sharief MK, Howard RS (1996). Infection-associated encephalopathies: their investigation, diagnosis, and treatment. *Journal of Neurology*, **253**, 833–45.

Davis LE and Greenlee JE (2003). Pneumococcal meningitis: antibiotics essential but insufficient. *Brain*, **126**, 1013–14.

Garcia HH, Evans CAW, Nash TE, *et al.* (2002). Current consensus guidelines for treatment of neurocysticercosis. *Clinical Microbiology Reviews*, **15**, 747–756.

Howard RS (2005). Poliomyelitis and the postpolio syndrome. *BMJ*, **330**, 1314–18.

Idro R, Jenkins NE, Newton CRJC (2005). Pathogenesis, clinical features, and neurological outcome of cerebral malaria. *Lancet Neurology*, **4**, 827–40.

National Institute for Health and Care Excellence (2010). Bacterial meningitis and meningococcal septicaemia: Management of bacterial meningitis and meningococcal septicaemia in children and young people younger than 16 years in primary and secondary care. NICE clinical guideline 102. <https://www.nice.org.uk/guidance/cg102>.

Rosenstein NE, Perkins BA, Stephens DS, Popvic T, Hughes JM (2001). Meningococcal disease. *New England Journal of Medicine*, **344**, 800–6.

Solomon T, Michael BD, Smith PE, *et al.* (2012). Management of suspected viral encephalitis in adults. Association of British Neurologists and British Infection Association National Guidelines. *Journal of Infection*, **64**, 347–373.

Thwaites GE (2002). The diagnosis and management of tuberculous meningitis. *Practical Neurology*, **5**, 250–61.

Thwaites G, Fisher M, Hemingway C, *et al.* (2009). British Infection Society guidelines for the diagnosis and treatment of tuberculosis of the central nervous system in adults and children. *Journal of Infection*, **59**, 167–187.

Van de Beek D, de Gans J, Tunkel AR, Wijdicks EFM (2006). Community-acquired bacterial meningitis in adults. *New England Journal of Medicine*, **354**, 44–53.

Demyelinating diseases

Multiple sclerosis

Multiple sclerosis (MS) is an inflammatory demyelinating disorder of the central nervous system (CNS).

Epidemiology

The prevalence of MS is $100-150/10^5$ population, with an annual incidence of new cases of $3.5-7/10^5$ population.

The incidence of multiple sclerosis worldwide tends to increase with increasing latitude.

Multiple sclerosis typically presents at 20–40 years of age.

Females are more susceptible than males by a factor of approximately 2:1.

Clinical course

Multiple sclerosis is characterized by lesions disseminated throughout the CNS, which may appear, disappear, or gradually worsen over time, and this is reflected in its clinical presentation and course. Presentation is variable, and the course and prognosis are unpredictable, although broad clinical categories of the disease are well recognized. Clinical disease activity in multiple sclerosis may manifest as relapses or insidious progression.

Clinically isolated syndrome. This is the first acute episode suggestive of CNS demyelination, and it may be the first presentation of multiple sclerosis. The average risk of developing multiple sclerosis, following a clinically isolated syndrome, is between 30% and 70%, although the risk increases with the length of follow-up. An abnormal MRI at first presentation has been consistently shown to confer a higher risk of conversion to multiple sclerosis.

- **Relapsing/remitting multiple sclerosis.** Approximately 85% of individuals present with an episode of acute or subacute neurological dysfunction, followed by relapses and remissions.
- **Secondary progressive multiple sclerosis.** Relapsing/remitting multiple sclerosis may evolve into a gradually progressive course, with accumulating irreversible neurological deficit and disability (i.e. secondary progressive multiple sclerosis). The proportion of people developing secondary progressive disease increases with length of follow-up.
- **Primary progressive multiple sclerosis.** This describes insidious disease progression from onset. It results in gradual accumulation of neurological deficit or disability, without relapse or remission. It accounts for approximately 10–15% of multiple sclerosis.
- **Benign multiple sclerosis** describes a disease course with accumulation of minimal or no disability at 10–15 years after disease onset.
- **Aggressive multiple sclerosis.** Rarely, an aggressive or malignant disease course may result from severe or frequent relapses, with little or no neurological recovery between episodes/relapses, or from rapid disease progression. However, aggressive disease is uncommon, and early death in multiple sclerosis is rare.

Natural history and prognosis

The natural history of multiple sclerosis is extremely variable. The spectrum of disease activity ranges from clinically asymptomatic demyelinating lesions, detected incidentally on imaging or at post-mortem, to an aggressive course with rapidly accumulating disability. The median time to reach a level of disability requiring assistance for walking is between 15 and 30 years. The age of onset does

not influence prognosis, and the rate of progression is similar in the primary and secondary progressive groups.

Factors affecting relapse activity include:

- **Infections.** Systemic infections may trigger a relapse or exacerbate existing symptoms of multiple sclerosis.
- **Pregnancy.** Relapse rate declines during pregnancy, especially in the third trimester, but increases during the first 3 months post-partum and then returns to pre-pregnancy rate.
- **Stress and vaccines.** These factors may trigger a relapse, but a causal association is not proven.

Clinical features

Multiple sclerosis can cause a wide variety of symptoms mirroring involvement of any part of the CNS. The spinal cord, optic nerves, and brainstem are the most commonly involved sites. The commonest clinical manifestations include:

- **Optic neuritis** presents with ocular pain and blurring of vision. The visual impairment may progress over a few days but not usually longer than 1–2 weeks. Colour vision and visual acuity are impaired, and a central scotoma may be detected. The optic disc may be normal, but swelling may be present, and pallor of the optic disc may develop later. A relative afferent pupillary defect is usually present.
- **Diplopia** is usually due to a sixth cranial nerve palsy (failure of abduction on the affected side) or an internuclear ophthalmoplegia (i.e. identified on conjugate contralateral gaze as impaired adduction on the side of the lesion and nystagmus of the abducting eye on the unaffected side).
- **Spinal cord syndrome.** Altered sensation in the lower limbs, spreading to the trunk and arms, with variable degrees of numbness and tingling.
- **Motor involvement.** Weakness is usually greater in the legs than the arms, and paraparesis is frequently asymmetrical. Spasticity may manifest as stiffness, clonus, or spasms.
- **Bladder and bowel disturbance.**
- **Cerebellar involvement** is evidenced by nystagmus, dysarthria, limb ataxia and intention tremor, and truncal ataxia.
- **Fatigue** is often worse during relapses, but disturbed sleep, drug therapy, and depression may also be contributory factors.
- **Heat sensitivity** may cause worsening motor and sensory symptoms.
- **Cognitive impairment** is usually mild in the early stages, but severe dementia may occur. Pain is common and is often due to myelopathy, spasticity, neuromuscular causes, or trigeminal neuralgia.
- **Lhermitte's symptom**, a brief electrical sensation, radiating down the back into the legs or arms, precipitated by neck flexion.

Diagnosis

Diagnosis depends on demonstrating CNS lesions disseminated in time and space:

- **Magnetic resonance imaging** (MRI). Plaques of white matter demyelination in multiple sclerosis are visualized on MRI. The characteristic locations for foci of demyelination occur in the periventricular region, corpus callosum, juxtacortical, brainstem, cerebellar white matter, and spinal cord. Gadolinium enhancement is invariable in new lesions in relapsing multiple sclerosis and last an average of 2–6 weeks.

- **Cerebrospinal fluid.** In clinically definite multiple sclerosis, intrathecally synthesized oligoclonal immunoglobulin G (IgG) bands are found in approximately 90% of patients. A parallel blood sample is required to demonstrate the intrathecal origin of bands. About two-fifths of patients have a mildly raised CSF white cell count (5–50 mononuclear cells/mm^3) and protein.
- **Evoked potentials**. Visual evoked potentials in MS may show a markedly delayed P100 wave of normal amplitude, which provides strong evidence for optic nerve demyelination.

Management

Acute relapse

Steroid therapy may accelerate the recovery from a relapse, although a long-term benefit has not been proven. Treatment is with intravenous methylprednisolone, 0.5–1 g/day, or high-dose oral methylprednisolone, 0.5–2 g/day, for 3–5 days.

Disease-modifying therapy

These therapies should be initiated and supervised by a neurologist.

- **Interferon-beta and glatiramer acetate.** All the interferon formulations and glatiramer acetate are licensed in the UK for ambulatory individuals with relapsing/remitting multiple sclerosis. Interferon-beta 1b is also licensed for secondary progressive multiple sclerosis with superimposed relapses. Treatment should be started and supervised by a consultant neurologist, after careful and informed discussion with the individual and, where available, with nurse specialist support.
- **Mitoxantrone.** Restricted to subjects with aggressive and rapidly progressing disease.
- **Natalizumab.** Licensed for individuals with rapidly evolving, severe relapsing/remitting disease, defined as at least two disabling relapses in 1 year.
- **New therapies.** Humanized monoclonal antibodies show great promise in the treatment of relapsing and remitting multiple sclerosis.

Symptomatic treatment

- **Fatigue.** Treatment is difficult and unsatisfactory. Treat underlying contributory factors, such as disturbed sleep patterns (e.g. nocturia, nocturnal spasms, depression). Fatigue management is the mainstay of treatment. Graded aerobic exercise programmes may be helpful. Drug therapy has included the use of amantadine, modafinil, 4-aminopyridine, and fluoxetine.
- **Spasticity.** Management incorporates education, physical therapy, drug therapy, and occasionally surgery. A multidisciplinary approach is required. Exacerbating factors, such as infection, constipation, pain, and pressure ulcers, should be reversed.

  Baclofen (e.g. 10 to >80 mg daily) is widely used to alleviate spasticity but limited by drowsiness and muscle weakness. Tizanidine (initially 2 mg daily, increased slowly, according to response, to a maximum of 24–36 mg daily in three divided doses) is also effective in reducing spasticity. It is not associated with an increase in weakness, but side effects include dizziness, drowsiness, dry mouth, fatigue, and hypotension. Dantrolene (muscle relaxant) acts peripherally and can be used as an adjunct to a centrally acting

drug but is limited by nausea, diarrhoea, weakness, fatigue, and hepatotoxicity. Benzodiazepines, such as diazepam and clonazepam, reduce muscle tone, but side effects include their sedative effects.

Locally administered agents, including intramuscular and intrathecal therapies, may be helpful. Intramuscular botulinum toxin may be used in the treatment of focal spasticity. For severe generalized spasticity, intrathecal administration of baclofen is an effective and well-tolerated treatment. However, adverse effects related to both the implanted device and the dosing are common and may rarely be life-threatening.

- **Weakness**. Treatment for weakness includes therapy-directed exercise programmes. Supportive measures include orthoses for focal weakness or specialist seating for postural weakness.
- **Ataxia.** Cerebellar ataxia is difficult to treat. Therapeutic options include physical therapy, drug therapy, and surgery, but all have limited efficacy. Physiotherapy and occupational therapy are first-line interventions and should address posture, seating, and aids to improve function and safety. Drug therapy is unrewarding. Stereotactic thalamotomy and thalamic electrostimulation are of benefit for tremor in very specific circumstances.
- **Bladder and bowel dysfunction.** In the bladder, this results from detrusor hyperreflexia and incomplete emptying. It is important to assess whether incomplete emptying is occurring before initiating treatment, as this may be exacerbated by drugs for detrusor instability. This is carried out by measuring the post-micturition residual by 'in-out' catheterization or simple ultrasound. If the residual is <100 mL, treatment is directed at detrusor hyperreflexia. This may be treated successfully with anticholinergic drugs (i.e. oxybutynin (2.5–5 mg three times daily), tolterodine (2 mg twice daily), and solifenacin).

  If the residual is >100 mL, techniques to manually empty the bladder should be used (e.g. clean intermittent self-catheterization).
- **Pain and paroxysmal symptoms.** Chronic pain is common and includes dysaesthetic extremity pain, painful leg spasms, and musculoskeletal back pain. Amitriptyline (10 mg daily), gabapentin (initial dose 300 mg, increasing in 300 mg steps to a maximum of 1.8 g daily), carbamazepine (100–200 mg three times daily), pregabalin, and other anticonvulsants may be used for dysaesthetic extremity pain. Painful leg spasms are best managed by treating the underlying spasticity.

  Musculoskeletal pain may result from abnormal posture and gait; physical therapy input is the first line of treatment, although anti-inflammatory drugs and other analgesics, electrical stimulation, and antidepressants may all have a role in treatment. Acute and paroxysmal neurogenic pain may be due to Lhermitte's symptom, tonic spasms, and trigeminal neuralgia. Carbamazepine and gabapentin may be effective for trigeminal neuralgia, and other anticonvulsants, tricyclic antidepressants, and misoprostol have been used.
- **Neurological rehabilitation.** Benefits gained from inpatient rehabilitation may be maintained for several months, but carry-over of benefits declines over time, reinforcing the need for continuity of care into the community. Physiotherapy alone improves mobility and well-being in multiple sclerosis, with similar effects seen for outpatient and home physiotherapy, although the benefit may only last a few weeks.

Neuromyelitis optica (Devic's disease)

Neuromyelitis optica (NMO) is an inflammatory demyelinating disease of the CNS which is now recognized as being immunologically and pathologically distinct from multiple sclerosis. The diagnosis is confirmed by finding NMO-IgG (aquaporin-4 Ab). The hallmark features of NMO are severe episodes of transverse myelitis and optic neuritis, without clinical involvement of other parts of the CNS. Acute attacks of NMO are often severe and necessitate early and aggressive immunomodulation. First-line treatment is high-dose intravenous corticosteroids, followed by maintenance oral steroids. The next line of treatment is plasma exchange or rituximab (a monoclonal antibody against the protein CD20, which is primarily found on the surface of immune system B cells).

Further reading

Association of British Neurologists (ABN) (2007, revised 2009). ABN guidelines for treatment of multiple sclerosis with β-interferon and glatiramer acetate. <http://www.theabn.org/abn/userfiles/file/ABN_MS_Guidelines_2009_Final(1).pdf>.

Clarke C, Howard R, Rossor M, Shorvon S (2009). Neurology—A Queen Square textbook. Wiley Blackwell, Oxford.

Cocco E, Marrosu MG (2014). The current role of mitoxantrone in the treatment of multiple sclerosis. Expert Review of Neurotherapeutics, 14, 607–16.

Coles AJ, Cox A, Le Page E, et al. (2006). The window of therapeutic opportunity in multiple sclerosis: evidence from monoclonal antibody therapy. Journal of Neurology, 253, 98–108.

Compston A, Confavreux C, Lassmann H, et al., eds. (2006). McAlpine's multiple sclerosis, 4th edn. Churchill Livingstone Elsevier, Philadelphia.

Department of Health (2005). The National Service Framework for long-term conditions. Department of Health, London. <https://www.gov.uk/government/publications/quality-standards-for-supporting-people-with-long-term-conditions>.

Kesselring J and Beer S (2005). Symptomatic therapy and neurorehabilitation in multiple sclerosis. Lancet Neurology, 4, 643–52.

Lassmann H, Bruck W, Lucchinetti CF (2007). The immunopathology of multiple sclerosis: an overview. Brain Pathology, 17, 210–18.

Miller D, Barkhof F, Montalban X, Thompson A, Filippi M (2005). Clinically isolated syndromes suggestive of multiple sclerosis. Part I. Natural history, pathogenesis, diagnosis, and prognosis. Lancet Neurology, 4, 281–8.

National Institute for Health and Care Excellence (2002). Beta interferon and glatiramer acetate for the treatment of multiple sclerosis. NICE technology appraisal guidance 32. <http://www.nice.org.uk/guidance/TA32>.

National Institute for Health and Care Excellence. (2007). Natalizumab for the treatment of adults with highly active relapsing–remitting multiple sclerosis. NICE technology appraisal guidance 127. <http://www.nice.org.uk/guidance/TA127>

National Institute for Health and Care Excellence (2014). Multiple sclerosis: management of multiple sclerosis in primary and secondary care. NICE clinical guideline 186. <https://www.nice.org.uk/guidance/cg186>.

Polman CH, O'Connor PW, Havrdova E, et al. (2006). A randomized, placebo-controlled trial of natalizumab for relapsing multiple sclerosis. New England Journal of Medicine, 354, 899–910.

Sweetland J, Riazi A, Cajo SJ, Playford ED (2007). Vocational rehabilitation services for people with multiple sclerosis: what patients want from clinicians and employers. Multiple Sclerosis, 13, 1183–9.

Turner-Stokes L, Sykes N, Silber E, Khatri A, Sutton L, Young E (2007). From diagnosis to death: exploring the interface between neurology and palliative care in managing people with long-term neurological conditions. Clinical Medicine, 7, 129–36.

Wingerchuk DM, Lennon VA, Pittock SJ, Lucchinetti CF, Weinshenker BG (2006). Revised diagnostic criteria for neuromyelitis optica. Neurology, 66, 1485–9.

Neuromuscular disease

Acute neuromuscular weakness may be caused by disease of muscle, neuromuscular junction, peripheral nerve, roots, or the CNS. The distinction between these sites of pathology can largely be made on clinical grounds, with supportive investigations where necessary (see Table 7.4).

Peripheral nerve

Diseases of the peripheral nerve can be genetic or acquired. The acquired neuropathies may be primary or secondary to other conditions. They may be symmetrical or multifocal and patchy. In addition, they can be predominantly sensory, motor, or, more commonly, mixed sensorimotor. They may be subdivided into axonal forms, in which degeneration of the nerve body develops distal to nerve damage, or demyelinating forms, in which the myelin sheath is denuded and conduction velocity is slowed. The pattern and rate of development often provides important clues to the aetiology, with inflammatory, vasculitic, and infective neuropathies developing over days or weeks.

Inflammatory neuropathies

These are characterized by inflammatory infiltration of the peripheral nerves, associated with destruction of myelin and/or axons.

Guillain–Barré syndrome (GBS) and its variants
Patients with GBS present with progressive ascending sensorimotor paralysis and areflexia affecting one or more limbs and reaching a nadir in <4 weeks. Pain, cranial nerve involvement, and autonomic disturbances, with arrhythmias and labile blood pressure, are common. Papilloedema may occur. Some patients progress to tetraparesis and require ventilation in as little as 48 hours. It is the commonest cause of acute generalized flaccid paralysis, with an incidence of ~1.7 per 100,000 of the population annually.

Pathophysiology
It is an acute inflammatory, demyelinating polyradiculoneuropathy, often occurring a few weeks after surgery, flu vaccination, or minor respiratory (45%) or gastrointestinal (20%) infections. Implicated organisms include *Campylobacter jejuni* (20–45%), CMV (10–20%), Epstein–Barr virus, and mycoplasma. Cross-reactivity between the immune response to an organism and peripheral nerves is the likely mechanism.

Investigations
Investigation excludes other causes of weakness (e.g. hypokalaemia). The CSF is acellular (<10 cells/mm^3). Nerve conduction studies show patchy proximal and distal demyelination with slowed motor nerve conduction velocities. Axonal changes without evidence of slowing are found in acute motor axonal neuropathy (AMAN) and acute motor and sensory axonal neuropathy (AMSAN), and these may indicate a worse prognosis. Hyponatraemia occurs in a proportion of patients caused by both the syndrome of inappropriate antidiuretic hormone (SIADH) and an excess of atrial natriuretic factor. Serology indicating a preceding *Campylobacter* infection is a poor prognostic feature.

Variants of GBS include:
- **AMAN/AMSAN** which form a spectrum of axonal GBS.
- **Fisher syndrome:** the triad of ataxia, areflexia, and ophthalmoplegia. This is the most common variant, accounting for between one-third and a half of atypical cases. It seldom progresses to requiring supportive or therapeutic treatment, although a Fisher/GBS overlap syndrome may progress to extensive neuropathic weakness.

Management
Respiratory monitoring is essential. Forced vital capacity (FVC) is recorded immediately on presentation and at least every 4 hours thereafter until the patient has begun to recover. Elective endotracheal intubation should be considered if the FVC falls below 15 mL/kg, with early conversion to a tracheostomy for comfort and prevention of complications.

An ECG should be recorded. Cardiac monitoring should be undertaken in all patients for arrhythmia and blood pressure fluctuations. Persistent or severe bradyarrhythmias may require the insertion of a pacemaker. Anticoagulation (low molecular weight heparin), pressure stockings, and calf massage devices, to prevent deep venous thrombosis (DVT), should be used routinely.

Physiotherapy should start immediately, with hand and foot splints to prevent contractures. Detection and treatment of issues related to pain, emotion, continence, nutrition, and mouth care are crucial.

Treatment
Specific treatments include:
- Plasma exchange may speed recovery if given early (<7 days). Typically, four to five 3 L exchanges are given over the course of 10 days.
- High-dose (intravenous) immunoglobulin therapy (IVIG) 2 g/kg over 5 days is as effective as plasma exchange and more likely to be completed, as it has fewer complications.
- Steroids are of no benefit and are not indicated in the treatment of GBS, except possibly for radicular (root)

Table 7.4 Differential diagnosis and investigation of acute neuromuscular diseases

Differential diagnosis	Investigations
Toxic (e.g. heavy metal)	**Blood tests:** haematology, biochemistry (e.g. K$^+$), serology, toxicology, ACR assays, autoimmune screen (e.g. ANA)
Biochemical (e.g. hypokalaemia)	
Metabolic (e.g. porphyria)	**Urine tests** (e.g. porphyrins)
Nutritional (e.g. neurotoxic fish)	**Microbiology/virology**
Connective tissue disease (e.g. SLE)	**CXR** (e.g. lung cancer)
Systemic disease (e.g. lymphoma)	**CSF fluid examination**
Infective (e.g. polio, tetanus, diphtheria, botulism, HIV)	**Edrophonium test** (e.g. myasthenia gravis)
Neuromuscular diseases (e.g. myasthenia gravis)	**Electromyography** (e.g. nerve conduction studies)
Malignancy-related Lambert–Eaton myasthenic syndrome (i.e. small cell lung cancer, breast)	**Nerve biopsies**

pain and in chronic inflammatory demyelinating polyradiculoneuropathy (CIDP; see section on chronic inflammatory neuropathies).

- Pain may be severe and is treated with combinations of high-dose anticonvulsants/analgesics (e.g. gabapentin, pregabalin, carbamazepine) and tricyclic antidepressants or selective serotonin reuptake inhibitors (SSRIs), in conjunction with opiates (e.g. fentanyl).

Outcome
About 30% require mechanical ventilation (MV) for a few days to >1 year. Neurological deficit usually peaks at ~14–21 days, followed by gradual recovery over weeks or months. Poor prognostic factors include advanced age, rapid onset, axonal degeneration, and ventilator dependence at the nadir of the illness. Even with the best medical care, 5–8% of patients die, and about one-third are left with significant disability.

Chronic inflammatory neuropathies
The chronic inflammatory neuropathies include the idiopathic and those associated with other diseases, e.g. the paraproteinaemias and the vasculitides.

- ***Chronic inflammatory demyelinating polyradiculoneuropathy*** (CIDP) is an acquired demyelinating neuropathy with progressive or relapsing proximal and distal weakness of the limbs, sensory loss, and/or cranial nerve involvement, reaching a nadir in more than 8 weeks, with absent or reduced reflexes in all limbs. Treatment for CIDP includes both oral steroids and IVIG or plasma exchange.
- ***Multifocal motor neuropathy with conduction block*** is a progressive immune-mediated demyelinating motor neuropathy which begins asymmetrically in the upper limbs. Weakness develops in the distribution of individual nerves with patchy loss of reflexes. Wasting and fasciculation occur later and may mimic motor neurone disease.

Other neuropathies
- ***Vasculitic neuropathies*** are uncommon, and, although often severe, they are treatable. Sequential progressive, painful sensorimotor neuropathies develop over days or weeks. The lower limb nerves tend to be affected first. Progression to confluence occurs, especially in polyarteritis nodosa (PAN) and Wegener's granulomatosis. Systemic involvement may present as fever, weight loss, myalgia, fatigue, and night sweats. The vasculitides may be treated with oral steroids or pulsed methylprednisolone. More aggressive treatment with other immunosuppressant agents may be necessary.
- ***Diabetes*** is the most common cause of neuropathy worldwide. The risk of neuropathy increases with duration of disease, poor control, height, male sex, and with other cardiovascular risk factors.
  - Distal symmetric sensory neuropathy is the most common of the diabetic neuropathies. It presents with a slowly progressive 'glove and stocking' sensory loss which may be painful. Small fibre symptoms may also be present. With severe neuropathy, neuropathic Charcot joints may be present.
  - Autonomic neuropathy is common and leads to postural hypotension, impotence, constipation, nocturnal diarrhoea, and fixed high heart rates.
- ***Toxic neuropathies.*** Most toxins cause axonal neuropathies, some of which have motor or sensory predominance. Heavy metal poisoning (e.g. lead, mercury, and thallium) may require specific treatment (see Chapters 9

and 18). Prolonged supportive therapy in ITU may be required (e.g. botulism, tetanus).

- ***Vitamin deficiency neuropathies*** are axonal (e.g. Vitamin B1 and B12 deficiencies). Some are associated with pain or ataxia and many with CNS involvement. Replacement of deficient vitamins by supplementation or providing an alternative metabolite can halt, and sometimes improve, the neuropathy.
- ***Critical illness polyneuropathy*** is an acute sensorimotor axonal neuropathy, which develops in the setting of systemic inflammatory response syndrome (SIRS), septic encephalopathy, and/or multiorgan failure. It is characterized by delayed weaning, severe distal flaccid wasting and weakness, areflexia, and sensory impairment in patients who are able to cooperate with the examination. Persisting weakness and sensory deficits are common in long-term survivors of protracted critical illness, even up to 4 years after discharge. No specific treatment of the neuropathy is known.

Focal and compressive neuropathies

Focal neuropathies are the result of local damage to individual nerve trunks. They may be single or multiple. Damage occurs most frequently because of nerve compression, usually as the nerve passes through a tissue tunnel (bone, ligament, aponeurosis, muscle) or against an underlying surface at an exposed site (e.g. the peroneal nerve as it passes around the head of the fibula). Compression may also occur with prolonged abnormal postures at atypical sites (e.g. radial paralysis in the 'Saturday night palsy' due to falling asleep with an arm hanging over the arm rest of a chair, compressing the radial nerve at the spiral groove). Diabetes, hereditary neuropathy with pressure palsies (HNPP), and alcohol overuse may render nerves more susceptible to the effects of otherwise non-damaging pressure. The most common focal neuropathies affect the median (carpal tunnel syndrome), ulnar, and common peroneal nerves.

Acute brachial neuritis
Acute brachial neuritis is characterized by acute deep aching pain affecting the neck, shoulder, and upper arm in a diffuse pattern. This may last from hours to 2 weeks or more and is followed by focal wasting and weakness, most commonly in the distribution of nerves originating from the upper plexus (deltoid, serratus anterior, supraspinatus and infraspinatus, and biceps). Sensory symptoms occur in about one-third of patients and signs in about two-thirds, most often sensory loss in the territory of the axillary nerve.

The cause is not known. It may be associated with immunization, infection, trauma, surgery, pregnancy, and childbirth, intravenous heroin usage, radiotherapy, and vasculitis. Steroids do not alter the outcome, and analgesics are necessary. About 90% of patients with a typical brachial neuritis will recover in 3 years.

Inherited neuropathies

The inherited neuropathies can be divided into those in which the neuropathy is the sole, or primary, part of the disease and those where the neuropathy is part of a more widespread neurological or multisystem disorder. The first group includes Charcot–Marie–Tooth (CMT) disease, also called hereditary motor sensory neuropathies (HMSN). The second group is a large, varied group of disorders that usually also involve the central nervous system (e.g. leukodystrophies, spinocerebellar ataxias) or those where systems, other than the nervous system, are significantly involved (e.g. mitochondrial disorders, porphyrias).

Charcot–Marie–Tooth and related disorders are a group of neuropathies that are clinically and genetically heterogeneous. They are characterized by distal muscle wasting and weakness, reduced reflexes, impaired distal sensation, and variable foot deformity. Neurophysiologically, they are associated with a motor and sensory neuropathy.

There is a wide variation in the age of onset and disease severity, depending on the underlying genetic defect. Classifications differentiate between CMT, which has both motor and sensory involvement, hereditary sensory autonomic neuropathy (HSAN), which has more sensory and autonomic features and less motor neuropathy, and distal hereditary motor neuropathy (dHMN), which only causes a motor neuropathy.

CMT is either demyelinating (CMT1) or axonal (CMT2), although intermediate forms occur.

- **CMT1.** About 90% of cases of CMT1 are either autosomal dominant or X-linked. The commonest cause CMT1A is associated with duplication on chromosome 17p of the peripheral myelin protein 22 gene (*PMP22*). CMT1B is less common and is caused by mutations in the myelin protein zero gene (*MPZ*). The X-linked form of CMT1 is caused by mutations in the gene which codes for the protein connexin 32. Hereditary neuropathy, with liability to pressure palsies (HNPP), is an autosomal dominant condition, in which patients present with episodic recurrent pressure palsies.
- **CMT2** is caused by a wide variety of genes, and the true prevalence is not known. An adult presenting with a long-standing mild axonal neuropathy, without an obvious family history and where an acquired case has not been identified, may have a CMT2.
- **Hereditary sensory autonomic neuropathy** is much rarer than CMT and is characterized by prominent sensory and autonomic neuropathy and less motor involvement.
- **Familial amyloid polyneuropathies** are dominantly inherited small-fibre neuropathies, associated with deposition of a fibrillar beta-pleated protein in the extracellular space of many organs.

Anterior horn cell diseases

Motor nerve diseases principally affect the anterior horn cell body and are usually neurodegenerative (e.g. motor neurone disease) or hereditary (e.g. spinal muscular atrophy).

Motor neurone disease

Motor neurone disease (MND) is a progressive neuronal degenerative disease that leads to severe muscle wasting, disability, and death. The annual incidence is 1.5–2/100,000 population and the prevalence approximately 4–8/100,000 population.

There is considerable variability in presentation, clinical course, and prognosis. The condition is divided into several different clinical subtypes.

- **Amyotrophic lateral sclerosis** (ALS) is the most common. It is characterized by upper and lower motor neurone involvement of the bulbar, upper, and lower limb territories. ALS causes progressive, often distal, muscle wasting, fasciculations, cramps, weakness, spasticity, brisk reflexes, and extensor plantar responses.

Bulbar involvement is characterized by dysarthria, tongue wasting, fasciculations, slow movement, absent jaw jerk, and dysphagia. Pseudobulbar involvement is associated with dysarthria, dysphagia, brisk jaw jerk, spastic 'stiff' tongue, increased gag-reflex, and pathological emotional lability in which there is excessive uncontrolled laughter or crying.

- **Progressive bulbar palsy** (PBP) presents with predominantly, or exclusively, bulbar weakness.
- **Primary lateral sclerosis** (PLS) in which there is exclusively upper motor neurone involvement.
- **Progressive muscular atrophy** (PMA) involves only lower motor neurones.

Investigation
Neurophysiology is essential in establishing the diagnosis. Needle EMG shows neurogenic changes of denervation and re-innervation.

Management
The management of MND involves the coordination of multidisciplinary care. Important aspects include:

- Riluzole (50 mg twice daily) is the only drug which has been shown to prolong survival in MND.
- Respiratory support, in particular, non-invasive ventilation, can provide symptomatic relief and increase life expectancy.
- Sialorrhoea is generally managed with anticholinergic agents, including atropine (0.4 mg 4–6-hourly) or amitriptyline (10–125 mg daily) taken orally, hyoscine (scopolamine) transdermally, or glycopyrronium bromide subcutaneously.
- Percutaneous endoscopic (or radiological) gastrostomy (PEG) should be considered for patients with severe swallowing difficulties, as an alternative or supplementary route for nutrition, hydration, and medication.
- Progressive dysarthria can occur, and speech becomes severely impaired or lost within a short time. Communication can be maintained with a variety of aids and devices, ranging from pointing boards to computerized speech synthesizers.
- Musculoskeletal pain is common and may respond to antispasticity agents, NSAIDs, and stronger analgesics, including opiates. Skin pressure pain, caused by immobility, may also occur.
- Cramps are usually nocturnal and may respond to quinine sulfate, diazepam, carbamazepine, or phenytoin.
- Stiffness is caused by spasticity and muscle or joint contracture. Tizanidine and baclofen may ease the pain of spasticity.
- Emotional lability can be distressing for patient and carers and may be relieved by amitriptyline or an SSRI.
- Palliative care should be introduced before the terminal stages of MND. Home care teams and day centres offer respite care to aid home carers. Close liaison between the family physician, community healthcare and hospice teams, and palliative care physicians is essential.
- Terminal care aims to alleviate psychological distress and the symptoms of bulbar weakness and respiratory failure.

Prognosis
The natural history of motor neurone disease is variable, and occasional prolonged periods of stability may occur. Patients with PBP have the worst prognosis because of the risk of aspiration, with a median survival of 2–2.5 years. In ALS, the mean disease duration is 3–4 years. Over 50% of patients die within 3 years and 90% within 5 years of the first symptom.

Spinal muscular atrophy

Spinal muscular atrophy (SMA) is a group of predominantly autosomal recessive disorders, characterized by the degeneration of anterior horn cells and bulbar nuclei.

- **SMA type I** (Werdnig–Hoffmann disease) develops in infancy, with failure to achieve a sitting posture and death by 2 years old.
- **SMA type II** (intermediate SMA) is associated with the development of muscle weakness after 6 months of age and manifests as delay in motor development. Independent sitting is achieved but not walking.
- **SMA type III** (juvenile SMA; Kugelberg–Welander disease) becomes symptomatic in early childhood (>18 months), and patients usually achieve mobility. Fasciculation, cramps, and a fine tremor are common, and there is proximal limb weakness and wasting which is more prominent in the lower limbs.
- **SMA type IV** (adult-onset SMA).
- **Several rare clinical variants** can occur, affecting the bulbar, limb girdle, musculature, and diaphragm, with variable patterns of inheritance.

Kennedy disease (X-linked bulbospinal neuronopathy)

The clinical pattern of Kennedy disease resembles MND but progresses more slowly, and respiratory muscle involvement is less common. It is caused by a CAG trinucleotide repeat expansion in the androgen receptor gene.

Disorders of the neuromuscular junction

Functional or structural abnormalities of the neuromuscular junction (NMJ) interfere with the transmission of neural impulses from motor nerves to muscles.

Myasthenia gravis

Myasthenia gravis (MG) is an autoimmune disorder, characterized by skeletal muscle fatigability and weakness. It is caused by antibodies directed against the post-synaptic acetylcholine receptors (AChR) in the muscle membrane.

About 20–25% of patients with clinical autoimmune MG are AChR antibody-negative. IgG autoantibodies to muscle-specific kinase (MuSK) have been identified in 70% of patients with ocular and generalized seronegative MG.

It affects $5/10^5$ population (M:F ratio 1:2). The thymus gland is abnormal in 75%, mainly thymic hyperplasia in young women and benign thymoma (~10%) in elderly males. MG is also associated with autoimmune disorders (e.g. hyperthyroidism, SLE), drugs (e.g. penicillamine), and thymic tumours.

Clinical features

MG occurs most commonly in women in the second and third decade of life. Men are predominantly affected in the sixth and seventh decades. MG usually develops insidiously over weeks. Presentation is with fatigable weakness in the ocular, cranial nerve, limb, or truncal musculature which recovers with rest. Extraocular muscles are most frequently involved, trunk muscles least. Ptosis and diplopia are the commonest presenting features, and MG is confined to the extraocular muscles in 20%. Bulbar muscle involvement causes dysphagia, aspiration, and a snarling smile (myasthenic facies). Selective diaphragm weakness is rare.

Drugs may precipitate or exacerbate myasthenic weakness. These include aminoglycoside antibiotics, beta-blockers, quinine, and penicillamine. The anti-MuSK phenotype causes predominantly facial, bulbar, and respiratory muscle weakness and often occurs in young female patients.

Diagnostic tests

Electrophysiological studies show the characteristic decline in muscle action potentials to repetitive stimulation at a rate of 3 Hz. AChR antibodies are detected in approximately 75% of patients with generalized myasthenia and 50% with pure ocular myasthenia. Anti-striated muscle antibodies are present in approximately 90% with concurrent thymoma. CXR and CT scans exclude thymoma.

The edrophonium (Tensilon®) test is diagnostic. Edrophonium prevents the breakdown of acetylcholine by acetylcholinesterase. Increased acetylcholine temporarily restores neuromuscular transmission, abolishing weakness, ptosis, and diplopia. However, AChR stimulation may cause autonomic side effects (e.g. sweating, bradycardia), requiring treatment with atropine. Initially, a test dose of edrophonium (2 mg) is injected, followed by a further 8 mg if the side effects are not excessive. Improved strength within 1 min, lasting several minutes, supports the diagnosis. Facilities for intubation must be available because excess acetylcholine inhibits neuromuscular transmission and may precipitate a cholinergic crisis (e.g. apnoea, paralysis, bulbar palsy, excessive secretions, colic).

Management

Supportive therapy involves monitoring respiratory function in patients with dyspnoea or difficulty swallowing. Assess swallowing in dysphagic patients, and start thromboembolic prophylaxis if immobile.

Specific treatments may be symptomatic (e.g. anticholinesterases), disease-modifying (e.g. immunosuppression with steroids, immunosuppressant drugs, immunoglobulins, or plasma exchange), and/or surgical (e.g. thymectomy).

- **Anticholinesterase drugs** (e.g. pyridostigmine; starting dose of 30 mg 8-hourly, maintenance 60–90 mg up to 4-hourly). Slowly increase the dose to achieve optimal symptomatic relief. Excessive therapy, in an attempt to abolish all weakness, may result in a cholinergic crisis. Anticholinergics are used to control muscarinic side effects (e.g. salivation, colic, diarrhoea).
- **Corticosteroids** (e.g. prednisolone starting <60 mg/day, with maintenance doses varying, according to response): are effective in improving weakness and establishing remission. Their use is limited by considerable toxicity, and they should be weaned to the lowest dosage possible to prevent glucocorticoid side effects.
- **Immunosuppressants.** Azathioprine (2.5 mg/kg daily) suppresses the disease and reduces the dosage of prednisolone required to maintain remission. Other immunosuppressant agents used in MG include mycophenolate, ciclosporin, cyclophosphamide, and rituximab.
- **Plasma exchange** produces valuable short-lived (~4 weeks), but marked, improvements in severe myasthenic weakness and may aid ventilator weaning. Unfortunately, difficulties and complications with venous access, biochemical derangements, and high overhead costs limit its use.
- **High-dose (intravenous) immunoglobulin therapy** (IVIG) is similar in efficacy to plasma exchange and is valuable in producing short-term improvement in myasthenic crisis.
- **Thymectomy** for non-thymomatous autoimmune MG increases the probability of remission or improvement and reduces mortality, compared to medical therapy alone.

Myasthenic crisis indicates the development of ventilatory failure, often precipitated by bronchopneumonia, systemic sepsis, medication, surgery, or inadequate treatment, which is often related to a rapid tapering of the steroid dosage. Rarely, cholinergic crisis or the commencement of high-dose corticosteroids is to blame.

Urgent elective tracheal intubation and ventilation should be undertaken when the vital capacity falls below 15 mL/kg (i.e. VC ~1L). It may be necessary to admit the patient to ITU, intubate and ventilate, and withdraw all anticholinergic medication.

Other causes of abnormal neuromuscular transmission
- Snake venoms, tick paralysis, and toxic agents, including organophosphates, may affect neuromuscular transmission.
- Organophosphates (OPs) are used as nerve agents but are also widely employed as pesticides; exposure may be occupational, food-borne, or as a consequence of suicide attempts. Acute exposure results in cholinergic crisis. Respiratory muscle weakness is resistant to atropine, and intubation is required.

Lambert–Eaton myasthenic syndrome (LEMS)
This is a rare disorder caused by impaired release of ACh by the presynaptic terminal of the NMJ. It is associated with underlying malignancy or autoimmune disease. LEMS is characterized by weakness and fatigue. Reflexes are reduced or absent, but, after a short period of sustained effort, they become brisker, showing the phenomenon of post-tetanic potentiation.

Treatment
Any underlying carcinoma must be appropriately addressed. Successful treatment often leads to improvement in LEMS. Pyridostigmine has a mild effect in enhancing neuromuscular transmission, but most patients require 3-4 diaminopyridine which increases quantal acetylcholine release. The response to plasma exchange and IVIG is less reliable than in MG. Prednisolone, azathioprine, and ciclosporin are all effective in LEMS.

Diseases of muscle
Inherited muscle diseases
The clinical practice and understanding of genetic muscle disease is changing rapidly as a direct result of the wealth of recent molecular genetic discoveries.

Muscular dystrophies
Many genes causing different muscular dystrophies have been discovered in recent years.
- **Xp21 dystrophies (dystrophinopathies).** Duchenne muscular dystrophy, an X-linked recessive condition, is an aggressive and lethal dystrophy affecting boys, in which there is a severe reduction in the amount of the dystrophin protein in muscle. Improved ventilatory support increases the quality of life and life expectancy.

  Becker muscular dystrophy is also an X-linked recessive disease, which presents as a limb girdle pattern of muscle weakness, with pseudohypertrophy of calf muscles. Cardiomyopathy is an important complication; occasionally, severe dilated cardiomyopathy may be the presenting feature.

  Diagnosis may be confirmed by genetic testing, but a muscle biopsy with dystrophin studies can be required. Genetic counselling, as for an X-linked recessive diseases, is important, but one-third of dystrophinopathy cases are new mutations without family history.
- **Limb girdle muscular dystrophy** (LGMD) patients have the common feature of a limb girdle pattern of muscular weakness without facial involvement. An array of proteins with different functions has been shown to cause the LGMD phenotype. The propensity to develop cardiomyopathy or respiratory muscle failure varies considerably between different forms.
- **Facioscapulohumeral muscular dystrophy** (FSHD) is an autosomal dominant condition in which the development of facial muscle weakness is followed by periscapular and humeral muscle involvement. Later in the disease course, lower limb weakness, particularly anterior tibial, and abdominal wall weakness may occur. The severity is variable, ranging from isolated asymmetrical scapular winging through to pronounced early-onset weakness and scoliosis, making the patient wheelchair-bound.
- **Oculopharyngeal muscular dystrophy** (OPMD) is an uncommon disorder, characterized by late-onset pharyngeal muscle weakness and ophthalmoplegia.
- **Emery–Dreifuss muscular dystrophy** is characterized by a scapulohumeroperoneal pattern of muscular weakness. It is often associated with strikingly thin muscles. Contractures of the cervical extensor muscles, as well as the biceps and long finger flexor tendons, are common. Cardiac conduction defects are also frequent, and cardiac screening is important.
- **Myotonic dystrophy** is an autosomal dominant multisystem disorder that affects men and women equally. Neuromuscular symptoms include facial weakness, mild distal myopathy, and myotonia. Additional features are cataracts, endocrine disturbance (e.g. diabetes mellitus), cardiomyopathy, hair loss (e.g. frontal balding), cognitive slowing, daytime somnolence, bowel dysmotility, and respiratory muscle weakness.
- **Congenital myopathies** are a group of uncommon muscle disorders, defined on the basis of distinctive morphological muscle biopsy features. They include central core disease and nemaline myopathy.

Skeletal muscle channelopathies
- **Human periodic paralyses and myotonias** are conditions in which there is a disturbance in skeletal muscle fibre membrane excitability. Periodic paralyses are related to changes in serum potassium levels during attacks, and patients experience focal or generalized episodes of muscle weakness of variable duration. In myotonia, patients experience muscle stiffness because of a failure of normal electrical inactivation of activated muscle.

Metabolic muscle disease
- **Mitochondrial respiratory chain diseases** have a varying phenotype which can include progressive external ophthalmoplegia, isolated proximal myopathy, or, less commonly, distal myopathy. Myopathy may occur in isolation or in combination with CNS involvement in mitochondrial encephalomyopathy with lactic acidosis and strokes (MELAS) and mitochondrial encephalomyopathy with ragged red fibres (MERRF).
- **Glycogenoses and lipid storage disorders.** Other metabolic disorders in muscle include defects in glucose metabolism (e.g. glycogen storage disorders) and defects in fat metabolism (e.g. lipid storage disorders). Patients with these autosomal recessive disorders generally develop muscle pain on exertion. Myoglobinuria, and sometimes fulminant rhabdomyolysis, may occur.

Acquired muscle disease
Inflammatory myopathies are the most commonly encountered acquired muscle diseases; three subtypes exist:

- **Dermatomyositis** (DM) includes inflammation of muscle and skin. It is a humorally mediated autoimmune disorder, in which the pathology is a microvasculopathy.

DM typically produces a subacute, progressive, proximal, and symmetrical weakness, affecting the lower limbs more than the arms. CK is usually raised. There is often some myalgia but not severe pain. The extraocular and facial muscles are typically spared, but dysphagia may be a problem in severe or advanced cases, while neuromuscular respiratory compromise is also well recognized. The classic skin lesion is the 'heliotrope' erythematous rash of the face (especially the eyelids) and upper trunk. DM may lead to calcinosis within affected tissues. There is a 20% association with malignancy, most commonly with adenocarcinoma and gynaecological tumours.

The prognosis of DM is worse in those with pulmonary or cardiac complications, underlying malignancy, arthritis, hypergammaglobulinaemia, or in acute or febrile presentations.

- **Polymyositis** (PM) is characterized by a progressive, proximal, and symmetrical weakness without the skin lesions. It is very rare in those under 20 years old and typically occurs in middle or later life. Although it can be rapidly progressive, the most frequent presentation is with slowly progressive weakness. Myalgia is common but rarely severe. Distal and facial weakness is rare, but respiratory muscle involvement can occur.
- **Inclusion body myositis** (IBM). Sporadic inclusion body myositis is more frequent than DM or PM. Typically, IBM occurs late in life. The onset of IBM is insidious and usually slower than seen with PM or DM. IBM causes a distinctive pattern of wasting and weakness, involving the quadriceps and deep finger flexors. Falls may occur relatively early because of buckling of the knees. Dysphagia occurs in 10–30%.

Treatment
Treatment of idiopathic inflammatory myopathies remains uncertain. No beneficial effect of treatment has been shown in IBM, although individual patients do show a response to steroids. DM and PM respond to treatment with steroids but often require the use of a second-line immunosuppressant, such as azathioprine, mycophenolate, or methotrexate.

Other forms of inflammatory myopathies

- **Systemic sclerosis** occurs in conjunction with a DM-like picture in approximately 10% of cases. Similarly, 5–10% of people with systemic lupus erythematosus (SLE) have a condition similar to PM.
- **Sjögren's syndrome** is occasionally seen, with features similar to either DM or IBM.
- **Common infections** (e.g. Coxsackie, EBV, CMV, influenza) have all been associated with acute and chronic muscle inflammation. A definite causative link has been established for the retroviruses HIV and human T lymphocyte virus (HTLV-1) and myositis. At seroconversion, HIV can lead to a polymyositis that can be explosive enough to provoke myoglobulinuria and which is steroid-responsive.
- **Lyme disease**, in addition to its more frequent CNS and nerve involvement, can unusually lead to myositis; this may be either a localized painful swelling or a rarer generalized dermatomyositis-like picture.

- **Granulomatous myopathies** present as a slowly evolving proximal weakness, possibly with dysphagia. The serum CK is typically elevated, and muscle biopsy demonstrates focal non-caseating granulomas. The differential includes sarcoidosis, autoimmune conditions (rheumatoid arthritis, mixed connective tissue disease, Wegener's disease, or in association with myasthenia gravis and thymoma) and some infections (fungal, mycobacterial, protozoal).

Myopathies associated with malignancy

Weakness may simply accompany tumour-induced cachexia, but cancers can cause a number of other muscle disorders. Dermatomyositis is associated with a range of malignancies (e.g. ovary, lung, gastrointestinal, non-Hodgkin's lymphoma). An aggressive necrotizing myopathy is rarely seen in older patients with cancer (e.g. lung, gastrointestinal, adenocarcinoma, breast). Steroids and treatment of the underlying tumour may help to arrest symptoms.

Endocrine myopathies

- **Hypothyroidism** frequently causes non-specific fatigue, myalgia and cramps, and a raised CK. Proximal symmetrical weakness can develop. Hyperthyroidism, when severe, is often associated with distal muscle wasting and weakness which may be acute and profound, mimicking MND.
- **Cushing's syndrome** leads to steroid myopathy, while Addison's disease (whether primary or iatrogenic) typically causes myalgia, cramps, and fatigue. Inadequate circulating levels of corticosteroids may lead to proximal weakness, which can lead to respiratory difficulty.
- **Parathyroid.** Both inadequate and excessive levels of parathyroid hormone may lead to a mild progressive proximal myopathy.
- **Acromegaly.** Untreated, excess growth hormone will cause a proximal weakness, sometimes with muscle hypertrophy and with an elevated CK.

Drugs and myopathy

Many drugs may cause a myopathy; the severity varies from an asymptomatic raised CK to profound weakness with rhabdomyolysis. Drugs may also worsen an existing muscle disease or, alternatively, unmask one that was previously hidden.

- **Statin myopathy.** There is an eightfold risk of myopathy in those taking statins, raised to 42-fold if a fibrate is taken concurrently. The risk of statin-induced myopathy is dose-dependent but higher in the elderly or those with diabetes, hypothyroidism, or concurrent renal or liver disease. The most common problem is of an asymptomatic elevation of CK, and the most frequent symptoms are of myalgia and cramps. Stopping the statin usually leads to improvement within a few weeks, but myalgia and raised CK may persist. Severe myopathy can leave permanent sequelae.
- **Steroid myopathy** is an insidious proximal weakness, especially of the quadriceps muscles. The incidence is highest with dexamethasone, betamethasone, triamcinolone, and high-dose prednisolone.

Rhabdomyolysis

Rhabdomyolysis is the breakdown of striated muscle fibres that leads to the release of muscle enzymes into the circulation. Myoglobinuria leads to a brownish discoloration of the urine, and acute renal failure may develop. It usually results from muscle injury, resulting from trauma or other external causes (e.g. medication or intoxication), but may also develop if there is an underlying muscle disorder.

Management is treatment of the underlying disorder, correction of fluid and electrolyte abnormalities, and prevention of renal failure (see Chapter 11). The development of compartment syndrome may require fasciotomy.

Neuromuscular respiratory failure

Respiratory insufficiency may develop during the course of many neurological disorders. It occurs most commonly as a consequence of neuromuscular weakness but may also accompany disturbances of brainstem function or interruption of descending respiratory pathways. Previously unsuspected respiratory insufficiency may present as failure to wean from elective perioperative mechanical ventilation.

Clinical presentation

Respiratory insufficiency may develop insidiously. There may be exertional dyspnoea, nocturnal hypoventilation, or sleep apnoea. Symptoms include insomnia, daytime hypersomnolence and lethargy, morning headaches, reduced mental concentration, depression, anxiety, or irritability. Patients with progressive diaphragm weakness develop orthopnoea which may prevent the patient lying flat. Nocturnal orthopnoea is usually severe and can mimic paroxysmal nocturnal dyspnoea. Diaphragmatic weakness or paralysis causes paradoxical movement of the abdominal wall, with inspiratory indrawing of the lower lateral rib margin when the patient is supine or near supine. As the condition progresses, the full picture of respiratory failure is present, and sudden unexpected death may then occur.

Investigations

Investigations in progressive neuromuscular disease should include:

- **Vital capacity** (VC) which gradually falls because of respiratory muscle weakness and/or fatigue and reduced chest wall and lung compliance due to microatelectasis and restriction of chest wall movement. Diaphragmatic weakness is associated with a marked fall (greater than one third) in VC when sitting or lying.

- **Arterial blood gases** are often virtually normal during the early stages of neurological respiratory insufficiency, even when significant nocturnal hypoventilation is occurring. As the condition progresses, daytime $PaCO_2$ rises due to increasing alveolar hypoventilation.

- **Oximetry** is the measurement of choice to detect periodic sleep apnoea.

Management

Patients with acute neurological diseases affecting the respiratory muscles (e.g. Guillain–Barré syndrome) are nursed in an intensive care unit and require conventional mechanical intermittent positive pressure ventilation (IPPV). If the underlying disease is readily reversible within a short period, IPPV can be delivered via a tracheal tube.

However, in the majority of cases, prolonged respiratory support is needed until adequate respiratory muscle function returns, and IPPV is best delivered via a tracheostomy which affords greater patient comfort, easier and more effective tracheobronchial suction, and results in less tracheal trauma.

As respiratory muscle function improves, the patient is gradually weaned from mechanical ventilation, using a variety of weaning techniques. In contrast, patients with chronic neuromuscular disease are often managed at home, with the choice of various methods of assisted ventilation including non-invasive positive pressure ventilation (NIV) (see 'Respiratory practical procedures' in Chapter 19).

Further reading

Auer-Grumbach M, Mauko B, Auer-Grumbach P, *et al.* (2006). Molecular genetics of hereditary sensory neuropathies. *NeuroMolecular Medicine*, **8**, 147–58.

Engel AG, Franzini-Armstrong C, eds. (2004). *Myology*, 3rd edn, pp. 1535–677. McGraw Hill, New York.

European Federation of Neurological Societies (2005). Guideline on management of chronic inflammatory demyelinating polyradiculoneuropathy. Report of a joint task force of the European Federation of Neurological Societies and the Peripheral Nerve Society. *Journal of the Peripheral Nervous System*, **10**, 220–8.

Guarantors of Brain (2000). *Aids to the examination of the peripheral nervous system*, 4th edn. WB Saunders, London.

Howard RS and Orrell RW (2002). Management of motor neurone disease. *Postgraduate Medical Journal*, **78**, 736–41.

Karparti G, Hilton-Jones D, Griggs RC (2001). *Disorders of voluntary muscle*. Cambridge University Press, Cambridge.

Lauria G (2005). Small fibre neuropathies. *Current Opinion in Neurology*, **18**, 591–7.

Leigh PN, Abrahams S, Al-Chalabi A, *et al.* (2003). The management of motor neurone disease. *Journal of Neurology, Neurosurgery & Psychiatry*, **74** (Suppl IV), 32–47.

Mastaglia FL (2006). Drug-induced myopathies. *Practical Neurology*, **6**, 4–13.

Newsom-Davis J and Beeson D (2001). Myasthenia gravis and myasthenic syndromes, autoimmune and genetic disorders. In G Karpati, D Hilton-Jones, R Griggs, eds. *Disorders of voluntary muscles*, 7th edn, pp. 660–75. Cambridge University Press, Cambridge.

National Institute for Health and Care Excellence (2010). Motor neurone disease: The use of non-invasive ventilation in the management of motor neurone disease. NICE clinical guideline 105. <https://www.nice.org.uk/guidance/cg105>.

National Institute for Health and Care Excellence (2016). Assessment and management of motor neurone disease. <https://www.nice.org.uk/guidance/indevelopment/gid-cgwave0680>. Due Feb 2016.

National Institute for Health and Care Excellence (2013). Neuropathic pain – pharmacological management: The pharmacological management of neuropathic pain in adults in non-specialist settings. NICE clinical guideline 173. <https://www.nice.org.uk/guidance/cg173>.

Schaublin GA, Michet J, Dyck PJ, Burns TM (2005). An update on the classification and treatment of vasculitic neuropathy. *Lancet Neurology*, **4**, 853–65.

Movement disorders (disorders of the extrapyramidal system)

Movement disorders are described as:
- **Akinetic rigid** where there is too little movement, as in the bradykinesia of Parkinson's disease.
- **Dyskinetic** where there is too much movement, as in the chorea of Huntington's disease. The dyskinesias are tremor, chorea, myoclonus, tics, and dystonia.

These are clinical descriptors, and patients may have more than one abnormal movement type in any one disease or syndrome; akinesia, tremor, and dystonia are seen together in Parkinson's disease. Similarly, each of these movement disorders may be a feature of a number of different diseases and conditions; chorea is seen in Huntington's disease, Sydenham's chorea, and may be an adverse effect of medication, such as phenytoin.

When a pathological substrate is identified for these movement disorders, it typically involves the basal ganglia; these comprise the caudate and putamen which together are called the striatum, the pallidum, substantia nigra, and subthalamic nucleus. These nuclei form closed and open circuits which project to the thalamus and onto the cortex which, in turn, projects back to the striatum. Patients with pure extrapyramidal disorders typically have normal power, sensation, and coordination.

When assessing a patient with movement disorder, it is useful to describe each abnormal movement in terms of what the movement looks like, when it is present (on action, at rest, on stimulation), its anatomical distribution, its age of, and the rapidity of onset, and then look for additional features and signs (Are there cerebellar signs? Is cognition normal?) before trying to formulate a differential diagnosis.

Akinetic rigid syndromes

Idiopathic Parkinson's disease is by far the commonest of the akinetic rigid syndromes, but there are important differential diagnoses which include drug-induced parkinsonism (and, in its most severe form, the neuroleptic malignant syndrome), vascular parkinsonism, post-encephalitic parkinsonism, and the so-called Parkinson's plus syndromes—progressive supranuclear palsy (PSP), multiple system atrophy (MSA), and corticobasal degeneration (CBD).

Idiopathic Parkinson's disease
Epidemiology
About 120,000 people in the UK have Parkinson's disease. It affects 2% of the over 80s but can present in early adult life. Most general practitioners will only have 2–3 patients with Parkinson's disease on their list. Young-onset Parkinson's disease is described as presenting in patients under 40 years old. A number of genes have been identified as causing Parkinson's disease, but the majority of cases are idiopathic and are likely to have genetic and environmental triggers.

Clinical features and diagnosis
There is no diagnostic test for Parkinson's disease. The diagnosis is clinical and is based on the presence of the classical clinical features, bradykinesia (obligatory), rigidity, and an asymmetric resting tremor (the latter two not being essential for the diagnosis). True bradykinesia describes the decremental amplitude of a repetitive motor task rather than just slowness of movement.

A pill-rolling tremor of 4–6 Hz is the presenting symptom in over half of patients. It may be re-emergent on posture, and there may, in addition, be a jaw, face, tongue, or leg tremor. Rigidity describes increased tone through the whole range of movement (compared to spasticity).

Patients with idiopathic Parkinson's disease do not fall early in the course of their disease and can often tandem-walk (toe to heel walking) at presentation. However, as the disease progresses, postural and gait impairment becomes a prominent feature. With advancing disease, patients exhibit freezing (getting stuck going through doorways) and choreiform dyskinesia. These features are often the consequence of sustained levodopa therapy (~4 years), and patients change rapidly from stages with good response to medication and few symptoms ('on' state), to phases with no response to medication and important motor symptoms ('off' state).

The levodopa-induced dyskinesias (e.g. chorea and dystonia; less commonly tics, myoclonus, stereotypy, or hemiballismus) are a major challenge in the late management of Parkinson's disease. They are classified into peak-dose dyskinesias which tend to occur early in the disease progression, when the antiparkinsonian effects of levodopa are maximal and the patient is 'on' and mobile. With longer duration of levodopa treatment the dyskinetic phase may expand to the whole 'on' period (termed square-wave dyskinesia) with the severity varying little throughout. Diphasic dyskinesia is less common and occurs at the beginning and end of the dosing period (as levodopa concentration rises and falls) and often presents in the legs as chorea and dystonia. The 'on-off' effect, which occurs when the levodopa dose behaves in an unpredictable way, describes the sudden onset and cessation of dyskinesia, like a light switch being turned on and off. Even during the 'off' state, brief episodes of dyskinesia may be provoked by stress and this 'off' dystonia is frequently painful and may present as leg cramps at night.

Patients in the later stages of Parkinson's disease can appear very different in terms of mood and mobility between the, 'on' and 'off' state. This can be difficult for carers and medical staff to understand and induces comments, such as 'she can walk when she wants to'. In the off state, patients may feel mentally bleak and despairing and may call out that they feel like they are dying or that they wish to die, only to rapidly recover ('jubilant thaws') to a euthymic state as the drugs start to work again.

Non-motor features
Non-motor features are becoming increasingly recognized as a major cause of morbidity in Parkinson's disease.
- **Constipation** is almost universal and can result in impaction and obstruction.
- **Urinary frequency and urgency** is secondary to detrusor hyperreflexia but is aggravated by bradykinesia. Concomitant prostate disease is common in the elderly.
- **Postural hypotension** may be due to autonomic failure and is aggravated by dopaminergic medication.
- **Cognitive dysfunction** is common, with the incidence of overt dementia increasing with patient age and patient age of onset. Parkinson's disease dementia is present in up to 80% of patients over the age of 80 years. Typical features include attentional and visuospatial deficits and fluctuating confusion. The MMSE is a poor measure of cognition in basal ganglia disorders, as it does not test frontal lobe function; it can be enhanced by asking the patient to draw a clock face and testing letter and category verbal fluency.

- **Anxiety depression** is very common; one study reported that restoring dopaminergic tone was as effective as antidepressants in the treatment of this.
- **Pain** is common and can be related to 'off' dystonia.
- **Sleep disturbance** is very common and has multiple causal factors, including restless legs, REM sleep behaviour disorder (shouting and fighting in sleep), problems related to turning 'off', including an inability to turn over, 'off' psychosis, painful dystonia, and being woken by nocturia.
- **Visual illusions and hallucinations** are a common cause of care giver distress but are frequently benign and not frightening to the patient.

Many of these non-motor symptoms are due to the underlying disease process, but some are aggravated by the treatments given for the motor disorder, and most are worsened by intercurrent illness or the disorientating effects of a new environment.

Treatments
- **Levodopa** (initially 125–500 mg daily) remains the mainstay of treatment for Parkinson's disease. It crosses the blood–brain barrier and is taken up into the substantia nigra and other neurones where it is converted to dopamine before being released into the synapse. It is combined with a dopa decarboxylase inhibitor to prevent its conversion to dopamine in the periphery. Co-careldopa (Sinemet®) or co-beneldopa (Madopar®) both have a number of different strengths and slow-release preparations. It is important to continue the correct preparation when patients are admitted to hospital and that these medicines are given at the right time and on time (which may be as often as 1–2-hourly). Patients admitted for surgery should continue to be given their oral medication and should not be left off their drugs because of a nil-by-mouth order.
  - **Duodopa®** is a gel preparation of levodopa which is delivered as a continuous infusion via jejunostomy. It has a role in the management of patients with dopa-induced severe dyskinesia and 'on'-'off' symptoms who are unsuitable for deep brain stimulation.
- **Stalevo®** is the combination of Sinemet® with entacapone (Comtess®) a COMT (catechol methyltransferase) inhibitor. Entacapone (200 mg) prolongs the plasma half-life of Sinemet® and reduces 'off' time. Its most common serious side effect is colitis.
- **Dopamine agonists** act on post-synaptic dopamine receptors and do not have the complex conversion steps of levodopa. Apomorphine (e.g. typical dose 3–30 mg daily by subcutaneous injection, given as 1 to 10 injections; maximum single dose 10 mg, maximum daily dose 100 mg) and the dopamine agonists ropinirole, pramipexole, and the rotigotine patch are non-ergot compounds and, therefore, are thought not to carry the risk of fibrosis (i.e. pulmonary, retroperitoneal, pericardial) and valvular heart disease, as reported with the ergot derivatives bromocriptine, cabergoline, lisuride, and pergolide.

The rotigotine patch and apomorphine have the advantage of having a non-enteral delivery route. Rotigotine has an increasing role in the palliative care of Parkinson's disease patients. The majority of inpatients with Parkinson's disease should be given their standard doses of medication, via an NG tube if necessary, on time, and at the right dose.

The dopamine agonists are associated with a number of serious side effects, including behavioural changes, such as hypersexuality and pathological gambling (impulse control disorder, a class of psychiatric disorders characterized by impulsivity).
- **Monoamine oxidase B (MAO-b) inhibitors** selegiline and rasagiline block the breakdown of dopamine to homovallinic acid intracerebrally.
- **Antimuscarinic (anticholinergic) drugs**, including orphenadrine (150–400 mg in divided doses), benzatropine (initially 0.5–1 mg nocte, increasing to a 1–4 mg maintenance dose daily in a single or divided dose), and procyclidine (7.5–30 mg daily in three divided doses), may reduce tremor but have little effect on the other symptoms of Parkinson's disease. They are poorly tolerated and frequently cause confusion in the elderly.
- **Amantadine** (initially 100 mg daily, increasing to 100 mg twice daily) has a number of different modes of action. It can be useful for reducing drug-induced dyskinesia and sometimes helps to reduce freezing.
- **Cholinesterase inhibitors** (e.g. rivastigmine) are increasingly used in the management of Parkinson's disease dementia (which is associated with a cholinergic deficit). They can worsen tremor.

Surgical treatments

Functional neurosurgery with deep brain stimulation has been used to treat Parkinson's disease for more than 20 years. Thalamic stimulation is effective in the management of severe Parkinson's disease and essential tremor. Internal pallidal stimulation is effective in the management of dyskinesia. The most common target currently in use is the subthalamic nucleus. In animal models this nucleus was shown to be overactive in Parkinson's disease, and high-frequency stimulation blocks this. Subthalamic deep brain stimulation improves dopa-responsive 'off' symptoms and allows for a reduction in dopa therapy which, in turn, may alleviate the dyskinesias. Speech and swallowing problems and mood disturbance are recognized side effects and are more common with bilateral stimulation.

Fetal cell striatal transplants and intrastriatal delivery of growth factors have been under investigation for a number of years, with variable results and reported side effects.

Cautions

Patients with Parkinson's disease and Lewy body dementia should never be given neuroleptic medication, as this will aggravate their akinesia and may induce a neuroleptic malignant syndrome

Prognosis

Before the discovery of levodopa in the 1960s, patients with Parkinson's disease had a relentless disease progression to akinesia and death over 10 years but with symptomatic treatments most patients continue to lead an active life for many years and have a near-normal life expectancy.

DaT SPECT is a nuclear imaging technique which is used to visualize the concentration of dopamine transporters in the basal ganglia. This is a surrogate measure of the integrity of substantia nigra pars compacta neurones.

DaT scans can be used to differentiate Parkinson's disease from essential tremor and drug-induced parkinsonism but cannot be used to make a diagnosis of idiopathic Parkinson's disease from the other Parkinson's plus syndromes.

Other akinetic rigid syndromes

Drug-induced Parkinson's disease

Dopamine receptor-blocking drugs, used to treat psychosis, nausea, and vertigo, can induce a parkinsonian state. Even the atypical neuroleptics olanzapine and risperidone induce extrapyramidal side effects and these drugs should not be given to patients with idiopathic Parkinson's disease or Lewy body disease. Clozapine does not induce parkinsonism but can cause neutropenia, a potentially life-threatening side effect, and is not widely used in the UK. Other drugs which induce parkinsonism include sodium valproate.

Encephalitis lethargica

Occasional sporadic cases occur and present subacutely with parkinsonism, behavioural disturbance, particularly compulsions and dystonias, such as oculogyric crises which are not seen in idiopathic Parkinson's disease.

Multiple system atrophy

Multiple system atrophy (MSA) is an akinetic rigid syndrome presenting with rigidity (with or without tremor and slow movement) resembling Parkinson's disease but characterized by cytoplasmic glial inclusions (due to accumulation of a protein, alpha synuclein) in the basal ganglia, brainstem, and cerebellum. As many as 10% of patients thought to have Parkinson's disease actually have MSA at autopsy. The course is rapidly progressive over 5–10 years without remissions. It may present with cerebellar ataxia (MSA-C; previously known as sporadic olivopontocerebellar atrophy (OPCA)), a severe progressive autonomic syndrome (MSA-A; previously known as Shy Drager syndrome) with postural hypotension, erectile dysfunction and urinary incontinence, or a Parkinsonism poorly responsive to levodopa (MSA-P; previously known as striatonigral degeneration).

In the later stages of the disease, the symptoms and signs converge so that many patients have a combination of these features, with additional pyramidal signs and symptoms. Cognition and behaviour are usually relatively unaffected. There may be respiratory stridor, sighing, REM sleep behaviour disorder, and sleep apnoea. Fixed antecollis, hypophonia, and a jerky side-to-side finger tremor are characteristic. Marked autonomic disturbance with severe postural hypotension may require fludrocortisone and midodrine as well as other interventions, such as raising the head of the bed and wearing support stockings.

Progressive supranuclear palsy

Patients with progressive supranuclear palsy (PSP) have a syndrome of akinesia, axial rigidity, and early falls; patients typically fall early in the course of the disease and backwards, in contrast to Parkinson's disease patients who fall late and tend to fall forwards. Pseudobulbar speech and swallowing difficulties, with emotional lability and frontal lobe cognitive impairment, are common.

The characteristic eye movement disorder consists of early impairment of vertical saccades, followed by restricted downgaze, with progression to impairment of smooth pursuit and a horizontal gaze palsy. Patients complain that they cannot look down at their dinner plate and they cannot scan to read a book. The impairment is of voluntary eye movements (supranuclear), and the brainstem reflex eye movements are normal on performing the doll's head manoeuvre (itself difficult to perform because of the marked axial rigidity). PSP is a tauopathy and microsopic features include tau-positive tangles and tufted astrocytes.

Vascular parkinsonism

A lacunar state in the basal ganglia or extensive small-vessel disease in the deep white matter can present with a parkinsonism which is poorly responsive to levodopa therapy. It is frequently symmetrical, with no tremor, an upright, rather than a stooped stance with marked retropulsion and a small-stepping gait.

The dyskinesias

Tremor

Tremor is characterized as rest (e.g. Parkinson's disease), postural (e.g. physiological, essential, or neuropathic (e.g. IgM gammopathy)), action or terminal (e.g. dystonia), and intention (e.g. cerebellar). Exaggerated physiological tremor is a postural tremor, commonly caused by thyrotoxicosis, alcohol, caffeine, and beta agonists.

Essential tremor is common. It is slower than physiological tremor at 8–12 Hz with a symmetrical postural vertical tremor, affecting the arms and later sometimes the head, legs, and voice. There should be no extrapyramidal rigidity or bradykinesia. A family history is present in up to half of patients, and a beneficial response to small doses of alcohol is characteristic. In a small number of affected individuals it is very disabling. Beta-blockers, primidone, gabapentin, and topiramate may be useful as symptomatic treatments. Weighted wrist bands and aids for daily living, such as cups with lids and kettle tippers, can be useful. Thalamic deep brain stimulation is valuable in severe cases.

Chorea

Chorea describes fidgety, writhing, flitting, fragmented movements, involving different body parts.

Acute and subacute onset of chorea may be:

- Drug-induced (e.g. neuroleptics, alcohol, phenytoin).
- Paraneoplastic or immune-mediated (e.g. anti-voltage-gated calcium channel antibodies, SLE, antiphospholipid antibody syndrome).
- Metabolic (e.g. hypernatraemia, hypoparathyroidism).
- Endocrine (e.g. thyrotoxicosis).
- Haematological (e.g. polycythaemia rubra vera).
- Structural (e.g. stroke, tumour, trauma, infection in the subthalamic nucleus).
- Post-infectious (i.e. commonly streptococcal-induced, as in Sydenham's chorea, chorea gravidarum, and chorea induced by the oral contraceptive pill).

Huntington's disease (HD) is the most common cause of chorea, both inherited and sporadic. There are a number of other rare inherited Huntington's disease look-alikes which should be sought in patients with a positive family history who are found not to carry the Huntington's disease gene mutation. Huntington's disease is an autosomal dominant inherited CAG (trinucleotide) repeat disorder which commonly presents in mid-adult life and which is slowly progressive, resulting in death over 10–20 years.

The clinical features include movement disorder (e.g. chorea, dystonia, tics), frontostriatal dementia, and psychiatric disturbance. It should be noted that patients who are mute or who have severe dysarthria may have relatively preserved cognition and capacity.

There are, as yet, no treatments which delay the onset or progression of the disease. For disabling chorea, patients are prescribed low doses of tetrabenazine, risperidone, olanzapine, or sulpiride. There are a variety of effective supportive interventions and symptomatic treatments and therapies. The UK Huntington's Disease Association employs regional care advisors to help support patients and families.

Tics

Tics are described as repetitive and stereotyped brief, rapid involuntary movements and vocalizations. They are suppressible through force of will by the patient but with an urge to let the movement happen and an inner tension, followed by a rebound exacerbation of the tic. Simple motor tics are common in children, with eye blinking and sniffing, and these usually disappear. In Gilles de la Tourette's syndrome, there are simple and complex (e.g. touching, etc.) multiple motor tics, including vocalizations. In addition to coughs, grunts, and barks, patients exhibit echolalia (meaningless repetition of speech), echopraxia (imitation of movements), and palilalia (involuntary repetition of words, phrases, or sentences). A majority of patients have psychiatric or behavioural problems, including obsessive–compulsive behaviour/disorder (OCD) and attention deficit disorder.

Symptomatic treatment for disabling tics includes risperidone, aripiprazole, and sulpiride and, for OCD, may include cognitive behavioural therapy (CBT) and or selective serotonin reuptake inhibitors (SSRI; e.g. sertraline, fluoxetine). Botulinum toxin injections into the vocal cords have been used in the management of disabling vocal tics.

Myoclonus

Myoclonus describes sudden, brief involuntary electric shock-like movements.

It is characterized as:

- Focal, multifocal, or generalized.
- Spontaneous, action, or reflex (triggered by a stimulus).
- Cortical, subcortical, or spinal.
- Physiological (hiccough and hypnic), essential (myoclonus dystonia), epileptic, or symptomatic.

Multifocal and generalized myoclonus is seen in a wide variety of neurological conditions: neurodegenerative (Alzheimer's disease, prion), Huntington's disease (HD), and dentatorubral-pallidoluysian atrophy (DRPLA), and is a common feature of metabolic disorders (e.g. uraemia, hyponatraemia, hepatic failure, hypoglycaemia, non-ketotic hyperglycaemia).

Epileptic myoclonus is a seizure type seen in the idiopathic generalized epilepsies and may be symptomatic of the neurodegenerative progressive myoclonic epilepsies. Postanoxic myoclonus (action) can be the main residual pathological feature following cerebral hypoxia.

Focal myoclonus is confined to a particular body part or segment and can arise from the cortex (epilepsia partialis continua), the brainstem (palatal), and spinal cord.

Dystonia

Dystonia is a term used to describe sustained involuntary (or spasmodic) co-contraction of agonist and antagonist muscles which leads to abnormal postures. Dystonia is seen in a wide spectrum of diseases and syndromes which vary greatly in their severity, from blepharospasm and writer's cramp (task-specific dystonia) to primary idiopathic torsion dystonia. Patients may exhibit a 'sensory trick' or *geste antagoniste*; this is commonly seen in patients with torticollis, whereby they might touch a finger to the jaw and the dystonia temporarily abates.

Dystonia is divided into primary dystonia, in which dystonia (and tremor) is the only feature, the dystonia-plus syndromes (dopa-responsive dystonia and myoclonus dystonia), secondary dystonia (symptomatic and heredodegenerative), and paroxysmal.

Secondary or symptomatic dystonia can result from manganese poisoning, cerebral palsy, cerebral anoxia, previous encephalitis, neuroleptic or structural lesions, e.g. stroke.

The most important heredodegenerative cause is Wilson's disease, a disorder of copper metabolism, as early recognition and treatment prevent progression.

Patients sometimes respond to levodopa, anticholinergics, baclofen, tetrabenazine, and clonazepam. Botulinum toxin is an effective symptomatic treatment for focal dystonia, and functional neurosurgery with stereotactic pallidotomy or deep brain stimulation can be an effective treatment for generalized dystonia, especially in children.

Further reading

Bates G, Harper PS, Jones L, eds. (2002). *Huntington's disease*, 3rd edn. Oxford University Press, Oxford.

Chaudhuri KR, Healy D, Schapira AH (2006). Non-motor symptoms of Parkinson's disease: diagnosis and management. *Lancet Neurology*, **5**, 235–45.

Cure PSP. <http://www.psp.org/>.

Multiple System Atrophy guide. <http://multiplesystematrophy.info/The%20Sarah%20Matheson%20Trust.pdf>.

National Institute for Health and Clinical Excellence (2006). Parkinson's disease: diagnosis and management in primary and secondary care . NICE clinical guideline 35. <http://www.nice.org.uk/CG035>.

National Institute of Neurological Disorders and Stroke. <http://www.ninds.nih.gov/>.

OMIM. <http://www.ncbi.nlm.nih.gov/omim/>.

Parkinson's UK. <http://www.parkinsons.org.uk/>.

PSP Association. <http://www.pspeur.org/>.

Quinn N, Bhatia K, Brown P, et al. (2009). Movement disorders. In C Clarke, R Howard, M Rossor, S Shorvon, eds. *Neurology: A Queen Square textbook*, pp. 159–87. Blackwell Publishing, Oxford.

Rosenblatt A, Ranen NG, Nance MA, Paulsen JS (1999). *A physician's guide to the management of Huntington's disease*, 2nd edn. Huntington's Disease Society of America, New York. <http://www.hdsa.org/images/content/1/1/11289.pdf>.

The Dystonia Society. <http://www.dystonia.org.uk/>.

Worldwide Education and Awareness for Movement Disorders. <http://www.wemove.org/>.

Neuro-oncology

Different tumour types present in different age groups. The most frequent tumours in adolescence are germ cell tumours and astrocytomas; those in middle life are astrocytomas, meningiomas, and pituitary adenomas and, in later life, malignant astrocytomas and metastases.

In childhood, primary intracranial tumours arise in the cerebellum and brainstem, specifically astrocytomas, ependymomas, and medulloblastomas.

Clinical features

Clinical features depend on location, rate of growth, and pathology. Raised intracranial pressure is most common with high-grade tumours and posterior fossa mass lesions. Low-grade tumours are infiltrative and present more frequently with a seizure disorder.

Severity of headache is not helpful in diagnosis, and the characteristic features of diurnal variation (i.e. morning headache, worse on waking) and associated nausea or vomiting are often absent. The most important feature is the gradual evolution of associated symptoms (i.e. focal deficit, seizures, ataxia, and vomiting). Seizures may be partial and/or generalized and are most often associated with slow-growing tumours. Stroke-like presentations may occur due to intratumoural haemorrhage. Progressive focal deficits occur typically in patients with high-grade tumours, for example, glioblastoma multiforme and brain metastases.

A minority of tumours present with cognitive symptoms, behavioural disorder, for example, abulia (absence of willpower or an inability to act decisively), and psychiatric symptoms, such as depression, paranoid delusions, and personality changes.

Pituitary and hypothalamic tumours present with endocrine disturbances due to anterior or posterior pituitary failure or oversecretion (e.g. acromegaly). They may also cause visual failure, typically commencing with bitemporal quadrantanopia or hemianopia as the optic chiasm is further compressed.

Types of cerebral tumour

Astrocytomas

Astrocytomas arise from neuroepithelial tissue but differ in their location, age distribution, and clinical course. They are subdivided into WHO grades I–IV, according to malignant potential. Low-grade tumours (I and II) tend to develop within the cerebral hemispheres, especially in the frontal and temporal lobes. Some diffuse grade II tumours may transform to higher grades. High-grade anaplastic astrocytomas (III) infiltrate the brain, and glioblastoma multiforme (grade IV) is the most frequent malignant primary CNS tumour.

Surgery remains the mainstay of treatment for astrocytomas, including stereotactic biopsy, open craniotomy, and tumour resection. The overall goals of surgery are to obtain histological diagnosis, relieve mass effect, and improve focal neurological deficit. Complete macroscopic excision is only realistic in a limited proportion of tumours. Combination of radiotherapy and surgery is standard practice in the palliative management of patients with high-grade gliomas. The degree of benefit varies between different prognostic groups, but it is typically modest and there is considerable associated morbidity. The role of chemotherapy in first-line treatment of high-grade gliomas remains uncertain, and it is usually given at first relapse.

Oligodendrogliomas

Oligodendrogliomas account for 10–15% of all gliomas and occur predominantly in adults. They comprise a continuous spectrum, ranging from well-differentiated tumours to highly malignant neoplasms.

Ependymomas

Ependymomas are slow-growing tumours, most common in the first and second decades of life. They occur at any site along the ventricular system, most commonly in the 4th ventricle, the cervical spine, or the conus medullaris (lower spinal cord). In adults, ependymomas account for about 2% of all intracranial tumours and are associated with a high survival rate, compared with other glial tumours. Overall survival correlates well with histological grade, extent of resection, age, and performance status.

Medulloblastomas

Medulloblastomas are malignant, invasive embryonal tumours, which arise in the cerebellum, and are the most common malignant brain tumour in children.

Meningiomas

Meningiomas are common extra-axial (external to the brain parenchyma) intracranial tumours which grow slowly, are well demarcated, and do not usually infiltrate the brain. They are most common in elderly patients, with a peak incidence in the 6th and 7th decades. Generally, they arise within intracranial, orbital, and spinal cavities, favouring the parasagittal area, convexities, sphenoid wing, tuberculum sellae, olfactory groove, and tentorium.

Dysembryoplastic neuroepithelial tumours

Dysembryoplastic neuroepithelial tumours are non-aggressive tumours of neuronal origin which arise in the cerebral cortex and cause intractable complex partial seizures.

Metastases

Metastases most commonly develop in the brain due to carcinoma of the lung, breast, and malignant melanoma. They are frequently associated with vasogenic oedema, often disproportionate to the size of the tumour. Treatment for most brain metastases is purely palliative and may involve surgical resection and radiotherapy. However, the MRI appearances of metastases may be indistinguishable from abscesses, inflammatory or infective lesions (such as neurocysticercosis), or gliomas.

Pituitary tumours

Pituitary tumours represent 10–15% of all intracranial neoplasms. They can be classified by biological behaviour (i.e. benign, invasive adenomas or carcinomas), size (i.e. microadenomas <10 mm or macroadenomas >10 mm in diameter), or histological and functional criteria. Clinical presentation is typically with chronic mass effects, particularly affecting visual structures, chronic headaches, endocrine abnormalities due to hormonal hypersecretion and/or hyposecretion, or a combination of these factors. Occasionally, acute pituitary apoplexy (bleeding into, or impaired blood supply to, the pituitary gland, usually in the presence of a pituitary tumour, although in 80% of cases this has not been diagnosed previously) occurs, particularly in pregnancy.

Craniopharyngiomas

Craniopharyngiomas are slow-growing, benign extra-axial cystic tumours in the parasellar region. The cysts contain thick proteinaceous material with a high content of cholesterol crystals. Gross total surgical removal is the treatment of choice but carries considerable morbidity because of the risks of incomplete removal, cyst rupture, and hypothalamic damage. Recurrence is common.

Primary CNS lymphoma

Primary CNS lymphoma (PCNSL) has greatly increased in incidence over the past two decades in both immunocompetent as well as in AIDS patients. The majority of PCNSL are high-grade B cell lymphomas. Anaplastic large cell and T cell variants may occur.

PCNSL usually presents as either solitary or multiple mass lesions, with raised intracranial pressure, progressive focal neurological deficit, and seizures. The tumour proliferates within the small vessels of the brain, spreading along intravascular spaces (intravascular lymphoma), and presents as multifocal cerebrovascular events or a subacute encephalopathy.

PCNSL is often extremely sensitive to steroids, but recurrence is inevitable. It may respond to high-dose methotrexate, with or without spinal or ocular radiotherapy. The prognosis is extremely poor.

Pineal region tumours

Pineal region tumours, including germ cell and pineal parenchymal tumours (pineocytoma, pineoblastoma), gliomas, and metastases. There are typical clinical syndromes, including obstructive hydrocephalus (i.e. with associated headache, nausea, vomiting, and obtundation), Parinaud's syndrome (i.e. vertical gaze palsy, light-near dissociated midpoint pupils, loss of convergence, and convergence retraction nystagmus), and ataxia due to involvement of the superior cerebellar peduncle.

Schwannomas

Schwannomas are tumours of Schwann cells and account for about 8% of primary intracranial tumours. They arise most commonly from the VIII nerve in the cerebellopontine angle, but they can occur on almost any cranial nerve, particularly the V, VII, and XII as well as on spinal nerve roots and peripheral nerves. Bilateral vestibular schwannomata are a hallmark of neurofibromatosis type II.

Neurological complications of cancer

Complications of neurological tumours are common, potentially disabling but occasionally treatable. Pain, confusion, headache, and weakness are the most common symptoms.

Direct effects

Direct effects are due to either direct invasion of the nervous system or metastatic spread. Infiltration occurs when a primary or secondary tumour or draining lymph node is in direct contact with a nerve, nerve root, spinal cord, or brain. Tumour invasion of nerve roots is often severely painful.

Common presentations of direct invasion include multiple cranial nerve palsies with nasopharyngeal carcinoma, brachial plexus lesions due to breast cancer in the axillary tail and lung cancer causing a T1 root lesion with Horner's syndrome (Pancoast's syndrome). Metastases involving the CNS develop by haematogenous spread, lymphatic dissemination, or by dissemination through the CSF, producing leptomeningeal involvement.

The prognosis is uniformly poor, unless a single, isolated metastasis can be completely removed.

Malignant meningitis

Malignant meningitis often occurs in the later stages of malignant disease, and occasionally presents in a patient with no known tumour. It is characterized by invasion of the leptomeninges and/or CSF by cancer cells. Tumours that commonly cause malignant meningitis are lung and breast cancer, melanoma, and leukaemia or lymphoma. It carries an extremely poor prognosis, and treatment is palliative.

Indirect effects

Indirect effects include toxic/metabolic encephalopathy due to medication (e.g. opioids, benzodiazepines, corticosteroids, chemotherapy), sepsis, hypoxia, electrolyte imbalance, endocrine or nutritional factors. Intracerebral haemorrhage may follow thrombocytopenia, caused by either tumour or leukaemic invasion of bone marrow, chemotherapy, or radiotherapy. A hypercoagulable state can lead to arterial or venous thrombosis. Non-bacterial thrombotic endocarditis (marantic) is a rare cause of ischaemic stroke in the cancer population.

Paraneoplastic neurological disorders

Paraneoplastic neurological disorders are uncommon but important because they frequently present before the malignancy becomes symptomatic. They cause severe neurological disability, and are associated with specific antineuronal antibodies. These include:

- **Paraneoplastic cerebellar degeneration** typically presents with increasing ataxia of gait, trunk, and limbs. There may be nystagmus (often downbeating), gaze palsies, dysphagia, and dysarthria. It occurs in a variety of tumours, most commonly ovarian, breast and lung cancer, and Hodgkin's disease. The diagnosis is often supported by finding antineuronal antibodies (e.g. anti-Yo and anti-Hu).

- **Paraneoplastic encephalomyelitis and limbic encephalitis** are characterized by multifocal inflammatory processes, with predilection for limbic and brainstem structures. Limbic encephalitis occurs with small cell lung cancer and testicular and breast cancer and presents with personality changes, irritability, depression, seizures, memory loss, and sometimes dementia.

- **Brainstem encephalitis** is characterized by cranial nerve palsies, long tract signs, and cerebellar ataxia. Less common features include movement disorders, such as parkinsonism, chorea, and myoclonus, and central alveolar hypoventilation may occur.

- **Other paraneoplastic syndromes** include encephalomyelitis with rigidity, opsoclonus-myoclonus, retinal degeneration, and necrotizing myelopathy.

- **Paraneoplastic sensory neuronopathy** causes subacute, rapidly progressive, asymmetric, and painful sensory symptoms, dominated by severe proprioceptive loss that affects upper limbs more than lower limbs. Other paraneoplastic neuropathies include sensory and sensorimotor axonal neuropathy, acute and chronic forms of inflammatory demyelinating polyradiculopathy, motor neuronopathy, and vasculitic neuropathy.

- **Dermatomyositis,** polymyositis, and acute proximal necrotizing myopathy with rhabdomyolysis may also occur.

Further reading

Behin A, Hoang-Xuan K, Carpetier AF, Delattre JY (2003). Primary brain tumours in adults. *Lancet*, **361**, 323–31.

Brain and Spine Foundation. <http://www.brainandspine.org.uk/>.

Cancer Research UK. <http://www.cancerhelp.org.uk>.

Candler PM, Hart PE, Barnett M, Weil R, Rees JH (2004). A follow-up study of patients with paraneoplastic neurological disease in the United Kingdom. *Journal of Neurology, Neurosurgery & Psychiatry*, **75**, 1411–15.

Grant R (2004). Overview: brain tumour diagnosis and management/Royal College of Physicians Guidelines. *Journal of Neurology, Neurosurgery & Psychiatry*, **75** (Suppl II), 37–42.

Graus F, Delattre JY, Antoine JC, *et al.* (2004). Recommended diagnostic criteria for paraneoplastic neurological syndromes. *Journal of Neurology, Neurosurgery & Psychiatry*, **75**, 1135–40.

International Brain Tumour Alliance. <http://www.theibta.org>.

Macmillan Cancer Support. <http://www.macmillan.org.uk>.

National Institute for Health and Clinical Excellence (2006). *Improving outcomes in brain and other central nervous system tumours. The Manual.* The Stationery Office, London.

National Institute for Health and Clinical Excellence (2012). Brain and central nervous system cancers: recognition and referral. Clinical knowledge summaries. <http://cks.nice.org.uk/brain-and-central-nervous-system-cancers-recognition-and-referral>.

Taphoorn MJB and Klein M (2004). Cognitive deficits in adult patients with brain tumours. *Lancet*, **3**, 159–68.

Young RJ and Knopp EA (2006). Brain MRI: tumor evaluation. *Journal of Magnetic Resonance Imaging*, **24**, 709–24.

Cranial nerve disorders

This chapter reviews some of the clinical patterns caused by lesions of individual cranial nerves.

Trigeminal nerve

Lesions of specific divisions and peripheral branches of the trigeminal nerve (e.g. V_1) produce well-demarcated areas of sensory loss on the face and sometimes considerable pain.

The ophthalmic (V_1; sensory only), maxillary (V_2; sensory only), and mandibular (V_3; motor and sensory) divisions may be individually affected at:

- **The skull base** by:
  - Malignant meningeal infiltration.
  - Infective or granulomatous meningeal processes.
  - Bony metastases.
- **Petrous tip** (i.e. associated with ipsilateral facial sensory disturbance and VI) by:
  - Trigeminal schwannomas.
  - Cerebellopontine angle syndromes (see section on 'Facial nerve').

Superior orbital fissure syndrome (SOF)

This typically presents with ophthalmoplegia (i.e. cranial nerves III, IV, VI), accompanied by sensory disturbance and often pain in the distribution of V_1, sometimes in combination with proptosis with large orbital lesions. Horner's syndrome and visual loss may also occur. It may be due to tumours, such as nasopharyngeal cancers, trauma, infections, (e.g. epidural abscesses, mucormycosis), and inflammatory disorders (e.g. sarcoidosis, Wegener's granulomatosis).

Cavernous sinus syndrome

This can be clinically indistinguishable from the SOF syndrome, except that V_2 as well as V_1 may be involved. Proptosis only occurs with carotid cavernous fistulas. Causes include metastases, meningiomas, nasopharyngeal carcinoma, aneurysms of the intracavernous portion of the carotid artery, carotid cavernous fistula, and granulomatous and inflammatory disorders. Cavernous sinus thrombosis is a serious condition that can follow infection of the face, paranasal sinuses (particularly the sphenoid sinus), or teeth.

Trigeminal nuclear lesions

These result from intrinsic brainstem pathology, such as tumour, inflammatory, or vascular lesions. They are commonly due to infarction of the lateral medulla (e.g. Wallenberg's lateral medullary syndrome).

Trigeminal neuralgia

Trigeminal neuralgia is the most common disorder of the trigeminal nerve. It is more common in women in the sixth and seventh decades; younger patients are more likely to have symptomatic trigeminal neuralgia (e.g. caused by MS or occasionally a mass lesion). Trigeminal neuralgia is frequently caused by neurovascular compression.

The pain is characteristic, consisting of excruciating, lancinating paroxysms in the face, lasting for a few seconds or a minute but occurring in bouts. Patients are usually pain-free between attacks, but, in some, a superimposed dull background pain may develop, often a sign of a poor response to treatment. Sensory triggering of pain by touching a specific affected part of the face or by talking, chewing, or even exposing the face to wind is characteristic. The mandibular and maxillary territories of the nerve are far more commonly affected than the ophthalmic division. Bilateral trigeminal neuralgia is rare (3%) and usually caused by intrinsic brainstem pathology, such as demyelination.

The main differential diagnoses of trigeminal neuralgia include dental disease, acute glaucoma, sinusitis, giant cell arteritis, temporomandibular joint dysfunction, and angina with referred jaw pain. Atypical facial pain is frequently mistakenly labelled as trigeminal neuralgia, but the pain tends to be constant (rather than paroxysmal), aching (rather than lancinating), diffuse, and poorly localized.

Management

A variety of effective medical and surgical treatments now exist. Carbamazepine (200–2,400 mg daily) is the first-line drug for trigeminal neuralgia, and it is effective, or partially effective, in 70% of cases. Oxcarbazepine (start as 600 mg daily, increasing to maintenance of 1,200–1,800 mg daily), is used increasingly, and other agents, used alone or in combination, include lamotrigine (400 mg/day), baclofen (40–80 mg/day), gabapentin (300 mg–3,600 mg/day), and topiramate (25 mg–400 mg/day).

Surgery is more effective if trigeminal neuralgia is resistant to medical therapy. Gasserian ganglion ablative techniques involve selective ablation of part of the trigeminal ganglion and have a low morbidity and immediate efficacy. Radiofrequency thermocoagulation is the most common modality used, and microvascular decompression of vascular loop compressing the nerve has a high long-term success.

Trigeminal sensory neuropathy

Facial sensory loss, in the absence of a defined lesion of the trigeminal nerve or its central connections, evolves gradually and without significant pain. The condition is associated with autoimmune connective tissue diseases (CTD; undifferentiated CTD, mixed CTD, scleroderma, and primary Sjögren's syndrome).

Herpes zoster ophthalmicus (HZO)

HZO particularly affects the elderly and immunocompromised. Pain and sensory disturbance often precedes the appearance of a rash over the side of the nose and medial to the eye. Ocular complications include keratopathy, episcleritis, corneal perforation, iritis, and retinal necrosis, each of which may result in blindness. Corneal anaesthesia may lead to secondary damage to the eye.

Treatment is with aciclovir, valaciclovir, or famciclovir as early as possible. Topical steroids may be indicated where there is anterior chamber inflammation. Steroids (oral and/or intravenous), in combination with antiviral drugs, reduce the duration of pain, accelerate healing, and may reduce the incidence of post-herpetic neuralgia.

Post-herpetic neuralgia is much more common in the elderly; treatment is usually with tricyclic antidepressants (e.g. amitriptyline) or anticonvulsants.

Facial nerve

Facial weakness caused by lesions of the upper motor neurones innervating the facial nucleus (e.g. following hemispheric stroke) is usually associated with ipsilateral limb weakness. There is relative sparing of the upper facial muscles because of their bilateral cortical representation. Dissociation between voluntary and emotional facial movements may be seen; impairment of voluntary movement, with relative sparing of emotional facial movements, is more common than the converse.

Vascular, inflammatory, and occasionally infiltrative brainstem lesions can affect the facial nerve nucleus within the pons or the intrapontine fascicle. This produces a lower motor neurone-type facial palsy, usually associated with other cranial nerve palsies.

Cerebellopontine angle (CPA) syndrome

Mass lesions in the CPA cause combinations of lesions of VIII (e.g. high-pitched tinnitus, progressive sensorineural deafness, and episodic vertigo), V (e.g. facial sensory loss), and VII (e.g. facial weakness). Progressive enlargement leads to involvement of the cerebellum, IX nerve, and descending motor pathways, eventually leading to hydrocephalus. Causes include VIII nerve schwannoma (i.e. acoustic neuroma), meningioma, cholesteatoma, metastasis, and internal carotid artery aneurysm.

The facial nerve or its branches can be damaged at, or distal to, its exit from the skull at the stylomastoid foramen. Parotid tumours or inflammatory parotitis, resulting from infection or granulomatous disease, such as sarcoidosis, may cause facial palsy. Individual branches of the nerve may be damaged by surgery to the parotid or face, carotid endarterectomy, facial trauma, or carotid dissection.

Bell's palsy

Bell's palsy is an acute idiopathic peripheral facial palsy which is common. It may occur in childhood, but the incidence increases steadily with age. A viral aetiology has been postulated on the basis that decompression of the nerve in the acute phase usually reveals swelling of the facial nerve.

The clinical picture is stereotyped, with rapid onset of facial weakness progressing over 48 hours (and occasionally up to 5 days), preceded or accompanied by diffuse retroauricular pain in the region of the mastoid. There is facial weakness and asymmetry, with drooling of liquids from the corner of the mouth on the affected side; all facial muscles are usually equally affected. The palpebral fissure (opening between the eyelids) is widened on the affected side; eye closure and blinking are reduced or absent (with a visible Bell's phenomenon on attempted eye closure). The extent of maximal facial weakness is variable but is severe in the majority. A vague alteration of sensation on the affected side of the face is relatively common in Bell's palsy, although the corneal reflex is preserved. Loss of taste and hyperacusis may occur.

Other causes of acute facial paralysis include the Ramsay–Hunt syndrome (e.g. varicella-zoster reactivation in the geniculate ganglion), local pathology, such as cholesteatoma or malignant otitis externa, parotid tumours, Lyme disease, HIV seroconversion, and skull base tumours.

Management and outcome

Complete, or almost complete, recovery, without recurrence, over 3–8 weeks is the norm in at least 85% of Bell's palsy cases, even without any treatment. Use of lubricating eye drops is often required, and patients should be shown how to tape the eye closed at night. Severe facial weakness, with complete inability to close the eye, requires urgent ophthalmological assessment.

The use of early treatment with corticosteroids (60–80 mg for a week) is standard practice for many clinicians, but the role of antiviral agents remains controversial (valaciclovir 1 g three times daily). Recovery follows axonal regrowth and may be delayed for 4–6 months, or even longer. Aberrant reinnervation of facial muscles and glands is common in late recovery, leading to synkinesis and the phenomenon of jaw-winking—involuntary eye closure with lip or mouth movement; lip movement may occur on blinking or watering of the eye when eating. Reconstructive facial surgery can be helpful.

Bilateral facial weakness

Bilateral facial weakness is rare and is much more likely to be a manifestation of a systemic disease, such as:

- Infections (e.g. bilateral mastoiditis, diphtheria, HIV seroconversion, Epstein–Barr virus (EBV), Lyme disease).
- Sarcoidosis.
- Trauma with skull base fracture.
- Pontine glioma, tumours, including bone metastases.
- Leukaemic deposits within the skull base.
- Malignant meningitis.
- Neuromuscular disease (e.g. Guillain–Barré syndrome, myasthenia gravis, dystrophies).

Hemifacial spasm

Hemifacial spasm is a benign, usually painless but often distressing condition, characterized by unilateral, involuntary, irregular tonic or clonic contractions of muscles supplied by the facial nerve. Movements are irregular in rhythm and degree but synchronous in all affected muscles. They may be spontaneous or triggered by voluntary facial movements, including chewing and speaking, and are made worse by stress or fatigue. Movements usually persist during sleep. Hemifacial spasm is usually caused by extrinsic compression of facial nerve, generally by vascular structures.

Botulinum toxin injection into affected muscles is the first-line treatment but needs to be repeated regularly. Drug treatment is rarely effective.

Other involuntary facial movements

- Myokymia of orbicularis oculi, an irritating twitch usually of the lower eyelid, is a normal phenomenon but sometimes a cause of anxiety.
- More extensive facial myokymia, with persistent worm-like wriggling of the chin and other facial muscles is caused by intrinsic brainstem pathology, such as MS or a pontine glioma.
- Tics and tardive dyskinesia frequently involve facial or perioral muscles.
- Blepharospasm is a form of focal dystonia, affecting orbicularis oculi.
- Fasciculation of facial muscles can develop in motor neurone disease.
- Focal motor seizures may affect facial muscles alone in some cases; epilepsy partilias continua is a cause of persistent clonic–tonic facial movements, which can be localized and difficult to recognize.

Glossopharyngeal neuralgia

Glossopharyngeal neuralgia is a rare condition characterized by unilateral intense and stabbing pain in the ear or throat, lasting for seconds or minutes. It is triggered by movement of neighbouring structures,, such as yawning or chewing. The cause often remains unknown, although structural lesions, demyelination, and possibly vascular loop compression of the posterior inferior cerebellar artery have been found. Carbamazepine and gabapentin may be effective. Microvascular decompression is usually curative.

Bulbar and pseudobulbar palsy

Bulbar and pseudobulbar palsy refer to impairment of lower cranial nerve function (including IX, X, XI, and occasionally XII). The nuclei of these nerves lie in the medulla (i.e. 'bulb') of the brainstem. These nuclei may be affected by lesions involving the descending corticobulbar pathways from the cortex to the nucleus (pseudobulbar palsy) or lesions of the nucleus, fasciculus, or cranial nerves themselves (bulbar palsy). There is no lateralization of pseudobulbar weakness, but bulbar weakness may be unilateral or, more commonly, bilateral. The most obvious manifestation of lower cranial nerve impairment is neurogenic dysphagia, but both bulbar and pseudobulbar palsy include a constellation of characteristic associated clinical features.

Bulbar palsy

Whilst bulbar palsy may be unilateral or bilateral, swallowing impairment usually only occurs with bilateral involvement. Bulbar weakness is associated with a nasal dysarthria, dysphagia with nasal regurgitation, wasted atrophic tongue with fasciculation and slow movement. There may also be associated facial weakness, dysphonia, and limited jaw movement. There is consistent absence of the palatal and pharyngeal reflexes in bulbar palsy, and unilateral pharyngeal wall paresis causes the paralysed side to move towards the healthy side.

A unilateral XII nerve lesion causes the tongue to deviate to the healthy side on retraction (i.e. unopposed action of the styloglossus) as well as to the affected side on protrusion (i.e. genioglossus). Impaired swallow may lead to poor dietary intake and dehydration, aspiration, and bronchopneumonia. Secretions may pool in the pharynx, leading to aspiration and bronchopneumonia.

Causes of bulbar palsy

- Lesions of cranial nerve nuclei in the medulla (but not involving corticobulbar pathways).
  - Cerebrovascular—infarction, haemorrhage.
  - Tumour—glioma.
  - Infection—poliomyelitis.
  - Inflammatory—multiple sclerosis, sarcoidosis.
  - Degenerative—motor neurone disease.
  - Structural—syringomyelia.
  - Rhomboencephalitis—Fisher syndrome.
- Lesions of the cranial nerves.
- Neuromuscular junction.
  - Myasthenia gravis.
  - Lambert–Eaton myasthenic syndrome.
- Muscle.
  - Inflammatory—polymyositis, inclusion body myositis.
  - Dystrophy—myotonic, Duchenne, oculopharyngeal.

Pseudobulbar palsy

Pseudobulbar palsy is an upper motor neurone pattern of weakness, affecting muscles innervated by the bulbar nuclei. It is usually due to bilateral involvement of the descending corticobulbar and corticopontine pathways anywhere from the insular cortex to the medulla.

Pseudobulbar palsy is characterized by spastic dysarthria, slow and limited tongue movements with no wasting or fasciculation, an exaggerated jaw jerk, and pharyngeal weakness. There may be complete anarthria, with an inability to open the mouth, protrude the tongue, swallow, or move the face at will or on command. Patients with pseudobulbar palsy show a striking incongruity with loss of voluntary movements of muscles innervated by the motor nuclei of the lower pons and medulla (inability to swallow, phonate, articulate, move the tongue forcefully, close the eyes) but preservation of reflex pontomedullary actions, yawning, coughing, throat clearing, spasmodic laughter, crying.

Pseudobulbar affect is associated with emotional lability and profound motor retardation. There may be associated frontal release signs and primitive reflexes; the jaw jerk, facial, and pharyngeal reflexes may be particularly brisk, with clonic jaw movements or clamping down on a tongue blade. Movement of the palate and pharynx on phonation are variable but are often reduced. Occasionally, these clinical features may occur in isolation, with no other manifestations of pseudobulbar palsy. In particular, isolated inappropriate spasmodic laughing or crying, unrelated to surrounding circumstances or stimulation and with no corresponding emotional feeling may be a first manifestation of pseudobulbar palsy.

Causes of pseudobulbar palsy

- **Cerebrovascular disease**—infarction, haemorrhage, vasculitis.
- **Inflammatory**—multiple sclerosis.
- **Degenerative**—motor neurone disease.
- **Inborn errors of metabolism.**

Further reading

Keane JR (1994). Bilateral seventh nerve palsy: analysis of 43 cases and review of the literature. *Neurology*, **44**, 1198–202.

Keane JR (2005). Multiple cranial nerve palsies. *Archives of Neurology*, **62**, 1714–17.

Rowlands S, Hooper R, Hughes R, Burney P (2002). The epidemiology and treatment of Bell's palsy in the UK. *European Journal of Neurology*, **9**, 63–7.

Zakrzewska JM and Lopez BC (2006). Trigeminal neuralgia. *Clinical Evidence*, **15**, 1827–35.

Spinal cord lesions

Many non-traumatic conditions affect the spinal cord, with characteristic anatomical and temporal patterns. Myelopathy refers to pathology of the spinal cord. If vascular in origin it is known as a vascular myelopathy, and if inflammatory it is a myelitis.

Transverse myelitis

Transverse myelitis is a segmental spinal cord injury caused by acute inflammation.

The most important causes are:

- *Idiopathic:* possibly an autoimmune response to a preceding infection.
- *Multiple sclerosis* (MS).
- *Neuromyelitis optica* (Devic's disease).
- *Connective tissue diseases* (e.g. SLE, mixed connective tissue disease, Sjögren's syndrome, scleroderma, antiphospholipid antibody syndrome).
- *Sarcoidosis.*
- *Acute viral myelitis* is usually associated with cytomegalovirus, varicella-zoster, herpes simplex virus, hepatitis C, and Epstein–Barr virus (EBV).

The inflammation of transverse myelitis is generally restricted to one or two segments, usually in the thoracic cord, and symptoms typically develop rapidly over several hours, leading to weakness and sensory disturbance below the level of the lesion. Pain and tingling are common, and bowel and bladder dysfunction develops. In Devic's disease, the lesion extends over many segments.

Magnetic resonance imaging (MRI) shows gadolinium-enhancing signal abnormality, usually extending over one or more cord segments, and the cord often appears swollen at these levels. Cerebrospinal fluid (CSF) shows an elevated protein level (usually 100–120 mg/100 mL), moderate lymphocytosis (usually <100/mm^3), and the presence of oligoclonal bands suggests multiple sclerosis.

Treatment is with intravenous and oral corticosteroid therapy. Most patients make a complete or significant recovery, but severe residual disability is common.

Epidural abscess

Presentation is with fever, spinal pain, and gradually evolving neurological deficit. Infection is usually a complication of spinal surgery, other invasive procedures, or contiguous spread. *Staphylococcus aureus* is the most common aetiological agent. Surgical decompression and drainage, with systemic antibiotic therapy, is the treatment of choice for most patients.

Infection of the spinal cord

Infections of the spinal cord include:

- *HIV infection:* causes a vacuolar myelopathy in the later stages of AIDS. It presents as a slowly progressive spastic paraparesis, with proprioceptive loss and sphincter involvement.
- *HTLV-1:* presents with a similar pattern to HIV infection (i.e. tropical spastic paraparesis).
- *Tertiary syphilis:* may lead to tabes dorsalis, in which patients present with sensory ataxia and lancinating pains due to posterior column and nerve root involvement.
- *Tuberculosis* may manifest as myelopathy due to direct bony involvement, causing tuberculous spondylitis (i.e. Pott's disease), which can lead to secondary cord compression. Tuberculomas within the intramedullary, intradural, and extradural space can also produce myelopathy.

Infarction of the spinal cord

Infarction of the spinal cord is rare. It is usually associated with aortic disease, surgery, or an embolic source but it can be due to severe systemic hypotension or cardiac arrest. Vascular impairment affects the anterior cord, causing pyramidal and radicular (motor) weakness, impairment in pain and temperature sensation, and sphincter involvement.

Vascular malformations of the spinal cord

These may be:

- *Dural arteriovenous fistula.* These lie on the dural surface and present as progressive myeloradiculopathy, often associated with neurogenic claudication.
- *Intramedullary arteriovenous malformations* (AVMs).

Subacute combined degeneration of the cord

Degeneration of the posterior columns and lateral white matter of the spinal cord leads to progressive pyramidal weakness, paraesthesiae, and sensory ataxia. This is classically caused by vitamin B$_{12}$ deficiency but may also be due to nitrous oxide abuse, copper deficiency (parenteral feeding, gastrointestinal surgery), and excessive zinc ingestion.

Radiation myelopathy

Radiation myelopathy may occur in two distinct patterns:

- A transient myelopathy, occurring 2 to 6 months after irradiation which is often mild and resolves spontaneously over several months.
- A late slowly progressive myelopathy, developing 6 to 12 months after irradiation.

Decompression sickness myelopathy

Decompression sickness myelopathy occurs as a complication of deep sea diving and is due to gas emboli. Thoracic cord involvement may lead to an acute paraparesis with sensory involvement. Early therapeutic recompression with hyperbaric oxygen is the treatment of choice.

Neoplasms of the spinal cord

Both benign and malignant tumours can produce a myelopathy as a result of external compression or intramedullary growth. Extradural compression (e.g. metastases) may cause painful, progressive weakness below the level of the lesion, with sensory and sphincter loss. Intramedullary spinal cord tumours are typically primary central nervous system tumours (ependymoma, astrocytoma) that produce a progressive myelopathy, often with central cord features (i.e. disproportionately greater motor impairment in upper compared to lower extremities, and a variable degree of sensory loss below the level of injury with bladder dysfunction and urinary retention).

Inherited and degenerative conditions of the spinal cord

These include:

- *Amyotrophic lateral sclerosis.*
- *Hereditary spastic paraplegias.* A group of genetically diverse inherited conditions, causing a slowly progressive spastic paraparesis with early sphincter involvement.

- **Adrenoleukodystrophy.** An X-linked recessive disorder, which is characterized by a slowly progressive spastic paraparesis and mild polyneuropathy.
- **Friedreich's ataxia.** An autosomal recessive degenerative condition, which presents in adolescence with progressive limb and gait ataxia, absent reflexes with extensor plantar responses and proprioceptive loss.

Others

Syringomyelia

A syrinx is a fluid-filled cavity lying within the spinal cord, (usually between C2 and T9) which can extend into the brainstem (syringobulbia).

There are several causes:

- Arnold–Chiari malformation type 1 (downward displacement of the cerebellar tonsils through the foramen magnum which may obstruct free flow of CSF).
- Congenital malformations.
- Post-infectious.
- Post-inflammatory (transverse myelitis, multiple sclerosis).
- Spinal neoplasms (especially ependymoma and haemangioblastoma).
- Post-traumatic.

Cervical spondylosis

Cervical spondylosis is the most common cause of myelopathy, particularly in older adults. The cervical cord is compressed by degenerative changes in the vertebral bodies, discs, and connecting ligaments. Presentation is with a slowly progressive spastic gait, with limb weakness, radicular involvement, and sensory loss. The diagnosis is made by MRI showing cord or root compression, and management may include physical therapy and surgical decompression.

Radiculopathy

Radiculopathy refers to any pathological process affecting the nerve roots. Compressive cervical radiculopathy is usually due to cervical spondylosis and disc herniation. In addition, there are many non-compressive causes of radiculopathy, including infection (e.g. herpes zoster and Lyme disease), infarction, root avulsion, infiltration by tumour or granuloma, and demyelination.

Diagnosis is based on clinical findings and MR imaging of the cervical spine. Most patients with compressive cervical radiculopathy improve without specific treatment. Conservative therapy is recommended for patients with radicular pain, sensory disturbance, and non-progressive deficits. Surgery is indicated if there is a significant motor deficit or myelopathy.

Further reading

Clarke C, Howard R, Rossor M, Shorvon S (2009). *Neurology—A Queen Square textbook*. Wiley-Blackwell, Oxford.

Toxic and nutritional disease

Toxic exposure and nutritional derangements can cause damage to the nervous system by a variety of mechanisms, leading to a wide spectrum of neurological disorders.

Toxins

Exposure to toxic substances may be either accidental or, in the context of substance abuse, deliberate and can cause encephalopathy, stroke, seizures, or neuropathy.

Heavy metals

Exposure to heavy metals or industrial toxins is usually cumulative as a consequence of environmental or occupational exposure. However, these agents may be acutely toxic, following accidental or deliberate ingestion of excessive amounts.

- **Acute exposure** often leads to encephalopathy, with confusion, attention deficit, and seizures.
- **Chronic involvement** is of a more insidious onset with mood disturbance, memory and cognitive impairment. Systemic features usually accompany neurological manifestations.

Solvents and toxins

Central nervous system (CNS) dysfunction can occur as a consequence of an accidental exposure to a high dose of industrial solvents or to more prolonged chronic exposure to moderate levels in the workplace or as a drug of abuse.

- **Prolonged exposure to solvent vapour** leads to long-term symptoms. These include progressive cognitive deficits affecting attention, memory, executive function, and associated visuospatial disturbance, with subsequent cerebellar or motor involvement.

Carbon monoxide (CO)

CO is a clear, colourless, and odourless gas. It is commonly used in attempted suicide, but exposure also occurs with faulty engine exhausts or incorrectly installed domestic gas-powered boilers.

- **Acute exposure** causes headache, dizziness, confusion, disturbance of consciousness, and behavioural change. Visual disturbance and progressive shortness of breath develop rapidly, with subsequent loss of consciousness, seizures, coma, and cardiac arrest.
- **Following acute exposure**, patients with initial transient choreiform movements may develop parkinsonian features, progressive dystonia, and urinary incontinence.
- **Delayed-onset encephalopathy** may develop after a period of apparent partial or complete recovery with cognitive and personality impairment, with memory dysfunction, apathy, mutism, and the progressive development of vegetative features.
- **Insidious, chronic low-grade exposure** to CO may be due to industrial exposure but, most frequently, occurs in poorly ventilated homes with faulty household heating appliances. The syndrome of chronic occult CO poisoning is manifest as headache, fatigue, dizziness, paraesthesiae, and visual disturbance. Chest pain, palpitations, and associated ventricular arrhythmias may also occur.

Treatment

Treatment of acute exposure is by removal from the source and the provision of 100% oxygen. Hyperbaric oxygen may enhance recovery from acute symptoms. However, the prognosis for neurological recovery after CO exposure is poor (see also Chapter 18).

Nutritional deficiencies

Nutritional deficiency is the most common worldwide cause of neurological disease and manifests as a number of well-characterized, usually reversible, but potentially serious, neurological disorders.

Vitamin deficiency

Vitamin A

Vitamin A deficiency leads to a variety of ophthalmic disorders, in particular, night blindness. Overdose and toxicity, associated with ingestion of proprietary treatments, may cause idiopathic intracranial hypertension.

Vitamin B_1 (thiamine)

Vitamin B_1 is found in most food and cereals, but reduced intestinal absorption occurs in alcoholism and malabsorption syndromes. Thiamine depletion may develop acutely and is a medical emergency because of the development of congestive cardiac failure and peripheral oedema, the syndrome of 'wet beriberi'. In addition, a sensory axonal neuropathy, termed 'dry beriberi', or Wernicke–Korsakoff syndrome, termed 'cerebral beriberi', may also occur.

Vitamin B_3 (niacin, nicotinic acid)

Vitamin B_3 deficiency leads to the syndrome of pellagra, characterized by dementia, diarrhoea, and dermatitis ('the three ds'). There may be mood changes, fatigue, malaise, lethargy, and confusion with progression to neuropsychiatric disturbances, including apathy, inattentiveness, and memory loss or the development of spastic paraparesis with startle myoclonus. The cognitive impairment is characterized by a defect in recent memory, visuospatial ability, abstract reasoning, and speed of information processing.

Vitamin B_6 (pyridoxine)

In adults, pyridoxine deficiency is usually secondary to medication, including isoniazid, hydralazine, and penicillamine. There may be peripheral neuropathy with distal weakness and painful sensory loss, absent tendon reflexes, and Romberg's sign. High-dose pyridoxine also causes a distal sensory axonal neuropathy with sensory ataxia.

Vitamin B_{12} deficiency

Vitamin B_{12} is abundant in meat, fish, and animal by-products. Neurological features occur in up to 40% of patients with B_{12} deficiency, evolving over several months or longer.

- Subacute combined degeneration of the spinal cord is characterized by the presence of a sensorimotor axonal neuropathy and myelopathy. Neuropathic manifestations include distal paraesthesiae, numbness, gait ataxia, and diminished proprioception in the lower limbs, while the myelopathic component leads to variable motor impairment due to pyramidal tract involvement.
- Central manifestations include confusion, depression, progressive hallucination, and mental slowing.
- Isolated cognitive or psychiatric disturbances may occasionally be the presenting feature in some patients, but the direct relationship between B_{12} and dementia remains unclear.
- Optic neuropathy may occur.

With adequate treatment, some of the deficits of B_{12} deficiency may be reversible, with most improvement occurring within the first 6 months of treatment. The myelopathy is least likely to make a complete recovery.

Vitamin D deficiency
Vitamin D deficiency is associated with malabsorption, dietary deficiency, or inadequate exposure to sunlight. Neurological presentation is as a proximal myopathy which may be associated with osteomalacia. There is proximal weakness, with a characteristic waddling gait, but no involvement of bulbar or ocular musculature.

Vitamin E deficiency
Vitamin E deficiency is usually secondary to malabsorption in cystic fibrosis, adult coeliac disease, or because of abnormalities of specific vitamin E receptors. There is progressive spinocerebellar degeneration, with limb ataxia and an axonal, predominantly sensory, peripheral neuropathy.

Alcohol abuse

Alcohol abuse is extremely common and is associated with important cultural, economic, and environmental factors; there is also a strong genetic component. It affects all socioeconomic strata of society.

Acute intoxication
The initial behavioural effects are of euphoria, social disinhibition, loss of restraint, and reduced psychomotor capacity. This is followed by behaviour disturbance, irritability, slurred speech, ataxic gait, aggression, and loss of control. Depressant effects include drowsiness, stupor, and eventually coma supervenes with the risk of vomiting, aspiration, and respiratory impairment.

Acute intoxication is associated with psychotic disturbances. These include an acute paranoid state, with auditory hallucinations, anxiety, agitation, outbursts of aggression, and inappropriate violent or destructive social behaviour, of which the patient may have no recollection after awaking from sleep.

Periods of amnesia, in which there is no ability to retain short-term memories, increase in duration and persist into periods when sober and fully conscious.

Effects of alcohol substitutes
Methyl alcohol (methanol)
Methyl alcohol is commonly used as a solvent and in antifreeze. It may be abused as a substitute for ethyl alcohol in 'meths'. It is directly toxic to the CNS (e.g. putamen and optic nerves).

Acute intoxication may be delayed for many hours. Delirium may develop at the onset, but rapid progression occurs to cause visual field loss, blindness secondary to retinal oedema, pseudobulbar palsy, and cognitive impairment. Severe toxicity culminates in metabolic acidosis and cerebral oedema. This leads to respiratory failure, coma, and death. In patients who recover from acute intoxication, there may be residual blindness and parkinsonian features.

Treatment involves reversing the acidosis with large doses of sodium bicarbonate, competitive inhibition of methanol using ethyl alcohol or fomepizole, which prevents further damage, and, where necessary, haemodialysis (see Chapter 9).

Ethylene glycol
Ethylene glycol (antifreeze) intoxication is associated with lethargy and progressive hypersomnolence, hyperventilation, with seizures and hypotension. There is a metabolic acidosis with an anion gap. Anuric renal failure develops which is also associated with seizures. With high levels,

there may be the delayed onset of a cranial neuropathy, which resolves slowly.

Treatment often requires haemodialysis. Intravenous sodium bicarbonate may be given and, if necessary, ethanol. Fomepizole (4-methylpyrazole) is also used as a competitive inhibitor of alcohol dehydrogenase and thiamine (see Chapter 9).

Withdrawal syndromes
The severity of withdrawal symptoms is proportional to the level of previous alcohol intake and the abruptness of cessation. Withdrawal of alcohol in the chronic abuser may lead to the development of delirium tremens with CNS hyperexcitability. This is initially characterized by tremulousness, with anxiety, insomnia, confusion, hyperactivity, hallucinations, and seizures. The symptoms progressively worsen over several hours before settling up to 72 hours after the last intake of alcohol. The tremor is generalized, present at rest and on action, and may involve the face and tongue. It is associated with irritability and is usually present in the morning but progressively worsens and increases in duration with prolonged withdrawal. Disturbing, vivid, auditory and visual hallucinations may develop.

The patient frequently awakes lucid and with no recollection of the acute delirious phase. Recurrence is common, and, in severe cases, death may supervene. It is essential to consider the possibility of alcohol withdrawal in patients who develop confusion, tremor, or seizures after being admitted to hospital for more than 12 hours.

Treatment
Treatment depends on severity:
- **Minor symptoms** can be managed with simple reassurance and nursing in a calm, quiet, well-lit environment, although benzodiazepines may be helpful.
- **Moderate symptoms**, including autonomic hyperactivity and irritability, necessitate an incremental dose of benzodiazepines (e.g. chlordiazepoxide).
- **Severe symptoms**, associated with confusion, poor cooperation, restlessness, and aggressive behaviour, may require intravenous diazepam, given by slow injection, and, if further treatment is necessary, haloperidol is the drug of choice.

Withdrawal seizures (rum fits)
These typically occur within the first 24–48 hours of withdrawal. They are generalized tonic-clonic seizures, which usually occur singly or in brief clusters, although status may develop. Even if status develops, the condition is usually self-limiting, and patients often do not require antiepileptic medication, although acute treatment with chlordiazepoxide, lorazepam, or diazepam may be necessary (see Chapter 9).

Disorders due to prolonged alcohol abuse
Wernicke–Korsakoff's syndrome
This is a complex of symptoms and signs resulting from an acquired nutritional deficiency of thiamine (vitamin B_1), rather than any direct toxic effect of alcohol. It may occur in 5–20% of chronic alcohol misusers.

Wernicke's encephalopathy
This may present as an acute or slowly evolving disorder. The classically described triad of acute confusion, ataxia, and ophthalmoplegia is only seen in about 10% of cases. The acute syndrome is characterized by:
- Apathy and acute confusion (80%).

- Ocular signs, including ophthalmoplegia, nystagmus, and conjugate gaze palsy (30%).
- Progressive trunk and gait ataxia is common, but the limbs are rarely involved (25%).
- Encephalopathy with hallucinations, perceptual disorder, and agitation.
- Progressive disturbance of behaviour, personality, orientation, and cognitive function may develop over days or weeks, leading to stupor, coma, and ultimately death.

Treatment

Wernicke's encephalopathy is reversible in the early stages if central nervous system vitamin B levels, in particular thiamine, are rapidly restored. Treatment should be initiated immediately when a diagnosis is suspected.

Initially give intravenous Pabrinex® (two pairs of ampoules three times daily for 3–7 days), followed by oral thiamine 100 mg three times a day and vitamin B compound strong 2 tablets once daily, for 14 days or until reviewed. All patients undergoing alcohol withdrawal should be treated prophylactically for Wernicke's encephalopathy with intravenous Pabrinex® one pair of ampoules three times daily for 1 day. There is a very small risk (five cases per million) of anaphylaxis with parenteral thiamine.

Untreated Wernicke's encephalopathy is associated with a significant mortality (17%) and results in permanent brain damage in 85% of survivors. With adequate treatment, the prognosis is good, and signs resolve rapidly.

Korsakoff's syndrome

This is a progressive and severe amnesic syndrome which is incompletely reversible.

- Memory is preferentially involved, in comparison to other cognitive functions, with a profound impairment of both retrograde and antegrade memory. The memory of recent past is usually more severely affected than distant past, while language and calculation abilities are well preserved.
- There is confabulation (i.e. deliberate attempts to hide the memory defect by fabricating events).

Treatment

Treatment requires urgent and high doses of thiamine replacement and should be continued until a noticeable improvement has occurred and for as long as clinical recovery continues. Improvement in memory function is slow and usually incomplete. Up to one-quarter of patients show no recovery while only slight improvement occurs in the remaining patients. Significant or complete recovery is rare.

Cerebellar ataxia

Chronic alcohol abuse is the most common cause of acquired cerebellar atrophy and is often associated with alcohol polyneuropathy. The ataxia may be so severe that the patient is unable to stand without support. Patients walk with a broad-based gait with slow, short steps, but limb ataxia and speech disturbance are minimal. Abstinence from alcohol leads to a slow and incomplete improvement.

Alcohol peripheral neuropathy

Sensorimotor axonal peripheral neuropathy is due to thiamine deficiency or because of direct alcohol toxicity. Rapid progression may occur, with motor impairment severe enough to affect gait. Autonomic involvement is manifest as impotence, sweating, pupillary abnormalities, and postural hypotension.

Alcoholic myopathy

Acute myopathy can occur with chronic alcohol abuse but may also follow binge intake. The onset is with acute and severe muscle pain, cramp, swelling, and a rise in the CK, evolving rapidly into focal or generalized myopathic weakness. A cardiomyopathy may coexist.

In chronic alcohol abuse, depressive illness is common, particularly on withdrawal. Some patients also have an anxiety disorder which may develop into frank psychotic symptoms during withdrawal.

Traumatic injury

Traumatic injuries to the head and peripheral nerves may occur during intoxication, causing parenchymal contusions, subdural or extradural haematoma, subarachnoid haemorrhage, and post-traumatic epilepsy.

Compressive neuropathies

The most common neuropathies occurring in alcohol abuse include compression of the radial nerve at the spiral groove, causing Saturday night palsies (failure of wrist extension with 'wrist drop'). The peroneal nerve may be trapped at the fibula head, leading to a foot drop, and the sciatic nerve may be compressed in the gluteal region.

Amblyopia

Amblyopia is associated with poor dietary and heavy tobacco intake and weight loss. Progressive optic nerve involvement leads to painless visual loss, affecting both eyes, with diminished visual acuity with centrocaecal scotoma and mild disc pallor. The treatment is with adequate diet and B vitamins, which generally leads to visual recovery.

Confusional state and dementia

Cortical atrophy and ventricular dilatation occur with prolonged alcohol intake. This is associated with a global confusion characterized by a progressive indifference to personal surroundings. Patients are easily aroused but are disorientated with cognitive deficits which may worsen and become fixed. This interferes with activities of daily living, before evolving into frank dementia which may persist, even after discontinuation of alcohol.

Alcoholic cirrhosis

The neurological effects of alcohol abuse run in parallel with systemic factors. Alcohol-related cirrhosis is the most common and serious manifestation. Patients may develop portosystemic encephalopathy, tremor, myoclonus, and asterixis.

Further reading

Clarke C, Howard R, Rossor M, Shorvon S (2009). *Neurology—A Queen Square textbook*. Wiley-Blackwell, Oxford.

Victor M, Adams RD, Collins GH (1989). *The Wernicke–Korsakoff syndrome and related neurologic disorders due to alcoholism and malnutrition*. FA Davis, Philadelphia.

Victor M and Ropper A (2001). *Principles of neurology*. McGraw-Hill, New York.

Ward PC (2002). Modern approaches to the investigation of vitamin B12 deficiency. *Clinics in Laboratory Medicine*, **51**, 435–45.

Gastroenterology and hepatology

Presentation, examination, and investigations

Introduction

Gastrointestinal disease may present in a variety of ways, including loss of appetite, weight loss, nausea, and vomiting, dysphagia, pain on swallowing (odynophagia), indigestion or heartburn, abdominal pain, diarrhoea, change of bowel habit (diarrhoea or constipation), bloating or abdominal distension, or passage of fresh blood or mucus in the stool, melaena or haematemesis, jaundice or dark urine, itching, or pale stools.

Abdominal pain

Abdominal pain is a common presentation and, in all cases, may be referred from an adjacent site and be from a non-gastrointestinal source, such as pleural, renal, or cardiac, etc.

Epigastric pain

- Peptic ulcer.
- Pancreatitis.
- Reflux oesophagitis.
- Acute gastritis.
- Malignancy: gastric or pancreatic.
- Functional disorders: non-ulcer dyspepsia, irritable bowel syndrome.

Central abdominal (periumbilical) pain

- Gastrointestinal: intestinal obstruction, early appendicitis, gastroenteritis.
- Vascular: abdominal aortic aneurysm (leaking, ruptured), mesenteric ischaemia (thrombosis, embolism, vasculitis, e.g. polyarteritis nodosa).
- Medical causes, e.g. diabetic ketoacidosis, uraemia.

Diffuse abdominal pain

- Gastroenteritis.
- Peritonitis.
- Intestinal obstruction.
- Inflammatory bowel disease.
- Mesenteric ischaemia.
- Medical causes (see further text).
- Irritable bowel syndrome.

Right upper quadrant pain

- Gall bladder pathology: cholecystitis (usually related to gallstones, occasionally may be acalculous), biliary colic, cholangitis.
- Liver pathology: hepatitis, hepatomegaly (congestive, e.g. in congestive cardiac failure, Budd–Chiari syndrome), hepatic tumours, hepatic/subphrenic abscess.
- Appendicitis, e.g. in a pregnant woman.
- Colonic cancer (hepatic flexure).
- Herpes zoster.

Right iliac fossa pain

- Gastrointestinal: appendicitis, mesenteric adenitis (*Yersinia*, in children), Meckel's diverticulum (in children), inflammatory bowel disease, colonic cancer, constipation, irritable bowel syndrome.
- Reproductive: mittelschmerz (pain with ovulation), ovarian cyst torsion/rupture/haemorrhage, ectopic pregnancy, pelvic inflammatory disease, endometriosis.
- Renal: urinary tract infection or renal stone.

- Pain from hip pathology, psoas abscess, rectus sheath haematoma.

Suprapubic pain

- Urinary retention.
- Cystitis.

Left iliac fossa pain

- Gastrointestinal: diverticulitis, inflammatory bowel disease, colonic cancer, constipation, irritable bowel syndrome.
- Reproductive: mittelschmerz (pain with ovulation), ovarian cyst torsion/rupture/haemorrhage, ectopic pregnancy, salpingitis/pelvic inflammatory disease, endometriosis.
- Renal pain: urinary tract infection, ureteric colic (renal stones).
- Pain from adjacent areas, such as hip pathology, psoas abscess, rectus sheath haematoma.

Left upper quadrant pain

- Splenic rupture, splenic infarction (e.g. sickle cell disease), splenomegaly.
- Subphrenic abscess.
- Colonic cancer (splenic flexure).
- Herpes zoster.

Loin pain

- Infection: urinary tract infection (pyelonephritis), perinephric abscess or pyonephrosis.
- Renal obstruction, e.g. stones, tumour, blood clots, prostatic/pelvic mass, retroperitoneal fibrosis.
- Renal carcinoma.
- Renal vein thrombosis.
- Polycystic kidney disease.
- Pain from vertebral column.

Groin pain

- Renal stones (pain radiating from loin to groin).
- Testicular pain, e.g. torsion, epididymo-orchitis.
- Hernia (inguinal).
- Hip pathology.
- Pelvic fractures.

Unusual causes of abdominal pain

- Cardiovascular/respiratory: MI, pneumonia, Bornholm's disease (Coxsackie B virus infection).
- Metabolic: diabetic ketoacidosis, Addisonian crisis, hypercalcaemia, uraemia, acute porphyria, phaeochromocytoma, lead poisoning.
- Neurological: herpes zoster.
- Haematological: sickle cell crisis, retroperitoneal haemorrhage, lymphadenopathy.
- Inflammatory: vasculitis (e.g. Henoch–Schönlein purpura, polyarteritis nodosa), familial Mediterranean fever.
- Infections: intestinal parasites, tuberculosis, malaria, typhoid fever.

Abdominal distension

- Fat (obesity).
- Fluid (ascites, fluid in an obstructed intestine).
- Flatus (intestinal obstruction).

- Faeces.
- Fetus.
- Massive organomegaly (e.g. an ovarian cystadenoma, hepatomegaly, lymphoma), large tumour.
- Large abdominal hernia.

Diarrhoea

Also see section on bloody diarrhoea.

Infection

- Viral (adenovirus, astrovirus, calciviruses (norovirus and related viruses), rotavirus). Bacterial (*Campylobacter*, *Salmonella*, *Shigella*, haemorrhagic *E. coli*, *Clostridium difficile*, *Yersinia enterocolitica*, *C. perfringens*, *Vibrio cholerae*, *Vibrio parahaemolyticus*). Parasites (cryptosporidia, *Giardia*, *Entamoeba histolytica*). HIV (AIDS enteropathy, cryptosporidia, microsporidia, cytomegalovirus (CMV)).
- Inflammatory bowel disease.
- Malabsorption: small intestine disease/resection, biliary or chronic pancreatic disease.
- Medication: laxatives, antibiotics.
- Overflow diarrhoea: secondary to constipation.
- Endocrine: thyrotoxicosis, VIPomas.

Note: *Staphylococcus aureus* and *Bacillus cereus* mainly present with vomiting 1–6 hours after ingestion of prepared food, e.g. salad, dairy, meat, and rice.

Bloody diarrhoea

- Infective colitis: *Campylobacter*, haemorrhagic *E. coli*, *Salmonella, Shigella, Entamoeba histolytica*, CMV in the immunocompromised.
- Inflammatory bowel disease.
- Ischaemic colitis.
- Diverticulitis.
- Malignancy.

Haematemesis

- Peptic ulcer (gastric/duodenal).
- Gastritis/gastric erosions, duodenitis, oesophagitis.
- Gastro-oesophageal varices.
- Mallory–Weiss tear.

- Medications: non-steroidal anti-inflammatory drugs (NSAIDs), anticoagulants, steroids, thrombolytics.
- Oesophageal/gastric cancer.

Rare

- Bleeding disorders (thrombocytopenia, haemophilia), hereditary haemorrhagic telangiectasia, Dieulafoy's gastric vascular abnormality, aortoduodenal fistulae, angiodysplasia, leiomyoma, pseudoxanthoma elasticum.

Jaundice

- Pre-hepatic: Gilbert's (bilirubin rarely >80 micromoles/L), haemolysis. Absence of bilirubin in urine.
- Hepatic: alcoholic hepatitis, viral hepatitis, autoimmune hepatitis, ischaemic hepatitis, primary biliary cirrhosis (PBC), primary sclerosing cholangitis (PSC), drug-induced hepatitis or cholestasis, end-stage cirrhosis. Rare infections—leptospirosis, Epstein–Barr virus (EBV) or CMV, severe sepsis (any cause, e.g. pneumonia). Overdose (paracetamol), toxins, vascular obstruction including Budd–Chiari syndrome.
- Post-hepatic: gallstones, pancreatic or biliary malignancy, congenital abnormalities of biliary tree, parasitic infection, obstruction from a large varix (portal hypertension).

Vomiting

- Drugs, poisoning, alcohol.
- Abdominal pathology (gastrointestinal, hepatic, gynaecological).
- Metabolic/endocrine: diabetic ketoacidosis, Addisonian crisis, hypercalcaemia, uraemia, pregnancy.
- Increased intracranial pressure (infection, space-occupying lesion, benign intracranial hypertension).
- Acute labyrinthitis.
- Acute angle closure glaucoma.

Further reading

British Society of Gastroenterology. Guidelines. <http://www.bsg.org.uk/clinical/general/guidelines.html>.

National Institute for Health and Clinical Excellence. Gastrointestinal diseases. <http://www.nice.org.uk/guidance/index.jsp?action=byTopic&o=7220>.

Acute upper GI bleeding

Upper gastrointestinal (GI) bleeding has an overall mortality of 11–14%. Good management will reduce the overall mortality significantly.

Causes of upper GI bleeding
See Figure 8.1.
- Peptic ulcer (60%).
- Gastro-oesophageal varices (10%).
- Gastroduodenal erosions (10%).
- Oesophagitis (5%).
- Mallory–Weiss tear (5%).
- Vascular malformations (5%):
  - Hereditary haemorrhagic telangiectasia.
  - Gastric antral vascular ectasia (GAVE).
  - Portal hypertensive gastropathy.
  - Angiodysplasia.
  - Dieulafoy's lesion.
- Rare miscellaneous (4%):
  - Hiatus hernia.
  - Meckel's diverticulum.
  - Crohn's disease.
  - Aorto-enteric fistula.
- Upper GI malignancy (1%).

Presentation
Haematemesis
Vomiting fresh blood or significant 'coffee grounds'; 29% of patients with coffee grounds in nasogastric aspirate have a significant high-risk lesion at endoscopy.

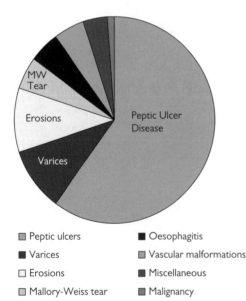

- ▨ Peptic ulcers
- ▨ Varices
- ☐ Erosions
- ▨ Mallory-Weiss tear

- ▉ Oesophagitis
- ▨ Vascular malformations
- ▉ Miscellaneous
- ▉ Malignancy

Figure 8.1 Causes of upper GI bleeding.

Melaena
Black, sticky, smelly stool. This occurs following bleeding proximal to the transverse colon. Blood is cathartic, with melaena appearing 4–6 h following a GI bleed and continuing for up to 2 days. Other causes of a dark stool include iron therapy, bismuth, liquorice, or drinks, such as Guinness and red wine.

Fresh rectal bleeding
11% of massive upper GI bleeds present in this way.

Shock
Weakness, sweating, palpitations, postural dizziness, fainting, collapse.

Management priorities are to:
1. Stabilize the patient: protect the airway, restore circulating volume.
2. Assess the severity.
3. Identify the source of the bleeding.
4. Stop the bleeding.

Initial management: stabilize the patient
Protect the airway
Position the patient on their left side if actively vomiting to minimize the risk of aspiration of blood.

Rapidly assess circulatory status
Feel the hands and feet. Does the patient look unwell? Is there pallor or sweating? Measure blood pressure (BP ± postural drop in BP) and heart rate.

IV access
Insert two large-bore intravenous cannulae (e.g. 16G/grey). Jugular, subclavian, or femoral vein cannulation may be necessary. If the patient is shocked (systolic <100 mmHg, HR >100) or has signs of hypovolaemia, such as pallor, sweating, cold peripheries, weak pulse, postural hypotension (>20 mmHg drop in systolic pressure on standing), then infuse 1 L of normal saline or Hartmann's solution over 15–30 minutes.

Blood tests
Request full blood count (FBC), urea and electrolytes (U&E), liver function tests (LFT), calcium and phosphate, glucose and clotting. Cross-match 4 to 8 units if the patient is shocked on admission. 'Group and save' serum only if the patient is stable and the history suggests 'coffee ground' vomit only. Measure arterial blood gases in severely ill patients.

Haemoglobin (Hb) and packed cell volume (PCV)
Hb and PCV do not fall until the plasma volume has been restored, but, if low at presentation, this suggests massive blood loss or acute-on-chronic bleeding. The white blood count may be elevated but is usually <15,000/mm³. If WCC is elevated, look for sepsis which can predispose to haemorrhage.

A low platelet count
This suggests hypersplenism and chronic liver disease, but thrombocytopenia of any cause may predispose to gastrointestinal bleeding.

An elevated plasma urea out of proportion to plasma creatinine indicates renal hypoperfusion or the absorption of blood proteins from the gut. It signifies a significant GI bleed or dehydration. A ratio of urea (mM) x 100, divided by creatinine (micromoles/L), >7.0 indicates that the urea is disproportionately high.

If there is massive haemorrhage, ask for 'O'-negative blood, which may be given without cross-matching: avoid doing this unless absolutely necessary, and remember to save serum for retrospective cross-matching.

History and examination
A brief history will probably already be available, but ask specifically about: use of NSAIDs and anticoagulants, symptoms suggestive of peptic ulcer disease, a history of alcohol abuse or liver disease, and previous GI bleeds or ulcers or surgery. Determine whether bleeding was spontaneous or followed retching and vomiting (occurs in 40% of Mallory–Weiss tears or variceal bleeds). Examine for stigmata of chronic liver disease, such as jaundice, spider naevi, hepatosplenomegaly, or ascites, which may suggest that the bleed is variceal. Rectal examination may reveal melaena or semi-fresh blood.

Restore the circulating volume
Tachycardia, hypotension, or a postural hypotension suggests low intravascular volume. Initially, give 1–2 L of crystalloid (saline or Hartmann's solution) stat. Colloid solutions should be considered second line therapy for resuscitation as there is no proven benefit, they are more expensive and may cause potential harm (see Chapter 2). If there are no signs of hypovolemia, use a slower rate of infusion. Continue infusing crystalloid to normalize the blood pressure until blood is available. Try to maintain the systolic BP >100 mmHg. There are no 'hard' rules about the rate of IV infusion. In general, if the patient is >70–75 years old, use a slower rate of infusion so as to avoid precipitating pulmonary oedema, but this has to be gauged against the degree of hypotension. Assess, infuse, and reassess again until you have a stable patient.

Central venous pressure (CVP) monitoring
This is primarily used to prevent 'overfilling' (i.e. excessive fluid administration). It should be considered in the elderly, those with chronic liver disease, or a history of heart failure following resuscitation after a large bleed. It is easier to place a central line once the patient has been resuscitated. A rapid drop in CVP (fall >5 cmH$_2$O) may indicate rebleeding, although this may also occur in patients with chronic liver disease due to abnormal venous compliance.

Blood transfusion
Indicated in massive haemorrhage, but not in moderate or minor haemorrhage (e.g. Hb >8 g/dL after fluid resuscitation). Give blood at 1 unit/h until the circulating volume is restored or the CVP is between 5 and 10 cm H$_2$O, as measured from the mid-axilla with the patient supine. 'O'-negative blood can be transfused immediately in massive bleeds. Serum calcium may fall after several units of citrate-containing blood. Give 10 mL (4.5 mEq) of 10% calcium gluconate for every 3–4 units transfused. Supplement magnesium and phosphate, as necessary (often low in alcoholics).

Monitor vital signs
Measure the BP (aim for a systolic BP >100 mmHg) and heart rate (aim for <100 beats/min) every 15 minutes initially, and then less frequently as the patient is stabilized. Although it is often not necessary to catheterize patients, monitor urine output (aim for >30 mL/h), and insert a urinary catheter if urine output is low. Oliguria may indicate inadequate fluid resuscitation. Watch for fluid overload (raised jugular venous pressure (JVP), or CVP, pulmonary oedema). Rapid transfusion may precipitate pulmonary oedema, even before the total lost volume has been replaced. Consider elective intubation in obtunded patients who cannot protect their airway.

Keep the patient nil by mouth
Inform the nursing staff to keep the patient nil by mouth for endoscopy. Inform the surgical team about the patient, especially if they remain unstable following endoscopy. If the patient is suffering a life-threatening bleed, make sure they are admitted to ITU/HDU or a suitable ward. Often such patients are best managed by both medical and surgical teams. If in doubt, seek advice from the senior surgeon on-call.

Commence intravenous (IV) proton pump inhibitors (PPI)
Patients with a significant GI bleed should be treated with a high-dose IV PPI, such as 80 mg omeprazole, followed by an infusion at 8 mg/h for 72 h which was demonstrated to reduce rebleed rates in patients shown to have high-risk lesions (active bleeding, visible vessel, adherent blood clot).

It may be is sensible to start this therapy at presentation, since a significant number of patients will have high-risk lesions. In the UK, pantoprazole 40 mg twice daily (bd) IV is often given. This can be converted to an oral PPI (e.g. omeprazole 20 mg bd) after 24–48 hours.

Management of suspected variceal bleeding
Until endoscopy, it is not possible to establish whether the bleeding is variceal, but you should assume that it is in any patient with signs or history of portal hypertension. Oesophageal and gastric varices develop in patients with portal hypertension of whatever cause. Bleeding from varices is typically vigorous and difficult to control and often occurs in the setting of abnormal clotting, thrombocytopenia, and bacterial infections. A history or stigmata of chronic liver disease or portal vein thrombosis makes it more likely that there is a variceal source of bleeding in which case:

If the patient is stable and not actively bleeding
Upper GI endoscopy
This should be arranged as soon as possible. It is inadvisable to delay endoscopy too long, since emergency endoscopy during acute bleeding is much more difficult, and the incidence of rebleeding is high.

When undertaking resuscitation with blood products and fluids, it is important to avoid overtransfusion, as this may increase portal pressure and the risk of rebleeding (aim for a CVP of 5 cmH$_2$O).

Treat presumed sepsis
Take blood, urine, and (if present) ascites for cultures ± microscopy. Ascitic fluid should be transported in blood culture bottles. Studies have shown that variceal bleeding is often associated with bacterial infections.

Start IV broad-spectrum antibiotics: a third-generation cephalosporin (e.g. ceftriaxone 1 g IV once daily (od)) or ciprofloxacin 400 mg IV stat, then 500 mg bd orally plus amoxicillin (500 mg three times daily (tds)). Treat for 5 days.

If the patient has bled within the last 24 hours, start terlipressin (2 mg initially, and then 1 mg IV 4-hourly for up to 72 hours). If the history suggests that their last episode of bleeding was >24 hours ago and they remain stable, it is probably safe to delay giving terlipressin until an endoscopy has been done, provided it will be carried out within the next 12 hours (see further text).

To prevent hepatic encephalopathy

Give lactulose 10–15 mL every 8 hours orally (PO) to prevent encephalopathy. Use magnesium or phosphate enemas for patients with severe encephalopathy.

To prevent Wernicke's

If the patient is alcoholic or malnourished, start Pabrinex® 1 & 2 IV tds for 3–5 days and oral thiamine at 200 mg PO od.

Active bleeding in the patient with suspected varices

The most important part of the management of these patients is airway protection and restitution of blood volume.

Give terlipressin, a synthetic analogue of vasopressin (2 mg initially, and then 1–2 mg IV every 4 hours for up to 72 hours). This is moderately effective in controlling variceal bleeding. It causes splanchnic vasoconstriction and reduces relative mortality by ~34%. Serious side effects occur in 4%, including cardiac ischaemia and peripheral vasoconstriction, which may produce significant hypertension, skin, and splanchnic ischaemia.

Arrange a therapeutic endoscopy as soon as possible, and continue with blood and volume resuscitation as described previously. Give vitamin K 10 mg IV once only, since it is important to correct any underlying vitamin K deficiency, assuming that the patient is NOT taking warfarin for another indication. Vitamin K normally has little or no effect in patients with cirrhosis. It may be necessary to give fresh frozen plasma (FFP) or platelets to some patients.

The use of somatostatin and octreotide is debated. A recent Cochrane review found that octreotide had no effect on mortality and had a minimal effect on transfusion requirements. Many liver centres do NOT use octreotide, since terlipressin is associated with a reduction in mortality, compared to placebo. If used, somatostatin (250 mcg bolus, followed by 250 mcg/h IVI for 5 days) is normally given.

General management of non-cirrhotic patients with upper GI bleeding

Correct any coagulopathy

For those patients taking warfarin, the risk of reversing anticoagulation should be weighed against the risk of continued bleeding without reversal. In general, active bleeding is more life-threatening than any of the conditions whose risk is increased by reversal of anticoagulation.

The annual risk of embolization in non-anticoagulated patients with prosthetic heart valves is 4% for aortic and 8% for mitral valves, with greater risk with caged ball valves, especially the Starr–Edwards type.

The annual risk of stroke in non-anticoagulated patients with AF is 3–5% (relative risk 2.5 to 3) but is much lower in those <75 years old without comorbidity.

Thrombocytopenia

Patients with active or severe gastrointestinal bleeding with a platelet count <40–50,000/mm^3 should be treated with platelet support (6–12 units of platelets).

Warfarin effect

For patients with prosthetic valves, correct the INR to <1.5 with fresh frozen plasma (2–4 units), or, if stable, inject a low dose of vitamin K (0.5–1 mg IV). This will correct the INR within a few hours. Avoid large doses of vitamin K, as this prolongs the time taken to re-anticoagulate once bleeding has stopped. For patients with prosthetic heart valves, it is important to prescribe antibiotic prophylaxis during endoscopy. For conditions in which the need for anticoagulation is less defined (e.g. anticoagulation for AF), give fresh frozen plasma and low-dose IV vitamin K (1 mg).

Heparin effect

Heparin can be reversed with protamine sulphate (1 mg IV neutralizes 100 units; bolus doses of more than 25 to 50 mg of protamine sulphate are seldom required, as the half-life of heparin is 30 to 60 minutes). Use protamine (1 mg/100 anti-Xa units) to neutralize low molecular weight heparin (LMW), but halve the dose if the LMW heparin was administered >8 h beforehand.

What should I do if the patient continues to bleed despite these simple measures?

There are no hard rules on what to do when patients continue to bleed despite attempts to correct the above. Clearly, the sooner they undergo urgent therapeutic endoscopy, the better. You can only use what is available. Unfortunately, Beriplex® or factor VIIa (see further text) are often not available. Below are various manoeuvres that may help. There are no right answers and no clear guidelines.

Transfusion of large volumes of blood leads to deficiency of various clotting factors, such as fibrinogen. Cryoprecipitate may be required if fibrinogen levels are low, indicative of widespread consumption of clotting factors.

Beriplex® is a mixture of clotting factors II, VII, IX, and X. It can be given to acutely reverse warfarin in massive, life-threatening bleeding: discuss with the haematology team (this treatment is expensive, so there may be reluctance to use it, but it should be requested if needed).

Recombinant factor VIIa (90 mcg/kg every 2 hours until haemostasis is achieved) may have a role in stabilizing the serum prothrombin time in massive variceal bleeding in patients with Child–Pugh B and C cirrhosis (this is an expensive treatment but may be lifesaving).

If the above are unavailable and coagulation needs to be corrected, then consider the following, but there are limited data on efficacy:

Give *aprotonin* if massive, life-threatening bleeding occurs, following thrombolysis for other conditions, (50–100 mL = 0.5–1 MU) as a slow IV bolus, followed by 20 mL/h until bleeding stops.

Tranexamic acid (0.5–1.5 g IV tds or 1–1.5 g tds PO) increases the levels of fibrinogen and can be given when bleeding is difficult to control in patients with renal failure. Likewise, desmopressin (0.3 mcg/kg in 50 mL normal saline (NS) over 30 min) may be useful in these patients by increasing the release of von Willebrand factor multimers from endothelial storage sites. It is said to be particularly effective in renal failure. Its effect lasts for 4 to 24 hours.

Assessment of severity

It is essential to categorize patients at the time of admission into high or low risk of death. Most deaths occur in the elderly with comorbid disease.

High-risk factors include:

- Age >60 years (30% risk of death if >90 years).
- Chronic liver disease.
- Other chronic disease (e.g. cardiac, respiratory, renal).
- Bleeding diathesis.
- Rebleed or bleeding whilst an inpatient for another reason (3-fold mortality).

- Decreased conscious level.
- Shock (systolic BP <100 mmHg in patients <60 years or <120 mmHg in patients >60 years; or heart rate >100).

The Rockall score (see Figure 8.2) can be used once the patient has been endoscoped to determine the mortality risk. Whilst there is much enthusiasm for scoring systems, in practice, they are not used very much, with most clinicians recognizing that a large bleed with a high urea, shock, and melaena is high risk which will require active treatment. Endoscopy allows for more accurate risk stratification but, more importantly, allows for definitive therapy.

Endoscopy

Diagnostic endoscopy
It is important to try and identify patients with portal hypertension, since these patients have a much higher mortality.

Consider 250 mg IV erythromycin
Two controlled studies have now shown that injection of 250 mg erythromycin IV 30–60 minutes before endoscopy gives much better endoscopic views in patients with haematemesis. A clear stomach was observed in 80% of patients given erythromycin, compared to 35% of controls. The use of erythromycin is not standard practice as yet.

Timing of endoscopy
Endoscopy should be performed as soon as possible in patients who need major resuscitation or those who remain haemodynamically unstable (i.e. still shocked after 4 L of fluid resuscitation) or in those in whom variceal bleeding is suspected. In all other patients, it should ideally be done within 12 hours of the bleed (especially in elderly patients or those with comorbidity) and certainly within 24 hours. Patients must be adequately resuscitated before endoscopy.

Contact the senior endoscopist on-call. In working hours liaise with the endoscopy unit, and inform them that you have a patient with a GI bleed who needs urgent endoscopy. Pregnancy or a recent MI are not necessarily contraindications to endoscopy (see Box 8.2). Young patients with an insignificant bleed, normal blood pressure, and normal haemoglobin can often safely be discharged from accident and emergency but should be endoscoped within 1 week.

Consenting the patient
Patients with capacity must provide at least verbal consent. If the bleed is life-threatening, endoscopy can proceed in the absence of consent, as long as the patient has not expressed a current or prior wish not to have the procedure. A doctor should provide consent in patients who lack capacity (in the UK, this is the Consent Form 4 <http://www.dhsspsni.gov.uk/ph_consent_form_4.pdf>).

Sedating the patient
Usually, patients are sedated using a short-acting benzodiazepine, such as midazolam (1–5 mg IV). Oxygen administration with oxygen saturation and pulse rate monitoring is mandatory. At least three trained individuals should be present when the endoscopy is performed. General anaesthesia should be considered for agitated patients, especially if there is a large haemorrhage.

Therapeutic endoscopy
It is important to perform quick, but thorough, endoscopy, and ideally someone experienced should undertake the procedure. Therapy can be applied once the bleeding lesion has been discovered (see following paragraph). The

absence of bleeding suggests mid- or hindgut haemorrhage, which has a lower mortality risk. Further investigations may be warranted in such situations (see section on obscure bleeding). If too much blood is present to determine the bleeding site, a repeat endoscopy after 6–12 hours should be performed, following IV erythromycin administration.

Endoscopic therapy for bleeding peptic ulcers
Bleeding peptic ulcers are the commonest cause of upper GI bleeding, accounting for 35–50% of all cases. The majority are caused by *Helicobacter pylori* whilst NSAIDs are the cause in ~30% of cases. It is said that upper GI bleeding in cirrhotic patients has a non-variceal origin in ~30% of cases. Without endoscopic therapy, there is a high risk of rebleeding in the case of:

- Active bleeding (90%).
- A visible vessel (50%).
- An adherent clot (25–30%).

The endoscopist should inject these lesions quadrantically and centrally with 0.5–1 mL 1/10,000 epinephrine, and also apply a second therapeutic modality (e.g. bipolar coagulation or endoscopic clips, see Box 8.3). This reduces the risk of rebleeding by ~50%. If an adherent clot obscures the bleeding lesion, experienced endoscopists should inject the clot as above before removing it using a 'cold' snare and then apply a second therapy. Low-risk lesions (clean ulcer base ± a red spot) do not require any endoscopic therapy, since their risk of rebleeding is low (<10%).

Endoscopic therapy for varices
Band ligation of the varices is the preferred method for elective variceal obliteration but can be technically more difficult in the setting of acute haemorrhage. In these patients intravariceal injection of sclerosant (e.g. 1 mL ethanolamine) can control the bleeding. However, initial treatment with a sclerosant is usually indicated for gastric varices, which are often harder to obliterate (ethanolamine, thrombin, or glue (cyanocrylate), e.g. histocryl). Serious side effects occur in 7%, mainly retrosternal pain and fever immediately post-injection, with subsequent mucosal ulceration.

Box 8.1 Relative indications for surgery in non-variceal bleeding

- Exsanguinating haemorrhage (too fast to replace)
  - Initial resuscitation with >6 units blood
  - Continued bleeding at >1 unit per 8 hours or
  - Persistent hypotension
- Rebleed in hospital uncontrolled by a second therapeutic endoscopy
- Lower thresholds in the elderly or with lesions at high risk of rebleeding, e.g. posterior duodenal ulcer (DU) with visible vessel or large gastric ulcer
- Special situations, e.g. patients with a rare blood group or patients refusing blood transfusion, should be explored earlier
- It is useful to invite a senior member of the surgical team to attend the endoscopy of patients who may need to undergo surgery

Adapted from Punit S. Ramrakha, Kevin P. Moore, and Amir Sam, *Oxford Handbook of Acute Medicine*, Third Edition, 2010, Box 3.2, page 231, copyright Punit S. Ramrakha and Kevin P. Moore, with permission.

Box 8.2 Risk of endoscopy in pregnancy or post-myocardial infarction

Risks of endoscopy during pregnancy. Guidelines have been published.[1] Endoscopy is safe in pregnancy, but deep sedation should be avoided and have a low threshold for anaesthetic involvement. Be careful of drugs and the fetus.

Risks of endoscopy post-myocardial infarction (MI). The overall risk of cardiovascular complications in upper GI endoscopy is ~0.3%.[2] In 200 patients undergoing upper GI endoscopy within 30 days of an MI, the risk of a significant cardiovascular complication was 7.5% exclusively in unwell patients or patients with ongoing hypotension.[3] There are no clear guidelines for endoscopy in patients within 7 days of an MI. The risks have to be balanced against the risk of no intervention in patients in whom therapeutic endoscopy may be lifesaving. There are data to show that even PEG placement is relatively safe in patients following a recent MI.[4]

[1] Qureshi WE, Rajan E, Adler DG, et al. (2005). ASGE Guideline: Guidelines for endoscopy in pregnant and lactating women. *Gastrointestinal Endoscopy*, 61, 357–62.

[2] Gangi S, Saidi F, Patel K, Johnstone B, Jaeger J, Shine D (2004). Cardiovascular complications after GI endoscopy: occurrence and risks in a large hospital system. *Gastrointestinal Endoscopy*, 60, 679–85.

[3] Cappell MS, Lacovone FM Jr (1999). Safety and efficacy of esophagogastroduodenoscopy after myocardial infarction. *American Journal of Medicine*, 106, 29–35.

[4] Cappell MS, Lacovone FM Jr (1996). The safety and efficacy of percutaneous endoscopic gastrostomy after recent myocardial infarction: a study of 28 patients and 40 controls at four university teaching hospitals. *American Journal of Gastroenterology*, 91, 1599–603.

Box 8.3 Endoscopic therapies

Injection therapy involves injection of epinephrine (1:10,000). Whilst epinephrine is good at achieving haemostasis initially, the rebleeding rate is 18% in the short term. Therefore, endoscopists follow this with either thermal coagulation or placement of a hemoclip (endoclip).

Thermal coagulation involves the application of a contact heater probe to the bleeding ulcer base. Bipolar thermal devices are preferred, as desiccated tissue limits the penetration of alternating current (e.g. 'gold' probe 15 W applied for 6 seconds, repositioned, as necessary). Use 30 J for four pulses before repositioning if using the 'heater' probe (direct current).

Endoclips are effective in Dieulafoy's lesions and small visible vessels but are of limited value for large ulcers.

Argon plasma coagulation (APC) is a thermoablative technique, with a limited penetration of the mucosa. The non-contact nature of application allows large areas to be treated rapidly, in contrast to contact thermal techniques, such as the heater probe. APC also allows the treatment of lesions that are not directly 'en face' or lesions behind folds. It is mainly used to treat gastric antral vascular ectasia (GAVE) (use 40 W).

Fibrin sealant can be injected into a bleeding ulcer. In one trial, this resulted in less rebleeding than injection of a sclerosant (polidocanol) and fewer treatment failures, although the differences were not large. It is not widely used.[1]

A meta-analysis[2] of 16 studies (1990–2002), containing 1,673 patients with severe bleeding stigmata, demonstrated that dual modality endoscopic treatment reduced rebleed and mortality rates from 18.4% to 10.6% and 5.1% to 2.6%, respectively.

[1] Rutgeerts P, Rauws E, Wara P, et al. (1997) Randomised trial of single and repeated fibrin glue compared with injection of polidocanol in treatment of bleeding peptic ulcer. *Lancet* 350, 692–96.

[2] Calvet X, Vergara M, Brullet E, Gisbert JP, Campo R (2004). Addition of a second endoscopic treatment following epinephrine injection improves outcome in high-risk bleeding ulcers. *Gastroenterology*, 126, 441–50.

Box 8.4 If non-variceal haemorrhage is not controlled by endoscopy

Rebleeding usually occurs in the first 24 h (defined as a reduction in haemoglobin concentration of >2 g/dL after allowing for haemodilution; or redevelopment of shock; or a fall in the CVP of >5 cmH$_2$O). It increases the mortality risk threefold (see Rockall score in Figure 8.2); therefore, consider admitting the patient to a high dependency unit. It is more common with ulcers on the incisura or posterior duodenal bulb. **Repeat therapeutic endoscopy** should be performed if the bleeding had been partially controlled, following the initial endoscopy.[1] If peptic ulcer bleeding is not controlled at all, following attempted therapeutic endoscopy, or is not sufficiently controlled, following a second attempt, ask the surgical team whether surgery is indicated. If surgery is declined, ask the interventional radiologists to undertake angiography of the coeliac axis and superior mesenteric artery, with selective embolization of the bleeding vessel. Intra-arterial vasopressin can effectively control haemorrhagic gastritis and is used if the collateral blood supply is poor, following previous surgery. Embolization with a biodegradable, long-acting gelatin sponge is used for other causes of upper GI bleeding, as long as the bleeding is brisk (0.5–1 mL/min). Both are effective in about 70%.

[1] Lau JY, Sung JJ, Lam YH, et al. (1999). Endoscopic treatment compared with surgery in patients with recurrent bleeding after initial endoscopic control of bleeding ulcers. *New England Journal of Medicine*, 340, 751–6.

Management of failed endoscopic therapy

There is no clear definition of endosopic failure for non-variceal bleeding, but, in general, it is regarded as an inability to control bleeding after two attempted therapeutic endoscopies by an experienced endoscopist (see Box 8.4). The indications for surgery are shown in Box 8.1. Continued bleeding from varices should be treated with the placement of a Sengstaken tube (see Box 8.5). If a second endoscopic procedure fails to prevent bleeding from the varices, patients should be referred to a liver unit where either there are more experienced endoscopists for bleeding varices or

Box 8.5 If variceal haemorrhage is not controlled by endoscopy

Severe ongoing bleeding from varices is treated with terlipressin ± balloon tamponade, pending TIPS (see below).

Balloon tamponade. A Sengstaken–Blakemore tube should be inserted if the patient continues to bleed despite therapeutic endoscopy. The tube should be removed from the fridge at the last moment possible to maintain its stiffness. The airway must be protected prior to insertion, which usually requires a general anaesthetic. After insertion, inflate the gastric balloon with 200 mL water, and apply traction. Fix the tube at the mouth by anchoring it between two tongue depressors taped together. The oesophageal balloon should not be inflated, unless the patient is known to be bleeding from a mid-oesophageal ulcer or varix (usually as a result of previous injection sclerotherapy). Arrange a repeat therapeutic endoscopy within 12 hours; otherwise, ischaemic ulceration may occur, a risk that may be increased by the co-administration of terlipressin. Major complications occur in 15%, of which the most lethal is oesophageal rupture.

Transvenous intrahepatic portosystemic shunting (TIPS) is available in specialized units to provide definitive treatment for uncontrolled variceal bleeding. The hepatic veins are cannulated, using a jugular or femoral approach, and an expandable stent is placed between the hepatic veins (low pressure) and the portal venous system (high pressure). The portal pressure should be decompressed to less than 12 mmHg. This has largely superseded surgical management (emergency portocaval shunting or oesophageal transection).

where they can carry out an emergency TIPS procedure. Emergency TIPS is successful in 90% of cases, with a 6-week survival of 60–90%. A recent study showed a marked improvement of survival with early TIPs for variceal bleeding in patients with Child C cirrhosis or persistent bleeding in Child B cirrhosis. Patients were randomized within 24 hours of admission and after endoscopy, to either continued vasoactive drug therapy, followed after 3 to 5 days by treatment with propranolol or nadolol and long-term endoscopic band ligation (EBL), or to treatment with a polytetrafluoroethylene-covered stent within 72 hours (i.e. early TIPS procedure). The 1-year actuarial probability of remaining bleeding-free was 50% in the pharmacotherapy-EBL group vs 97% in the early-TIPS group (P <0.001). The 1-year actuarial survival was 61% in the pharmacotherapy-EBL group vs 86% in the early-TIPS group (P <0.001).

Endoscopic therapy for other conditions

Mallory–Weiss tear
This is characterized by a longitudinal tear in the mucosa at the gastro-oesophageal junction, following severe retching, and is particularly common following large bouts of alcohol. It can be precipitated by any increase in intra-abdominal pressure, such as vomiting, straining at stool, coughing, lifting, or convulsions. Many patients have a hiatus hernia (>40%). The first vomit is usually normal and then becomes bright red. There may be associated back or abdominal pain. Most stop bleeding spontaneously. Endoscopic therapy can be applied, as described for peptic ulcer disease, if bleeding is ongoing at the time of endoscopy. Endoscopic clips may be particularly effective. Tamponade with a Sengstaken–Blakemore tube has been used with very severe bleeding.

Erosive gastritis or oesophagitis
This usually presents as relatively minor bleeds but may be significant in patients with a bleeding diathesis. They may occur due to 'stress' in the critically ill patient or in those with a long-term nasogastric tube. At endoscopy, there is commonly a generalized ooze of blood from the inflamed mucosa. Endoscopic therapy is not beneficial. If the bleeding continues, partial gastric resection may be necessary, but this is very rare. The overall mortality rate is very low.

Ongoing management after the endoscopy
Following endoscopy patients with high-risk lesions or varices should be kept nil by mouth until reviewed the next morning, in case a repeat endoscopy is needed. If stable (no haemoglobin drop and observations stable), they should be fed and possibly discharged 24 hours later. If the endoscopy demonstrates a low-risk lesion, the patient can probably be safely discharged the same day as the endoscopy with anti-ulcer therapy (see Rockall score in Figure 8.2).

Post-discharge management of non-variceal haemorhage
Treat all patients with a proton pump inhibitor (PPI), such as omeprazole 40 mg od for 6–8 weeks. This may need to be continued in patients who had sustained life-threatening bleeding (especially the elderly) and should be continued in those requiring ongoing treatment with steroids, non-steroidals, or aspirin.

Patients with a gastric or duodenal ulceration not associated with NSAID use should receive an H. pylori eradication regimen. In patients taking steroids, non-steroidals, and probably aspirin, a biopsy should be taken at the original endoscopy for the H. pylori urease test. As patients are usually on PPI therapy by this time, also check for H. pylori using another method (e.g. serology, faecal antigen testing). Eradicate H. pylori in those patients found to be colonized.

Repeat endoscopy for gastric ulcers at 6–8 weeks to ensure the ulcer was not malignant. Duodenal ulcers do not usually need to be reviewed endoscopically. Endoscopic surveillance should be considered in those requiring ongoing treatment with steroids, non-steroidals, or aspirin, although, if possible, such treatments should be stopped. Of the NSAIDs, ibuprofen has one of the lowest risks of causing bleeding.

Post-discharge management of variceal haemorrhage
Treat all patients with a PPI, such as omeprazole 40 mg od for 6–8 weeks; this reduces the risk of early loosening of variceal bands.

Banding ligation is normally carried out at weekly intervals until variceal obliteration and then considered at 3-monthly intervals or longer. It is more effective and rapid than injection sclerotherapy (39 days vs 72 days) and has fewer complications (2% vs 22%). Following a banding programme, some centres obliterate any remaining varices with injection sclerotherapy, although this technique is no longer used for the primary obliteration of varices.

Propranolol (e.g. 20 to 40 mg tds PO): this reduces the rate of bleeding and rebleeding from varices and portal hypertensive gastropathy. Aim for a 25% reduction in resting heart rate or a rate of 50–60 beats/min. Ideally, a reduction of portal pressure should be confirmed by measurement of wedged hepatic venous pressure gradient in specialist centres. Do NOT give propranolol to patients with refractory ascites, as this increases mortality in the short to medium term.

TIPS provides a more definite cure, and bleeding tends to recur only when the shunt blocks, but there is an increased incidence of chronic hepatic encephalopathy (about 20%).

Prognosis
Overall mortality of non-variceal bleeding is <10% but can be estimated by the Rockall score. Mortality is reduced by early surgery in high-risk patients. Overall mortality following variceal haemorrhage is 30%. This is highest in those with severe liver disease (Child's grade C). Terlipressin controls bleeding in about 70%, which is increased to about 80–85% if combined with injection sclerotherapy or band ligation. Balloon tamponade has a similar efficacy (see Box 8.5), although it is only a temporary measure.

Uncommon causes of upper GI bleeding
Dieulafoy's lesion
A Dieulafoy's lesion is a dilated aberrant blood vessel, which erodes through the gastric lining in the absence of an ulcer. They are usually located in the upper stomach along the lesser curvature near the oesophagogastric junction and can be hard to locate endoscopically. They are thought to be congenital in origin, but bleeding tends to occur in men with cardiovascular disease, renal disease, or alcohol abuse. Rebleeding is common (10–35%). Hemoclips are said to reduce the risk of rebleeding, but there has only been one randomized study. Others recommend injection of epinephrine with bipolar or heater probe thermal coagulation or banding.

Table 8.1 Risk assessment after acute upper GI bleeding

Variable	0	1	2	3
Age		60–79	>80	
Shock		HR >100	SBP <100	
Comorbidity			CVS; GI cancer	Renal or liver failure or metastases
Endoscopic diagnosis	Mallory–Weiss tear	Other	Malignancy	
Stigmata of recent haemorrhage			Clot or bleeding or visible vessel	

Reproduced from *Gut*, TF Rockall *et al.*, 'Risk assessment after acute upper gastrointestinal haemorrhage', 38, 3, pp. 316–321, copyright 1996, with permission from BMJ Publishing Group Ltd.

Gastric antral vascular ectasia (GAVE)
GAVE or watermelon stomach is a rare cause of GI bleeding. There are longitudinal rows of reddish stripes radiating from the pylorus to the antrum due to the presence of ectatic mucosal vessels. The cause is unknown, but it is more common in cirrhosis or systemic sclerosis. Bleeding is rarely massive. Therapy is by thermal or argon plasma coagulation. It does not respond to TIPS.

Portal hypertensive gastropathy
Bleeding from portal hypertensive gastropathy is rare and is generally due to oozing, rather than haemorrhage from a specific point. The risk of portal hypertensive gastropathy seems to increase post-sclerotherapy. Bleeding can be prevented by TIPS or thermal coagulation.

Haemobilia
Bleeding from the hepatobiliary tract is very rare and suggests hepatic or biliary tract injury, often caused by liver biopsy. Bleeding can occur up to 2 weeks following a procedure. It often causes pain, GI bleeding, and jaundice. Treatment may require surgical resection or angiography. Rarely, bleeding also occurs from the pancreatic duct due to chronic pancreatitis or tumours.

Aorto-enteric fistulae
These rare lesions tend to occur in the third or fourth portion of the duodenum. They cause massive GI bleeding and have a high mortality. The most common cause is secondary to an atherosclerotic aortic aneurysm, usually following its repair with a prosthetic graft which has become infected, but they can occur due to syphilis or tuberculosis. A small 'herald' bleed can occur. Therefore, a low threshold for organizing a CT scan is required in such patients. The vascular team should review the scan, as the changes can be subtle.

Post-ERCP bleeding
This is relatively rare (1–2%) and usually occurs following sphincterotomy. Risk is increased by thrombocytopenia, prolongation of the prothrombin time, and renal failure. It is occasionally life-threatening and should be treated seriously. Patients should be endoscoped and undergo endoscopic therapy with injection of adrenaline (epinephrine) or fibrin sealant or application of a hemoclip. Other therapeutic modalities can be used, but, as a last resort, patients may need angiography or surgery.

Risk scores
Rockall score
This is a validated risk score that predicts mortality. The maximum score is 11 (see Table 8.1).

The Rockall score (see Figure 8.2) can predict patient outcome. For example, patients with scores of 2 or less have a rebleed and mortality rate of 4.3% and 0.1%, respectively. Usually, they can safely be discharged from hospital the same day as the endoscopy.

Blatchford score
The Blatchford score is useful in predicting patients who do not need intervention, in that, if the score is zero, then endoscopic intervention is very unlikely (see Table 8.2). The higher the score, the higher the need for intervention, with at least 30% of patients requiring intervention if the score is 4 or greater.

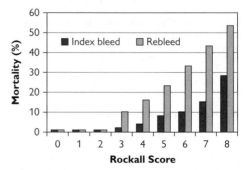

Figure 8.2 The Rockall score. Reproduced from *Gut*, TF Rockall *et al.*, 'Risk assessment after acute upper gastrointestinal haemorrhage', 38, 3, pp. 316–321, copyright 1996, with permission from BMJ Publishing Group Ltd.

Table 8.2 Low-risk upper GI bleeding

Blood urea (mmol/L)	
6.5–8.0	2
8.0–10.0	3
10.0–25.0	4
>25	6
Haemoglobin (men) (g/dL)	
12–13.0	1
10–12.0	3
<10.0	6
Haemoglobin (women)	
10-12.0 g/dL	1
<10 g/dL	6
SBP (mmHg)	
100–109	1
90–99	2
<90	3
Other markers	
HR >100 bpm	1
Presentation with melaena	1
Presentation with syncope	2
Hepatic disease	2
Cardiac failure	2

Reprinted from *The Lancet*, 373, AJ Stanley *et al.*, 'Outpatient management of patients with low-risk upper-gastrointestinal haemorrhage: multicentre validation and prospective evaluation', pp. 42–47. Copyright 2009, with permission from Elsevier.

Further reading

Barkun AN, Bardou M, Kuipers EJ, *et al.* (2010). International consensus recommendations on the management of patients with nonvariceal upper gastrointestinal bleeding. *Annals of Internal Medicine*, **152**, 101–13.

Bernard B, Grangé JD, Khac EN, Amiot X, Opolon P, Poynard T (1999). Antibiotic prophylaxis for the prevention of bacterial infections in cirrhotic patients with gastrointestinal bleeding: a meta-analysis. *Hepatology*, **29**, 1655–61.

Calvet X, Vergara M, Brullet E, Gisbert JP, Campo R (2004). Addition of a second endoscopic treatment following epinephrine injection improves outcome in high-risk bleeding ulcers. *Gastroenterology*, **126**, 441–50

Cannegieter SC, Rosendaal FR, Briët E (1994). Thromboembolic and bleeding complications in patients with mechanical heart valve prostheses. *Circulation*, **89**, 635–41.

Evans G, Luddington R, Baglin T (2001). Beriplex P/N reverses severe warfarin-induced overanticoagulation immediately and completely in patients presenting with major bleeding. *British Journal of Haematology*, **115**, 998–1001.

Frossard JL, Spahr L, Queneau PE, *et al.* (2002). Erythromycin intravenous bolus infusion in acute upper gastrointestinal bleeding: a randomized, controlled, double-blind trial. *Gastroenterology*, **123**, 17–23.

Garcia-Altes A, Jovell AJ, Serra-Prat M, Aymerich M (2000). Management of Helicobacter pylori in duodenal ulcer: a cost-effectiveness analysis. *Alimentary Pharmacology & Therapeutics*, **14**, 1631–8.

García-Pagán JC, Caca K, Bureau C, *et al.* (2010). Early use of TIPS in patients with cirrhosis and variceal bleeding. *New England Journal of Medicine*, **362,** 2370–9.

Gøtzsche PC and Hróbjartsson A (2005). Somatostatin analogues for acute bleeding oesophageal varices. *Cochrane Database of Systematic Reviews*, **1**, CD000193.

Jensen DM, Kovacs TO, Jutabha R, *et al.* (2002). Randomized trial of medical or endoscopic therapy to prevent recurrent ulcer hemorrhage in patients with adherent clots. *Gastroenterology*, **123**, 407–13.

Lau JY, Sung JJ, Lee KK, *et al.* (2000). Effects of intravenous omeprazole on recurrent bleeding after endoscopic treatment of bleeding peptic ulcers. *New England Journal of Medicine*, **343**, 310–6.

National Institute for Health and Clinical Excellence (2012). Acute upper gastrointestinal bleeding: management. NICE clinical guideline 141. <http://www.nice.org.uk/nicemedia/live/13762/59549/59549.pdf>.

Park CH, Sohn YH, Lee WS, *et al.* (2003) The usefulness of endoscopic hemoclipping for bleeding Dieulafoy lesions. *Endoscopy*, **57**, 388–92.

Rockall TA, Logan RF, Devlin HB, Northfield TC (1996). Selection of patients for early discharge or outpatient care after acute upper gastrointestinal haemorrhage. National Audit of Acute Upper Gastrointestinal Haemorrhage. *Lancet*, **347**, 1138–40.

Sanyal AJ, Freedman AM, Luketic VA, *et al.* (1996). Transjugular intrahepatic portosystemic shunts for patients with active variceal hemorrhage unresponsive to sclerotherapy. *Gastroenterology*, **111**, 138–46.

Scottish Intercollegiate Guidelines Network (2008). Guideline 105: Management of acute upper and lower gastrointestinal bleeding. <http://www.sign.ac.uk/guidelines/fulltext/105/>.

Stiegmann GV, Goff JS, Michaletz-Onody PA, *et al.* (1992). Endoscopic sclerotherapy as compared with endoscopic ligation for bleeding esophageal varices. *New England Journal of Medicine*, **326**, 1527–32.

Acute gastroenteritis

Introduction
Acute gastroenteritis may present with vomiting or diarrhoea or both. Food poisoning is an acute attack of abdominal pain, diarrhoea ± vomiting, 1–40 hours after ingesting
contaminated foodstuffs, and lasting 1–7 days. With the
exception of an acute attack of inflammatory bowel disease
and mesenteric ischaemia (see 'Bloody diarrhoea'), the
majority of acute onset diarrhoea has an infective aetiology.
However, drugs or various foods (e.g. sorbitol in sugar-free
sweets) can cause acute diarrhoea, although the latter tends
to be self-limiting (see Table 8.3).
  Diarrhoea is defined as:
- Acute: ≤14 days in duration.
- Persistent diarrhoea: >14 days in duration.
- Chronic: >30 days in duration.

  The major causes of acute infectious diarrhoea include
viruses, bacteria, and rarely protozoa, although, in most
cases, the cause remains undiagnosed. Bacterial causes
account for the majority of severe diarrhoea. Thus, nearly
90% of cases of acute diarrhoea associated with >4 stools
per day are due to bacterial organisms, most commonly E.
coli. Persistent diarrhoea is most frequently associated with
Giardia, Cryptosporidium, Entamoeba histolytica, or Cyclospora
infection.
  Investigation and culture of stools should be carried out if
there are any of the following:
- Profuse watery diarrhoea with signs of hypovolaemia.
- Passage of several small-volume stools containing blood
  and mucus per day.
- Bloody diarrhoea.
- Fever >38°C.
- Passage of >6 unformed stools for >48 h.
- Recent use of antibiotics.
- Severe diarrhoea in pregnancy.
- The elderly.

  Take a full history, including ingestion of unusual or unpasteurized foods and whether relations or friends are affected.
  Symptoms that begin within 6 hours suggest ingestion of
a pre-formed toxin, such as Staphylococcus aureus or Bacillus
cereus toxin.

Table 8.3 Differential diagnosis of acute diarrhoea

Common	
Gastroenteritis (bacterial, viral, protozoal)	Food intolerance/allergy (e.g. lactase deficiency)
Clostridium difficile diarrhoea (pseudomembranous colitis)	Drugs, e.g. ACE-I, mycophenolate, colchicine
Inflammatory bowel disease	
Uncommon	
Coeliac disease	Pancreatic insufficiency
Tumour (benign or malignant)	Bile salt enteropathy
Carcinoid syndrome	Hyperthyroidism
Bacterial overgrowth	Autonomic neuropathy

Symptoms that begin at 8 to 16 hours suggest infection
with Clostridium perfringens.
  Symptoms that begin at more than 16 hours may be secondary to viral or bacterial infection (e.g., contamination of
food with enterotoxigenic or enterohaemorrhagic E. coli).
  Syndromes that begin with diarrhoea, but progress to
fever and more systemic complaints, such as headache,
muscle aches, and neck stiffness, may suggest infection
with Listeria monocytogenes.

Presenting features
Ask specifically about:
- Recent eating habits, especially restaurants and food prepared by caterers. Anyone else (e.g. family/friends) with
  similar symptoms?
- Time interval between eating any suspicious substance
  and onset of symptoms. Early onset of vomiting or
  diarrhoea (i.e. 6–12 h) suggests ingestion of pre-formed
  toxin (e.g. Staphylococcus exotoxin). Enterotoxin-
  producing organisms may take 1–3 days to produce
  symptoms.
- Recent travel (i.e. associated with enterotoxigenic E. coli,
  Salmonella, Giardia, or amoeba)?
- Recent medication, including antibiotics (i.e. associated
  with C. difficile)?
- Past medical history, including gastric surgery or immunosuppression (e.g. drugs or HIV).
- Anal intercourse increases the risk of amoebiasis, giardiasis, shigellosis, rectal syphilis, rectal gonorrhoea,
  Chlamydia trachomatis, and herpes simplex virus (HSV)
  infection of rectum and perianal area.
- The gross appearance of the diarrhoea may help: frank
  bloody stool, Campylobacter or Shigella; watery, 'rice-
  water stool', classically secretory diarrhoea due to cholera, enterotoxigenic E. coli, or neuroendocrine tumours.
  Typhoid produces greenish 'pea-soup' diarrhoea.
- Abdominal pain may be present, usually cramp-like, or
  tenesmus.
- Fever: common with the severe bacterial diarrhoeas and
  acute exacerbations of Crohn's or ulcerative colitis.

When to use antibiotics early
Unless shiga toxin-producing E. coli is suspected, it is reasonable to give antibiotics (e.g. ciprofloxacin) to all patients
with an increased risk of fatal or severe diarrhoea. These
include frail elderly patients with achlorhydria (including patients on PPIs, such as omeprazole), inflammatory bowel
disease, poor haemodynamic reserve, or the immunocompromised.

Investigations
See Table 8.4.

General approach to treat acute diarrhoea
See Table 8.5.

Travellers' diarrhoea
Travel through developing countries is commonly associated with self-limiting acute diarrhoeal illness transmitted
through food and water. The most frequent pathogen is
enterotoxigenic E. coli (40% of cases). The illness lasts 3–5
days with nausea, watery diarrhoea, and abdominal cramps.
Oral rehydration is usually sufficient. Antimotility agents

Table 8.4 Investigations for acute diarrhoea

FBC	↑ WBC; ↑ haematocrit (dehydration)
U&E	↑ urea (dehydration); ↓ K$^+$
Blood cultures	Systemic infection may occur
Stool cultures	Fresh samples, mandatory for wet mount microscopy for ova, cysts and parasites, culture, and antibiotic sensitivities. WBC in stool implies intestinal inflammation (mucosal invasion, toxin, inflammatory bowel disease, ischaemic colitis)
Clostridium difficile toxin	Specifically request this for all patients who have recently taken antibiotics
Sigmoidoscopy and rectal biopsy	Useful for persistent bloody diarrhoea (>4–5 days) without diagnosis or improvement

(e.g. loperamide) may be used with caution. Antibiotic treatment (ciprofloxacin 500 mg bd) may help patients with more protracted illness. Alternatives include doxycycline or co-trimoxazole. Diarrhoea that persists for more than 7 days requires further investigation, including stool microscopy and culture, serology, sigmoidoscopy, and biopsy (see Table 8.4). A 3–5-day course of a broad-spectrum antibiotic, such as ciprofloxacin, may terminate the illness.

Norovirus and viral gastroenteritis

In addition to diarrhoea, upper respiratory tract infection (URTI)-like symptoms, abdominal cramps, headache, and fever may occur. The causative agent is usually not found, but many viruses can be implicated (e.g. echovirus, norovirus, and adenoviruses). It tends to be a self-limiting illness (3–5 days).

Management

Management with oral fluids along with restricting solid foods and dairy product intake usually suffice.

Norovirus (formerly termed the Norwalk agent) is an RNA virus that is thought to be responsible for around 50–85% of non-bacterial outbreaks of gastroenteritis around the world. It is probably responsible for most food-borne outbreaks of gastroenteritis in the western world and affects people of all ages. Noroviruses are transmitted directly from person to person and indirectly via contaminated water and food. They are highly contagious, and very low exposure can lead to illness. Other causes included the rotavirus, as well as adenovirus and astrovirus, with rotavirus

Table 8.5 General approach to treat acute diarrhoea

Severity of symptoms	Management
Mild (1–3 stools/day)	Oral fluids only
Moderate (3–5 stools/day)	Oral fluids, loperamide
Severe (>6 stools/day, fever)	Fluids (± IVI), antimicrobial agent

Note: avoid using loperamide, unless you have excluded infectious causes of diarrhoea. IVI, intravenous infusion.

predominating in children. Transmission occurs through ingestion of contaminated food and water and by person-to-person spread. Transmission is predominantly faecal-oral but may be airborne due to aerosolization of vomit. The viruses continue to be shed for up to several weeks after symptoms have subsided.

Following infection, there is incomplete and temporary immunity to norovirus. Outbreaks of norovirus infection often occur in closed or semi-closed communities where the infection spreads very rapidly, either by person-to-person transmission or through contaminated food.

Symptoms appear after 1–2 days, with either febrile symptoms and diarrhoea or more constitutional symptoms, such as vomiting, headache, diarrhoea, myalgia, and lethargy. There is no treatment. Patients should be isolated to prevent cross-infection.

Bacterial gastroenteritis

E. coli is the head of the bacterial family Enterobacteriaceae, the enteric bacteria, which are facultative anaerobic Gram-negative rods that live in the intestinal tracts of man. The commensal *E. coli* strains that inhabit the large intestine of man comprise <1% of the total bacterial mass. Over 700 serotypes of *E. coli* are recognized, based on O, H, and K antigens. Thus, the serotype O157:H7 (O refers to somatic antigen; H refers to flagellar antigen) is uniquely responsible for causing haemolytic uraemic syndrome (HUS). Five classes (virotypes) of *E. coli* that cause diarrhoeal illness are recognized: enterotoxigenic *E. coli* (ETEC), enteroinvasive *E. coli* (EIEC), enterohaemorrhagic *E. coli* (EHEC), enteropathogenic *E. coli* (EPEC), and enteroaggregative *E. coli* (EAEC).

Enterotoxigenic E. coli (ETEC)

ETEC is an important cause of diarrhoea in travellers to underdeveloped countries. The symptoms range from minor discomfort to a severe cholera-like syndrome without fever. ETEC are acquired by ingestion of contaminated food and water. ETEC may produce a heat-labile enterotoxin (LT) or a heat stable toxin (ST) that is resistant to boiling for 30 minutes.

Enteroinvasive E. coli (EIEC)

EIEC resemble *Shigella* in their mechanism of action and the clinical illness they produce. EIEC penetrate and multiply within epithelial cells of the colon, causing widespread cell destruction. The clinical syndrome is identical to *Shigella* dysentery and includes a dysentery-like diarrhoea with fever. Like *Shigella*, EIEC are invasive organisms. They do not produce any toxins. The primary source for EIEC appears to be infected humans.

Enteropathogenic E. coli (EPEC)

EPEC induce a profuse watery, sometimes bloody, diarrhoea. They are a leading cause of infantile diarrhoea in developing countries. Outbreaks are linked to contaminated drinking water as well as some meat products. Enteroaggregative *E. coli* (EAEC) are associated with persistent diarrhoea in young children.

Enterohaemorrhagic E. coli (EHEC)

EHEC are the primary cause of haemorrhagic colitis or bloody diarrhoea, which can progress to the potentially fatal haemolytic uraemic syndrome (HUS). Infection is usually from contaminated meat/burgers. EHEC are characterized by the production of verotoxin or shiga toxins. O157:H7 is the commonest cause for haemolytic uraemic syndrome. HUS complicates up to 9% of EHEC infections. The incubation period is ~5 days. Stools become bloody over 24–48 hours, secondary to a diffuse colitis. Most patients recover over 5–7 days without treatment. However, some, especially children, may go on to develop HUS with tiredness, microangiopathic anaemia, thrombocytopenia, renal failure, and encephalopathy. Most recover with supportive care. Antibiotics are relatively contraindicated, as some antibiotics are thought to increase shiga toxin production and exacerbate or cause the development of HUS.

Salmonella spp. may produce acute gastroenteritis (e.g. *S. enteritidis*, ~70–80% of cases), enteric fever (*S. typhi* and *S. typhimurium*), or asymptomatic carriage. Acute gastroenteritis often occurs in epidemics and is derived from poultry, eggs or egg products, and occasionally pets (e.g. terrapins). Symptoms occur 8–48 hours after ingestion, with headache, vomiting (worse than either *Shigella* or *Campylobacter*), fever, and diarrhoea lasting 2–4 days (rarely bloody with mucus). Reactive arthritis may occur (e.g. in HLA-B27-positive patients).

The involvement of *Salmonella enterica* (serotypes *typhi* and *paratyphi*) in enteric fever (typhoid fever) is discussed below in the section on 'Enteric fever'.

Clostridium perfringens (type A)
This accounts for 15–25% of cases of bacterial food poisoning. Spores are heat-resistant and may germinate during reheating or slow cooking of meats. Enterotoxin is released when sporulation occurs in the intestine. Incubation occurs over 8–22 hours. Symptoms include diarrhoea, abdominal pain, and nausea (although vomiting is rare). Fever does not occur. It usually lasts 12–24 hours. Management is supportive.

Campylobacter
These infections are common (5–10% of patients with acute diarrhoea). The incubation period is 3–7 days, with symptoms lasting for 1–2 weeks. Presentation often follows eating contaminated poultry. Symptoms include a flu-like illness, followed by headache, myalgia, abdominal pain (continuous, then colicky), diarrhoea, and occasionally rectal bleeding. Rarely, it is complicated by reactive arthritis (1–2%), Guillain–Barré syndrome, or Reiter's syndrome. Management is supportive, as it is usually self-limiting in <5 days. Active treatment is with either erythromycin or tetracycline therapy. Antidiarrhoeals are contraindicated.

Staphylococcus aureus
Staphylococcus aureus (2–5% of cases) can multiply at room temperature in foods rich in carbohydrates and salt (dairy products, cold meats, mayonnaise). A heat-stable exotoxin produces nausea, vomiting, and diarrhoea 1–6 hours after ingestion. Fever is uncommon. Treatment is supportive.

Bacillus cereus
This is associated with slow-cooking foods and reheated rice (fast food takeaways). It produces a toxin that causes vomiting within 1–5 hours, and diarrhoea 8–16 hours later. Treatment is supportive.

Vibrio parahaemolyticus
This produces epigastric pain (compared with those above), diarrhoea, vomiting, and fever 12–18 hours after ingestion of raw seafood (shellfish). Symptoms may last up to 5 days. *Vibrio cholerae* is uncommon in Western nations. It produces profuse secretory diarrhoea. The disease is usually self-limiting (i.e. 5–7 days), but tetracyclines may be used.

Yersinia enterocolitica
This has an incubation period of 4–10 days after contact with infected animals, water, or ice cream. Symptoms include diarrhoea (80%), abdominal pain (80%), fever (40%), bloody stool in 10%, mesenteric adenitis, lymphadenopathy, and reactive arthritis. It is diagnosed by serology, rather than culture. Management is supportive.

Enteric fever (typhoid fever)
Epidemiology and presentation
Salmonella enterica serotype *typhi* and serotype *paratyphi* (less severe) have a widespread distribution, including Africa, South America, and the Indian subcontinent. Typhoid fever has an incubation period of 5–21 days, and presents as a febrile illness 5 to 21 days after ingestion of the causative microorganism (i.e. *Salmonella enterica* serotype *typhi* and serotype *paratyphi*) in contaminated food or water. It is very rare to develop enteric fever >1 month after return from an endemic area. Untreated mortality is 10–15%. However, with adequate therapy, mortality is <1% in the UK. The relapse rate is 1–7%.

Symptoms develop in stages.

- Week 1 is characterized by rising fever and bacteraemia. Non-specific symptoms (e.g. anorexia, myalgia, headache, malaise, fever, chills, and sweats) are common. Remittent temperature gradually rising during the first week to >40°C with a relative bradycardia.
- Week 2 is associated with abdominal pain and rash (i.e. rose spots, faint pink macules on the trunk and abdomen). Rose spots are 2–4 mm erythematous maculopapular lesions, blanch with pressure, and occur in crops of ~10 lesions on the upper abdomen, lasting only a few hours. They occur in 10–30% of cases and are easily missed. Abdominal pain (30–40%), diarrhoea and vomiting (40–60%), or constipation (10–50%) may all be seen.
- Week 3: an acute abdomen may occur in the later stages (e.g. perforation of bowel). Splenomegaly (40–60%), hepatomegaly (20–40%), and intestinal bleeding may develop.
- Respiratory symptoms are common, including sore throat and cough.
- Neurological manifestations, including encephalopathy, coma and meningism (± seizures), are seen in 5–10% of cases.
- A fulminant, toxaemic form occurs in about 5–10% of cases, with rapid deterioration in cardiovascular, renal, hepatic, and neurological function. In other patients, onset may be insidious. In the first 7–10 days after infection, bacteraemia occurs with seeding into the Peyer's patches of the gut, leading to ulceration and necrosis (weeks 2–3).

Investigations
- During the initial week of illness the white cell count (WBC) may be increased or decreased or normal. There may be elevated hepatic enzymes. Blood cultures are positive in 80–90% of cases.
- During the second and third weeks of illness, anaemia, leucocytosis, and thrombocytopenia may occur due to marrow suppression. Blood cultures become negative, whilst urine and stool cultures become positive. Marrow culture may be positive. Abdominal X-rays and imaging are indicated if there is abdominal pain.
- Serology is unhelpful at discriminating active infection from past exposure or vaccination.

Complications
Complications are all uncommon with prompt diagnosis and therapy.

- Toxaemia: Acute complications include hyperpyrexia, renal and hepatic dysfunction, bone marrow failure, and myocarditis.
- Gastrointestinal: Late complications due to breakdown in Peyer's patches, including gastrointestinal haemorrhage and perforation.
- Metastases: Meningitis, endocarditis, osteomyelitis, liver/spleen.
- Chronic carriage: The development of a chronic carrier state is increased in the elderly, immunocompromised, and patients with gallstones. Chronic carriage occurs in 1–3% beyond 1 year.

Management
Enteric fever is usually self-limiting after 2–5 days, and treatment is supportive for most cases. Some antibiotics can prolong carriage of the illness and make clinical relapse more likely.

- Supportive care. If toxaemic, admit to ICU. A central venous line to monitor central venous pressure (CVP) may be required to manage fluid balance. Insert a urinary catheter as renal support may be indicated.
- Antibiotics. Multiple drug resistance has become a problem, and ampicillin and amoxicillin (4–6 g/day + probenecid 2 g/day) can no longer be used for empirical treatment. Quinolones (e.g. ciprofloxacin, 750 mg bd orally for 14 days or 400 mg bd IV) may be used, but resistance has been described, and ceftriaxone 2 g daily is an alternative until sensitivities are known. If the organism is sensitive to the antibiotic used, then 4 weeks' administration will clear the organism in 80–90% of patients, falling to 20–50% if the patient has gallstones. Cholecystectomy may eradicate carriage but is not usually indicated if carriage is asymptomatic.
- Steroids are indicated for the severe toxaemic form. They have reduced acute mortality but with a small increase in relapses. Give high-dose dexamethasone 3 mg/kg, followed by 1 mg/kg 6-hourly for eight doses.
- Surgery is essential for bowel perforation (add metronidazole).
- Infection control. These cases are notifiable. Spread is faecal/oral, and individuals should not prepare food until follow-up stool cultures (off antibiotics) are negative.

Giardiasis

Giardia lamblia (syn. *Giardia intestinalis*) is a flagellate protozoan that colonizes the lumen of the small intestine. It is acquired by ingesting cysts of the parasite, typically in water or food, with faeco-oral transmission. Strains of the parasite that can infect humans are harboured by various mammals, including domestic dogs and cattle.

Risk factors include recent travel, immunosuppression, homosexuality, and achlorhydria. Clinical features include watery diarrhoea, abdominal discomfort and distension, weight loss, and malabsorption. The infection is typically persistent and severe in individuals with genetic impairment of antibody production. Giardiasis often leads to a chronic diarrhoeal illness.

Diagnosis is by faecal examination for evidence of *G. intestinalis* infection, including: (1) cysts—by microscopy, including immunofluorescence microscopy with fluorescent antibodies; (2) antigen—by enzyme-linked immunoassay; or (3) DNA—by polymerase chain reaction (PCR) amplification. If negative, consider a blind therapeutic trial.

Management
Metronidazole is the treatment of choice, 400 mg tds for 5 days orally. Alternatives include tinidazole (2 g single dose) or nitazoxanide 500 mg bd for 3 days, or quinacrine 100 mg tds for 5 days. Lactose intolerance post-infection may persist for up to 6 weeks.

Microsporidiosis

Microsporidia are obligate intracellular parasites. Spores are shed into the environment by infected hosts and infect others. HIV-infected patients and the immunocompromised are most susceptible to infection.

Clinical features include watery diarrhoea, weight loss, and occasionally fat malabsorption in HIV-infected patients with intestinal microsporidiosis. Symptoms of sinusitis, cough, and dyspnoea have been reported in patients with microsporidian infection of the paranasal sinuses and respiratory tract.

Microsporidia infection of the conjunctiva and corneal epithelium causes keratoconjunctivitis sicca (i.e. sensation of a foreign body in the eye, with ocular discomfort and redness, photophobia, blurred vision ± reduced visual acuity). Infection of the cornea reduces visual acuity ± corneal ulceration. Clinical features in patients with cerebral microsporidiosis include headache, cognitive impairment, nausea, vomiting, and epileptic seizures. Symptoms of myositis (i.e. muscle pain, tenderness, weakness, and wasting) have been described in patients with microsporidian infection of skeletal muscles.

Bloody diarrhoea
Causes
- Acute infectious colitis:
  - Pseudomembranous colitis.
  - Bacillary dysentery (*Shigella* spp.).
  - Salmonellosis.
  - *Campylobacter.*
  - Haemorrhagic colitis (shiga-like toxin-producing *E. coli*).
- Inflammatory bowel disease (IBD; for example, ulcerative colitis (UC) or Crohn's disease).

The causes of lower GI bleeding include:
- Diverticular disease (30%).
- Gastroenteritis (15%).
- Colonic ulcers (10%).
- Anorectal (e.g. haemorrhoids, anal fissures, rectal ulcers) (10%).
- Neoplasia (e.g. polyps and cancers) (7%).
- Ischaemia (5%).
- Small bowel bleed (5%).
- Inflammatory bowel disease (3%).
- Angiodysplasia (1%).
- Radiation colitis (1%).
- Rectal varices (1%).
- Other (10%).
  See Figure 8.3.

Presenting features
- Ask about the duration of symptoms and recent eating habits. Have others been affected? Discuss recent travel (enterotoxigenic *E. coli*, *Salmonella*, *Giardia*, or amoeba) and medications, including antibiotics (i.e. associated with *C. difficile* infection).

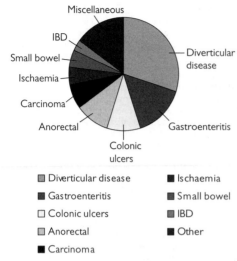

Figure 8.3　Causes of lower GI bleeding.

- The gross appearance of the stool may help. Inflammatory bowel disease can result in rectal bleeding (fresh red blood) in patients with disease largely confined to the rectum and sigmoid colon. Diffuse disease tends to be associated with diarrhoea. Infectious colitis results in frank bloody stools (e.g. *Campylobacter* or *Shigella*).
- Abdominal pain may be present: usually cramp-like or tenesmus.
- Vomiting is uncommon in acute inflammatory bowel disease.
- Systemic features, such as general malaise and lethargy, dehydration, electrolyte imbalance, or fever, are seen with the severe bacterial diarrhoeas and acute exacerbations of Crohn's disease or UC. Skin, joints, and eyes may be involved in either IBD or following acute infection.
- Previous altered bowel habit, weight loss, smoking history, vascular disease (mesenteric infarction) and mesenteric angina may be relevant.

Examination
Look for:
- Fever, signs of dehydration (e.g tachycardia, postural hypotension), abdominal distension. Abdominal tenderness or rebound over affected colon (e.g. IBD) may indicate colonic dilatation or perforation. An abdominal mass may indicate tumour or inflammatory mass.
- Mouth ulcers and perianal disease are common in active IBD.
- Erythema nodosum and pyoderma gangrenosum occur in IBD; *Yersinia* may produce erythema nodosum. Rose spots indicate typhoid fever.
- Joint involvement (often an asymmetrical, non-deforming synovitis, involving large joints of the lower limbs) may occur in active IBD, but also in infectious colitis (e.g. *Campylobacter*, *Yersinia*).
- Uveitis is associated with both IBD and acute infectious colitis.

Investigations
- Microbiology: Stool M,C&S, blood cultures, *Clostridium difficile* toxin
- Sigmoidoscopy: May help to distinguish between acute infectious colitis and IBD (increased risk of perforation during colonoscopy)
- Imaging: Plain AXR may help monitor colonic dilatation. Contrast studies are contraindicated in the acute phase.

Practice point
- Always test for *C. difficile* in patients with new-onset bloody diarrhoea.
- Unexplained extreme leucocytosis (e.g. WBC >35,000), consider *Clostridium difficile* infection.

Clostridum difficile
Pseudomembranous colitis is caused by two necrolytic toxins (A and B) produced by *Clostridium difficile*. It is the commonest cause of hospital-acquired diarrhoea. Infection typically follows antibiotic therapy. Diarrhoea may occur during, or up to, 4 weeks following cessation of treatment and may recur despite successful treatment.

Symptoms
Diarrhoea is usually profuse, watery, and without blood (may be bloody in ~5%). It is commonly associated with abdominal cramps and tenderness, fever, and an elevated white cell count.

Diagnosis
Diagnosis is based on detection of *Clostridium difficile* toxin in the stool. Culture of the organism itself is unhelpful; ~5% of healthy adults carry the organism. Sigmoidoscopy is not diagnostic but may show mucosal inflammation, together with multiple yellow plaques.
Note: occasionally patients with *C. difficile* infection exhibit marked increases in the white blood count (e.g. >40,000), and the patient may have few symptoms.

Management
Patients should be isolated and barrier-nursed. Rehydrate, and correct electrolyte abnormalities. Mild disease responds to oral metronidazole (500 mg tds). Oral vancomycin (250 mg qds) for 7–14 days is an alternative. Severe disease requires intravenous therapy. Faecal transplant has emerged as the optimal therapy for this condition. Complications include toxic megacolon and colonic perforation.

Bacterial dysentery
This is due to infection with *Shigella* (*S. dysenteriae, S. flexneri, S. boydii, S. sonnei*) or some shigella-like *E. coli* (0157:H7). Transmission is by the faeco-oral route.

Symptoms
- It may cause a spectrum of illness from mild diarrhoea to severe systemic illness between 1 and 7 days following exposure.
- Fever (usually resolves in 3–4 days).
- Abdominal cramps with tenesmus.
- Watery diarrhoea, nausea, and vomiting (which usually resolves by day 7). Bloody diarrhoea occurs later (after 24–72 hours) due to invasion of the mucosa.
- Diagnosis is by stool culture. *E. coli* infections may be complicated by haemolytic uraemic syndrome.

Management
- Patients may require intravenous fluid replacement.
- Antibiotics should be reserved for the most severe cases. Ampicillin (250 mg PO qds for 5–10 days) is usually effective, but, in resistant cases, co-trimoxazole or ciprofloxacin may be used.
- Antimotility agents, such as loperamide and codeine, are contraindicated, as they prolong carriage and worsen symptoms.

Amoebic dysentery
Entamoeba histolytica can produce intermittent diarrhoea or a more severe illness that resembles inflammatory bowel disease (see also Chapter 6). There is an increased risk in homosexuals and in those with recent travel to Third World countries. It is transmitted by the faeco-oral route.

Symptoms
- Diarrhoea or loose stool (± blood), abdominal discomfort, and mild fever. In severe cases, liver abscess may occur.
- Fulminant attacks present abruptly with high fever, cramping abdominal pain, and profuse bloody diarrhoea.
- Marked abdominal tenderness may be present.
- Diagnosis is made by identifying amoebic cysts on stool microscopy.
- May be complicated by late development of amoebic liver abscess.

Treatment
- Initial therapy is aimed at replacement of fluid, electrolytes, and blood loss, with eradication of the organism.
- In acute invasive intestinal amoebiasis oral metronidazole (800 mg tds for 5–10 days) is the treatment of choice. Tinidazole (2 g daily for 2–3 days) is also effective. This should be followed with oral diloxanide furoate (500 mg tds for 10 days) to destroy gut cysts.
- Metronidazole (or tinidazole) and diloxanide furoate are also effective for liver abscesses. Ultrasound (USS) guided aspiration may help to improve penetration of the drugs and shorten the illness.
- Diloxanide furoate is the treatment of choice for asymptomatic patients with *E. histolytica* cysts in the stool, as metronidazole and tinidazole are relatively ineffective.

Further reading
Thomas PD, Forbes A, Green J, *et al.* (2003). Guidelines for the investigation of chronic diarrhoea, 2nd edition. *Gut,* **52** (Suppl V), v1–15.

World Gastroenterology Organisation. Acute diarrhoea. <http://www.worldgastroenterology.org/assets/.../guidelines/01_acute_diarrhoea.pdf>.

Jaundice

Assessment

The presence of jaundice generally requires urgent investigation and diagnosis. It may herald the onset of a severe hepatitis and acute liver failure or it may indicate an obstructive jaundice which can be complicated by cholangitis and septicaemia. Drug-induced hepatitis leading to jaundice is associated with a 10% mortality, and any potential drugs should be stopped immediately. Pancreatic or biliary carcinoma (20%), gallstone disease (13%), and alcoholic liver cirrhosis (10%) are the most frequent causes of jaundice. Gilbert's syndrome (present in 5% of the population) causes unconjugated hyperbilirubinaemia, although the level of jaundice rarely exceeds 80 micromoles/L and other liver function tests are usually normal, unless there is coexisting fatty liver disease (common) or other liver pathology.

History

- Non-specific symptoms include anorexia, pruritus, malaise, lethargy, drowsiness, confusion, or coma.
- Dark urine and pale stools may be features of either obstructive jaundice or hepatitis.
- Colicky right upper quadrant (RUQ) pain, previous biliary colic, or known gallstones suggests gallstone disease. Fever, rigors, abdominal pain, and fluctuating jaundice should raise the suspicion of cholangitis. Painless jaundice and weight loss suggest pancreatic or bile duct malignancy.
- Take a detailed drug history, including homeopathic or proprietary preparations. Ask specifically about the use of paracetamol and alcohol. Be aware of inadvertent paracetamol overdose in chronic alcoholics.
- Risk factors for viral hepatitis include IV drug use, unprotected sex and travel. There is an increased risk of viral hepatitis from blood transfusion, unprotected anal sex, ingestion of shellfish, and in patients from Eastern Europe or Asia.
- Ask about a history of gallstones, including family history (e.g. hereditary spherocytosis).

Examination

- Note the degree of jaundice, and look for stigmata of chronic liver disease (spider naevi or telangiectasia, palmar erythema, Dupuytren's contractures, etc.). Lymphadenopathy may reflect malignancy.
- Hepatic encephalopathy results in falling conscious level and a liver flap and suggests chronic liver disease.
- Note the blood pressure: the mean arterial pressure (signified by low diastolic pressure) falls with liver failure, leading to oliguria or shock.
- Examine for pleural effusions (may occur with ascites).
- Examine the abdomen for ascites, hepatomegaly, splenomegaly (secondary to portal hypertension or intravascular haemolysis), or masses.
- Test the urine for bilirubin. Absent bilirubin in a jaundiced patient suggests Gilbert's or haemolysis.

Practice points

1. The urine is dark in both hepatitic and cholestatic jaundice.
2. Itching suggests either extrahepatic (e.g. gallstones or pancreatic mass) or intrahepatic cholestasis (e.g. primary biliary cirrhosis (PBC) or primary sclerosing cholangitis (PSC)).

3. Severe haemolysis, sepsis with disseminated intravascular coagulation (DIC), or rhabdomyolysis can mimic an acute severe hepatitis.
4. Ischaemic hepatitis occurs when there is hypotension in a hypoxic patient, with a raised jugular venous pressure (JVP) and congested liver.
5. The only causes of a very high transaminase (>10,000 U/L) are paracetamol overdose, herpes simplex hepatitis, and severe hepatic ischaemia.
6. A very high bilirubin, with other liver function tests being nearly normal, include massive haemolysis (usually sickle cell disease), Weil's disease, or intra-abdominal sepsis.
7. Severe alcoholic hepatitis may have a normal alanine transaminase (ALT), although the aspartate transaminase (AST) is usually elevated (60–200 U/L), and clotting is often deranged. The transaminases are never >400 U/L in alcoholic hepatitis, and rarely >200 U/L, and the AST always exceeds the ALT.
8. Jaundice in middle-aged women with high transaminases (>2,000 U/L) suggests autoimmune or non-A non-B hepatitis.
9. Acute hepatitis A can cause a marked fever (40°C).
10. Muscle injury or excessive exercise can increase both AST and ALT. Rhabdomyolysis is often mistaken for liver disease, since it may also cause mild jaundice.

The investigations in Tables 8.6 and 8.7 will delineate between a hepatitic cause of jaundice or cholestasis. Haemolysis is a rare cause of jaundice, without being obvious. Imaging will determine whether there is biliary obstruction, portal hypertension, or a pancreatic mass.

Table 8.6 Urgent investigations for jaundice

U&E, LFTs	Exclude renal failure (hepatorenal syndrome). Determine whether pattern of LFTs suggest cholestasis or hepatitis or are non-specific.
Glucose	Diabetes is common in haemochromatosis or pancreatic carcinoma; hypoglycaemia occurs in acute liver failure.
PT	Raised in severe liver injury or DIC.
FBC	Decreased platelet count (chronic liver disease with hypersplenism, alcoholism, paracetamol overdose, or malaria, etc.); leucocytosis (sepsis, alcoholic hepatitis).
Urinalysis	Absence of bilirubin in the urine in a jaundiced patient suggests haemolysis or Gilbert's or a conjugation defect.
CXR	Tumour or metastases. Pleural effusions are associated with ascites.
USS scan, CT/MRI scan	If the patient is unwell or septic, exclude biliary obstruction which may require urgent decompression. Note spleen size (portal hypertension) and any masses in the liver.
Paracetamol levels	If overdose is suspected or possible. Paracetamol overdose may cause very high transaminase levels (>10,000 U/L).

Table 8.7 Semi-urgent investigations for jaundice

Viral serology	Anti-hepatitis A IgM, HBsAg and anti-HBc, anti-HCV, anti-HEV, EBV, CMV serology.
Immunology	ANA, ANCA, anti-smooth muscle antibodies (autoimmune hepatitis, sclerosing cholangitis), anti-mitochondrial antibodies (primary biliary cirrhosis), and immunoglobulins.
Ferritin, iron	Ferritin increases in any acute inflammatory disease (e.g. alcoholic hepatitis).

Box 8.6 and Figure 8.4 give an approximation of the relative frequency of different causes of jaundice. Inner cities will see more viral hepatitis. The presence of a high bilirubin, but normal or modestly elevated liver enzymes, raises the possibility of Gilbert's syndrome, with or without fatty liver.

Viral hepatitis

Hepatitis A, hepatitis B, or delta co-infection of hepatitis B virus (HBV) carriers can cause an acute hepatitis with jaundice. Acute hepatitis C can present with jaundice, but this is unusual. Epstein–Barr virus (EBV) infection frequently causes abnormal liver function tests, including mild or moderate jaundice, and is often associated with splenomegaly during the acute phase. Patients should be asked about intravenous (IV) drug use, recent tattoos, sexual contacts, and any family or contact history for jaundice or hepatitis.

Viral hepatitis is characterized by a prodromal 'flu-like' illness and very high transaminase (up to ~4,000 U/L), with a small increase in alkaline phosphatase activity.

If there is no coagulopathy, encephalopathy, or renal failure, send the patient home, and await virology results. Advise the patient to avoid alcohol. Arrange repeat liver function tests (LFT) and clotting at 2–3-day intervals, and review the results (but not necessarily the patient). See the patient again within a week. Instruct the patient and carers to return if increasingly unwell or drowsy.

Hepatitis A

Patients with acute hepatitis A (anti-HAV IgM-positive) require no specific treatment, but all household and school contacts should be referred to the local Health Protection Unit (HPU), who will assess each case as to who may benefit from post-exposure prophylaxis (NICE 2014). This may include hepatitis A virus (HAV) vaccination, if not immune, or human normal immunoglobulin (HNIG). Patients with acute hepatitis A may rarely develop acute liver failure, although the prognosis is relatively good in those that do develop acute liver failure (>80% survival), with conservative management. Acute hepatitis A may be associated with a high fever (40°C).

Hepatitis B

Most adults (>95%) clear hepatitis B virus following an acute infection, and few become carriers. Hepatitis B surface antigen (HBsAg) appears in serum 1 to 10 weeks after an acute exposure to hepatitis B and prior to the onset of symptoms or increased ALT. As HBsAg disappears from serum, hepatitis B surface antibody (HBsAb) appears, and there may be a period when both are negative. The detection of anti-hepatitis B core

Box 8.6 Causes of jaundice

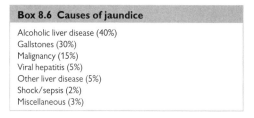

Alcoholic liver disease (40%)
Gallstones (30%)
Malignancy (15%)
Viral hepatitis (5%)
Other liver disease (5%)
Shock/sepsis (2%)
Miscellaneous (3%)

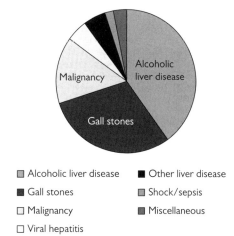

☐ Alcoholic liver disease   ■ Other liver disease
■ Gall stones   ☐ Shock/sepsis
☐ Malignancy   ■ Miscellaneous
☐ Viral hepatitis

Figure 8.4 Causes of jaundice.

IgM (anti-HBc IgM) is usually regarded as an indication of acute hepatitis B virus (HBV) infection; however, anti-HBc IgM may remain detectable up to 2 years after the acute infection, and anti-HBc IgM may increase to detectable levels during exacerbations of chronic hepatitis B.

In patients who subsequently recover, HBsAg usually becomes undetectable after 4 to 6 months. Persistence of HBsAg for more than 6 months suggests chronic infection. The probability of progression from acute to chronic hepatitis B is less than 1–5% for adult-acquired infection. Patients with acute HBV do not require antiviral treatments, as these are unproven. However, many hepatologists do treat patients with a severe hepatitis (e.g. those who develop a coagulopathy (INR >1.5)) or those with a protracted course (such as persistent symptoms or marked jaundice for >4 weeks after presentation). In addition, patients who are immunocompromised, have concomitant infection with hepatitis C or D, have pre-existing liver disease, or who are elderly, as well as those who develop acute liver failure, are also treated since this may improve prognosis (unproven) and reduce the likelihood of reinfection post-liver transplant.

Subjects infected in childhood are much more likely to become chronic carriers and HBeAg-positive, which is associated with a high viral load and high infectivity.

For HBsAg-positive patients, family and close contacts should be tested for HBsAg, HBsAb, and anti-HBc IgM. Prophylactic-specific hepatitis B immunoglobulin ('HBIG' 500 units intramuscularly (IM)) is protective if given within 10 days of exposure to HBV; however, it should only be used for persons with a clear exposure to HBsAg-contaminated material (needle-stick or sexual contacts who are HBsAb-negative). Follow up these cases for at least 6 months to ensure viral clearance in those that do develop acute hepatitis B (i.e. now HBsAg –ve, HBsAb +ve).

Treatment of hepatitis B

Most acute hepatitis B infection does not require treatment and most adults clear the infection spontaneously. However, early antiviral treatment may be required in <1% of people with aggressive acute infection (fulminant hepatitis) and the immunocompromised. Treatment of chronic infection may be necessary to reduce the risk of cirrhosis and liver cancer. Chronically infected individuals with persistently elevated serum ALT and HBV DNA levels and those with current cirrhosis may benefit from therapy which usually lasts 6–12 months, depending on medication and genotype. Although none of the available drugs can clear the infection, they prevent the virus from replicating and reduce liver damage. The World Health Organization recommended a combination of tenofovir and entecavir as first line agents but other medications licensed for treatment of hepatitis B infection include lamivudine, adefovir, and telbivudine, and the two immune system modulators interferon alfa-2a and pegylated interferon alfa-2a (peginterferon alfa-2a).

Hepatitis C

Hepatitis C virus (HCV) RNA is usually detectable in serum by PCR within 8 weeks, following HCV exposure, but may be much earlier. Transmission is predominantly through blood exposure. Sexual or perinatal transmission is rare (<5% risk). Acute hepatitis C accounts for up to 20% of cases of acute viral hepatitis in the USA, although the figure is much lower (<5–10%) in the UK. Most cases are asymptomatic; less than 25% develop any discernible jaundice, and serum ALT is usually <1,000 U/L. The presence of HCV RNA in serum is the first evidence of HCV infection and is detectable within days to 2 months, following exposure. Anti-HCV ELISA tests become positive as early as 8 weeks after exposure but may take many months. Approximately 50% of patients presenting with acute hepatitis C have anti-HCV antibodies at presentation.

About 80% of patients develop chronic HCV, but a significant number clear the virus. All patients with diagnosed HCV should be followed up and treated once it is established that they have chronic disease.

Treatment of acute hepatitis C with pegylated interferon

In a study of 40 patients with proven acute hepatitis C who were treated with either pegylated interferon monotherapy or pegylated interferon plus ribavirin for 24 weeks, there was a sustained virological response rate of 80–85%, compared to 35% in 14 untreated subjects with acute hepatitis C.

For anti-HCV-positive patients, attempt to determine the source. Check LFTs and HCV RNA, and follow up, since the majority of untreated patients will need treatment with pegylated interferon and ribavirin.

Telaprevir, simeprevir, and sofosbuvir are three of the newest hepatitis C medications recommended by NICE in 2012 and 2015 for specific genotypes of hepatitis C, and in combination with pegylated interferon and ribavirin. They also work by stopping the hepatitis C virus from replicating.

Hepatitis E

Hepatitis E virus (HEV) is transmitted via the faecal-oral route and is endemic throughout tropical and subtropical countries. Epidemics are caused by contamination of water supplies. Sporadic cases of viral hepatitis E infection also occur in the UK, particularly in the south-west (e.g. Cornwall). Hepatitis E is the most common cause of acute liver failure in India and Pakistan and South East Asia, including China. Sporadic cases with increasing frequency are being reported in the UK, with evidence suggesting a porcine origin.

Mortality rates from acute hepatitis E viral infection are low (<1%), with a worse outcome in elderly patients and those with established chronic liver disease. Infection appears to be more common in pregnant women and may be associated with a higher mortality. Vertical transmission of hepatitis E from women with acute infection results in acute liver failure in >50% of neonates.

Hepatitis E viral infection typically results in a hyperacute pattern of liver failure, although the course may be indolent. Acute hepatitis E may result in chronic disease in the immunocompromised.

Needle-stick injuries: prophylaxis or treatment for hepatitis B and hepatitis C

Post-exposure prophylaxis can only be given for hepatitis B, although it is worth treating patients with acute hepatitis C with tenofovir or pegylated interferon and ribavirin.

Ideally, all sources of a needle-stick injury should be tested for HCV, HBV, and HIV by requesting HCV antibody and HCV RNA, HBsAg and HBV DNA, and HIV antibodies and HIV RNA levels. See also section 'Post-exposure prophylaxis for prevention of HIV infection' in Chapter 13.

Hepatitis B

Patients known to be at risk or known carriers

What is the risk of catching HBV from patients who are known to be carriers of hepatitis B? For a fresh needle-stick injury (i.e. the needle is coated in fresh blood), the risk is partly dependent on the degree of viraemia. The risk is high following exposure to patients who are HbeAg-positive and who have a high level of viraemia. For many, the potential risk is unknown or guessed. For those exposed to a known risk of HBV, ideally prophylaxis should be commenced within hours of exposure, although it should be considered up to 1–2 weeks later.

Potential exposure to known or suspected hepatitis B carrier

If the source is known to have significant risk factors for HIV or HBV infection, it is best to commence treatment immediately and then reassess later. Subjects will either be vaccinated or unvaccinated. Vaccinated persons should ideally know whether they responded and developed adequate anti-HBs antibodies.

• Unvaccinated: give HBIG, and initiate vaccination.
• Known HBsAb responders: no action required.
• Known HBsAb non-responders: give HBIG x2, and re-vaccinate.
• Unknown response: test and decide.

Potential exposure to known or suspected hepatitis C carrier

If someone is subjected to a needle-stick injury from a patient with chronic hepatitis C, the risk of transmission of the infection is dependent on how fresh the blood is and the degree of viraemia. Staff who have had significant exposures to hepatitis C infection from a patient known to be infected with HCV should be offered hepatitis C testing for HCV by PCR at 6 weeks and testing for anti-HCV at 12 and 24 weeks. Unless there is a risk of hepatitis B and HIV, it is not necessary to advise staff to have only protected sexual intercourse during the follow-up period or to discontinue breastfeeding or to avoid pregnancy.

All subjects should be tested for anti-HCV antibodies and HCV RNA immediately and at 4, 6, and 8 weeks, and 12 weeks, if necessary. An early negative HCV PCR appears to have a high negative predictive value.

Serum aminotransferases become elevated approximately 6 to 12 weeks after exposure (range 1 to 26 weeks). Serum ALT levels are variable but generally are <1,000 U/L.

For subjects who develop acute hepatitis C, treatment with pegylated interferon monotherapy (seek advice from an expert) results in 80–95% cure.

Alcoholic liver disease

Alcoholism

Taking an alcohol history

There is a tendency to diagnose alcoholic liver disease when all other causes have seemingly been excluded, despite the fact that an alcohol drinking history may be absent. Some patients drink a lot of alcohol but are not alcoholic, and these are the patients most amenable to treatment. Patients generally need to drink 100 units per week for at least 10 years to develop alcoholic liver disease (a bit less in women and a bit more in men). If a patient denies alcohol abuse and their partner confirms this, believe them, and look for another cause. Ask what alcohol they drink, and, if they drink beer, what beer and what percentage (%) of alcohol it contains, whether they drink every day, whether they ever drink in the morning, whether they ever feel guilty about drinking, and whether it ever affects their work. Be wary of the patient who boldly states the number of units they drink per week. Most people do not know how to calculate this and do not care.

Use the following four questions to assess alcohol risk

Ask the patient: have they felt the need to reduce their alcohol intake; do they get irritated when their alcohol consumption is questioned; are they concerned about their alcohol intake, or do they find they have to take a drink first thing in the morning to avoid anxiety and tremors? A positive response to at least two questions is seen in most patients with alcoholism, and to all four questions in about 50%. In comparison, over 80% of non-alcoholic patients have a negative response to all four questions, and virtually none has a positive response to more than two questions.

Wernicke's encephalopathy and Korsakoff's psychosis

If a patient is confused, a bit somnolent at times, but with no features of encephalopathy and has a disturbed gait or nystagmus, consider Wernicke's encephalopathy or Korsakoff's psychosis.

Wernicke's encephalopathy is characterized by disorientation, indifference, and inattentiveness with memory impairment. These patients may have impaired oculomotor function and gait ataxia. Less than 10% have a depressed level of consciousness, although, if untreated, patients will progress to stupor, coma, and death. Nystagmus, lateral rectus palsy, and conjugate gaze palsies may all occur in Wernicke's.

Korsakoff's psychosis is characterized by marked deficits in short-term memory, apathy, but an intact sensory system, and relative preservation of long-term memory and other cognitive functions.

Treatment is with high-dose thiamine (Pabrinex® IV for 5 days and oral thiamine (200 mg/day continued)), and, although success in reversing presenting features is poor, it may prevent further progression.

Alcoholic hepatitis

Presentation and diagnosis

Acute alcoholic hepatitis may be asymptomatic or present with jaundice on a background of anorexia, nausea, vomiting, and rarely right upper quadrant (RUQ) pain. Fever may reflect severe liver damage, but infection needs to be excluded.

Acute alcohol withdrawal is unusual, since most patients have stopped drinking alcohol shortly before presentation. The majority of patients who present with alcoholic hepatitis have cirrhosis at presentation.

On examination, most patients are malnourished, with clinically evident jaundice and stigmata of chronic liver disease, including multiple spider naevi, palmar erythema, and a hyperdynamic circulation. The liver is usually obviously or markedly enlarged. It is unusual to be able to palpate the spleen, and cirrhotic patients often have ascites, with thin skin and visible superficial veins over the abdomen. The presence of xanthelasmata suggests PBC. Approximately 15% of patients have hepatic encephalopathy at presentation, with confusion, somnolence, and a hepatic flap (asterixis).

The most common cause for hepatic decompensation and development of jaundice in stable cirrhosis (of any cause) is bacterial infection (acute-on-chronic liver failure). If the liver is not palpable, then consider whether the patient is developing end-stage liver failure, i.e the liver is just failing. In general, most cases of liver failure have a precipitating cause of infection.

Investigations

The term alcoholic hepatitis is a misnomer, since the transaminases rarely exceed 200 U/L and are always <500 U/L. The AST is always higher than the ALT. Serum gamma glutamyl transferase (GGT) is often grossly elevated, and, in those that stop drinking, it takes about 1 month for levels to halve. Bilirubin may be up to 1,000 micromoles/L, albumin is often decreased, and a prolonged prothrombin time (PT) usually signifies underlying cirrhosis. The full blood count (FBC) often shows macrocytosis with a leucocytosis ± left shift (even without infection), anaemia, and thrombocytopenia. Thrombocytopenia suggests cirrhosis but may be a direct result of alcohol abuse. Renal failure (i.e. hepatorenal syndrome) occurs in 20–40% of patients with severe alcoholic hepatitis (GAHS >9; see further text).

Screen for bacterial or fungal infections (e.g. blood, urine, ascitic microscopy, and culture).

Table 8.8 The Glasgow alcoholic hepatitis score

Score given	1	2	3
Age	<50	>50	–
WCC (10⁹/L)	<15	>15	–
Urea (mmol/L)	<5	>5	–
PT ratio or INR	<1.5	1.5–2.0	>2.0
Bilirubin (micromoles/L)	<125	125–250	>250

Reproduced from *Gut*, Forrest EH et al., 'Analysis of factors predictive of mortality in alcoholic hepatitis and derivation and validation of the Glasgow alcoholic hepatitis score', 54, 8, pp. 1174–1179, copyright 2005, with permission from BMJ Publishing Group Ltd.

INR, international normalized ratio; PT, prothrombin time; WCC, white cell count. Each variable is given a score, and then a combined score of between 5 and 12 is obtained. A score ≥9 is associated with a mortality of ~50% at 28 days. A score of 8 or less is associated with a survival of 85% or more at 28 days.

Assessing the severity of alcoholic hepatitis

• **Glasgow alcoholic hepatitis score (GAHS)**

This is now considered to be the best scoring system for alcoholic hepatitis in the UK (see Table 8.8).

• *Discriminant index*

The classic way to calculate the severity of alcoholic hepatitis is to calculate the discriminant index (DI): a DI >32 indicates ~50% mortality.

DI = serum bilirubin/17 + (prolongation of PT x 4.6), e.g. bilirubin = 340 micromoles/L, PT = 17 s (control 12 s). The DI would score 43.

$$(340/17) + ((17 - 12) \times 4.6)) = 20 + 23 = 43$$

Treatment of alcoholic hepatitis

Since alcoholic hepatitis may be associated with a high short-term mortality, it is best to admit most patients to hospital, unless mild (bilirubin <50 micromoles/L, normal PT) and the patient is in an abstinent environment. Those who are not admitted should be seen within 1 week. Many patients with alcoholic hepatitis are malnourished, and some may also be deficient in thiamine. Prescribe intravenous Pabrinex® and oral thiamine (200 mg/day), folic acid, and multivitamins. Monitor and correct potassium, magnesium, phosphate, and glucose. Start a high-calorie, high-protein diet. Low-protein diets are contraindicated. Consider enteral feeding overnight for those with severe malnutrition, and consider the possibility of refeeding syndrome, and start slowly in very malnourished patients or those that have not eaten for 3 days or more.

If an infection is clinically suspected (e.g. pyrexial and leucocytosis), start broad-spectrum antibiotics (e.g. cefotaxime), and give fluconazole (100 mg IV daily or equivalent oral dose) as prophylaxis against fungal infections. Many patients with alcoholic hepatitis have a fever and leucocytosis that does not respond to antibiotics and antifungal agents.

Delirium tremens or severe agitation does not seem to be a major problem with these patients, since many have stopped drinking by the time they present to hospital. If they do become symptomatic, they should be managed with oral clomethiazole or low-dose diazepam. In recent years, we have avoided clomethiazole, since the intravenous preparation was used inappropriately in some patients. However, the oral preparation is probably safer than chlordiazepoxide, which should be avoided in patients with cirrhosis, since the half-life is up to 150 hours in patients with cirrhosis and is not easily cleared if the patient becomes drowsy. Treat seizures in the standard way.

Drug therapy for alcoholic hepatitis. Until recently, patients with severe alcoholic hepatitis (GAHS >9 or DI >32) were treated with prednisolone at 40 mg/day for 4 weeks. A recent study showed that prednisolone and acetylcysteine combined decreased 1 month-mortality from 24% to 8%. Prednisolone should be given at 40 mg/day for 4 weeks. Intravenous acetylcysteine should be given on day 1 at a dose of 150 mg per kg of body weight over 4 hours, and then acetylcysteine at 100 mg/kg 12-hourly for 24 hours, and then 100 mg/kg per 24 hours thereafter for 5 days. This is a slight, but safer and simpler, variation on the published regime and delivers a similar amount of acetylcysteine in the first 24 hours to the published study.

The only practical contraindication is untreated sepsis. If there is doubt, then give broad-spectrum antibiotics for 24–48 hours prior to steroids and acetylcysteine. For patients with a GAHS greater than or equal to 9, the 28-day mortality for corticosteroid-treated patients was 22%, with untreated patients having a mortality of 48%. A discriminant index of >32 is associated with a 30% mortality and should be treated with prednisolone 40 mg/day for 4 weeks.

An alternative treatment is pentoxifylline at 400 mg three times daily for 4 weeks. Two studies have shown this improved survival and was associated with a decreased occurrence of the hepatorenal syndrome; however, its use has not been readily accepted.

Drug-induced hepatitis

Drug-induced jaundice is always of significant concern. Patients with drug-induced jaundice should be monitored at least three times per week or more frequently, depending on the clinical context, until the liver injury is clearly resolving as many cases are serious and may not resolve, requiring liver transplantation. Hepatitic drug reactions with jaundice are generally far more serious (10% mortality) than cholestatic drug reactions (e.g co-amoxiclav). Paracetamol-induced liver injury is considered separately and is discussed in Chapter 9 and later in this chapter.

The most important action when drug-induced liver injury is suspected is to withdraw the suspected drug or drugs, and observe. Look for rash and eosinophilia and exclude other causes. Some of the more common drugs causing jaundice are listed in Table 8.9. Drugs causing a rise in transaminases, but rarely causing jaundice, are not listed. All drug-induced causes of jaundice should be reported to the CSM (yellow pages at the back of the *BNF*) or to the national drug monitoring board.

Drug-induced liver injury is broadly classified into intrinsic and idiosyncratic types; intrinsic drug-induced liver injury is dose-dependent and predictable (e.g. paracetamol or acetaminophen toxicity), whereas idiosyncratic drug-induced liver injury is rare, unpredictable, and not dose-dependent. Its pathogenesis is poorly understood but can be subdivided into hypersensitivity or immunoallergic reactions, and those that are metabolic-idiosyncratic. It is likely to arise from complex interactions among genetic and non-genetic host susceptibility, and environmental factors.

Table 8.9 Common drugs that may cause jaundice

Hepatitic	Cholestatic	Mixed
Paracetamol	Co-amoxiclav	Sulfonamides
Isoniazid	Flucloxacillin	Sulfasalazine
Pyrazinamide	Azathioprine	Carbamazepine
NSAIDs	Anabolic steroids	Co-amoxiclav
Allopurinol	Chlorpromazine	Ranitidine
Rifampicin	Penicillamine	Amitriptyline
Hydralazine	Erythromycin	Nitrofurantoin
Fluoxetine	Captopril	Dapsone
Khat	Oral contraceptive	Amiodarone
Chinese herbs		Duloxetine
Statins		
Methyldopa		
Phenytoin		
Propylthiouracil		

Idiosyncratic drug-induced liver injury is rare, even amongst individuals who are exposed to drugs that are known to be hepatotoxic. It can occur in 1 in 5,000 to 1 in 100,000 individuals.

Although there is little supporting science, it appears that, if you take a drug at a lower dose, you are much less likely to have a fatal outcome (i.e. <10 mg/day compared to 50 mg/day or greater).

The US Acute Liver Failure Study Group recently reported their experience using intravenous acetylcysteine to treat acute liver failure as a result of causes other than acetaminophen. In this prospective, double-blind trial, patients with acute liver failure (non-paracetamol) were randomized to receive acetylcysteine or a placebo for 72 h. They observed that the transplant-free survival was significantly better in patients with drug-induced liver injury randomized to receive acetylcysteine (40 vs 27%, P <0.05). The benefits of acetylcysteine were primarily seen in patients in the early phase of the disease with coma grades I–II (52 vs 30% transplant-free survival) but not in those with advanced coma grades III–IV at randomization.

Table 8.9 shows recorded causes, but it should be recognized that all new and existing drugs have hepatotoxic potential which should be reported if it occurs.

Khat is a form of tobacco chewed by Somalians and other African nationals. In susceptible individuals, it can cause an acute hepatitis, commonly associated with anti-smooth muscle antibody positivity, but with little response to steroids.

There are a number of host factors that may enhance susceptibility to drug-induced liver disease. These include:

- **Females**—halothane, nitrofurantoin, sulindac.
- **Male**—amoxicillin-clavulanic acid (co-amoxiclav).
- **Elderly**—paracetamol (acetaminophen), halothane, isoniazid, amoxicillin-clavulanic acid.
- **Children**—salicylates, valproic acid, propylthiouracil.
- **Fasting or malnutrition**—paracetamol (acetaminophen).
- **Obesity**—halothane.
- **Diabetes**—methotrexate, nicotinic acid.
- **Renal failure**—tetracycline, allopurinol.
- **AIDS**—dapsone, co-trimoxazole, and paracetamol.
- **Pre-existing liver disease**—niacin, tetracycline, methotrexate, probably paracetamol, and specifically hepatitis C may enhance ibuprofen, ritonavir, and flutamide-induced liver injury.

Autoimmune hepatitis

Autoimmune hepatitis is a chronic hepatitis of unknown aetiology that occurs in adults (as well as children) of all ages, although it tends to occur more frequently in young and middle-aged women. Patients generally have circulating autoantibodies, and 60% have other autoimmune diseases. There is generally a good response to corticosteroid therapy.

In about 30% of cases, the onset is indistinguishable clinically from acute viral hepatitis, with anorexia, nausea, hepatic discomfort, and the development of jaundice. However, it may present as an acute or fulminant hepatitis or as advanced liver disease with cirrhosis, with a long-standing asymptomatic stage before presentation. It is characterized by the presence of circulating autoantibodies and high serum globulin concentrations. Biochemically, the patient may present with an acute hepatitis, transaminases of 500–1,500 U/L or lower and an elevated bilirubin. If serum total protein is measured, it will be elevated due to increased levels of total globulins (total protein minus albumin). If the total globulins (total protein minus albumin) is >45 g/L, con-

sider autoimmune hepatitis. This should be confirmed by liver biopsy. Minocycline can rarely cause an autoimmune-like reaction with positive anti-dsDNA antibodies, which may also be found in autoimmune hepatitis.

There are two types of autoimmune liver disease. Type 1 autoimmune hepatitis is the commonest form and characterized by circulating antinuclear antibodies (ANA) and anti-smooth muscle antibodies (SMA). Type 2 autoimmune hepatitis is characterized by the presence of anti-liver/kidney microsomal antibodies (anti-LKM). Other autoantibodies may be positive, and there is an overlap syndrome with primary sclerosing cholangitis (PSC).

Diseases commonly seen with autoimmune hepatitis include haemolytic anaemia, idiopathic thrombocytopenic purpura, type 1 diabetes mellitus, thyroiditis, coeliac disease, and ulcerative colitis (which is more frequently associated with PSC). A polyglandular autoimmune syndrome may occur in children with type 2 autoimmune hepatitis.

Diagnostic criteria[1]

1. Autoantibodies:
- Score 1: ANA or SMA is ≤1:40.
- Score 2: ANA or SMA is ≥1:80 (or if the LKM ≥1:40).

2. Immunoglobulin G:
- Score 1: if IgG is > upper limit of normal (ULN).
- Score 2: if the IgG is >1.10 x ULN.

3. Liver histology:
- Score 1 point: if the histological features are compatible with autoimmune hepatitis.
- Score 2 points: if the histological features are typical of autoimmune hepatitis.

4. Absence of viral hepatitis:
- Score 2 points: if viral hepatitis is excluded.

If the total score is ≥6, there is 88% sensitivity and 97% specificity for a diagnosis of autoimmune hepatitis.

Differential diagnosis

The differential diagnosis includes viral and drug-induced hepatitis, autoimmune cholangiopathy (see following paragraph), as well as Wilson's disease and alpha-1-antitrypsin deficiency. Some alcoholic patients may manifest histological appearances overlapping with autoimmune hepatitis.

Autoimmune cholangiopathy: up to 10% of cases may show mixed autoimmune hepatitis and immune biliary disease, generally PBC and less frequently PSC. The disease may also coexist with autoimmune cholangitis (which resembles PBC but is anti-mitochondrial antibody-negative). In children, the overlap with autoimmune primary sclerosing cholangitis is more common, and patients frequently evolve from hepatitis to sclerosing cholangitis.

Treatment

Treat patients with severe disease with prednisolone or budesonide which reduces inflammation in 80–90% of cases, decreases the chance of progression to cirrhosis if it has not already occurred, and prolongs survival. Initial therapy aims to markedly decrease inflammation of the liver. Prednisolone 30–40 mg od for 2 weeks, followed by azathioprine (75 or 100 mg/day) as a steroid-sparing agent, and thereafter decreasing the dose of prednisolone fairly rapidly over 2–4 months to 7.5 mg/day is effective in 85% of cases. If there is failure to respond in a young patient

---

[1]Adapted with permission from Hennes EM et al., 'Simplified Criteria for the Diagnosis of Autoimmune Hepatitis', *Hepatology*, 48, 1, pp. 169–176, published by Wiley, © 2008 American Association for the Study of Liver Diseases.

(<30 years), consider Wilson's disease. Thereafter, therapy is a judgement call, but most clinicians attempt a trial of withdrawal of immunosuppression, usually slowly after 2 years or more of successful immunosuppression, based on transaminases, serum globulins, and occasionally repeat liver biopsy. Alternative steroids include budesonide, and alternatives to azathioprine include mycophenolate (~500 mg bd is usually sufficient).

Transplantation
End-stage cirrhosis due to autoimmune hepatitis and acute non-responsive autoimmune hepatitis, leading to acute or subacute liver failure, provide firm indications for orthotopic liver transplantation. Failure to achieve an early response in acute disease, with a shrinking liver volume, should prompt consideration of transplantation. Overall, the prognosis after transplantation is good, with 5-year survival rates in excess of 80%.

Acholuric jaundice: haemolysis and Gilbert's syndrome
Haemolysis
This is characterized by the absence of bilirubin in the urine. It may be due to any cause of increased haemolysis, including haemolytic anaemia, malaria, rhabdomyolysis, hereditary spherocytosis, etc. (see Chapters 6 and 15). Note the patient's past medical history, splenomegaly, reticulocytosis, and excess urinary urobilinogen. It should be noted that increased chronic haemolysis (e.g. hereditary spherocytosis) is associated with an increased risk of pigment gallstones and, therefore, an increased risk of obstructive jaundice.

Gilbert's syndrome
The other group of causes includes congenital disorders of conjugation, of which Gilbert's syndrome, affecting at least 5% of population, is the most common. It is sometimes termed benign familial unconjugated hyperbilirubinaemia.

Gilbert's syndrome is caused by reduced activity of UDP-glucuronosyltransferase 1A1 (UGT1A1), an enzyme which conjugates bilirubin and other lipophilic molecules to glucuronide. Conjugation renders the bilirubin water-soluble, after which it is excreted in bile into the duodenum. The gene responsible for decreased enzyme activity is termed UGT1A1, and it is located on human chromosome 2. UGT1A1 (*)28, the main genetic abnormality, leading to Gilbert's syndrome, is found in approximately 40% of Caucasoid individuals. Over 100 UGT1A1 variants have been reported, causing a spectrum of disorders, ranging from mild hyperbilirubinaemia to life-threatening jaundice. Gilbert's syndrome is also associated with abnormalities of other glucuronosyltransferases, including UGT1A6 and UGT1A7. Because of its effects on drug and bilirubin breakdown and because of its genetic inheritance, Gilbert's syndrome can be classified as a minor inborn error of metabolism.

Overall, Gilbert's syndrome is generally considered asymptomatic, although occasional patients attribute many non-specific symptoms to its presence. There are data to suggest that Gilbert's syndrome is associated with a decreased risk of coronary artery disease. Symptomatically, patients may have adverse drug reactions when the drug is conjugated by the same enzyme (UDP-glucuronyltransferase 1A1). Thus, impaired glucuronidation in Gilbert's syndrome impacts drug therapy, including irinotecan and atazanavir.

Mild jaundice may appear during exertion, stress, fasting, and infections, but the condition is otherwise usually asymptomatic.

> **Box 8.7 Factors predisposing to ischaemic hepatitis**
>
> 1. Decrease in arterial pressure
> 2. Congested liver secondary to right-sided heart failure
> 3. Hypoxaemia

Fasting (<400 calories) for 48–72 hours (or 50 mg of intravenous nicotinic acid) will increase serum unconjugated bilirubin in patients with Gilbert's syndrome (although the bilirubin is rarely >80 micromoles/L). The other liver function tests are usually normal, although haemolysis may increase serum AST (present in RBC) as well as lactate dehydrogenase.

Investigations should include screening for haemolysis, including a blood film (ask about travel abroad, and consider malaria), reticulocyte count, serum haptoglobin, and a direct Coomb's test.

Ischaemic hepatitis
Ischaemic hepatitis may be due to acute hepatic arterial occlusion or, more commonly, due to a decrease in hepatic blood inflow in a patient with cardiac failure. There are three factors which predispose an individual to the development of ischaemic hepatitis. These are reported in Box 8.7 and include the combined need for a reduced arterial pressure in a patient with a congested liver and significant hypoxaemia.

In its mildest form, it manifests as mildly deranged LFTs (i.e. hepatitic picture with increased PT) in a patient with congestive cardiac failure (CCF). In its most severe form, it may present as acute liver failure. It should be noted that the prothrombin time (PT) may increase very rapidly, but equally it tends to recover quite quickly during recovery of the ischaemic insult to the liver.

Look for evidence of hypoxia, hypotension (which may have normalized by the time of assessment), and signs of right ventricular failure. Ischaemic hepatitis may cause confusion or hepatic encephalopathy. Exclude other causes of hepatitis.

Management
Most ischaemic hepatitis will respond to correction of the underlying aetiology. Aim to restore the blood pressure and circulation (see Chapters 1 and 4), and give oxygen to correct hypoxia. The prognosis is poor if the hepatic artery or coeliac axis is occluded but it depends on the extent of hepatic necrosis. Usually, age and extent of disease preclude salvage surgery. Discuss ongoing management with a specialist centre if signs of severe (acute) liver failure develop.

The liver in sepsis
Patients with bacterial sepsis frequently present with deranged LFTs in the absence of evidence of direct liver infection. They account for up to 20% of jaundiced patients in hospital. Patients with chronic liver disease who develop bacterial sepsis frequently decompensate and develop acute-on-chronic liver failure.

Jaundice is particularly common in patients with pneumococcal pneumonia. It usually occurs on days 4–5 of illness, especially in right lower lobe pneumonias. Typically, bilirubin is <100 micromoles/L, and liver transaminases and ALP are normal. The cause is unknown, but it may be due to endotoxin and cytokine-mediated repression of hepatic transporters and enzymes.

Deranged LFTs are also a feature of Legionnaire's disease, in which AST, ALT, and alkaline phosphatase (ALP) may all be elevated. Hyperbilirubinaemia is less common and tends to be seen only in patients who are severely ill.

Cholestasis of sepsis occurs primarily in children and adults with Gram-negative infections. Pruritus is not a major feature. LFTs typically reveal a mild conjugated hyperbilirubinaemia (<100 micromoles/L), with elevated ALP (usually <3-fold ULN).

The evaluation of jaundiced patients should follow the guidelines set out in the section on jaundice and is directed at excluding other treatable causes. Unconjugated hyperbilirubinaemia should prompt an evaluation for haemolysis and conjugated hyperbilirubinaemia, imaging of the liver and biliary tree to rule out hepatic abscesses and cholangitis. Liver biopsy is not helpful.

Management of the jaundiced patient with sepsis is directed at treatment of the underlying infection. There is no evidence to support treatment aimed primarily at ameliorating liver dysfunction, such as N-acetylcysteine or ursodeoxycholic acid.

Neither the presence of jaundice nor its severity influences survival outcomes or overall prognosis. There is usually complete resolution of hepatic dysfunction and cholestasis, following sepsis.

Bacterial infections, such as severe pneumonia, tend to cause only modest elevations of serum bilirubin (<100 micromoles/L). Exclude other causes, and treat infection with antibiotics or surgical drainage, as indicated.

For leptospirosis, see Infections and the liver.

Sepsis in patients with pre-existing cirrhosis

Up to 40% of patients admitted with cirrhosis develop a bacterial infection whilst in hospital. These infections are associated with a high mortality and consequently, a high index of suspicion is required.

Suspect bacterial infection in a patient with cirrhosis if they develop any of the following (WHEU):

1. **W**orsening liver function tests.
2. **H**epatorenal syndrome.
3. **E**ncephalopathy.
4. **U**pper GI bleeding.

Sepsis appears to be the predominant precipitant of most complications of liver disease, and patients with pre-existing cirrhosis who develop sepsis are at increased risk of developing acute-on-chronic liver failure and associated complications. Thus, a patient with ascites who develops spontaneous bacterial peritonitis (SBP) has a 30% chance of developing hepatorenal syndrome or acute kidney injury unless treated appropriately. Secondly, a patient with cirrhosis who develops a bacterial infection is more likely to develop worsening jaundice and coagulopathy and hepatic encephalopathy.

Causes of severe jaundice and relatively normal liver enzymes

Occasionally, patients present with an extremely high serum bilirubin (500–1,000 micromoles/L), and yet virtually all other liver function tests are normal (see Box 8.8). This is particularly so if the laboratory does not measure the serum AST, which can be increased in haemolysis or alcoholic hepatitis, with a relatively normal ALT.

Further reading
Bauer M, Press AT, Trauner M (2013). The liver in sepsis: patterns of response and injury. *Current Opinion in Critical Care*, **19**, 123–7.

> **Box 8.8 Causes of severe jaundice and relatively normal liver enzymes**
>
> 1. Alcoholic hepatitis
> 2. Sickle hepatopathy
> 3. Intra-abdominal sepsis after major liver surgery
> 4. Small for size liver resection
> 5. Leptospirosis
> 6. Severe haemolysis, including malaria

Booth JCL, O'Grady J, Neuberger J (2001). Clinical guidelines on the management of hepatitis C. <http://www.bsg.org.uk/pdf_word_docs/clinguidehepc.pdf>.

British Association for Sexual Health and HIV (2008). United Kingdom national guideline on the management of the viral hepatitides A, B & C. <http://www.bashh.org/documents/1927.pdf>.

British Society of Gastroenterology. Chronic management: viral hepatitis. <http://www.bsg.org.uk/clinical/commissioning-report/viral-hepatitis.html>.

Ewing JA (1984). Detecting alcoholism: the CAGE questionnaire. *JAMA*, **252**, 1905–7.

Gleeson D and Heneghan MA (2011). Guidelines for the management of autoimmune hepatitis. *Gut*, **60**, 1611–29.

Kamal SM, Ismail A, Graham CS, et al. (2004). Pegylated interferon alpha therapy in acute hepatitis C: relation to hepatitis C virus-specific T cell response kinetics. *Hepatology*, **39**, 1721–31.

Lamers MM, van Oijen MG, Pronk M, et al. (2010). Treatment options for autoimmune hepatitis: a systematic review of randomized controlled trials. *Journal of Hepatology*, **53**, 191–8.

Manns MP, Czaja AJ, Gorham JD, et al. (2010). Diagnosis and management of autoimmune hepatitis. *Hepatology*, **51**, 2193–213.

Metha N, Ozick LA, Gbadehan E (2012). Drug-induced hepatotoxicity. <http://emedicine.medscape.com/article/169814-overview>.

National Institute for Health and Clinical Excellence (2010). Alcohol-use disorders: Diagnosis and clinical management of alcohol-related physical complications. <http://www.nice.org.uk/cg100>.

National Institute for Health and Clinical Excellence (2012). Telaprevir for the treatment of genotype 1 chronic hepatitis C. NICE technology appraisal guidance 252. <https://www.nice.org.uk/guidance/ta252>.

National Institute for Health and Clinical Excellence (2014). Hepatitis A. Clinical knowledge summaries. <http://cks.nice.org.uk/hepatitis-a>.

National Institute for Health and Clinical Excellence (2015). Sofosbuvir for treating chronic hepatitis C. NICE technology appraisal guidance [TA330]. <https://www.nice.org.uk/guidance/ta330>.

Nguyen-Khac E, Thevenot T, Piquet MA, et al. (2011). Glucocorticoids plus N-acetylcysteine in severe alcoholic hepatitis. *New England Journal of Medicine*, **365**, 1781–9.

O'Shea RS, Dasarathy S, McCullough AJ (2010). Alcoholic liver disease. *American Journal of Gastroenterology*, **105**, 14–32.

Roche SP and Kobos R (2004). Jaundice in the adult patient. *American Family Physician*, **69**, 299–304.

Ryder SD and Beckingham IJ (2001). ABC of diseases of liver, pancreas, and biliary system: acute hepatitis. *BMJ*, **322**, 151–3.

Theodossi A (1985). The value of symptoms and signs in the assessment of jaundiced patients. *Journal of Clinical Gastroenterology*, **14**, 545–57.

World Health Organization (2015). Guidelines for the prevention, care and treatment of persons with chronic hepatitis B infection. <http://www.who.int/hiv/pub/hepatitis/hepatitis-b-guidelines/en/>.

Complications of cirrhosis

Ascites

The majority of patients (75%) who present with ascites have cirrhosis and portal hypertension. About 10% will have malignancy, and the remainder will have other rarer causes, such as constrictive pericarditis, cardiac failure, tuberculosis, pancreatitis, hepatic vein thrombosis (Budd–Chiari syndrome), or nephrotic syndrome.

Investigations

- **Blood tests.** U&E, glucose, FBC, PT, LFTs, blood cultures, amylase.
- **Ascitic tap.** An ascitic tap should be carried out in all patients, unless a diagnosis of malignant ascites is known. Inoculate blood culture bottles, and send fluid in a sterile pot for microscopy and WBC.
- **Imaging.** Plain abdominal X-ray (AXR) shows a ground glass pattern, with loss of the psoas shadow. Ultrasound scan (USS) can detect as little as 30 mL ascites. Note the size and texture of the liver and spleen; check the patency of hepatic veins. A CT scan may be required.
- **Urine.** Urine sodium (cirrhotic ascites), 24-hour protein.

Management

Admit all patients with symptomatic ascites, and treat the underlying cause.

Cirrhotic ascites

Do not start diuretics if there is renal impairment, and salt restrict to 90 mmol/day. Paracentese tense or moderate ascites: drain all ascites as quickly as possible (maximum 25 L in 5 hours), and then give 6–8 g albumin per litre of ascites removed as 20% albumin. Start spironolactone 50–100 mg/day, increasing to 400 mg/day and then add furosemide 40 mg/day if the response is poor. If there is renal impairment (creatinine >140 micromoles/L), give an extra crystalloid volume challenge (e.g. Hartmann's solution 500 mL over 1 hour, followed by 1 L over 4 hours). There is no hurry to commence diuretics which can be started once the patient has settled, following the paracentesis. More harm than good is done by diuresing patients who are hypovolaemic.

Malignant ascites

Treatment is palliative and may include total paracentesis to make the patient more comfortable. Specialist advice should be sought for future management of the malignancy.

Pancreatic ascites

This is usually associated with a pancreatic pseudocyst and should be managed in consultation with surgical colleagues.

Spontaneous bacterial peritonitis (SBP)

SBP occurs in up to ~15% of patients admitted with cirrhotic ascites and is frequently asymptomatic. It rarely, if ever, occurs in non-cirrhotic ascites. The risk is increased with low ascitic protein. Over 90% will yield positive ascitic cultures if inoculated into blood culture (BC) bottles. The ascitic fluid should be inoculated into BC bottles at the bedside. Initial diagnosis is based on an ascitic white cell count (WCC) >250 PMN/mm^3. If the cultures are positive, but the ascitic WCC is low, repeat the tap for microscopy, and treat if the WCC is >250 PMN/mm^3. Treat with a broad-spectrum antibiotic for enteric organisms and Gram-positive cocci (e.g. cefotaxime). Suspect tuberculous (TB) ascites if there is a predominant lymphocytosis.

Table 8.10 Causes of acute decompensation of chronic liver disease

• Intercurrent infection, including spontaneous bacterial peritonitis, pneumonia, skin infections, etc.	• Drugs, e.g. sedatives, narcotics, diuretics
• Acute viral hepatitis	• Metabolic derangement, including hypoglycaemia, and electrolyte disturbance
• Acute GI haemorrhage	• Major surgery
• Additional hepatotoxic insult, e.g. paracetamol overdose	• Constipation
• Alcoholic binge	• Progression of disease
• Hepatotoxic drugs	

In patients with spontaneous bacterial peritonitis, the administration of intravenous albumin (1.5 g/kg) at the time of diagnosis of infection, and a second dose of 1.0 g/kg on day 3 of antibiotic therapy has been shown to reduce the incidence of renal impairment and mortality.

Acute-on-chronic liver failure

Patients with chronic liver disease from cirrhosis may present with acute decompensation due to a variety of causes, but bacterial infection is the most common (see Table 8.10).

Clinical features

- Patients usually have signs of chronic liver disease.
- Examine specifically for features of hepatic decompensation including encephalopathy (confusion, 'liver flap'), ascites (see Figure 8.5), oedema, jaundice, or fever.

Investigations

Assuming that the cause of liver disease is known, the most important aspect of investigation is multiple cultures, looking for any evidence of infection.

Management

As for patients with acute liver failure, the mainstay of treatment is supportive. The decision as to how aggressively the patient is managed (i.e. admission to ICU, invasive monitoring, etc.) depends on the previous diagnosis, on the presence of a reversible element to the acute insult, and whether the patient is a candidate for liver transplantation. In general, unless the patient is well known, or if this is a first presentation, then it should be managed aggressively initially. However, when all the information is known and for the sake of the patient's dignity, it is important to de-escalate therapy if you believe that the prognosis is very poor.

Sepsis

Start 'blind' treatment if there is a fever, an increased WCC, or a high C-reactive protein (CRP) (e.g. IV cefotaxime), and be guided by culture results when available. Add intravenous fluconazole as an antifungal agent.

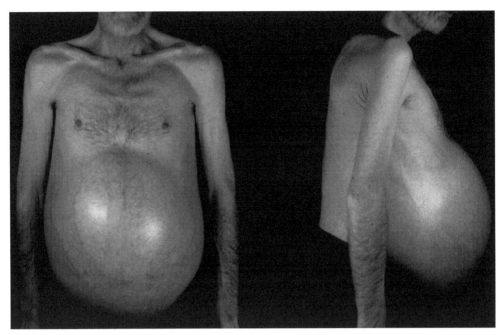

Figure 8.5 Ascites.

Hepatic encephalopathy

Hepatic encephalopathy is a neuropsychiatric disturbance of cognitive function in a patient with acute-on-chronic liver disease (see 'Acute-on-chronic liver failure'). It is often suggested that patients with cirrhosis do not develop cerebral oedema. This is not true, and patients with cirrhosis may rarely develop signs of cerebral oedema, following an acute insult, e.g. variceal haemorrhage.

There is increasing evidence that the development of hepatic encephalopathy is associated with subclinical sepsis; therefore, all patients should be screened and treated for presumed bacterial infection in the acute stage.

Clinically, there is usually an altered conscious level, asterixis (liver flap), abnormal EEG, impaired psychometric tests, and an elevated arterial ammonia concentration. Patients may present with Parkinsonian features. However, in patients with chronic liver disease, it may be subclinical, with subtle changes in awareness or attention span. It is graded, as described in Acute liver failure.

The aim of treatment is to improve symptoms.

- Exclude other causes of confusion (see Chapters 7 and 14).
- Identify and correct the precipitating causes, e.g. infection (including spontaneous bacterial peritonitis), hypovolaemia, hypokalaemia, hypoxia, hypoglycaemia, gastrointestinal bleeding, constipation, drugs (sedatives or tranquillizers), or rarely hepatoma or hepatic or portal vein thrombosis.

- Give lactulose. This semi-synthetic disaccharide is poorly absorbed. It is digested in the large bowel and undergoes fermentation. This alters faecal pH and nitrogen utilization by bowel flora. Lactulose enemas can be given if the patient cannot take lactulose orally.
- Rifaximin is a non-systemic antibiotic, and very little of the drug passes from the gastrointestinal tract into the circulation.
- Lactitol has a similar action to lactulose but has fewer side effects.
- Phosphate enemas help to purge the large bowel, most useful in the context of an acute food load (e.g. GI bleeding).
- Ensure adequate calorie intake.
- There are other drugs, such as ornithine aspartate or sodium benzoate, but these are rarely used.

Further reading

Jalan R, Gines P, Olson JC, et al. (2012). Acute-on chronic liver failure. *Journal of Hepatology*, **57**, 1336–48.

Kashani A, Landaverde C, Medici V, et al. (2008). Fluid retention in cirrhosis: pathophysiology and management. *QJM*, **101**, 71–85.

Laleman W, Verbeke L, Meersseman P, et al. (2011). Acute-on-chronic liver failure: current concepts on definition, pathogenesis, clinical manifestations and potential therapeutic interventions. *Expert Review of Gastroenterology and Hepatology*, **5**, 523–37.

Moore KP and Aithal GP (2006). Guidelines on the management of ascites in cirrhosis, British Society of Gastroenterology. *Gut*, **55**, 1–12.

Acute liver failure

Assessment

Acute liver failure (fulminant hepatic failure) is defined as a potentially reversible severe liver injury, with an onset of hepatic encephalopathy within 8 weeks of the appearance of the first symptoms and in the absence of pre-existing liver disease.

A more recent classification is:

- Hyperacute liver failure: encephalopathy within 7 days of jaundice.
- Acute liver failure: encephalopathy within 8–28 days of jaundice.
- Subacute liver failure: encephalopathy within 29–84 days of jaundice.

Presentation

The history may point to a cause (see Tables 8.11, 8.12, and 8.13). Ask specifically about recent viral illnesses, paracetamol, alcohol, and drug history (see Figure 8.6). Signs of chronic liver disease are typically not present (unless 'acute-on-chronic'). Splenomegaly does not occur. If present, consider an acute presentation of Wilson's disease, autoimmune chronic active hepatitis, or lymphoma. Frequently, the presenting feature is a complication of liver failure. Patients with paracetamol overdose may present with severe abdominal pain and retching. Be aware that acute hepatitis E, although relatively uncommon, does occur in the UK, particularly in the west country.

Fluid balance

At presentation, many patients with acute liver failure have significant depletion of their circulating intravascular volume. Intravenous fluid repletion, often guided by invasive monitoring, should commence immediately after presentation, and may improve outcome. Hartmann's and other physiologically balanced solutions which contain sodium are suitable resuscitation fluids.

Encephalopathy

This is present in all cases (by definition) and conventionally divided into four grades (see Table 8.14). In acute liver failure, hepatic encephalopathy ranges from minor confusion and disorientation to frank coma with cerebral oedema and intracranial hypertension. In patients with acute liver failure,

the progression of hepatic encephalopathy may be rapid and can quickly impair airway control. Therefore, any patient with developing hepatic encephalopathy should be sedated, intubated, and ventilated prior to transfer. The development of intracranial hypertension as a consequence of cerebral oedema may occur abruptly. Staff involved in the transfer of such patients should be specifically warned and instructed on the importance of frequent pupillary examinations and the appropriate therapeutic interventions, should it develop. Cerebral oedema accounts for 20–25% of deaths. Survival without transplantation for patients with acute liver failure is poor in those with severe encephalopathy, and the risk of significant cerebral oedema and intracranial hypertension is greatest in those with hyperacute or acute presentations. In patients with subacute liver failure, the presence of modest hepatic encephalopathy is a sign of poor outcome.

Cerebral oedema is heralded by spikes of hypertension and disconjugate eye movements. Papilloedema is rare. Unless treated, it progresses to decerebrate posturing (i.e. the back, arms, and legs are rigid and extended (with internal rotation of the arms and legs), the hands are flexed and progression leads to opisthotonus (hyperextension of the head, neck, and spinal column)), and brainstem coning.

Metabolic disturbances

Hypoglycaemia and hyponatraemia are common. Other abnormalities include hypokalaemia, respiratory alkalosis, and severe hypophosphataemia. Lactic acidosis carries a poor prognosis.

Cardiovascular abnormalities

Spikes of systolic hypertension may reflect cerebral oedema. The diastolic BP falls as disease progresses with a vasodilated hyperdynamic circulation (reduced SVR, increased cardiac output).

Circulatory dysfunction is frequently present in patients with acute liver failure, and its severity is closely related to outcome. In addition to fluid depletion, hypotension may be secondary to vasodilation and the development of a high cardiac output state with low systemic vascular resistance. Relative adrenal insufficiency is common in patients with acute liver failure.

Table 8.11 Causes of acute liver failure

Country	Drugs		Viral			Unknown	Other
	Paracetamol (acetaminophen)	Non-Paracetamol	HAV	HBV	HEV		
UK	57%	11%	2%	5%	1%	17%	7%
Spain	2%	17%	2%	32%		35%	12%
Sweden	42%	15%	3%	4%		11%	25%
Germany	15%	14%	4%	18%		21%	28%
USA	39%	13%	4%	7%		18%	19%
Australia	36%	6%	4%	10%		34%	10%
India	0%	1%	2%	15%	44%	31%	7%
Pakistan	0%	2%	7%	20%	60%	7%	4%

Reprinted from The Lancet, 376, W Bernal et al., 'Acute liver failure', pp. 190–201, Copyright 2010, with permission from Elsevier.

Table 8.12 Typical features of different forms of acute liver failure

	Hyperacute	Acute	Subacute
Jaundice to encephalopathy time	0–1 week	1–4 weeks	4–12 weeks
Increase in prothrombin time	Marked	Moderate	Mild to moderate
Severity of jaundice	Moderate	Moderate	Severe
Intracranial hypertension	Severe	Moderate	May occur
Survival without liver transplantation	Good	Moderate	Fair
Typical causes	Paracetamol, hepatitis A and E	Hepatitis B	Non-paracetamol drug-induced liver injury

Reprinted from *The Lancet*, 376, W Bernal *et al.*, 'Acute liver failure', pp. 190–201, Copyright 2010, with permission from Elsevier.

Early restoration of an appropriate circulating fluid volume, systemic perfusion, and oxygen delivery are crucial to the successful management of the patient with acute liver failure. Hypotensive patients with acute liver failure should receive an early volume challenge as described previously. Failure to respond to a fluid challenge should be regarded as an indication for other forms of haemodynamic assessment and monitoring.

In general, a cardiac index of less than 3.5 L/min/m², with evidence of inadequate tissue perfusion despite apparent euvolaemia, is treated with vasopressor/inotropic agents. A target mean arterial pressure of 65–80 mmHg is generally sought, and noradrenaline (norepinephrine) should be used as the primary vasopressor. In all patients who require vasopressor or volume support, adrenal function should be assessed via a short Synacthen® (tetracosactide) test and replacement doses of oral or intravenous hydrocortisone administered, as appropriate.

Table 8.13 Causes of acute liver failure in the UK

Drug-induced hepatitis (68%)	Paracetamol overdose. Less commonly halothane, isoniazid, sulfonamides, NSAIDs, phenytoin, valproate, penicillins, MAOIs, ecstasy, sulfasalazine, disulfiram, ketoconazole
Viral hepatitis (9%)	Hepatitis A , B, delta co-infection in HBsAg positive carrier, NANB (not HCV in UK), E, less commonly CMV, EBV, and HSV
Toxins (2%)	*Amanita phalloides* (these mushrooms are available in the UK), herbal remedies, khat (form of tobacco chewed by Somalis and other ethnic groups)
Malignancy (1%)	Lymphoma, malignant infiltration
Vascular (1%)	Budd–Chiari syndrome, veno-occlusive disease, ischaemic injury (shock and hypotension)
Miscellaneous (2%)	Wilson's (not strictly acute, as many are cirrhotic, but in all clinical respects similar), autoimmune hepatitis, malignant hyperthermia (incl. ecstasy), fatty liver of pregnancy, PET/HELLP syndrome, Reye's syndrome
Unknown (17%)	

Respiratory failure
Hypoxia is relatively common and may be worsened by localized infection, aspiration, or atelectasis. Non-cardiogenic pulmonary oedema is seen in ~10%.

Acute kidney injury
The development of renal failure or acute kidney injury generally indicates a worse prognosis. Paracetamol overdose may cause acute renal failure directly.

Bleeding problems
The prothrombin time (PT) is prolonged and reflects progression of the disease. There is no indication for the prophylactic administration of clotting factors to patients with acute liver failure despite marked abnormalities of coagulation. Overt haemorrhage is uncommon. Low-grade DIC may occur with bleeding from the GI tract (e.g. gastritis) or elsewhere. Subconjunctival haematoma is common in paracetamol-induced liver failure.

Infections
Bacterial and fungal infections (septicaemia, pneumonia, peritonitis, urinary tract infections) are more frequent due to impaired neutrophil function and multiple invasive procedures. They may be difficult to diagnose, as the usual clinical signs of infection may be absent.

The development of infection is of major prognostic importance, since it retards hepatic regeneration and is associated with progression of hepatic encephalopathy and possibe renal failure. In particular, it reduces the rate of successful liver transplantation, increasing mortality and morbidity.

Investigations

- Blood tests (daily): U&E, glucose (and 2-hourly BM stix), FBC, PT, LFTs, phosphate, arterial blood gases.
- Blood tests on admission: viral serology (HAV IgM, HBsAg, HBcore Ab IgM, diagnosis delta if HBsAg +ve, EBV, CMV, HSV), drug screen (especially paracetamol), plasma caeruloplasmin. Blood group and cross-match.
- Bacteriology: blood cultures, urine and sputum M,C&S daily initially (including fungal cultures). Throat and vaginal swabs.
- USS (liver): to assess hepatic veins, portal vein patency, vein size (if possible), spleen size, nodes (lymphoma).
- ECG/CXR: repeat CXR daily initially (infection/ARDS).
- EEG: may be helpful in the assessment of hepatic encephalopathy though not widely used.
- Liver biopsy: for suspected lymphoma, malignancy, or bizarre presentation.

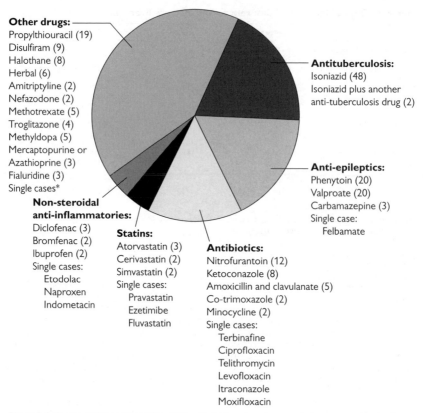

Other drugs:
Propylthiouracil (19)
Disulfiram (9)
Halothane (8)
Herbal (6)
Amitriptyline (2)
Nefazodone (2)
Methotrexate (5)
Troglitazone (4)
Methyldopa (5)
Mercaptopurine or
Azathioprine (3)
Fialuridine (3)
Single cases*

**Non-steroidal
anti-inflammatories:**
Diclofenac (3)
Bromfenac (2)
Ibuprofen (2)
Single cases:
    Etodolac
    Naproxen
    Indometacin

Statins:
Atorvastatin (3)
Cerivastatin (2)
Simvastatin (2)
Single cases:
    Pravastatin
    Ezetimibe
    Fluvastatin

Antibiotics:
Nitrofurantoin (12)
Ketoconazole (8)
Amoxicillin and clavulanate (5)
Co-trimoxazole (2)
Minocycline (2)
Single cases:
    Terbinafine
    Ciprofloxacin
    Telithromycin
    Levofloxacin
    Itraconazole
    Moxifloxacin

Antituberculosis:
Isoniazid (48)
Isoniazid plus another
anti-tuberculosis drug (2)

Anti-epileptics:
Phenytoin (20)
Valproate (20)
Carbamazepine (3)
Single case:
    Felbamate

Figure 8.6 Causes of drug-induced liver failure. Anti-tuberculous drugs remain the commonest cause of non-paracetamol drug-induced liver failure (parentheses indicate numbers of cases, * = many but not listed individually). Reprinted from *The Lancet*, 376, 9736, W Bernal, G Auzinger, A Dhawan, and J Wendon, 'Acute liver failure', pp. 190–201, copyright 2010, with permission from Elsevier.

The mainstay of treatment is supportive until the acute insult resolves. Box 8.9 lists the key points in the management of acute liver failure. If a patient fulfils criteria for liver transplantation (see Tables 8.15 and 8.16) on, or during, their admission, they should be referred to a centre where liver transplantation is available.

It is vital to discuss all cases of severe liver injury with one of the regional liver transplant centres, even though patients may not fulfil the criteria above, as it generally takes up to 48 hours to obtain an emergency graft, and delay in referral can result in failure to procure an adequate graft. All of these centres are also experienced in managing this serious illness. None of the known causes of acute liver failure respond well to medical therapy. Steroids may be of benefit in

Table 8.14 Grades of hepatic encephalopathy

Grade 1	Drowsy but coherent; mood change
Grade 2	Drowsy, confused at times, inappropriate behaviour
Grade 3	Very drowsy and stuporous but rousable; alternatively restless, screaming
Grade 4	Comatose, barely rousable

Data from Conn H, Lieberthal M, *The hepatic coma syndromes and lactulose*, Baltimore: Williams & Wilkins; 1979. p. 7.

patients with lymphoma or autoimmune hepatitis, but, by the time most patients present, it is usually too late. All patients should be admitted to a high dependency or intensive therapy unit.

Paracetamol overdose

Give acetylcysteine. The benefit of acetylcysteine may be evident up to 48 hours after paracetamol ingestion and possibly longer. When given within 24 hours of paracetamol ingestion, acetylcysteine can prevent or reduce liver damage, even after large overdoses. Early randomized trials suggested reductions in mortality from late administration of acetylcysteine, and intervention studies showed improvements in systemic and cerebral haemodynamics and oxygen uptake. A multicentre, double-blind, randomized trial of acetylcysteine in non-paracetamol acute liver failure showed that acetylcysteine was well tolerated and associated with improved non-transplanted survival, but only in patients treated early in the course of disease and with low-grade encephalopathy.

- **General measures**. Nurse supine (not at 45°, as often stated). Keep in a peaceful environment. Insert an arterial line and CVP line for monitoring.
- **Coagulopathy**. The PT is the best indicator of liver function. Avoid giving fresh frozen plasma (FFP), unless there is bleeding or if the patient is undergoing surgical procedures or line insertion. Factor concentrates may precipitate

Table 8.15 King's College criteria for selection of recipients of emergency liver transplants

Paracetamol

1. Arterial pH less than 7.3, following adequate volume resuscitation
2. Combination of encephalopathy grade 3 or more, creatinine >300 micromoles/L, and international normalized ratio (INR) more than 6.5

Non-paracetamol

1. Any grade encephalopathy and INR >6·5
2. Three of: INR >3.5, bilirubin >300 micromoles/L, age <10 years or >40 years, unfavourable cause (drug-induced liver injury, seronegative disease)

This criteria was published in *Gastroenterology*, **97**, 2, John G O'Grady *et al.*, 'Early indicators of prognosis in fulminant hepatic failure', pp. 439–445, Copyright American Gastroenterological Association, 1989.

DIC. The PT may rise and fall precipitously and should be measured twice daily if deteriorating. Give intravenous vitamin K 10 mg once only. Give platelet support if thrombocytopenic and bleeding.

- **Encephalopathy**. Patients are often given lactulose, although this has no effect on outcome, and the development of encephalopathy is dependent on liver function which will either respond to treatment with acetylcysteine or deteriorate.
- **Cerebral oedema**. Cerebral oedema develops in 30–50% of patients with grade 4 encephalopathy. Intracerebral pressure (ICP) monitoring is used in some centres. If signs of cerebral oedema are present, then give mannitol (100 mL of 20% mannitol); if in renal failure,

Table 8.16 Current UK criteria for registration for emergency liver transplantation in adults

Paracetamol overdose

1. Paracetamol overdose: pH <7.25 after fluid resuscitation
2. Paracetamol overdose: lactate >3.5 mmol/L on admission or >3.0 mM after fluid resusicitation at least 24 hours after paracetamol overdose
3. Paracetamol overdose: coexisting INR >6.5 or 100 seconds, and serum creatinine >300 micromoles/L and grade 3–4 encephalopathy
4. Paracetamol overdose: two of three of the criteria from (3) above, with clinical evidence of deterioration (e.g. increased ICP, or increased FiO_2 requirements, or increasing inotrope requirements in the absence of sepsis)

Non-paracetamol overdose

1. Seronegative hepatitis, hepatitis A, hepatitis B, or idiosyncratic drug reaction, with prothrombin time >100 s or INR >6.5 and any grade of encephalopathy
2. Seronegative hepatitis, hepatitis A, hepatitis B, or idiosyncratic drug reaction, with any three of the following: PT >50 s or INR >3.5, jaundice to encephalopathy time >7 days, serum bilirubin >300 micromoles/L, and age >40 years
3. Acute presentation of Wilson's disease or Budd–Chiari syndrome with both a coagulopathy and encephalopathy
4. Hepatic artery thrombosis <21 days after liver transplantation

Reproduced from 'Liver Transplantation: Selection Criteria and Recipient Registration', Policy POL195/2, created by the Liver Advisory Group on behalf of NHSBT, available at http://www.odt.nhs.uk/pdf/liver_selection_policy.pdf. Accessed 21st May 2014. With permission from NHS Blood and Transplant.

Box 8.9 Key points: management of acute liver failure

Discuss all cases with the **regional liver transplant** centre.

Nurse supine, and keep patient in a peaceful environment.

Correct hypovolaemia (colloid or blood) **and electrolyte disturbances** (e.g. hypokalaemia, hypophosphataemia). Avoid fluid overload. Persistent hypotension may respond to noradrenaline or vasopressin infusion.

Encephalopathy: observe

Cerebral oedema: if signs of cerebral oedema (e.g. hypertension) are present, give mannitol (100 mL of 20% mannitol).

Coagulopathy: monitor PT. Give vitamin K (10 mg IV once only). Avoid FFP unless if bleeding or undergoing surgical procedures. Platelet support if thrombocytopenic and bleeding.

Hypoglycaemia: monitor blood glucose level 2-hourly, and treat with 10% or 50% glucose to keep glucose >3.5 mmol/L.

Hepatorenal syndrome: terlipressin and intravenous albumin with early renal support.

Sepsis: prophylactic antibiotics/antifungals (e.g. cefotaxime and fluconazole).

Treat the underlying cause: for example, in paracetamol overdose: acetylcysteine; stop the suspected drug.

Monitor: pulse rate, BP, oxygen saturations, CVP, urine output/fluid balance, grade of encephalopathy, and renal function closely in the high dependency or intensive therapy unit.

watch for fluid overload. Hyperventilation decreases ICP at the expense of cerebral blood flow and should be avoided. Epoprostenol and N-acetylcysteine may decrease ICP. Hypertension is almost always secondary to raised ICP and should be treated with mannitol as above; antihypertensive drugs may precipitate brainstem coning. Seizures should be treated in the usual way.

- **Haemodynamic support**. Correct hypovolaemia with crystalloid fluids (as above) or blood, but avoid fluid overload (keep CVP ~8 cm). Persistent hypotension may respond to noradrenaline or terlipressin infusion.
- **Metabolic changes**. Monitor glucose 2-hourly, and give 10% or 50% glucose to keep glucose >3.5 mmol/L. Monitor serum phosphate (often very low), and replace with intravenous supplements (9–18 mmol/24 h) if less than 0.4 mmol/L. Ensuring adequate nutrition may be difficult as an ileus is usually present. However, most units attempt initial enteral nutrition and amend to parenteral nutrition if this fails.
- **Renal failure** (see Chapter 11). Monitor renal function (renal failure occurs in ~70% cases). Treat by haemodiafiltration, rather than haemodialysis.
- **Respiratory support**. Monitor oxygen saturations continuously, and give oxygen by face mask if SaO_2 <90%. Ventilate when grade 3 or 4 encephalopathy is present (avoid ET tube ties which compress the internal jugular veins).
- **Infection**. Start prophylactic antibiotics and antifungal agents (e.g. cefotaxime and fluconazole).
- **Wilson's disease**. Consider penicillamine and intravenous vitamin E.

Further reading

Bernal W and Wendon J (1999). Acute liver failure; clinical features and management. *European Journal of Gastroenterology and Hepatology*, **11**, 977–84.

Lee WM, Larson AM, Stravitz T (2011). AASLD position paper: the management of acute liver failure: update 2011. American Association for the Study of Liver Diseases, Baltimore. <http://www.guidelines.gov/content.aspx?id=36894>.

Infections and the liver

Liver abscesses

Bacterial abscesses may arise from systemic infection or local portal phlebitis. Common associations include obstructive biliary tree disease (30–40%, often causing multiple abscesses), intra-abdominal infection (15–25%, particularly diverticular disease, appendicitis, inflammatory bowel disease, and colonic malignancy), systemic infection (15–20%, especially infective endocarditis), and direct trauma. Pre-existing liver lesions constitute a significant risk, especially with prior instrumentation or tumour necrosis, e.g. following chemoembolization or radiofrequency ablation of a hepatocellular carcinoma.

Infections are often polymicrobial, with gut-derived Gram-negative bacteria (*Escherichia coli*, *Klebsiella*), Gram-positive organisms (enterococci, *Streptococcus milleri*), and anaerobes (*Bacteroides*). *Staphylococcus aureus* is common in children.

Presentation

- Liver abscesses commonly present with fever and night sweats, weight loss, or right upper quadrant (RUQ) or intercostal pain.
- The underlying cause (e.g. appendicitis) may be silent or barely noticed. Ask about recent abdominal pain, altered bowel habit, diarrhoea, biliary colic, rectal bleeding, or inflammatory bowel disease.
- The travel history, occupation (farming is a risk factor for amoebiasis), or contact with infected persons (TB) may help.
- Examine for jaundice, hepatomegaly, pleural effusions (commonly right-sided), intercostal tenderness (characteristic of amoebic abscesses), abdominal masses (tumour or inflammatory mass), and lymphadenopathy. Perform a rectal examination for pelvic tumour.
- Severe infection may be associated with septic shock (see Chapter 2).

Causes

- Pyogenic organisms (appendicitis, diverticulitis, carcinoma, biliary).
- Amoebic abscess (*Entamoeba histolytica*).
- Hydatid cyst (*Echinococcus granulosus*).
- Tuberculosis (TB, very rare).

Investigations

Biochemistry including U&Es detects renal impairment due to sepsis. LFTs typically show an elevated ALP and reduced albumin. Non-specific LFTs are usually due to cholestasis and may be normal with amoebic abscess. Inflammatory markers (WCC, CRP, and ESR) are often raised. Blood cultures are positive in 50–80%.

- Prothrombin time may be prolonged with multiple abscesses.
- FBC (leucocytosis, eosinophilia, non-specific anaemia).
- Blood cultures, CRP, ESR.
- Amoebic and hydatid serology. ELISA for *E. histolytica* should be performed in travellers from endemic regions.
- Stool may contain amoebic cysts or vegetative forms.
- CXR (looking for effusion or pulmonary TB). CXR may demonstrate a raised right hemidiaphragm, pleural effusion, or right lower lobe consolidation.
- USS of liver, biliary tree, and abdomen (iliac fossae, in particular). Ultrasound has a sensitivity of 80–90%. The main differential is a simple cyst; abscesses appear as hypoechoic masses with irregular borders. Ultrasound also allows close evaluation of the rest of the biliary tree.
- CT scan with contrast, looking for masses, and sensitivity is almost 100%. Both pyogenic and amoebic abscesses tend to be thick-walled; hydatid cysts are thin-walled, and there may be daughter cysts. Solid tumours are echodense but may have necrotic hypodense centres.
- Gallium scans (or indium-111 labelled WBC scans) will show up pyogenic foci in the liver and elsewhere (e.g. terminal ileitis); amoebic abscesses do not take up the label.
- Aspirate large abscesses, and send the aspirate/pus for Gram stain and culture. If there is a suspicion of hydatid disease, aspiration is contraindicated (see Chapter 6).
- The primary site of infection should be carefully sought, with a low threshold for echocardiogram and colonoscopy.

Management

- Antibiotics should initially be given empirically to cover the broad spectrum of organisms above (e.g. cefuroxime and metronidazole, or piperacillin-tazobactam), then adjusted, according to sensitivities. Treatment should be continued for 2 weeks intravenously, then 6 weeks orally.
- Aspirate any large abscesses under USS. It is pointless to try and drain multiple abscesses. If there is a continuing intra-abdominal source, it is virtually impossible to eradicate liver abscesses without removing or dealing with the source (e.g. appendix).
- Pyogenic abscess: perform percutaneous aspiration of any large abscesses. Commence broad-spectrum antibiotics (e.g. cefotaxime and metronidazole).
- Amoebic abscess: treat with metronidazole (or tinidazole), followed by diloxanide furoate. USS-guided aspiration may help to improve penetration of the drugs and shorten illness (see Chapter 6). Secondary bacterial infection occurs in up to 20%.
- Hydatid disease: open surgical drainage is the treatment of choice. Albendazole may help to reduce the risk of recurrence post-surgery or be used in inoperable cases (see Chapter 6).
- Anti-tuberculous therapy for tuberculous abscesses.
- Surgery is rarely required but may be indicated for abscesses that are >5 cm, multiloculated, or ruptured.

Complications

- Sepsis.
- Empyema.
- Peritonitis.
- Endophthalmitis (particularly with *Klebsiella* bacteraemia).

Prognosis

Treatment is successful in 80–90%, although abscesses may take weeks to months to resolve. Be guided clinically, rather than radiologically. Nonetheless, mortality is high in children and the elderly, as well as those with severe comorbidity or delayed diagnosis.

Amoebic liver abscess

Entamoeba histolytica is the major pathogenic amoebic species infecting humans. Asymptomatic or convalescent carriers are the principal sources, and cysts remain viable in the environment for up to 2 months. Incidence is particularly high in South America, West Africa, and South East Asia.

Cysts are ingested and colonize the caecum and proximal colon. Tissue invasion subsequently occurs, and organisms reach the liver via the portal vein. They then progressively and continuously extend, causing hepatocyte necrosis, liquefaction, and liver abscess (see Chapter 6).

Presentation
Fewer than 50% of patients give a history of preceding dysentery, and the latent period can be several months. The main symptoms are fever, sweating, liver or diaphragmatic pain, and weight loss. The onset is insidious, although pain may be abrupt. Fever is characteristic, with prominent evening spikes, associated rigors, and profuse sweating. Painful dry cough due to diaphragmatic irritation is common.

On examination, patients are often anaemic. Localized, tender hepatomegaly may occur; if involving the left lobe, this can present as an epigastric mass.

Amoebic brain abscesses are extremely rare (<0.1% cases) but arise exclusively alongside hepatic disease. The usual presentation is with sudden-onset headache, vomiting, changes in mental state, and seizures.

Investigations
Blood tests
They typically show normochromic normocytic anaemia, neutrophilia and an elevated CRP and ESR. LFTs are usually normal. Serology is >95% sensitive and specific although it does not distinguish between current and past infection. False negatives can occur early in infection, but rising titres will be seen on repeating the test.

Radiology
As for pyogenic abscesses. Most lesions are solitary (70%), though multiple abscesses are commoner in children and patients with concurrent dysentery.

Diagnostic aspiration
A therapeutic trial of an amoebicide (see 'Treatment' section) is generally preferable to diagnostic aspiration. When performed, the classic description is of a pink-brown 'anchovy sauce' aspirate (see Figure 6.4, Chapter 6). Diagnosis is made on observation of cysts or trophozoites on wet mounts of this material.

Gastrointestinal investigations
Stool culture or colonoscopy may reveal unsuspected luminal involvement, even in the absence of dysentery. Microscopic examination of stool alone cannot differentiate E. histolytica from non-pathogenic E. dispar.

Treatment
Antibiotics are mandatory, with metronidazole 800 mg three times daily (tds) or tinidazole 2 g once daily for 5 days. This should be accompanied by 10 days of diloxanide 500 mg tds to eliminate luminal bowel infection, as relapse is common, unless parasitological cure is achieved. Ultrasound monitoring of lesions is helpful, although no change is expected within the first 2 weeks. The criteria for aspiration and surgery are the same as those for pyogenic abscesses. Additionally, patients whose pain and fever does not subside within 72 h have a high risk of rupture or antibiotic failure and should generally undergo therapeutic aspiration.

Abscesses that rupture always require laparotomy. Those that extend into pleural or pericardial cavities necessitate drainage of these structures as well as liver lesions.

Complications
- Extension into pleura, peritoneum and pericardium.
- Extension to skin, with sinus formation.
- Subphrenic rupture.
- Empyema.
- Obstructive jaundice, secondary to compression of the biliary tree.
- Portal hypertension, secondary to compression of the portal vein.
- Metastatic abscesses (i.e. lung and brain).
- Rupture into biliary tree, presenting as haemobilia.
- Hepatobronchial fistulation, presenting with 'anchovy sauce' sputum.

Prognosis
Treatment is successful in 85%, although median time for complete resolution is 8 months.

Hydatid disease
Cystic hydatid disease is a zoonotic infection caused by the tapeworm *Echinococcus granulosus*. There are numerous endemic regions, and it is most common in rural communities. Adult tapeworms infest the small intestine of definitive hosts, usually canines. Eggs pass into faeces and contaminate soil, remaining viable for long periods before ingestion by intermediate hosts that include sheep, cattle, and man. They then hatch in the bowel into oncospheres, which penetrate the intestinal mucosa and disseminate through the bloodstream and lymphatics to generate cysts in the liver (60%), lung (25%), and rarely bone, brain, and kidney (see Chapter 6).

Incubation is highly variable and may be prolonged for several years. Cyst growth is also unpredictable, ranging from static to >5 cm/year.

Presentation
Most cysts are asymptomatic, though symptoms can arise from mass effects (e.g. palpable RUQ mass, abdominal pain, or obstructive jaundice) or complications (e.g. rupture, with anaphylaxis or secondary infection).

Extrahepatic cysts may present as:
- Lung: dyspnoea, cough ± haemoptysis, pneumothorax, or empyema.
- Peritonitis.
- Bone: pathological fracture or deformity.
- Central nervous system (CNS): raised intracranial pressure, fits, spinal cord compression.

Investigation
- **Blood tests.** FBC may be normal, though eosinophilia occurs in 25%. LFTs may be normal or deranged. Serology is 90% sensitive.
- **Imaging.** CXR detects coexistent lung lesions. Ultrasound can delineate hepatic cysts, although CT is the gold standard, with 95% accuracy and high sensitivity for demonstrating characteristic daughter cysts.
- **Casoni skin test.** This is now obsolete, as the sensitivity is low and there is the potential for anaphylaxis.

Treatment
Surgery is the first-line treatment, as only 30% are cured with medical therapy alone. Options include limited cystectomy or partial organ resection. During the procedure, sterilization of the cyst, with 20% hypertonic saline or 90% alcohol, and prevention of spillage by prior evacuation of contents are essential. Accidental release of scolices into the peritoneal cavity can cause anaphylaxis or secondary peritoneal hydatidosis.

An alternative in patients where surgery is unsuitable is percutaneous aspiration, injection, and re-aspiration (PAIR). Cysts are punctured under ultrasound guidance and contents withdrawn. A protoscolicidal agent is injected (usually hypertonic saline), left for 15 min, then re-aspirated.

Albendazole 10–15 mg/kg daily should be given for at least 1 month during the perioperative/procedural period. Mebendazole is an alternative treatment but less effective. FBC and LFTs should be monitored every 2 weeks. Prophylactic antihistamines are helpful.

Prognosis
Generally good, although recurrence occurs in up to 30%.

Bacterial infections
The liver may be involved during infection with spirochaetes (*Leptospira* and *Borrelia*), actinomycetes, and mycobacteria.

Leptospirosis (Weil's disease)
Weil's disease refers to the 10% of infections with *Leptospira interrogans* (previously termed *Leptospira icterohaemorrhagiae*) that result in clinical hepatitis (see also Chapter 6). It is endemic in the tropics but, in the west, is mainly carried by rats. Infection occurs through direct contact with contaminated soil, water, or urine. It enters the skin through cuts or abrasions. Diagnosis requires a careful history to elicit possible exposures. Occupational and recreational risk factors include:

- Farm workers, veterinarians, and abattoir workers.
- Plumbers.
- Sewage workers.
- Military and naval personnel.
- Sports, including caving and those involving water contact.

Leptospirosis is caused by infection with the spirochaete *Leptospira interrogans*, of which there are many subtypes (serovars). Leptospira are spiral-shaped aerobic spirochaetes, best visualized by dark field microscopy, silver stain, or fluorescent microscopy. *L. interrogans* can be grown from clinical specimens, including blood, urine, and cerebrospinal fluid (CSF), but special media are required for isolation, so you should discuss this with the laboratory before samples are sent. Growth may take up to 3 months.

The commonest cause of leptospirosis in the UK is contact with rat urine, although cases have been seen in pig farmers and fisheries.

Investigations
These should include FBC, U&E, LFTs, PT, CPK, CXR, urinalysis and cultures, *Leptospira* serology and blood cultures with a specific request to culture *Leptospira*.

Laboratory findings
There may be a leucocytosis, sterile pyuria, severe jaundice (bilirubin >1,000 micromoles/L), with other liver function tests being virtually normal (transaminases, especially AST, may increase up to 200 U/L), increased serum creatinine indicative of renal failure, increased creatinine kinase (CPK) due to muscle injury (50%), hyponatraemia, and abnormal CXR with a ground glass appearance.

Treatment
Patients should be treated with either benzylpenicillin or doxycycline, although these probably do not affect outcome.

Presentation
Following a 7–14-day (up to a month) incubation period, *Leptospirosis* tends to present with an abrupt onset of a 4–7-day septicaemic phase, characterized by flu-like symptoms, including fever, rigors, muscle aches, dyspnoea and headache in 75–100% of patients. Sometimes patients are suspected of having meningitis and undergo lumbar puncture which is then attributed to viral meningitis, since there tends to be a CSF lymphocytosis, a small or modest increase in CSF protein, and no organisms seen (aseptic meningitis). As organisms are cleared, there is a period of clinical improvement. Within the next 1–2 weeks, there follows a second phase of illness, which is immune-mediated. Features include recurrence of fever, meningeal irritation, iritis, skin haemorrhagic lesions (e.g. petechiae, purpura, and ecchymoses), renal failure with acute tubular necrosis, and jaundice with hepatomegaly, as part of the biphasic illness. The pathogenesis of jaundice remains unexplained: neither haemolysis nor hepatocellular necrosis are prominent, and it is difficult to demonstrate many organisms within the affected tissue.

Approximately 25% have a non-productive cough, and 50% have nausea, vomiting, and diarrhoea. Abdominal pain is rare.

Physical examination may reveal jaundice and a rash, as well as conjunctival suffusion, at least in the early stages and sometimes later stages too. Patients may also have hepatomegaly (60%), muscle tenderness, splenomegaly, lymphadenopathy, and pharyngitis.

Leptospirosis has a variable clinical course. Most cases are mild to moderate with subclinical or self-limited systemic infection. However, severe, potentially fatal illness complicated by multiorgan failure, including renal failure, jaundice, haemorrhage, uveitis, ARDS, myocarditis, and rhabdomyolysis may occur. Liver failure and death are rare but do occur. Vasculitis with necrosis of extremities is also rare.

Investigation
Blood tests
FBC (usually Hb and platelets low, with neutrophilia), U&E (K^+ often low due to renal wasting), LFTs (elevated bilirubin and ALT/AST more than ALP), and clotting (prolonged PT). The degree of jaundice has no prognostic significance. CK and aldolase are elevated during the first week in >50%, with liver disease as a consequence of coexistent muscle damage. Blood cultures give a high yield in the first phase. Serology is highly sensitive and specific.

Urinalysis
Urinalysis is frequently positive for protein, WBCs, and RBCs. Dark field microscopy of serially diluted urines for spirochaetes becomes positive in the second phase and remains so for several weeks. Yield is high, but culture usually takes too long to be beneficial.

CSF
Look for pleocytosis and presence of leptospires. There is a high yield during the first week in the presence of meningitic symptoms. This becomes negative in the second phase.

Imaging
The CXR may show patchy snowflake-like infiltrates in the periphery.

Treatment
Antibiotics are highly effective if administered early. Give doxycycline 100 mg twice daily (bd) orally or amoxicillin 500 mg–1 g four times daily (qds) orally or IV (depending on

severity) for 1 week. Jarisch–Herxheimer reaction may occur, which should be managed supportively.

Complications

- Pulmonary haemorrhage. Consider prompt intubation and ventilation.
- Renal failure. Usually secondary to hypovolaemia that responds rapidly to intravenous fluids but interstitial nephritis can develop. May require renal replacement therapy, as renal failure is the commonest cause of death.
- Coagulopathy. Bleeding principally occurs into the skin or lung.
- Meningitis. Immune-mediated. Clinically evident in up to 50%.
- Myopathy.
- Myocarditis. First-degree heart block is common and reversible.

Prognosis

This is excellent if treated early, although overall mortality remains 5–10%, usually due to renal or cardiorespiratory failure. Liver involvement is rarely fatal, and patients demonstrate no residual liver dysfunction or pathological structural changes. Meningeal involvement is typically fully reversible.

Lyme disease

Lyme disease results from infection with *Borrelia burgdorferi*, transmitted to humans via the *Ixodes* tick. There is a tick-vertebrate cycle, involving white-footed mice in North America, and a variety of small mammals and birds in Europe. The disease is most prevalent in America, Canada, Northern Europe, and North Asia. It affects all ages, though incidences are highest in 5–9 year olds and adults >30 years old.

Presentation

The illness is triphasic, starting with erythema migrans, a red macule or papule, appearing at the site of a bite incurred 7–10 days earlier (see Figure 6.1, Chapter 6). This rash expands over days to weeks (3–30 days), with or without central clearing. Systemic involvement occurs in the second phase, including fatigue, myalgia, arthralgia, headache, fever, and regional lymphadenopathy. The third phase is marked by carditis (with conduction defects), cranial neuropathies, and/or meningitis.

Gastroenterological symptoms and signs are common during the early stages. Predominant findings include anorexia (20%), nausea (15%), vomiting (10%), abdominal pain (8%), hepatomegaly (5%), splenomegaly (5%), and diarrhoea (2%). Approximately 10% have symptoms suggestive of hepatitis, with biochemical evidence of mild hepatocellular injury in up to 30%. The usual pattern is mildly elevated transaminases, although these may also derive from myositis (see Chapter 6).

Treatment

Most manifestations resolve spontaneously, although antibiotics hasten recovery. Doxycycline 100 mg bd orally or amoxicillin orally for 2–3 weeks are effective. Jarisch–Herxheimer reactions may occur.

Prognosis

Prognosis is excellent. Almost all manifestations resolve with antibiotics.

Actinomycetes

Actinomycetes are subacute to chronic granulomatous suppurative inflammatory diseases, with slowly progressive formation of multiple abscesses. They are caused by polymicrobial infection with various facultative anaerobes, principally *Actinomyces* (most commonly *israelii* or *gerencseriae*) and *Propionibacterium*. There is frequently co-infection with other gut organisms. Many actinomycetes derive from commensal oral flora. Active tissue invasion typically occurs during times of reduced organ perfusion. Immunodeficiency does not specifically predispose.

Presentation

Abdominal actinomycoses are rare and usually originate from perforating disease, e.g. appendicitis, diverticulitis, or trauma. Most present as slow-growing tumours and can directly extend into other organs, including the liver. Haematogenous liver abscesses are also seen, particularly accompanying genital actinomycoses (associated with salpingitis and long-term use of intrauterine devices or vaginal pessaries).

Investigation

Diagnosis relies on bacteriological examination of pus or affected tissue and demonstration therein of pathognomonic sulphur granules. Radiology is non-diagnostic but may delineate organ invasion.

Treatment

Infection is always polymicrobial, so antibiotics should cover all causative and concomitant organisms. Suitable regimes are:

- Co-amoxiclav + metronidazole + gentamicin.
- Ampicillin + clindamycin + clarithromycin.

Treatment needs to be prolonged (at least 3 weeks). Surgical drainage may be indicated for non-resolving abscesses or acute compression of adjacent structures.

Prognosis

Good with early diagnosis, but complications can otherwise be severe.

Tuberculosis

Mycobacterium tuberculosis affects the liver in various forms. Mycobacteria reach the liver through haematogenous spread, direct extension from the lung, or via the portal tract. Five main pathological patterns are seen:

- **Miliary TB.** Occurs as part of systemic infection. There are rarely symptoms or signs directly relevant to the liver.
- **Granulomatous hepatitis.** Presents with unexplained fever, mild jaundice ± hepatomegaly. Biopsy shows caseating granulomas. There is improvement with antituberculosis therapy.
- **Localized disease.** Includes tuberculomas, abscesses, and solitary or multiple nodules.
- **Cholangitis.** Secondary to portal lymphadenopathy or inflammatory strictures of intrahepatic ductal epithelium. Very rare.
- **Abnormal LFTs.** Liver function tests may be slightly abnormal, usually cholestatic in any patient with TB.

Presentation

Abdominal pain (mostly RUQ) is the main symptom of hepatobiliary TB, although it may be asymptomatic. Nodular hepatomegaly is present in 50%, and splenomegaly in 25%. Jaundice occurs in up to 35% and is usually obstructive in nature. The differential diagnosis is from other infections, granulomatous disorders, and neoplasia.

Similar presentations can be seen in:

• Brucellosis, syphilis, toxoplasma, leishmaniasis, schistosomosis, toxocara, or coccidiomycoses.
• Sarcoidosis or Hodgkin's lymphoma.

Investigation
Radiology

CXR demonstrates concurrent pulmonary abnormalities in 65% of cases. Abdominal X-ray (AXR) may show liver calcification (50%). Ultrasound can delineate focal lesions.

Percutaneous aspiration and biopsy

This may be radiologically guided for localized lesions, or blind for miliary or granulomatous hepatitis.

Treatment

Antibiotic therapy is similar to pulmonary disease, although treatment is often protracted for up to 1 year. Obstructive jaundice requires ERCP, with stenting or percutaneous transhepatic drainage.

Prognosis

Two-thirds of patients respond well, but mortality is high in the remainder due to variceal bleeds related to portal hypertension and cholangitis. Hepatic failure, in itself, is rarely the cause of death.

Parasitic infections

The hepatobiliary system may be involved in a number of parasitic infections, including visceral leishmaniasis, schistosomiasis, and ascaris.

Leishmaniasis

The *Leishmania* parasite can cause visceral (kala-azar) or cutaneous disease, depending on subspecies. The former results from infection with *L. donovani* in India and Africa and *L. major* in the Middle East, Asia, and Mediterranean littoral. Epidemics may also occur, usually in 15–20 year cycles, particularly around the Ganges and Brahmaputra rivers in India and Bangladesh. Parasites are carried by sandflies, which live in rodent burrows (see also Chapter 6).

It is estimated that, for every clinical case of visceral leishmaniasis, approximately 30 are subclinical and undiagnosed. The disease shows a male predominance of 4:1, and, although all ages are affected, children <5 years old are particularly predisposed. Risk occupations include hunters, soldiers, and non-immune tourists. In immunocompromised individuals, leishmaniasis can develop as an opportunistic infection, in which the presentation may be atypical.

Presentation

The incubation period is 2–8 months. Onset is typically insidious but can be rapid in non-immune tourists during epidemics. The main initial presentation is fever that classically spikes twice daily, without rigors. Abdominal left upper quadrant (LUQ) pain and distension can result from massive splenomegaly; rupture is a rare, but critical, complication. The liver is moderately enlarged in one-third. Malabsorption leads to weight loss and diarrhoea. Hypoalbuminaemia can be profound, accompanied by oedema and leuconychia.

The clinical picture can vary, according to geographic location. In Africa, generalized lymphadenopathy is common. In India, 20% of patients experience increased pigmentation (kala-azar) of the face and extensor surfaces during recovery. This may resemble lepromatous leprosy.

Investigation
Blood tests

FBC typically shows normochromic normocytic anaemia, without reticulocytosis; leucopenia, and thrombocytopenia occur secondary to hypersplenism. Albumin is often <20 g/L, although other LFTs are usually normal. Serology is 80–100% sensitive in the absence of HIV infection.

Parasitology

Definitive diagnosis is made by observing the organism within affected reticuloendothelial tissues. Splenic aspiration is the most sensitive (95%), though complications are serious. Alternative sources are liver biopsy or bone marrow aspirate.

Leishmanin skin test

This delayed hypersensitivity reaction seen in cutaneous leishmaniasis is negative with visceral disease.

Treatment

The treatment of choice is liposomal amphotericin 2–3 mg/kg IV daily for 7–10 days. This is costly and in endemic regions alternatives include the antimony compounds sodium stibogluconate and megluminate antimoate. The dose is 10–20 mg/kg antimony for 21 days. LFTs and amylase must be monitored, along with ECG (long QT and non-specific T wave changes). Miltefosine is the first effective oral drug and has superseded traditional antimony injections in areas of high prevalence (e.g. North Bihar, India) where resistance has developed. Response is best determined clinically by monitoring fever, spleen size, haemoglobin level, albumin, and weight. Parasitological proof of cure is not required but helpful to determine relapse.

Nutritional deficiencies and intercurrent infections should be treated as they arise. Transfusion is rarely necessary.

Prognosis

Mortality in untreated cases is 15–25%, although there is generally a rapid response if treated early, with cure rates >90%. Relapse is not uncommon, particularly amongst HIV-infected individuals. Monitoring for parasites at 6 weeks and 6 months aids early detection.

Schistosomiasis

Schistosoma mansoni and *japonicum* are two of the commonest causes of hepatic infection worldwide. They are endemic in Africa, South America, the Middle East, China and Southeast Asia. Parasites are acquired from fresh water, where they reproduce in snails. They penetrate the skin to enter the bloodstream, and mature and migrate to the bowel. They can subsequently enter the portal system, where eggs induce an immune response, peri-portal fibrosis and granuloma formation, the severity of which correlates with disease duration and parasite load.

Presentation

A pruritic rash (cercarial dermatitis, 'swimmers itch') occurs at the entry site within 24 h. A hypersensitivity reaction can also manifest with a pruritic maculopapular eruption, lasting up to 2 weeks, and is more intense with repeat exposures.

In primary infection, an acute toxaemia can arise (Katayama fever). Patients present with fever, myalgia, and lethargy. This may mimic a viral illness, and the diagnosis is often missed. A history of exposure to contaminated freshwater is key.

Chronic infection leads to gastrointestinal symptoms and signs. Abdominal discomfort and diarrhoea are most common, although severe dysentery is rare. On examination, there may be tender hepatomegaly (particularly left lobe), with or without signs of portal hypertension, ascites, splenomegaly, and generalized lymphadenopathy. The lungs, kidneys, and CNS (including spinal cord) can also be involved.

Co-infection with hepatitis B or C is associated with particularly aggressive hepatic disease.

Investigations
Blood tests
May show anaemia and eosinophilia. LFTs are typically normal. Serology is unreliable.

Parasitology
Diagnosis is made by demonstrating eggs or schistosomes in the stool or affected liver.

Imaging
Ultrasound is helpful for grading fibrosis and portal hypertension.

Treatment
The drug of choice is praziquantel, which is effective against all schistosomes affecting man. The doses are:
- *S. mansoni*: 40 mg/kg in two divided doses over 24 h.
- *S. japonicum*: 60 mg/kg in three divided doses over 24 h.

Prognosis
Liver fibrosis is reversible if treatment is initiated early, although presentation is often delayed. Complete cure is achieved in 85%, and egg burden reduced by >95% in other patients. The most common cause of death is massive upper GI haemorrhage from oesophageal varices, present in approximately 80% of patients with hepatic disease.

Ascariasis
Ascaris lumbricoides is a nematode worm acquired from ingestion of contaminated soil. It has a widespread geographic distribution but is most prevalent in rural tropics. The disease is relatively more common in children, who also carry higher worm loads.

Eggs hatch in the small intestine, then penetrate the intestinal wall into the portal circulation. From the liver, they are carried haematogenously to the lungs, from where they migrate up the bronchial tree and over the epiglottis back into the digestive tract. They can also migrate to ectopic sites in patients who are febrile or in whom the gastrointestinal tract has been irritated, e.g. by drugs, anaesthesia, or surgical manipulation.

Adult worms have a lifespan of 1 year, after which they are spontaneously expelled from the bowel.

Presentation
Most cases are asymptomatic, although the presentation may include fever, malaise, nausea, vomiting, intestinal colic, or diarrhoea. The migratory phase can cause a hypersensitivity eosinophilic pneumonitis, with urticaria and bronchospasm (Loeffler's syndrome), lasting on average 7–10 days. In severe disease, a large number of worms can entangle to form obstructing boluses. Depending on location, these can cause intestinal obstruction, acute appendicitis, pancreatitis, or ascending cholangitis with obstructive jaundice. The latter is often associated with multiple liver abscesses, caused

by the disintegration of trapped worms or eggs and secondary bacterial infection.

Investigation
Blood tests
FBC is usually normal, apart from eosinophilia during the migration phase. LFTs and amylase are useful if obstruction of the biliary tree or pancreatic duct is suspected. Serology is not helpful for diagnosis.

Imaging
CXR may show transient mottling or opacities during the migratory phase but is otherwise normal. AXR is usually normal although it can show a large bolus of worms (particularly during contrast studies) or obstruction with extremely heavy loads. Ultrasound will reveal obstruction of the biliary tree and the presence of hepatic abscesses.

ERCP
This is indicated for diagnosis if there is evidence of cholangitis or pancreatitis, and for the therapeutic removal of worms.

Treatment
Antihelminth agents are indicated in all cases, irrespective of the presentation or worm load, as the consequences of a single episode of ectopic migration are severe. Treatment should, however, be avoided during active pulmonary migration or infection, as the risks of pneumonitis from dying worms are high. Suitable choices include:
- Albendazole 400 mg orally, single dose.
- Mebendazole 100 mg bd for 3 days.
- Pyrantel pamoate 11 mg/kg (maximum total dose 1 g), single dose.
- Piperazine salts 75 mg/kg (maximum total dose 3.5 g) once daily for 2 days.
- These agents are unsuitable for pregnant women and children, and expert advice should be sought in such cases. Pyrantel pamoate and piperazine are paralysing agents and should not be used in intestinal obstruction, as they may exacerbate the blockage.

Supportive treatment is required for other complications. ERCP is indicated for cholangitis or pancreatitis. Intestinal obstruction should be managed, as described in the section on acute abdominal pain, and may require surgical intervention.

Prognosis
Medical therapy is curative in >90% patients.

Further reading
Chen SC, Lee YT, Yen CH, *et al.* (2009). Pyogenic liver abscess in the elderly: clinical features, outcomes and prognostic factors. *Age and Ageing*, **38**, 271–6.

Hughes MA and Petri WA Jr (2000). Amebic liver abscess. *Infectious Disease Clinic of North America*, **14**, 565–82.

Mazza OM, Fernandez DL, Pekolj J, *et al.* (2009). Management of non-parasitic hepatic cysts. *Journal of the American College of Surgeons*, **209**, 733–9.

Nazir NT, Penfield JD, Hajjar V (2010). Pyogenic liver abscess. *Cleveland Clinic Journal of Medicine*, **77**, 426–7.

Stanley SL Jr (2003). Amoebiasis. *Lancet*, **361**, 1025–34.

Complications in liver transplant recipients

It is important to refer all patients who present with complications of liver transplantation back to the original or local transplant centre. Nevertheless, sometimes it is necessary to investigate and treat patients locally. It is assumed that all patients would have been managed locally for the first 2–4 weeks in their liver transplant unit. The complications that may bring a patient to their local unit are the following:

1. Jaundice.
2. Abdominal pain.
3. Fever.
4. Ascites.
5. Incidental finding of abnormal bloods.
6. Vascular complications.

Jaundice

The commonest causes of jaundice in immediate post-transplant recipients are biliary complications or acute rejection. Occasionally, patients transplanted for acute non-A non-B hepatitis develop recurrent acute viral hepatitis. For longer-term patients (e.g. transplanted >1 year previously), there may be recurrent disease, leading to graft dysfunction, including hepatitis C, hepatitis B (if immune prophylaxis has not been taken), alcoholic liver disease, autoimmune hepatitis, primary biliary cirrhosis, or primary sclerosing cholangitis. Occasionally, patients transplanted for paracetamol overdose re-take an overdose.

Biliary complications

These occur in 10–30% of patients and can range from minor complications, such as contained bile leaks, to biliary strictures, biliary leaks that cause generalized peritonitis, stones, or biliary necrosis secondary to hepatic artery thrombosis. Most biliary complications occur within the first 3 months following liver transplantation, but may occur late when arterial complications are present.

Biliary leak may present with acute abdominal pain, fever, or, if the bile tracks down to the pelvis, patients may present with dysuria and lower abdominal discomfort or pain. Biliary strictures usually cause jaundice ± cholangitis.

Investigations to diagnose biliary problems include triple-phase CT scan of the liver, magnetic resonance cholangiopancreatography (MRCP), or ERCP. A HIDA (hepatobiliary iminodiacetic acid) scan is sometimes useful.

Bile leaks are generally treated by stenting. Biliary strictures due to poor arterial flow are more complicated and need to be managed in the transplant centre.

Acute liver rejection

Acute liver rejection tends to occur early, although it may occur in patients many years after liver transplantation. It is associated with an increasing serum bilirubin, together with increasing serum aminotransferases. Fever may also be present. There may be a mild elevation in eosinophil count.

Management of acute rejection

In general, it is better to avoid giving immunosuppressive drugs (pulsed methylprednisolone), unless the diagnosis is confirmed. All patients should have an ultrasound scan, including Doppler of the hepatic artery. Patients ideally should have a liver biopsy before commencing treatment, and this may be done transjugularly if the patient is on aspirin, warfarin, or tinzaparin.

Unless acute rejection is confirmed or highly suspected, avoid giving further immunosuppression unless recommended by a liver transplant unit. Further immunosuppression increases the risk of opportunistic infections as well as the later complication of lymphoproliferative disease or malignancy.

Initial treatment is with methylprednisolone 1 g IV daily for 3 days.

Vascular complications

Vascular complications may occur and can be diagnosed by Doppler imaging of the hepatic artery or magnetic resonance angiography. If there is impaired blood supply to the liver, the patient will need to be managed by the local or original liver transplant unit.

Recurrent disease

Recurrent disease is best managed by the liver transplant unit. Rarely, there may be an acute hepatitis secondary to CMV infection.

CMV hepatitis

CMV hepatitis is relatively rare following liver transplantation (<2%), but may occur.

Abdominal pain

Abdominal pain may be due to the following:

1. Biliary leak (as described previously).
2. Gastroenteritis.
3. Adhesions.
4. Localized infection (see 'Fever' section).
5. Infected ascites.
6. Constipation secondary to analgesia.
7. Other.

Occasionally, patients develop a localized infection or a collection below the wound, following liver transplantation. This should be treated conventionally, with opening up of the wound if there is a collection or simple administration of antibiotics (e.g co-amoxiclav).

There may also be an intra-abdominal collection or even a false aneurysm, causing abdominal pain.

Fever

Fever may be due to the following:

1. Localized or systemic infection.
2. Acute rejection.
3. Biliary complications.
4. CMV infection.
5. Infected ascites.
6. Other.

Most of these causes are covered above. CMV infections occur in up to 30% of liver transplant patients who are not given prophylaxis, primarily during the first 3 months when immunosuppression is most intense. CMV infection occurs in up to 80% of patients who are CMV-negative, but receive a CMV-positive graft, and they should be given prophylaxis.

Cytomegalovirus infection may cause fever, hepatitis, neutropenia, thrombocytopenia, pneumonitis, gastrointestinal disease ± diarrhoea, and retinitis.

Most CMV infections are picked up by routine screening and are rare in units that use CMV prophylaxis.

Treatment includes intravenous ganciclovir, foscarnet, or oral valganciclovir. Take advice, based on viral load from local liver transplant unit.

Ascites

Ascites may recur, following liver transplantation, particularly in patients with severe or refractory ascites prior to liver transplantation. It usually resolves, although diuretic treatment may be required for the first 2–3 months post-liver transplantation.

Also consider veno-occlusive disease which, although rare, may occur in the post-liver transplant setting. A TIPS (transjugluar intrahepatic portosystemic shunt) insertion may occasionally be required.

Incidental finding of abnormal bloods

In practice, these only include acute graft dysfunction (covered under jaundice above) or renal impairment. Occasionally, a patient may present with known CMV infection for treatment with ganciclovir or foscarnet (seek advice). For renal impairment, the most important aspect of practical management is to ensure adequate drug levels of tacrolimus or ciclosporin. Whilst there are therapeutic ranges for each of these drugs, most liver transplant units operate on the lowest possible drug regime that enables normal graft function without renal dysfunction.

If a patient presents with significant renal dysfunction, you should ensure that they are adequately hydrated, and withhold tacrolimus or ciclosporin until levels are known. In liver transplant recipients, levels are run quite low and, in the absence of liver dysfunction, serum levels are allowed to go below the therapeutic level if liver function tests are relatively normal at 3 months and beyond post-liver transplantation.

Check for fever, sepsis, and CRP. If these are positive, then take blood and urine cultures, and treat with antibiotics, as appropriate. Otherwise, simply withhold tacrolimus or ciclosporin until levels are known.

Vascular complications

Acute hepatic arterial thrombosis may cause an acute hepatitis (rise in liver transaminases) or, rarely, liver failure. If hepatic arterial thrombosis is subclinical, it may lead to liver abscess formation in the infarcted segment of liver or late biliary strictures.

All patients with hepatic arterial thrombosis need to be referred back to the liver transplant centre.

Further reading

Hirschfield GM, Gibbs P, Griffiths WJ (2009). Adult liver transplantation: what non-specialists need to know. *BMJ*, **338**, 1670.

Nadalin S, Malagò M, Radtke A, *et al.*. (2007). Current trends in live liver donation. *Transplant International*, **20**, 312–30.

Thuluvath PJ, Pfau PR, Kimmey MB, Ginsberg GG (2005). Biliary complications after liver transplantation: the role of endoscopy. *Endoscopy*, **37**, 857–63.

Pregnancy and the liver

Liver function in pregnancy

During the first trimester, there is a decrease in serum albumin due to haemodilution. As pregnancy progresses, there is an increase in serum alkaline phosphatase, mainly of placental origin (placental isoenzyme of alkaline phosphatase). Gamma GT tends to decrease throughout pregnancy.

Most pregnancy-specific liver disorders occur in the third trimester, including cholestasis of pregnancy, pre-eclampsia, and HELLP syndrome, although these may all occur in the second trimester (see Chapter 21). Acute fatty liver and hepatic rupture only occur in the third trimester. Hyperemesis gravidarum occurs in the first trimester only.

Hyperemesis gravidarum

Intractable severe vomiting, causing dehydration and ketosis, occurs in 0.2–1% of pregnancies. It arises during the first trimester and typically resolves by 18 weeks' gestation. It is more common in younger women, non-smokers, primiparas, and multiple or molar pregnancies. A twofold reversible increase in serum aminotransferases occurs in 50%, with minor elevation of ALP and bilirubin in 10%. The aetiology of the deranged LFTs is unclear, as is their significance.

Management is of fluid and electrolyte deficiencies. Give thiamine 200 mg daily orally or 100 mg intravenously weekly to prevent Wernicke's encephalopathy; total parenteral nutrition (TPN) may be required, if severe. Antiemetics are helpful (metoclopramide 10 mg tds or cyclizine 50 mg tds), as is acid suppression. Steroids have been beneficial in uncontrolled trials and should be tapered, but not stopped until after delivery. Pregnancy outcomes do not differ.

Cholestasis of pregnancy

Cholestasis of pregnancy usually manifests as generalized pruritus in the third trimester of pregnancy. It accounts for 20% of jaundice in pregnancy and affects 0.5–1% of women usually of North European, Chinese, or Chilean descent. It is rare in black or Asian women. The cause is due to a mutation of the MDR3 biliary transporter and is familial. It occurs in 50% of patients who have developed cholestasis due to oral contraceptive pill use. It is relatively benign for the mother but has negative consequences for the fetus: prematurity is increased 3-fold, and rates of fetal distress and stillbirth are higher. Intrahepatic cholestasis recurs in 65% of subsequent pregnancies.

Onset can be at any time, although the third trimester is most common. The main presentation is generalized pruritus, particularly severe on the palms and soles. Jaundice is uncommon (<25%) and typically occurs 1–4 weeks later, associated with pale stools and dark urine. Subclinical steatorrhoea may be detectable, accompanied by fat malabsorption and vitamin K deficiency. LFTs show elevated bilirubin and aminotransferases, but ALP and gamma GT are within the normal range for pregnancy. Serum bile acids rise. An ultrasound is necessary to exclude gallstone disease, and magnetic resonance cholangiopancreatography (MRCP) may be helpful. Liver biopsy is not required.

Treatment is symptomatic, using ursodeoxycholic acid (10–15 mg/kg/day), which relieves pruritus and may improve fetal outcomes. Colestyramine should be used with caution, as it may exacerbate vitamin K deficiency. In general, elective delivery is recommended at 38 weeks to minimize fetal complications, although some advocate careful observation and induction of labour only if fetal distress intervenes. Perinatal mortality is 35%. Cholestasis recurs in up to 60%.

Acute fatty liver of pregnancy

Acute fatty liver of pregnancy is a microvesicular steatosis, caused by mitochondrial dysfunction that complicates 1 in 14,000 pregnancies. It predominantly occurs during the third trimester (particularly between 34 and 37 weeks), although it may manifest earlier or post-partum. Risk factors include being primagravida, male fetus, and twin pregnancy. Up to 40% have associated pre-eclampsia or HELLP syndrome or have an overlap syndrome.

Initial symptoms include nausea, vomiting, and abdominal pain. Headache may be present. At its worse, those affected develop liver failure, encephalopathy, renal failure, pancreatitis, haemorrhage, and DIC.

In severe cases, jaundice (conjugated bilirubin >100 micromoles/L) develops within 2 weeks. Urine is dark, and stools are pale. Progression to acute liver failure may be rapid, with encephalopathy and death over a course of days. Serum aminotransferases are usually elevated to 200–750 IU/L. Hypoglycaemia is common, and the blood film commonly shows neutrophilia, normoblasts, thrombocytopenia, target cells, and giant platelets. DIC is relatively common. Upper gastrointestinal haemorrhage, acute renal failure, pancreatitis, and transient diabetes insipidus may occur. Hyperuricaemia is present in 80%. Ultrasound may reveal steatosis, although a CT scan is more sensitive. Fetal and maternal mortality is within the range of 10–20%.

Symptoms and signs in acute fatty liver
- Nausea and vomiting (100%).
- Severe dyspepsia (35%).
- Abdominal pain (60%).
- Jaundice (90%).
- Oedema (60%).
- Hypertension (65%).

Biochemistry and haematology in acute fatty liver
- Increased serum bilirubin without haemolysis.
- Hypoglycaemia.
- Elevated urea and uric acid (80%).
- Elevated transaminases.
- Proteinuria (60%).
- Elevated prothrombin time.
- Leucocytosis (90%).
- Thrombocytopenia (75%).

Liver biopsy may rarely be required to differentiate acute fatty liver from acute viral hepatitis and pre-eclampsia, which may be important for assessing prognosis in future pregnancies. Histology demonstrates microvesicular fat deposition with rare hepatocyte necrosis and minimal inflammation, similar to Reye's syndrome.

Management involves early delivery. Extreme caution with careful monitoring is advised if expectant management is employed, as deterioration can be sudden and unpredictable. Careful fluid balance is required, as the risk of pulmonary or cerebral oedema is increased. Hypoglycaemia is prevented, using intravenous dextrose. Aggressive correction of coagulopathy has been recommended. Liver transplantation is rarely required. With specialist care, maternal mortality is <1%, and perinatal mortality 7%. These values may increase without close monitoring and early intervention. The risk of recurrence is <15%.

Although most cases are idiopathic, acute fatty liver of pregnancy may arise in heterozygous mothers carrying fetuses with long-chain 3-hydroxyacyl-CoA dehydrogenase (LCHAD) deficiency. These infants may present after birth with non-ketotic hypoglycaemia, Reye's syndrome, or sudden infant death. Diagnostic testing for the G1528C mutation is, therefore, recommended in all mothers with this presentation.

Pre-eclampsia

The triad of peripheral oedema, proteinuria, and hypertension (BP >140/90 mmHg, or >30/15 mmHg above baseline) occurs in 3% of pregnancies. It arises from the end of the second trimester. Risk factors include being primagravida, extremes of age, multiple gestation, and family history. Deranged LFTs occur in 25% of mild disease and 80% of severe presentations. The most common abnormality is raised serum aminotransferases, usually <150 IU/L. Jaundice complicates severe cases. Ultrasound and CT scans demonstrate a combination of parenchymal infarcts and haemorrhage. The management of liver disease is that of pre-eclampsia, with urgent delivery alongside blood pressure control (first-line antihypertensive medications include labetalol, hydralazine, and nifedipine) and magnesium sulfate to prevent convulsions. LFTs then typically improve, although a late cholestatic phase, with a rise in ALP and gamma GT, is common.

HELLP syndrome

The syndrome of haemolysis, elevated liver enzymes, and low platelets is a thrombotic microangiopathy, affecting 0.2–0.6% of pregnancies. It occurs in 20% of patients with severe pre-eclampsia, although it can be diagnosed in its absence. Risk factors include older age, Caucasian ethnicity, and multiparity. Diagnostic criteria are:

- Haemolysis on peripheral blood film.
- LDH >600 U/L.
- ALT or AST >70 U/L.
- Platelets <100 x 10^9/L.

Symptoms begin from the second trimester (usually weeks 27–36) but can occur post-partum. Malaise and fatigue are followed by headache, nausea, and vomiting. Epigastric and RUQ pain and massive LFT derangement are ominous signs, particularly when accompanied by right shoulder tip pain. These indicate liver infarction or haematoma, with pending rupture, confirmed by ultrasound or CT scan.

In addition to the laboratory abnormalities above, the blood film picture is of a microangiopathic haemolytic anaemia (MAHA), with schistocytes, echinocytes and spherostomatocytes, and depleted serum haptoglobin. This picture may also be seen in, and needs to be differentiated from, haemolytic uraemic syndrome (HUS) and thrombotic thrombocytopenia purpura (TTP). Severity may be graded, using the Mississippi classification. It is graded as severe if the platelet count is <50 x 10^9, moderate if 50–100 x 10^9, and mild if >100 x 10^9. Haematological and LFT abnormalities usually resolve from 2 days post-partum. Liver biopsy is rarely indicated.

Maternal complications occur in up to 50%, often requiring blood transfusion and correction of coagulopathy. Up to 25% develop DIC (high D-dimer predicts severity), and 20% manifest pleural effusions or pulmonary oedema. Renal failure secondary to acute tubular necrosis arises in up to 8%.

Thrombocytopenia predisposes to placental abruption (16%), subcapsular liver haematomas (1%), wound haematomas following Caesarean section, and retinal detachment (1%). Eclampsia is twice as common in these patients.

Although conservative supportive treatment has been advocated in mild disease, indications for urgent delivery include maternal or fetal distress and persistent severe RUQ pain or shoulder tip pain with hypotension. Dexamethasone may temporally improve maternal disease and promote fetal maturation, reducing complications of premature delivery. Maternal mortality is 1%, but perinatal mortality is up to 30%. Raised urate is an independent predictor of poor outcome. Liver transplantation has been used successfully.

Close observation is required for at least 48 h, following delivery. HELLP recurs in 5% of patients.

Spontaneous hepatic rupture

Spontaneous rupture of the liver is at the extreme end of a spectrum of complications of the toxaemias of pregnancy. It complicates 1 in 100,000 pregnancies, almost exclusively in the late third trimester, and is life-threatening. Approximately 80% arise in association with severe pre-eclampsia or HELLP, and 20% with acute fatty liver of pregnancy, hepatic neoplasia, or liver abscess. The right lobe is most commonly affected.

The classic presentation is sudden-onset RUQ pain, nausea and vomiting, shock, and abdominal distension. Peritonitis may ensue. The diagnosis can be confirmed by ultrasound or CT scan; differential diagnoses include aortic dissection and diaphragmatic rupture. Current treatment is angiography with hepatic artery embolization or laparotomy and surgical haemostasis. Delivery should be by Caesarean section.

Gallstones in pregnancy

Gallstones develop in 10% of pregnancies, and existing stones grow more rapidly. Less than 0.3% are symptomatic with acute abdominal pain. ERCP with sphincterotomy or stenting is indicated for common bile duct (CBD) stones, which are sensitively and safely detected by magnetic resonance cholangiopancreatography, without risk of radiation to the fetus. Surgery can usually be deferred until after delivery, although those presenting early risk recurrence. Laparoscopic cholecystectomy can be considered in the second trimester.

Pancreatitis in pregnancy

Pancreatitis occurs most frequently in the third trimester or immediately post-partum. Management is as described in the section on acute abdominal pain. Most cases in pregnancy are as a result of gallstone disease. Diagnosis can be more difficult, as there is a physiological increase in serum amylase during pregnancy, though a rise >1,000 U is still essentially diagnostic. Serum lipase may be helpful. TPN should be considered to protect the fetus.

Budd–Chiari syndrome

High oestrogen states increase prothrombotic tendency, related to diminished concentrations of antithrombin III. This can be associated with thrombosis of the hepatic veins or inferior vena cava. RUQ pain, hepatomegaly, and maternal ascites should suggest the diagnosis, which is confirmed by ultrasound.

Anticoagulation, with therapeutic dose of low molecular weight heparin twice daily, should be commenced. In patients who do not respond, further treatment options include hepatic venous balloon dilatation or insertion of a transjugular intrahepatic shunt, although data on their use in pregnancy are limited. Maternal mortality is high (>70%).

Viral hepatitis in pregnancy

Acute viral hepatitis remains the commonest cause of jaundice in pregnancy. The presentation, course and management are largely unchanged.

Hepatitis A

The course of acute hepatitis A is generally the same in pregnancy, except that, when acquired late in pregnancy, there is a much higher risk of gestational problems, such as premature contractions, placental separation, vaginal bleeding, or premature rupture of membranes.

Hepatitis B

The course of acute hepatitis B is generally the same in pregnancy as under normal conditions. Severe hepatitis B may need treatment with lamivudine, which appears to be safe in pregnancy.

Vertical transmission occurs in 50% of cases of acute hepatitis B, rising to 70% in the third trimester. Transmission is less common with chronic carriage, but varies with viral replication rate, and is up to 90% in patients who are e antigen-positive. This can be prevented by immunization of the neonate with hepatitis B IVIG at birth and vaccination within the first week post-partum with boosters at 1, 2, and 12 months.

Hepatitis C

Transmission in chronic carriers occurs in 5–10%, correlating with viral load and, to some extent, with vaginal delivery. The risk of vertical transmission is much higher in HIV co-infected mothers. 80% of infected children become chronic carriers.

Hepatitis E

This is an RNA virus that causes acute hepatitis. It occurs predominantly in the Middle East and Asia, often in water-borne epidemics, and is transmitted via the faeco-oral route. In pregnancy, mortality is 15–20% due to acute liver failure in the third trimester. Fetal mortality is high (~50%). Vertical transmission is rare. Diagnosis is by IgM anti-HEV serology, and treatment is supportive.

Further reading

Beaulieu DB and Kane S (2011). Inflammatory bowel disease in pregnancy. *World Journal of Gastroenterology*, **17**, 2696–701.

Hay JE (2008). Liver disease in pregnancy. *Hepatology*, **47**, 1067–76.

Milkiewicz P, Elias E, Williamson C, *et al.* (2002). Obstetric cholestasis. *BMJ*, **324**, 123–4.

Royal College of Obstetricians and Gynaecologists (2011). Obstetric cholestasis. <http://www.rcog.org.uk/womens-health/clinical-guidance/obstetric-cholestasis-green-top-43>.

Inflammatory bowel disease

Introduction

Inflammatory bowel disease (IBD) includes Crohn's disease and ulcerative colitis (UC) (see Table 8.17). Crohn's disease (CD) is a chronic inflammatory disease, characterized by patchy, transmural granulomatous inflammation, which may affect any part of the gastrointestinal tract. It may be defined by age of onset, location, or behaviour. UC is characterized by diffuse mucosal inflammation, limited to the colon. It is classified according to the maximal extent of inflammatory disease of the colon observed at colonoscopy. It always affects the rectum and extends proximally to affect a variable extent of the colon. The prevalence of UC is 0.1–0.2% of the population, and, for Crohn's, it is 0.05–0.1%. The aetiologies of both UC and CD remain unknown. Both diseases seem to occur as a response to environmental triggers (e.g. infection, drugs, or other agents) in genetically susceptible individuals. The genetic component is stronger in CD than in UC. Smoking increases the risk of CD but decreases the risk of UC through unknown mechanisms. The most recent UK guidelines on inflammatory bowel disease in adults are available (see 'Further reading' section).

Ulcerative colitis

Presentation
- Gradual onset of increasingly severe symptoms.
- Diarrhoea is dependent on disease activity and extent. Nocturnal diarrhoea and urgency are common symptoms of severe UC.
- Mucus and frank pus, or blood are often mixed in with the stool.

Table 8.17 Features distinguishing Crohn's disease from ulcerative colitis

	Crohn's disease	Ulcerative colitis
Clinical features		
Bloody diarrhoea	Uncommon	Common
Perianal disease	Common	Uncommon
Abdominal mass	Common	Rare
Endoscopy or radiology		
Rectal inflammation	Uncommon	Defining feature
Distribution	Patchy	Continuous
Ulceration	Pleiomorphic, deep	Superficial, fine
Strictures/fistulae	Characteristic	Rare
Histology		
Depth	Transmural	Superficial
Infiltrate	Lymphocytes, macrophages, plasma cells	Neutrophils, plasma cells, eosinophils
Granulomata	Characteristic	Confined to ruptured crypts

Reproduced from David Warrell et al., *Oxford Textbook of Medicine* Fifth edition, 2010, Table 15.11.1, page 2364, with permission from Oxford University Press.

- Occasionally, abdominal pain occurs (but is not a prominent feature, although lower abdominal cramping pain, relieved by defecation, is common. Intense abdominal pain suggests a severe attack, with acute bowel dilatation or perforation, or ischaemic colitis).
- Urgency and tenesmus.
- In aggressive disease, there is severe diarrhoea (>6 motions/day), abdominal cramps, fever, nocturnal diarrhoea, anorexia, and weight loss. Blood loss may be considerable and require blood transfusion.
- Aphthous ulcers (also present in Crohn's).
- Ask about recent cessation of smoking (precipitant).

Examination
Look for fever, signs of dehydration (i.e tachycardia, postural hypotension), and abdominal distension. Abdominal tenderness (± rebound) may indicate colonic dilatation or perforation. This may be masked if the patient is on steroids. An abdominal mass may indicate a tumour or an inflammatory mass. Systemic features: examine for extra-intestinal manifestations.

Crohn's disease

Presentation
- Diarrhoea (80%).
- Abdominal pain (50%). Colic and vomiting suggest ileal disease.
- Weight loss (70%) and fever (40%).
- Obstructive symptoms (e.g. colic, vomiting).
- Rectal bleeding (50%) is commoner in colonic disease but is present in 50% with ileal disease. Colonic disease is associated with perianal disease in 30%.
- Extra-intestinal manifestations, such as erythema nodosum (5–10%), arthropathy (10%), or eye complications (5%).
- Symptoms of anaemia (e.g. iron, B12, or folate deficiency) or nutritional deficiencies.

Markers of a severe attack of IBD

- >6 bloody stools/day.
- Systemically unwell: pyrexia and tachycardia.
- Hb <10 g/dL.
- Albumin <30 g/L.
- Toxic dilatation (colon >6 cm).
- CRP markedly elevated.
- Weight loss.

Truelove and Witt suggested that >6 stools/day, together with any of the following: temperature >37.8°C, large amounts of rectal bleeding, heart rate >90 beats per minute, haemoglobin of <10.5 g/dL, or an erythrocyte sedimentation rate (ESR) >30 mm/h would warrant admission to hospital.

Although the presence of the above symptoms, signs, or findings may indicate severe inflammatory bowel disease, it should be noted that severe Crohn's disease may be present in the absence of any of the above symptoms or signs and may present in a variety of ways, including the extra-intestinal manifestations listed in Tables 8.18 and 8.19.

The differential diagnosis of anyone presenting with the above symptoms includes ischaemic colitis, infective gastroenteritis (e.g. *Campylobacter*, *Salmonella*, *Shigella*, *C. difficile*,

Table 8.18 Common extra-intestinal manifestations of inflammatory bowel disease

Musculoskeletal: arthritis—ankylosing spondylitis (4%) and sacroiliitis (15%), hypertrophic osteoarthropathy with clubbing and periostitis. Also osteoporosis, aseptic necrosis, polymyositis, osteomalacia

Skin and mouth: erythema nodosum (5%), pyoderma gangrenosum (0.5%), aphthous ulcers (20%), vesiculopustular eruption, necrotizing vasculitis, Sweet's syndrome, fissures and fistulas, oral Crohn's disease, drug rashes. Nutritional deficiency—acrodermatitis enteropathica (zinc), purpura (vitamin C), glossitis (vitamin B), hair loss, and brittle nails. Associated diseases include vitiligo, psoriasis, amyloid, epidermolysis bullosa acquisita

Hepatobiliary: primary sclerosing cholangitis (PSC) and cholangiocarcinoma with ulcerative colitis. Gallstones. Autoimmune hepatitis, granulomatous involvement of liver in Crohn's disease, fatty liver, gallstones associated with ileal Crohn's disease

Ocular: uveitis iritis, episcleritis, scleromalacia, corneal ulcers, retinal vascular disease, gastrobulbar neuritis, Crohn's keratopathy

Entamoeba histolytica, Yersinia, or mycobacterium), CMV colitis, carcinoid, drug-induced diarrhoea (e.g. NSAIDs), and radiation colitis.

Investigations
Blood tests
Laboratory investigations should include full blood count, urea and electrolytes, liver function tests, and erythrocyte sedimentation rate or C-reactive protein, ferritin, transfer-

Table 8.19 Rare extra-intestinal manifestations of inflammatory bowel disease

Blood and vascular: anaemia due to iron, B12, or folate deficiency, anaemia of chronic disease, autoimmune haemolytic anaemia, thrombocytopenic purpura.
A hypercoagulable state exists in IBD, leading to both venous and arterial thromboembolism. Patients may also develop polyarteris nodosa, Takayasu's arteritis, cutaneous vasculitis, anticardiolipin antibody, and hyposplenism.

Renal: urinary calculi (oxalate stones in ileal disease), local extension of Crohn's disease involving ureter or bladder, amyloidosis, drug-related nephrotoxicity, renal tubular injury.

Neurological: up to 3% of patients may develop peripheral neuropathy, myelopathy, vestibular dysfunction, myasthenia gravis, and cerebrovascular disorders, pseudotumour cerebri. These complications tend to appear a few years after the onset of inflammatory bowel disease and are often associated with other extra-intestinal manifestations.

Cardiac: pericarditis, myocarditis, endocarditis, and heart block (more common in ulcerative colitis than in Crohn's disease), cardiomyopathy. Pericarditis may also occur from sulfasalazine/5-aminosalicylate.

Lung disease: pulmonary fibrosis, vasculitis, bronchitis, acute laryngotracheitis, interstitial lung disease, sarcoidosis. Abnormal pulmonary function tests occur in up to 50% of cases.

Pancreas: acute pancreatitis is more common in Crohn's disease than in ulcerative colitis. Risk factors include drug therapy, duodenal Crohn's disease.

rin saturation, vitamin B12, and folate. Serological markers, such as pANCA (antineutrophil cytoplasmic antibodies), ASCA (anti-*Saccharomyces cerevisiae*) antibodies are present in a significant proportion of patients with IBD.

Anaemia may be present if the colitis is acute and florid. Iron deficiency may occur. Leucocytosis and thrombocytosis are common in severe disease. Hypokalaemia may follow frequent diarrhoea. There may be an element of pre-renal dehydration. In extensive colitis, albumin often falls to 20–30 g/L. ESR and CRP reflect disease activity but are often not elevated in distal (rectal) disease. They are useful to monitor therapy.

Stool culture and microscopy
To exclude infective causes of diarrhoea.

Supine AXR and erect CXR
To look for bowel wall thickening (moderate to severe) and mucosal oedema, with loss of haustration and colonic dilatation (severe cases). Colonic diameter >6 cm indicates toxic dilatation, with a risk of perforation. The extent of the disease can be indirectly assessed as distal colitis is often associated with proximal faecal loading. In the acute stages of a severe attack, abdominal films should be performed daily, or twice daily if there is borderline toxic dilatation. Free air under the diaphragm on an erect CXR indicates perforation.

Gallium or white cell scan
111 indium-labelled WBC accumulate in areas of active inflammation and are a useful adjunct to a plain AXR to assess the extent of active disease. Crohn's typically shows patchy uptake and involvement of the small bowel while UC is commonly limited to colon.

Sigmoidoscopy and colonoscopy
Bowel preparation is unnecessary and may cause reddening of the mucosa. Flexible sigmoidoscopy has a lower risk of bacteraemia and is easier than rigid sigmoidoscopy. Nonspecific findings, such as hyperaemia and contact or spontaneous bleeding, are common. Ulceration suggests acute disease; pseudopolyps and atrophy of the bowel mucosa indicate chronic UC. Rectal biopsy from the posterior wall below 10 cm should be taken from all patients (where there is less risk of perforation).

Drugs used in inflammatory bowel disease
Aminosalicylates
These are available as oral tablets, sachets or suspension, liquid or foam enemas, or suppositories. They act on epithelial cells by a variety of mechanisms to moderate the release of lipid mediators, cytokines, and reactive oxygen species.

Oral formulations include:
1. pH-dependent release/resin-coated (eg Asacol®, Salofalk® or Ipocol®, Octasa®).
2. Time-controlled release (Pentasa®).
3. Delivery by carrier molecules, with release of 5-aminosalicylate (5-ASA) after splitting by bacterial enzymes in the large intestine (sulfasalazine (eg Salazopyrin®), olsalazine (Dipentum®), balsalazide (Colazide®)).

The main action of 5-ASA is to maintain remission in ulcerative colitis, although these drugs have some efficacy in Crohn's colitis. All 5-ASA derivatives show comparable efficacy to sulfasalazine, but, in a meta-analysis, the parent compound had a modest therapeutic advantage for maintaining remission. The choice of which 5-ASA formulation to use is debated and is influenced by tolerability (i.e. mesalazine is tolerated by 80% of those unable to tolerate sulfasalazine), dose schedule (i.e. twice-daily dosing is associated with better compliance), and cost. Efficacy depends more on adherence with the prescribed dose than the delivery system.

Side effects
Side effects of sulfasalazine occur in 10–45%, depending on the dose. Headache, nausea, epigastric pain, and diarrhoea are the most common and are dose related. Serious idiosyncratic reactions (including Stevens–Johnson syndrome, pancreatitis, acute liver failure, agranulocytosis, or alveolitis) are rare. Mesalazine intolerance occurs in up to 15%. Diarrhoea (3%), headache (2%), nausea (2%), and rash (1%) are reported. Acute intolerance (3%) may resemble a flare of colitis, as it includes bloody diarrhoea. Recurrence on rechallenge provides the clue. Renal complications, such as interstitial nephritis and nephrotic syndrome, are rare.

Other drugs

Steroids
Oral prednisolone (starting at 40 mg daily) induces remission in 75% of patients with mild to moderate disease within 2 weeks, compared with 48% treated with 8 g/day sulfasalazine. A combination of oral and rectal steroids is better than either alone.

Azathioprine
This is sometimes used as a steroid-sparing drug in both UC and Crohn's disease and is effective at preventing relapse. FBC should be monitored for the first 4 weeks and thereafter at 3-monthly intervals. The most common cause of intolerance (affecting up to 20%) is flu-like symptoms (myalgia, headache, diarrhoea) that characteristically occur after 2–3 weeks and cease rapidly when the drug is withdrawn. Profound leucopenia can develop suddenly and unpredictably between blood tests in 3%. Hepatotoxicity and pancreatitis are uncommon (<1%).

Ciclosporin
Intravenous ciclosporin is rapidly effective as a salvage therapy for patients with refractory colitis, who would otherwise face colectomy, but its use is controversial because of toxicity and long-term failure.

Methotrexate
Methotrexate (MTX) is effective for inducing remission or preventing relapse in CD. At present, the role of MTX is in the treatment of active or relapsing CD in those refractory to, or intolerant of, azathioprine.

Anti-TNF therapy
Infliximab (IFX;) is a chimeric anti-TNF monoclonal antibody with potent anti-inflammatory effects, possibly dependent on apoptosis of inflammatory cells. There are now several other anti-TNF agents available, although most experience is with infliximab. Numerous controlled trials have demonstrated its efficacy in both active and fistulating CD. Guidelines for the use of infliximab have been produced by the National Institute for Health and Care Excellence.

Management of ulcerative colitis

Symptoms in patients with ulcerative colitis typically remit and relapse. The aims of therapy are to induce remission and to prevent relapse (see Box 8.10). The mainstay drugs of choice are the 5-aminosalicylates (5-ASA) and topical steroids. Mild and moderate disease can usually be managed

as an outpatient, whereas patients with severe disease require admission to hospital.

Mild disease
Patients with mild disease (<4 motions per day and who are not systemically unwell) can usually be managed with local therapy, using 5-aminosalicylic acid and/or steroids as an enema, as a foam, or as a suppository, depending on the extent of disease. Local therapy is given once or twice daily until remission and then less frequently, generally at night before retiring.

Ulcerative colitis is generally divided into distal or more extensive disease. Topical management is often appropriate for patients with active proctitis even if the disease extends into the sigmoid colon. For patients with more extensive disease, oral or parenteral therapy is the mainstay of treatment, although many patients may get additional benefit from topical therapy.

Active left-sided or extensive UC
Left-sided disease extends proximal to the sigmoid descending junction up to the splenic flexure. Extensive ulcerative colitis extends beyond, or proximal to, the splenic flexure. Disease activity should be confirmed by sigmoidoscopy and infection excluded, although treatment should not wait for microbiological analysis.

For the treatment of active left-sided or extensive UC
Oral mesalazine, 2.4–4.8 g daily in once-daily or divided doses, is effective first-line therapy for mild to moderately active disease. Balsalazide, 6.75 g daily which delivers 2.4 g mesalazine, is also effective. Topical mesalazine, combined with oral mesalazine, tends to be more effective than oral mesalazine alone. There used to be a trend to use sulfasalazine in patients with a reactive arthropathy, but this is no longer recommended.

Prednisolone 20–40 mg daily is appropriate for patients with moderately active disease. Once initiated, the dose of prednisolone should be reduced gradually, according to disease severity and patient response, generally over 8 weeks. Long-term treatment with steroids is always undesirable.

Patients with steroid-dependent disease, i.e. flares occur if steroids are stopped, should be treated with azathioprine 2–2.5 mg/kg/day or mercaptopurine 0.75–1.5 mg/kg/day. Topical agents (either steroids or mesalazine) can be used, and, although they are unlikely to be effective alone, they may benefit patients with rectal symptoms.

Active distal UC (predominantly proctitis)
The term distal colitis applies to disease up to the sigmoid descending junction, including proctitis, and means disease limited to the rectum. Patient preference has a big influence on management, since much is about quality of life.

For the treatment of active distal UC
In mild to moderate disease, topical mesalazine 1–2 g daily (in an appropriate form dependent on the extent of disease) may be effective alone but may require oral mesalazine 2–4 g daily or balsalazide 6.75 g daily.

Topical steroids are less effective than topical mesalazine and should be reserved as second-line therapy for patients who cannot tolerate topical mesalazine.

Patients who have failed to improve on a combination of oral mesalazine with either topical mesalazine or topical steroids should be treated with oral prednisolone 40 mg daily, and prednisolone should be reduced gradually, according to the severity and patient response, generally over 8 weeks.

For patients with proximal faecal loading, a non-stimulant laxative may be helpful.

Acute severe ulcerative colitis

Patients who fail to respond to maximal oral treatment, with a combination of mesalazine and/or steroids with or without topical therapy, or those who present with severe disease, defined by the Truelove and Witts' criteria (>6 bloody stools/day and signs of systemic illness (HR >90, temperature >37.8°C, Hb <10.5 g/dL) and ESR >30), should be admitted to hospital. Monitoring of pulse rate, stool frequency, ESR, C-reactive protein, and plain AXR helps to identify those who need urgent colectomy. Close liaison with a surgeon who specializes in the management of patients with UC is ideal. Acute-onset UC is sometimes difficult to distinguish from infective colitis, but treatment with corticosteroids should not be delayed until stool microbiology results are available.

The approach to treatment of severe UC involves:

- Daily physical examination to evaluate abdominal tenderness and rebound tenderness. Joint medical and surgical management.
- Check for *Clostridum difficile* infection (you need four stool samples to detect 90% of cases). Consider CMV infection.
- Record vital signs 4–8 times daily, with a stool chart to record the number and character of stools, including the presence or absence of blood or liquid.
- Intravenous fluid and electrolyte replacement (e.g Hartmann's solution) to prevent dehydration or electrolyte imbalance, with blood transfusion to maintain a haemoglobin >10 g/dL.
- Intravenous hydrocortisone 400 mg/day or methylprednisolone 60 mg/day.
- Measurement of FBC, ESR or CRP, serum electrolytes, serum albumin, and liver function tests daily.
- Daily AXR looking for colonic dilatation (transverse colon diameter >5.5 cm or caecum >9 cm).
- Subcutaneous heparin to reduce the risk of thromboembolism (this may make rectal bleeding worse).
- Nutritional support (by enteral or parenteral route) if the patient is malnourished.
- Avoid antimotility and opiate drugs (such as loperamide and codeine) and anti-spasmodics, as they cause proximal constipation and may precipitate paralytic ileus and megacolon.
- In reality, if the patient has not responded to current therapy, they should now be under the care of a specialist who will consider rescue therapy, with ciclosporin at 2 mg/kg/day or infliximab if there has been no improvement by day 3. Following induction of remission, oral ciclosporin for 3–6 months is appropriate. Measure magnesium when starting ciclosporin, as very low levels (magnesium <0.5 mmol/L) or significant hypocholesterolaemia (cholesterol <3 mmol/L) may be associated with more side effects. Infliximab is used at a dose of 5 mg/kg at 0, 2, and 6 weeks.
- Continue treatment with oral mesalazine once oral intake resumes, although the efficacy of this in severe disease is unknown.
- Immediate surgical referral is required if there is evidence of toxic megacolon (transverse colon diameter >5.5 cm or caecum >9 cm). The urgency with which surgery is undertaken after recognition of colonic dilatation

---

Box 8.10 Key points: management of severe IBD

IV fluids: rehydrate patient, and correct any electrolyte imbalance (e.g. hypokalaemia). Correct anaemia.

Corticosteroids: IV hydrocortisone 100 mg qds (+ rectal steroids in acute UC or Crohn's with distal colonic disease). Prophylactic heparin (5,000 units SC bd).

Metronidazole for colonic Crohn's disease.

Avoid antimotility drugs, opiates, and anti-spasmodics (cause proximal constipation and may precipitate paralytic ileus and megacolon).

Inform and discuss the patient with surgical colleagues.

Nutrition: a low-residue diet and early institution of TPN may be of benefit, especially if the patient is likely to come to surgery.

---

depends on the condition of the patient. The greater the dilatation and the greater the degree of systemic toxicity, the sooner surgery should be undertaken, but signs may be masked by steroid therapy. In selected patients with mild dilatation, there needs to be joint management. Any significant clinical, laboratory, or radiological deterioration may suggest the need for immediate colectomy.

- Objective re-evaluation should be undertaken on the third day of intensive treatment. A stool frequency of >8/day or CRP >45 mg/L at 3 days appears to predict the need for surgery in 85% of cases. Surgical review and input from a specialist colorectal nurse or stomatherapist is appropriate at this stage. There is no benefit from intravenous steroids beyond 7–10 days.

Consider colectomy or intravenous ciclosporin (as described previously) if there is no improvement during the first 3 days. Intravenous ciclosporin alone may be as effective as methylprednisolone, but potential side effects mean that it is rarely an appropriate single first-line therapy.

Indications for surgery

- Failure of symptoms to resolve after 5–10 days is an indication for proctocolectomy.
- Colonic perforation, uncontrollable bleeding, toxic megacolon, and fulminating disease require urgent proctocolectomy; ~30% of all patients with UC will require a colectomy at some stage.
- Toxic dilatation prior to treatment is not an indication for surgery (although failure of the colonic diameter to decrease after 24 hours suggests surgery is indicated). The development of dilatation during treatment is an indication for surgery.
- Surgery in Crohn's disease is not 'curative' and is only indicated for perforation, obstruction, abscess formation, and fistulae (enterocutaneous or enterovesical). There is a high recurrence rate after surgery.

Management of acute Crohn's disease

The severity of CD is more difficult to assess than UC. The general principles are to consider the site (ileal, ileocolic, colonic, other), pattern (inflammatory, stricturing, fistulating), and activity of the disease before treatment decisions are made in conjunction with the patient (see Box 8.10). An alternative explanation for symptoms, other than active disease, should be considered (such as bacterial overgrowth, bile salt malabsorption, fibrotic strictures, dysmotility, gallstones) and disease activity confirmed (usually by CRP or

ESR) before starting steroids. Individuals with CD have many investigations over their lifetime, and imaging (e.g. colonoscopy, small bowel radiology) should not be repeated, unless it will alter management or a surgical decision depends on the result.

Active ileal, ileocolonic, or colonic Crohn's disease
- In mild ileocolonic CD, high-dose mesalazine (4 g/daily) may be sufficient initial therapy.
- For patients with moderate to severe disease or those with mild to moderate ileocolonic CD that has failed to respond to oral mesalazine, oral corticosteroids, such as prednisolone 40 mg daily, are appropriate.
- Prednisolone should be reduced gradually, according to severity and patient response, generally over 8 weeks. More rapid reduction is associated with early relapse.
- Budesonide 9 mg daily is appropriate for patients with isolated ileocaecal disease with moderate disease activity but is marginally less effective than prednisolone.
- Intravenous steroids (e.g. hydrocortisone 400 mg/day or methylprednisolone 60 mg/day) are appropriate for patients with severe disease. Concomitant intravenous metronidazole is often advisable because it may be difficult to distinguish between active disease and a septic complication.
- Elemental or polymeric diets are less effective than corticosteroids but may be used to induce remission in selected patients with active CD who have a contraindication to corticosteroid therapy or who would themselves prefer to avoid such therapy.
- Total parenteral nutrition may be an appropriate adjunctive therapy in complex, fistulating disease.
- Sulfasalazine 4 g daily is effective for active colonic disease but cannot be recommended as first-line therapy in view of the high incidence of side effects. It may be appropriate in selected patients.
- Metronidazole 10–20 mg/kg/day, although effective, is not usually recommended as first-line therapy for CD in view of the potential for side effects. It has a role in selected patients with colonic or treatment-resistant disease or those who wish to avoid steroids.
- Topical mesalazine may be effective in left-sided colonic CD of mild to moderate activity.
- Azathioprine 1.5–2.5 mg/kg/day or mercaptopurine 0.75–1.5 mg/kg/day may be used in active CD as adjunctive therapy and as a steroid-sparing agent. However, its slow onset of action precludes its use as a sole therapy.
- Infliximab 5 mg/kg is effective but is best avoided in patients with obstructive symptoms.
- Surgery should be considered for those who have failed medical therapy and may be appropriate as primary therapy in patients with limited ileal or ileocaecal disease.

Fistulating and perianal disease
Active perianal disease or fistulae are often associated with active CD elsewhere in the gastrointestinal tract. The initial aim should be to treat active disease and sepsis. For more complex, fistulating disease, the approach involves defining the anatomy, supporting nutrition, and potential surgery. For perianal disease, MRI and examination under anaesthetic are particularly helpful. Treatment options include:
- **Metronidazole** 400 mg tds and/or ciprofloxacin 500 mg bd are appropriate first-line treatments for simple perianal fistulae.
- **Azathioprine** 1.5–2.5 mg/kg/day is potentially effective for simple perianal fistulae or enterocutaneous fistulae where distal obstruction and abscess have been excluded.
- **Infliximab** (three infusions of 5 mg/kg at 0, 2, and 6 weeks) should be reserved for patients whose perianal or enterocutaneous fistulae are refractory to other treatments and should be used as part of a strategy that includes immunomodulation and surgery.
- **Surgery**, including Seton drainage, fistulectomy, and the use of advancement flaps, is appropriate for persistent or complex fistulae, in combination with medical treatment.
- **Elemental diets or parenteral nutrition** have a role as adjunctive therapy, but not as sole therapy.

Further reading

Carter MJ, Lobo AJ, Travis SPL (2004). Guidelines for the management of inflammatory bowel disease in adults. *Gut*, **53**, v1–16.

CORE (Digestive Disorders Foundation). <http://www.corecharity.org.uk>.

Crohn's and Colitis Foundation of America. <http://www.ccfa.org>.

Crohn's and Colitis UK. <http://www.nacc.org.uk>.

Mowat C, Cole A, Windsor A, et al. (2011). Guidelines for the management of inflammatory bowel disease in adults. *Gut*, **60**, 571–607.

National Institute for Health and Clinical Excellence (2010). Infliximab (review) and adalimumab for the treatment of Crohn's disease. NICE technology appraisal guidance 187. <http://www.nice.org.uk/nicemedia/live/12985/48687/48687.doc>.

National Institute for Health and Clinical Excellence (2010). Ulcerative colitis: Management in adults, children and young people. NICE clinical guideline 166. <https://www.nice.org.uk/guidance/cg166>.

National Institute for Health and Clinical Excellence (2011). Colonoscopic surveillance for prevention of colorectal cancer in people with ulcerative colitis, Crohn's disease or adenomas; NICE clinical guideline 118. <http://guidance.nice.org.uk/CG118>.

National Institute for Health and Clinical Excellence (2012). Crohn's disease. Management in adults, children and young people. NICE clinical guideline 152. <http://www.nice.org.uk/nicemedia/live/13936/61001/61001.pdf>

Stange EF, Travis SP, Vermeire S, et al. (2006). European evidence based consensus on the diagnosis and management of Crohn's disease: definitions and diagnosis. *Gut*, **55** (Suppl 1), 1–15.

Truelove SC and Witts LJ (1955). Cortisone in ulcerative colitis; final report on a therapeutic trial. *British Medical Journal*, **2**, 1041–8.

Acute pancreatitis

Acute pancreatitis is generally managed by surgeons, but occasionally by physicians. Intensive care physicians are often involved in the care of these patients.

Clinical features (e.g. abdominal pain and vomiting), together with elevation of plasma levels of pancreatic enzymes (i.e amylase and lipase), are the cornerstones of diagnosis (see Box 8.11). Pancreatic enzymes are released into the circulation during an acute attack, peak early, and decline over 3–4 days. Measurement of plasma lipase activity is more sensitive and more specific than serum amylase. The incidence of acute pancreatitis is 150–400 cases per million of the general population. The overall mortality is <10% but rising to 30% in severe acute pancreatitis.

Presentation
- Abdominal pain is epigastric or generalized and of rapid onset. It may occur anywhere (including chest) and is usually dull, constant, and boring. The pain may radiate to the back or between the scapulae and is often relieved by leaning forward (differential diagnosis is leaking aortic aneurysm).
- Nausea, vomiting, and dehydration (± jaundice) often occur.
- Peritonitis may be present with epigastric tenderness, localized rebound tenderness, or generalized abdominal rigidity. An abdominal mass may indicate a pancreatic pseudocyst or abscess. Bowel sounds are usually absent.
- Tachycardia and hypotension may progress to shock and collapse. Respiratory failure due to ARDS may occur in severe cases (especially in the elderly).
- Very rarely there may be signs of bleeding in the pancreatic bed with Grey–Turner's sign (bruising in the flanks) or Cullen's sign (periumbilical bruising). Occasionally tender red skin nodules are present (due to subcutaneous fat necrosis).
- Hypocalcaemia ± tetany may occur.

Causes of acute pancreatitis
Common (80%)
- Gallstones (60%) and alcohol (20%).

Rare (20%)
- Iatrogenic (ERCP or any form of abdominal surgery).
- Trauma (even minimal trauma).
- Infections: viral (mumps, rubella, Coxsackie B, EBV, CMV, hepatitis A and B); bacterial (mycoplasma); parasitic (ascaris, flukes (*Clonorchis sinensis*)).
- Drugs (e.g. thiazides, furosemide, NSAIDs, sulfonamides, azathioprine, tetracyclines, and valproate; possibly steroids).
- Hypertriglyceridaemia (serum amylase falsely low).
- Hypothermia.

Box 8.11 Causes of abdominal pain and elevated serum amylase

Acute pancreatitis	Acute liver failure
Stomach or small bowel perforation	Acute cholecystitis or cholangitis
Perforated peptic ulcer	Renal failure (modest elevation)
Mesenteric infarction	Diabetic ketoacidosis

- Hypercalcaemia or IV calcium infusions.
- Systemic vasculitis (SLE, polyarteritis nodosa, etc.).
- Pancreatic carcinoma (3% present with acute pancreatitis).
- Miscellaneous: anatomical abnormalities (pancreas divisum, duodenal or peri-ampullary diverticulae), scorpion bites, cystic fibrosis.
- Unknown (10%).

Investigations
- Amylase: is elevated but not specific. A persistently raised amylase (several days to weeks) may indicate the development of a pancreatic pseudocyst.
- Lipase: elevated lipase is a more specific test for pancreatitis than serum amylase.
- FBC: raised haematocrit and leucocytosis.
- U&E: urea may be raised with hypovolaemia.
- Glucose: may be raised.
- LFTs: AST and bilirubin are often elevated, especially in gallstone pancreatitis. Disproportionately elevated gamma GT may indicate an alcohol aetiology.
- Calcium: hypocalcaemia (unless the precipitant was hypercalcaemia) tends to occur late.
- CRP: is elevated and used to monitor progression of the attack.
- ABGs: are mandatory and may reveal hypoxia ± metabolic acidosis.
- AXR: detects generalized ileus or sentinel loops (dilated gas-filled loops in the region of the pancreas). Look for evidence of pancreatic calcification or biliary stone.
- CXR: may show a pleural effusion, elevated diaphragm, or pulmonary infiltrates.
- USS: may confirm the diagnosis and detect gallstones ± biliary obstruction, pseudocysts, and abscesses, as well as aneurysms. A swollen pancreas is only observed in 25–50% of cases.
- CT scans of the abdomen and pancreas: dynamic contrast-enhanced scans are reliable at detecting pancreatic necrosis and in grading severity.

Assessment of severity
The severity of disease has no correlation with the elevation of serum amylase or lipase. Several prognostic indices have been published, but it takes 48 hours to fully appreciate disease severity (see Table 8.20).

The mortality from acute pancreatitis is approximately 10% and rises to 40% in those developing a pancreatic abscess. The mortality is highest in those with a first episode of pancreatitis. Around 15% of patients presenting with acute pancreatitis will have recurrent disease.

Other features that may suggest or predict a severe attack include a body mass index >30, pleural effusion on CXR at admission, APACHE II score >8, and C-reactive protein >150 mg/L and rising, as well as the development of multiple organ failure.

Audit standards, as defined in the British Society of Gastroenterology guidelines are:

1. Mortality should be <10% overall and <30% in severe pancreatitis.
2. The diagnosis of acute pancreatitis should be made in all patients within 48 hours.

Table 8.20 Markers of severity in acute pancreatitis

At presentation	At 48 hours
Age >55 years	Haematocrit fall >10%
WBC >16 x 10^9/L	Urea rise >10 mmol/L
Glucose >10 mmol/L (non-diabetic)	Serum Ca^{2+} <2.0 mmol/L
LDH >350 IU/L	Base excess >4 mmol/L
AST >250 IU/L	PaO_2 <8 kPa Serum albumin <32 g/L Estimated fluid sequestration >6 L

Mortality:
0–2 criteria = 2%
3–4 criteria = 15%
5–6 criteria = 40%
>7 criteria = 100%

3. The aetiology of acute pancreatitis should be determined in at least 80% of cases.
4. Severity stratification should be made in all patients within 48 hours.
5. Patients with persisting organ failure, signs of sepsis, or deterioration in clinical status 6–10 days after admission should have computed tomography, using a dedicated pancreatic protocol.
6. All patients with severe acute pancreatitis (>4 criteria) should be managed in a high dependency unit or intensive therapy unit.
7. Antibiotic prophylaxis against infection of the necrosis should not be given for more than 14 days without positive cultures.
8. All patients with biliary pancreatitis should undergo definitive management of gallstones during admission.
9. Patients with extensive necrotizing pancreatitis or with other complications should be managed in, or referred to, a specialist unit.
10. Facilities and expertise should be available for ERCP to be performed at any time for common bile duct evaluation, followed by sphincterotomy and stone extraction or stenting, as required.

Management

The principles of management are (see Box 8.12):
1. Liaise with or transfer care to surgeons.
2. Supportive measures: most subside in 3–10 days.
3. Monitor for the development of complications (see Table 8.21).
4. Identify the cause.

Supportive treatment

- Establish intravenous access. If there is shock, markers of moderate to severe pancreatitis, elderly patient, hypoxia, or other coexistent disease, insert a CVP line to help control fluid balance.
- Adequate prompt fluid resuscitation is crucial in the prevention of systemic complications and to maintain urine output >0.5 mL/kg body weight. Since patients are usually severely volume-depleted, give prompt fluid replacement with a balanced salt solution, such as Hartmann's or

Box 8.12 Key points: management of acute pancreatitis

- Liaise with surgeons.
- Give IV fluids.
- Normal feeding or by NG tube is successful in 80%.
- Analgesia with pethidine.
- Antibiotic prophylaxis (e.g. cefuroxime) decreases secondary infections.
- Oxygen should be given if there is hypoxia on air.
- Gallstone pancreatitis: ERCP within 72 h in severe cases.
- Monitor urine output, oxygen sats, blood glucose, and CVP (if there is shock or markers of moderate to severe pancreatitis).
- Careful observation for the development of complications.

0.9% saline. Monitor urine output, and insert a urinary catheter, if required.
- Oxygen should be given if there is hypoxia on air. Use pulse oximetry continuously in severe cases, otherwise, at 6-hourly intervals for the first 48 hours to monitor for respiratory failure.
- Keep nil by mouth initially (although current data suggest that unless patients cannot tolerate food due to nausea and vomiting, normal feeding has no adverse effect on outcome). Once settled, if enteral nutrition is required, nasogastric (NG) feeding is effective in 80% of cases. Occasionally, nasojejunal (NJ) feeding is preferred if an ileus is present.
- Monitor blood glucose regularly, and treat with insulin if elevated.
- Pethidine, if used for pain relief, causes the least spasm of the sphincter of Oddi.
- Antibiotic prophylaxis (e.g. cefuroxime) is associated with fewer deaths. In an ad hoc analysis of previous studies, there were 26 deaths in the control group of 177 patients, compared to only 10 in a similar sized group (n = 177) treated with antibiotics (i.e. a reduction from 14.7% to 5.7 % mortality).
- Octreotide: no proven benefit.
- Peritoneal lavage: no proven benefit.
- H_2-receptor antagonists have not been shown to affect mortality.

Septic complications

Sepsis is the most common cause of death. This should be suspected when there is a persistent fever, leucocytosis,

Table 8.21 Complications (seen in <20%)

Local	Systemic
• Abscess	• Electrolyte imbalance
• Pseudocyst ± infection	• $\downarrow Ca^{2+}$, $\downarrow Mg^{2+}$
• Biliary obstruction	• Acute renal failure
• Ascites, pleural effusion	• Shock
• Fistula	• Respiratory failure
• Splenic, portal, or mesenteric vein obstruction	• Sepsis

pain/tenderness, an overall clinical deterioration, and a rising CRP. These signs are an indication for multiple blood cultures and an abdominal CT scan. Pancreatic pseudocysts are more common in alcoholic pancreatitis (15% vs 3% in gallstones), but infection is more common in gallstone pancreatitis.

Gallstone-induced pancreatitis

Urgent ERCP and sphincterotomy within 72 hours of presentation reduces complications and mortality in patients with severe gallstone pancreatitis. The benefit has not been demonstrated in mild cases. There is a growing vogue for the use of MRCP (magnetic resonance cholangiopancreatogaphy) to diagnose biliary disease prior to ERCP.

All patients with signs of cholangitis require ERCP sphincterotomy.

Patients with gallstone pancreatitis should undergo definitive treatment for gallstones before discharge from hospital or within 2 weeks.

Indications for surgery

Most patients with acute pancreatitis do not require surgical treatment of the inflamed pancreas, although many will subsequently undergo cholecystectomy.

Patients with persistent symptoms for more than 7 days and >30% pancreatic necrosis, and those with smaller areas of necrosis and a clinical suspicion of sepsis, should undergo image-guided fine needle aspiration (FNA) to obtain material for culture. FNA is safe and has very few complications, and has a high sensitivity and specificity for the detection of infection. Infected pancreatic necrosis or a pancreatic abscess requires drainage.

Thorough debridement of necrotic tissue is essential during any surgical intervention. Following this, the abdomen may be either closed over drains; packed and left open; or closed over drains and the pancreatic cavity irrigated. There is no clear evidence to support one technique over the others. The choice of surgical technique for necrosectomy, and subsequent post-operative management, depends on individual features and locally available expertise. Radiologically guided percutaneous drainage may be preferred to surgery for pancreatic pseudocysts.

Further reading

Banks PA and Freeman ML (2006). Practice guidelines in acute pancreatitis. *American Journal of Gastroenterology*, **101**, 2379–400.

British Society of Gastroenterology (2005). UK guidelines for the management of acute pancreatitis. *Gut*, **54** (Suppl 3), iii1–9.

Malnutrition and chronic gastrointestinal disease

Anorexia and bulimia nervosa

Eating disorders result from a severe preoccupation with food and body image leading to disturbed eating habits, resulting in impaired physical health and/or psychosocial functioning.

Anorexia nervosa is characterized by a set of adverse attitudes to body shape and weight, in which self-worth is largely determined by these parameters. It predominates in women between the ages of 16–25 years. Body image is frequently distorted, with active maintenance of extreme low body weight (<85% ideal weight or BMI <17.5 kg/m^2). There may be associated bulimic behaviours.

Bulimia nervosa is a syndrome of episodic uncontrolled overeating (binges), followed by extreme, maladaptive weight control behaviours designed to correct for caloric intake. These include intense dieting, overexercising, and purging with self-induced vomiting or diuretic or laxative misuse. It affects 2–5% of adolescent females. Hallmark personality features include loss of control, low self-esteem, and guilt. Most bulimic individuals are of normal weight and perceive their behaviour as problematic, in contrast to anorexia nervosa. Clinically, these patients may have marks on their teeth from frequent vomiting (vomit is acidic and affects the enamel).

Clinical features

Patients with severe anorexia nervosa may present with hypothermia, bradycardia, hypotension, acrocyanosis, or lanugo hair (fine, downy hair). Those with bulimia nervosa may manifest parotid hypertrophy, dental enamel erosion, excoriations or calluses on finger knuckles of the dominant hand (Russell's sign), and chronic pharyngitis; these result from digitally induced vomiting. Post-menarchal women may have amenorrhoea.

Complications of both disorders include electrolyte disturbances and consequent cardiac arrhythmias and seizures, malabsorption syndromes and nutritional deficiencies, osteoporosis, growth retardation, subfertility, and predisposition to infection. Gastrointestinal complications include constipation, oesophagitis, Mallory–Weiss tears, peptic ulceration, melanosis coli, and deranged LFTs. Exclude pancreatitis if abdominal pain is present.

Ask about coexistent depression (up to 50%) and suicide risk. Explore both home and social circumstances.

Investigation

Biochemistry may reveal hypokalaemia, hyponatraemia (from excessive water intake or purging), hypomagnesaemia, hypocalcaemia, and hypophosphataemia. There may be multiple endocrine abnormalities. Check amylase in all patients with abdominal pain. Exclude pregnancy as a cause of recurrent vomiting. ECG should be performed in those with electrolyte disturbances and risk of dysrhythmias. Exclude a prolonged QT interval.

Management

Treatment requires a multidisciplinary approach (medical and psychiatric teams need regular communication) to address the underlying psychosocial determinants, as well as the consequent nutritional deficiencies and other medical complications. Treatment can be provided on an outpatient, day patient, or inpatient basis. Cognitive behavioural therapy forms the basis of psychological treatment.

Indications for admission include:

- Suicide risk.
- Adverse home circumstances.
- Failure of outpatient treatment.
- Severe low weight (BMI <13.5 kg/m^2).
- Rapid weight loss.
- Severe electrolyte disturbance, dehydration, hypoglycaemia, or oedema.
- Cardiac abnormalities (significant bradycardia, hypotension, or long QTc).
- Intercurrent infection.

Admission can be to a general medical ward or psychiatric unit with good access to general medical advice and assistance. Outcomes are better in units with staff experienced in the management of eating disorders. Inpatient therapies include intravenous or high-dose oral thiamine; calcium/vitamin D and multivitamins as ongoing supplementation, daily measurement of calcium-phosphate, magnesium, and potassium (i.e to correct any abnormalities). Consider cardiac monitoring if the ECG is abnormal and the BMI <13.5 kg/m^2. Reduce the initial calorie intake to prevent refeeding syndrome (e.g. 33% of basal metabolic requirement on day 1, increasing by 33% each day and taking dietetic advice as to the final threshold). See Table 8.22 for indicators predicting the risk of refeeding syndrome. Be aware that such patients often try to divide teams, and the therapeutic plan must be clear and understood by all care givers. Ideally, only one person should make changes to this plan. Also be aware that those admitted are often devious in their strategies to avoid being fed.

The legal and ethical arguments relating to non-consensual treatment in anorexia nervosa are complex and based on the following:

- Restriction of autonomy is justified only when a person is likely to do themselves considerable harm.
- Anorexia can cause considerable harm and lead to death.
- Being severely underweight produces cognitive distortion, providing a legal reason to administer non-consensual therapies.
- Therefore, patients with severe anorexia can be detained for assessment and treatment (of the mental condition anorexia).
- If informed consent is not provided, forced (tube) feeding can be provided until the severe phase of anorexia has passed.

Table 8.22 Predicting risk of refeeding syndrome

≥1 of:	or ≥2 of:
BMI <16 kg/m^2	BMI <18.5 kg/m^2
>15% weight loss in 3–6 months	>10% weight loss in 3–6 months
Minimal nutritional intake for 10 days	Minimal nutritional intake for 5 days
Pre-existing electrolyte disturbance	Alcohol or drug misuse, use of antacids or diuretics

Outcomes

Early mortality is 5%, but late mortality can be as high as 20%, largely attributable to suicide, cardiac arrhythmias, and infection. Inpatients can be discharged if their physical state has normalized, which usually takes at least 1–2 weeks of inpatient feeding. Consider the need for hormone replacement therapy (HRT) at discharge.

Acute presentations of gastrointestinal malignancy

Although uncommon, gastrointestinal malignancy can present acutely. Symptoms, often consciously ignored, usually predate the acute presentation and include:

- Weight loss (>5%).
- Abdominal pain.
- Anorexia, nausea.
- Change in bowel habit.
- Abdominal distension.

Investigation is directed towards the dominant symptom. Request standard blood tests (FBC, creatinine and elecrolytes, LFT, calcium and phosphate, CRP, glucose). Tumour markers should not be used to make a diagnosis, although CA-125, CEA, and alpha-fetoprotein are appropriate if there is a high index of suspicion for ovarian, colonic, or liver cell cancer, respectively. More specific tests are related to symptomatology and include:

- Haematemesis, nausea, or vomiting—gastroscopy.
- Jaundice—abdominal ultrasound or (preferably) pancreatic protocol abdominal CT scan or MRCP/ERCP if the bile ducts are dilated.
- Weight loss, abdominal pain—CT scan of the abdomen; then consider gastroscopy and colonoscopy.
- Iron-deficient anaemia—gastroscopy and colonoscopy.
- Change in bowel habit—colonoscopy.
- Abdominal distension—abdominal ultrasound or (preferably) CT scan, and pelvic ultrasound.

Gastric tumours
Presentation

Haematemesis, gastric outlet obstruction (vomiting), or anaemia.

Emergency management

Gastroscopy to control bleeding (diathermy, clips), stenting to prevent obstruction, or (often with limited success) argon plasma coagulation or laser to prevent chronic bleeding.

Small bowel tumours
Presentation

Abdominal pain, rectal bleeding or melaena, anaemia, bowel obstruction.

Emergency management

Urgent surgery is required if there is bowel dilatation proximal to the obstruction (as peritonitis due to perforation is usually fatal) or if there is severe bleeding. If the patient is too frail for surgery, bleeding can be controlled angiographically.

Colorectal tumours
Presentation

Nausea and vomiting can accompany impending bowel obstruction, haemorrhage and perforation can lead to limited or generalized peritonitis.

Emergency management

If available, consider urgent (within 24 h) colonic stenting in patients with rapid colonic dilatation (i.e. rate of change is more important than absolute diameter). A transverse diameter of >6 cm on a supine film is abnormal. Stenting reduces surgical mortality, in part, by allowing primary anastomosis. NICE guidelines recommend chest, abdominal, and pelvis CT scan before stenting to confirm the diagnosis of mechanical obstruction, and to determine whether the patient has metastatic disease or colonic perforation. Alternatively, request urgent surgery. Haemorrhage usually predicates urgent surgery, or interventional angiography if patients are too frail for surgery.

Pancreatico-biliary tumours
Presentation

These are relatively uncommon. They include pancreatic tumours presenting with weight loss and back pain; head of pancreas tumours or cholangiocarcinoma presenting with jaundice; and gall bladder cancer presenting with biliary colic, weight loss and possibly jaundice.

Emergency management

Urgent (ideally within 24 h) ERCP is indicated for an obstructed biliary system if the patient is septic. In the absence of sepsis, ERCP should be performed within a few days, but only if the serum bilirubin is rapidly rising, to allow pigtail catheter placement, which facilitates bile drainage. If ERCP fails to provide drainage, percutaneous drainage is required, which can be internalized radiographically or as a combined procedure (with radiologist and endoscopist).

Liver tumours
Presentation

Weight loss, right upper quadrant pain, jaundice, and hepatomegaly.

Emergency management

This is rarely required, although haematobilia can be prevented with angiographic techniques.

Lymphoma
Presentation

Weight loss, abdominal pain, and 'B' symptoms (e.g. fever, night sweats).

Emergency management

As for small bowel tumours (described previously).

Gastroparesis

Gastroparesis in patients receiving nutritional support may either occur transiently in the critically unwell or post-operative surgical patient, or be related to an underlying medical disorder (typically neuropathic). It may present as nausea, vomiting, early satiety, bloating, epigastric pain, or aspiration of large volumes of undigested feed through a NG or a percutaneous endoscopic gastrostomy (PEG) tube. Dehydration, weight loss, and vitamin (± mineral) deficiencies may develop long-term.

Management is stepwise, initially with conservative measures. Electrolyte disturbances should be corrected (including magnesium). Stop medications that inhibit gastric emptying, particularly anticholinergics, opiates, calcium channel blockers, phenothiazines, and tricyclics. Intake can be modified to include multiple small volume feeds, with more liquid consistency and lower fat content.

Should symptoms persist, prokinetic agents may be helpful. The most frequently used are metoclopramide 5–20 mg tds, erythromycin 125–250 mg tds, or domperidone 5–20 mg tds. Start at a low dose, then escalate. There is no strong clinical evidence to differentiate these agents. If gastroparesis is severe and not ameliorated by the above measures, nasojejunal (NJ) feeding, jejunostomy, or TPN are indicated, depending on the clinical scenario.

Phosphate replacement
Infuse 500 mL of polyfusor phosphate (which contains 50 mmoles of phosphate) if serum phosphate falls below 0.4 mmol/L. A single infusion is adequate in 35% of patients, but 65% of patients require a second infusion to correct serum phosphate levels.

Magnesium replacement
If serum magnesium is less than 0.5 mmol/L, then infuse 24 mmoles of magnesium over 6–12 hours, and replace, as necessary.

Short bowel syndrome
This is defined as an inadequate length of functional small bowel, resulting in electrolyte and calorie deficiencies. If local staff are not experienced in managing such patients, consider discussing their care with a specialist centre.

Critical lengths of normal small intestine have been defined that guide the likely mode of future food and fluid replacement (see Table 8.23). Optimal management often requires several weeks of inpatient care, with changes made every few days so as to tailor therapy to each patient.

Initial assessment
- Ensure accurate fluid balance is recorded. Weigh patients daily.
- Measure baseline blood tests (FBC, urea and electrolytes (U&E), LFT, bone profile, glucose, thyroid function tests, CRP, clotting, haematinics, coeliac screen, vitamin A, vitamin D, zinc, magnesium).
- Request daily U&E, magnesium; twice-weekly FBC, bone profile, LFT.
- Measure urine sodium concentration weekly: <10 mmol/L suggests dehydration.

Initial management
- Keep nil by mouth for the first 48 h to assess basal output (e.g. from jejunostomy). High output, defined as >1 L, is associated with the development of dehydration and electrolyte abnormalities; <1 L is unlikely to require the stringent management outlined here.

Table 8.23 Likely outcomes post-small bowel resection

	Small bowel length	Likely treatment
Jejunostomy	<75 cm	HPN
	<100 cm	HPE ± HPN
	<150 cm	EN
	<200 cm	Fluid restriction and oral ORS
Jejunocolic anastomosis	<50 cm	HPN
	<100 cm	EN
	<150 cm	Fluid restriction and ORS

HPN, home parenteral nutrition; HPE, home parenteral electrolytes; EN, enteral nutrition; ORS, oral rehydration solution.

- Then restrict oral intake to 1,500 mL (at least 1 L being an oral rehydration solution, such as 'St. Mark's solution'; give cold, and add cordial if unpalatable). Replace excess fluid loss with intravenous normal saline, ensuring urine output >800 mL/day.
- Explain to the patient that hypotonic oral intake promotes Na^+ secretion in the proximal small bowel, leading to increased fluid output and dehydration in patients without a functioning colon to resorb fluid. Patients, and some doctors, find this hard to comprehend, often leading to conflicting advice being given, and to patients surreptitiously drinking fluids to quench an increasing thirst. Prescribe loperamide, 4 mg four times daily (qds) orally to be taken 30 minutes before meals. Prescribe double-dose vitamins/minerals, one tablet twice daily (bd) orally.
- Recommend six small meals/day, predominantly dry foods, avoiding fluids for 30 minutes before or after meals. Nasogastric or intravenous nutrition may be necessary initially. Oral calorific intake needs to be 2–3 times the likely energy expenditure if the output is high. Liquid feeds should contain >100 mmol/L sodium, with osmolarity >300 mOsm/kg.

Highly osmotic fatty foods or sorbitol can exacerbate diarrhoea if the colon remains *in situ*. Recommend high carbohydrate intake, but see the long term management section relating to carbohydrate and starch-induced D-lactic acidosis in patients with short functional small bowel anastomosed to the colon. Salt can be added, as desired. Avoid foods containing excess oxalate (e.g. spinach, rhubarb, beetroot, nuts, chocolate, tea, wheatbran, strawberries), as calcium oxalate renal stones occur in 25% of such patients.

The following can then be tried:
- Codeine phosphate, 30–60 mg qds orally.
- Increase each loperamide dose by 2 mg, up to 12 mg, as necessary.
- If there is a high-output jejunostomy, prescribe high-dose proton pump inhibitors to lower gastric secretion. Then consider subcutaneous octreotide (then depot octreotide intramuscularly, if effective). If there is electrolyte imbalance, try oral replacement with up to 24 mmol magnesium glycerophosphate, and slow sodium or potassium supplements, as necessary. For colecalciferol use 10,000 to 20,000 units per week until levels are replete, and continue as necessary. Routine medication doses may need to be increased.
- Consider colestyramine if >60 cm of terminal ileum has been resected, with small bowel anastomosed to colon, to prevent bile acid-associated diarrhoea. This can exacerbate steatorrhoea. Vitamin B12 and fat (and, therefore, fat-soluble vitamins) malabsorption is likely in the longer term.
- Parenteral fluids will be required if, following treatment optimization, daily jejunostomy output is >1.5 L. If the output is 1–1.5 L, then administer 1 L normal saline, containing 4 mmol magnesium sulfate. This can be infused subcutaneously overnight if you wish to avoid IV fluids.

Parenteral nutrition is indicated if >10% weight loss occurs, despite optimal enteral nutrition, and should be anticipated if the amount of remaining small intestine is limited (see Table 8.23).
- Infuse 25 calories/kg ideal body weight, including 0.5–1.0 g protein/kg/day (critically ill patients need up to double this amount) and 1 g lipid/kg/day.

- Excessive parenteral calories cause hyperglycaemia, associated with increased rates of infection.
- Reduce the protein content if there is evidence of significant renal or hepatic disease.

Long-term management
- Initially, measure FBC, U&E, magnesium, LFT, bone profile, CRP, and urine sodium weekly, then less often. Annually, measure zinc, selenium, vitamin A, vitamin D, vitamin B12, red cell folate, and clotting. Bone density should be measured biennially.
- Weigh weekly. Consider overnight enteral, instead of parenteral, feeding if there is weight gain (possible in 20% of patients due to intestinal adaptation, enhancing absorption).
- Increased output can be caused by medication, excess drinking, sepsis, obstruction, and disease (e.g. coeliac, Crohn's). Consider bacterial overgrowth if the colon is *in situ*.
- Gallstones occur in up to 50–100% of patients with short bowel syndrome. The highest incidence of gall bladder disease, from previous reports, is seen in patients with terminal ileal disease or resection. Ursodeoxycholic acid can be tried to prevent recurrence, but a prophylactic cholecystectomy should be considered, since gallstone disease is an important cause of mortality in the longer term.
- In addition to bile acid diarrhoea and calcium oxalate renal stones, patients with short functional small bowel anastomosed to the colon can develop D-lactic acidosis. Glucose and starch are metabolized by colonic bacteria into D-lactic acid. This is absorbed but not broken down by L-lactate dehydrogenase.
  - Episodic metabolic acidosis occurs after high carbohydrate intake.
  - Ataxia, slurred speech, and confusion occur (i.e. patients appear drunk).
  - The anion gap is increased, acidosis present, but the lactate levels are normal (because the assay only measures L-lactate).
  - Treat D-lactic acidosis by giving sodium bicarbonate to correct the acidosis; sterilize the bowel with metronidazole or neomycin; avoid probiotics (because lactobacilli produce D-lactate), and decrease carbohydrate intake.

Other causes of malnutrition
Usually, in-hospital malnutrition is multifactorial. One of the most significant causes is poor dietary intake (often iatrogenic), partly caused by regular interruption of feeding for investigations (e.g. X-rays) which get cancelled and rescheduled. Take a dietetic history, and monitor nutritional replacement in those staying in hospital for more than 1 week.
Other causes of malnutrition include:
- Cardiac cachexia.
- Infections:
  - AIDS.
  - Tuberculosis.
- Thyroid disease.
- Malabsorption:
  - Coeliac disease, tropical sprue.
  - Whipple's disease.
  - Pancreatic disease.
  - Bacterial overgrowth.
  - Amyloid, etc.

- Starvation:
  - This should be considered in thin, elderly patients, particularly if they need help with feeding or there is evidence of neglect at home. Two clinical syndromes occur:
  - Kwashiorkor—inadequate protein intake leads to muscle atrophy but fat stores are maintained due to adequate caloric intake. Signs include decreased muscle mass, diarrhoea, irritability, poor quality hair, hepatomegaly, and dermatitis.
  - Marasmus—wasting of muscles and fat due to inadequate intake of protein and fat. Patients are very thin.

Syndromes resulting from lack of essential nutrients
- Beriberi is due to a lack of thiamine (vitamin B1). Most foods are enriched with vitamin B1, so this is rare, except in alcoholics (who eat less and have malabsorption) and those on dialysis.
  - Dry beriberi presents with neurological symptoms, including nystagmus and confusion (i.e. Wernicke's encephalopathy, leading to Korsakoff's psychosis. The latter is often permanent).
  - Wet beriberi presents with congestive cardiac failure.
- Megaloblastic anaemia: consider in patients with diarrhoea, headache, loss of appetite, and a sore tongue. Screen for low B12 or folic acid.
- Osteomalacia (or rickets in infancy/childhood): follows a chronic deficiency of vitamin D, calcium, or phosphate. Consider in patients with inadequate sun exposure (<10 min/day), especially in lactose-intolerant vegetarians. Presentation includes bony pain, muscle weakness, and poor appetite.
- Pellagra: is due to a deficiency of niacin (B3) or tryptophan. This is well remembered by the '4 Ds': diarrhoea, dermatitis, dementia, and death. More common in alcoholics and those who eat large amounts of corn.
- Scurvy: is due to vitamin C deficiency. Signs include anaemia, gingivitis, pinpoint bleeding at the base of hair follicles, and 'corkscrew' hairs.

Indications for nutritional support
It is important to recognize that the best route of nutrition is always through the gastrointestinal tract (GIT). This has important implications for immune function, viability of the GIT, and overall well-being.
The only indication for parenteral nutrition is the failure of enteral nutrition. This can be due to contraindications to enteral feeding or failure of enteral feeding to maintain weight (even if feasible but failing because of multiple interruptions to enteral feeding).
Intravenous nutrition carries certain complications, most of which relate to sepsis, some to atrophy of the gut mucosa, and some to the simple relative inefficiency of the system.

Complications of nutritional support
- Venous catheter-related problems:
  - Use of central or peripheral catheters.
  - Line sepsis.
  - Line occlusion.
  - Venous thrombosis.
- Problems with enteral tubes:
  - PEG.
  - Jejunal extension tubes.
- Refeeding syndrome.
- Short bowel syndrome.
- Gastroparesis.

Venous catheter-related problems

Central or peripheral feeding?
Central venous feeding is preferred, as this avoids thrombophlebitis from hyperosmolar feeds. Well-managed catheters can be left *in situ* for a long time.

Peripheral feeding with midline catheters (i.e. tip in the proximal portion of the arm) is limited by an excessive rate of catheter dysfunction. Narrow-gauge peripheral cannulae can be used but require low calorie regimes (i.e. osmolarity needs to be <900 mOsm/L), so only useful short-term (e.g. <5 days) or supplemental to enteral intake.

Line sepsis
Line-related bloodstream infections are potentially lethal. Two-thirds are due to coagulase-negative staphylococci. *S. aureus*, Gram-negative bacilli, *Candida* species, and *Pseudomonas* cause most of the remainder and carry the worst prognosis. Line infection (significant growth from the line of $>10^3$ colony-forming units (CFU)) should be differentiated from localized exit site cellulitis. One-third of patients with bacteraemia develop major complications, including septic shock, suppurative thrombophlebitis, metastatic infection, or endocarditis. Mortality is 10%.

Risk factors
• Site: femoral lines are at much greater risk of infection than internal jugular lines, which are at greater risk than subclavian lines. Leg lines are at much greater risk than arm lines.
• Technique and setting: a venous cut-down is a greater risk for infection than an emergency procedure, which is a greater risk than an elective procedure.
• Use: parenteral nutrition is a greater risk than other uses.
• Number of hubs: a multilumen line is a greater risk than a single lumen line.
• Duration of insertion for >5 days increases the risk of infection (but a well-managed central feeding catheter can be left *in situ* ad infinitum).

Meticulous asepsis should be practised during insertion, using full barrier precautions, with skin decontaminated with 2% chlorhexidine. Lines should be routinely monitored and changed if infection is confirmed or suspected in an unwell patient. Central feeding catheters should not be routinely changed. Peripheral feeding catheters are changed every 5 days; use gauze dressings which are only changed if apparently dirty. Administration sets should be changed at least every 72 hours. Antimicrobial-impregnated catheters are associated with less risk of infection.

Making the diagnosis
Bloodstream infection typically manifests with spiking fevers and rigors or complications. There may be associated exit site cellulitis. Take peripheral and central blood cultures. Definitive diagnosis requires identification of the microorganism from blood obtained from the feeding catheter. Infections may be polymicrobial. All patients with *S. aureus* should have an echocardiogram, and those with fungaemias require ophthalmological review.

When to remove the line
Clinical studies suggest that routine line removal results in the loss of many lines that are sterile, with no outcome benefits. They should not be exchanged over guidewires. Lines should only be withdrawn if:
• The patient is in septic shock.
• Infection is strongly suspected in a temporary line/catheter.

• Tunnelled central line infection recurs at least twice.
• There are signs of venous thrombosis.
• New endocarditis.
• There is significant purulence and erythema at the insertion site despite careful nursing care.

Management
Give empiric antibiotics if the patient is too ill to wait for definitive microbiology or a highly virulent organism is suspected. A glycopeptide (usually intravenous vancomycin 500 mg bd for 7 days) is appropriate, with a prolonged course of >4 weeks if there is deep-seated infection. In critically ill patients, it is appropriate to cover Gram-negatives and *Pseudomonas* (e.g. intravenous piperacillin-tazobactam 4.5 g tds or meropenem 1 g tds) and fungi (e.g. intravenous fluconazole 400 mg daily). Exit site abscesses may need surgical drainage or debridement.

Infection of tunnelled central feeding lines is managed using central antibiotic administration (as per sensitivities) and cessation of feeding for 7 days, with subsequent demonstration of sterile central cultures.

Line occlusion
Central feeding lines can be flushed with streptokinase. Seek expert advice from the nutrition team. Peripheral lines are usually removed if flushing with saline is not effective.

Venous thrombosis
The feeding catheter is removed and anticoagulation provided for 3–6 months. Vein patency is confirmed by Doppler ultrasound before further feeding catheters are inserted, which should be heparin-bonded if used long-term, in which case anticoagulation should be continued.

Problems with enteral tubes

Percutaneous endoscopic gastronomy (PEG) tubes
Complications directly related to the procedure include damage to surrounding structures (e.g. viscera and blood vessels), resulting in haemorrhage, perforation, or peritonitis. These occur more in the elderly or patients with comorbidity. The procedure has a directly attributable 30-day mortality of about 1 in 150, serious morbidity of 1 in 30, and minor morbidity of 1 in 8.

Procedural risks are much higher in patients with advanced dementia, in whom PEG placement is contraindicated (30-day mortality >50%). Prior abdominal surgery does not preclude a PEG but has a higher risk of colonic perforation. PEG is probably contraindicated in patients with ascites. Some complications can be easily prevented by careful technique and patient/carer education. The product instructions should be followed, correct traction applied, and importantly, 10 days following insertion, the external fixation plate must be loosened by 1-2 cm at the skin surface. Thereafter, the tube should be rotated 360° weekly to prevent tissue overgrowth.

Immediate complications—major: bleeding
Before placement, correct the full blood count (FBC) and clotting profiles, as necessary. Bleeding is uncommon but can be life-threatening if due to vascular injury at the time of PEG insertion. Localized vessel damage may respond to tamponade by tightening the intragastric flange against the skin (e.g. moving the marker at the skin surface from 4 cm to 3 cm). The bolster must be released within 48 hours to avoid mucosal pressure necrosis. If bleeding is persistent or life-threatening, consider interventional angiography or surgery.

Immediate complications—major: perforation

Perforation usually involves the catheter passing through an anterior-placed transverse colon. This can present with abdominal pain, peritonitis, or feed passing per rectum. It is diagnosed by ultrasound. Emergency laparotomy is indicated if the patient is peritonitic. Otherwise, the PEG tube should not be used and the patient placed on antibiotics for 4 weeks, at which time it can be removed endoscopically. The fistulous tract will gradually close, requiring only simple dressings (also see following paragraphs).

Immediate complications—major: peritonitis

Peritonitis not due to colonic perforation should usually be treated conservatively with intravenous antibiotics. PEG feeding must not be given until resolved. Necrotizing fasciitis is a rare, serious infection that requires immediate surgical debridement.

Immediate complications—minor

Pneumoperitoneum is common after PEG placement and is of no consequence in the absence of other worrying features. Surgical emphysema has also been described without any mishap having occurred.

Ileus may occur. Exclude perforation with a contrast study. Aspirate excess gastric air or fluid from the PEG. Resume feeding once resolved.

Long-term PEG tube complications: catheter occlusion

This is common (up to 45%). The catheter may be re-opened by vigorous flushing with warm water (consider prior instillation of pancreatic enzymes in bicarbonate) or manually with a brush or balloon catheter. Wires should be avoided, as they may cause perforation. Tubes can be used immediately. To avoid recurrence, advise flushing before and after feeds and medications (which should be fully dissolved or in liquid form), using 30 ml water. Avoid saline as it may crystallize.

Dislodged feeding tubes

Replace the feeding catheter within 5 days to maintain nutrition. If dislodged within 1 month of the original placement, relocate endoscopically to avoid peritoneal siting. By contrast, mature tracks are easily re-cannulated: maintain the tract patency by placing a Foley catheter in the tract within 12 hours (this may be successful for up to 5 days; if in doubt, this can be performed using screening). Definitive tube replacement can then be endoscopic or radiological. If dislodgement is recurrent, review PEG care, and consider a larger catheter, larger balloon, or more durable silicone tube.

Leakage

This is usually due to excessive tube motion, overtight fixation of the PEG to the skin surface (causing pressure necrosis), or an incorrectly placed external fixation plate. Partial obstruction should be excluded. Treat malnutrition, diabetes, and skin infection . Ensure the correct position of external fixation plates. Larger catheters are ineffective (i.e. tissue growth and healing are more important). Removal of the PEG tube for 24–48 hours to allow partial tract closure has been reported to be successful when established tracts leak, but often a new puncture site will be required.

Cellulitis

Peristomal cellulitis is common and usually presents as localized erythema and tenderness. Systemic upset is rare. Infections are most commonly due to *S. aureus* and/or beta-haemolytic streptococci. Candidal superinfection may occur. Treatment requires stoma care, culture, and oral antibiotics (e.g. co-amoxiclav 625 mg tds or clindamycin 250 mg qds if the patient is penicillin-allergic). The PEG tube may need to be removed and the infection treated before a new PEG tube is replaced. Patients with MRSA should have nasopharyngeal decontamination prior to PEG (re)-placement.

Bleeding

Late occuring bleeds are most frequently due to oesophagitis or gastric ulcers. These should be visualized and treated endoscopically, together with the use of proton pump inhibitors.

Obstruction

Gastric outlet obstruction occurs if the internal flange lodges in the pylorus or duodenum, most frequently after replacement. It presents as proximal small bowel obstruction, with prominent reflux of stomach contents through the PEG. Diagnosis is by contrast studies. Management involves withdrawing and fixing the tube at the skin surface with 2 cm of 'play'. Often 'partial obstruction' represents gastroparesis (see further text).

Diarrhoea

The usual cause is intolerance to the feed preparation. Try feeds with a reduced osmolarity or with a lower fibre content. Small doses of loperamide may be beneficial.

The rare complication that should be excluded is gastrocolic fistula. Patients may be asymptomatic for months, and the PEG may function normally. It often presents when a PEG tube is inadvertently replaced into the bowel lumen. The characteristic symptom is transient diarrhoea, occurring within minutes of the feed, associated with passage of undigested feed per rectum or faecal material through the PEG. Most cases can be managed by removal and re-siting of the PEG; the residual track closes within days. Tubes may require laparoscopic replacement, at which any residual fistula can be excised (see as described previously).

Buried bumper syndrome

This is a rare and under-recognized complication, in which gastric mucosa overgrows and seals the internal tube lumen. It is thought to arise due to excessive tension between the inner and outer bolsters. Presentation is with mechanical failure to deliver feed, associated with abdominal pain during feeding and associated leakage. Endoscopic examination confirms blockage and allows the bumper to be released (techniques include snare cautery, laser, simple traction, 'push/pull technique'). All symptomatic patients should have their tubes replaced. Rotating the tube every few days following placement, and releasing tube traction at 10 days, once the tract has formed can aid prevention.

Jejunal extension tubes

Reflux and aspiration

Reflux and aspiration are common with long-term PEG feeding, particularly in patients with gastroparesis (e.g. after CVA, multiple sclerosis, Parkinson's disease). Pulmonary aspiration is likely if feed is aspirated from the mouth (this can be clarified by injecting blue ink through the PEG) or if chest infections recur. If suspected, avoid opiates and agents that predispose to constipation; correct electrolytes (K^+, Na^+, Mg^{2+}); reduce the rate of feed; avoid feeding if the patient is supine, and prescribe prokinetics (e.g. domperidone linctus). Endoscopic jejunal extension tubes (JET) can be used but often kink. Radiological JETs are wider gauge and more effective.

PEG use in pregnancy

PEG feeding has been successfully conducted in pregnancy, and the associated complications are similar to those outlined in the previous paragraphs. Intractable hyperemesis gravidarum may require conversion to a (radiological) JET.

Refeeding syndrome

Refeeding syndrome is characterized by severe fluid and electrolyte shifts in severely malnourished individuals, in whom nutritional support has commenced. It occurs following the introduction of both enteral or parental nutrition. High-risk factors are shown in Table 8.22.

The principal pathogenetic mechanism in refeeding syndrome involves the insulin response to the reintroduction of carbohydrates. Glycogen, lipid, and protein synthesis is stimulated, processes that deplete phosphate, magnesium, and thiamine. Insulin also drives potassium intracellularly. Fluid shifts occur due to osmotic gradients.

Clinical features

- Fluid shifts.
- Disordered sodium balance.
- Hypokalaemia.
- Hypomagnesaemia.
- Hypophosphataemia. Serum inorganic phosphate <0.5 mmol/L predisposes to rhabdomyolysis, immunosuppression, cardiorespiratory failure, hypotension, muscle weakness, cardiac arrhythmia, and seizures.
- Hypocalcaemia.
- Wernicke's encephalopathy. This presents with confusion, ocular signs, and ataxia, and may lead to Korsakoff's psychosis.

NICE guidelines recommend starting refeeding at no more than 50% of energy requirements (25% if very high risk). This does not need to wait for the correction of fluid and electrolyte imbalances, which can be done concurrently. Parenteral vitamin supplementation should be commenced immediately and continued for the first 3–5 days of refeeding. Electrolytes and electrocardiogram should be monitored daily for 1 week, then three times the following week. Inspect daily for oedema, heart failure, and confusion.

Management

1. Identify at-risk patients (e.g. chronic alcoholics, anorexia, neglected patients).
2. Check potassium, magnesium, phosphate, and calcium.
3. Prior to feeding, administer intravenous thiamine (Pabrinex® 1 + 2), continued three times daily for 3–5 days; oral thiamine 200–300 mg od is an alternative. Long-term supplementation, with oral vitamin B co-strong 1–2 tablets daily, thiamine 100 mg daily, and multivitamin supplements one tablet daily, is recommended.
4. Start feeding at 20 kcal/kg/day, and increase by 100–200 kcal/day.
5. Rehydrate cautiously; supplement and correct potassium, phosphate, magnesium, and calcium, as required.

Further reading

Elia M and Russell CA, eds. (2009). *Combating malnutrition: recommendations for action.* A report from the Advisory Group on Malnutrition, led by BAPEN. BAPEN, Redditch.

Holt PR (2001). Diarrhoea and malabsorption in the elderly. *Gastroenterology Clinics of North America*, **30**, 427–44.

Malhi H, Thompson R (2014). PEG tubes: dealing with complications. *Nursing Times*, **110**, No 45, 18–21.

Milne AC, Potter J, Vivanti A, et al. (2009). Protein and energy supplementation in elderly people at risk from malnutrition. *Cochrane Database of Systematic Reviews*, **2**, CD003288.

Morris J and Twaddle S (2007). Anorexia nervosa. *BMJ*, **334**, 894–8.

National Institute for Health and Clinical Excellence (2006). Nutrition support in adults: oral nutrition support, enteral tube feeding and parenteral nutrition. NICE clinical guideline CG32. <http://guidance.nice.org.uk/CG32>.

National Institute for Health and Care Excellence (2011). The diagnosis and management of colorectal cancer. NICE clinical guideline CG131. <https://www.nice.org.uk/guidance/cg131>.

Sundaram A, Koutkia P, Apovian CM (2002). Nutritional management of short bowel syndrome in adults. *Journal of Clinical Gastroenterology*, **34**, 207–20.

Thomas PD, Forbes A, Green J, et al. (2003). Guidelines for the investigation of chronic diarrhoea. *Gut*, **52** (Suppl V), v1–15.

Treasure J, Claudino AM, Zucker N (2010). Eating disorders. *Lancet*, **375**, 583–93.

Chapter 9

Drug overdoses

Overdoses: general approach

Drug overdoses account for 15% of acute medical emergencies, and 50% of patients will have taken alcohol as well. Thirty per cent of self-poisonings involve multiple drugs, and the majority of the drugs (65%) involved belong to the patient, a relative, or friend.

The history may be unreliable. Question any witnesses or family about where a patient was found and any possible access to drugs. Examination may reveal clues as to the likely poison (e.g. pinpoint pupils with opiates) and signs of solvent or ethanol abuse, and IV drug use should be noted (see Table 9.1).

Management

Priorities are:

1. Resuscitate the patient.
2. Reduce absorption of the drug, if possible.
3. Give specific antidotes, if available.

Secure their airway (place in the recovery position), and monitor breathing, BP, temperature, acid-base balance, and serum electrolytes. Treat seizures or dysrhythmias. Intubate if the Glasgow Coma Scale (GCS) is less than 8 and not reversible with naloxone. Flumazenil should not be used diagnostically in the unconscious patient.

Take account of any active medical problems that the patient may have, e.g. intravenous (IV) drug users may have concurrent septicaemia, hepatitis, subacute bacterial endocarditis (SBE), pulmonary hypertension, or HIV-related disease.

Measures to reduce gut absorption

Gastric lavage should not be employed routinely, if ever, in the management of drug overdose. The amount of drug removed by gastric lavage is variable and diminishes with time. Gastric lavage should not be considered, unless a patient has ingested a potentially life-threatening amount of a poison and the procedure can be undertaken within 60 minutes of ingestion. Even then, clinical benefit has not been confirmed in controlled studies. Risks of the procedure include hypoxia, dysrhythmias, laryngospasm, perforation of the GI tract or pharynx, fluid and electrolyte abnormalities, and aspiration pneumonitis. It is contraindicated if corrosive substances or hydrocarbons have been ingested. Unless a patient is intubated, gastric lavage is contraindicated if airway protective reflexes are lost.

Activated charcoal (50 g as a single dose) will adsorb many drugs if given within 1 hour of ingestion, although its effectiveness falls off rapidly thereafter. Drugs not adsorbed by charcoal include iron, lithium, salts, alkalis, acids, ethanol, methanol, ethylene glycol, and organic solvents.

Multiple dose activated charcoal (50 g every 4 hours) may also accelerate whole body clearance of some drugs by interrupting enterohepatic cycling, e.g. phenobarbital (INN), phenytoin, carbamazepine, digoxin, paraquat, dapsone, quinine, and slow-release preparations, such as theophylline. Charcoal is rather unpleasant to drink repeatedly and will be more reliably taken if given down a nasogastric (NG) tube.

Table 9.1 Assessment of poisoning in the unconscious patient

Sign	Consider
Hypoventilation	Opiates, ethanol, benzodiazepines
Hyperventilation	Metabolic acidosis (aspirin, paracetamol, ethylene glycol), gastric aspiration, carbon monoxide
Pinpoint pupils	Opiates, organophosphates
Dilated pupils	Methanol, anticholinergics, tricyclics, LSD
Bradycardia	Beta-blockers, digoxin, opiates
Tachyarrhythmias	Tricyclics, theophylline, anticholinergics, caffeine, lithium, digoxin
Hyperthermia	Ecstasy, amphetamines, anticholinergics
Pyramidal signs, ataxia, hypotonia, hyperreflexia, and extensor plantars	Tricyclics, anticholinergic agents
Hypertension	Cocaine, amphetamines, ecstasy

Adapted from Punit S. Ramrakha, Kevin P. Moore, and Amir Sam, *Oxford Handbook of Acute Medicine*, Third Edition, 2010, Box 14.1, page 693, copyright Punit S. Ramrakha and Kevin P. Moore, with permission.

PEG bowel lavage. In whole bowel irrigation, Klean-Prep®, a solution of polyethylene glycol (not to be confused with ethylene glycol), is given orally or by NG tube at 2 L/h in adults. It is continued until the rectal effluent becomes clear. It is used, following ingestion of sustained-release or enteric-coated preparations of toxic drugs, such as calcium channel blockers and lithium. Percutaneous endoscopic gastrostomy (PEG) bowel lavage may be used in body packers to hasten the passage of packets of illicit drugs. Contraindications include bowel obstruction, perforation, ileus, or in the seriously ill patient, e.g. haemodynamic instability.

Ipecacuanha-induced emesis is no longer used.

For uncommon overdoses, always seek advice from the National Poisons Information Service (listed inside the front cover of the *British National Formulary* (*BNF*) and on telephone number 0844 892 0111 in the UK). The US National Capital Poisons Center can be contacted on 1-800-222-1222. Advice about poisoning is also available on TOXBASE (<http://www.toxbase.org>).

Occasionally, patients present where poisoning is suspected but not known. Even where the history suggests self-poisoning, be aware that serious underlying disease may be present. For example, patients who feel very ill will often self-medicate with aspirin and paracetamol.

Table 9.2 gives an immediate indication of specific therapies that are currently available.

Table 9.2 Summary of therapies and antidotes for specific overdose episodes

Drug	Action	Antidote/therapy
Antidepressants	Activated charcoal	Diazepam for convulsions, cardiac monitoring
Aspirin	Activated charcoal Gastric emptying if <1 h	Alkaline diuresis, haemodialysis
Benzodiazepines	Protect airway	Flumazenil if severe
Beta-blockers	Check ABC	Atropine (3 mg), glucagon 7mg IM, consider pacing
Calcium antagonists	Calcium gluconate	Anticholinergics
Carbon monoxide	Give 100% oxygen	Hyperbaric oxygen
Cyanide	Give 100% oxygen	Sodium thiosulfate, dicobalt edetate
Digoxin	Check K⁺ and ECG	Digibind® (digoxin-binding antibody)
Ethylene glycol	Check acid-base	Infuse ethanol or fomepizole (4 methyl pyrazole)
Heavy metals	Ask NPIS/NCPC (below)	Chelating agents are occasionally recommended
Iron tablets	Charcoal is ineffective	Desferrioxamine
Lithium	Gastric emptying If >4 g and <60 min	Adequate hydration and dialysis Activated charcoal is of NO value
Methanol	Monitor U&E, glucose	Infuse ethanol, phenytoin for seizures, dialysis if severe
Organophosphorus insecticides	Gastric aspiration if <4 h. Remove clothes, and decontaminate	Atropine, pralidoxime. Consult NPIS/NCPC
Opiates	Check respiration	Naloxone
Paracetamol	Activated charcoal if <4 h	acetylcysteine (or methionine)
Paraquat	Activated charcoal	Fuller's earth (or bentonite or activated charcoal), vitamin E

NPIS, National Poisons Information Service; telephone UK (+44) (0) 844 892 0111 or the NCPC; US National Capital Poisons Center; telephone US 1-800-222-1222 (or other appropriate national poisons centre).

Adapted from Punit S. Ramrakha, Kevin P. Moore, and Amir Sam, *Oxford Handbook of Acute Medicine*, Third Edition, 2010, Table 14.1, page 694–695, copyright Punit S. Ramrakha and Kevin P. Moore, with permission.

Drugs

Amphetamines

This agent (and its cogener methamphetamine) is widely abused for its effects on CNS arousal. A number of its methylenedioxy derivatives (e.g. 'ecstasy' or methylenedioxy-methamphetamine (MDMA)) are also available on an illicit basis and have additional hallucinogenic actions (LSD-like).

Presentation

Sympathomimetic effects

- Mydriasis.
- Hypertension.
- Tachycardia.
- Skin pallor.

Central effects

- Hyperexcitability.
- Agitation.
- Talkativeness.
- Paranoia (especially with chronic use).

Complications

- Intracranial (and subarachnoid) haemorrhage; although attributed to its hypertensive effect, this can occur after a single dose.
- Vasospasm may be seen on angiography ('string of beads').
- Ecstasy is associated with a heatstroke-like syndrome (see 'Thermal disorders' Chapter 18).

Poor prognostic features

- Hyperpyrexia (>42°C).
- Rhabdomyolysis.
- Disseminated intravascular coagulation.
- Acute renal failure.
- Acute liver failure.

Management

- Sedate agitated patients with a benzodiazepine (e.g. 5–10 mg diazepam IV or 1–2 mg lorazepam IM/IV). Psychotic patients may require haloperidol (5–10 mg IM). Haloperidol may decrease the seizure threshold.
- Monitor core temperature at least hourly initially.
- Seizures should be controlled with diazepam (5–10 mg IV stat). New focal signs should prompt urgent CT scanning, looking for evidence of intracranial bleeding.
- Significant hypertension (diastolic >120 mmHg) may respond to sedation with diazepam. If not, it should be controlled with intravenous nitrates, e.g. GTN 1–2 mg/h, titrating to response, or IV labetalol if in a high dependency unit.
- Hyperpyrexia requires prompt cooling with tepid sponging or even chilled IV fluids, as necessary. Aim to keep the rectal temperature <38.5°C. Chlorpromazine (25–50 mg IM) will decrease the core temperature but may cause sedation and hypotension. Dantrolene can also decrease hyperpyrexia.
- Acidification of the urine substantially increases drug elimination but can exacerbate electrolyte and pH disturbances and is best avoided.

Antipsychotic drugs

Chlorpromazine, haloperidol, risperidone, olanzapine

All of these drugs have antipsychotic activity with dopamine receptor antagonist activity. Their management is similar.

Presentations

Deep sleep, coma, extrapyramidal symptoms, abnormal involuntary muscle movements, and hypotension and occasional fitting. Most antipsychotic drugs may cause prolongation of the QT interval and torsade de pointes, but this is most likely with amisulpride.

Management

This is symptom-directed, supportive, and includes essential general overdose strategies.

Consider activated charcoal (50 g for adults) if the patient presents within 1 hour of ingestion of a toxic amount.

- Treat hypotension with IV fluids and raising the foot of the bed. Some patients may need an inotropic support.
- Seizures usually respond to diazepam (5–10 mg IV; may be repeated every 15 minutes; maximum 30 mg) or to phenytoin.
- Cardiac arrhythmias often respond to IV phenytoin (15 mg/kg, up to 1 g total dose) while other antiarrhythmics may be used. Administer IV magnesium sulfate (INN) for torsade de pointes.
- Treat extrapyramidal symptoms, e.g. acute dystonic reactions, with anticholinergic agents, e.g. procyclidine (5–10 mg IV) or benzatropine mesilate (1–2 mg IV or IM). Benzatropine may not be readily available. These agents are usually effective within 2–5 minutes but may take up to 30 minutes.

Haloperidol

Haloperidol is rapidly absorbed. Peak plasma levels are reached 2–6 hours after ingestion, with a half-life of 13–35 hours. Serious toxicity is uncommon. The most common problems are drowsiness and the development of acute dystonic reactions of the type seen with phenothiazines. These include oculogyric crises, torticollis, trismus, orolingual dyskinesia, and a feeling that the tongue is swelling. Rarely, hypotension (or, conversely, hypertension), tachycardia or bradycardia, QT prolongation, ventricular arrhythmias (torsade de pointes), convulsions, hypokalaemia, hypothermia, acute renal failure, and coma may develop. Ventricular arrhythmias have been reported in adults after ingestion of >200 mg haloperidol, and survival has been reported in overdoses up to 1,000 mg.

Benzodiazepines

Deliberate overdose with this group of compounds is very common. Unless combined with other sedatives (e.g. alcohol or tricyclics), the effects of overdosing are generally mild.

Presentation

- Drowsiness.
- Slurred speech.
- Nystagmus.
- Hypotension (mild).
- Ataxia.
- Coma.
- Respiratory depression.
- Cardiac arrest.

The elderly and patients with severe chronic obstructive airways disease are generally more susceptible to cardio-respiratory depression with benzodiazepine overdose.

Peak plasma concentrations occur within 30–90 minutes after taking tablets. The elimination half-life of diazepam is 24 to 48 hours, and a number of active agents are produced from metabolism, in particular desmethyldiazepam with a half-life up to 5 days. When co-ingested with alcohol and other central nervous system depressants, the effects of benzodiazepines are potentially more severe. Severe effects in overdose also include rhabdomyolysis and hypothermia.

Management

If patients present within 1 hour, give 50 g activated charcoal. Ensure the patient can protect their airway. No further intervention is usually required for pure benzodiazepine overdoses. Hypotension should be treated with intravenous fluids and inotropes, if needed.

Flumazenil, a benzodiazepine antagonist, may be used to reverse significant cardiorespiratory depression in severe overdose. It is given as an IV bolus of 0.2 mg. If no response, give further IV bolus doses of 0.3 and thereafter 0.5 mg every 30 seconds to a maximum of 3 mg until the patient is rousable. Most benzodiazepines have a substantially longer duration of action than flumazenil, and an IV infusion of 0.1–0.4 mg/h will be needed to prevent early re-sedation.

Flumazenil should not be used diagnostically in comatose patients where the diagnosis is uncertain, as it may cause fits or death.

Avoid giving excess flumazenil to completely reverse the effect of a benzodiazepine. In chronic benzodiazepine abusers, this can cause marked agitation.

Flumazenil is contraindicated when patients have ingested multiple medicines, especially after co-ingestion of a benzodiazepine and a pro-convulsant (e.g. dextropropoxyphene, theophyllines, and tricyclics). This is because the benzodiazepine may be suppressing seizures induced by the second drug; its antagonism by flumazenil can reveal severe status epilepticus that is very difficult to control.

Contraindications to flumazenil include features suggestive of a tricyclic antidepressant ingestion, including a wide QRS or large pupils. Its use in patients post-cardiac arrest is also contraindicated. It should be used with caution in patients with a history of seizures, head injury, or chronic benzodiazepine use.

Beta-blockers

These agents competitively antagonize the effects of endogenous catecholamines. They cause profound effects on atrioventricular conduction and myocardial contractility, and their effects are predictable, based on their known pharmacology.

Presentation

- Sinus bradycardia.
- Hypotension.
- Cardiac failure.
- Cardiac arrest.
- Bronchospasm (rare in non-asthmatics).
- Fits (especially with propranolol).
- Drowsiness.
- Hallucinations.
- Coma.
- Hypoglycaemia.

Prognostic features

- Patients with pre-existing impaired myocardial contractility are less likely to tolerate an overdose of beta-blockers.
- The ECG may provide some indication as to the severity: first-degree heart block occurs with mild overdose; widening of the QRS and prolongation of the corrected QT interval (particularly after sotalol) with moderate to severe overdose.

Management

- Establish IV access.
- Check a 12-lead ECG, and then monitor ECG continuously.
- Record HR and BP regularly (at least every 15 minutes).
- Consider activated charcoal (50 g for adults) if the patient presents within 1 hour of ingestion.
- Hypotension. Seek expert help early. Treat with IV glucagon (50–150 mcg/kg, followed by an infusion of 1–5 mg/h). This peptide is able to exert an inotropic effect, independent of beta-receptor activation, by raising myocardial cAMP levels. Inotropes, such as dobutamine, may be used, and use of an intra-aortic balloon may provide an adequate cardiac output whilst the drug is metabolized and excreted.
- Bradycardia may respond to atropine alone (3 mg IV bolus). Isoprenaline infusions (5–50 mcg/min) may be tried but are often ineffective. If the bradycardia persists and the patient is in cardiogenic shock, they may need pacing (see Chapter 4).
- Convulsions. Give diazepam 5–10 mg IV initially (see Chapter 7).
- Bronchospasm. Treat initially with high-dose nebulized salbutamol (5–10 mg or higher). If nebulized bronchodilators are ineffective, an aminophylline infusion should be used (e.g. 0.5 mg/kg/min).
- Monitor blood glucose regularly (hourly BMs). If hypoglycaemia develops, give 50 mL of 50% glucose, followed by an IV infusion of 10% glucose, adjusting the rate, as necessary.

Calcium channel blockers

Nifedipine and amlodipine

The most important effects are on the cardiovascular system. Dihydropyridine calcium antagonists, including nifedipine and amlodipine, cause severe hypotension secondary to peripheral vasodilatation. This may be associated with reflex tachycardia. Bradycardia and AV block may be present in severe poisoning.

Features include nausea, vomiting, dizziness, agitation, confusion, and occasionally coma in cases of severe poisoning. Metabolic acidosis, hyperkalaemia, hypocalcaemia, and hyperglycaemia may be present.

Other reported features include seizures, pulmonary oedema, paralytic ileus, acute pancreatitis, hepatotoxicity, and mesenteric infarction.

Consider activated charcoal (50 g for adults) if the patient presents within 1 hour of ingestion of a toxic amount.

Monitor blood pressure and cardiac rhythm. Check serum urea and electrolytes (U&E), calcium, glucose, and arterial blood gases.

Perform a 12-lead ECG and further ECGs if a slow release preparation has been ingested or there is a fall in heart rate or blood pressure.

Asymptomatic patients should be observed for at least 12 hours after ingestion.

Correct hypotension by raising the foot of the bed and by giving an appropriate fluid challenge.

Give atropine for symptomatic bradycardia (1 mg for an adult). Repeat doses may be needed.

In severe cases, an insulin and dextrose infusion may improve both myocardial contractility and systemic perfusion. It is particularly useful in the presence of acidosis. Such patients should be managed in an HDU/ICU setting. An infusion of 10–20% glucose should be given with an infusion of insulin at 0.5–1.0 unit/kg/h. Monitor serum glucose and potassium levels.

If hypotension fails to respond to the above, consider an epinephrine (adrenaline) infusion or a combination of dobutamine and norepinephrine (noradrenaline). Both regimes may improve cardiac dysfunction and systemic vascular resistance.

Verapamil and diltiazem

These have a profound cardiac depressant effect, causing hypotension. They also have effects on the AV node, causing bradyarrhythmias, including junctional escape rhythms, second-degree and complete heart block, and asystole. They also cause peripheral vasodilatation.

Other non-cardiac effects include nausea, vomiting, dizziness, agitation, confusion, and occasionally coma in cases of severe poisoning. Metabolic acidosis, hyperkalaemia, hypocalcaemia, and hyperglycaemia may be present. Seizures are rare. Management is as for nifedipine and amlodipine.

Carbon monoxide

See Toxic inhalation injury (Chapter 18). The commonest sources are smoke inhalation, poorly maintained domestic gas appliances, and deliberate inhalation of car exhaust fumes. It causes intense tissue hypoxia by two mechanisms. Firstly, it interrupts electron transport in mitochondria. Secondly, it reduces oxygen delivery by competing with oxygen (O_2) for binding to haemoglobin (Hb) (its affinity for Hb is 220-fold that of O_2), and by altering the shape of the HbO_2 dissociation curve (making it shift to the left).

Presentation

Patients present with signs of hypoxia without cyanosis. Skin and mucosal surfaces may appear 'cherry-red' (most obvious at post-mortem). Carboxyhaemoglobin (COHb) levels correlate poorly with clinical features. In general, levels of COHb below 30% cause only headache and dizziness, whilst levels of 50–60% produce syncope, tachypnoea, tachycardia, and fits. Levels over 60% cause increasing risk of cardiorespiratory failure and death.

Complications

These are the predictable result of local hypoxia. Sites at particular risk are CNS, affecting cerebral, cerebellar, or midbrain function, e.g. parkinsonism and akinetic mutism; the myocardium, with ischaemia and infarction; skeletal muscle, causing rhabdomyolysis and myoglobinuria; and skin involvement which ranges from erythema to severe blistering.

Prognostic features

Anaemia, increased metabolic rate (e.g. children), and underlying ischaemic heart disease all increase susceptibility to carbon monoxide toxicity. Neurological recovery depends on the duration of the hypoxic coma; complete recovery has been reported in young patients (<50 years) after up to 21 hours, as compared to 11 hours in older subjects.

Management

An arterial blood gas should be taken. Although PaO_2 may be normal, it is essential to measure the COHb concentration. Most ITUs have a carboxyhaemoglobinometer. Note that monitoring O_2 saturation with a pulse oximeter is unhelpful since it will not distinguish between HbO_2 and COHb (hence, the apparent oxygen saturation will be falsely high).

Apply a tight-fitting face mask, and give 100% O_2. Check a 12-lead ECG, and continuously monitor rhythm. Take blood for FBC, U&E, creatine phosphokinase (CPK), and cardiac enzymes.

If the patient is comatose, they should be intubated and ventilated with 100% FiO_2 (this reduces the half-life of COHb to 80 minutes, compared with 320 minutes on room air). This should also be considered in all patients who are severely acidotic or who show evidence of myocardial ischaemia.

Fits should be controlled with IV diazepam (5–10 mg). The metabolic acidosis is best treated by increasing tissue oxygenation, and IV sodium bicarbonate ($NaHCO_3$) is best avoided.

Hyperbaric oxygen will shorten the washout of COHb, but lack of easy access to a hyperbaric chamber makes this difficult. Consider: (1) if the patient has been unconscious, (2) if COHb is >30%, (3) if there are neurological or psychiatric signs, and (4) if there is a significant metabolic acidosis. Ensure medical follow-up, as the neuropsychiatric sequelae may take many weeks to evolve.

Cocaine

Cocaine is rapidly absorbed when applied intranasally ('snorting') or smoked (free-basing 'crack'). Occasionally, it presents as massive overdosing when the swallowed packets of illicit, smuggled cocaine rupture. Its subjective and sympathomimetic actions are often indistinguishable from amphetamine.

Presentation

- Hypertension.
- Seizures (common).
- Tachycardia.
- Skin pallor.
- CNS depression (with high doses).
- Ventricular arrhythmias.
- Paranoid delusions (chronic use).
- Cardiorespiratory failure.

Complications

- Vasoconstrictor effects on the coronary circulation can cause myocardial ischaemia and infarction, even in patients with normal vessels.
- Cerebrovascular accident.
- Psychotic reactions may occur.

Prognostic features

- The lethal dose of pure cocaine by ingestion is approximately 1 g, but regular users tolerate larger doses.
- Cocaine can cause seizures in epileptics in 'recreational' doses. Presentation in status epilepticus in non-epileptics implies massive overdose and carries a poor prognosis.
- Rhabdomyolysis, hyperpyrexia, renal failure, severe liver dysfunction, and DIC have been reported and have high mortality.
- Patients with pseudocholinesterase deficiency are thought to be at particular risk of life-threatening cocaine toxicity.

Management

- General measures: establish IV access, and take blood for U&E and CPK levels. Ensure the airway is clear. If GCS ≤8, consider intubation and mechanical ventilation. Agitation may require diazepam (5–10 mg IV). Monitor ECG continuously for arrhythmias.
- Perform a 12-lead ECG for evidence of myocardial ischaemia, infarction, or dysrhythmias.
- Narrow complex tachycardias. If these do not settle after treatment with diazepam, give verapamil (5–10 mg IV).
- Ventricular arrhythmias. Treat with IV 8.4% sodium bicarbonate (50 mmol). Lidocaine IV may be used cautiously if there is no response.
- Monitor core temperature for evidence of hyperpyrexia. If necessary, start cooling measures (see 'Thermal disorders', Chapter 18), e.g. tepid sponging or chilled IV fluids, as necessary, to keep the temperature below 38.5°C. Chlorpromazine 25–50 mg IM may be useful, however, it may cause sedation and hypotension.
- Significant hypertension (diastolic >120 mmHg) should be controlled initially with diazepam (5–10 mg IV); if it remains high, start an IV infusion of GTN (1–2 mg/min, titrating to response). Alternatively, use calcium channel blockers, combined alpha- and beta-blockers (e.g. IV phentolamine) or IV sodium nitroprusside. Beta-blockers may worsen the hypertension through unopposed alpha effects.
- Chest pain should be treated with diazepam and nitrates (sublingual or intravenous). Myocardial infarction due to cocaine should be managed conventionally (see Chapter 4).
- Seizures should be controlled with diazepam (10–30 mg IV stat and, if necessary, an IV infusion of up to 200 mg/24h). Presentation with focal seizures after cocaine ingestion usually implies ischaemic or haemorrhage stroke. In these circumstances arrange an urgent brain CT scan.

Cyanide

Poisoning is most commonly seen in victims of smoke inhalation (hydrogen cyanide (HCN) is a combustion product of polyurethane foams). Cyanide derivatives are, however, widely employed in industrial processes and fertilizers. Children may also ingest amygdalin, a cyanogenic glycoside, contained in kernels of almonds and cherries. Cyanide has a high affinity for ferric ions, and reacts readily with the ferric ions of mitochondrial cytochrome oxidase irreversibly blocking mitochondrial electron transport.

Presentation

Cyanide gas can lead to cardiorespiratory arrest and death within a few minutes. Onset of effects after ingestion or skin contamination is generally much slower (up to several hours). Early signs are dizziness, chest tightness, dyspnoea, confusion, and paralysis. Cardiovascular collapse, apnoea, and seizures follow. Cyanosis is not a feature. The classical smell of bitter almonds is unhelpful (it is genetically determined, and 50% of observers cannot detect it). Pulmonary oedema and lactic acidosis are common in severe poisoning.

Prognostic features

- Ingestion of a few hundred milligrams of a cyanide salt is usually fatal in adults. Absorption is delayed by a full stomach and high gastric pH (e.g. antacids).
- Patients surviving to reach hospital after inhalation of HCN are unlikely to have suffered significant poisoning.
- Acidosis indicates severe poisoning.

Management

- Do not attempt mouth-to-mouth resuscitation. Give 100% O_2 through a tight-fitting face mask or intubate and ventilate if necessary.
- Establish IV access.
- Check arterial blood gases. Lactic acidosis indicates severe poisoning.
- Skin contamination requires thorough washing of the affected area with soap and water.
- If signs of moderate to severe cyanide toxicity are present, give 300 mg of dicobalt edetate (Kelocyanor®) IV over 1 minute, followed immediately by 50 mL of 50% glucose. If there is no response in 1 minute, repeat the dose. Further doses may cause cobalt toxicity. However, be aware that dicobalt edetate is very toxic and may be fatal in the absence of cyanide poisoning. Alternatively in less severe cyanide poisoning, give sodium nitrite (10 mL of a 3% solution) followed by sodium thiosulfate (25 mL of 50% solution). Sodium nitrite reacts with haemoglobin to form methaemoglobin (MetHb), to which cyanide preferentially binds, restoring cytochrome oxidase activity. As cyanide dissociates from the MetHb, it is converted to relatively non-toxic thiocyanate by the enzyme rhodanese. The lack of a suitable sulphur donor is the rate-limiting step for this reaction, and the provision of sulphur by sodium thiosulfate administration enhances this endogenous cyanide detoxification. Treatment with sodium nitrite is not without risk as MetHb cannot carry oxygen and may cause significant tissue hypoxia. Consequently, MetHb levels should be measured if sodium nitrite is given.
- Hydroxocobalamin 5 g (Cyanokit®), infused over 15–30 minutes, is also available for use when cyanide poisoning is suspected (e.g. smoke inhalation). It binds cyanide to form harmless cyanocobalamin.

Digoxin

Deliberate overdosing with digoxin is unusual. Significant toxicity is, however, a common adverse drug reaction in patients taking digoxin therapeutically (up to 25% of patients in some series). It is particularly common when renal impairment occurs (digoxin is almost totally cleared by the kidneys) and is exacerbated by hypokalaemia.

Presentation

- Nausea, vomiting, confusion, and diarrhoea.
- Visual disturbance (blurring, flashes, disturbed colour vision).
- Cardiac dysrhythmias (tachyarrhythmias or bradyarrhythmias).

Complications

- Hyperkalaemia.
- Cardiac dysrhythmias (see Chapter 4). The initial effect is usually a marked sinus bradycardia which is vagally mediated. This is followed by atrial tachyarrhythmias (with/without heart block), accelerated junctional rhythms, ventricular ectopy, and finally VT or VF.

Prognostic features

- Digoxin level >10 ng/mL and hyperkalaemia represent a severe overdose.
- Susceptibility to digoxin toxicity is increased by renal impairment, electrolyte disturbance (K^+ or Mg^{2+}), and hypothyroidism.

Management

- Take blood for a digoxin level (in patients not normally on digoxin, this should be at least 6 hours post-ingestion) and U&E.
- Perform a baseline 12-lead ECG and continuous ECG monitoring.
- Gastric lavage should be attempted if seen within 1 hour of overdose, followed by activated charcoal (50 g stat). Activated charcoal (25 g) may be repeated every 2 hours, provided the patient is not vomiting.
- Sinus bradyarrhythmias and AV block usually respond to atropine (0.6 mg IV, repeated to a total of 2.4 mg). Asymptomatic ventricular ectopics do not require specific treatment.
- Ventricular tachyarrhythmias should be treated with magnesium sulphate (8–10 mmol IV).
- Patients with haemodynamic instability, resistant ventricular tachyarrhythmias, or high K$^+$ require treatment with digoxin-binding antibody fragments (Fab, Digibind®). Dose: (number of vials) = 1.67 amount ingested (mg). If the latter is unknown, give 20 vials (infused over 30 minutes). The neutralizing dose for patients intoxicated during chronic therapy: (number of vials) = digoxin level (ng/mL) × weight (kg) × 0.01. Half this dose should initially be given and repeated if there is recurrence of toxicity. Fab therapy will terminate VT in 20–40 minutes. The K$^+$ and free serum digoxin levels should be monitored for 24 hours after Fab therapy. A substantial hypokalaemia can develop, and, not infrequently, there is a rebound in digoxin levels which may require administration of additional Fab. In patients with renal impairment, this rebound is delayed, and monitoring should be extended to 72 hours.
- Patients with severe renal failure are obviously unable to clear the Fab-digoxin complexes. Plasmapheresis is indicated to clear the bound digoxin.
- If Digibind® is not available, insert a transvenous pacing wire, and try to control arrhythmias with a combination of overdrive pacing, DC shock, and drugs (see Chapter 4).

Ecstasy

Ecstasy, 'E', and 'XTC' are street names for MDMA (methylenedioxy-metamphetamine). Ecstasy may be combined with LSD, ketamine, caffeine, or sildenafil ('sextasy'). Ketamine causes pain-free floating sensations with vivid dreams.

It produces a positive mood state, with feelings of increased sensuality and euphoria. Side effects with chronic use include anorexia, palpitations, jaw stiffness, grinding of teeth, sweating, and insomnia. It can cause dehydration with hyperthermia, agitation, and fits. Other features include hyponatraemia, cerebral infarction, cerebral haemorrhage, and vasculitis. Most deaths from ecstasy result from disturbance of thermo- and osmoregulation, leading to hyperthermia and increased plasma osmolality. MDMA also causes life-threatening cardiac dysrhythmias, abnormal liver function tests, acute liver failure and has been associated with cerebral infarction and haemorrhage.

Severe hyperthermia may occur within hours of ingestion and often follows intense physical activity. Features include core temperature >40°C, severe metabolic acidosis, muscle rigidity, disseminated intravascular coagulation (DIC), and rhabdomyolysis.

Management

Hyperthermia

Consider other causes of hyperthermia. Patients should be treated with dantrolene 1 mg/kg, up to a maximum of 10 mg/kg. Dantrolene inhibits release of calcium from the sarcoplasmic reticulum in cells. Rhabdomyolysis should be

treated in the usual way (see 'Acute kidney injury', Chapter 11).

Ethanol: acute intoxication

Patients may present with acute intoxication including withdrawal and/or nutritional deficiency syndromes, or with chronic toxicity (e.g. cirrhosis, neurological impairment, peripheral neuromyopathy, etc.).

Ethanol is rapidly absorbed from the GI tract. Adults absorb 80–90% of ingested alcohol within 1 hour and metabolize it at a rate of 7–15 g per hour (reducing blood concentrations by approximately 15–20 mg/dL per hour).

The fatal dose in adults is approximately 5–8 g/kg body weight (6–10 mL/kg absolute ethanol) and 3 g/kg body weight (4 mL/kg absolute ethanol) in children.

A blood concentration of 180 mg/dL would usually cause intoxication, and concentrations of 350 mg/dL are associated with stupor and coma. Concentrations of >450 mg/dL are often fatal.

Presentation

Alcohol intoxication results in disinhibition, euphoria, incoordination, ataxia, stupor, and coma. Chronic alcoholics require higher blood alcohol levels than 'social' drinkers for intoxication. Obtain a history from friends or relatives. Examine the patient for signs of chronic liver disease, trauma, or signs of infection.

- Mild—concentration <180 mg/dL. Impaired visual acuity, reaction time and coordination, and emotional lability.
- Moderate—concentrations 180–350 mg/dL. Slurred speech, diplopia, blurred vision, ataxia, incoordination, blackouts, sweating, tachycardia, nausea, vomiting, and incontinence. Alcoholic ketoacidosis or lactic acidosis, hypoglycaemia, and hypokalaemia may occur. Hypoglycaemia may be delayed up to 36 hours in previously fasted or malnourished individuals.
- Severe—concentrations 350–450 mg/dL. Cold clammy skin, hypothermia, hypotension, stupor, coma, dilated pupils, depressed or absent tendon reflexes. Severe hypoglycaemia, convulsions, respiratory depression, and metabolic acidosis may occur. Cardiac arrhythmias, such as atrial fibrillation and atrioventricular block, have been recorded.
- Potentially fatal—concentration >450 mg/dL. Deep coma, respiratory depression or arrest, and circulatory failure.

Other complications

- Acute gastritis causes nausea and vomiting, abdominal pain, and GI bleeding.
- Accidental injury, especially head injury (subdural).
- Rhabdomyolysis and acute renal failure.
- Infection (septicaemia, meningitis).

Management

- Mild to moderate intoxication usually requires no specific treatment; the need for admission for rehydration and observation depends on the individual patient. Admit all patients with stupor or coma.
- Check the airway is clear of vomit and the patient is able to protect their airway. Nurse the patient on their side in the recovery position. Ipecacuanha, gastric lavage, or charcoal are not indicated.
- Take blood for U&E, CPK, glucose, amylase and ethanol (and methanol) levels, arterial blood gas (acidosis), lactate, ammonia. Analyse urine (myoglobin). Consider the possibility of other drug overdoses.

- Monitor closely for respiratory depression, hypoxia, cardiac arrhythmias and hypotension, and withdrawal syndromes.
- Check blood glucose levels. In comatose patients, there is a good argument for giving 25–50 mL of 50% glucose immediately for presumed hypoglycaemia because this will usually not cause any harm. Follow with an IV infusion of 10% glucose, if necessary.
- The only concern is that glucose replacement/infusion may precipitate Wernicke's encephalopathy in malnourished individuals. Consequently some clinicians favour giving a bolus of thiamine 1–2 mg/kg IV and Pabrinex® (high-dose multivitamins) before glucose administration.
- Rehydrate with intravenous fluids, and monitor urine output.
- Naloxone reduces the effects of alcohol toxicity but is not standard.
- Rarely, haemodialysis is used if intoxication is very severe (ethanol >450 mg/dL) or if there is acidosis.
- Observe adults with features of moderate or severe toxicity for a minimum of 4 hours.
- After recovery from the acute episode, arrange for a psychiatric or medical assessment and follow-up. Consider referral to an alcohol rehabilitation programme, if appropriate. Treatment for alcohol withdrawal and delirium tremens (DTs) may be required following recovery.

Equivalents and conversions
- 1 mL of pure ethanol = 798 mg ethanol.
- 1 g ethanol = 21.7 mmol ethanol.
- 1 L of spirits at 40% proof = 400 mL alcohol = ~320 g ethanol.
- 1 bottle of wine (13% alcohol by volume) = ~90 g ethanol.
- 500 mL of beer (5% alcohol) = 25 g ethanol.

Ethylene glycol

Intake is usually 'accidental' when it is ingested as an ethanol 'substitute'. It is present in radiator 'antifreeze' and degreasing agents. Ethylene glycol (EG) is rapidly absorbed from the gut. Peak concentrations occur 1 to 4 hours after ingestion. The elimination half-life of ethylene glycol is approximately 3 hours but is prolonged to 17–18 hours, following inhibition of alcohol dehydrogenase. The fatal dose for a 70 kg adult is approximately 100 g of ethylene glycol (about 90 mL of pure ethylene glycol), but it may be fatal in doses as low as 30 g. Ethylene glycol is first metabolized to glycolaldehyde by the enzyme alcohol dehydrogenase, which then undergoes further oxidation to glycolic, glyoxylic, and oxalic acids which are responsible for the majority of its toxic effects. Glycolic acid is cleared by the kidney and is largely responsible for the marked acidosis seen in severe cases. Calcium oxalate monohydrate crystals are thought to be the cause of cerebral oedema and renal failure. This metabolic route is blocked by competitive antagonism with ethanol.

Early treatment with an antidote will prevent the production of toxic metabolites and prevent a rise in the anion gap. Delay in commencing treatment with an antidote will result in greater toxicity.

Presentation
Stages of ethylene glycol toxicity
Typically, after a brief period of inebriation due to the intoxicating effects of ethylene glycol itself, metabolic acidosis develops. This is followed by tachypnoea, coma, seizures, hypertension, the appearance of pulmonary infiltrates, and oliguric renal failure. Untreated, death from multiorgan failure occurs 24 to 36 hours after ingestion.

- Stage 1 (30 minutes to 12 hours after ingestion). The patient appears intoxicated with alcohol (but no ethanol on breath) and there may be accompanying nausea and vomiting (± haematemesis), coma, and convulsions (often focal). Nystagmus, ataxia, ophthalmoplegia, papilloedema, hypotonia, hyporeflexia, myoclonic jerks, tetanic contractions, and cranial nerve palsies may occur. Metabolic acidosis develops.
- Stage 2 (12–24 hours after ingestion). This is associated with increased respiratory rate, sinus tachycardia, hypertension, pulmonary oedema, and congestive cardiac failure.
- Stage 3 (24–72 hours after ingestion). Includes the development of flank pain, renal tenderness, acute tubular necrosis, hypocalcaemia (as a consequence of calcium complexing with oxalate), calcium oxalate monohydrate crystalluria, hyperkalaemia, and hypomagnesaemia.

Prognostic features
- It is often taken with ethanol which is actually protective by blocking the metabolism of glycol to toxic metabolites.
- Renal failure can be averted if specific treatment is started early.
- Plasma levels of ethylene glycol >500 mg/L (8 mmol/L) indicate severe overdose.
- The degree of acidosis is the best indicator of likely outcome.

Complications
- Oliguric renal failure (crystal nephropathy).
- Cerebral oedema.
- Hypotension.
- Non-cardiogenic pulmonary oedema.
- Myocarditis.

Management
Delay in commencing treatment with an antidote will result in a more severely poisoned patient.

Perform gastric lavage if the patient presents within 1 hour of ingestion. This will also enable confirmation that EG has been taken as commercial 'antifreeze' often contains fluoroscein which is easily detected with a UV light source (also detectable in urine).

Establish IV access, and take blood for U&E, glucose, biochemical profile, including serum Ca^{2+} levels, plasma osmolality, and ethanol and EG levels.

Check arterial blood gases to assess the degree of acidaemia. Calculate the anion and osmolar gap. Patients will develop a high osmolar gap, as they absorb the glycol over the first few hours. Thereafter, as the glycol is metabolized to acids, the osmolar gap will fall while the patient's anion gap increases and the acidosis worsens.

A high anion gap metabolic acidosis suggests that the presentation is late and that a substantial amount of ethylene glycol has been metabolized. The high anion gap usually occurs, as the serum bicarbonate falls with progressive development of metabolic acidosis.

A high anion gap metabolic acidosis is not specific to ethylene glycol ingestion and can occur with toxic alcohol ingestion (e.g. methanol, isopropanol) or with other clinical conditions (e.g. diabetic or alcoholic ketoacidosis, renal failure, multiorgan failure).

Microscope a fresh urine sample. Needle-shaped crystals of calcium oxalate monohydrate are pathognomonic.

Fomepizole is an inhibitor of alcohol dehydrogenase (see below), and, unlike ethanol, it does not cause CNS depression. It is expensive but easier to use than ethanol. It is given as a loading dose of 15 mg/kg in 100 mL saline over 30 minutes, followed by 12-hourly maintenance doses. Increase the frequency of maintenance doses if haemodialysis is needed.

The half-life of EG is short (3 hours). If fomepizole is unavailable, then an ethanol infusion should be started as soon as possible (see below). The infusion should be continued until plasma EG is undetectable. Infusion of ethanol will cause intoxication.

Indications for dialysis

Severe acidosis (declining vital signs, an ethylene glycol level >500 mg/L) or oliguria requires haemodialysis. Normal renal function is generally restored in 7–10 days, although chronic renal failure may follow. Haemodiafiltration is less effective than dialysis, but high-flow haemodiafiltration should be considered if haemodialysis is unavailable.

Using fomepizole

Fomepizole is a competitive inhibitor of alcohol dehydrogenase which prevents metabolism of EG to glycolaldehyde (see above) and is licensed for use in ethylene glycol poisoning. There is emerging evidence of its benefit in the management of methanol poisoning.

Fomepizole is preferred to ethanol as an antidote in the following situations:

1. Patients with depressed conscious level.
2. Patients taking disulfiram or metronidazole.
3. Liver disease.
4. Inability of local laboratory to measure ethanol concentrations out of hours.
5. Lack of a facility to monitor the patient closely, such as an intensive care or high dependency unit.

Fomepizole is supplied in ampoules of 5 mg/mL. If solid, the solution should be liquefied by running the vial under warm water. Aseptically draw the appropriate dose from the vial with a syringe, and inject into at least 100 mL of sterile sodium chloride injection or 5% glucose injection. Mix well.

Adult dose

All doses should be administered as a slow intravenous infusion for 30 minutes. The loading dose is 15 mg/kg IV, diluted in 100 mL saline or glucose, and given over 30 minutes.

This is followed by a maintenance dose of 10 mg/kg IV in 100 mL saline or glucose given over 30 minutes every 12 hours (starting at 12 hours after the loading dose is given) for a maximum of four doses. Liaise with the appropriate National Poisons Centre (e.g. UK National Poisons Information Service or US National Capital Poisons Center), as it is sometimes necessary to continue with longer and larger doses.

Using ethanol as an antidote

Ethanol should be used with caution in the following circumstances:

1. Patients with depressed conscious level.
2. Co-ingestion of other drugs that may cause CNS depression (e.g. opioids, sedatives, antidepressants, anticonvulsants, antihistamines, hypnotics, muscle relaxants).
3. Patients taking disulfiram or metronidazole—may cause hypotension and flushing (in such patients, fomepizole may be a better choice).
4. Pregnancy—the use of alcohol in the first trimester is controversial.

Give an oral loading dose equivalent to 800 mg/kg absolute (100%) ethanol. This can be given in the form of whisky, gin, or vodka (40% ethanol) in a dose of 2.5 mL/kg body weight (about 175 mL spirits for a 70 kg adult). Note: if using gin, check the ethanol concentration, as this may be less than 40% v/v.

Ethanol infusion is an alternative to fomepizole. Give IV as a 10% solution in 5% glucose or normal saline (i.e. take 50 mL normal saline from a 500 mL bag, and replace with 50 mL absolute ethanol). A loading dose of 10 mL/kg of the 10% solution should be given, followed by an IV infusion of 1–1.5 mL/kg/h for non-drinkers (regular drinkers 2 mL/kg/h). Titrate to a plasma ethanol level of 1–1.5 g/L (21.7–32.6 mmol/L). Continue the ethanol IV infusion until the acidosis or systemic toxicity resolves.

How long should you continue fomepizole or ethanol?

Once initiated, an antidote should be continued until the plasma ethylene glycol concentration is <50 mg/L (0.05 g/L; 0.8 mmol/L).

Treatment with either fomepizole or ethanol decreases the rate at which ethylene glycol is metabolized. Treatment may be required for several days whilst ethylene glycol is eliminated from the body. Intensive monitoring may be required during this period, particularly for patients treated with ethanol. The decision to discontinue an antidote should be guided by measurement of the ethylene glycol concentration.

Flunitrazepam

Flunitrazepam (Rohypnol®) is sometimes referred to as the 'date rape' drug. It is used as a short-term treatment for insomnia, as a sedative hypnotic, and a pre-anaesthetic. It has similar effects to diazepam but is 710 times more potent. For guidance, see the section on diazepam.

Flunitrazepam intoxication impairs judgement and motor skills and can make a victim unable to resist a sexual attack. It also causes retrograde amnesia. The combination of alcohol and flunitrazepam has a more marked effect than flunitrazepam alone. Effects begin within 30 minutes, peak by 2 hours, and can persist for up to 8 hours. It is commonly reported that individuals intoxicated on a combination of alcohol and flunitrazepam have 'blackouts', lasting 8–24 hours following ingestion. Adverse effects of flunitrazepam include decreased blood pressure, memory impairment, drowsiness, visual disturbances, confusion, dizziness, gastrointestinal disturbances, and urinary retention. Manage as for benzodiazepine overdose.

Gamma hydroxybutyric acid (GHB) or liquid ecstasy

This drug is dissolved in water and consumed until a high is reached. GHB acts as an agonist at GABA receptors in the brain, leading to drowsiness, seizures, hypoventilation, and unconsciousness. It acts synergistically with ethanol, leading to CNS and respiratory depression. GBL (gamma-butyrolactone) and 1,4-butanediol (1,4-BD) are precursor molecules of gamma hydroxybutyrate (GHB) and, once ingested, are rapidly metabolized in the body by peripheral lactonases and alcohol and aldehyde dehydrogenase to form GHB. Absorption is rapid. The onset of effects occurs within 15–60 minutes after ingestion. They usually resolve spontaneously within 24 hours. The maximum reported duration is 96 hours. Features in mild/moderate toxicity include nausea, vomiting, diarrhoea, drowsiness, headache, ataxia, dizziness, confusion, amnesia, urinary incontinence, tremor, myoclonus, hypotonia, agitation, euphoria, and hypothermia.

In severe cases, there may be coma, convulsions, bradycardia, and other ECG abnormalities, such as U waves, hypotension, Cheyne–Stokes respiration, and respiratory depression leading to respiratory arrest.

The effects are potentiated by ethanol, benzodiazepines, antipsychotics, and other CNS depressants.

Ibuprofen

Ibuprofen is a non-steroidal anti-inflammatory analgesic (NSAID), which has relatively low toxicity.

In adults, those who have ingested less than 100 mg/kg are unlikely to require treatment. The half-life in overdose is 1.5–3 hours.

Most patients who have ingested clinically important amounts of NSAIDs will develop no more than nausea, vomiting, epigastric pain, or, more rarely, diarrhoea. Tinnitus, headache, and gastrointestinal bleeding are also possible.

In more serious poisoning, toxicity is seen in the central nervous system, with drowsiness, excitation, and disorientation or coma. Occasionally, patients develop convulsions. Metabolic problems in serious poisoning may include acidosis and an increase in INR, probably due to interference with the actions of clotting factors in the circulation. Acute renal failure and liver injury may occur but are rare. Exacerbation of asthma is a possible side effect in asthmatics.

Management

Consider activated charcoal (50 g for adults) if the patient presents within 1 hour of ingestion of a potentially toxic amount.

Observe patients for at least 4 hours after ingestion of potentially toxic amounts or 8 hours after sustained-release preparations. Ensure adequate hydration.

Single, brief convulsions do not require treatment. If frequent or prolonged, control with intravenous diazepam or lorazepam (4 mg in an adult). Give oxygen, and correct acid-base and metabolic disturbances, as required. Phenytoin (loading dose 15 mg/kg IV infusion in adults) may be useful if convulsions are unresponsive to the above measures. Give slowly (over 20–30 minutes), with BP and ECG monitoring.

Iron

Accidental ingestion is almost exclusively a problem in children. In overdose, iron-binding mechanisms are rapidly saturated, leading to high concentrations of free iron. The latter catalyses the widespread generation of free radicals which is the basis of the toxic manifestations of iron overdose. Ingestion of 20 mg/kg elemental iron is potentially toxic, and 200–250 mg/kg elemental iron is potentially fatal.

Presentation

- Iron is extremely irritant and causes prominent abdominal pain, vomiting and diarrhoea, haematemesis, and rectal bleeding.
- Usually, the initial GI symptoms subside before secondary signs develop 12–24 hours after ingestion. Hepatic failure, jaundice, fits, and coma may occur.
- Very large overdose can cause early cardiovascular collapse and coma.
- In children, 1–2 g of iron may prove fatal. Patients alive 72 hours after ingestion usually make a full recovery.
- Late sequelae of gastric fibrosis and pyloric obstruction have been occasionally reported.

Management

- Gastric lavage should be considered, following ingestion of more than 60 mg/kg elemental iron within 1 hour, provided the airway can be protected. A plain abdominal

x-ray (AXR) may be useful within 2 hours of ingestion to assess the number of tablets ingested.
- Establish IV access. Take blood for U&E, LFTs, FBC, serum iron levels and transferrin saturation.
- Take blood for urgent measurement of the serum iron concentration, preferably at 4 hours after ingestion, but do not wait for the results before administering chelation therapy. After 6 hours, the peak level will have passed, and interpretation is more difficult. The use of desferrioxamine will prevent interpretation of subsequent iron concentrations. Do not delay therapy for repeat measurements in symptomatic patients. If the serum iron concentration is between 55 and 90 micromoles/L, repeat after 2 hours.
- Parenteral chelation therapy is indicated if the serum iron concentration is >90 micromoles/L (5 mg/L), or in shocked patients.
- Give desferrioxamine IV at a rate of 15 mg/kg/h for a maximum daily dose of 80 mg/kg (i.e ~5 hours infusion) (although, if the patient tolerates it and it is indicated by the serum iron concentration, higher doses may be given). The IV infusion is continued until the serum iron level falls below the total iron-binding capacity (TIBC).
- Dialysis. Haemodialysis is indicated for very high serum iron levels that respond poorly to chelation therapy or if the urine output is not maintained during chelation therapy, as the iron chelate is only excreted in the urine.
- Exchange transfusion has also been used successfully for very severe intoxication.
- Managing iron overdose is complex, and we recommend that all physicians contact their national poisons centre (e.g. the National Poisons Information Service, UK or the National Capital Poisons Center, USA).

Lithium

A single acute overdose usually carries low risk, and patients tend to show mild symptoms only, irrespective of their serum lithium concentration. However, more severe symptoms may occur after a delay if lithium elimination is reduced because of renal impairment. With sustained-release tablets, absorption is variable, peak plasma concentrations occuring after 4–5 hours. Half-life ranges from 8 to 45 hours (mean 24 hours); this may be prolonged in overdose.

If an acute overdose has been taken by a patient on chronic lithium therapy, this can lead to serious toxicity, occurring even after a modest overdose, as the extravascular tissues are already saturated with lithium.

Lithium (Li^+) has a low therapeutic index, and accidental toxicity can, and does occur, much more frequently than deliberate self-administration. Toxicity is commonly precipitated by administration of diuretics, NSAIDs, or intercurrent dehydration, e.g. following vomiting or a febrile illness.

Presentation

Mild toxicity

Thirst, polyuria, diarrhoea, nausea, vomiting, and fine resting or coarse tremor are common. Blurred vision, light-headedness, muscular weakness, and drowsiness may also occur.

Moderate toxicity

Increasing confusion, blackouts, fasciculation, and increased deep tendon reflexes. Myoclonic twitches and jerks, choreoathetoid movements, urinary or faecal incontinence, hypernatraemia, and increasing restlessness followed by stupor.

Severe toxicity

Coma, convulsions, cardiac dysrhythmias, including sino-atrial nodal block, cerebellar signs, sinus and junctional bradycardia, and first-degree heart block. Hypotension, or rarely hypertension, peripheral vascular collapse, and renal failure.

Prognostic features

Features of toxicity are usually associated with Li^+ levels of >1.5 mmol/L. However, Li^+ enters cells relatively slowly so that the levels taken shortly after a large overdose may be very high, with the patient showing few, if any, signs of toxicity. Levels >4 mmol/L will probably require haemo- or peritoneal dialysis. Patients who are lithium-naive may tolerate higher levels, following an overdose.

Risk factors

The risk of toxicity is greater in those with coexisting hypertension, diabetes, congestive heart failure, chronic renal failure, schizophrenia, and Addison's disease.

Management

- Patients presenting within 1 hour of ingestion of a large overdose should undergo gastric lavage. Many slow/sustained release preparations are too large to pass up the lavage tube. If slow-release preparations are involved, whole bowel irrigation with PEG is useful. (Note: activated charcoal does not adsorb lithium).
- Check serum Li^+ level (ensure the tube used does not contain lithium-heparin anticoagulant), and repeat 6-hourly.
- Check U&E. If serum sodium is elevated, check serum osmolality.
- Stop any diuretic (especially thiazides) or other drug likely to alter renal handling of Li^+ (e.g. NSAIDs).
- Correct any fluid or electrolyte deficits, and ensure adequate hydration. Forced diuresis should not be undertaken.
- Patients on chronic lithium therapy with levels >4 mmol/L or who have neurological features should be treated with haemodialysis. Although Li^+ can be effectively cleared from the extracellular compartment with dialysis, movement out of cells is much slower. Dialysis should be continued until Li^+ is not detected in the serum or dialysate. Levels should be measured daily for the next week in case Li^+ rebounds due to slow release from intracellular stores.
- All patients should be observed for a minimum of 24 hours.
- Repeat measurements of lithium concentration are helpful in timing the re-institution of chronic therapy, following an episode of toxicity. The usual target range is approximately 0.4–1.0 mmol/L 12 hours post-dose.

Methanol

Poisoning usually follows ingestion of contaminated alcohol beverages or 'methylated spirits'. Toxicity can occur through ingestion, inhalation, and skin absorption. Ingestion of 10 mL of pure methanol has resulted in blindness; 30 mL has resulted in death. Intoxication in industrial settings follows absorption across the skin or lung. Methanol is slowly metabolized by alcohol dehydrogenase to formaldehyde. This is oxidized to toxic formic acid in the liver and follows zero order kinetics. Approximately 3% of a methanol dose is excreted through the lungs or excreted unchanged in the urine. The half-life of methanol is prolonged to 30–50 hours during antidote therapy. Methanol is an alcohol and will cause the features of intoxication. Its main toxicity is secondary to its metabolic products, formaldehyde and formic acid, which are responsible for the most serious effects, including metabolic acidosis and blindness.

Ocular toxicity results from formic acid accumulation and is made worse by acidosis.

Absorption of methanol is rapid, but the onset of metabolic toxic features may be delayed for several hours, particularly if co-ingested with ethanol which competitively delays methanol metabolism.

The mainstay of early treatment is the inhibition of methanol metabolism through administration of an antidote, such as ethanol or fomepizole. Early treatment with an antidote minimizes the production of high concentrations of toxic metabolites.

Presentation

Ataxia, drowsiness, dysarthria, and nystagmus may occur within 30 minutes of methanol ingestion, followed by a latent period of 12–24 hours, before metabolic toxicity becomes apparent.

Severe, but reversible cardiac failure, and ECG abnormalities have been described.

- Significant ingestion causes nausea, vomiting, and abdominal pain.
- Its effects on the CNS resemble those of ethanol, although, in low doses, it does not have a euphoric effect.
- Visual symptoms present with falling visual acuity, photophobia, and the sensation of 'being in a snow storm'.

Central nervous system

Headache, confusion, and vertigo occur with mild to moderate methanol toxicity. Convulsions and coma are seen in severe toxicity.

Extrapyramidal features may develop in patients who survive severe toxicity. This is due to necrosis in the putamen and subcortical white matter, which can often be shown by an MRI scan.

Visual

Common features include blurred vision, with the appearance of a 'snow field', and photophobia. Optic disc and retinal oedema occur with diminished pupillary light response. The extent of these features appears to correlate with the severity of toxicity.

Patients may be left with persistent visual impairment, including optic atrophy, diminished visual acuity, loss of colour vision, central scotoma, or blindness. Blindness is usually permanent, but, in some cases, a degree of recovery may occur over a period of months.

Gastrointestinal

Common features include nausea, vomiting, and abdominal pain. Acute pancreatitis can occur, and a small, transient rise in liver transaminases may be seen.

Metabolic

A severe metabolic acidosis, with an increased anion and osmolar gap, is usually seen. Tachypnoea is common. Hyperglycaemia may occur. Renal failure may develop in severe cases.

Complications

- Up to 65% of patients have a raised amylase, but this does not necessarily represent pancreatitis (usually salivary gland amylase). If pancreatitis is suspected clinically, measure serum lipase (haemorrhagic pancreatitis has been reported at post-mortem).

- Seizures are seen in severe intoxication. CT scanning usually shows cerebral oedema or even necrosis in the basal ganglia.
- Patients with visual symptoms may develop irreversible visual impairment, even with aggressive intervention.
- Rhabdomyolysis and acute renal failure.
- Hypoglycaemia.

Prognostic features

- 10 mL of methanol can cause blindness, and 30 mL can be fatal.
- Peak plasma methanol measurement is useful; >0.2 g/L (6.25 mmol/L) indicates significant ingestion, and 0.5 g/L (15.6 mmol/L) is severe.
- Arterial pH correlates with formate levels; a pH <7.2 indicates severe intoxication.
- Poor prognostic features include convulsions, coma, shock, persistent acidosis, bradycardia, and kidney failure.

Management

- Early treatment with an antidote will minimize the production of toxic metabolites which cause metabolic acidosis and blindness. For patients with methanol intoxication, early administration of fomepizole or ethanol will minimize the metabolism of methanol and the development of these clinical and metabolic complications. Take blood for U&E, CPK, glucose, amylase and ethanol/methanol levels, plasma osmolality, and arterial blood gases to assess acidosis. Calculate the anion and osmolar gap. Check urine for myoglobin; see 'Acute Renal Failure' Chapter 11.
- Seizures should be treated initially with diazepam (5–10 mg IV) and subsequently with phenytoin (250 mg IV over 5 minutes). Exclude hypoglycaemia.
- Antidote therapy with fomepizole should be given to all patients with methanol levels >0.2 g/L (6.25 mmol/L), patients with a high osmolar gap (>10 mOsm/kg H$_2$O) or metabolic acidosis (pH <7.3). *Fomepizole* is an inhibitor of alcohol dehydrogenase and has the advantage that, unlike ethanol, it does not cause CNS depression. It is easier to use than ethanol. It is given as a loading dose of 15 mg/kg in 100 mL saline over 30 minutes, followed by 12-hourly maintenance doses of 10 mg/kg (see section on ethylene glycol). *Ethanol infusion* is an alternative to fomepizole. Give IV as a 10% solution in 5% glucose or normal saline (i.e. take 50 mL normal saline from a 500 mL bag, and replace with 50 mL absolute ethanol). A loading dose of 7.5 mL/kg of the 10% solution should be given, followed by an IV infusion of 1 mL/kg/h for non-drinkers (regular drinkers 2 mL/kg/h). Titrate to a plasma ethanol level of 1–1.5 g/L (21.7–32.6 mmol/L). Continue the ethanol IV infusion until the acidosis or systemic toxicity resolves or the methanol level is undetectable.
- Metabolic acidosis should be corrected with IV sodium bicarbonate.
- Haemodialysis is reserved for those patients with renal failure, any visual impairment, CNS toxicity, metabolic acidosis not responsive to sodium bicarbonate, or a plasma methanol level of >0.5 g/L (15.6 mmol/L). The ethanol infusion rate should be doubled during dialysis.

Isopropanol

Isopropanol is present in car screenwash. As a cause of poisoning with alcohols, this is second after ethanol.

Presentation

Clinical features include:

- Gastrointestinal: burning sensation in the mouth and throat, nausea, vomiting, dysarthria, acetone on the breath, abdominal pain, gastritis, haematemesis, and melaena.
- CNS: ataxia, headache, dizziness, drowsiness, stupor, hallucinations, areflexia, and muscle weakness. In severe poisoning, CNS and respiratory depression may occur, leading to deep coma, cyanosis, and convulsions.
- Cardiovascular: initially tachycardia. In severe cases, myocardial depression may develop, leading to bradycardia, hypotension, and dysrhythmias.
- Other complications may include hypoglycaemia or hyperglycaemia, red blood cell haemolysis, ketonuria, renal tubular acidosis, hepatic dysfunction, rhabdomyolysis, and bronchopneumonia.
- Skin contact may cause paraesthesiae and erythema. Prolonged skin contact or inhalation may also result in systemic features. Accidental inhalation may cause mild irritation to the eyes, nose, and throat but would be unlikely to cause systemic effects.
- A high serum or urinary acetone concentration, without metabolic acidosis, is strongly suggestive of isopropyl alcohol poisoning.

Isopropanol has twice the potency of ethanol on the CNS (its major metabolite is acetone), and isopropanol-induced coma can last >24 hours. Effects are seen within 30–60 minutes of ingestion, and large overdoses cause coma and hypotension as the major effect. Haemodialysis is indicated if the hypotension fails to respond to IV fluids, vital signs decline, or blood levels are >4 g/L (66.7 mmol/L). Monitor for hypoglycaemia and myoglobinuria.

Olanzapine

See section on antipsychotic drugs.

Opiates

Overdosing with opiates usually occurs in regular drug users where the most commonly abused agent is diamorphine (heroin). It may be taken intravenously, by skin-popping, smoked, or snorted. A number of other opiates have been similarly abused. Opiates, such as dextropropoxyphene and dihydrocodeine (present in combination formulations with paracetamol), are often taken with alcohol by non-addicts with suicidal intent.

Presentation

Pinpoint pupils, severe respiratory depression ± cyanosis, and coma are typical. The depressive effects are exacerbated by alcohol. BP may be low but is often surprisingly well maintained. Although some opiates, e.g. dextropropoxyphene and pethidine, increase muscle tone and cause fits in overdose, in general, opiates cause marked hypotonia.

Prognostic features

- Non-cardiogenic pulmonary oedema carries a poor prognosis.
- Patients with underlying ischaemic heart disease may be more susceptible to haemodynamic disturbance after naloxone is given.
- Renal impairment reduces the elimination of many opiates and prolongs their duration of action.

Management

- Monitor respiratory rate, depth of respiration, and pulse oximetry. Give oxygen by mask. Monitor ECG continuously for arrhythmias.
- Establish IV access; take blood for U&E and CPK. If paracetamol and opiate combinations have been ingested, measure paracetamol level (see later in this chapter).
- Any patient who is comatose or has respiratory signs requires a chest x-ray (CXR) (for signs of infection, septic emboli, and interstitial shadowing).
- The specific antidote is naloxone (a pure opiate antagonist) which should be given IV in boluses of 0.4 mg at 2–3 minute intervals until the patient is rousable and any evidence of respiratory depression corrected. Doses of up to 2 mg (and above) may be required, but, if no response is seen at this level, then the diagnosis of opiate overdose should be revised.
- The duration of action of naloxone is shorter than many opiates, hence an infusion should be started to avoid re-sedation (starting with two-thirds of the dose required to initially rouse the patient per hour and adjusted, as necessary). In the case of overdose with long-acting opiates, such as methadone, infusion of naloxone may be necessary for 48–72 hours.
- Avoid giving sufficient naloxone to completely reverse the effect of opiates in an opiate-dependent subject. This is likely to precipitate an acute withdrawal reaction. If this occurs and hypertension is marked (diastolic >120 mmHg), then give diazepam (5–10 mg initially IV), and, if it persists, commence IV GTN (1–2 mg/h, titrating until the BP is controlled). Note that marked hypertension, acute pulmonary oedema, and VT/VF have been observed in non-addicts given naloxone to reverse the effects of high therapeutic doses of opiates for pain.
- Convulsions which are opiate-induced (usually pethidine or dextropropoxyphene) may respond to IV naloxone. Additional anticonvulsant therapy may be required.
- Pulmonary oedema, present on admission, requires oxygen, CPAP, or mechanical ventilation (see 'Respiratory practical procedures' Chapter 19). It does not respond to naloxone.
- For rhabdomyolysis and acute renal failure, see Chapter 11.

Complications

- All opiates can cause non-cardiogenic pulmonary oedema, although it is most frequently seen with IV heroin.
- Rhabdomyolysis is common in opiate-induced coma and should be looked for in all cases.
- The substances used to dilute ('cut') illicit opiates may also carry significant toxicity when injected (e.g. talc and quinine).
- IV drug users may develop right-sided endocarditis and septic pulmonary emboli (seen as localized infiltrates on CXR).
- Ingestion of paracetamol-containing preparations (e.g. co-dydramol) may cause renal or hepatic failure.

Important points

1. Dextropropoxyphene, in combination with alcohol, can cause marked CNS depression. Respiratory arrest can evolve rapidly within <30 minutes of ingestion. Give naloxone, even if the patient is only mildly drowsy. Dextropropoxyphene also causes an acute cardiotoxicity due to its blockade of cardiac membrane sodium channels, with arrhythmias, decreased contractility and conduction due to the resulting membrane-stabilizing effects, and toxicity similar to that seen with Class 1c antiarrhythmics (naloxone ineffective).
2. The respiratory depressant effects of buprenorphine are not fully reversed by naloxone. Doxapram has been used in milder cases of buprenorphine overdose as a respiratory stimulant (1–4 mg/min), but mechanical ventilation is preferable in severe cases.

Paracetamol

Assessment

In therapeutic doses, only a minor fraction is oxidized to the reactive/toxic species, N-acetyl-p-benzoquinone imine (NABQI), which is detoxified by conjugation with glutathione. In overdose, normal metabolic routes become saturated; therefore, an increased fraction is metabolized via the cytochrome p450 system to toxic metabolites, which are detoxified by hepatic glutathione which becomes depleted in severe overdose.

Presentation following overdose

- Apart from mild nausea, vomiting, and anorexia, patients presenting within 24 hours of ingestion of a paracetamol overdose are generally asymptomatic.
- Hepatic necrosis becomes apparent in 24–36 hours, with right subchondral pain/tenderness, jaundice (and acute liver failure), vomiting, and symptoms of neuroglycopenia (confusion).
- Encephalopathy may worsen over the next 72 hours.
- Oliguria and renal failure.
- Lactic acidosis: either <12 hours (very rare) or late (10% of patients with ALF).

Complications

- Acute liver failure (ALF, see 'Acute Liver Failure' Chapter 8), with hypoglycaemia, cerebral oedema, and GI bleeding.
- Severe metabolic (lactic) acidosis.
- Pancreatitis (alone or with liver failure).
- Some 10% of patients develop acute kidney injury (AKI) from acute tubular necrosis in the absence of liver failure.
- Very rarely, patients with G6PD deficiency develop methaemoglobinaemia and haemolysis.

Investigations

- Paracetamol levels that are detectable 24 hours after overdose indicate a severe overdose or a staggered overdose.
- Measure levels at least 4 hours post-ingestion, and plot on the graph, as shown in Figure 9.1. If the time of overdose is not known, measure paracetamol 4 hours later, but commence acetylcysteine if in doubt.
- Biochemistry (U&E): AKI may be the predominant abnormality and is obvious by day 3.
- Glucose: this may fall with progressive liver failure. Give IV dextrose (25–50 mL of 50% dextrose), if necessary.
- FBC: thrombocytopenia may be severe.
- Liver function tests (LFTs): transaminases may rise by 24 hours.
- Prothrombin time (PT): is the best indicator of the severity of liver injury. It may be normal with high transaminases.

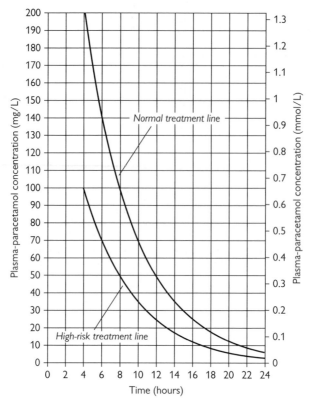

Figure 9.1 Determining the treatment for paracetamol overdoses This Crown copyright material is reproduced by permission of the Medicines and Healthcare products Regulatory Agency (MHRA) under delegated authority from the Controller of HMSO. Available at: <http://www.mhra.gov.uk/home/groups/pl-p/documents/drugsafetymessage/con184396.pdf>. Accessed 30th September 2013.

• ABGs: to assess whether there is a severe metabolic acidosis (poor prognosis).

Risk factors

1. Poor nutrition: if the patient is malnourished, has nutritional deficiency and/or a chronic debilitating illness and is, therefore, likely to be glutathione-deplete, e.g. acute or chronic starvation (patients not eating for a few days, e.g. due to recent febrile illness in children, or dental pain in adults), eating disorders (anorexia or bulimia), children with 'failure to thrive', cystic fibrosis, AIDS, cachexia, alcoholism, and hepatitis C.
2. Hepatic enzyme-inducing drugs or evidence of ongoing liver injury, e.g. the patient is on long-term treatment with drugs, such as carbamazepine, phenobarbital, phenytoin, primidone, rifampicin, rifabutin, efavirenz, nevirapine, St John's wort, or other drugs that induce liver enzymes. Regular consumption of ethanol in excess of recommended amounts. Fatal overdose may occur with <10 g (usually in alcoholics, epileptics, or patients on enzyme-inducing drugs). The cause of death is usually acute liver failure. Chronic alcoholics or patients on hepatic enzyme-inducing drugs are more susceptible to developing hepatotoxicity and nephrotoxicity.

Prognostic features

If the patient has ingested less than 150 mg/kg paracetamol (i.e. 10–12 g total) and has no risk factors, it is unlikely that serious toxicity will occur. If the patient has risk factors (as described previously), consider treatment following a lower ingested dose (75 mg/kg).

All patients with acidosis (pH <7.32) and coagulopathy (INR >1.5) should be discussed with a liver unit.

If a patient develops a further elevation of PT on day 4, then they have a >90% chance of dying with conservative management. In one study of 150 patients with acute liver failure due to paracetamol overdose, the overall mortality was ~50%; 92% of 37 patients with a peak prothrombin time of ≥180 seconds died, with 50% mortality in those with a PT of 130–179 seconds. Patients with a continuing rise in prothrombin time (n = 42/150) between days 3 and 4 after overdose had a poor prognosis (93% died), compared with 21 of the 96 (22%), in whom the prothrombin time fell.

Management

• Give activated charcoal 50 g to patients presenting within 1 hour of ingestion.
• Acetylcysteine should be given to all patients who present with a paracetamol overdose irrespective of the plasma paracetamol level in circumstances where the

Table 9.3 Specific treatment for paracetamol poisoning

Acetylcysteine infusion
- 150 mg/kg in 200 mL 5% glucose over 60 minutes, followed by
- 50 mg/kg in 500 mL 5% glucose over 4 hours, and finally
- 100 mg/kg in 1 L 5% glucose over 16 hours.
- Up to 10% of patients have a rash, bronchospasm, or hypotension during the infusion. Stop the IV infusion and give chlorphenamine (10 mg IV), and restart later when symptoms have settled.

Oral methionine
- Only use if patient is truly allergic to acetylcysteine. Give 2.5 g stat and three further doses of 2.5 g every 4 hours.

overdose is staggered or there is doubt over the time of paracetamol ingestion; or
- Paracetamol overdose with a timed plasma paracetamol concentration on or above a single treatment line joining points of 100 mg/L at 4 hours and 15 mg/L at 15 hours on the nomogram (see Figure 9.1), regardless of the risk factors of hepatotoxicity.
- All patients with a large overdose of paracetamol (>10 g) who present 8–24 hours after ingestion should be treated with acetylcysteine until levels are available (see Figure 9.1).
- Mild reactions to acetylcysteine occur in 10–15% of patients but can be effectively treated with an antihistamine. Acetylcysteine can be restarted at a slower rate once the reaction subsides. True allergic reactions are extremely rare.
- Measure paracetamol levels at least 4 hours post-ingestion and ideally 4 hours later, and plot on the nomogram (see Figure 9.1).
- All patients on or above the treatment line (and presenting up to 24 hours after ingestion) should be given acetylcysteine (see Table 9.3). Hypersensitivity to acetylcysteine infusion as evidenced by vasodilatation and mild bronchospasm is no longer considered a contraindication to treatment with acetylcysteine.
- Patients on enzyme-inducing drugs (e.g. phenytoin, carbamazepine, rifampicin, St John's wort), as described previously, or with a history of high alcohol intake or low glutathione stores (anorexics, cachexia, AIDS) may develop toxicity at lower plasma concentrations.
- If the initial levels indicate no treatment is necessary, repeat the paracetamol levels 4 hours later. If there is uncertainty about the timing of ingestion, or if other drugs delay gastric emptying, or slow-release preparations have been taken, give acetylcysteine.
- Give acetylcysteine to all severe overdoses (>10 g) that present within 72 hours with symptoms or deranged LFTs and PT.
- There are few data on the length of time for which acetylcysteine should be administered. If the patient has evidence of liver injury or a detectable plasma paracetamol concentration >24 hours after ingestion, continue administration of acetylcysteine. Blood tests should initially be monitored approximately 8-12-hourly to assess progression of liver injury and the need for referral to a liver unit. All patients should receive a full course of acetylcysteine. The best prognostic parameters are the INR and plasma creatinine, but transaminase (ALT or AST) rise is the most sensitive marker of liver injury. acetylcysteine may be discontinued if the patient is not considered to be at risk of liver damage; the INR, plasma creatinine, and

Box 9.1 Indication for liver transplantation in paracetamol overdose

- Late acidosis (>36 hours post-overdose) with arterial pH <7.3.
- PT >100 s.
- Serum creatinine >300 micromoles/L.
- Grade 3 encephalopathy (confused, distressed, barely rousable).

transaminase are normal; and the patient is asymptomatic. Such patients do not normally need to be followed up or have repeat blood samples checked.
- Monitor U&E, FBC, PT, LFTs, glucose, and arterial blood gases daily. Monitor glucose with BM stix at least 6-hourly.
- Give vitamin K IV 10 mg (as a single dose, in case body stores are deficient), but avoid giving FFP, unless there is active bleeding. The PT is the best indicator of the severity of liver failure and FFP may only make management decisions (e.g. liver transplantation) more difficult. Patients with encephalopathy or with a rapidly rising PT should be referred to a liver unit.
- If AKI occurs in isolation (no coagulopathy but transaminase levels high), then refer to a renal unit.
- Management of acute liver failure, see 'Acute Liver Failure' Chapter 8. Box 9.1 lists the indications for liver transplantation.
- All patients should be assessed, following recovery, for risk of further self-harm by a psychiatrist or specialist.

Practice point
Patients with paracetamol OD often develop subconjunctival haematoma due to vomiting, coagulopathy, and thrombocytopenia.

Paraquat

Paraquat or weed killer is sold as granules (Weedol®) to the general public. These products contain an emetic, and vomiting is usual following ingestion. Local symptoms in the mouth and stomach are common. In addition, most patients develop diarrhoea. Paraquat concentrate (which is not on sale to the general public) is a more readily toxic form of paraquat. Ingestion of small quantities of paraquat concentrate (<15 mL) can cause a burning sensation in the mouth, throat, and chest. Buccal burns appear (paraquat solutions are strongly alkaline), with dysphagia, dysphonia, and difficulty in clearing saliva and bronchial secretions. Oesophageal perforation and mediastinitis have been reported. Buccal burns are also seen after paraquat concentrate is taken into the mouth and then spat out. A rise in serum creatinine usually occurs within 36 hours and indicates paraquat-induced kidney injury. Hepatocellular jaundice may also occur. A pneumonitis develops within a few days, leading to the development of progressive pulmonary fibrosis. The onset of pulmonary fibrosis may be delayed for several weeks in less severe cases. The lung lesion is usually, but not invariably, fatal, though death can be delayed for 2 or 3 weeks. Death is usually due to delayed pulmonary fibrosis and respiratory failure. The mechanism is thought to be due to the generation of cytotoxic oxygen radicals.

Presentation
- Nausea and vomiting are seen within a few hours of ingestion.
- Mouth and oesophageal ulceration are common.

- Oliguric renal failure develops with doses >2 g within 12 hours of ingestion.
- Very high doses (e.g. 50–100 mL 20% solution, i.e. >10 g) may cause acute dyspnoea, with an ARDS-like picture and rapid multiorgan failure.
- Insidious pulmonary fibrosis develops in the second week after exposure (often as the oliguria is resolving). This is not reversible, and occasional survivors invariably have a severe handicap.
- Liver failure and myocarditis are also reported and are thought to reflect the same free radical-mediated cell damage.

Prognostic features

- The dose ingested is a good predictor of outcome; death has been reported after only 10–15 mL of the 20% solution (3 g) of paraquat and is universal after 50 mL (10 g).
- Plasma levels of paraquat, e.g. >2 mg/L at 4 hours or 0.1 mg/L at 24 hours, are associated with a poor prognosis.
- A low WBC on admission carries a poor prognosis.

Management

- Patients presenting within 1 hour of ingestion should receive activated charcoal (50–100 g).
- Take blood for FBC, U&E, LFT, and paraquat levels.
- Perform a baseline CXR and arterial blood gases.
- Monitor urine output (catheterize, if necessary).
- Supplemental oxygen increases toxicity and should be avoided unless required to relieve dyspnoea in distressed patients.
- IV fluids (but not a forced diuresis) are indicated when oesophageal ulceration is severe enough to produce dysphagia.
- Haemoperfusion and haemofiltration have been used to remove circulating paraquat, but there are no data on efficacy, and this has largely been abandoned. Haemodialysis may be needed, independently of drug elimination, if renal failure develops.
- Options to prevent or slow the process of pulmonary fibrosis should be considered. Some have advocated the use of steroids or cyclophosphamide, but there are no data.

Phenytoin

Phenytoin is an anticonvulsant which inhibits voltage-dependent sodium channels. Deaths after acute ingestion are rare.

The half-life in overdose may be markedly prolonged because of saturation of metabolism (zero order kinetics). In naive adults, symptoms are unlikely if they have taken less than 1 g.

Presentation

Nausea, vomiting, ataxia, and fine, rapid nystagmus on lateral gaze occur with phenytoin overdose. Less frequently, dysarthria, with increasing incoordination of the limbs and trunk which, after gross overdosage, may be so severe that the patient cannot lift the head or body from the bed. Divergent gaze, impairment of consciousness, hypotension, apnoea, and respiratory depression may also occur. Permanent cerebellar dysfunction has been reported.

Cardiovascular toxicity may follow rapid IV injection (bradycardia, hypotension, and arrhythmia) but is rarely seen after poisoning by the oral route.

Management

1. Consider activated charcoal (50 g for adults) if the patient presents within 1 hour of ingestion of more than 20 mg/kg body weight. Give further doses of oral activated charcoal, provided the patient is not vomiting and the airway is protected. Evidence suggests it may increase the elimination of phenytoin.
2. An urgent phenytoin concentration is helpful if the diagnosis is in doubt, e.g. in patients with coma, respiratory depression, or arrhythmias. The usual target range for phenytoin is 8–15 mg/L (32–59 micromoles/L). Symptomatic toxicity is usually associated with concentrations in excess of 20 mg/L (79 micromoles/L), while concentrations >40 mg/L (159 micromoles/L) suggest serious toxicity.
3. Observe for at least 4 hours. Monitor BP, pulse, respiratory rate, and conscious level. Perform a 12-lead ECG. Patients who have not developed symptoms by 4 hours are unlikely to do so.
4. Give intravenous fluids if vomiting is severe.
5. Correct hypotension by raising the foot of the bed and by giving an appropriate fluid challenge. Where hypotension is thought to be secondary to negative chronotropic and inotropic effects, with little evidence of systemic vasodilatation, then beta-adrenergic agonists, such as dobutamine, or low-dose dopamine (2–10 mcg/kg/min) may be helpful.
6. If the patient is epileptic, monitor plasma phenytoin concentrations daily in order to decide when to restart therapeutic doses.

Risperidone

See sections (earlier in this chapter) on antipsychotic drugs and haloperidol.

Salicylates

Aspirin is one of the commonest drugs to be ingested deliberately in overdose. Occasionally, poisoning follows the topical application of salicylic acid in keratolytics or ingestion of methyl salicylate ('oil of wintergreen'). Its primary toxic effect is to uncouple oxidative phosphorylation.

Presentation

- The typical features of moderate salicylate toxicity are sweating, vomiting, epigastric pain, tinnitus, and blurring of vision.
- In adults, there is also an early increase in respiratory rate, causing an alkalosis that precedes the later development of a metabolic acidosis (children do not develop the early respiratory alkalosis).
- In severe overdose, the acidosis reduces the ionization of salicylic acid which enhances tissue penetration. In the CNS, this presents as agitation, tremor, fits, coma, and respiratory depression.

Complications

- Disturbance of electrolytes (hypokalaemia and either hyper- or hyponatraemia) and blood glucose (hyper- or hypoglycaemia) are common.
- Pulmonary oedema (non-cardiogenic, ARDS).
- Acute renal failure.
- Abnormal clotting due to hypoprothrombinaemia is very rare.
- Significant GI bleeds are surprisingly infrequent.

Prognostic features

- Therapeutic levels of salicylate are generally <300 mg/L (2.2 mmol/L). Levels of 500–750 mg/L represent a moderate overdose, and >750 mg/L (5.4 mmol/L) is severe.
- Children (<10 years old) and elderly (>70 years old) patients are at higher risk of severe toxicity and have a lower threshold for treatment.
- Severe metabolic acidosis is associated with a poor outcome.

Management

- Gastric lavage should be attempted, following a large overdose (>500 mg/kg body weight) within 1 hour of ingestion.
- Give oral activated charcoal (50 g for adults) to patients with salicylate overdoses >150 mg/kg body weight, for unknown dosages, after gastric lavage in large overdoses (>500 mg/kg body weight), and to those presenting more than 1 hour after ingestion of a large overdose or who are unsuitable for gastric lavage.
- Take blood for U&E, PT, and salicylate (and paracetamol) levels on admission. Ideally, repeat the salicylate (and paracetamol) levels 4 hours later to access continued absorption, as tablets may adhere to form large masses in the stomach and some preparations are enteric-coated.
- Further doses of oral activated charcoal may be given to patients with rising salicylate levels to prevent late absorption.
- Check arterial blood gases to assess the degree of acidosis.
- Monitor blood glucose regularly (laboratory and/or BM stix every 2 hours).
- Mild or moderate salicylate overdose (serum salicylate levels <600 mg/L) requires only oral or IV rehydration, with particular attention to K$^+$ supplements.
- Marked signs or symptoms of salicylism, or serum salicylate levels >600 mg/L need specific elimination therapy (below, in order of use):
  - Urinary alkalinization, e.g. 1 L 1.26% NaHCO$_3$, over 4 hours, and repeat, as necessary, to a maximum of ~4 L/day to keep urine at pH 7.5–8.5. This may cause hypokalaemia. Check serum potassium every 2–3 hours. Forced alkaline diuresis is no more effective and is potentially dangerous.
  - Haemodialysis is indicated for levels >700 mg/L (5.1 mmol/L), persistent or progressive acidosis, deteriorating level of consciousness, renal or cardiac failure.
- Pulmonary oedema may indicate either fluid overload or increased vascular permeability. Admit to the ICU, and insert a pulmonary artery catheter for measuring wedge pressures. Non-cardiogenic pulmonary oedema may require CPAP or mechanical ventilation (see 'Respiratory practical procedures' Chapter 19).

SSRIs

The selective serotonin reuptake inhibitors (SSRIs) include paroxetine, fluoxetine, citalopram, fluvoxamine, and sertraline as well as other drugs.

Presentations

Most SSRIs have similar toxic effects, leading to sedation, nausea, vomiting, hepatic dysfunction, sinus tachycardia, ataxia, coma, urinary retention, acute renal failure, dilated pupils, and ECG abnormalities (QT prolongation). The maximal effect on QT prolongation occurs ~8 hours after ingestion. Uncommon features include left bundle branch block, supraventricular tachycardia, and torsade de pointes.

Features of the 'serotonin syndrome' may occur in severe poisoning. These include hyperpyrexia, muscle rigidity, and elevation of serum creatine kinase activity.

Management

1. Maintain a clear airway and ensure adequate ventilation if consciousness is impaired.
2. Consider oral activated charcoal (50 g) in adults who have ingested more than 3 mg/kg body weight within 1 hour.
3. Observe asymptomatic patients for at least 6 hours. Patients with ECG abnormalities should be observed until these resolve. Monitor pulse, blood pressure, temperature, level of consciousness, and cardiac rhythm. Assess QRS and QTc durations. If these are prolonged, administer sodium bicarbonate. Monitor the ECG and pulse oximetry.
4. Correct hypotension by fluid challenge and raising the foot of the bed. Beta-adrenergic agonists, such as dobutamine, may be beneficial. The dose of inotrope should be titrated against blood pressure.
5. Control convulsions with IV diazepam (5–10 mg in adults) or lorazepam (2–4 mg in adults).
6. If metabolic acidosis persists, despite correction of hypoxia and adequate fluid resuscitation, correct with 250 mL of 1.26% sodium bicarbonate IV.
7. Ventricular arrhythmias are best treated with IV amiodarone (5 mg/kg over 30–60 minutes) or IV disopyramide (2 mg/kg over 5 minutes). Avoid lidocaine or mexiletine since they may exacerbate convulsions.
8. Haemodialysis or haemofiltration may be required for cases of acute renal failure or severe hyperkalaemia.

Theophylline

Intoxication can be deliberate or iatrogenic due to the low therapeutic index of theophylline.

Presentation

- The features of acute ingestion reflect the local irritant gastrointestinal (GI) effects of theophylline, i.e. nausea, vomiting, abdominal cramps, and diarrhoea. GI bleeding is also well recognized.
- Features of systemic toxicity include cardiac arrhythmias, hypotension, and seizures.

Complications

- Acid-base disturbance: an initial respiratory alkalosis, which gives way to a secondary metabolic acidosis.
- Marked hypokalaemia is common.
- Theophylline-induced fits carry a high mortality (up to 30%) and usually reflect serum theophylline levels of >50 mg/L (0.28 mmol/L).

Management

- Gastric lavage should be attempted if the patient is seen within 1 hour of ingestion. Multiple-dose activated charcoal should also be given both to prevent further absorption and to enhance systemic clearance (50–100 g stat, then 50 g 4-hourly), although this may not be practical in the presence of severe nausea and vomiting.
- Take blood for U&E and a theophylline level.
- Hypokalaemia should be corrected aggressively with IV supplements (40–60 mmol/h may be needed).

- Record a 12-lead ECG, and then monitor the ECG continuously for arrhythmias.
- Verapamil (10 mg IV) and propranolol (2–5 mg IV) are useful for treating supraventricular and ventricular tachyarrhythmias, respectively. Lidocaine appears to have little effect on ventricular ectopy and should be avoided.
- GI bleeding should be managed in the usual way (see 'Acute upper and lower GI bleeding' Chapter 8). Avoid cimetidine which substantially inhibits theophylline metabolism (ranitidine is safe, e.g. 50 mg IV tds).
- Seizures should be controlled with diazepam (10 mg IV prn).
- Haemoperfusion (charcoal or resin) should be considered in severe overdoses, particularly those with recurrent seizure activity or intractable vomiting. The latter represents direct stimulation of the area postrema (a medullary structure in the brain that controls vomiting) and generally responds poorly to antiemetics, e.g. metoclopramide and prochlorperazine, but ondansetron is effective (4–8 mg IV).

Tricyclic antidepressants

First-generation agents (e.g. amitriptyline, imipramine, and desipramine) are the most likely to cause lethal intoxication. The newer second-generation tricyclics (e.g. lofepramine) and tetracyclics are generally much safer in overdose.

Presentation

- Anticholinergic features are prominent early on, with dry mouth, dilated pupils, blurred vision, sinus tachycardia, urinary retention, myoclonic jerking, agitation, and hallucinations (anticholinergic mnemonic: 'Blind as a bat, mad as a hatter, red as a beet, hot as Hades, dry as a bone, the bowel and bladder lose their tone, and the heart runs alone').
- Cardiac arrhythmias due to a quinidine-like effect on the heart. Profound hypotension, convulsions, and coma follow.

Complications

- Severe toxicity causes coma, with respiratory depression, hypoxia, and a metabolic acidosis.
- Neurological signs include a temporary loss of oculocephalic and oculovestibular reflexes, long tract signs (upper motor neuron syndrome), and internuclear ophthalmoplegia.
- Hypothermia, skin blistering (compared with barbiturates), and rhabdomyolysis are also reported.

Prognostic features

- Death may follow ingestion of as little as 1,000 mg of a tricyclic.
- Prolongation of the QRS to >100 ms suggests significant intoxication with a high risk of convulsion; a QRS >160 ms is generally seen before ventricular arrhythmias develop. Patients with ischaemic heart disease (especially post-MI) and conduction defects are particularly at risk.

Management

- Patients with CNS depression should be monitored closely, preferably on an ICU or a high dependency area.
- Gastric lavage should be attempted if the patient is seen within 1 hour of ingestion. Activated charcoal should be given orally (50 g).
- Record a 12-lead ECG, and monitor for up to 48 hours.
- Respiratory failure may require intubation and ventilation.

- Alkalinization with boluses of 50 mmol IV 8.4% sodium bicarbonate, aiming for an arterial pH of 7.45–7.55, is the initial treatment for patients with prolonged QRS duration, metabolic acidosis, hypotension, or arrhythmias.
- Severe hypotension may be treated with IV glucagon or vasopressors, e.g. noradrenaline (norepinephrine) (see Chapters 1, 2, and 4).
- Control seizures with diazepam (5–10 mg IV).
- Arrhythmias that do not compromise cardiac output do not need treatment. If the blood pressure is falling, then correct acidosis or hypoxia before giving antiarrhythmics. Most class I antiarrhythmic agents are ineffective. Magnesium sulfate is used for unresponsive ventricular dysrhythmias.
- Tricyclic coma may last 24–48 hours. In many patients, recovery is marked by profound agitation and florid visual and auditory hallucination. Sedation may be necessary.

Valproate

Sodium valproate is an anticonvulsant used in the treatment of tonic-clonic seizures, particularly in primary generalized epilepsy, generalized absence, and myoclonic seizures.

- In mild to moderate overdoses most patients experience mild drowsiness, but in severe cases, unconsciousness may occur if over 200 mg/kg body weight of valproate has been ingested. Doses of less than 5,000 mg in adults are unlikely to cause toxicity. Fatalities have been reported after ingestion of more than 20 g.
- Toxic effects are frequently associated with blood concentrations over 100 mg/L. The time to peak plasma concentration depends on the pharmaceutical formulation. It is 1–2 hours for liquid or plain tablets, and 3–8 hours for enteric-coated tablets. In therapeutic doses, the half-life of valproate is 8–14 hours. In overdose, the half-life may be prolonged to more than 20 hours.
- Drowsiness is the commonest feature. Hypotension, nausea, vomiting, diarrhoea, and abdominal pain may also occur. In more severe poisoning, myoclonic movements, seizures, coma, and respiratory or circulatory failure can occur. Cerebral oedema may develop at 12–72 hours post-ingestion. Haemorrhagic pancreatitis can also occur. Diplopia and nystagmus are rarely seen. Metabolic abnormalities include metabolic acidosis, hypernatraemia, hypoglycaemia, hyperammonaemia, and hypocalcaemia.
- Observe for at least 12 hours after ingestion.
- Monitor pulse, BP, and conscious level at least hourly. Check blood glucose, U&E, LFTs, and amylase. Measure arterial blood gases and ammonia in severely poisoned patients.
- Consider the use of naloxone in patients with a reduced level of consciousness, as rapid improvement has been reported with its use in moderately severe toxicity (but not severe toxicity).
- Correct hypotension by raising the foot of the bed and by giving an appropriate fluid challenge. Where hypotension is thought to be mainly due to decreased systemic vascular resistance, drugs with alpha-adrenergic activity, such as noradrenaline, or high-dose dopamine (10–30 mcg/kg/min) may be beneficial. The dose of inotrope should be titrated against blood pressure.
- Consider giving levocarnitine to patients who have taken a massive valproate overdose and have hyperammonaemia or hepatotoxicity (deficiencies in dietary intake and endogenous production of levocarnitine increase the risk of developing hyperammonaemia, and the associated encephalopathy, following valproic acid exposure).

Endocrinology and metabolic disorders

Diabetes and diabetic coma

Diabetic ketoacidosis

Diabetic ketoacidosis (DKA) is an acute metabolic complication of diabetes mellitus, characterized by hyperglycaemia, metabolic acidosis, and ketosis. This condition has a mortality of 2–5%, and this is largely preventable. Many deaths occur due to delays in presentation and initiation of treatment, with a mortality rate of up to 50% in the elderly. The most common triggers for DKA are discontinuation/missing insulin treatment, underlying infection, and new onset of diabetes mellitus. The groups most usually affected are patients with known type 1 diabetes or those with type 2 diabetes of Afro-Caribbean or Hispanic origin (also known as 'ketosis-prone type 2 diabetes mellitus').

Patients with DKA usually present to emergency departments or medical assessment units and are often managed by non-specialist teams, particularly during the critical first 24 hour period. Therefore, proformas and protocols may be helpful in the management of these patients, reducing the time spent in ICU/HDU by up to 30% in some studies. However, the early involvement of specialist diabetes teams is associated with a better outcome.

Diagnosis

This is usually based on a collection of biochemical abnormalities, namely:

- **Hyperglycaemia:** >11.1 mmol/L (usually >27.8 mmol/L and <44.4 mmol/L, although, with starvation or pregnancy, the glucose may be only mildly elevated).
- **Metabolic acidosis:** arterial pH <7.3, serum bicarbonate (HCO_3) <15 mmol/L, base excess <−10.
- **Ketonuria.** Some dip-testing methods (e.g. Ketostix®) only check for acetoacetate and acetone, but not beta-hydroxybutyrate (beta-OHB) which can be the main ketone body found in the urine initially. Captopril can also give a false positive test for urinary acetone, and serum ketones may also interfere with some creatinine assays and give falsely high readings. If in doubt, and if available, measure capillary ketone levels (normal <1.0 mmol/L, ketonaemia >3 mmol/L) using, for example, the Optium Xceed™ meter which measures up to 8 mmol/L.

In addition, the serum anion gap is a clinically useful estimate of the quantity of unmeasured anions in the serum, such as albumin, lactate, drugs, alcohol, and, in DKA, ketones. Patients with DKA usually present with a serum anion gap >20 mEq/L. It is calculated using the formula:

Serum anion gap = (sodium + potassium) − (chloride + bicarbonate)

There is also an uncommon condition of euglycaemic ketoacidosis (in 1–3% of cases at most) when ketones are produced early on in patients with a reduced carbohydrate intake (in particular, consider this possibility in pregnancy and in pre- or post-operative surgical patients who are being starved and whose insulin has been withheld). Typically, blood glucose is <17 mmol/L, acidosis is marked, and dehydration is not usually severe. Treatment is to initiate oral carbohydrate intake and monitor the need for IV insulin/fluids, as in full-blown hyperglycaemic ketoacidosis.

Some units grade the level or degree of DKA, as this will determine whether a person is managed in a medical admissions or assessment unit/MAU (mild), a high dependency unit/HDU (moderate), or an intensive care unit/ICU (severe). This classification is based on the degree of acidosis,

Table 10.1 Example of a subclassification for severity/degree of ketoacidosis

Degree of ketoacidosis	Mild	Moderate	Severe
Blood pH	7.25–7.34	7.00–7.24	<7.00
Serum bicarbonate	15–18	10–14.9	<10

not the level of hyperglycaemia, and the facilities available (see Table 10.1).

Epidemiology

Diabetic ketoacidosis is common in patients with type 1 diabetes, with 1 in 11 subjects in the European IDDM (insulin dependent diabetes mellitus) complications study (EURODIAB) reporting hospitalization for this over a 12-month period. The incidence is 5–8/1,000 diabetic patients per year, usually in patients with known type 1 diabetes, but up to 25% of cases are patients with newly diagnosed/presenting diabetes, some of whom subsequently obtain adequate control with oral agents or diet alone. These 'ketosis-prone type 2 patients' are typically, but not exclusively, of Afro-Caribbean, sub-Saharan, or Hispanic origin. In 30–40% of people, DKA occurs because of an intercurrent infection, and this needs to be looked for in all patients. The remainder of cases are triggered by omission of insulin/poor compliance, and other stresses, such as myocardial infarction, stroke, surgery, alcohol, pancreatitis, pregnancy, and drugs (in particular, clozapine, olanzapine, cocaine, lithium, and terbutaline) (see Table 10.2). Do not forget that insulin needs to be stored carefully. In hot weather, some cases of DKA may be due to a problem with the insulin itself, not because of a compliance issue. If this is suspected, remember to destroy the old insulin, and change to a new vial which has been stored correctly (at <30°C if not refrigerated at 2–8°C).

Pathogenesis

Diabetic ketoacidosis occurs as a result of insulin deficiency and counter-regulatory hormone excess. Insulin deficiency results in excess mobilization of free fatty acids from adipose tissue. This provides the substrate for ketone production in the liver. Ketones (beta-hydroxybutyrate, acetoacetate, and acetone) are excreted by the kidneys and buffered in the blood initially, but, once this system fails, acidosis develops. Hyperglycaemia also occurs, as the liver produces glucose from lactate and alanine, which are generated by muscle proteinolysis. This is exacerbated by the reduced peripheral glucose utilization associated with insulin deficiency.

Hyperglycaemia and ketonuria cause an osmotic diuresis and hypovolaemia, with both intracellular and extracellular

Table 10.2 Precipitants of diabetic ketoacidosis

Infection	30–40%
Non-compliance with treatment	25%
Inappropriate alterations in insulin (i.e. errors by either patient or doctor)	13%
Newly diagnosed diabetes	10–25%
Myocardial infarction	1%

dehydration. Glomerular filtration is reduced, and blood glucose levels, therefore, rise even further, as do the levels of counter-regulatory hormones, such as glucagon. The metabolic acidosis due to ketone accumulation leads to widespread cell death which, combined with hypovolaemia, can be fatal, if untreated.

Clinical features
Polyuria, polydipsia, and weight loss are often seen. Muscle cramps, abdominal pain, and shortness of breath (air hunger or Kussmaul's breathing, with deep regular rapid breaths, suggesting acidosis) can also occur. Subsequent nausea and vomiting can worsen both the dehydration and electrolyte losses which often precede the onset of coma (occurring in about 10% of cases). Remember to consider other causes of coma and a raised blood glucose, such as head injury, alcohol, and drug overdoses. If there is any doubt about the cause of the acidosis, always check serum lactate and salicylate levels.

On examination, the breath can smell of ketones (acetone is like nail varnish remover—but, due to genetic differences some people are less able, or unable, to smell ketones). Postural hypotension (exacerbated by peripheral vasodilatation due to acidosis) and hypothermia are also frequently seen. The vasodilatation due to acidosis may also mask a fever in these cases. Infection and trauma can precipitate hypotension and should be carefully looked for, especially in the unconscious patient.

Hypovolaemia (fluid deficit) at presentation is usually at least 5–6 L, accompanied by electrolyte losses of 300–700 mmol of sodium, 200–700 mmol of potassium, and 350–500 mmol of chloride. The normal daily intake of both sodium and potassium is ~60 mmol, so the severity of this is apparent.

Management
Initial management is guided by the severity of symptoms at presentation. Assess the need for immediate resuscitation by examining the airway, breathing, and circulation (ABC), and if the patient is self-ventilating, the GCS score. Determine the volume status (e.g. hypotension, low JVP, decreased skin turgor, and dry mucosal membranes) and commence fluid resuscitation with an IV infusion of 0.9% normal saline. Take a history and examine the patient to look for obvious precipitants, such as surgery, trauma, sites of infection, or myocardial infarction. The first steps are intravenous access, fluid and electrolyte replacement, and insulin therapy. Initial investigations will be modified by the history, examination, and suggested site of infection but should include:

- Laboratory blood glucose measurement.
- Blood for urea/electrolytes (note potential ketone/creatinine assay interaction).
- Full blood count (a leucocytosis can occur without infection).
- Arterial blood gases (PaCO$_2$ will be low due to hyperventilation, with a metabolic acidosis—check pH and bicarbonate).
- Cultures of blood and urine (and other bodily fluids, if indicated).
- Chest radiograph and ECG.
- In the 'older' patient (>40 years), also consider cardiac markers, such as troponin I, even if asymptomatic.

Replacement of fluids, electrolytes, and insulin is the mainstay of treatment, along with therapy for any precipitant, such as infection. Central venous access and urinary catheterization are often necessary to monitor treatment. A nasogastric tube may be useful, especially in the unconscious patient. In the elderly and those with a cardiac history or autonomic neuropathy, central venous access is imperative.

Fluid therapy
Most clinicians start with 0.9% normal saline IV infusion, switching to 5% glucose once the blood glucose has fallen <15 mmol/L. Aim to replace half the fluid deficit over the first 24 hours and the rest over the next 72 hours. The 0.9% normal saline helps to expand the intravascular and extravascular fluid space and replaces electrolyte losses as well as diluting the plasma glucose and encouraging clearance and excretion of any circulating counter-regulatory hormones. Typically, fluid is given rapidly, but overenthusiastic replacement may lead to marked osmotic shifts, and risks acute respiratory distress syndrome (ARDS), particularly in the elderly with comorbidities, such as congestive cardiac failure, or possibly cerebral oedema in the young. It is thought that cerebral oedema occurs in 5 per 1,000 episodes of DKA in those under 15 years of age. In view of this potential risk, some centres suggest a conservative fluid replacement regimen in those aged 16–25 years as well as in children, although no studies are available to confirm or refute the need for this. In this modified regimen, these young adults aged 16–25 years old are given 3 L of fluid/0.9% normal saline in the first 6 hours (e.g. 0.9% normal saline 500 mL/hour for the first hour, then 0.9% normal saline with 40 mmol/L potassium chloride at 500 mL/hour, as long as the serum potassium is <5.5 mmol/L and the patient is passing urine), rather than the more standard 3 L in the first 3 hours (e.g. 1 L 0.9% normal saline over 30 minutes with no potassium, unless this is low on the arterial blood gas measurement, and then 2 × 1 L 0.9% normal saline with added potassium over 2 hours, then 2 × 1 L 0.9% normal saline with added potassium over 4 hours, followed by 2 × 1 L normal saline with added potassium over 6 hours). There is no evidence that colloid offers any benefit over crystalloid as the replacement fluid of choice. Serum potassium is usually depleted in patients with DKA, and, once the serum potassium level is known, the 0.9% normal saline will have potassium added to it, based on that serum level, i.e. if potassium level is >5.5 mmol/L, none is added; if serum potassium is 3.5–5.5 mmol/L, add 40 mmol/L of potassium, and if <3.5 mmol/L, add 60 mmol/L of potassium. Some guidelines suggest 20 mmol/L of potassium if the serum level is 4.0–5.4 mmol/L and 40 mmol/L <4 mmol/L, but all regimens lack significant randomized trial evidence and rely on regular repeated measurements of the serum potassium level with appropriate adjustments of infused potassium.

In patients with euglycaemic DKA, remember that, as the serum glucose level falls <15 mmol/L, the temptation is to switch to 5% glucose, instead of continuing with 0.9% normal saline, even though the patient's dehydration may not have been adequately corrected and the 0.9% normal saline is needed to correct this. Continuing with both 0.9% normal saline and 5% glucose via separate intravenous lines may avoid this potential problem, but care must be taken not to fluid-overload the elderly or post-MI patients.

Insulin therapy
Insulin is needed in DKA to reduce the serum glucose level and to prevent gluconeogenesis by the liver, therefore, switching off the production of free fatty acids and ketones. Typically, this is given as 50 units of a short-acting insulin,

Table 10.3 Example of an IV sliding scale insulin regimen for use when pH >7.30

Capillary glucose level (mmol/L)	Insulin infusion rate (units per hour or mL/hour)
<4.0	0.5
4.0–6.0	1
6.1–8.0	2
8.1–10.0	3
10.1–15.0	4
>15.0	6

diluted in 50 mL of 0.9% normal saline, administered via a syringe driver as 1 unit per mL. If there is likely to be a significant delay in preparing/giving this intravenous insulin infusion, a 10 unit dose of intramuscular soluble insulin can be given initially. Aim to start the intravenous infusion at a rate of 0.1 unit/kg per hour, which is a rate of 6 units/hour in a 60 kg patient or 8 units/hour in an 80 kg patient. The aim is to drop the blood glucose level by 3–5 mmol/L per hour until the pH is >7.30, and the capillary blood glucose level is <15 mmol/L. The intravenous fluid is then changed to 5% glucose. The insulin administration rate is subsequently adjusted using a 'sliding scale' as shown in Table 10.3, depending on the capillary blood glucose level. If, however, after the first 2 hours, the capillary blood glucose has failed to fall adequately, the infusion rate should be increased by 1–2 units/hour and the sliding scale may need to be adjusted. Once the patient is ketone-free and eating and drinking, they can be transferred back to standard subcutaneous insulin.

An alternative regime for the treatment of diabetic ketoacidosis is the GKI (glucose, potassium, and insulin) infusion, also known as the 'Alberti regime'. This method requires that variable amounts of insulin and potassium are added to 0.9% normal saline, 5% glucose, or 10% glucose solutions for infusion. For example, when the blood glucose level is >15 mmol/L, 50 units of insulin and 40 mmol of potassium are added to a 500ml bag of 0.9% normal saline, and the infusion is run initially at 80–100 mL/hour, reducing to a maintenance dose of 30–60 mL/hour. Although not as popular as the above 'sliding scale', 'syringe driver' continuous regimen, this method does have the advantage of the insulin, potassium, and fluid (with or without glucose) being given together so reducing the risk of insulin being given on its own (i.e. reduces the risk of potential hypokalaemia). Once the capillary blood glucose level falls <15 mmol/L, the concentrations of infused insulin and potassium should be adjusted. This is achieved by adding 20 units of soluble insulin and 40 mmol of potassium (adjusted for serum potassium level) to 500 mL of 5% glucose. This mixture is then infused at 100 mL/hour (which equates to 4 units of insulin per hour initially). Measure capillary blood glucose levels hourly initially, aiming for glucose levels of 7–11 mmol/L ideally, and 5–15 mmol/L at worst. If >15 mmol/L or <5 mmol/L, adjust the amount of insulin added, and also review the serum potassium level and adjust the potassium concentration and administration rate of the infused solution accordingly. After each alteration, recheck blood glucose levels after 1 hour, and adjust further, if required. Once stable, reduce the capillary blood glucose level checks to 2-hourly. As with any IV regimen, convert to regular therapy

once the patient is eating. There is no evidence that this regimen has any advantage or disadvantage compared to a 'sliding scale' continuous intravenous insulin infusion with separate 0.9% normal saline or glucose.

Monitoring

Once treatment has commenced, monitor fluid balance carefully, avoiding fluid overload. Check capillary blood glucose hourly, with serum potassium, sodium, and glucose 2-hourly and arterial blood gases 2–4-hourly, depending on response. Once stabilized reduce the frequency of tests, e.g. monitor capillary glucose and ketones hourly, with serum potassium and venous pH checked at 2, 4, 8, 16, and 24 hours. Then check electrolytes at least daily for the first 72 hours. Continuous ECG monitoring will also aid the detection of hypo- and hyperkalaemia in the acute phase. Magnesium levels should also be checked, as low levels may increase the risk of cardiac arrhythmias. Consider magnesium therapy if serum magnesium is <0.7 mmol/L when checked at 12–24 hours. In addition, whole body and serum phosphate levels are also often low and can take several days to correct after resolution of DKA. Current guidelines (NICE 2015, Joint British Diabetes Societies guideline 2011) do not recommend routine phosphate replacement, as prospective studies have shown no benefit from doing so. However, in the presence of respiratory and skeletal muscle weakness, phosphate measurement and replacement may be considered.

Pulse oximetry may be a useful indicator of deteriorating oxygen saturation due to fluid overload and/or acute respiratory distress syndrome (ARDS), especially in those patients with comorbidities.

Additional therapies

- Intravenous bicarbonate therapy is only rarely indicated, as it can cause hypokalaemia, paradoxically worsen intracellular acidosis, and potentially increase the risk of cerebral oedema. Several clinical trials using small numbers of patients have shown no clinical benefit, even with a pH of 6.8. If used, give only when the pH is <6.8, by administering 250 mL of 1.26% bicarbonate, initially infusing it over 30–60 min, whilst monitoring arterial blood gases to assess response. Aim for the pH to be no greater than 7.1. This should only be administered in an intensive care setting. Do not use 8.4% bicarbonate, as its high sodium load can alter electrolyte levels too rapidly and precipitate pulmonary oedema as well as cause local tissue necrosis if it extravasates.

- Inotropic support may be required for severe hypotension that is unresponsive to crystalloid fluid replacement therapy. However, dopamine, dobutamine, and adrenaline will all exacerbate insulin resistance, necessitating a more aggressive insulin replacement, sliding scale regime.

- Low molecular weight heparin in subcutaneous prophylactic doses can be given in the unconscious or immobile patient, especially if there are vascular comorbidities.

- Prophylactic broad-spectrum, intravenous antibiotics should be administered if no obvious precipitant is found. Use appropriate antibiotics if a likely site of infection is found.

- Cerebral oedema typically presents 8–24 h after starting IV fluids, with a declining conscious level, and may carry a mortality as high as 90%. If this occurs, dexamethasone (12–16 mg/day) and mannitol (1–2 g/kg body weight as a 20% solution, e.g. 5 mL/kg over 20 minutes) may be given. A CT brain scan is required to exclude other causes for the altered conscious level.

Subsequent treatment

Once the ketoacidosis has settled, and the blood glucose is within a range of 7-11 mmol/L with the patient eating and drinking normally, change the insulin administration from an intravenous to a standard subcutaneous regime. Overlap the intravenous and first subcutaneous dose by 2 hours. Stabilize on this therapy before discharge from hospital. Maintain potassium supplements orally for at least 48 hours following cessation of intravenous potassium, monitoring serum levels regularly.

In view of the potential for poor compliance as a precipitant, it is important to undertake patient education prior to discharge. This enables the patient to be aware of the cause for the DKA episode, which may help avoid future occurrences, or alert the patient to 'herald' signs and symptoms prompting an earlier presentation.

Hyperosmolar hyperglycaemic coma (HHC)

(previously known as hyperosmolar non-ketotic hyperglycaemia or HONK)

This is characterized by hyperglycaemia with a high serum plasma osmolality without significant ketonuria or acidosis. It is a more sinister complication than ketoacidosis, with a mortality as high as 50%, and is said to be found in 11–30% of adult hyperglycaemic emergencies. Typically it affects an older population (middle-aged or elderly, e.g. >60 years of age) than diabetic ketoacidosis and 40–67% of cases are in patients with previously undiagnosed diabetes. Its insidious onset with vague symptoms, such as confusion and drowsiness, can be mistaken for many other conditions, including a stroke.

Diagnosis

This is a biochemical diagnosis:
- Hyperglycaemia (usually 30–70 mmol/L).
- Raised serum osmolality (>350 mOsm). This can be calculated using the following equation: osmolality = 2(sodium + potassium) + glucose + urea (result is in mOsm) if not available from the laboratory.
- No acidosis, arterial pH 7.35–7.45, serum bicarbonate >15 mmol/L, but remember that lactic acidosis with infection or a myocardial infarction may alter this.
- No ketonuria (e.g. <++ on standard urine dip-testing strips, as a single + can occur with starvation and vomiting); capillary blood ketone measurements are available with some blood glucose meters and can help to clarify this (normal <1.0 mmol/L, ketonaemia >3 mmol/L).

Epidemiology

This occurs in an older age group of insulin-producing type 2 diabetic patients, a large proportion (40–67%) of whom will not previously be known to have diabetes. Ingestion of high sugar-containing drinks, intercurrent infection, and myocardial infarction are all commonly seen as precipitants of this condition. Drugs, such as glucocorticoids, cimetidine, phenytoin, thiazide, and loop diuretics, have all been implicated in the pathogenesis of this problem.

Pathogenesis

This occurs from a combination of insulin deficiency and counter-regulatory hormone excess, with the insulin that is present stopping ketone production, but in insufficient quantities to prevent worsening hyperglycaemia.

Clinical features

There is normally an insidious onset, with several days of ill health and profound dehydration at presentation (equivalent to a 9–10 L deficit). Confusion is not uncommon nor is drowsiness or coma (coma is especially common once serum osmolality >440 mOsm), and occasionally fits occur. Gastroparesis and associated vomiting with gastric erosions and subsequent haematemesis can occur. These patients are also hypercoagulable, and venous thromboses and cerebrovascular events are important to exclude. It is important to look for a precipitating cause, such as infection/sepsis and myocardial infections.

Management

Initial investigation and treatment is the same as for ketoacidosis, with fluid, electrolyte, and insulin replacement, although there are a few important exceptions, as these are older patients, and paradoxically these patients can be quite insulin-sensitive.
- The fluid regime should be less rapid/vigorous. Central venous access for monitoring is more often required, e.g. 1 L of 0.9% normal saline over the first hour, 1 L 2-hourly for the next 2 h, then 1 L 4–6-hourly.
- If hypernatraemic (serum sodium >155 mmol/L), consider 0.45% saline, rather than 0.9%, although this may increase the risk of cerebral oedema if serum sodium or osmolality is lowered too rapidly, and has a mortality as high as 70%. However, as 0.9% normal saline is relatively hypotonic compared to the patient's own serum, many units use only 0.9% normal saline in all patients and avoid 0.45% saline in this situation due to this risk.
- Prophylactic subcutaneous low molecular weight heparin should be considered, although recent evidence suggests more formal anticoagulation carries a high risk of upper gastrointestinal bleeding.
- A gentler insulin regime is needed, with 3–6 units per hour of soluble insulin IV, aiming to reduce the blood glucose by a maximum of 5 mmol/L per hour to avoid precipitating cerebral oedema.
- A more aggressive use of IV antibiotics is encouraged.

Subsequent treatment

Continue IV fluids and insulin for at least 24 hours after initial stabilization, and then convert to maintenance therapy, such as subcutaneous insulin or oral hypoglycaemic agents. Patient education is advisable to avoid further episodes.

Hypoglycaemia

This complication of diabetic treatment should be excluded in any unconscious or fitting patient. If prolonged, it can result in death. Most insulin-treated patients can expect to experience hypoglycaemic episodes at some time, with up to 1 in 7 having a more severe episode each year and 3% suffering recurrent episodes. Of particular concern is the loss of hypoglycaemic awareness occurring in 25% of people on long term insulin. Nocturnal hypoglycaemic episodes with a hyperglycaemic response the next morning (due to increased counter-regulatory hormones—the Somogyi phenomenon), which tend to occur in younger insulin-treated patients, should not be overlooked and may only present with morning headaches or a 'drunken' feeling.

Diagnosis

This is a biochemical diagnosis from a blood glucose <2.5 mmol/L but is often first recognized by the patient, their family, or their doctor from the presenting clinical features (as described below). Saving serum before treatment for blood glucose, insulin, and C-peptide levels will confirm the diagnosis and may help to determine the cause. In any patient not known to have diabetes, a detailed screen should be undertaken to determine the cause.

In such cases, consider at least performing tests or saving samples for:

- Laboratory blood glucose.
- Insulin and C-peptide (if high insulin and no C-peptide, consider exogenous insulin).
- Beta-hydroxybutyrate.
- Sulfonylurea screen.

Pathogenesis

Hypoglycaemia results from an imbalance between glucose supply, glucose utilization, and insulin levels, resulting in more insulin than is needed at that time. A reduced glucose supply occurs when a meal or snack is missed or as a late effect of alcohol. It can also be due to delayed gastric emptying with autonomic neuropathy or be associated with coeliac disease, Addison's disease, or an acute illness such as gastroenteritis. Increased utilization occurs with exercise and high insulin levels, mostly with sulfonylurea or exogenous insulin therapy. The net result of this imbalance is hypoglycaemia.

Human insulin therapies have a slightly faster onset of action and a shorter duration of action than their animal predecessors, and many patients report alterations in hypoglycaemic awareness when they switch from one to the other. Even so, no definite evidence of specific hypoglycaemic alterations due to human insulin itself has been reported. Likewise, the shorter-acting insulin analogues may have a similar effect in some patients, compared to standard human insulin therapies.

Sulfonylurea therapy can cause hypoglycaemia due to beta cell stimulation. This is most commonly seen with glibenclamide, especially in the elderly and those with reduced renal excreting ability, but can occur in anyone who takes this therapy and fasts.

Other secretagogues (a substance that causes another substance to be secreted) can have a similar effect to sulfonylureas, such as the meglitinides (e.g. nateglinide and repaglinide), as can insulin-sensitizing agents, such as the ACE-Is (angiotensin-converting enzyme inhibitors) and the thiazolidinediones (e.g. rosiglitazone and pioglitazone). However, the biguanide metformin and the alpha-glucosidase inhibitor acarbose are unlikely to precipitate hypoglycaemia.

In patients without known diabetes, who are not taking drugs known to cause hypoglycaemia, other causes need to be sought. These are typically split into either fasting hypoglycaemia (occurring >5 hours after food) or reactive/postprandial hypoglycaemia (typically occurring 2–5 hours after food). The main conditions to consider/exclude in these patients are:

- Drug–induced:
  - Exogenous insulin or sulfonylurea therapy (either deliberate or accidental).
  - Alcohol (impairs gluconeogenesis and alters glycogen stores).
  - Salicylates (alters hepatic glucose efflux).
  - Quinine (causing hyperinsulinaemia).
- Infections:
  - Septicaemia with high metabolic requirements and reduced energy intake, e.g. Gram-negative septicaemia or meningococcus.
- Tumours:
  - Insulinoma.
  - Other non-islet cell tumours (e.g. large mesenchymal tumours, such as fibrosarcomas).

- Hormone deficiency:
  - Addison's disease.
  - Hypopituitarism.
  - Growth hormone deficiency.
- Organ failure:
  - Acute liver failure.
  - Chronic renal failure.
- Starvation:
  - Anorexia nervosa or kwashiorkor.
- Autoimmune:
  - Anti-insulin antibodies causing hypoglycaemia is a rare condition which is commonest in Japanese patients (IAS—insulin autoimmune syndrome or Hirata's disease is strongly associated with HLA-DR4).
  - Insulin receptor-activating antibodies (again rare but commonest in middle-aged women).
- Inborn errors of metabolism:
  - Glycogen storage disease.
  - Hereditary fructose intolerance.
  - Maple syrup disease.
- Post-surgery:
  - Post-gastrectomy, e.g. 'dumping' with rapid gastric emptying, giving a greater than normal insulin response than is needed and a subsequent hypoglycaemic episode 2–3 hours postprandially.

Clinical features

The features of hypoglycaemia can be divided into two main groups: autonomic symptoms and neuroglycopenic symptoms. The autonomic symptoms usually occur first (when the blood glucose is <3.6 mmol/L), but some drugs, such as the non-selective beta-blockers and alcohol may mask these, with neuroglycopenia (at blood glucose <2.6 mmol/L), then causing confusion with no warning. Some patients lose these predominantly autonomic warning symptoms and are, therefore, at higher risk of injury. Typically, there is a deterioration in neuropsychological performance as the blood glucose falls to 3.0–3.5 mmol/L, then a subjective perception of hypoglycaemia as it falls to 2.7–2.9 mmol/L. Note that EEG changes become evident when the blood glucose falls to 2.0 mmol/L.

Signs and symptoms of hypoglycaemia

- **Autonomic:**
  - Sweating.
  - Pallor.
  - Anxiety.
  - Nausea.
  - Tremor.
  - Shivering.
  - Palpitations.
  - Tachycardia.
- **Neuroglycopenia:**
  - Confusion.
  - Tiredness.
  - Lack of concentration.
  - Headache.
  - Dizziness.
  - Altered speech.
  - Incoordination.
  - Drowsiness.

- Aggression.
- Coma.

Management

In the conscious patient, oral carbohydrate (usually 20 g) is often sufficient to resolve the problem. This can be given as either:

- 7 glucose tablets.
- 4 Jelly babies.
- 6 wine gums.
- 15–20 Jelly beans.
- 115 mL Lucozade (310 mL of Lucozade Sport).
- 180 mL Coca Cola.
- 150 mL Fanta.
- 144 mL of a carton of Ribena.
- 200 mL of milk.

Having raised the sugar rapidly, maintain the normal blood glucose level by providing the patient with a carbohydrate source that is absorbed more slowly, such as a sandwich or two digestive biscuits. In the confused patient, buccal gels (e.g. a 30% glucose gel) are an alternative, although this should not be used in the unconscious patient, as there is a risk of aspiration.

The unconscious, hypoglycaemic patient should be treated with 1mg of IM glucagon, or 25–50mL of IV 50% glucose, once a blood sample has been taken. However, glucagon mobilizes glycogen from the liver and will not work, even if given repeatedly, in starved patients with no glycogen stores. In this situation or if prolonged treatment is needed, IV glucose is better (50% initially, then 10%). In view of the possibility of tissue necrosis due to extravasation of 50% glucose, some units use 20% glucose initially and convert to 5% or 10% glucose for continuation therapy. The potential need for larger fluid loads to give the same amount of glucose at lower concentration does not appear to be a problem in this situation but should be tailored to the individual patient.

Subsequent management

Having corrected the acute event, determine why it happened, especially if the patient is not known to have diabetes or to take therapy known to be associated with hypoglycaemic episodes. If possible, then alter treatment or address their lifestyle to prevent it recurring. Extreme exercise may require an alteration in insulin doses for 24 hours afterwards. Alcohol causes not only an initial hyperglycaemia, but also a degree of hypoglycaemia 3–6 h after ingestion, and may alter insulin requirements the next morning. Education to avoid precipitating hypoglycaemic episodes in these situations is advisable. A severe hypoglycaemic episode may be associated with a deterioration in the patient's ability to respond as well to a subsequent hypoglycaemic episode in the next few days, and education regarding care to adjust therapy and lifestyle to avoid this risk is important. Recurrent hypoglycaemic events may also herald a deterioration in renal or liver function, and these should be excluded.

During an acute hypoglycaemic event, patients on long-acting sulfonylureas who experience hypoglycaemia will need careful monitoring, as the drug may last longer than the glucose, or glycogen given to correct it and repeated hypoglycaemic episodes may occur. A continuous IV glucose infusion is, therefore, often required for 24 hours, particularly in overdose with these agents.

Further reading

EURODIAB IDDM Complications Study Group (1994). Microvascular and acute complications in IDDM patients: the EURODIAB IDDM Complications Study. *Diabetologia*, **37**, 278–85.

Joint British Diabetes Societies Inpatient Care Group (2012). The management of the hyperosmolar hyperglycaemic state (HHS) in adults with diabetes. <http://www.diabetologists-abcd.org.uk/JBDS/JBDS_IP_HHS_Adults.pdf>.

National Institute for Health and Care Excellence (2009). Type 2 diabetes: The management of type 2 diabetes. NICE clinical guideline 87. <https://www.nice.org.uk/guidance/cg87>.

National Institute for Health and Care Excellence (2015). Diabetes (type 1 and type 2) in children and young people: diagnosis and management. NICE guideline 18. <https://www.nice.org.uk/guidance/ng18>.

National Institute for Health and Care Excellence (2015). Type 1 diabetes in adults: diagnosis and management. NICE guideline 17. <https://www.nice.org.uk/guidance/ng17>.

National Institute for Health and Care Excellence (2015). Diabetes in pregnancy: management of diabetes and its complications from preconception to the postnatal period. NICE guideline 3. <https://www.nice.org.uk/guidance/ng3>.

Savage MW, Dhatariya KK, Kilvert A, *et al.* (2011). Joint British Diabetes Societies guideline for the management of diabetic ketoacidosis. Diabetes UK Position Statements and Care Recommendations. *Diabetic Medicine*, **28**, 508–515.

Abnormalities of sodium and potassium

Sodium

Pathophysiology

Sodium is the predominant cation within the extracellular fluid, with normal serum levels of 135–145 mmol/L. Only 10 mmol/L is contained within the intracellular fluid. Sodium homeostasis is regulated by thirst, ADH secretion, the renin-angiotensin-aldosterone system, and renal handling of filtered sodium. The majority of filtered sodium is reabsorbed in the proximal tubule of the loop of Henle. The tiny percentage of filtered sodium remaining (0.5%) is reabsorbed or excreted in the distal tubule or collecting ducts under the influence of ADH which inhibits sodium reabsorption and the release of renin and aldosterone. ADH is produced in the hypothalamus and stored in the posterior pituitary, from where it is released in response to rising osmolality and hypovolaemia. Nausea, pain, fear, and hypoxia also cause ADH to be released. Alcohol inhibits ADH release.

Hyponatraemia

Hyponatraemia is the most commonly encountered electrolyte abnormality, being seen in up to 6% of patients in hospital. It is observed most frequently in the very young and the elderly due to an inability to regulate fluid intake independently and a reduced sense of thirst. Acute hyponatraemia (developing in <48 hours) requires urgent identification and correction to prevent cerebral oedema that occurs due to the development of an osmotic gradient between the intracellular and extracellular fluid, resulting in water entering cells. The development of cerebral oedema is less marked in chronic hyponatraemia (>48 hours) due to the ability of the brain to compensate for a gradual change in the osmotic gradient. In acute or profound chronic hyponatraemia, seizures and central pontine myelinolysis are the main causes of morbidity and mortality.

History and clinical signs

Symptoms, signs, and examination findings vary, depending on the severity and the duration of hyponatraemia. Mild hyponatraemia is usually asymptomatic. Initial symptoms of nausea and malaise are observed at serum sodium concentrations <130 mmol/L. Below 120 mmol/L, lethargy, headache, muscle cramps, restlessness, and disorientation can occur. Patients with acute or severe chronic hyponatraemia can present with seizures, coma, irreversible brain damage, brainstem herniation, and death.

Examination findings may be normal. However, the GCS, Abbreviated Mental Test (AMT), and seizure activity, should be assessed to determine the extent of neurological involvement. Coma, fixed dilated pupils, decorticate or decerebrate posturing, hypertension, and respiratory arrest would suggest brainstem herniation.

Investigations

1. Urinary sodium.
2. Renal function.
3. Glucose.
4. Lipids.
5. Thyroid function.
6. Urine and plasma osmolality.
   Normal serum osmolality = (Na + K) x 2 + urea + glucose = 285–295 mOsm/kg.
7. Short Synacthen® test.
8. CXR or CT scan may be indicated.

Causes/treatment

Assessing volume status and measurement of urinary sodium are important when trying to establish a cause (see Tables 10.4, 10.5, and 10.6).

Central pontine myelinolysis typically occurs 1 to 3 days after serum sodium correction. Some patients are more susceptible:

- Alcoholics.
- Malnourishment.
- Burns.
- Elderly females taking thiazide diuretics.
- Hypokalaemia.

Pseudohyponatraemia is due to hyperlipidaemia or hyperproteinaemia and is associated with a normal serum osmolality.

Table 10.4 Euvolaemic hyponatraemia

Clinical signs	Causes (urine sodium >30 mmol/L)
Normal	Psychogenic polydipsia
	Hypotonic fluid replacement
	Syndrome of inappropriate ADH secretion (SIADH)
	Glucocorticoid deficiency
	Hypothyroidism
	Drugs
	– Psychoactive agents, e.g. haloperidol, 'ecstasy'
	– Anti-cancer drugs, e.g. vincristine, cyclophosphamide
	– Carbamazepine, bromocriptine, vasopressin

Treatment

Fluid restriction (<1 L/day)
Demeclocycline (600–1,200 mg/day) for SIADH when fluid restriction alone insufficient

Table 10.5 Hypovolaemic hyponatraemia

Clinical signs	Extrarenal cause (urine sodium <30 mmol/L)	Renal cause (urine sodium >30 mmol/L)
Dry mucous membranes	Vomiting	Diuretics
Reduced skin turgor	Diarrhoea	Salt-wasting nephropathy
Reduced JVP	Fistula	Cerebral salt-wasting syndrome
Tachycardia	Pancreatitis	Mineralocorticoid deficiency
Postural hypotension	Burns	Proximal RTA
	Trauma	Osmotic diuresis (↑ urea, glucose)

Treatment

Volume replacement with intravenous normal (0.9%) saline.
Slow correction of serum sodium concentration reduces the risk of central pontine myelinolysis. Correct at a rate of no greater than 8–12 mmol/day. Requires close monitoring of serum sodium concentration.

RTA, renal tubular acidosis; JVP, jugular venous pressure.

Table 10.6 Hypervolaemic hyponatraemia

Clinical signs	Urine sodium <30 mmol/L	Urine sodium >30 mmol/L
Elevated JVP	Congestive	Chronic renal
Gallop rhythm	cardiac failure	failure
Crepitations on chest auscultation	Liver cirrhosis with ascites	
Ascites	Nephrotic syndrome	
Peripheral oedema		

Treatment
Treat underlying cause
Fluid restriction ± demeclocycline

Syndrome of inappropriate ADH secretion (SIADH)

In SIADH, inappropriately high serum levels of ADH are found and occur independently of serum osmolality (for causes, see Table 10.7). Hyponatraemia results from an excess of water (i.e. dilutional hyponatraemia). SIADH is a diagnosis of exclusion and requires specific clinical and biochemical criteria to be met. Serum sodium should be low (<125 mmol/L) with a decreased serum osmolality <260 mOsm/kg. Urine should be concentrated with high urine sodium concentration (>20 mmol/L) and osmolality (>500 mOsm/kg). Renal, adrenal, and thyroid function should be normal. Diuretic use should also be excluded. Clinical examination confirms the absence of oedema or hypovolaemia.

Treatment

Choice of treatment depends upon the underlying cause, the duration, and the presence of symptoms and clinical signs.

Specific treatments for hyponatraemia are included in Tables 10.4, 10.5, and 10.6. In addition, the pharmacological therapy for SIADH includes demeclocycline (600–1,200 mg/day). Furthermore, many non-peptide vasopressin antagonists have been discovered in the past decade. This group of drugs (the vaptans) may be V_{1a} selective antagonists, V_{1b} selective antagonists, or V_2 selective antagonists. There is also an intravenous dual V_{1a}/V_2 antagonist. The potential benefits of these drugs include the predictability of their effect, rapid onset of action, and limited urinary electrolyte excretion. These medications should be initiated in a closely monitored setting to prevent rapid correction of serum sodium, which can result in central pontine myelinolysis. These agents may also be used in the case of hypervolaemic hyponatraemia.

In acute severe hypernatraemia, e.g. marathon runners, or post-neurosurgery, hypertonic saline may be considered but should be reserved for individuals who have been previously well but are now symptomatic with seizures, coma, or other new focal neurological signs, in association with a serum sodium concentration of 110–120 mmol/L. Administer 3% or 5% saline intravenously, and aim to raise the serum sodium concentration by 10–12 mmol/L per 24 hours. This usually requires management in a critical care environment.

Hypernatraemia

This is observed in approximately 1% of hospital inpatients and often develops after admission.

Symptoms/signs

Symptoms are usually non-specific. Early symptoms include nausea, vomiting, and restlessness. This is followed by lethargy, irritability, confusion, and subsequently coma. Other symptoms include muscle twitching, hyperreflexia, ataxia, tremor, and seizures.

Causes

Hypernatraemia results from either inadequate water intake, excessive salt intake, or a combination of both. Similar to hyponatraemia, volume status should be assessed when trying to establish the underlying cause (see Tables 10.8, 10.9, and 10.10).

Investigations

The initial tests required are listed. Further tests may be required to establish an underlying cause.

1. Renal function.
2. Urine and plasma osmolality.
3. Consider CT or MRI of the brain and adrenal glands.
4. Consider a water deprivation test or a desmopressin test for investigation of diabetes insipidus.

Treatment

Whenever possible, treat with oral fluids, and treat/remove the underlying cause.

Hypernatraemia that has developed over hours can be corrected rapidly (reducing serum sodium concentration by 1 mmol/L per h) with 5% glucose.

Slower correction is required (reduction in serum sodium concentration by 0.5 mmol/L per h) in hypernatraemia of longer duration due to the risk of cerebral oedema.

Potassium

Pathophysiology

Potassium is predominantly an intracellular ion, with only 2% contained within the extracellular fluid. Normally, serum concentration is kept between 3.5 and 5.0 mmol/L. It is obtained in the diet from foods, such as fruits, vegetables, nuts, and meats. Potassium is required by excitable tissues, such as nerve and muscle, to generate an action potential, and Na^+/K^+-ATPase maintains the concentration gradient across the cell membrane. Potassium homeostasis is mainly controlled by aldosterone. About 90% of excess potassium is excreted via the kidneys, with the remainder being excreted through

Table 10.7 Causes of SIADH

Malignancy	CNS disorders	Pulmonary disease	Metabolic disease	Drugs
Small cell lung	Head injury	TB	Porphyria	Opiates
Pancreas	Infections	Pneumonia	Trauma	Psychotrophics
Prostate	Haemorrhage	Abscess		SSRIs
Lymphoma	Stroke	Aspergillosis		Cytotoxics
	Guillain–Barré			
	Vasculitis			

Table 10.8 Euvolaemic hypernatraemia

Clinical signs	Causes
Normal	Cranial diabetes insipidus
	Nephrogenic diabetes insipidus
	Hypodipsia
	Insensible losses—fever, hyperventilation

Treatment

Treat underlying cause

Calculate free water deficit (see Box 10.1)

Best replaced with water orally but consider intravenous 5% dextrose or 0.45% saline

Table 10.9 Hypovolaemic hypernatraemia

Clinical signs	Extrarenal cause	Renal cause
Dry mucous membranes	Vomiting	Loop or osmotic diuretics
Reduced skin turgor	Diarrhoea	Post-obstruction
Reduced JVP	Excessive sweating	Intrinsic renal disease
Tachycardia	Burns	
Postural hypotension	Fistulae	

Treatment

Treat underlying cause

Saline to correct hypovolaemia/hypotension

Calculate free water deficit (see Box 10.1)

Best replaced with water orally, but consider intravenous 5% dextrose or 0.45% saline

Table 10.10 Hypervolaemic hypernatraemia

Clinical signs	Causes
Elevated JVP	Salt ingestion
Gallop rhythm	Iatrogenic (hypertonic saline, sodium bicarbonate, parenteral nutrition, hypertonic dialysate)
Crepitations on chest auscultation	
Ascites	Conn's syndrome
Peripheral oedema	Cushing's syndrome

Treatment

Treat the underlying cause

Combination of 5% dextrose and diuretics

Dialysis may be required if associated with renal failure

the gastrointestinal tract and sweat glands. Within the kidneys, potassium is secreted in the distal tubule and collecting ducts. A rise in extracellular concentrations of potassium stimulates the adrenal cortex to release aldosterone which

---

Box 10.1 Free water deficit

Free water deficit = body weight (kg) × % of total body water (TBW) × ([serum Na/140] – 1)

% of total body water (TBW) is:
- 0.6% for young males
- 0.5% for young females and elderly males
- 0.4% for elderly females

Add a further 900 mL for insensible losses. Total volume is infused over 48 hours.

---

results in increased potassium secretion from the kidneys. The converse applies when extracellular potassium is low.

The transport of potassium into cells and the renal handling of potassium can be affected by other factors. Insulin, adrenaline, aldosterone, and falling pH (due to the presence of non-organic acids) result in increased potassium movement into cells. Aldosterone, glucocorticoids, volume expansion, pH, and diuretics influence renal handling of potassium.

Hyperkalaemia

Urgent treatment is required when the serum potassium is greater than 6.5 mmol/L or for those with ECG changes.

History and clinical signs

Hyperkalaemia is usually asymptomatic and is frequently discovered on routine laboratory tests. Symptoms are non-specific and are predominantly cardiac or neurological. They include muscle weakness and fatigue, palpitations, and paraesthesiae.

Establish, from the history, any predisposing factors which include renal failure (acute or chronic), trauma, including crush injuries or burns, diabetes, adrenal insufficiency, or medications.

Examination is usually normal. Some patients present with arrhythmias or bradycardia due to heart block. There may be muscle weakness, flaccid paralysis, and depressed or absent tendon reflexes. Rarely, examination may reveal hypoventilation due to respiratory muscle weakness or presentation may be with sudden death.

Causes

Hyperkalaemia may be spurious (pseudohyperkalaemia) or can be caused by increased potassium intake, decreased potassium excretion, or potassium shifting from the intracellular to extracellular space.

Investigations

Tests are aimed at identifying an underlying cause or an abnormality which may further predispose to arrhythmia:

1. Recheck the potassium to exclude spurious hyperkalaemia unless it is associated with ECG changes.
2. Urea and creatinine.
3. Glucose.
4. Calcium (hypocalcaemia can increase the risk of arrhythmia).
5. Consider arterial blood gas if acidosis is suspected.
6. ECG. Progressive changes may be observed, paralleling serum potassium levels. Early changes include tall tented T waves, short QT interval, and ST segment depression. This is followed by the development of small P waves, increased PR interval, and wide QRS complexes. Untreated, the QRS complex becomes sinusoidal, followed by ventricular fibrillation or asystole. Many

patients, however, have no ECG changes, while others rapidly progress to life-threatening arrhythmias.

Treatment
Choice of treatment depends upon urgency. Not everyone will need all of the treatments available, for example, patients with mild hyperkalaemia and no ECG changes may only require treatment with a cation exchange resin.
1. Calcium Resonium® (calcium polystyrene sulfonate) 15 g qds orally or 30 g rectally.
   Cation exchange resins can be administered via the oral or rectal route. They act by exchanging potassium for sodium in the extracellular fluid which is then lost via the gut.
2. 20 units soluble insulin + 50 mL 50% glucose intravenously.
3. Nebulized salbutamol 2.5 mg qds.
   Insulin and beta-2 agonists rapidly decrease serum potassium by moving potassium from the extracellular to the intracellular space by stimulating the Na^+/K^+ pump.
4. 10 mL 10% calcium gluconate intravenously over 2 minutes, with continuous ECG monitoring.
   Calcium gluconate does not alter serum potassium levels. It acts by stabilizing the myocardium, allowing time for the other treatments to take effect. ECG changes can be observed after a few minutes, and its effects last for 30 to 60 minutes.
5. Dialysis is required for severe life-threatening hyperkalaemia, unresponsive to medical therapy, or when the underlying cause cannot be corrected without this form of treatment.

Hypokalaemia
Urgent treatment is required if serum potassium levels are less than 2.5 mmol/L.

History and clinical signs
As with hyperkalaemia, these patients are often asymptomatic or symptoms are non-specific and associated with muscle or cardiac function. Muscle weakness can manifest as fatigue, skeletal muscle weakness/paralysis, muscle cramps, abdominal cramps, and constipation. Palpitations may be described.
   Examination is usually normal. There may be arrhythmias, signs of a paralytic ileus, respiratory muscle weakness, decreased muscle strength, hypotonia, fasciculations, tetany, or decreased tendon reflexes.

Causes
Hypokalaemia can be caused by poor intake (uncommon), increased excretion, or potassium movement from the extracellular to the intracellular space (uncommon).
   Vomiting causes hypokalaemia due to a variety of mechanisms. A small amount is lost directly from gastric fluid. Secondary hyperaldosteronism is precipitated by volume depletion, while hydrogen ion loss, and resulting metabolic alkalosis, increases potassium secretion from the distal nephron (in exchange for hydrogen ion uptake).
   Medications which cause hypokalaemia include diuretics, beta-adrenoceptor agonists (e.g. salbutamol), insulin, steroids, theophylline, aminoglycosides, laxative abuse, some penicillins and antifungals, and cisplatin.

Investigations
The initial tests required are listed. Further tests may be required to establish an underlying cause.
1. Urea and creatinine.
2. Glucose.
3. Sodium, calcium, and magnesium.
4. Consider arterial blood gas if alkalosis is suspected.
5. Consider digoxin levels, as hypokalaemia potentiates digoxin toxicity.
6. ECG may show a prolonged PR interval, small or inverted T waves, prominent U wave, ST segment depression, and atrial or ventricular arrhythmias.

Treatment
Therapy depends upon the severity of hypokalaemia. Sometimes, in less severe cases, treatment of the underlying cause is sufficient.
   Mild hypokalaemia (serum potassium >2.5 mmol/L) can be treated with oral potassium supplements.
   Severe hypokalaemia (serum potassium <2.5 mmol/L) is treated with intravenous potassium. This should be administered at a rate not exceeding 20 mmol/h and a concentration not exceeding 40 mmol/L. Rapid rates of infusion can cause hyperkalaemia, with subsequent cardiac arrhythmia and death, while high concentrations can cause local pain and phlebitis.
   As a general rule, potassium should not be administered to oliguric patients.
   Hypokalaemia is often associated with low serum magnesium levels and can be difficult to treat, unless the magnesium has been replaced.

Further reading
Adrogue HJ and Madias NE (2000). Primary care: hypernatremia. *New England Journal of Medicine*, **342**, 1493–9.
Adrogue HJ and Madias NE (2000). Primary care: hyponatremia. *New England Journal of Medicine*, **342**, 1581–9.
Clayton JA, Le Jeune IR, Hall IP (2006). Severe hyponatraemia in medical in-patients: aetiology, assessment and outcome. *QJM*, **99**, 505–11.
Evans KJ and Greenberg A (2005). Hyperkalaemia: a review. *Journal of Intensive Care Medicine*, **20**, 272–90.
Gennari FJ (1998). Current concepts: hypokalaemia. *New England Journal of Medicine*, **339**, 451–8.
Gill G and Leese G (1998). Hyponatraemia: biochemical and clinical perspectives. *Postgraduate Medical Journal*, **74**, 516–23.
Kumar S and Berl T (1998). Sodium. *Lancet*, **352**, 220–8.
National Institute for Health and Care Excellence (2015). Hyponatraemia. Clinical knowledge summaries. <http://cks.nice.org.uk/hyponatraemia>.
Nyirenda MJ, Tang JI, Padfield PL, Seckl JR (2009). Hyperkalaemia. *BMJ*, **339**, b4114.
Reynolds RM, Padfield PL, Seckl JR (2006). Disorders of sodium balance. *BMJ*, **332**, 702–5.
Semenovskaya Z (2013). Hypernatraemia in emergency medicine (at eMedicine). <http://emedicine.medscape.com/article/766683-overview>.
Spasovski G, Vanholder R, Allolio B, et al. (2014). Clinical practice guideline on diagnosis and treatment of hyponatraemia. *European Journal of Endocrinology*, **170**, G1–G47.
UK Renal Association (2014). Treatment of acute hyperkalaemia in adults. Clinical practice guidelines. <http://www.renal.org/guidelines/joint-guidelines/treatment-of-acute-hyperkalaemia-in-adults#sthash.23mylSiq.qTWyVZOP.dpbs>.

Calcium, magnesium, and phosphate metabolism

Calcium

Calcium (Ca^{2+}) is the most abundant mineral in the body, with 98% stored in bone. Plasma Ca^{2+} (normal serum concentration ($[Ca^{2+}]$) range 2.25–2.65 mmol/L) is either bound to albumin ($\pm$ other proteins; ~40%) or anions (e.g. bicarbonate; ~10%) or is in the free ionized form and physiologically active (~50%). It has important roles in muscle contraction and relaxation, regulation of clotting, maintenance of cell membrane integrity, nerve cell transmission, control of cell signalling, stimulation of hormone secretion, maintenance of skeletal, bone, and dental structures and enzyme activity.

Calcium homeostasis

The gastrointestinal tract, bone, and kidneys are the key organs involved in calcium homeostasis, maintaining calcium concentration within a narrow range (i.e. <2% variability). The main calcium regulators are parathyroid hormone (PTH) and 1,25-$(OH)_2$ vitamin D. PTH secretion depends on a critical magnesium concentration, and, consequently, severe hypomagnesaemia may prevent PTH release, even in severe hypocalcaemia.

- The gastrointestinal tract normally absorbs about 40% (i.e. 10 mmol) of the daily dietary calcium intake of 25–30 mmol, but this can be greatly increased if required. Calcium absorption is either active or passive. Active transport is a saturable process, regulated by 1,25-$(OH)_2$ vitamin D. It involves attachment of calcium to calbindin (a calcium-binding protein) and transport by an active Na^+/Ca^{2+}-ATPase and Na^+/Ca^{2+} exchanger. Passive absorption is driven by the concentration gradients between the gut lumen and the serosal surfaces. Calcium absorption can be inhibited by drugs (e.g. theophyllines), citrates, and phytates.
- The renal proximal convoluted tubule (PCT) reabsorbs ~65% of filtered calcium, and this process is closely associated with sodium and water balance, rather than hormonal regulation, whereas PTH regulates the reabsorption of filtered calcium in the loop of Henle (~25%) and the distal convoluted tubule (DCT; ~10%). PTH also stimulates the formation of 1,25-$(OH)_2$ vitamin D in the kidney which increases intestinal calcium and phosphate absorption.
- Bone metabolism is also regulated by PTH and 1,25-$(OH)_2$ vitamin D. Normally formation and resorption are in balance, with no net movement of calcium from bone. Osteoclastic activity and bone resorption are increased by 1,25-$(OH)_2$ vitamin D deficiency and hyperparathyroidism.

Hypocalcaemia

Hypocalcaemia is severe when the serum Ca^{2+} concentration ($[Ca^{2+}]$) is <1.75 mmol/L. Clinical features of hypocalcaemia are determined by the rate of fall and severity of the hypocalcaemia. Hypokalaemia, hypomagnesaemia, and alkalosis often coexist with hypocalcaemia and may worsen the clinical picture. Many patients are completely, or relatively, asymptomatic, but they may also present with acute life-threatening manifestations.

- Acute hypocalcaemia is associated with perioral numbness and paraesthesiae, muscle and abdominal ($\pm$ biliary) cramps, tetany in muscles supplied by long nerves, laryngospasm ($\pm$ bronchospasm), myopathy, seizures, Trousseau's sign (i.e. carpopedal spasm after inflation of

an upper arm blood pressure cuff for 3 minutes), and Chvostek's sign (i.e. facial muscle twitching/spasm on tapping the facial nerve).
- Chronic hypocalcaemia also causes depression, irritability, dementia, movement disorders, papilloedema, prolongation of the QT interval on the ECG, syncope ($\pm$ occasional heart failure or angina), dry/brittle skin, alopecia, rickets, cataracts, and basal ganglia calcification. It may be associated with alkalosis, hypokalaemia, and hypomagnesaemia.

Causes

Causes of hypocalcaemia (see Table 10.11) include:
- **25-$(OH)_2$ vitamin D deficiency:** due to poor intake (e.g. the elderly in nursing homes, vegetarians), lack of sunlight and/or people with more pigmented skin living in temperate climates, anticonvulsants (e.g. phenytoin), and malabsorption of fat-soluble vitamins (e.g. Crohn's disease, chronic pancreatitis, and hepatobiliary disorders). In nephrotic syndrome, loss of vitamin D-binding proteins may cause vitamin D deficiency.
- **1,25-$(OH)_2$ vitamin D deficiency:** is most commonly associated with chronic kidney disease (CKD) with a GFR <30 mL/min or, less commonly, inherited disorders (e.g. vitamin D-dependent rickets types I and II are due to 1-alpha-hydroxylase deficiency and end-organ resistance to 1,25-$(OH)_2$ vitamin D, respectively). It leads to osteomalacia.
- **Acute or chronic kidney disease** impairs renal vitamin D hydroxylation (i.e. formation of 1,25-$(OH)_2$ vitamin D from 25-$(OH)_2$ vitamin D) and promotes phosphate retention which depresses serum Ca^{2+}. Secondary hyperparathyroidism follows, with osteoclast activation and

Table 10.11 Causes of hypocalcaemia

Deficient vitamin D
No sunlight
Malabsorption (e.g. chronic pancreatitis)
Liver/renal disease
Anticonvulsants (e.g. phenytoin)
Genetic syndromes

Ca^{2+} deficiency
Rhabdomyolysis
Recurrent blood transfusions
Pancreatitis
Dietary deficiency

Hypoparathyroidism
Autoimmune
Post-surgery
Infiltrative
Congenital (e.g. parathyroid aplasia)

Hyperphosphataemia
Renal failure
Rhabdomyolysis
Tumour lysis syndrome
Excess administration (e.g. enemas)

Other
Sepsis, burns, critical illness
Hungry bone syndrome
Drugs (e.g. excess bisphosphonate)

characteristic bone and X-ray findings in the hands, skull (i.e. 'pepper-pot'), and spine (i.e. 'rugger jersey'). Treatment is with vitamin D and phosphate binders. If untreated, parathyroid hyperplasia, with autonomous PTH production, causes tertiary hyperparathyroidism and hypercalcaemia.

- **Hyperphosphataemia:** (see section on phosphorus below) due to CKD, rhabdomyolysis, tumour lysis syndrome, or excess phosphate absorption (e.g. enemas).
- **Hypoparathyroidism:** after parathyroid or thyroid surgery, associated with infiltrative disorders, congenital (e.g. parathyroid aplasia), and pseudohyperparathyroidism.
- **Idiopathic autoimmune parathyroid failure:** is rare and associated with vitiligo, parathyroid antibodies, and autoimmune conditions.
- **Other:** severe magnesium deficiency, drugs (e.g. excess bisphosphonates in CKD), acute pancreatitis, sepsis, and burns.

Treatment
Initially, correct the underlying cause. Subsequent treatment depends on the severity, symptoms, and rate of onset of the hypocalcaemia.

- Acute symptomatic hypocalcaemia (i.e. $[Ca^{2+}]$ <1.75 mmol/L) is managed with a 10 mL bolus of intravenous (IV) 10% calcium gluconate, with ECG monitoring. This may be followed by an infusion (i.e. 20 mL 10% calcium gluconate over 6 h) and then oral calcium and vitamin D supplements. Coexisting hypomagnesaemia, hyperphosphataemia, and hypokalaemia should be treated cautiously (see following sections), especially in CKD.
- Chronic hypocalcaemia is treated with vitamin D metabolites (e.g. alfacalcidol) and oral calcium. In CKD, the aim is to prevent metabolic bone disease and vascular mineralization due to secondary hyperparathyroidism by maintaining a normal $[Ca^{2+}]$.

Hypercalcaemia
Hypercalcaemia affects 5–50/10,000 population. It may be mild (2.6–3 mmol/L), moderate (3–3.5 mmol/L), or severe (>3.5 mmol/L). The key factors in diagnosis are parathyroid hormone (PTH) level, clinical picture, and biochemical tests.

Causes
Causes of hypercalcaemia (see Table 10.12) include:

- **Primary hyperparathyroidism**: is the commonest cause of hypercalcaemia (>50%), but 50% are asymptomatic. About 85% of cases are due to a single adenoma; 15% are multiglandular or associated with multiple endocrine neoplasia (MEN; types I and 2a), and ~1% are due to parathyroid carcinoma. The female:male ratio is 2:1, and >90% of patients are >50 years old. PTH is raised. In mild asymptomatic hypercalcaemia, no therapy, other than simple observation, may be required. Definitive treatment involves surgical resection, with the adenoma located by the surgeon during surgery. Post-operative hypocalcaemia is usually transient and treated with calcium supplements and vitamin D.
- **Malignancy.** Hypercalcaemia occurs in ~30% of all cancers (e.g. 35% lung, 25% breast, 14% haematological malignancies (e.g. myeloma)). It is usually due to bony metastases (>75%), and symptoms relate to the cancer and the associated rapid rise in Ca^{2+}. However, hypercalcaemia may also be due to tumour release (e.g. most commonly from squamous cell lung cancer) of PTH-related peptides (PTHrP), which have N-terminals similar to PTH or cytokines (e.g. IL-6,

Table 10.12 Causes of hypercalcaemia

Primary hyperparathyroidism (accounts for >50% of hypercalcaemia)
Adenoma 85%, multiglandular 15%, carcinoma (<1%)

Malignancy (~30% of cancers)
>75% due to bone metastases
Tumour release of parathyroid hormone-related peptide (PTHrP) and cytokines (IL-6, TNF-alpha)
Lymphoma cells may promote 1,25-$(OH)_2$ vitamin D production and associated hypercalcaemia

Endocrine disease
Thyrotoxicosis, acromegaly, Addison's disease

Granulomatous disease
Sarcoidosis, tuberculosis

Drugs
Thiazide diuretics, lithium

Toxicity
Vitamin A toxicity
Vitamin D toxicity
Aluminium toxicity

Other
Tertiary hyperparathyroidism
Immobilization
Milk alkali syndrome
Familial hypocalciuric hypercalcaemia
Parenteral nutrition

TNF). Lymphomas are associated with the production of 1,25-$(OH)_2$ vitamin D from 25-$(OH)_2$ vitamin D, with associated hypercalcaemia. Malignant causes of hypercalcaemia are usually associated with low PTH levels.
- **Sarcoidosis and other granulomatous disease** (e.g. tuberculosis) are associated with steroid-sensitive hypercalcaemia.
- **Other causes** include drugs (e.g. thiazide diuretics, lithium), vitamin A and D toxicity, aluminium toxicity, tertiary hyperparathyroidism due to CKD, endocrine disease (e.g. thyrotoxicosis, Addison's disease, acromegaly), familial hypocalciuric hypercalcaemia, milk alkali syndrome, and immobility.

Clinical features
Presentation depends on $[Ca^{2+}]$ and rapidity of onset. Many cases (~80%) are asymptomatic. Mild and moderate cases experience lethargy, cognitive impairment, depression, nausea, vomiting, abdominal discomfort, constipation, thirst, and polyuria due to calcium-induced nephrogenic diabetes insipidus (DI).

- Acute, severe hypercalcaemia is associated with confusion, drowsiness, and coma. Arrhythmias, hypertension, and acute pancreatitis also occur.
- Chronic hypercalcaemia is associated with renal stone and bone disease.

Management
The decision to treat depends on symptoms, hypercalcaemia severity ($[Ca^{2+}]$ >3 mmol/L), rate of onset, chronicity, and the underlying cause which should be corrected when possible.

- **Acute, symptomatic hypercalcaemia** (i.e. $[Ca^{2+}]$ >3.5 mmol/L) is a medical emergency. Initially, treatment is with aggressive rehydration, using 0.9% normal saline

(2–6 L over 24 h). Loop diuretics are added, following adequate hydration, which reduce $[Ca^{2+}]$ by about a further 0.5 mmol/L. Intravenous bisphosphonates are effective, whatever the cause (e.g. pamidronate 30–90 mg over 2–4 h), but must be used with caution in CRF and may take up to 4 days to achieve normocalcaemia. Persistent or recurrent hypercalcaemia may require repeat bisphosphonate infusions at 3–4 week intervals and risk causing paradoxical hypocalcaemia. Steroids are usually effective in haematological malignancies (e.g. myeloma), granulomatous disorders, and vitamin D-related hypercalcaemia. A 10-day trial of steroid therapy should be considered in these cases. Calcitonin acts within minutes but is only effective for ~48 h due to tachyphylaxis. It may help in Paget's disease.

• **Chronic hypercalcaemia** is managed by ensuring adequate hydration and avoiding thiazide diuretics. Use non-Ca^{2+}-based phosphate binders in CKD and address tertiary hyperparathyroidism (i.e. consider parathyroidectomy or cinacalcet (a drug that reduces PTH)).

Magnesium

Magnesium (Mg^{2+}) is the second most abundant intracellular cation. It is stored mainly in muscle, bone, and soft tissues. Less than 1% is in extracellular fluid (range 0.7–1 mmol/L). About 50% of extracellular Mg^{2+} is in the physiologically active ionized form and ~50% is bound to proteins (mainly albumin) and serum anions (e.g. phosphate, bicarbonate). Mg^{2+} modulates functions dependent on intracellular Ca^{2+} (e.g. muscle contraction, insulin release) and is an essential cofactor in many clotting, neuromuscular, and enzyme (e.g. metalloenzymes, ATP metabolism) systems.

Magnesium balance is regulated by intestinal absorption and renal excretion. Metabolic function is closely linked to Ca^{2+} and phosphate homeostasis. About a third of dietary Mg^{2+} is absorbed (10–15 mmol) daily, mainly in the small intestine, but can increase to >80% in deficient states. The TRPM6 protein cation channel regulates both intestinal and renal tubular Mg^{2+} reabsorption, with mutations causing severe Mg^{2+} and Ca^{2+} deficiency. About 1 mmol Mg^{2+} is secreted into the intestinal lumen daily, and this may increase during diarrhoeal illness, leading to significant losses.

Active and passive renal paracellular transport, partially regulated by ADH, glucagons, and parathyroid hormone, results in reabsorption of >95% of the 100 mmol Mg^{2+} that is filtered by the kidneys daily. About 20% is reabsorbed in the renal PCT, 70% in the thick ascending limb (TAL) of the loop of Henle (inhibited by loop diuretics, osmotic diuresis, hypercalcaemia, and saline infusions), and 10% in the DCT. Magnesium reabsorption can be severely reduced by renal impairment or hypermagnesaemia.

Inherited disorders of magnesium handling are also associated with disturbed Ca^{2+} and Mg^{2+} homeostasis (e.g. TAL transporter mutations (Bartter's syndrome), claudin 16 TAL protein defects (e.g. familial hypomagnesaemia, hypercalciuria, and nephrocalcinosis), and Gitelman's syndrome (i.e. hypomagnesaemia due to an abnormal renal NaCl transporter).

Hypomagnesaemia

Hypomagnesaemia is defined as a serum Mg^{2+} concentration ($[Mg^{2+}]$) <0.7 mmol/L. However, total body Mg^{2+} stores may be depleted by over 20% despite a normal $[Mg^{2+}]$. Routinely measured 'total' Mg^{2+} is affected by serum albumin, and about 50% of extracellular Mg^{2+} is protein-bound. Hypomagnesaemia occurs in the chronically ill, elderly care home residents (~30%), alcoholics (~30%), post-operatively, following ischaemic ventricular tachyarrhythmias, or with refractory hypokalaemia or hypocalcaemia. It may be severe ($[Mg^{2+}]$ <0.5 mmol/L) in ~10% of hospital patients and up to 65% of the critically ill. Table 10.13 lists the causes.

Clinical features

Hypomagnesaemia is associated with hypokalaemia in 60% of cases and hypocalcaemia in 15–50%. It is usually asymptomatic but may cause cardiac, muscular, or neurological dysfunction. Neuromuscular irritability, tremors, hypokalaemia, and hypocalcaemia occur at $[Mg^{2+}]$ of 0.5–0.7 mmol/L, whereas fits, tetany, cardiac arrhythmias, and sudden death are commoner at $[Mg^{2+}]$ <0.5 mmol/L. ECG changes are similar to those in hypokalaemia (i.e. PR interval prolongation, widening of QRS complexes, and ST depression). Magnesium has membrane-stabilizing properties, and some arrhythmias (e.g. atrial/ventricular fibrillation, torsade de pointes) may only respond to magnesium replacement. Other features of low $[Mg^{2+}]$ include hypertension, coronary vasospasm, muscle weakness (including respiratory), confusion, fatigue, vertigo, vertical nystagmus, Wernicke's encephalopathy, and coma.

Treatment

Therapy depends on the underlying cause and the severity of symptoms. If asymptomatic, use oral magnesium ~10–30 mmol/daily in divided doses. In patients with tetany, seizures, or ventricular arrhythmias, give 4–8 mmol intravenously over 10–30 min, with close cardiac monitoring, followed by a 12–90 mmol Mg^{2+} infusion over 24 h to maintain $[Mg^{2+}]$ >0.5 mmol/L. Reduce infusion rates by

Table 10.13 Causes of hypomagnesaemia

Gastrointestinal causes

Malnutrition

Malabsorption syndromes, coeliac disease

Chronic alcoholism

Inflammatory bowel disease

Vomiting, diarrhoea, nasogastric loss

Acute and chronic pancreatitis

Biliary, intestinal fistulae

Small bowel bypass syndrome

Drugs

Thiazide and loop diuretics

Aminoglycosides ($\downarrow Mg^{2+}$, $\downarrow K^+$, $\downarrow Ca^{2+}$ may last weeks)

Ciclosporin

Amphotericin

Pentamidine

Cisplatin ($\downarrow Mg^{2+}$ common)

Renal causes

Diuretic phase of acute tubular necrosis

Post-renal transplantation

Renal tubular acidosis

Tubulointerstitial nephropathies

Post-obstructive diuresis

Diabetic ketoacidosis, diabetes

Hyperthyroidism, hypoparathyroidism

Congenital Mg^{2+} wasting

Other causes

Insulin infusion

Major burns, excessive sweating

Hungry bone syndrome after parathyroidectomy

Inappropriate ADH secretion

~50% in renal impairment, and monitor $[Mg^{2+}]$ more frequently. In severe deficiencies, up to 160 mmol may be required over ~5 days. Treat hypokalaemia and hypocalcaemia, as necessary. Amiloride may help to reduce diuretic-induced and renal Mg^{2+} loss due to nephrotoxicity (e.g. cisplatin) or Bartter's and Gitelman's syndromes.

Hypermagnesaemia

Hypermagnesaemia is defined as a $[Mg^{2+}]$ >1.0 mmol/L and is relatively uncommon (~4–5% of hospital patients). Generally, the kidney excretes 3–5% of filtered Mg^{2+} but can increase this to >95%, if necessary.

Causes

Hypermagnesaemia occurs in acute and chronic renal impairment (GFR <30 mL/min), particularly when Mg^{2+} intake is raised (e.g. laxatives, enemas, antacids, Epsom salts). Hypothyroidism, Addison's disease, rhabdomyolysis, tumour lysis syndrome, lithium therapy, and familial hypocalciuric hypercalcaemia also cause moderate hypermagnesaemia.

Clinical features

Hypermagnesaemia is usually asymptomatic if $[Mg^{2+}]$ is <2.0 mmol/L but causes cardiovascular, metabolic, and neuromuscular toxicity above this. Lethargy, nausea, vomiting, drowsiness, and flushing occur between 2.0 and 2.9 mmol/L; bradycardia, hypotension, ECG changes (widened QRS and prolonged PR/QT intervals), and progressive tendon reflex suppression between 2.9 and 5.0 mmol/L. Coma, apnoea, ventricular arrhythmias, cardiac arrest, and paralysis occur at levels >5 mmol/L. Parasympathetic inhibition with fixed dilated pupils, ileus, urinary retention, complete heart block, and variable degrees of hyperkalaemia and mild hypocalcaemia also occur.

Treatment

In asymptomatic hypermagnesaemia, avoid further administration (e.g. Mg^{2+}-containing laxatives). Patients with cardiovascular toxicity or respiratory depression are given calcium gluconate to antagonize the effects of hypermagnesaemia (10 mL of 10% solution intravenously over 10 min, repeated as necessary). Volume expansion with 0.9% saline will also greatly increase the renal filtrate fractional Mg^{2+} excretion. In renal impairment, dialysis with low Mg^{2+} dialysate will reduce $[Mg^{2+}]$ by up to 50% in 4 h. Monitor serum K^+.

Phosphorus

Phosphate is the most abundant intracellular anion. About 80% is in bone and teeth as hydroxyapatite; ~20% is in viscera and skeletal muscle, and only 0.1% is in the extracellular compartment. Phosphate is essential for adenosine triphosphate (ATP) production and metabolism, oxygen binding to haemoglobin, bone mineralization, buffering, signalling pathways utilizing protein phosphorylation, and as a component of phospholipids, nucleoproteins, and lipid membranes.

Phosphorus is ubiquitous in food, and ~40 mmol is absorbed daily in the upper intestine (mainly by an active, saturatable sodium phosphate (NaPi) cotransporter). Vitamin D directly increases absorption, as do low serum phosphate and raised PTH indirectly through vitamin D. The kidney controls phosphate homeostasis, filtering ~180 mmol/day, with the renal NaPi cotransporters reabsorbing >80–95% in the proximal tubule, as required. Renal dysfunction, PTH, PTH-related peptide (PTHrP), steroids, hypokalaemia, volume expansion, and chronic hypocalcaemia reduce renal reabsorption, causing hypophosphataemia.

Table 10.14 Factors affecting formation and resorption of bone

	Formation	Resorption
Calcium-regulating hormones		
- Parathyroid hormone	↑	↓
- 1,25-$(OH)_2$ vitamin D	↑/↓	↑
- Calcitonin		↓
Systemic hormones		
- Glucocorticoids	↓	↑
- Insulin	↑	
- Growth hormone	↑	
- Growth factor	↑	
- Thyroxine	↑	↑(excess)
Other factors		
Interleukin-1	↑	
Interleukin-6		↓
PTHrP	↑	↑
Prostaglandin E2		↑

Vitamin D, insulin, thyroid and growth hormones, and a high calcium intake stimulate increased renal phosphate reabsorption. Table 10.14 illustrates factors associated with bone formation and resorption.

Hypophosphataemia

The normal serum phosphate concentration ($[PO_4^-]$) is 0.8–1.4 mmol/L. It refers to the inorganic phosphate moiety and varies with age, sex, and intake. A $[PO_4^-]$ <0.3 mmol/L is considered severe hypophosphataemia and is associated with a fourfold increase in mortality. Patients at risk include those with malnutrition, sepsis, trauma, diabetic ketoacidosis, COPD, and alcohol dependency.

Causes

Causes include vitamin D deficiency or resistance, raised PTH (or PTHrP), volume expansion, diuretics or osmotic diuresis, steroid excess, gastrointestinal factors (e.g. malabsorption, prolonged vomiting, phosphate-binding antacids); renal factors (e.g. renal impairment, renal tubular dysfunction (e.g. Fanconi syndrome), and genetic defects (e.g. autosomal dominant hypophosphataemic rickets). Internal redistribution (rather than deficiency) can cause hypophosphataemia in refeeding syndrome, treated diabetic ketoacidosis, respiratory alkalosis, or increased cell turnover (e.g. acute leukaemia).

Clinical features

The clinical features of hypophosphataemia are associated with reduced intracellular ATP and impaired tissue oxygenation (i.e. secondary to an increased affinity of haemoglobin for oxygen which reduces oxygen delivery at the tissue level). Musculoskeletal effects include muscle weakness, osteomalacia with bone pain, proximal myopathy, and diaphragmatic weakness with associated respiratory failure. In acute hypophosphataemia, rhabdomyolysis may occur, particularly in malnourished or alcoholic patients. Cardiac contractility can be reduced and platelet function impaired. Neurological features include paraesthesiae, confusion, metabolic encephalopathy, polyneuropathy (e.g. similar to Guillain–Barré syndrome), seizures, and coma. Renal consequences include glycosuria, hypercalciuria (due to increased bone turnover), increased Mg^{2+} excretion, and hyperchloraemic metabolic acidosis.

Treatment
Therapy depends on the cause and severity. Severe or symptomatic hypophosphataemia often requires treatment, particularly in the critically ill, to improve metabolic function, respiratory muscle strength, and tissue oxygen delivery. Infusions of sodium phosphate 10–20 mmol over 1–2 hours have been shown to be safe in the critically ill. Doses of up to 60 mmol/24 h may be given, but monitor serum $[Ca^{2+}]$, phosphate, K^+, and Mg^{2+} closely to avoid calcium precipitation, hypocalcaemia, fatal arrhythmias, and renal impairment. Consider oral supplementation (~30 mmol/day) when $[PO_4^-]$ >0.6 mmol/L.

Refeeding syndrome
Refeeding syndrome occurs within 3–4 days of restarting feed in malnourished patients. These patients may present with significant intracellular phosphate depletion despite a normal $[PO_4^-]$. The increase in insulin secretion on restarting feeding stimulates glucose, phosphate, K^+, and Mg^{2+} cellular uptake and may cause life-threatening hypophosphataemia (<0.3 mmol/L). Patients may develop symptoms requiring intravenous phosphate replacement at slightly higher phosphate levels (i.e. $[PO_4^-]$ <0.5 mmol/L). Patients at risk of refeeding syndrome include those with no food intake for >10 days, weight loss of >15% over 3–6 months, and a BMI <16–18 kg/m². In those at risk of refeeding syndrome, both oral and intravenous nutrition should start at 5–10 kcal/kg/day and increase slowly over 7 days.

Hyperphosphataemia
Plasma calcium ($[Ca^{2+}]$) and phosphate ($[PO_4^-]$) concentrations are closely correlated. It is usually recommended that $[Ca^{2+}] \times [PO_4^-]$ should be <4.2 mmol²/L².

Causes
Hyperphosphataemia is most common in acute and chronic kidney disease (CKD) and is almost universal with a GFR of <30 mL/min. Other causes are due to release from the intracellular compartment (e.g. rhabdomyolysis, tumour lysis, haemolysis), endocrine (e.g. hypoparathyroidism, acromegaly, thyrotoxicosis, steroid deficiency), excess intake (e.g. absorption of phosphate in enemas, vitamin D intoxication), and miscellaneous (e.g. tumour calcinosis, metabolic or respiratory acidosis).

Clinical features
Hyperphosphataemia has no specific symptoms but may present with features of hypocalcaemia. Elevation of the $[Ca^{2+}] \times [PO_4^-]$ product (i.e. >4.8 mmol²/L²) leads to ectopic calcification in the medial walls of blood vessels (and may occur in the myocardium and heart valves) causing hypertension. Calcium deposition in skin, subcutaneous, and joint tissues can cause painful necrosis. Asymptomatic corneal calcification and conjunctivitis also occur. Secondary hyperparathyroidism follows persistent hyperphosphataemia.

Treatment
Therapy depends on the speed of onset and severity of the hyperphosphataemia.

- *Acute, severe hyperphosphataemia* is potentially life-threatening, especially when associated with significant hypocalcaemia. If renal function is intact, increased phosphate excretion can be achieved with 0.9% normal saline infusion, but monitor for potential hypocalcaemia. Haemodialysis may be required in patients with renal impairment and symptomatic hypocalcaemia.
- *Chronic hyperphosphataemia* is usually associated with CKD (stages 3–5) and requires ongoing therapy. Restrict dietary intake to <1,000 mg phosphate/day and calcium to <2g/day (i.e. renal dietetic involvement). Oral phosphate binders are used to prevent absorption, and the choice is determined by the associated calcium requirements. Measure PTH every 3 months in stage 5 CKD, and aim to keep PTH levels <2–4 times normal. Less frequent measurement is required in stages 3 and 4 of CKD.

Further reading

Baker SB and Worthley LIG (2002). The essentials of calcium, magnesium and phosphate metabolism: Parts 1 and 2. *Critical Care and Resuscitation*, **4**, 301–15.

Body J and Boullon R (2003). Emergencies in calcium homeostasis. *Reviews in Endocrine and Metabolic Disorders*, **4**, 167–75.

Brunelli SM and Goldfarb S (2007). Hypophosphataemia: clinical consequences and management. *Journal of the American Society of Nephrology*, **18**, 1999–2003.

Davison AM, Cameron JS, Grunfeld J-P, et al. (2005). Hypo-, hypercalcaemia. In *Oxford textbook of clinical nephrology*, Vol 1, pp. 269–86. Oxford University Press, Oxford.

Davison AM, Cameron JS, Grunfeld J-P, et al. (2005). Hypo-, hypermagnesaemia. In *Oxford textbook of clinical nephrology*, Vol 1, pp. 309–19. Oxford University Press, Oxford.

Fulop T (2013). Hypomagnesaemia. <http://www.emedicine.com/emerg/topic274.htm>.

Gaasbeek A and Meinders E (2005). Hypophosphataemia: an update on its aetiology and treatment. *American Journal of Medicine*, **118**, 1094–101.

Geerse DA, Bindels AJ, Kuiper MA, Roos AN, P Spronk PE, Schultz MJ (2010). Treatment of hypophosphatemia in the intensive care unit: a review. *Critical Care*, **14**, R147.

Ketteler M (2009). The control of hyperphosphatemia in chronic kidney disease: which phosphate binder? *International Journal of Artificial Organs*, **32**, 95–100.

National Kidney Foundation: K/DOQI clinical practice guidelines for bone metabolism and disease in chronic kidney disease. <http://www.kidney.org/professionals/kdoqi/guidelines_bone/index.htm>.

The Renal Association. Clinical Practice Guidelines (2007). <http://www.renal.org/guidelines/index.html>.

Topf JM and Murray PT (2003). Hypomagnesaemia and hypermagnesaemia. *Reviews in Endocrine and Metabolic Disorders*, **4**, 195–206.

Acid-base balance

Introduction

Maintenance of a stable hydrogen ion (H$^+$) concentration ([H$^+$]) at ~35–45 nmol/L or pH 7.35–7.45 is essential for organ function, cellular metabolism, and, in particular, intracellular enzyme action. Normally, acids are generated by:

- **Metabolic processes.** These 'metabolic' or non-volatile acids include phosphoric or sulphuric acid from protein metabolism and breakdown, and lactic acid from anaerobic glucose metabolism.
- **Hydration of carbon dioxide (CO$_2$).** The volatile 'respiratory acids' (i.e. carbonic acid) are generated mainly from the aerobic metabolism of carbohydrate, the end result of which is the production of CO$_2$ and water.

The normal requirement for H$^+$ excretion is 70–100 mmol daily. This is derived from food breakdown (i.e. the dietary acid load) and partly from the end-products of the metabolism of endogenous body tissues. During starvation, the exogenous dietary acid load is reduced, but the endogenous tissue metabolic acid load increases by an equal, or greater amount due to catabolism.

Acid-base homeostasis is achieved by the integration of several physiological processes, including intracellular/ extracellular buffering and renal/respiratory compensatory mechanisms. Overall control of the homeostasis of acid-base status and acid excretion is dependent largely on the kidneys, which also reclaim filtered bicarbonate. The respiratory system acts as a temporary physiological buffer, in which the lungs facilitate CO$_2$ excretion.

The most important buffer at physiological pH (7.4) is bicarbonate (see section on control of acid-base balance).

Most changes in bicarbonate are the result of metabolic processes, whereas those of CO$_2$ concentration are due to respiratory (ventilatory) adjustments. Respiratory causes of acid-base disturbance are compensated/corrected by the kidneys, whilst metabolic causes are compensated/corrected by lung ventilatory adaptations.

In disease states, [H$^+$] can rise due to lactate production (e.g. ischaemia), ketoacid generation (e.g. diabetes), alcohol ingestion (e.g. methanol), or failure of normal excretion (e.g. renal, respiratory, or liver failure). Loss of H$^+$ (e.g. vomiting) or bicarbonate (HCO$_3^-$; e.g. diarrhoea) also has profound effects on acid-base balance.

Control of acid-base balance

The body prevents pH changes by regulating two pathways for eliminating acid: respiratory and renal. However, ~100 times more acid equivalents are expired each day in the form of CO$_2$/carbonic acid than are excreted as fixed acids by the kidneys.

Intracellular and extracellular buffers attenuate the changes that could occur, with retention of either acids or bases. These buffers bind to, or release, H$^+$, according to the pH, and limit the change in pH that would occur when an acid or a base is added. The relationship between the amount of acid added to a buffer-containing solution and the change in pH is described visually by the buffer line (see Figure 10.1).

The major buffer systems comprise:

- A base (H$^+$ acceptor). This is predominantly bicarbonate (HCO$_3^-$).
- An acid (H$^+$ donor). This is predominantly carbonic acid.

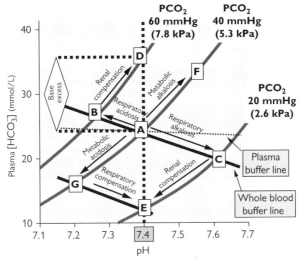

Figure 10.1 The relationship between pH, HCO$_3^-$, and PCO$_2$. The line BAC is the **buffer line** for whole blood; changes in PCO$_2$ alter HCO$_3^-$ and pH along this line. Point A represents normal conditions (pH 7.4, HCO$_3^-$ 24 mmol/L, PCO$_2$ 5.3 kPa). An acute rise in PCO$_2$ (e.g. hypoventilation) decreases the HCO$_3^-$:PCO$_2$ ratio and hence pH. This **respiratory acidosis** is represented by a move from A to B. A to C represents a **respiratory alkalosis** (e.g. hyperventilation). Sustained respiratory acidosis (e.g. chronic respiratory failure) is compensated for by renal HCO$_3^-$ reabsorption and H$^+$ excretion. The HCO$_3^-$:PCO$_2$ ratio is restored, and pH returns to normal. This **renal compensation** is described by the arrow B to D. Conversely, a respiratory alkalosis may be compensated for by increased renal excretion of HCO$_3^-$ (C to E). **Metabolic acidosis** (G) may be partially compensated by increased ventilation and a reduction in PCO$_2$ (G to E). There is little respiratory compensation of **metabolic alkalosis** (F). Reproduced from Jeremy P.T. Ward et al., The Respiratory System at a Glance, Third Edition, Wiley, Copyright 2009, with permission.

The bicarbonate buffer system

Carbonic anhydrase

$$CO_2 + H_2O \leftrightarrow H_2CO_3 \leftrightarrow HCO_3^- + H^+$$

The Henderson–Hasselbach equation

$\rightarrow$ $K = [HCO_3^-] \times [H^+] / [H_2CO_3]$

From the law of mass action
K = dissociation constant

$\rightarrow$ $K_A = [HCO_3^-] \times [H^+] / [H_2CO_3]$

At equilibrium $[CO_2] \propto [H_2CO_3]$
K_A = corrected dissociation constant

$\rightarrow$ $\log K_A = \log [H^+] + \log ([HCO_3^-] / [CO_2])$

$\rightarrow$ $-\log [H^+] = -\log K_A + \log ([HCO_3^-] / [CO_2])$

$\rightarrow$ $pH = pK_A + \log ([HCO_3^-] / [CO_2])$

(Henderson–Hasselbach equation)

Figure 10.2 The bicarbonate buffer system and the Henderson–Hasselbach equation.

Following addition or generation of an acid or alkali, buffer systems attenuate the change in pH but do not remove the underlying acid/alkali from the body; this is achieved by the kidneys or lungs. Buffers are most effective when the pH of the environment in which they are acting is close to their pK_A (log of the dissociation constant K_A).

Physiological buffer systems include:

1. **Bicarbonate.** This is the most important plasma and extracellular buffer system in man. The regulation of PCO_2 by the respiratory system and the control of the bicarbonate concentration ($[HCO_3^-]$) by the kidney constitute the regulatory processes that together act with the other buffer systems to control pH.

   HCO_3^- accepts H^+ to form carbonic acid (H_2CO_3), thus mopping up free H^+. This prevents an increase in $[H^+]$ and the associated acidosis/fall in pH. The H_2CO_3 slowly dissociates into CO_2 and water. This reaction is catalysed by carbonic anhydrase. The addition of an acid to the buffer system leads to the conversion of bicarbonate to CO_2, and, subsequently, for the pH to be maintained, CO_2 must be removed by the lungs.

   This relationship between pH, PCO_2, and $[HCO_3^-]$ is described by the Henderson–Hasselbach equation (see Figure 10.2). In order for acid-base homeostasis to be maintained, the correct ratio of $[HCO_3^-]$ to PCO_2 (~5:1) is needed. In normal blood, $[HCO_3^-]$ is 24 mmol/L, $PaCO_2$ 5.3 kPa, and pH calculates to 7.4. Although the pK_A of the bicarbonate system (6.1) is further away from the blood pH (7.4) than would appear ideal for a buffer, the fact that PCO_2 and HCO_3^- can be independently controlled by ventilation and the kidneys, respectively, means that, in practice, it makes an effective buffer system.

2. **Haemoglobin (Hb)** is an effective buffer, particularly when deoxygenated. The red blood cell buffering system acts a temporary aid to HCO_3^- replenishment. It significantly improves the buffering capacity in whole blood when compared with plasma. Other blood proteins have <20% of the buffering capacity of Hb.

3. **Organophosphate complexes.**

4. **Bone apatite.**

The respiratory system in acid-base balance

The respiratory system (i.e. lungs) regulates the elimination of CO_2 produced by metabolism. The CO_2 generated in the tissues passes into red blood cells, which are rich in carbonic anhydrase, down a concentration gradient and combines with water to form carbonic acid. The carbonic acid (H_2CO_3) dissociates into HCO_3^- and H^+. The H^+ are buffered by anion sites (replacing Na^+) on reduced haemoglobin (Hb) to form HHb. The HCO_3^- passes back into the plasma in exchange for chloride (Cl^-; a process termed the chloride shift), restoring plasma $[HCO_3^-]$. In the lungs, the process is reversed, and H^+ bound to Hb recombines with HCO_3^- to form water and CO_2 which diffuses into the alveoli and is breathed out as expired gas. This process reduces the plasma HCO_3^- again.

Note that, in this process, the red cells act as a temporary buffering system between the tissues and the lungs, acting as a 'sink' for H^+, which would otherwise limit the buffering capacity of HCO_3^- (because it would run out). The restoration and regeneration of HCO_3^- occurs mainly in the kidneys.

Metabolic acidosis (due to an increase in non-volatile acids) lowers pH and $[HCO_3^-]$ which stimulates ventilation, increasing alveolar ventilation and lowering $PaCO_2$. A mixed respiratory-metabolic acid-base disorder should be suspected when $PaCO_2$ is too high or too low for a given abnormal serum $[HCO_3^-]$.

Respiratory compensation does not usually correct pH completely, and the kidneys provide the principal route for excretion of non-volatile acids.

The kidneys in acid-base balance

The role of the kidneys in acid-base balance includes:

- Excretion of H^+ buffered by phosphate (i.e. the dihydrogen phosphate/monohydrogen phosphate buffer pair) or ammonia (i.e. the ammonia/ammonium buffer pair) in the renal tubule (see further text).
- Reclamation of large quantities of filtered HCO_3^-.
- Regeneration of the HCO_3^- used in the buffering of volatile (i.e. the kidney makes HCO_3^- to compensate for HCO_3^- lost as CO_2 through the lungs) and non-volatile acids.

The kidneys reabsorb ~97% of the ~4,000 mmol HCO_3^- that is filtered by the kidneys daily. About 70–80% is reabsorbed in the proximal convoluted tubule (PCT) and the remainder in the thick ascending limb (TAL) of the loop of Henle (10–20%), with a minor amount taken up in the distal convoluted tubule (DCT; ~5%). In the PCT, H^+ is excreted

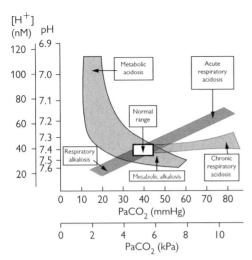

[H⁺] (nM) pH

Figure 10.3 Flenley acid-base nomogram. Reproduced from Richard M. Leach, Acute and Critical Care Medicine at a Glance, second edition, Figure d, Chapter 18, page 44, Wiley, Copyright 2009, with permission.

by the Na^+/H^+ exchanger into the lumen where it combines with filtered HCO_3^- to form H_2CO_3 (see Figure 10.4). Carbonic anhydrase in the luminal brush border catalyses dissociation into water (which is excreted in the urine) and CO_2 which diffuses back into the tubular cell. In the tubular cell, the CO_2 combines with hydroxyl ions (OH^-) to form HCO_3^- (see Figure 10.4) and diffuses back into the extracellular fluid. This HCO_3^- reclamation process prevents excessive loss of HCO_3^- but does not excrete acid. Reabsorption is influenced by pH, PCO_2, and peritubular [HCO_3^-] such that a raised $PaCO_2$ or potassium depletion stimulate HCO_3^- reabsorption, whereas hypocapnia, PTH, and phosphate depletion inhibit reabsorption. A decrease in extracellular volume enhances HCO_3^- reabsorption and vice versa.

The kidneys must excrete the H^+ produced from the dissociation of H_2CO_3. These excreted H^+ are bound in the renal tubule by urinary buffers, including phosphate (~50%) and ammonia (~50%), before being excreted. Only a very small amount of free H^+ is excreted in the urine. Phosphate buffers are responsible for excretion of ~20–30 mmol of H^+ daily, a process limited by the fixed amount of phosphate that is filtered into the renal tubule. Ammonia, generated in the renal tubule from glutamine and other amino acids, buffers a further 20–40 mmol of H^+ daily (to form ammonium). Net H^+ excretion in the DCT is affected by the electrical gradient in the tubule cells/renal lumen, with Na^+ reabsorption enhancing H^+ secretion. Aldosterone and other buffers (e.g. phosphate) enhance this effect.

Depending on the acid load that needs to be excreted, urine pH can vary from about 4.5 to 8. The PCT and DCT can maintain pH gradients of 1 and 3 units, respectively, resulting in a minimum urine pH (i.e. maximum acidity) of ~4.5. This acidification process is impaired in distal renal tubular acidosis.

Disorders of acid-base balance

Disturbances of acid-base balance are due to:

- Production or retention of an excess of H^+ (acidosis).
- Retention of HCO_3^- (alkalosis).

If these processes are severe, the following may occur:

- An increase in arterial [H^+] (acidaemia; blood pH <7.35).
- A reduction in arterial [H^+] (alkalaemia: blood pH >7.45).

These disturbances are due to respiratory (i.e. altered ventilation changing $PaCO_2$) or metabolic causes.

The relationship between pH, HCO_3^-, and PCO_2 is illustrated using Davenport diagrams (see Figure 10.1). Sudden, acute CO_2 changes cause respiratory acidosis or alkalosis. When CO_2 changes persist (e.g. type 2 respiratory failure in COPD), pH is slowly corrected by renal compensation (i.e. increased [HCO_3^-]). Metabolic acidosis and alkalosis describe the changes in acid-base status due to altered HCO_3^-, rather than CO_2, for example, as a result of renal disease or increased H^+ production (e.g. diabetic ketoacidosis). A metabolic acidosis can be partially compensated by an increase in ventilation. However, there may be relatively little respiratory compensation for a metabolic alkalosis, as this may require unsustainable reductions in ventilation. Mixed metabolic and respiratory acid-base disorders can occur. For example, respiratory acidosis due to respiratory failure (i.e.

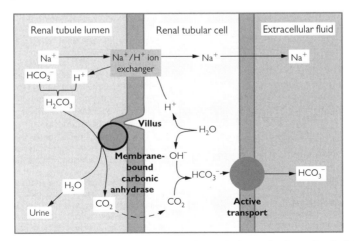

Figure 10.4 Reclamation of HCO3– is driven by the Na+/H+ exchanger in the proximal convoluted tubule and by the proton pump in the distal tubule. There is no net loss of H+ in this process.

increased $PaCO_2$) may be combined with a metabolic acidosis due to the associated hypoxaemia and resulting tissue lactic acidosis. The Flenley nomogram (see Figure 10.3) is a useful and simple diagnostic aid to determine the type of acidosis (i.e. metabolic, respiratory), as only one type of disturbance is likely if pH and PCO_2 fall within a specific band.

Metabolic acidosis

Metabolic acidosis is associated with a low arterial pH (i.e. acidaemia), reduced serum $[HCO_3^-]$, and reduced PCO_2 due to the associated increase in alveolar ventilation.

The causes of metabolic acidosis (see Table 10.15) include:

- Impaired excretion of the daily dietary H^+ load:
  Renal impairment (GFR <15–20 mL/min).
  Type 1 (distal) and type 4 renal tubular acidosis (RTA).
- Excessive loss of renal or gastrointestinal (GI) tract HCO_3^-:
  Renal (acetazolamide (carbonic anhydrase inhibitors); type 2 (proximal) RTA).
  GI tract (pancreatic/biliary fistulae, diarrhoea, urinary-GI tract fistulae).
- Increased acid (H^+) production:
  Lactic acidosis (anaerobic metabolism).
  Ketoacidosis (diabetic or alcohol excess).
  Poisoning (e.g. salicylate, iron, ethylene glycol, paraldehyde, methanol).
  Inborn errors of metabolism (e.g. propionic aciduria).

Table 10.15 Disorders of acid-base balance

1. Metabolic acidosis

Normal anion gap (= hyperchloraemic acidosis)
- Renal HCO_3^- loss: proximal RTA, tubular damage (e.g. heavy metals)
- Loss of HCO_3^- from the gut: diarrhoea, ileostomy, hyperparathyroidism
- Decreased renal H^+ secretion: distal RTA, hypoaldosteronism

Increased anion gap; organic acid accumulation
- Lactic acidosis: type A (sepsis, cardiac arrest, hypotension, methanol), type B (insulin deficiency, metformin, decreased hepatic metabolism)
- Ketoacidosis: insulin deficiency (e.g. diabetic ketoacidosis), starvation
- Exogenous acids: salicylates

2. Metabolic alkalosis
- H^+ loss: vomiting, renal loss (with hypokalaemia, hyperaldosteronism), diuretics, low Cl^- states
- HCO_3^- gain: sodium HCO_3^- (excess antacid), lactate, citrate administration

3. Respiratory acidosis
- Airways obstruction, pneumonia, ARDS, pulmonary oedema
- Respiratory muscle weakness: myasthenia, Guillain–Barré, polio
- Trauma: flail segment, lung contusion
- Respiratory depression: head trauma, opiates

4. Respiratory alkalosis
- High levels of anxiety or pain
- Altitude
- Excessive mechanical ventilation
- Respiratory stimulants: salicylate overdose
- Pulmonary embolism, asthma, oedema

HCO_3^-, bicarbonate; H^+, hydrogen ion; RTA, renal tubular acidosis; Cl^-, chloride; ARDS, acute respiratory distress syndrome.

Clinical features

The symptoms and signs associated with metabolic acidosis depend on the rate and size of the pH reduction and the underlying cause:

- Cardiovascular: tachycardia/bradycardia, impaired cardiac contractility, with hypotension and heart failure, arrhythmias, and chest pain.
- Respiratory: hyperventilation, Kussmaul ventilation.
- Gastrointestinal: diarrhoea, nausea and vomiting, abdominal pain, and gastric distension.
- Neurological: confusion, progressing to coma.
- Bone: increased osteoclast function, decreased osteoblast function, PTH secretion, and hypercalciuria.
- Nutritional: insulin resistance and protein catabolism.
- Metabolic: natriuresis, leucocytosis, systemic inflammation and leucocytosis.

Evaluation

1. Initially, measure the blood pH on an arterial blood gas to confirm the acidosis, and determine the effect of respiratory compensation.
2. Then determine the anion gap ($Na^+ - (HCO_3^- + Cl^-)$; range 10–20 mmol/L). The anion gap will either be normal due to the presence of an acid in which the anion is chloride (i.e. hyperchloraemic metabolic acidosis; e.g. diarrhoea, pancreatic fistulae, ileal conduit, toluene, RTA types 1, 2, and 4) or high due to the presence of an acid in which the anion is not chloride (e.g. diabetic ketoacidosis, starvation, lactic acidosis, toxins like ethylene glycol or methanol, and renal failure).
3. Further investigations to define the cause include urea and electrolytes, full blood count, blood glucose, liver function tests, plasma lactate, laboratory measured (e.g. freezing point depression osmometer) plasma osmolality (mOsm/kg) or calculated plasma osmolarity ($2 \times (Na^+)$ + glucose + urea (all in mmol/L) mOsm/L), urine pH, toxin assays, plasma lactate, cultures, and imaging, as appropriate.
4. Serum osmolal gap (the difference between measured osmolality and calculated osmolality) is normally <10 mOsm/kg. An increased gap indicates the presence of additional osmotically active solutes not taken into account in the calculated osmolality. A gap >10 mOsm/kg occurs in ketoacidosis and lactic acidosis and, if associated with an increased anion gap (= $([Na^+] + [K^+]) - ([Cl^-] + [HCO_3^-])$; normal range 8–16 mEq/L), raises the possibility of methanol or ethylene glycol ingestion (although ethanol also causes an increase). In general, an osmolal gap >25 mOsm/kg, with a high anion gap metabolic acidosis in the absence of diabetic ketoacidosis or lactic acidosis, requires treatment for methanol/ethylene glycol intoxication with an ethanol infusion whilst awaiting results of toxicology studies.

Treatment in metabolic acidosis

Patients with metabolic acidosis are often very unwell, and severe metabolic acidosis should be managed in a critical care unit, in liaison with a toxicology service when appropriate.

The underlying cause of the acidosis must be established and treated. In diabetic ketoacidosis, administer fluids, electrolyte replacement, and insulin. Correct hypovolaemia with fluid resuscitation in lactic acidosis. Some toxins require specific therapies. For example, ethanol is used in methanol or ethylene glycol poisoning, and/or haemodialysis is required in salicylate, methanol, ethylene glycol, and lithium poisoning. Haemodialysis may be required in renal failure.

Use of sodium bicarbonate infusions in metabolic acidosis is controversial. It can be associated with a variety of complications, including hypernatraemia, hypokalaemia, hypocalcaemia, and volume overload. However, it should be given in:

- Methanol or ethylene glycol poisoning to maintain pH >7.2.
- Salicylate poisoning to maintain blood pH >7.4 to promote renal excretion of salicylate and to reduce salicylate penetration into tissues.

Renal tubular acidosis

The hallmark of renal tubular acidosis (RTA) is a hyperchloraemic, normal anion gap metabolic acidosis. It results from a defect in tubular function that reduces HCO_3^- reabsorption or net tubular H^+ secretion. There are three main types (Type 3 is rarely used as a classification as it is thought to be a combination of types 1 and 2):

- **Type 1** (distal): is primarily due to failure of acid secretion by the distal tubule and collecting duct. The resulting systemic acidosis is more severe than in type 2 or 4 RTA. It may be familial, genetic (e.g. Ehlers–Danlos syndrome), immunological (e.g. SLE, primary biliary cirrhosis), or due to hyperparathyroidism or drugs (e.g. lithium). Serum potassium and bicarbonate are low and chloride high. Urine pH is >5.5, and the fractional bicarbonate excretion is >5%. It is associated with nephrocalcinosis, rickets, and osteomalacia. Response to treatment (i.e. high fluid intake with oral bicarbonate (1–2 mmol/kg) and potassium supplements (usually as potassium bicarbonate)), is good.
- **Type 2** (proximal): is due to the failure of the proximal tubule to reabsorb filtered bicarbonate. It may be familial or associated with inherited systemic diseases (e.g. Fanconi-like syndromes, galactosaemia), hyperparathyroidism, drugs (e.g. lead poisoning, gentamicin), multiple myeloma, amyloidosis, and nephrotic syndrome. Serum potassium is low or normal, bicarbonate low, and chloride high. Urine pH is <5.5 (as the distal tubules can still acidify the urine), and the fractional bicarbonate excretion is >10–15%. It is associated with rickets, osteomalacia, nephrolithiasis, and hypercalciuria. Response to treatment (i.e. oral bicarbonate (10–15 mmol/kg) and potassium supplements (usually as potassium bicarbonate) and a thiazide diuretic) is moderate.
- **Type 4**: is due to a lack of aldosterone which reduces potassium and hydrogen ion secretion (i.e. it is not a primary tubular disorder). It may be associated with hyper-reninaemic hypoaldosteronism (e.g. Addison's disease, drugs (e.g. angiotensin-converting enzyme (ACE) inhibitors), congenital adrenal hyperplasia), hypo-reninaemic hypoaldosteronism (e.g. diabetes, drugs (e.g. NSAID), gout, interstitial nephritis), drugs (e.g. spironolactone, amiloride), or distal tubular dysfunction. Serum potassium is high, bicarbonate low, and chloride high. Urine pH is <5.5 or >5.5, and the fractional bicarbonate excretion is >5–10%. It is associated with hypercalciuria, but nephrolithiasis does not occur. Response to treatment is poor and is mainly aimed at controlling the hyperkalaemia with a loop diuretic. In most cases mineralocorticoid supplementation is also required.

Metabolic alkalosis

Metabolic alkalosis is characterized by an arterial blood pH >7.45 (alkalaemia), increased serum $[HCO_3^-]$, and an increased $PaCO_2$ due to respiratory compensation. Often the clinical consequences are related to coexisting problems like hypovolaemia, hypokalaemia, hypophosphataemia, chloride depletion, and reduced ionized calcium concentration.

The causes of metabolic alkalosis (see Table 10.15) include:

- **Exogenous alkali administration:**
  Antacids, milk alkali syndrome.
  Sodium bicarbonate, acetate, or citrate administration.
  Gluconate administration.
  Massive blood transfusion.
- **Accumulation of HCO_3^- due to excessive loss of H^+ (acid):**
  Gastrointestinal loss (e.g. vomiting, NG tube loss, laxatives).
  Renal loss (e.g. diuretics, steroid excess, hypercalcaemia, Mg^{2+} deficiency).
- **H^+ redistribution into cells/HCO_3^- retention:**
  Hypokalaemia.

Clinical features

The systemic features associated with metabolic alkalosis are:

- Cardiovascular: impaired cardiac contractility, arrhythmias, vasodilation.
- Respiratory: hypoventilation, impaired distal oxygen unloading/delivery (i.e. oxygen dissociation curve shifted to the left).
- Nervous system: neuromuscular excitability, confusion, lethargy, seizures (due to reduced cerebral blood flow).
- Renal: increased tubular reabsorption of calcium.

Evaluation

The diagnosis is made, following biochemical investigation, but may be suspected on the basis of the clinical and drug history and the physical features, including the presence of hypertension.

Routine investigations should include arterial blood gas analysis (i.e. to confirm the alkalaemia and to exclude respiratory acidosis as a cause for the high serum $[HCO_3^-]$), serum urea, electrolytes, creatinine, chloride, and bicarbonate. Urine sodium, chloride, potassium, and pH should be measured and the ECG reviewed.

Specific investigations include serum cortisol and ACTH concentrations; plasma renin activity, aldosterone concentrations, and toxicology for laxatives and diuretics.

Diagnosis can be determined by assessing whether the metabolic alkalosis is:

- **Chloride-sensitive alkalosis,** i.e. urine chloride <10 mmol/L.

  In normotensive patients with a low urine chloride, the alkalosis is likely to be due to diuretics, potassium deficiency, diarrhoea, vomiting (or nasogastric fluid loss), and non-absorbable antacid ingestion.
- **Chloride-resistant alkalosis,** i.e. urine chloride >20 mmol/L.

  In normotensive or hypotensive patients, likely causes for the alkalosis include severe potassium or magnesium deficiency, diuretics, and Bartter's or Gitelman's syndromes.

In hypertensive patients, the likely causes include primary hyperaldosteronism (Conn's syndrome), Cushing's syndrome, mineralocorticoid excess, renin-producing tumours, and congenital adrenal hyperplasia.

Treatment of metabolic alkalosis
Initial management requires identification and treatment of the underlying cause which is partly determined by whether it is a chloride-sensitive or resistant metabolic alkalosis. Particular attention should be paid to correcting hypovolaemia and hypochloraemia. Severe metabolic alkalaemia (pH 7.6), especially if associated with fluid overload, may require haemodialysis or haemofiltration.

- ***Chloride-sensitive alkalosis***, with a low urinary chloride <10 mmol/L, suggests significant renal chloride reabsorption and an associated cause. Volume-depleted patients should be treated with 0.9% normal saline until urinary chloride is >25 mmol/L and the urine pH has returned to normal. Associated hypokalaemia should be corrected with potassium supplements. If the patient is oedematous, 0.9% normal saline should not be given, and the alkalosis should be corrected with potassium-sparing diuretics (e.g. spironolactone, amiloride) or carbonic anhydrase inhibitors (e.g. acetazolamide).
- ***Chloride-resistant alkalosis***, with a urinary chloride >20 mmol/L, suggests a chloride-resistant cause that is unlikely to respond to volume expansion. In these cases, the treatment will depend on the underlying cause (e.g. primary hyperaldosteronism may be treated with aldosterone antagonists, adrenal adenomas with surgery).

Respiratory acidosis
Respiratory acidosis is associated with a low arterial blood pH (<7.35), elevated $PaCO_2$ (hypercapnia), and a normal or increased serum $[HCO_3^-]$ due to renal compensation.

Respiratory acidosis usually occurs when there is alveolar hypoventilation, which lowers the HCO_3^-/PCO_2 ratio and blood pH, or when there is an imbalance between the production of PCO_2 by the tissues and elimination by the lungs. It may be acute, as occurs in sudden ventilatory failure, or chronic, as in chronic obstructive pulmonary disease (COPD).

The causes of respiratory acidosis (see Table 10.15) include:

- Severe pulmonary disease:
  COPD, emphysema, asthma.
  Pulmonary oedema, ARDS.
  Interstitial lung disease, pneumoconiosis.
  Aspiration, laryngospasm, bronchitis, infection.
  Chest trauma with flail chest, haemothorax.
  Inadequate mechanical ventilation.
- Neuromuscular disease with respiratory muscle fatigue:
  Multiple sclerosis, myopathy, poliomyelitis.
  Myasthenia gravis, Guillain–Barré syndrome.
  Diaphragmatic paralysis, muscle relaxant drugs.
  Tetanus, toxins (e.g. snakebites).
- Central nervous system diseases that suppress the respiratory control centre and ventilatory drive:
  Strokes, CNS haemorrhage, trauma, tumours.
  Drugs (e.g. opioids, sedatives, alcohol, anaesthetics).
  CNS infection, encephalitis.
  Primary alveolar hypoventilation.

- Other causes:
  Obesity hypoventilation syndrome.
  Cervical spinal cord lesions.
  Cardiac arrest with cerebral hypoxia.

Clinical features
Severity of hypoxaemia, the underlying cause, and the duration determine the clinical features associated with respiratory acidosis. Following immediate cellular buffering in acute respiratory acidosis, renal compensation raises serum $[HCO_3^-]$ over a period of 3–4 days, during which time renal HCO_3^- reabsorption and H^+ secretion are increased. The acidosis increases ionized calcium levels and causes an extracellular shift of potassium, although both these effects are relatively minor.

- Acute-onset hypercapnia is often associated with anxiety, confusion, hallucinations, reduced tendon reflexes, and psychosis. If severe it may cause coma, seizures, and death.
- Chronic hypercapnia symptoms are usually less severe and associated with daytime sleepiness, headaches (due to the vasodilator effects of CO_2), memory impairment, and motor effects, including tremor and myoclonic jerks.
- Cardiac effects include vasodilation with warm, flushed skin, bounding pulses, sweating, systemic hypotension, cor pulmonale, arrhythmias, peripheral oedema, and renal impairment.
- In renal failure, mixed acid-base abnormalities may occur.

Evaluation
A good history, careful examination, and arterial blood gas analysis to confirm the acidosis and exclude metabolic alkalosis as the cause of the high HCO_3^- are the best aid to diagnosis of respiratory acidosis. The pH on arterial blood gases may be normal in chronic conditions and haemoglobin raised (polycythaemia) on the full blood count. Electrolytes, renal function, bicarbonate, drug screens, lung function tests, chest X-rays, and other chest and brain imaging (e.g. CT scans, MRI) may help to confirm the underlying cause.

Treatment of respiratory acidosis
Treatment depends on the underlying cause, the speed of onset, and the severity. The aim is to restore adequate alveolar ventilation which may require non-invasive or mechanical ventilation. In chronic lung conditions, smoking cessation, bronchodilators, inhaled steroids, and diuretics may be necessary.

In ~10% of COPD patients, normal CO_2-mediated ventilatory drive is impaired, and, in these cases, caution must be taken to avoid excessive oxygen therapy which may reduce alveolar ventilation, increase CO_2 retention, and cause potentially harmful deterioration of the respiratory acidosis.

Rapid correction of chronic hypercapnia and the associated compensated respiratory acidosis may precipitate arrhythmias and seizures (due to reduced cerebral perfusion).

Respiratory alkalosis
Respiratory alkalosis is associated with a high arterial blood pH (<7.45), reduced $PaCO_2$ (hypocapnia), and a normal or reduced serum $[HCO_3^-]$ due to renal compensation.

Respiratory alkalosis occurs when there is alveolar hyperventilation, which increases the HCO_3^-/PCO_2 ratio and blood pH, or when there is an imbalance between the production of PCO_2 by the tissues and elimination by the lungs (e.g. hyperventilation syndrome with excessive ventilation and normal CO_2 production). It is commonly associated with mechanical ventilation, many cardiopulmonary disorders, and, in the critically ill, it tends to be associated with a worse prognosis, particularly if severe.

Within hours, acute respiratory alkalosis is associated with increased bicarbonate excretion and reduced renal acid secretion. In chronic hypocapnia, the serum $[HCO_3^-]$ rarely falls below ~12 mmol/L.

The causes of respiratory alkalosis (see Table 10.15) include:

- Hypoxaemia:
  Pneumonia, pulmonary oedema, high altitude, severe anaemia, cardiac shunts, ARDS.
- Drugs:
  Salicylates, methylxanthines, nicotine.
- Central nervous system diseases that stimulate the respiratory control centre and ventilatory drive:
  Pain, anxiety, psychological.
  Fever, meningitis, encephalitis.
  Strokes, trauma, tumour, head injury.
  Endogenous compounds (e.g. chronic liver disease, toxins, sepsis (cytokines), progesterone in pregnancy).
- Pulmonary causes:
  Pneumonia, pneumothorax, pulmonary embolism, pulmonary oedema, ARDS, interstitial lung disease.
- Other causes:
  Mechanical ventilation.
  Septicaemia, thyrotoxicosis, hyperthermia.

Clinical features
The clinical features depend on severity, duration, and underlying cause.

- Cardiovascular effects. Reduced cardiac contractility occurs in hypocapnia but has minimal effect in well, awake patients but may be significant in mechanically ventilated or anaesthetized patients (i.e. due to the associated effects of sedation and anaesthetic drugs on the circulation). Arrhythmias are more common in patients with ischaemic heart disease due to impaired tissue oxygen delivery caused by the left shift of the oxygen dissociation curve.
- Cerebral effects. Acute hypocapnia may cause cerebral vasoconstriction, leading to reduced blood flow and a variety of symptoms, including perioral paraesthesiae, carpopedal spasm, seizures, syncope, dizziness, and confusion.

- Respiratory alkalosis reduces ionized calcium and causes an intracellular shift of potassium and phosphate, but these effects are rarely significant.

Evaluation
A good history, careful examination, and arterial blood gas analysis (to confirm the alkalosis and exclude metabolic acidosis) aid diagnosis. Electrolytes, renal function, bicarbonate, drug screens, chest X-rays, and additional imaging (e.g. CT scans, MRI), as required, may help to confirm the underlying cause.

In suspected hyperventilation syndrome, pulmonary embolism, ischaemic heart disease, and hyperthyroidism should be excluded.

Treatment of respiratory acidosis
Treatment should focus on determining and alleviating the underlying cause, as respiratory alkalosis is rarely serious.

Hyperventilation syndrome is frequently managed with breathing techniques and by encouraging the patient to rebreathe from a paper bag which provides reassurance and emphasizes the psychological nature of the condition.

Further reading
Dublin A, Menises MM, Masevicius FD, *et al.* (2007). Comparison of three different methods of evaluation of metabolic acid-base disorders. *Critical Care Medicine*, **35**, 1264–70.

Figge J, Jabor A, Kazda A, Fenci V (1998). Anion gap and hypoalbuminaemia. *Critical Care Medicine*, **26**, 1807–10.

Gluck SL (1998). Acid-base. *Lancet*, **352**, 9126.

Hood VL and Tannen RL (1998). Mechanisms of disease: protection of acid-base balance by pH regulation of acid production. *New England Journal of Medicine*, **339**, 819–26.

Kopple JD, Kalantar-Zadeh K, Mehrotra R (2005). Risks of chronic metabolic acidosis in patients with chronic kidney disease. *Kidney International*, **67**, 521–7.

Kraut JA and Kurtz I (2001). Use of base in the treatment of severe acidaemic states. *American Journal of Kidney Diseases*, **38**, 703–27.

Morgan TJ (2004). What exactly is the strong anion gap and does anybody care? *Critical Care and Resuscitation*, **6**, 155–9.

National Kidney Foundation: K/DOQI clinical practice guidelines for bone metabolism and disease in chronic kidney disease. <http://www.kidney.org/professionals/kdoqi/guidelines_bone/index.htm>.

The Renal Association. Clinical practice guidelines (2007). <http://www.renal.org/guidelines/index.html>.

Wagner CA, Kovacikova J, Stehberger PA, Winter C, Benabbas C, Mohebbi N (2006). Renal acid-base transport: old and new players. *Nephron Physiology*, **103**, 1–6.

Thyroid emergencies

Thyrotoxic crisis

Thyrotoxic crisis or storm is the most severe form of hyperthyroidism with a significant mortality rate. Although serum thyroid hormone concentrations are usually markedly elevated, there is no biochemical threshold for making the diagnosis which depends upon clinical judgement and is, therefore, subjective. Affected patients invariably have Graves' disease, an autoimmune disease, due to the development of cross-reacting, thyroid-stimulating autoantibodies. The cause is unclear but is thought to involve a combination of genetic and environmental factors. The associated hyperthyroidism in Graves' disease is more marked than in patients with nodular thyroid disease. Given the current ready access to accurate tests of thyroid function and, therefore, earlier diagnosis of thyroid dysfunction, thyrotoxic crisis is a rare condition and might be seen by an endocrinologist in a large centre once every 5 years or so. In the past, thyrotoxic crisis would be precipitated by an infection or trauma in a patient with long-standing severe, poorly controlled or unrecognized hyperthyroidism. Now it is more likely to develop within hours of thyroid surgery or days of iodine-131 therapy in a patient with Graves' disease with a large vascular goitre due to release of preformed thyroid hormone by manual handling or radiation-induced thyroiditis, respectively. In both situations, the patient will have been poorly controlled with antithyroid drugs beforehand.

Clinical features

There is likely to be a large goitre with an overlying bruit and bilateral exophthalmos, but these features may be absent, particularly in older patients. There is pyrexia, usually in excess of 39°C, with profuse sweating. Characteristically, the patient is agitated and tremulous, and there may be confusion and even psychosis. Reduced conscious level and coma are poor prognostic signs.

There is a sinus tachycardia (130–140 beats per minute), with a raised systolic blood pressure of around 160 mmHg due to increased cardiac output and a reduced diastolic pressure of approximately 70 mmHg due to peripheral vasodilatation with a resultant full volume and, occasionally, collapsing pulse. If there has been a significant reduction in intravascular volume due to the salt and water depletion of excessive perspiration, there may be hypotension. In patients over the age of 40, there may be atrial fibrillation, with an uncontrolled ventricular rate of 150–160 beats per minute, associated with cardiac failure. There is marked proximal muscle weakness and difficulty in swallowing due to weakness of the bulbar muscles.

Investigations

Serum concentrations of thyroid hormones are usually markedly elevated, e.g. free T4 of greater than 60 pmol/L (normal 10–23) and total T3 of more than 10 nmol/L (normal 1.0–2.4). Serum TSH concentration is undetectable and the TSH receptor antibody in patients with Graves' disease is usually significantly elevated. Liver function tests are frequently deranged as a consequence not only of the hyperthyroidism, but also from the hepatic congestion of cardiac failure and/or infection. Serum calcium concentration may be slightly elevated at 2.7–2.9 mmol/L as a consequence of dehydration. There may be modest hyperglycaemia due to increased glycogenolysis and an elevated white blood cell count, even in the absence of infection.

Treatment

Supportive

It is essential that the patient with thyrotoxic crisis is managed in a monitored bed, preferably in an intensive care area. Salt and water depletion will necessitate intravenous fluid replacement. In the absence of recent surgery or iodine-131 therapy, it should be assumed that there is underlying infection and empirical treatment given with a broad-spectrum antibiotic. Cardiac failure should be treated initially with intravenous furosemide 80 mg.

Reducing the tachycardia

A beta-adrenoceptor antagonist, such as propranolol, should be given in a dose of 80 mg orally every 4–6 hours. A significant reduction in tachycardia will be evident within 12–24 hours. More rapid reduction in heart rate can be achieved with propranolol 1 mg intravenously over 10–15 minutes and repeated every 4 hours until oral propranolol is effective or can be initiated.

In the presence of atrial fibrillation, digoxin is unlikely to be effective. There is not only reduced sensitivity of the heart to digoxin in hyperthyroidism, but also increased renal clearance.

Reducing thyroid hormone concentrations

Although propranolol, but not other beta-adrenoceptor antagonists, inhibits the peripheral conversion of T4 (thyroxine) to T3 (triiodothyronine), with a rise in the serum concentration of a metabolically inactive reverse T3, the changes are minor and confer no clinical benefit. Carbimazole, its active metabolite, methimazole, and propylthiouracil (PTU) act by inhibiting thyroid hormone synthesis. Carbimazole should be given in a high dose of 40 mg 12-hourly. No intravenous preparation is available, but the drug has been shown to be effectively absorbed if given rectally. The dose of PTU is ten times that of carbimazole. It has the theoretical, if not necessarily practical, advantage of inhibiting, to some extent, the peripheral conversion of thyroxine (T4) to triiodothyronine (T3). Antithyroid drugs take 10–14 days to begin to affect serum thyroid hormone concentrations. In the interim, it is important to inhibit the release of stored thyroid hormones with potassium iodide 60 mg 8-hourly orally or Lugol's solution (iodine 5%, potassium iodide 10%, in purified water, freshly boiled and cooled and, therefore, not immediately available) in a dose of 0.1–0.3 mL three times daily, well diluted with milk or water. It is important that no iodine is administered for at least 1 hour after the first dose of carbimazole, as the excess iodine will increase thyroid hormone synthesis in the absence of the inhibiting antithyroid drug. This combination of carbimazole or PTU and potassium iodide leads to a significant reduction in thyroid hormone concentrations at 5–7 days.

The most effective treatment in the days before antithyroid drugs are effective is the oral cholecystographic agent iopanoic acid. This has the dual role of inhibiting thyroid hormone release and conversion of thyroxine to triiodothyronine, resulting in a reduction of serum T3 concentrations by 70% within 48 hours. The dose of iopanoic acid is 500 mg twice daily. It should not be given for more than 14 days because of the likelihood of worsening hyperthyroidism in the longer term. Unfortunately, iopanoic acid is not widely available.

Antithyroid drugs and potassium iodide are of no value in the patient who develops a thyrotoxic crisis within hours or days of surgery, or in the patient receiving iodine-131 therapy for Graves' disease, as the worsening hyperthyroidism is due to the release of preformed thyroid hormones. In addition to supportive measures and in the absence of iopanoic acid, the only effective treatment is with a beta-adrenoceptor antagonist, such as propranolol. Fortunately, in these situations, the severe hyperthyroidism is relatively short-lived, lasting 2–3 days.

Amiodarone-induced thyrotoxic crisis

The commonest cause of thyrotoxic crisis currently is probably the result of amiodarone therapy for cardiac dysrhythmias in patients with unrecognized underlying Graves' disease or nodular thyroid disease. By taking amiodarone, the patient is effectively consuming large amounts of iodine which, as one of the building blocks of thyroid hormones, results in severe hyperthyroidism which is difficult to control (type I amiodarone-induced hyperthyroidism). As amiodarone is stored in fat, hyperthyroidism may develop many months after the drug has been withdrawn. Most patients in iodine-replete areas of the world, in whom hyperthyroidism is induced by amiodarone, do not develop thyrotoxic crisis.

In areas of iodine deficiency, however, severe hyperthyroidism is not uncommon. Treatment with carbimazole alone is not usually effective and should be combined with potassium perchlorate, a competitive inhibitor of thyroid iodine transport, in an initial dose of 200 mg three times a day. Amiodarone may also cause a destructive thyroiditis (type II amiodarone-induced hyperthyroidism), with release of preformed thyroid hormones. It may be difficult to distinguish between these two types, and indeed they may coexist. The pragmatic approach, therefore, is to add to the antithyroid drugs prednisolone, which inhibits the thyroiditis, in a dose of 30 mg daily for 2 weeks, gradually withdrawing over a period of 3 months.

Myxoedema coma

This is an increasingly rare condition, given the low threshold in primary care for requesting thyroid function tests for non-specific complaints, such as tiredness, with the detection of thyroid failure early in its development. Myxoedema coma is best considered as the most severe form of hypothyroidism, in which there is type II respiratory failure with hypoxia and CO_2 narcosis, leading to confusion, somnolence, and ultimately coma. There is a decreased hypoxic respiratory drive and a decreased ventilatory response to hypercapnia, but reduced lung volumes due to obesity, ascites, and pleural effusions contribute to the impaired respiratory effort. Sedation and significant hyponatraemia due to water intoxication contribute to the reduced level of consciousness.

It is important to recognize that coma in a patient with hypothyroidism may not be a consequence of the degree of thyroid failure, but the result of an unrelated condition, such as cerebral haemorrhage or encephalitis.

Clinical features

The characteristic features of severe hypothyroidism will be present, such as dry and flaky skin, non-pitting oedema of periorbital tissues, hands, and feet, erythema abigne, macroglossia, delayed relaxation phase of the tendon jerks, and loss of body hair. Hypothermia is constant, and the core temperature is usually less than 34°C. There is sinus bradycardia, hypotension, and infrequently cardiac failure. Ascites and pleural effusions are well recognized. The presence of a thyroidectomy scar is invaluable in differentiating between primary and secondary hypothyroidism before thyroid function tests are available.

Investigations

There will be a low serum free T4 concentration <5 pmol/L and a raised serum TSH concentration at >50 mU/L. Measurement of serum T3 concentration should not be requested, as it is an inaccurate indicator of hypothyroidism. In the rare secondary form of hypothyroidism due to pituitary or hypothalamic disease, serum free T4 concentration is undetectable, but serum TSH may be low, normal, or slightly elevated in the range of 5–8 mU/L.

Hypoventilation leads to a type II pattern of respiratory failure, with a typically low PO_2 of around 5–6 kPa and raised PCO_2 of 10 kPa. Chest X-ray may reveal pleural effusions, cardiomegaly due to a combination of dilatation and pericardial effusion, and pneumonia as the precipitating event. ECG may reveal a sinus bradycardia with low voltage complexes.

Serum sodium concentration is likely <130 mmol/L and often below 120 mmol/L. Other non-specific abnormalities which may be present include a normochromic, macrocytic anaemia which may, or may not, be due to pernicious anaemia, reduced eGFR, raised serum creatine kinase, and hypercholesterolaemia.

Treatment

Supportive

The patient with myxoedema coma requires assisted ventilation in an intensive care area. Hyponatraemia is due to water intoxication, and it is important that fluid replacement with 0.9% saline and 5% glucose is managed carefully. Intravenous furosemide will promote proportionately greater loss of water and sodium and should be given as a single bolus of 40 mg intravenously. The temperature will begin to rise within 3–4 hours of initiating triiodothyronine therapy, and aggressive rewarming in the interim should be avoided, as it may provoke vasodilatation and hypotension. Underlying infection should be assumed, usually respiratory or urinary tract, and a broad-spectrum antibiotic administered intravenously.

Thyroid hormone replacement

There are no infallible guidelines for the form or speed of thyroid hormone replacement. In the UK, levothyroxine is not available for intravenous administration. It is customary, therefore, to give triiodothyronine 10–20 mcg (20 mcg per vial) intravenously, followed by 10 mcg intravenously every 6–8 hours for 48 hours. At this stage, it should be possible to change to oral replacement with levothyroxine in a dose of 50 mcg daily, increasing after 2 weeks to 100 mcg daily. Retesting thyroid function some 6–8 weeks later is needed before making further minor adjustments to the dose of thyroxine, such that free thyroxine is in the upper part of its reference range, and TSH in the lower part of its reference range. More aggressive initial replacement, especially in the elderly who may have concomitant and significant ischaemic heart disease, runs the risk of precipitating ventricular fibrillation.

Hydrocortisone

Treating a patient with myxoedema coma due to pituitary or hypothalamic disease with thyroid hormones alone is likely to lead to a fatal outcome. In the absence of thyroid function test results, unless there is a thyroidectomy scar or unequivocal evidence of previous treatment with iodine-131, it is essential that hydrocortisone is given in a dose of 100 mg 8-hourly intravenously at the same time as treatment is started with triiodothyronine.

Non-thyroidal illness

Thyroid function tests may be altered in non-thyroidal illness and mimic biochemical hyperthyroidism. Several mechanisms are involved and include:

- Suppression of TSH release due to increased concentrations of dopamine, cytokines, cortisol, and somatostatin.
- Reduction in the extrathyroidal conversion of T4 to T3, also a feature of treatment with amiodarone.
- Displacement of thyroid hormones from plasma proteins by drugs, such as furosemide in the management of cardiac failure.
- Changes in the affinity characteristics and in the serum concentrations of thyroid hormone-binding proteins and methodological problems associated with free T3 and T4 measurements.

The finding of a suppressed serum TSH with a raised free T4 of 25–40 pmol/L is not an uncommon finding in patients with significant non-thyroidal illness, such as atrial fibrillation and cardiac failure. Indeed, in a large series of hospitalized patients, a low serum TSH concentration was three times as likely to be due to non-thyroidal illness as to hyperthyroidism. In most patients with significant non-thyroidal illness, serum total T3 will be low normal but, if in the upper part of the reference range, may be due to a fall from a previously elevated concentration in a patient with hyperthyroidism due to impaired T4 to T3 conversion. In this situation, measurement of the TSH receptor antibody and isotope imaging may be helpful in detecting Graves' disease or impalpable nodular thyroid disease. If doubt remains, a trial of antithyroid drugs for a period of 3–6 months may be indicated.

However, in the absence of clinical pointers to hyperthyroidism, such as goitre, ophthalmopathy, or unexplained atrial fibrillation, the wisest course is not to measure thyroid function tests, as an abnormal result may lead to inappropriate therapy. If they are measured, no action should be taken and the tests repeated some 6–8 weeks later. At that stage, during recovery from the non-thyroidal illness, serum TSH may be transiently elevated.

Further reading

Bahn RS, Burch HB, Cooper DS, et al. (2011). Hyperthyroidism and other causes of thyrotoxicosis: management guidelines of the American Thyroid Association and American Association of Clinical Endocrinologists. *Thyroid*, **21**, 593–646.

Beckett GJ and Toft AD (2008). Thyroid dysfunction. In WJ Marshall, SK Bangert, eds. *Clinical biochemistry. Metabolic and clinical aspects*, pp 394–421. Churchill Livingstone Elsevier, Philadelphia.

Bogazzi F, Bartalena L, Cosci C, et al. (2003). Treatment of type II amiodarone-induced thyrotoxicosis by either iopanoic acid or glucocorticoids: a prospective randomized study. *Journal of Clinical Endocrinology and Metabolism*, **88**, 1999–2002.

Franklyn JA, Boelaert K (2012). Thyrotoxicosis. *Lancet*, **379**, 1155–1166.

Garber JR, Cobin RH, Gharib H, et al. (2012). Clinical practice guidelines for hypothyroidism in adults: co-sponsored by the American Association of Clinical Endocrinologists and the American Thyroid Association. *Endocrine Practice*, **18**, 988–1028.

Martino E, Lombardi-Aghini F, Mariotti S, et al. (1986). Treatment of amiodarone associated thyrotoxicosis by simultaneous administration of potassium perchlorate and methimazole. *Journal of Endocrinological Investigation*, **9**, 201–6.

National Institute for Health and Care Excellence (2011). Hypothyroidism. Clinical knowledge summaries. <http://cks.nice.org.uk/hypothyroidism>.

National Institute for Health and Care Excellence (2013). Hyperthyroidism. Clinical knowledge summaries. <http://cks.nice.org.uk/hyperthyroidism>.

Spencer C, Eigen A, Shen D, et al. (1987). Specificity of sensitive assays for thyrotropin (TSH) used to screen for thyroid disease in hospitalized patients. *Clinical Chemistry*, **33**, 1391–6.

Pituitary emergencies

Pituitary emergencies are rare. The most important condition for acute care physicians is pituitary apoplexy, with its clinical similarities to the more commonly encountered subarachnoid haemorrhage and meningitis. Prompt administration of glucocorticoids to a patient with pituitary apoplexy may be lifesaving.

Pituitary apoplexy

Definition
Pituitary apoplexy is defined as acute haemorrhage into, or ischaemic infarction of, a pituitary tumour. It may occur in people with previously diagnosed or undiagnosed pituitary macroadenomas.

Incidence
Acute apoplexy occurs in up to 5% of those requiring surgery for a pituitary adenoma. However, subclinical pituitary tumour haemorrhage is common and found in 25% of surgical specimens from patients without clinical features of apoplexy.

Causes and risk factors
The main risk factor for apoplexy is the presence of a pituitary adenoma whose abnormal structure and vascular supply predispose to spontaneous haemorrhage or infarction.
Reported additional risk factors include:
• Sudden head trauma.
• Hypertension.
• Diabetes mellitus.
• Bleeding disorders.
• Anticoagulants.
• Cardiac surgery.
• Oestrogens.
• Dopamine agonists (bromocriptine or cabergoline).
• Pituitary function testing with TRH (thyrotropin-releasing hormone) or GnRH (gonadotropin-releasing hormone).
• Pituitary radiotherapy.

Clinical features
First described in 1898, Brougham described the characteristic syndrome in a series of five patients in 1950 and coined the term pituitary apoplexy. Typically, the patient experiences sudden onset of headache (may be thunderclap in type), vomiting, visual disturbance (loss of vision or visual field loss), ophthalmoplegia, and altered consciousness. Series of more than ten patients are unusual, but the clinical features of 143 patients from four recent UK series are summarized in Figure 10.5, and two illustrative cases are shown in Figures 10.6 and 10.7.
Assessment of patients with features consistent with pituitary apoplexy should include an endocrine history to reveal possible symptoms of hypopituitarism (e.g. amenorrhoea, impotence) or excessive hormone secretion (e.g. growth hormone producing acral enlargement). A full physical examination should include cranial nerves and visual fields by confrontation.

Differential diagnosis
The sudden onset of headache may lead to confusion with subarachnoid haemorrhage (see Box 10.2). The presence of neck stiffness and fever may suggest meningitis. It should be noted that adrenal insufficiency due to ACTH hyposecretion is not usually associated with significant hypotension, as is common in primary adrenal failure.

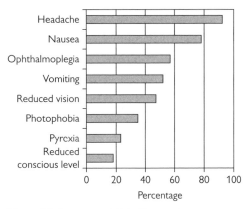

Figure 10.5 Frequency of clinical features in acute pituitary tumour apoplexy. Data derived from Ayuk et al. 2004, Gruber et al. 2006, Randeva et al. 1999, and Sibal et al. 2004.

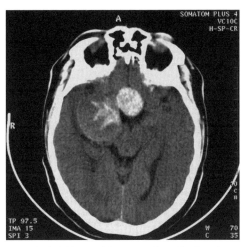

Figure 10.6 A 30-year-old man on cabergoline for a large prolactinoma presented acutely with frontal headache, vomiting, and loss of vision in one eye. Emergency non-contrast-enhanced cranial CT showed high signal (arrow) within the suprasellar extension of his tumour, diagnostic of acute haemorrhage.

Investigations
Urgent blood samples should be drawn for electrolytes, renal function, liver function tests, clotting screen, full blood count, free T4, TSH, and random cortisol. Urgent CT scan will usually identify a pituitary mass and evidence of haemorrhage (either within the mass or in the subarachnoid spaces). If a pituitary mass is confirmed, MRI should be performed for better delineation of the local structures, particularly the optic pathways. Lumbar puncture (if performed) often shows red blood cells, caused by the tumour haemorrhage rupturing into the subarachnoid space.

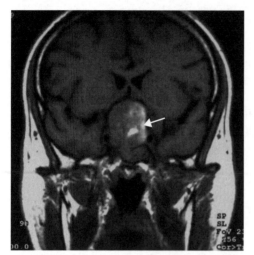

Figure 10.7 A 50-year-old man presented as a medical emergency with headache, vomiting, reduced conscious level, meningism, and visual disturbance. MRI revealed a heterogeneous and previously unsuspected pituitary mass (arrow)—histology confirmed infarction and haemorrhage within a pituitary adenoma. He responded well to surgical decompression but has needed long-term pituitary hormone replacement therapies.

Management

Early referral should be made to a multidisciplinary neuroendocrine team, including experts in neurosurgery, endocrinology, and ophthalmology.

Indications for empirical steroid therapy include haemodynamic instability, altered conscious level, reduced visual acuity, and visual field loss. Patients with pituitary apoplexy without the above indications, but with serum cortisol <600 nmol/L, should also receive steroid support. Appropriate therapy is with either hydrocortisone (100 mg IV stat, followed by 50 mg tds, then tapered) or dexamethasone (10 mg IV stat, followed by 4 mg tds, then tapered).

Intravenous fluids should be administered cautiously; pituitary hypothyroidism impairs the ability to excrete a water load. Diabetes insipidus should be excluded but is rare in pituitary apoplexy.

Box 10.2 Clinical scenario

Emergency medical admission with . . .
- Thunderclap headache
- Vomiting
- Meningism
- Visual impairment
- Diplopia
- Reduced conscious level
- Haemorrhage on CT brain (± blood in CSF)

Ask. . . could this be pituitary apoplexy, rather than aneurysmal SAH?
Is there a pituitary mass on scan?
If yes:
- Check urgent serum cortisol
- Start hydrocortisone replacement
- Urgent referral to specialist neuroendocrine team
- Request MRI pituitary

The decision to manage conservatively or to intervene with surgical decompression (usually transsphenoidal) should be made by the specialist pituitary team. Early surgery (usually within a week) is recommended for severe visual disability or for deteriorating vision. A conservative course may be recommended for those patients without neuro-ophthalmic signs or with mild/stable signs. Daily monitoring of visual acuity and visual fields plus general neurological status is essential.

Outcome

Visual deficits improve in the majority of patients after surgical decompression, although complete blindness in one or both eyes is less likely to reverse. Minor visual dysfunction may recover in patients treated conservatively (tumour shrinkage often being demonstrable on MRI scans 3–6 months after the acute event). Some patients will have permanent hormonal deficits after pituitary apoplexy, but all should be re-evaluated by an endocrinologist 6–8 weeks after the event. Some endocrine deficits recover when the normal pituitary is decompressed (after either surgical or conservative treatments).

Acute hypopituitarism in a patient with a previously normal pituitary gland

Acute or subacute hypopituitarism may occur in a patient with a normal pituitary gland if there is disruption of its fragile blood supply or if there is pituitary haemorrhage due to a coagulopathy. The following clinical situations warrant consideration of hypopituitarism.

Post-partum haemorrhage

Significant hypotension due to post-partum haemorrhage may lead to infarction of the hyperplastic pituitary in a pregnant woman (Sheehan's syndrome). The incidence of this complication has fallen with improved standards of obstetric care, but the condition remains an important cause of endocrine morbidity and mortality in the developing world.

Head trauma

A major shear force due to head trauma may disrupt the vascular and neural connections between the brain and the pituitary gland. Anterior hypopituitarism of all grades may result. Diabetes insipidus is common but usually transient.

Disseminated intravascular coagulation (DIC)

DIC is a complication of severe underlying illness (particularly sepsis, trauma, and extensive surgery) that produces both thrombosis and haemorrhage. Pituitary haemorrhage may result in hypopituitarism.

Venomous snakebite

Some snakebites produce a coagulopathy similar to DIC, and victims may develop pituitary haemorrhage. Hypopituitarism is not uncommon in survivors of Russell's viper envenomation in India and South East Asia.

Clinical features

There are usually no diagnostic clinical features in patients with recent-onset anterior hypopituitarism, so a high level of clinical suspicion should be maintained. However, excess thirst and the production of large volumes of dilute urine in a head injury patient suggest the possibility of cranial diabetes insipidus.

Investigations

Urgent blood samples should be drawn for electrolytes, glucose, random cortisol, and thyroid profile.

Interpretation

If a patient judged to be at risk of hypopituitarism is severely unwell and the serum cortisol level is <600 nmol/L, steroid replacement should be given without delay (see next section). Definitive endocrine diagnosis can be delayed until after recovery. If serum cortisol is >600 nmol/L, the patient does not require steroid support, but ongoing cortisol monitoring every 1–2 days should be undertaken. It should be remembered that the thyroid profile of any acutely ill patient is likely to reflect the adaptations seen in non-thyroidal illness (typically, low free T3, low free T4, and variable TSH)—such a profile does not require immediate thyroid hormone replacement. Similarly, gonadotrophins may be downregulated and prolactin elevated due to non-endocrine factors in acute illness.

Management of a patient with known hypopituitarism during acute intercurrent illness

Patients with known hypopituitarism (usually a result of previous treatment for a pituitary adenoma) may develop unrelated acute illnesses, and questions frequently arise about appropriate hormone replacement protocols, particularly if the patient is unable to take medications by mouth.

Corticosteroids

Most patients will be on routine treatment with oral hydrocortisone, 15–30 mg daily, in divided doses. In the acute setting, a stat IV dose of 100 mg should be administered, followed by 50 mg tds IV. The dose can be reduced as the patient recovers, but, if there is ongoing illness-related stress, a dose of 20 mg tds (IV or oral) can be maintained.

Thyroid hormones

Levothyroxine has a half-life of 1 week, so there is no concern if a patient misses medication for 2–3 days. Crushed T4 tablets can be administered via a nasogastric tube in usual dosage. Parenteral T3 administration is rarely necessary.

Growth hormone and sex steroids

These should be stopped temporarily during severe intercurrent illness.

Vasopressin

Most patients on routine treatment for cranial diabetes insipidus will be taking either intranasal (10–20 mcg bd) or oral (100–200 mcg tds) desmopressin. This can be exchanged for 1–2 mcg, twice daily intravenously during intercurrent illness.

Fluids

Patients with inadequately replaced cortisol and thyroid hormone deficiencies are less able to excrete a water load. Particular care with intravenous fluids is, therefore, required in sick patients with hypopituitarism. Careful fluid balance and daily monitoring of electrolytes is essential.

Pituitary emergencies after elective pituitary surgery

Patients may present as acute medical emergencies during the early weeks after pituitary tumour surgery. Urgent input from the neuroendocrine MDT is recommended in all cases.

SIADH

Transient diabetes insipidus is common during the early days after surgery for pituitary adenoma (both transsphenoidal and transcranial). In some patients, this is followed,

1–2 weeks later, by release of endogenous vasopressin from damaged hypothalamo-neurohypophyseal neurones, resulting in water retention and acute symptomatic hyponatraemia. Patients are euvolemic and should be treated with fluid restriction. Any treatment with desmopressin should be withdrawn, at least, temporarily.

Cerebral salt wasting (CSW)

SIADH should be distinguished from cerebral salt wasting, a much less common condition that may also occur in the first few weeks after pituitary surgery. Blood and urine chemistries are similar in the two conditions, but CSW is distinguished by clinical evidence of hypovolemia (particularly hypotension) and should be treated with intravenous saline.

CSF rhinorrhoea

CSF leakage is a recognized complication of transsphenoidal pituitary surgery. The amount of CSF loss is rarely excessive, but the leak usually needs surgical correction to prevent ascending infection. CSF glucose level is similar to blood glucose, and this helps to distinguish CSF from secretions originating from the nasal passages. Early neurosurgical consultation is essential.

Meningitis

Any patient presenting with headache, fever, and meningism shortly after pituitary surgery should be fully evaluated for bacterial meningitis.

Pituitary situations that are not true emergencies

The following are not true emergencies but do warrant prompt neuroendocrine referral.

Visual failure due to pituitary tumour

Large pituitary tumours commonly expand superiorly and compress the optic chiasm, producing classically a bitemporal hemianopia. This used to be regarded as a neurosurgical emergency requiring surgery within hours/days. Apart from pituitary apoplexy (as previously described), this is no longer necessary. Measurement of serum prolactin is the most important investigation. A massively elevated level (>10x upper limit) is diagnostic of macroprolactinoma; most patients respond to primary dopamine agonist therapy (e.g. cabergoline), with rapid tumour shrinkage and visual improvement. Patients with acromegaly and minor visual impairment may be similarly treated with primary somatostatin analogue therapy (e.g. octreotide). Other tumour types should undergo surgical decompression within a few weeks of diagnosis.

Diabetes insipidus

A patient newly presenting with polydipsia and polyuria should have routine biochemistry to exclude diabetes mellitus, renal impairment, hypokalaemia, and hypercalcaemia. A patient with true cranial diabetes insipidus may pass well over 5 L of poorly concentrated urine in 24 hours. Provided the patient has an intact thirst mechanism, is conscious, and has access to oral fluids, adequate hydration can usually be maintained. Early outpatient referral to an endocrinologist for definitive diagnosis and treatment is recommended. However, for a patient with reduced consciousness (e.g. post-head injury), there is a high risk of serious water depletion, and urgent inpatient management is required.

Further reading

Ayuk J, McGregor EJ, Mitchell RD, Gittoes NJL (2004). Acute management of pituitary apoplexy—surgery or conservative management? *Clinical Endocrinology*, **61**, 747–52.

Gruber A, Clayton J, Kumar S, Robertson I, Howlett TA, Mansell P (2006). Pituitary apoplexy: retrospective review of 30 patients—is surgical intervention always necessary? *British Journal of Neurosurgery*, **20,** 379–85.

Nawar RN, AbdelMannan D, Selman WR, Arafah BM (2008). Pituitary tumor apoplexy. *Journal of Intensive Care Medicine*, **23,** 75–90.

Randeva HS, Schoebel J, Byrne J, Esiri M, Adams CBT, Wass JAH (1999). Classical pituitary apoplexy: clinical features, management and outcome. *Clinical Endocrinology*, **51,** 181–8.

Rajasekaran S, Vanderpump M, Baldeweg S, *et al.* (2011). UK guidelines for the management of pituitary apoplexy. *Clinical Endocrinology*, **74**, 9–20.

Semple PL, Jane JA, Laws ER (2007). Clinical relevance of precipitating factors in pituitary apoplexy. *Neurosurgery*, **61,** 956–62.

Sibal L, Ball SG, Connelly V, *et al.* (2004). Pituitary apoplexy: a review of clinical presentation, management and outcome in 45 cases. *Pituitary*, **7,** 157–63.

Adrenal emergencies

Introduction
Adrenal emergencies may be related to either disease of the adrenal cortex or medulla. The cortex produces cortisol, aldosterone, and androgens. The adrenal medulla secretes epinephrine (adrenaline; ~80%) and norepinephrine (noradrenaline; ~20%).

Pathophysiology
Cortisol
Cortisol is produced from two hydroxylations of 17-alpha-hydroxyprogesterone. Cortisol, also termed hydrocortisone, is ~90% protein-bound, mainly to corticosteroid binding globulin. Glucocorticoids are non-specific cardiac stimulants. They also activate vasoactive factors. In the absence of corticosteroids, stress causes shock, hypotension, and potentially death. Glucocorticoid actions include:

- Stimulation of gluconeogenesis and reduced cellular glucose utilization, inhibition of the effects of insulin, mobilization of fatty and amino acids, and ketogenesis.
- Elevation of red blood cell and platelet levels.
- Inhibition of inflammation by inhibition of macrophage cytokine (e.g. IL-2) production, depletion of eosinophils and circulating lymphocytes (e.g. T cells), stimulation of polymorphonuclear neutrophil (PMN) leucocytosis, prevention of macrophage adherence to the endothelium, impaired capillary permeability, and maintenance of normal vasoconstrictor vascular responses.

Aldosterone
Aldosterone, a mineralocorticoid, is produced by hydroxylation of deoxycorticosterone and is ~60% protein-bound. Aldosterone release is stimulated by the renin-angiotensin system. Serum potassium elevation stimulates aldosterone secretion, whereas reduction in serum potassium and chronic adrenocorticotrophic hormone (ACTH) deficiency inhibit production. Aldosterone acts on the kidneys, gastrointestinal tract, and sweat/salivary glands to maintain electrolyte balance. The kidneys stimulate sodium reabsorption and potassium/hydrogen excretion and depend on the intake of these ions (i.e. increased sodium intake causes potassium excretion). Excess aldosterone results in sodium retention, hypokalaemia, and alkalosis, whereas deficiency results in sodium loss, hyperkalaemia, and acidosis.

Persistent aldosterone excess causes atrial natriuretic factor release and renal haemodynamic changes for compensation. Hyperkalaemia stimulates aldosterone secretion to aid potassium excretion and is the first-line defence against hyperkalaemia.

Diseases of the adrenal cortex
Diseases of the adrenal cortex result in failure of secretion of, or excess production of, adrenal cortical hormones.

Adrenal failure
Adrenocortical insufficiency describes failure of the adrenal cortex to produce normal amounts of glucocorticoid and mineralocorticoid hormones. It may be primary or secondary. Primary adrenocortical failure is due to disease of the adrenal gland. Secondary adrenocortical failure is due to failure of ACTH production by the pituitary gland and may be due to pituitary or hypothalamic disease. Rare congenital conditions are due to specific enzyme deficiencies in the corticosteroid synthetic pathway (e.g. congenital adrenal

hyperplasia). Causes are listed in Table 10.16, and clinical features are shown in Figure 10.8.

Primary adrenal insufficiency
Primary adrenal insufficiency (PAI) follows adrenal damage due to autoimmune 'adrenalitis' ('Addison's disease') or local destruction of the adrenal gland (e.g. tuberculosis, fungal infection, lymphoma, haemorrhage). It may be acute or chronic. PAI may also be due to metabolic adrenal failure or inhibition (i.e. insufficient hormone production) due to congenital adrenal hyperplasia, enzyme inhibitors (e.g. metyrapone), or cytotoxic agents (e.g. mitotane).

Autoimmune destruction of the adrenal cortex (Addison's disease) is the commonest cause of PAI (~70–80%). Antibodies to the adrenal cortex are found in ~70% of cases. It may be associated with vitiligo, premature ovarian failure, and hypothyroidism. Consider other polyglandular autoimmune (PGA) disorders like Schmidt's syndrome (i.e. autoimmune thyroid and adrenal disease, and insulin-dependent diabetes mellitus, which usually presents with adrenal insufficiency). Tuberculosis accounts for ~20%, and rare destructive causes ~5% of cases. Waterhouse–Friderichsen syndrome is due to destruction of the adrenal cortex by haemorrhage associated with meningococcal infection and causes acute adrenal insufficiency.

PAI is an uncommon disorder and has a prevalence of ~50/million population in the West. Idiopathic autoimmune PAI is most often discovered in the third to fifth decades of life, but PAI can occur at any age. Autoimmune PAI is also more common in females (2–3:1), but overall the male to female ratio is equal. There may be a family history of Addison's disease or autoimmune diseases. Local prevalence of tuberculosis is important, as it suggests the possibility of adrenal gland destruction by the disease.

Secondary adrenal insufficiency
Secondary adrenal insufficiency is due to adrenocorticotrophic hormone (ACTH) deficiency, following pituitary or hypothalamic damage. Abrupt withdrawal of therapeutic steroids also presents as adrenal insufficiency because ACTH secretion remains depressed after clearance of

Table 10.16 Causes of adrenal insufficiency

Adrenal gland destruction
Autoimmune adrenalitis (Addison's disease)
Surgical adrenalectomy, infarction
Infection (e.g. TB, fungal, histoplasmosis, HIV)
Infiltration (e.g. tumour, leukaemia, amyloidosis)
Haemorrhage (e.g. anticoagulation, septicaemia)

Secondary (reduced pituitary ACTH secretion)
Pituitary damage (e.g. adenoma, trauma)
Pituitary infarction (e.g. post-partum haemorrhage)
Pituitary haemorrhage (e.g. anticoagulation)
Sudden exogenous steroid withdrawal

Rarely hypothalamic (reduced ACTH synthesis)
Hypothalamic destruction (e.g. tumour, granuloma)

Drugs
Inhibit steroid production (e.g. ketoconazole)
Increase hepatic metabolism (e.g. rifampicin, phenytoin)

Relative adrenal insufficiency
Critical illness

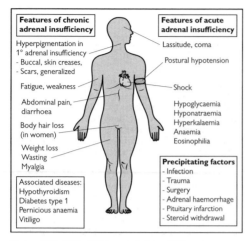

Figure 10.8 Clinical features of adrenal failure.

exogenous steroid. Secondary adrenocortical insufficiency due to steroid withdrawal is much more common and may affect very large numbers of patients on steroid therapy, particularly during times of stress.

Clinical presentation

Early symptoms of adrenal insufficiency are often vague and include lethargy, weakness, or anorexia. Later, there is weight loss, postural hypotension, nausea, vomiting, and abdominal pain. Hyperpigmentation, another late sign due to raised ACTH levels, has a characteristic distribution and is most evident in exposed skin and areas affected by pressure or irritation. Oral pigmentation, on the inside of the cheek or gums and on the lips, is characteristic.

Presentation of adrenal insufficiency may be either acute or chronic.

• **Acute (Addisonian) crises** are precipitated by stress (e.g. surgery, intercurrent infection, trauma) in patients with unrecognized chronic adrenal insufficiency or it may follow adrenal haemorrhage in critical illness (e.g. meningococcal septicaemia) and pituitary infarction after post-partum haemorrhage (Sheehan's syndrome). Acute adrenal insufficiency is a medical emergency and should always be suspected in shock with hyponatraemia (± hyperkalaemia and hypoglycaemia) if the cause is not apparent. Other characteristic features include nausea, vomiting, apathy, confusion, postural hypotension, and coma. In critical illness, relative adrenal insufficiency is common, and steroid supplementation may be beneficial.

• **Chronic deficiency** (e.g. autoimmune adrenal insufficiency) presents with fatigue, weakness, weight loss, fever, and nausea. In PAI, hyperpigmentation is caused by excess pituitary melanocyte-stimulating hormone and/or ACTH. Body hair loss in females is due to reduced adrenal androgen production. It may coexist with other autoimmune disorders like thyroid disease and premature ovarian failure.

Investigation

Initial investigations should include full blood count, routine biochemistry, and blood sugar. Hyponatraemia and

Table 10.17 ACTH stimulation test

Pituitary adrenal axis	Cortisol level	
	Baseline	**Post-ACTH**
Normal	Normal	Increased
Primary adrenal failure	Low	Low
Secondary adrenal failure	Low	Increased
Critical illness	Low/normal	Poor response

hyperkalaemia are features of aldosterone reduction in PAI. Hypoglycaemia, hypercalcaemia, lymphocytosis, eosinophilia, and volume depletion, with raised blood urea occur in all forms of autoimmune insufficiency. Immunology may reveal adrenal autoantibodies. Blood cultures and occasionally adrenal biopsy cultures may detect an infective cause. Adrenal CT scans may be helpful in non-autoimmune disease (e.g. tuberculosis).

Adrenal function tests must not delay cortisol replacement. A low baseline cortisol confirms adrenal insufficiency. Cortisol levels taken at 0, 30, and 60 minutes after a 250 mcg IV ACTH injection (short Synacthen® (tetracosactide) test) normally show a rise of >200–550 mmol/L. If there is an impaired response, a long Synacthen® test is performed. This involves giving 1 mg ACTH IM for 3–5 consecutive days and measuring the cortisol. In Addison's disease, there is no response. If the initial poor response to the short Synacthen® test is due to partial adrenal atrophy due to pituitary or hypothalamic disease, the cortisol levels will gradually rise (see Table 10.17). ACTH is high in PAI and low in secondary adrenal insufficiency.

Management

Addisonian crisis: acutely ill patients need immediate therapy. Do not await the results of investigations. Give hydrocortisone 100 mcg 6-hourly for 48 hours. Treat hypotensive shock with aggressive fluid therapy (e.g. 4–5 L of 0.9% normal saline and/or a more physiologically balanced solution over 12–24 h), and provide inotropic support, if required. Hyperkalaemia corrects rapidly with fluid and steroids, and hypoglycaemia with glucose supplements. Treat infection with antibiotics. When stable, convert to maintenance glucocorticoid and mineralocorticoid (e.g. aldosterone) therapy, as required.

Stress can increase cortisol levels tenfold, and high-dose hydrocortisone (or dexamethasone which does not interfere with serum cortisol assays) may be needed. Mineralocorticoid replacement (e.g. fludrocortisone) is only needed in PAI.

Less severe Addison's disease is treated with oral therapy from the onset and aims to mimic the normal circadian rhythm of cortisol control (hydrocortisone 20 mg a.m. 10 mg p.m.; and fludrocortisone (mineralocorticoid) 0.1–0.2 mg/day). In Addison's disease, therapy is lifelong and must never be stopped. Therapy should be increased during periods of stress. A steroid card should be issued and should document appropriate details of the underlying condition and therapy.

Intercurrent stress requires an increase in therapy. For minor surgery, a single oral or intravenous/intramuscular injection of hydrocortisone 100 mg may be adequate. For major procedures requiring a general anaesthetic, give 100 mg hydrocortisone intravenously 6-hourly until oral medication can be restarted.

Prognosis
Acute adrenal insufficiency may be difficult to diagnose, as many of the presenting signs and symptoms are non-specific (e.g. post-operative fever may be treated as an infection or inflammatory response). Untreated adrenal insufficiency has a poor prognosis (80% mortality within 2 years) and, during acute stress, may be considerably worse. Treatment must be started as soon as possible if the diagnosis is suspected. Delays whilst awaiting diagnostic confirmation cannot be justified.

Cushing's syndrome
Cushing syndrome is characterized by prolonged exposure to an excess of adrenocortical hormone production. The commonest cause is iatrogenic exposure to prolonged steroid therapy. Endogenous hypersecretion is rare (~2/100,000 population) but with a higher incidence in patients with diabetes, hypertension, obesity, or osteoporosis. Young adults (25–45 years old) are most often affected by adrenal or pituitary adenomas, whereas ectopic ACTH-related syndromes tend to occur later in life. Cushing's disease due to an adrenal or a pituitary tumour is more common in females (5:1 female:male), and Cushing's syndrome due to ectopic ACTH production is more common in males.

Cushing's syndrome (percentage of overall cases in brackets) may be:
- **ACTH-dependent:**
  - Pituitary adenoma (Cushing's disease); female:male ratio 4:1 (70%).
  - Ectopic ACTH (14%): bronchial small cell carcinoma, carcinoids of thymus, lung, or gastrointestinal tract.
- **ACTH-independent:**
  - Adrenal adenoma (10%).
  - Adrenal carcinoma (5%).
  - Adrenal hyperplasia (1%).
- **Other causes**
  - Pseudo-Cushing's syndrome due to alcoholism, obesity, poorly controlled diabetes, or depression.

Clinical features
Characteristic features include a plethoric 'moon' face, centripetal distribution of body fat, obesity, buffalo hump, and a protuberant abdomen. The arms and legs often look thin due to muscle wasting, with proximal weakness. The skin is thin and easily bruised, with abdominal striae. Back pain results from osteoporosis (~50%) and vertebral collapse. Women are often hirsute, with greasy skin and acne. Hypertension (~50%), diabetes mellitus (~10%), and hypokalaemia (e.g. arrhythmias, muscle weakness) are common. Psychiatric features occur in up to 90% of cases, including depression (common), hypomania, and frank psychosis (rare). Irregular menses, oedema, thirst, polyuria, impaired immune function (e.g. impaired wound healing), and nephrolithiasis may also occur.

Cushing's syndrome must be differentiated from chronic alcoholism (alcoholic pseudo-Cushing's syndrome), requiring a careful history of alcohol use.

Investigation
Routine full blood count, biochemistry, and blood sugar are required. Polycythaemia, leucocytosis, and a low eosinophil count are common. There may be hypernatraemia and hypokalaemia. Glucose intolerance is common (insulin resistance of excess steroid).

Specific Cushing's syndrome tests include:
- **Plasma ACTH** defines Cushing's syndrome as either ACTH-dependent or independent. ACTH levels are low in autonomous adrenal production of glucocorticoids (e.g. adrenal adenoma), normal or slightly high in Cushing's disease (e.g. pituitary-dependent disease), and very high in ectopic ACTH production (e.g. cancers).
- **Diurnal rhythm of cortisol secretion** is lost in Cushing's syndrome, with raised midnight cortisol levels.
- **The overnight low-dose dexamethasone suppression test** is useful in the outpatient setting for suspected Cushing's syndrome. Dexamethasone 1 mg is taken orally at bedtime and a plasma cortisol taken at 9 a.m. the next morning. Normally, plasma cortisol is suppressed (<100 nmol/L), but, in Cushing's syndrome, it is not, although false positives do occur in obese or depressed patients.
- **The low-dose dexamethasone suppression** test also confirms a diagnosis of Cushing's syndrome. Dexamethasone is given at a dose of 0.5 mg 6-hourly for 48 hours. Normally, this suppresses plasma cortisol levels, but, in Cushing's syndrome, cortisol levels are not suppressed. However, Cushing's syndrome and, in particular, Cushing's disease may be intermittent, leading to diagnostic difficulty and requiring repeated tests.
- **The high-dose dexamethasone suppression test** differentiates pituitary-dependent Cushing's disease from Cushing's syndrome. Dexamethasone 2 mg 6-hourly for 48 hours suppresses plasma cortisol and urinary metabolites by 50% in 90% of patients with Cushing's disease. Rarely, it causes suppression of ectopic ACTH syndrome, particularly in slow-growing tumours.
- **Metyrapone test:** metyrapone (750 mg 4-hourly for 24 h) inhibits the final step in cortisol synthesis. It reduces feedback on ACTH production and increases urinary glucocorticoid metabolites. In Cushing's disease, there is an exaggerated response to the metyrapone test.
- **Response to corticotrophin-releasing factor** (CRF): ACTH levels are measured, following CRF injection. In Cushing's disease (pituitary-dependent), CRF causes an excessive rise in plasma ACTH; whereas ectopic ACTH-related disease is associated with a flat response.
- **Urinary free cortisol** is raised in a 24-hour urinary collection in Cushing's syndrome (>250 nmol in men; >400 nmol in women). False positives can occur with pregnancy, exercise, alcohol, and anorexia.
- **Imaging** may detect adrenal adenomas or tumours. Cushing's disease is usually due to microadenomas of the pituitary which may not always be visible on CT or MRI scans. CT scans of the chest or abdomen may detect ectopic sources of ACTH.

Management
Treatment is determined by the cause and may include surgery, radiotherapy, or pharmacological therapies.

Cushing's disease
Transsphenoidal adenomectomy is the treatment of choice, aiming to remove the adenoma (if it can be localized), with preservation of normal pituitary tissue. It produces remission in >70% of cases. Pituitary radiotherapy is a useful adjunct to surgery if this fails to control the raised cortisol levels but is only slowly effective without surgery.

Bilateral adrenalectomy has been used to treat Cushing's disease in the past and requires lifelong replacement therapy. However, adrenal surgery can cause significant morbidity and mortality in Cushing's disease, which can be reduced by pre-treatment with metyrapone before surgery. Bilateral adrenalectomy is associated with an increased risk of Nelson's syndrome, with very high levels of ACTH, skin pigmentation, and an enlarging pituitary tumour. Pituitary radiotherapy may help prevent Nelson's syndrome.

Occasionally, long-term metyrapone to suppress corticol synthesis may be a useful therapeutic option.

Adrenal adenomas and carcinoma
Operative removal of adrenal tumours, following pre-treatment with metyrapone, is the treatment of choice. Radiotherapy is given post-operatively for malignant tumours. In adrenal carcinoma, drug treatment with mitotane, an adrenolytic agent, can be helpful.

Ectopic ACTH production
Aim to surgically remove the ACTH-producing tumour, if possible; otherwise, consider metyrapone therapy or bilateral adrenalectomy.

Prognosis
Untreated Cushing's syndrome is associated with 50% mortality at 5 years due to cardiovascular disease, thromboembolism, or bacterial infection. Rare adrenocortical carcinomas have a 5-year survival rate <30%.

Hyperaldosteronism
Primary hyperaldosteronism (Conn's syndrome)
Primary hyperaldosteronism results from the excessive secretion of aldosterone which acts on the distal renal tubule to promote sodium, and consequently water retention, which causes volume expansion and hypertension. There is also potassium excretion, causing hypokalaemia.

The cause may be a solitary adrenal adenoma (70–80%; Conn's syndrome), bilateral adrenal hyperplasia (BAH; 15–25%) or occasionally an adrenal carcinoma, or steroid therapy. Unilateral adrenal hyperplasia is rare. Familial hyperaldosteronism also occurs and may be glucocorticoid-remedial aldosteronism (GRA; type 1) which is associated with early-onset hypertension, cerebral aneurysms, and haemorrhagic strokes. Type 2 familial hyperaldosteronism is characterized by inherited aldosterone-producing adenomas or inherited BAH.

It is an uncommon condition, with a peak incidence between the ages of 30 and 50 years old. The prevalence is unclear but probably about 0.2% in unselected hypertensive patients. It is more common in females.

Clinical features
Hyperaldosteronism is characterized by hypertension due to sodium and water retention. Hypokalaemia (potassium <3.5 mmol/L) may only occur in 30% of cases (i.e. 70% of patients may be normokalaemic). Sodium is often at the high end of the normal range. It may also cause metabolic alkalosis, with associated tetany. Other features include polyuria, polydipsia, headaches, and lethargy. Hypokalaemia is associated with muscle weakness (e.g. post-operative ventilatory impairment). Diagnosis involves a high index of suspicion and exclusion of other causes of hypokalaemia.

Investigation
The diagnosis is confirmed by high plasma aldosterone and low plasma renin concentrations when off diuretics for at least 4 weeks, beta-blockers and calcium channel inhibitors for at least 2 weeks, and steroids, laxatives, and potassium supplements have been stopped. This confirms autonomous aldosterone production, with feedback suppression of renin. A high renin level virtually excludes the diagnosis of primary hyperaldosteronism. Urinary potassium is also increased.

The salt loading test can be used for further confirmation of primary hyperaldosteronism. Sensitivity of adenoma aldosterone production to ACTH is the most useful test to differentiate between adenoma and hyperplasia.

Diagnostic imaging includes CT scans of the adrenal glands, although adenomas may be too small for identification. Radiolabelled cholesterol scans may distinguish hyperplasia from adenoma due to bilateral uptake in hyperplasia and unilateral uptake in adenoma. Renal vein blood sampling for aldosterone under imaging control may also help to locate the adenoma.

Management
Treatment depends on the underlying cause. Surgery is usually recommended for an adenoma, as it will often cure the associated hypertension. Potassium replacement is essential before surgery and is achieved by pre-treatment with specific aldosterone antagonists like spironolactone and occasionally by potassium supplementation.

Bilateral adrenal hyperplasia is best treated medically with spironolactone which controls both the hypertension and the hypokalaemia. Side effects include tender breast enlargement in men and decreased libido. Additional antihypertensives may be required to control the hypertension. Alternative aldosterone antagonist therapies include amiloride and triamterene.

Secondary hyperaldosteronism
Secondary hyperaldosteronism is the result of excessive renin in the circulation, which stimulates the adrenals to produce aldosterone. The causes are diuretics, congestive cardiac failure, hepatic failure, nephritic syndrome, renal artery stenosis, and malignant hypertension. Investigation and treatment should be directed towards the underlying cause.

Prognosis
The long-term cure rate for adenoma-induced hyperaldosteronism is ~80%. However, up to 50% of patients will continue to require antihypertensive therapy. Excessive aldosterone has harmful effects on cardiac function due to myocardial fibrosis. This can be offset with aldosterone antagonists (e.g. spironolactone), which markedly reduce mortality in patients with congestive cardiac failure.

Diseases of the adrenal medulla
The normal adrenal medulla secretes adrenaline (~85%) in response to neural control. Phaeochromocytomas are rare tumours that secrete catecholamines and are derived from chromaffin cells. These tumours are not innervated, and the stimulus for secretion is unknown, but they may secrete constantly or intermittently. They can arise anywhere in the sympathetic chain but are usually located in the adrenal medulla (~90%). Some authors define phaeochromocytomas as arising only from the adrenal medulla and label similar tumours located in other areas of the sympathetic chain as paragangliomas.

Phaeochromocytoma
The name phaeochromocytoma is of Greek derivation (phios means dusky; chroma means colour, and cytoma means tumour) and refers to the colour of tumour cells when stained with chromium salts.

The prevalence of phaeochromocytoma is unknown but is ~0.2% in the hypertensive population. It presents in adults aged 25–55 years old, about 10% present in children, and there is no sex difference or racial predisposition.

About 10–15% of phaeochromocytomas are malignant; 10% are bilateral, 18% extra-adrenal, and ~20% familial. Inherited familial forms can be inherited alone or in combination.

- Multiple endocrine neoplasia (MEN type 2), a familial autosomal dominant trait with coexisting medullary carcinoma of the thyroid and hyperparathyroidism (and mucosal neuromas in MEN type 3). Phaeochromocytomas are bilateral in ~70% of MEN syndromes.
- Neurofibromatosis (von Recklinghausen's disease) has a 1% incidence of phaeochromocytoma.
- Phaeochromocytosis is also associated with hereditary cerebellar ataxia (Sturge–Weber disease), cerebello-retinal haemangioblastomatosis (von Hippel–Lindau syndrome), and renal cell carcinoma.

'Sporadic' adrenal phaeochromocytomas secrete both adrenaline (epinephrine) and noradrenaline (norepinephrine) whereas those arising in the sympathetic chain only secrete noradrenaline. Malignant tumours also secrete dopamine. Familial forms tend to produce mainly noradrenaline.

Clinical features
The typical features are the result of the catecholamines released into the circulation. Symptoms are usually intermittent/paroxysmal and may be precipitated by emotion, postural changes, abdominal examination, surgery, general anaesthesia, beta-blockade, certain foods (e.g. cheese), and physical exercise. Attack frequency varies between once a month to several times a day and can last from a few minutes to many hours. They are characterized by palpitations, severe headache, profuse sweating, flushing, nausea, vomiting, anxiety (sense of doom), and tremors. There may be discomfort or pain in the chest and abdomen. The diagnosis should be suspected in any hypertensive patient, especially if the hypertension is paroxysmal, those with postural hypotension, arrhythmias, pallor, or fever, and particularly if they also have glycosuria.

Investigations
Investigation is aimed at demonstrating catecholamine overproduction and locating the source and cause.

Blood tests
Haemoglobin may be elevated due to reduced circulating volume; blood glucose is often raised, and calcium may be elevated. Plasma catecholamines (measured after 30-min rest) and plasma metanephrines (the methylated metabolites of catecholamines) are both used in diagnosis.

Urine tests
24-hour urine collections for total catecholamines, vanillyl mandelic acid (VMA), and metanephrines are measured, although various drugs (e.g. tricyclic antidepressants, alcohol, levodopa, sotalol, benzodiazepines) and dietary factors (e.g. cheese) may affect these tests. VMA has a false positive rate in excess of 15%, and metanephrine measurement is usually the most reliable. The collection bottle should be dark, acidified, and kept cool to prevent degradation of the catecholamines. Ideally, the urine collection should occur after a crisis.

Imaging
After biochemical confirmation of the presence of a phaeochromocytoma, imaging is necessary to locate it. About 90% are in the adrenal medulla and 98% within the abdomen. Extra-adrenal tumours can occur anywhere in the sympathetic chain (i.e. chromaffin tissue) from the base of the brain to the bladder. Common extraneal locations include the mediastinum, carotid body, heart, bladder wall, and the origin of the inferior mesenteric artery.

MRI scans best locate adrenal tumours. CT scans are less sensitive and detect ~80% of adrenal tumours >1 cm in diameter.

If CT/MRI scans do not detect a biochemically confirmed tumour, a metaiodo-benzylguanidine (MIBG) scan, using labelled iodine, is performed to help locate the site of origin. MIBG is similar to norepinephrine and concentrates in adrenal or extra-adrenal tumours. Labelled pentetreotide is an alternative if MIBG is not concentrated by the phaeochromocytoma. Arteriography, with selective venous sampling, is occasionally necessary to locate tumours in difficult cases.

Genetic testing allows early diagnosis and follow-up in the management of susceptible relatives.

Provocation tests (e.g. glucagon, tyramine) and phentolamine suppression testing are rarely used now due to the risk of precipitating dangerous hypertensive or hypotensive crises, respectively.

Histopathology
Removed surgical tissue shows large pleomorphic chromaffin cells and is graded using the PASS system to differentiate benign (PASS <4) from malignant (PASS >6) tumours.

Management
Surgical resection of the tumour is the treatment of choice and usually results in the cure of the hypertension (surgical mortality rates are <2%, and complete resection is usually possible). Preoperative therapy with alpha- and beta-blockers is required to control blood pressure and prevent intraoperative hypertensive crises. Alpha-blockade with phenoxybenzamine should start at least 7–10 days before the operation and aids expansion of the circulating volume. Only when this is achieved should a beta-blocker be started, as early beta-blockade with unopposed alpha stimulation can precipitate a hypertensive crisis. Calcium channel blockers can also be helpful.

In malignant phaeochromocytomas, palliative care can be achieved with radiotherapy and chemotherapy. For example, MIBG at therapeutic doses may be helpful in some cases with metastatic disease. Targeted therapies (i.e. directed at specific tumour cells), such as tyrosine kinase inhibitors (e.g. sunitinib), which inhibit the signal required for metastatic phaeochromocytomas to grow, may have an important role in future treatment.

Prognosis
The 5-year survival rate is >95% for non-malignant phaeochromocytomas but is <50% for malignant tumours. Recurrence after surgery is <10%, and the surgical cure rate for hypertension is ~75%.

Further reading
Arnaldi G, Angeli A, Atkinson AB, *et al.* (2003). Diagnosis and complications of Cushing's syndrome: a consensus statement. *Journal of Clinical Endocrinology and Metabolism*, **88**, 5593–602.

Douma S, Petidis K, Douma M, *et al.* (2008). Prevalence of primary hyperaldosteronism in resistant hypertension: a retrospective observational study. *Lancet*, **371**, 1921–6.

Fishbein L, Orlowski R, Cohen D (2013). Pheochromocytoma/Paraganglioma: Review of perioperative management of blood pressure and update on genetic mutations associated with pheochromocytoma. *Journal of Clinical Hypertension*, **15**, 428–434.

Hahner S and Allolio B (2009). Therapeutic management of adrenal insufficiency. *Best Practice & Research: Clinical Endocrinology & Metabolism*, **23**, 167–79.

Hahner S, Loeffler M, Bleicken B, *et al.* (2010). Epidemiology of adrenal crisis in chronic adrenal insufficiency: the need for new prevention strategies. *European Journal of Endocrinology*, **162**, 597–602.

Manger WM and Eizenhofer G (2004). Phaeochromocytoma: diagnosis and management update. *Current Hypertension Reports*, **6**, 477–84.

Marik PE, Pastores SM, Annane D, *et al.* (2008). Recommendations for the diagnosis and management of corticosteroid insufficiency in critically ill adult patients: consensus statements from an international task force by the American College of Critical Care Medicine. *Critical Care Medicine*, **36**, 1937–49.

Muiatero P, Amar, Chatellier G (2010). Evaluation of primary aldosteronism. *Current Opinion in Endocrinology, Diabetes and Obesity*, **17**, 188–93.

Newell-Price J, Bertagna X, Grossman AB, *et al.* (2006). Cushing's syndrome. *Lancet*, **367**, 1605–17.

Trilos NA and Biller BM (2012). Advances in medical therapies for Cushing's syndrome. *Discovery Medicine*, **13**, 171–9.

Westphal SA (2005). Diagnosis of a phaeochromocytoma. *American Journal of the Medical Sciences*, **329**, 18–21.

Toxin-induced hyperthermic syndromes

Toxin-induced hyperthermic syndromes is the preferred nomenclature for the group of conditions that are triggered by medications which share the following key features:

- Fever.
- Muscle rigidity.
- Disruption of normal thermogenic mechanisms.
- Activation of the sympathetic nervous system.
- Muscular overactivity.

Confusion, agitation, and altered levels of consciousness are also common.

All syndromes are potentially fatal if untreated and include neuroleptic malignant syndrome (NMS), malignant hyperthermia (MH), serotonin syndrome (SS), and parkinsonism-hyperpyrexia syndrome (PHS) (see Table 10.18). Malignant catatonia and stiff man syndrome are related disorders, although medication tends not to be implicated in their pathogenesis. Although there are many similarities in the clinical presentations, important differences exist among their triggers and treatments. Given that failure to recognize and treat such syndromes may result in death from multiorgan failure, careful history and examination, a high index of suspicion, and early aggressive therapy are crucial to management.

Clinical approach

The approach outlined is to distinguish between the syndromes.

History: key points

- Medication. Establish the use of psychoactive drugs, such as antidepressants, antipsychotics, and anti-parkinsonian medication. Anticholinergics, antiemetics, analgesics herbal treatments (e.g. St John's wort) and other centrally acting drugs are also important, particularly in combination with psychoactive drugs. Temporal relationships between the use of drugs, especially starting or changing medication, and the onset of symptoms are important. Onset in SS mostly occurs within 24 h of beginning treatment or overdose; onset in NMS is 1–3 days, while PHS is more insidious in onset (up to 7 days). These syndromes are usually triggered by a change in the medication regime, but SS, NMS, and PMS can occur in patients seemingly stable on medication.
- Exposure to anaesthetic agents. MH is seen almost exclusively in patients exposed to volatile anaesthetics and depolarizing neuromuscular agents. Previous uneventful anaesthesia does not exclude a diagnosis of MH. Masseter muscle spasm at induction is highly suggestive of MH.
- History of psychiatric disorder and severity.
- History of Parkinson's disease or parkinsonian syndrome, such as Shy–Drager, multisystem atrophy, Lewy body dementia.
- Histories of central core disease, King Denborough syndrome, and Evans myopathy are associated with MH.
- Other triggers. Dehydration, reduced food intake, intercurrent illness, stress, and weather factors are implicated in NMS and PHS.
- Family history. Family history of anaesthetic-related deaths is strongly associated with MH.
- History of heat stroke, exercise, or drug-induced rhabdomyolysis is associated with MH.

Examination: key points

- Hyperthermia is a key feature in all conditions. However, its absence does not preclude the diagnosis, as it may be a late sign of fulminant disease.
- Tachycardia and tachypnoea are common.
- Blood pressure. May be labile—initial hypertension may be followed by cardiovascular collapse.
- Pupils. Mydriasis occurs only in SS.
- Skin. Sweating can occur in all conditions. Mottled appearance suggests MH, while pallor suggests NMS.
- Mental state. Psychomotor agitation occurs in SS and MH, while mutism, bradykinesia, stupor, and altered GCS characterize PHS and NMS.
- Coma. A late feature in all syndromes.
- Neuromuscular tone. Increased in SS, especially in lower limbs; lead pipe rigidity in NMS; rigor mortis-like rigidity in MH. In PHS, rigidity is also axial and present without muscle stretch (as opposed to resistance to passive stretch, usually found in Parkinson's).
- Masseter muscle spasm. Strongly suggests MH.
- Reflexes. Hyperreflexia and clonus are found in SS; bradyreflexia in NMS; hyporeflexia in MH.
- Ocular clonus is a key sign in establishing SS.
- Bowel sounds. Often increased in SS; normal or decreased in other syndromes. Ileus may occur in PHS.

Special investigations

All toxin-induced syndromes are diagnosed primarily by history and examination, as there is no single diagnostic test. Other conditions, such as central nervous system infection, heavy metal poisoning, lithium toxicity, anticholinergic overdose, cocaine or ecstasy use, heat stroke, sepsis, thyrotoxicosis, phaeochromocytoma, and withdrawal states (alcohol, benzodiazepines, barbiturates), need to be excluded.

- Full blood count. Leucocytosis is common in all syndromes.
- Electrolytes. Hyperkalaemia is common, reflecting the degree of muscle breakdown and acidosis.
- Creatinine. Acute kidney injury is a poor prognostic sign.
- Liver function tests. May be elevated.
- Creatinine kinase (CK). Elevated in all conditions and must be tracked—rhabdomyolysis is potentially fatal.
- Urinary myoglobin.
- Coagulation studies. Disseminated intravascular coagulation (DIC) marks a poor outcome.
- Iron studies. Serum iron is often low in NMS and PHS.
- Blood gases. Respiratory and/or metabolic acidosis may be present.
- Blood cultures.
- Lumbar puncture, CT head, and EEG should be considered.
- In patients with suspected MH, an MH *in vitro* contracture test (IVCT) should be undertaken at a later time. This is performed on a fresh muscle biopsy and measures contraction in response to halothane and caffeine. Test results are categorized as MH-susceptible, equivocal or not susceptible.
- Genetic screening for MH can be offered in a limited capacity, looking for mutations of the RYR1 gene.

Table 10.18 Toxin-induced hyperthermic syndromes

	Neuroleptic malignant syndrome	Malignant hyperthermia	Serotonin syndrome	Parkinsonian-hyperthermia syndrome
Underlying illness	Schizophrenia Depression	Central core disease King Denborough syndrome Evans myopathy	Depression Anxiety disorders Personality disorders	Parkinson's disease Parkinsonian syndromes
Medication history	Dopamine antagonists (antipsychotics, antidepressants)	Volatile anaesthetics agents (e.g. halothane) Depolarizing muscle relaxants (succinylcholine)	Pro-serotonergic drugs (SSRIs, MAOIs)	Withdrawal of dopamine agonists (levodopa, bromocriptine)
Time to onset	1–3 days	30 min–24 h	<12 h	1–7 days
Pupils	Mydriasis	Normal	Normal	Normal
Tone	Increased (lead pipe)	Increased (rigor mortis-like)	Increased (esp. in lower limbs)	Increased (present without muscle stretch)
Reflexes	Bradyreflexia	Hyporeflexia	Hyperreflexia Clonus	Bradyreflexia
Mental status	Stupor Mutism Coma	Agitation	Agitation Coma	Stupor Mutism Coma
Other key clinical features		Masseter muscle spasms	Hyperactive bowel sounds Ocular clonus	
Clinical course	Onset often rapid, but may be insidious	Onset rapid and highly progressive if left untreated	Onset often rapid May present as subacute/chronic May progress rapidly	Onset usually insidious More slowly progressive
Pathophysiology	Blockade of D2 dopamine receptors	Dysregulation of calcium release in skeletal muscle	Hyperstimulation of 5-HT receptors	Dopaminergic hypostimulation
Genetic basis	Unclear	Autosomal dominant RYR1 (ryanodine receptor) mutations	No	No
Supportive treatment	Aggressive	Aggressive	Aggressive	Aggressive
Treatment	Mild: benzodiazepines Moderate: dopamine agonists ± dantrolene Severe: consider ECT	Dantrolene	Benzodiazepines 5-HT2A antagonists (cyproheptadine, chlorpromazine)	Restart anti-Parkinsonian drugs Consider IV prednisolone/ECT for severe cases
Time to resolution	7–21 days	36–48 hours	2–5 days	7–21 days
Outcomes	Early intervention usually effective Severe neuropsychiatric complications in small number of patients	Early intervention almost always effective	Early intervention almost always effective	2/3 full recovery; 1/3 do not return to previous level of function

SSRI, selective serotonin re-uptake inhibitors; MAOI, monoamine oxidase inhibitors; ECT, electroconvulsive therapy.

However, ~3% false negative rate means IVCT remains the definitive test.

Differential diagnoses

Neuroleptic malignant syndrome

- The Diagnostic and Statistical Manual of Mental Disorders criteria for NMS require the presence of both muscle rigidity and elevated temperature and at least two of the following: diaphoresis, dysphagia, tremor, incontinence, changes in level of consciousness, mutism, tachycardia, elevated or labile blood pressure, leucocytosis, or elevated CK.
- Incidence is up to 3% of patients taking first-generation antipsychotics but thought to be less frequent with second-generation drugs.
- The use of antidepressants, including monoamine oxidase inhibitors and selective serotonin reuptake inhibitors (SSRIs), has been implicated, as have other agents, such as metoclopramide, promethazine, and droperidol.

- All medications implicated in NMS have dopamine D2 receptor antagonist properties. The clinical syndrome is thought to be secondary to decreased dopamine availability, either through primary blockade of the D2 receptors or decreasing dopamine levels. SSRIs increase serotonin levels and inhibit dopamine release in the ventral tegmentum area and the substantia nigra.
- This syndrome usually occurs within 1–3 days of commencing or increasing the medication. Of patients who develop NMS, 90% do so within 10 days of regime change.

Malignant hyperthermia
- This is an autosomal dominant condition characterized by disturbed skeletal muscle calcium release in response to specific triggers, such as volatile anaesthetic agents or depolarizing muscle relaxants.
- The incidence is 1:15,000 anaesthetics for children and adolescents, and 1:50,000–1:150,000 anaesthetics for adults. Prevalence is estimated at 1:2,000.
- About half of all cases occur in patients who previously have had an uneventful anaesthetic.
- The primary defect in MH-susceptible patients is in the ryanodine receptor (RYR1), a skeletal muscle calcium release channel. Various mutations are thought to make the RYR1 channel sensitive to lower concentrations of agonists, leading to uncontrolled calcium release from the sarcoplasmic reticulum upon exposure to trigger agents. The result is sustained muscle contraction and accelerated anaerobic metabolism.
- The first signs of MH are a rising end-tidal CO_2 and an unexplained persistent tachycardia during anaesthesia.
- About 50–80% cases are diagnosed with muscle rigidity.
- Hyperthermia is a late sign or may be absent.
- Some patients do not present until after the completion of the anaesthetic, leading to delays in diagnosis.

Serotonin syndrome
- Serotonin syndrome (SS) describes the triad of mental state changes, autonomic hyperactivity, and neuromuscular abnormalities in patients on pro-serotonergic medications.
- In a small proportion of patients (0.4–0.8%), SS occurs as a severe reaction to SSRIs. However, this syndrome is seen in 14–16% of patients who overdose on SSRIs.
- SS is the result of overstimulation of the 5-HT receptors in the central grey nuclei and medulla. In severe cases, peripheral receptors are also involved.
- Revised criteria for SS include at least four major symptoms or three major and two minor ones. Major symptoms include: confusion, elevated mood, coma or semi-coma, fever, hyperhydrosis, myoclonus, tremors, rigidity, and hyperreflexia. Minor symptoms include: agitation and nervousness, insomnia, tachycardia, tachypnoea and dyspnoea, diarrhoea, altered blood pressure, impaired coordination, mydriasis, and akathisia.
- Onset is usually rapid, with 60% of patients presenting within 6 hours of initial use of medication, change in dosage, or overdosage.
- This may present as a subacute or chronic condition, and requires a high index of suspicion.
- Severe cases, e.g. after overdose, may progress rapidly towards death.

Parkinson-hyperpyrexia syndrome
- Features consist of worsening Parkinsonism, with a marked increase in muscle tone, hyperpyrexia, altered consciousness, and autonomic dysfunction, usually in the context of withdrawal of dopaminergic agents, such as levodopa, bromocriptine, pergolide, or amantadine.
- True incidence is unclear—most cases are often previously misdiagnosed as a form of NMS.
- Underlying pathogenesis is dopaminergic hypofunction in the striatoniagral, hypothalamic, and mesocortical systems, although the exact mechanisms are yet to be delineated.
- Onset is often insidious. Fever alone is the most common presentation. May present as worsening of Parkinsonism without any other features in the early stages.
- Elevation in CK may help to differentiate PHS from other non-toxic diagnoses.

Malignant catatonia
Malignant catatonia is difficult to differentiate from a toxin-induced hyperthermic syndrome, particularly PHS or NMS. Malignant catatonia is defined as a life-threatening febrile neuropsychiatric disorder, characterized by psychosis with autonomic instability, hyperactivity, mutism, and stuperous exhaustion. Careful history may help to clarify the diagnosis.

Management
The key to successful management in all syndromes is early recognition, with aggressive supportive therapy.

General recommendations
- Patients should be cared for in a suitable environment, with access to high-level monitoring.
- In the case of MH, NMS, and SS, the offending agent must be immediately stopped. In MH manifesting intraoperatively, switch to non-triggering anaesthetic agents immediately, and terminate surgery as quickly as safely possible.
- Intravenous fluids should be commenced, with the goal to correct vital signs.
- Cool the patient as needed. Forced air and circulating water should be tried as first-line measures. Peritoneal lavage, ice water immersion, and cold intravenous fluids should be considered if the initial response is poor.
- In patients with severe hyperthermia (>41.1°C), consideration should be given to paralysis and ventilation.
- Agitation may respond to use of benzodiazepines.
- Hyperkalaemia should be treated with glucose, insulin, and calcium gluconate, as per local protocols.
- Life-threatening acidosis can be managed with sodium bicarbonate.
- Rhabdomyolysis should be aggressively treated with forced diuresis and urinary alkalinization. Dialysis may be necessary for severe acute renal failure.
- DIC treatment should be discussed with the haematologists and corrected with fresh frozen plasma, cryoprecipitate, and platelet transfusion, as required.
- Acute respiratory failure, usually secondary to either aspiration pneumonia or pulmonary embolism, should be treated with appropriate ventilatory support (e.g. NIV, intubation).

Specific treatments
Neuroleptic malignant syndrome
A stepped approach is recommended, depending on severity.

- Mild cases can be treated initially with benzodiazepines alone.
- Dopamine agonists, such as bromocriptine, amantidine, and levodopa, appear to decrease mortality and shorten the course of the episode. Bromocriptine: 7.5–30 mg/day PO in three divided doses (max 100 mg/day). Amantidine: 100–300 mg PO bd. Levodopa/carbidopa: 25/250 mg PO tds/qds.
- Dantrolene has been used for NMS. However, a recent review suggests that dantrolene monotherapy is associated with higher mortality rates. As an adjunct to dopamine agents the suggested dosage is 1–3 mg/kg IV initially, followed by 10 mg/kg/day PO/IV in divided doses.
- Electroconvulsive therapy has been used safely in patients with very severe NMS, in those in whom antipsychotics cannot be withdrawn, and in cases where it was not possible to distinguish between malignant catatonia and NMS.

The syndrome may last up to 21 days with oral neuroleptics and longer in patients receiving depot injections.

Malignant hyperthermia
- Prognosis is markedly affected by the time between the onset of symptoms and the administration of dantrolene. The starting dose is 2.5–3 mg/kg IV. Low-dose dantrolene may exacerbate the syndrome.
- Repeated dantrolene dosing may be required every 5–10 minutes until the metabolic derangement is reversed.
- When symptoms subside, a dantrolene infusion should be continued at 0.25 mg/kg/hour for a further 24 hours.
- In patients in whom the symptoms are not reversed with >20 mg/kg, the diagnosis should be reconsidered.
- Dysrhythmias should NOT be treated with calcium channel blockers—these may cause cardiac arrest. Lidocaine or beta-blockers are most appropriate.

Serotonin syndrome
- Control of agitation with benzodiazepines is essential.
- 5-HT2A antagonists are recommended. Cyproheptadine 12 mg initially, then 2 mg every 2 hours while symptoms continue. Maintenance dosing is 8 mg qds.
- Parenteral chlorpromazine 50–100 mg IM may be considered in patients unable to swallow, but careful monitoring is needed.

Parkinsonian-hyperpyrexia syndrome
- Therapeutic doses of anti-parkinsonian drugs should be started immediately.
- Bromocriptine, starting at 5–10 mg tds PO, appears most effective.
- Intravenous levodopa infusion can be commenced in patients with ileus, 50–100 mg over 3 hours, 3–4 times a day; 50 mg of IV levodopa corresponds to 100 mg oral.
- Dantrolene is used, but there are no good trial data.
- One study found that methylprednisolone 1 g per day for 3 days, in addition to oral levodopa and bromocriptine, shortened illness duration and improved symptoms.
- ECT has also been successfully used in severe cases.

Outcomes
- Untreated, mortality in toxin-induced hyperthermia syndromes is as high as 80%.

- Mortality is related to the development of rhabdomyolysis, renal failure, and aspiration pneumonia.
- With appropriate treatment, mortality in MH has been reduced to 1.4%.
- Mortality in SS appears low (two attributed deaths per million prescriptions in the UK).
- In PHS, mortality is ~4%, and 15–20% in NMS.
- Most patients with MH and SS experience no long-term complications, but only 66% of patients with PHS return to their previous level of function, and ~3% of patients with NMS suffer from neuropsychiatric complications.

Prevention
- In MH, NMS, and SS, the trigger medication should be avoided. Underlying conditions should be carefully reassessed and medication regimes reconsidered. Polypharmacy should be avoided.
- In patients with MH, IVCT should be considered, as should family counselling and testing.
- There is no evidence for the use of dantrolene preventatively in patients with MH undergoing anaesthesia.

Further reading
Ali SZ, Taguchi A, Rosenberg H (2003). Malignant hyperthermia. *Best Practice & Research Clinical Anaesthesiology*, **17**, 519–33.
American Malignant Hyperthermia Association hotline (24/7). Tel: +1 315 464 7079.
American Psychiatric Association (2004). Diagnostic and statistical manual of mental disorders: DSM-IV. American Psychiatric Association: Washington.
Boyer EW and Shannon M (2005). The serotonin syndrome. *New England Journal of Medicine*, **352**, 1112–20.
British Malignant Hyperthermia Association. <http://www.bmha.co.uk>. Emergency hotline: +44 (0)7947 609 601.
Cheeta S, Schifano F, Oyefeso A, et al. (2004). Antidepressant-related deaths and antidepressant prescriptions in England and Wales, 1998–2000. *British Journal of Psychiatry*, **184**, 41–7.
Hu SC and Frucht SJ (2008). Emergency treatment of movement disorders. *Current Treatment Options in Neurology*, **9**, 103–14.
Krause T, Gerbershagen MU, Fiege M, et al. (2004). Dantrolene—a review of its pharmacology, therapeutic use and developments. *Anaesthesia*, **59**, 364–73.
Larach MG, Brandom BW, Allen GC, et al. (2008). Cardiac arrests and deaths associated with malignant hyperthermia in North America from 1987 to 2006. *Anesthesiology*, **108**, 603–11.
Malignant Hyperthermia Association of the United States. <http://www.mhaus.org>.
Parkinson's UK. <http://www.parkinsons.org.uk>.
Radomski JW, Dursun SM, Revely MA, Kutcher SP (2000). An exploratory approach to the serotonin syndrome; an update of clinical phenomenology and revised diagnostic criteria. *Medical Hypotheses*, **55**, 218–24.
Reulbach U, Duetch C, Biermann T, et al. (2007). Managing an effective treatment for neuroleptic malignant syndrome. *Critical Care*, **11**, R4.
Robinson RL, Anetseder MJ, Brancadoro V, et al. (2003). Recent advances in the diagnosis of malignant hyperthermia susceptibility: how confident can we be of genetic testing? *European Journal of Human Genetics*, **11**, 342–8.
Rusyniak DE and Sprague JE (2005). Toxin-induced hyperthermic syndromes. *Medical Clinics of North America*, **89**, 1277–96.
Sato Y, Asoh T, Metoki N, Satoh K (2003). Efficacy of methyl-prednisolone pulse therapy in neuroleptic malignant syndrome in Parkinson's disease. *Journal of Neurology, Neurosurgery & Psychiatry*, **74**, 574–6.

Renal diseases and emergencies

Renal emergencies

Clinical symptoms
Patients with renal disease may present with specific complaints, ranging from renal colic and loin pain to macroscopic haematuria, dysuria, nocturia, urinary frequency, and reduced urine output. Non-specific symptoms include malaise, weight loss, anorexia, nausea, exertional dyspnoea, and peripheral oedema. In addition, some cases may have manifestations of systemic disease. However, the majority of patients with chronic kidney disease (CKD) are asymptomatic and identified on routine biochemical screening.

History
There may be a family history of renal disease, heart disease (cardiorenal syndrome), or relevant industrial, toxin, and/or drug exposure, in particular, non-prescription and recreational drug use. Renal disease may occur as a complication of hypertension, atherosclerosis, diabetes mellitus, vasculitis, amyloid, myeloma, HIV, HBV, or HCV infection, liver disease, sickle cell disease, bacterial endocarditis, or sarcoidosis. A list of conditions associated with secondary renal disease is shown in Table 11.1.

Examination
A detailed clinical examination is required since kidney disease, particularly CKD, has systemic manifestations, and renal disease may also occur in patients with vasculitis or other conditions. A list of some associations is shown in Tables 11.2 and 11.3.

Calciphylaxis affects dialysis patients and may present with ulceration, typically involving the lower limbs. Vasculitic rashes, affecting the hands, elbows, and lower limbs, may be present in patients with SLE, Wegener's granulomatosis, rheumatoid and seronegative arthritides. Typically, cryoglobulinaemic rashes affect the lower legs, with the lesions being papular, rather than macular, whereas, in cases of Henoch–Schönlein purpura, the vasculitic rash is typically over the buttocks. Sometimes, the lower limb rashes associated with the peripheral cholesterol emboli syndrome can be very similar to typical vasculitic rashes.

Patients with diabetes may have typical diabetiform skin lesions, and those with Fabry's disease small purplish papules, termed angiokeratoma, in the bathing trunk area.

Table 11.1 Conditions associated with secondary renal disease

Condition	Secondary renal disease
Hypertension	Hypertensive nephrosclerosis
Atherosclerosis	Renal cholesterol emboli
Diabetes mellitus	Diabetic nephropathy
Cirrhosis	Hepatorenal syndrome
Amyloid	Renal amyloid
Multiple myeloma	Myeloma kidney
Sickle cell disease	Glomerulonephritis
HIV infection	HIV nephropathy
Hepatitis B or C	Glomerulonephritis
Ventriculoatrial shunt	Gomerulonephritis
Bacterial endocarditis	Glomerulonephritis
Vasculitis	Glomerulonephritis
Sarcoid	Chronic kidney disease
Malignancy	Glomerulonephritis
Fabry's disease	Glomerular disease

Table 11.2 Facial sign on clinical examination and associated disease or therapy

Facial appearance	Associations
Butterfly rash	SLE
Microstomia	Scleroderma
Sunken nasal ridge	Wegener's
Dark aural cartilage	Alkaptonuria
Facial lipodystrophy	Mesangiocapillary GN type 2
Moon facies/acne	Steroid therapy
Psoriatic plaques	Psoriasis
Hair loss	SLE/heparin

Patients with tuberous sclerosis may have a shagreen patch. Scleroderma may lead to subcutaneous deposits of calcium, particularly around the finger tips, leading to digital ischaemia and infarction. More recently, another fibrosing skin condition has been recognized, termed nephrogenic sclerosing dermopathy, which follows the use of gadolinium contrast agents in patients with CKD.

Nails
In CKD, patients may develop the classic half and half nail where the distal portion of the nail has a brown red band above a white band. Previous episodes of illness may leave white or Beau's lines, and chronic hypoalbuminaemia, due to persistent nephrotic syndrome, may also lead to white nails. Both CKD and renal transplant patients may have fungal nail infections. Splinter haemorrhages and nail infarcts may be found in patients with vasculitis and bacterial endocarditis.

Patients with the nail-patella syndrome often have dystrophic nails and are at risk of developing CKD. In severe cases of tertiary hyperparathyroidism, pseudoclubbing may occur due to resorption of the terminal phalanx. Periungual fibromas may be associated with tuberous sclerosis.

Table 11.3 Hand and skin examination findings and associated clinical renal conditions

Hands and skin	Associations
Pitting oedema	Fluid retention/nephrotic
Calciphylaxis	Dialysis
Decreased skin turgor	Hypovolaemia
Dry pruritic skin	CKD
Itchy calcium deposits	Dialysis patients
Sallow yellowish hue	Uraemia
Extensive bruising	Uraemia/steroids
Gouty tophi	CKD
Skin cancers ± warts	Renal transplant patients
Drug-related skin rash	Interstitial nephritis
Sarcoid manifestations	Interstitial nephritis/GN
HIV-related skin rash	Renal involvement
Syphilitic rash	Renal involvement
T cell lymphoma	Renal involvement
Amyloid	Nephrotic syndrome
Myeloma	Renal failure
Vasculitis	See below
Fabry's disease	See below
Scleroderma	See below

Joints

Gout gout may cause acute monoarthritis, in patients with CKD and renal transplantation treated with diuretics, whereas gouty arthritis is relatively uncommon in dialysis patients. However, dialysis patients are at increased risk of periarticular calcium deposition, particularly in tendons. This limits shoulder movements and causes pseudogout due to intra-articular calcium deposition. Degenerative joint disease is increased in CKD patients due to underlying renal bone disease, which ranges from adynamic renal osteodystrophy to osteomalacia and hyperparathyroidism.

Tertiary hyperparathyroidism, typically in dialysis patients, is associated with increased risk of tendon rupture, so patients may present with acute Achille's and/or patella tendon rupture. Similarly, CKD patients are more likely to develop partial supraspinatus and biceps tendon tears. This may explain the increased risk of tendon damage with quinolone antibiotics in CKD patients.

Skeleton

Renal osteodystrophy is common in CKD patients, leading to increased degenerative changes. Treatment with peritoneal dialysis alters the postural centre of gravity, predisposing patients to increased lower back pain. Thus, many patients with CKD complain of generalized bone pains.

Central venous catheters are associated with an increased risk of staphylococcal infection, with secondary spread leading to osteomyelitis and discitis, which can result in paraplegia.

In long-standing dialysis patients, beta-2 microglobulin accumulates and deposits in the lower cervical and lumbar vertebrae. This can lead to local inflammation, bone destruction, and vertebral collapse. Beta-2 microglobulin accumulation can also occur in the shoulder joint. Aluminium accumulation in dialysis patients can lead to fracturing renal osteodystrophy.

Muscles

Muscle weakness is a common finding in CKD patients with low vitamin D3 levels, and patients typically develop a proximal myopathy, which can be exacerbated by steroid therapy.

Eyes

CKD patients may develop perilimbal calcification, and long-term dialysis patients often suffer with deposits of calcium in the sclera, which lead to the development of ptyergia and pingueculae, typically with a localized vascular reaction. Staphylococcal infection in the dialysis patient can cause endophthalmitis. Immunosuppressed renal transplant patients may be at risk of cytomegalovirus (CMV) retinitis.

Patients with sarcoid and Sjögren's syndrome may develop a keratoconjunctivitis sicca syndrome. Small-vessel vasculitis can cause subconjunctival haemorrhage, uveitis, and/or retinal changes. Patients with SLE and antiphospholipid may suffer retinal venous and/or arterial thrombosis. In addition, fundoscopy can show the characteristic changes of malignant phase or chronic hypertension, diabetic retinopathy, and the CMV retinitis associated with HIV disease.

Lenticonus may be found in some cases of Alport's syndrome, and cataracts are common in renal transplant patients and those treated with steroids. Some childhood conditions like Lowe's syndrome and Bardet–Biedl are also associated with cataracts, and the latter also with retinitis pigmentosa. Slit light examination may show cystine deposits in cystinosis. Patients with Fabry's disease may have distinctive corneal deposits, and treatment with desferrioxamine can also lead to corneal and retinal deposits, with blue-yellow colour blindness

Ears

Since the same ion transporters/channels are present in both the middle ear and the renal tubule, some renal tubular transport disorders, such as Gitelman's syndrome, are associated with deafness. Deafness due to nerve damage typically occurs with Wegener's granulomatosis but may occur with other vasculitides and sarcoid. Previous exposure to aminoglycoside antibiotics and desferrioxamine can also result in VII and VIII nerve damage. Deafness may be associated with Alport's syndrome.

Cardiovascular system

Patients with large-vessel vasculitis may have missing pulses or arterial bruits. Thus, it is important to feel both radial pulses and to check blood pressure in both arms. Carotid and femoral bruits and a palpable aortic aneurysm increase the likelihood of macrovascular renal artery disease.

Left ventricular hypertrophy is a common finding in CKD patients. Cardiac murmurs may be due to increased flow, secondary to anaemia, or the valvular calcification commonly associated with hyperparathyroidism. Murmurs also occur with vasculitis (typically SLE and Wegener's granulomatosis) and bacterial endocarditis, which has an increased prevalence in haemodialysis patients.

Pericarditis typically presents acutely with chest pain and a pleuropericarditic rub in the setting of untreated progressive uraemia or following a preceding viral infection in an established dialysis patient. Tamponade may develop, necessitating pericardial drainage. CKD patients with SLE and tuberculosis (TB) are more prone to develop pericardial effusions.

Respiratory system

The sinuses and upper respiratory tract are typically affected by Wegener's granulomatosis. Haemoptysis may occur with community-acquired pneumonia, and *Legionella*, pneumococcal, and staphylococcal pneumonia may all lead to acute kidney injury (AKI), but haemoptysis may also occur due to the pulmonary renal syndromes (see Box 11.1), tuberous sclerosis, and other conditions with pulmonary vascular abnormalities.

Patients with end-stage CKD and uraemic metabolic acidosis may have chronic compensatory hyperventilation. Shortness of breath in a renal transplant patient may herald a community-acquired or opportunistic pneumonia, without the classic signs.

Dyspnoea may be caused by anaemia, asthma in Churg–Strauss syndrome, or a pleural effusion which develops, following a lower respiratory tract infection, as part of a cardiorenal syndrome, or due to extracellular fluid overload. Uraemia per se and SLE and/or other connective tissue diseases can also cause pleural effusions. Patients treated by peritoneal dialysis may develop a unilateral pleural effusion due to the transdiaphragmatic leak of peritoneal dialysis fluid.

Box 11.1 Pulmonary renal syndromes

Goodpasture's syndrome
Wegener's granulomatosis
Microscopic polyangiitis
Systemic lupus erythematosus
Henoch–Schönlein purpura
Churg–Strauss syndrome

Pulmonary emboli are more common in CKD dialysis patients than the general population. Pleural rubs may be due to emboli but can also occur in patients with serositis, such as those with SLE, and uraemia per se.

Abdomen

In adults, polycystic kidneys and the liver may well be palpable, as may a recently obstructed kidney. Acute haemorrhage into a renal cyst, pyelonephritis, or an infected cyst may lead to severe localized tenderness to palpation.

An enlarged bladder may be associated with multiple sclerosis or diabetic neuropathy, and prostatic hypertrophy or malignancy in males. Thus, it is important that rectal or vaginal examination (in women) is completed to exclude obstructive causes.

Peritoneal dialysis patients may present with an acute abdomen, with guarding, tenderness, and absent bowel sounds due to bacterial infection, and this has to be distinguished from an intra-abdominal infection, such as appendicitis or diverticulitis.

Nervous system

Untreated uraemia can cause an axonal peripheral neuropathy, typically sensory, although motor involvement may occur. This can progress with central nervous system involvement, leading to confusion and coma. Many dialysis patients also suffer with neurological symptoms, ranging from restless legs to sleep disturbances and obstructive sleep apnoea.

Cerebral infections may occur in the immunosuppressed patient, with atypical organisms, such as *Cryptococcus* which often have an indolent course. Similarly, confusion in the renal transplant recipient may be due to viral encephalitis or even a post-transplant lymphoproliferative disorder.

Peripheral nervous system involvement may be due to underlying diabetes mellitus, mononeuritis multiplex due to vasculitis, sarcoid, leprosy, and drug toxicities. The central nervous system is also affected by a variety of conditions, which also cause renal damage, including vasculitides (SLE), infections (HIV, malaria), malignant hypertension, and haemolytic uraemic syndrome/thrombotic thrombocytopenic purpura. Some antibiotics, including extended-spectrum penicillins, may accumulate and cause fitting.

Investigations

Assessment of renal function

Many factors modify the relationship between serum creatinine concentration and glomerular filtration rate (GFR), including sex, age, ethnicity, muscle mass, physical activity, certain drugs, recent meat intake, heavy proteinuria, endstage kidney disease, and the method of analysis. The simplified Modification of Diet in Renal Disease (MDRD) equation adjusts for three of these variables (age, sex, and ethnicity for African Americans) to generate an improved, but imperfect, estimate of GFR from the serum creatinine concentration.

$$\text{GFR mL/min/1.73m}^2 = 186 \times (\text{Se creat} \\ [\text{micromole/L}]/88.4)^{-1.154} \times (\text{age})^{-0.203} \times \\ (0.742 \text{ if female}) \times (1.21 \text{ if black race})$$

In the UK, all National Health Service laboratories now report an estimate of GFR (eGFR), using this equation. Based on this eGFR reporting system, patients are now classified, according to a stage of CKD, with a suffix of (p) to denote the presence of proteinuria (see Table 11.24). The rationale behind this classification is to detect patients with CKD at an early stage to allow potential targeting of treatments, such as

blood pressure control, to prevent or reduce progression of underlying renal disease. It is accepted that the accuracy of the eGFR system is limited, certainly when eGFR >60 mL/min, and it should also be noted that there is correction for the natural reduction in GFR with age in the CKD staging system (see Table 11.24). The eGFR is not designed for patients with changing renal function, in particular those with acute kidney injury (AKI). There are some groups (e.g. South Asians and diabetics) for whom the eGFR overestimates true renal function. More recently, there has been an association described between myosin heavy chain type 2 isoforms (MYH9) and increased serum creatinine in African Americans.

Isotopic methods

Isotopic methods can also be used to estimate GFR, using a single bolus injection technique, typically with chromium-labelled ethylene-diamine-tetra-acetic acid ($[^{51}\text{Cr}]\text{EDTA}$) or $[^{125}\text{I}]$ iothalamate. Below 30 mL/min, the accuracy of the isotopic GFR is reduced, as there is some renal tubular reabsorption. Accuracy is improved by taking a delayed (24-hour) plasma sample.

Urine appearance

- Red: haematuria, haemoglobinuria, beetroot, rifampicin, senna, porphyria.
- Brown: haematuria, haemoglobinuria, myoglobinuria, jaundice, chloroquine, carotene.
- Black: haematuria, haemoglobinuria, myoglobinuria, alkaptonuria (black on standing).
- Green: triamterene, propofol.
- Darkens on standing: porphyria (fluorescence in UV light), metronidazole, imipenem/cilastin.

Urine odour

- Urinary sepsis: pungent odour.
- Diabetic ketonuria: sweet odour.
- Hypermethioninaemia: fishy odour.
- Isovaleric acidaemia: sweaty feet odour.
- Maple syrup disease: maple syrup odour.
- Phenylketonuria: mousy odour.

Urine dipstick testing

Normal urine pH is 4.8–7.6, and patients with type 1 (distal) renal tubular acidosis consistently fail to produce urine with a pH ≤5.5.

UK NICE guidelines advocate urine dipstick testing to detect haematuria, but, although specificity is high, the sensitivity is relatively low, with positive tests occuring with haemoglobin, myoglobin, and bacterial infections (*Enterobacter*, streptococci, and staphylococci).

UK NICE guidelines do not advocate urine dipstick testing to detect proteinuria, unless the stick can quantitate the ratio of albumin/creatinine.

Both leucocyte esterase and nitrite sticks are used to detect the presence of bacterial infection in urine. Leucocyte esterase is preferred, as false negatives usually only occur with heavy proteinuria (>5 g/L) or glycosuria (>20 g/L) and cephalosporins (see Box 11.2).

Box 11.2 Teaching point

Several bacteria, including *Pseudomonas*, *Enterococcus*, and *Staphylococcus albus* which cannot reduce nitrate to nitrite, have false negative dipstick tests for nitrite.

Urinary protein excretion
Normal urine contains <150 mg protein/24 hours. Most centres use simple spot urine samples, which are expressed as a ratio of albumin or protein to creatinine to compensate for diurnal patterns in protein excretion.

Significant proteinuria is taken as an albumin/creatinine ratio of ≥30 mg/mmol, which is approximately equivalent to a protein/creatinine ratio of ≥50 mg/mmol (≥0.5 g/24h). Urine electrophoresis can be used to detect urinary paraproteins in myeloma.

Urinary microscopy
UK NICE guidelines do not support urine microscopy for general screening purposes due to the degeneration of urinary cellular elements with time. Thus, fresh urine is required for microscopy and should be examined by experienced operators.

Lower urinary tract red blood cells (RBC) are similar to those in peripheral blood (isomorphic), whereas those due to glomerular damage are dysmorphic. The typical dysmorphic cell is the acanthocyte, which appears as a circular red cell with little blebs of membrane attached. If acanthocytes are not present, then at least three differently shaped RBC are required. Normal urine contains ≤2 RBC/per high-powered field.

Eosinophils may be identified in cases of interstitial nephritis and fat-laden macrophages in nephrotic syndrome. Neutrophils may be present in cases of urinary infection and both interstitial and glomerular renal disease.

The distal renal tubule secretes Tamm–Horsfall protein, and this forms an impression of the tubule in acidic urine, termed a cast. Simple acellular casts are termed hyaline casts and those with adherent leucocytes granular casts. Erythrocyte casts incorporate red blood cells, as in cases of glomerular haematuria, and are characteristic of nephritic urinary sediment. Lipid droplets may be present in cases of proteinuria.

Urinary microscopy can be helpful in characterizing urinary crystals. Most crystals are not pathological. However, hexagonal crystals are associated with cystine stones. Several drugs can cause transient crystalluria, including aciclovir, indinavir, triamterene, vitamin C, amoxicillin, naftidrofuryl, primidone, and sulfonamide sulfadiazine. Acute precipitation can lead to AKI, e.g. uric acid following tumour lysis syndrome, oxalate following ethylene glycol (antifreeze), and, more recently, calcium phosphate following high phosphate cathartics used for bowel preparation. Microscopy may also detect bacteria and fungi and the eggs of *Schistosoma haematobium*.

Urine culture
Positive urine cultures are defined as a single culture with >10^5 colony-forming units (CFU)/mL. Thus, mixed growths and those with <10^5 CFU/mL are typically reported as no significant growth. However, patients may have lower urinary tract symptoms at lower CFU values, and the better test is urinary leucocyte esterase. Urinary cytospin or cytology preparations may be helpful in confirmation.

Urine cytology
Urine cytology may be useful in the diagnosis of malignancy of the renal tract.

Specialized testing of distal renal tubular function
Renal-induced hyper- and hyponatraemia. Patients with primary or secondary nephrogenic and/or cranial diabetes insipidus or with primary polydipsia may present with polyuria. A plasma osmolality of >295 mOsm/kg and a serum sodium of >143 mmol/L exclude a diagnosis of primary polydipsia.

Water deprivation test. Admit patient to a metabolic ward on the evening prior to the test; weigh, and take baseline samples for plasma osmolality, chemistries, and arginine vasopressin (AVP; also known as antidiuretic hormone (ADH)). After midnight, no oral fluids are allowed until completion of the test. If the early morning urine osmolality is >800 mOsm/kg (normal value), then the test can be stopped. Thereafter, the weight and both plasma and urine osmolality and plasma AVP concentration should be regularly recorded. If weight loss exceeds 5% body weight, then the test should be stopped to prevent further dehydration. Once urine osmolality reaches a plateau (hourly increase of <30 mOsm/kg for 3 consecutive hours), then 5 units of vasopressin is administered subcutaneously and both urine and plasma osmolality measured after 30 minutes and at 1 hour. Comparison of the last urine osmolality prior to the administration of vasopressin and the maximum osmolality following vasopressin helps to categorize patients. Patients with nephrogenic diabetes insipidus will produce a urine osmolality of <300 mOsm/kg, with no response to exogenous vasopressin, and have high AVP levels. In comparison, those with severe cranial diabetes insipidus will respond with dilute urine <300 mOsm/kg but respond to exogenous vasopressin by increasing urine osmolality by 50% or more, accompanied by low endogenous AVP levels. Both cranial and nephrogenic diabetes insipidus can occur as partial forms, which show some response to dehydration, but can be separated by analysing the relative changes in endogenous AVP and the urinary and plasma osmolalities. Patients with primary polydipsia do not show pituitary suppression and have little or no response to exogenous vasopressin.

Hyponatraemia may occur in patients with a reduced effective circulating plasma volume and also those with the syndrome of inappropriate ADH secretion (SIADH). Patients with reduced renal perfusion, such as those with cardiac failure, chronic liver disease, nephrotic syndrome, or pre-renal acute renal failure, will have a reduced fractional excretion of sodium (FE_{Na}) of <1% (normal 1–2%), where FE_{Na} % = $[Na]_{urine}$/ $[Na]_{plasma}$ × $[Cr]_{plasma}$/ $[Cr]_{urine}$ × 100. These patients develop hyponatraemia, as they have free access to water, and the kidney retains both salt and water, resulting in increased extracellular fluid, whereas those with SIADH preferentially retain water and have a normal FE_{Na}. The FE_{Na} is affected by diuretic administration and chronic renal failure.

Both groups have impaired free water excretion, which can be tested by giving the patient 20 mL/kg of water to drink after voiding. More than 75% of the water load should be excreted within 3 hours, and the urine osmolality should fall to <100 mOsm/kg. This test can be affected by gastrointestinal disease, smoking, and emotional factors. Additionally, the free water clearance can be calculated as the difference between the urine volume (mL/min) and [osmolality]$_{urine}$/ [osmolality]$_{plasma}$ × urine volume (mL/min). A positive free water clearance urine is when the urine is more dilute than plasma, and, conversely, a negative free water clearance is when the urine is more concentrated.

Salt wasting may occur in Addison's disease or following a subarachnoid haemorrhage or pituitary surgery.

Renal potassium handling. To determine whether there is a renal tubular cause for potassium disturbances, the transtubular potassium gradient (TTKG) can be calculated, as this attempts to estimate the potassium concentration in the cortical collecting duct, using TTKG = [potassium]$_{urine}$ × osmolality plasma/urine. A TTKG of <2 suggests a non-renal cause of hypokalaemia, whereas a high TTKG is associated with mineralocorticoid excess, Liddle's syndrome, or drugs, such as acetazolamide, fludrocortisone, and amphotericin. A TTKG of >10 implies a non-renal cause of hyperkalaemia, and a low TTKG is found in cases of potassium-sparing diuretics, hypoaldosteronism, and pseudohypoaldosteronism.

Hypokalaemia can also occur in Bartter's and Gitelman's syndromes. These syndromes result in a metabolic alkalosis with hypokalaemia and hypomagnesaemia. Whereas Bartter's syndrome characteristically is associated with hypocalciuria, urinary calcium excretion is normal in Gitelman's syndrome.

Further reading

Feehally J, Floege J, Johnson E, eds. (2007). *Comprehensive clinical nephrology*. Mosby, St Louis.

National Institute for Health and Clinical Excellence (2013). Acute kidney injury: Prevention, detection and management of acute kidney injury up to the point of renal replacement therapy. NICE clinical guideline 169. <https://www.nice.org.uk/guidance/cg169/resources/guidance-acute-kidney-injury-pdf>.

National Institute for Health and Clinical Excellence (2014). Chronic kidney disease: early identification and management of chronic kidney disease in adults in primary and secondary care. NICE clinical guideline 182. <https://www.nice.org.uk/guidance/cg182/resources/guidance-chronic-kidney-disease-pdf>.

Investigation of the renal tract

Radiology

Plain abdominal X-rays may demonstrate opaque renal stones, nephrocalcinosis, and the renal outlines. Ultrafast non-contrast CT scanning with three-dimensional reconstruction has replaced nephrotomograms for detecting low-opacity renal stones.

Simple chest X-rays may be helpful in determining fluid status by demonstrating the cardiac silhouette and any lung pathology, such as pulmonary haemorrhage and cavitation. Multiple rib fractures may suggest multiple myeloma.

Hyperparathyroidism typically causes trabecular bone loss. It is, therefore, picked up earlier with PIXIE scans which assess bone mineral content at the wrist and calcaneus, then DEXA scans which assess cortical bone in the femoral neck and lower lumbar spine.

Intravenous urography (IVU) has been replaced by ultrafast CT scanning, as this detects other pathologies which mimic renal colic. The calyces and papillae are well demonstrated, which may be diagnostic of medullary sponge kidney, papillary necrosis, and sloughed papillae. Similarly, intraluminal radiolucent foreign bodies may be demonstrated surrounded by contrast, typified by radiolucent stones, blood clots, fungal ball, tumour, or sloughed papillae. Abnormalities of the ureteric wall, such as localized thickening of the wall, may be found in transitional cell carcinoma, oedema, tuberculosis, and parasitic granuloma. The CT-IVU may also demonstrate external compression, due to aberrant blood vessels in the upper tract, retroperitoneal fibrosis affecting the middle ureter, or prostatic pathology in the lower tract.

Further information about the site and nature of an obstruction can be obtained by ureteropyelography. This may be performed antegradely by percutaneous puncture of the renal pelvis and the obstruction relieved by nephrostomy or by retrograde cystoscopy which allows direct visualization of the ureter distal to the obstruction and the possibility of removing an obstructing stone or passing double JJ stents to relieve the obstruction.

Renal ultrasound examination

The normal adult kidney is 10–12 cm long, with a thin bright capsule, surrounded by highly reflective perinephric fat. In CKD, renal size decreases, with reduced cortical thickness and increased reflectivity. In some conditions, the renal ultrasound appearances are characteristic; these include focal segmental glomerular sclerosis secondary to HIV infection, in which the kidney is large and the cortex uniformly of a high reflectivity (i.e. greater than that of the renal sinus).

Ultrasound is useful in the assessment of renal masses. Benign cysts have a smooth outline with demarcated borders and an echo-free centre, whereas renal tumours are usually irregular with heterogeneous echo reflectivity. Most tumours are vascular with high flow on colour Doppler scanning, and there may be renal vein extension with adenocarcinomas. Renal transitional cell carcinomas are not readily detected, as ultrasound does not visualize individual calyces.

Adult polycystic kidney disease may present with loin pain, haematuria, or renal failure. Typically, the kidneys are enlarged with multiple bilateral cysts. Hepatic cysts may also be present. Haemorrhage into a cyst, infection, or malignant change may all result in complex echoes within the cyst.

In acute urinary obstruction, ultrasound examination may appear normal. However, the colour Doppler scan may show a reduced diastolic flow due to increased intrarenal pressure and also the absence of the pulsatile jets of urine from the ureter into the bladder on the side with acute obstruction. When the obstruction has been present for some time, there is distension of the calyces. The cause of obstruction is not usually determined by ultrasound examination but it may detect para-aortic nodes, a bladder mass, prostatic enlargement, or a ureterocele.

Renal stones appear on ultrasound as a bright echogenic focus with a distal acoustic shadow. Nephrocalcinosis may result in an increase in medullary echoreflectivity due to calcium deposition, which usually affects all the medulla, whereas calcification from papillary necrosis has an appearance more like that of a renal stone.

Colour Doppler can be used to investigate renal arterial and venous disease, in particular thrombotic disease, with absent vessel flow and changes to the intrarenal blood flow. Colour Doppler scanning is also being used as a screening test for major renovascular disease. The changes at the site of renal artery stenosis are characterized by an increase in the peak systolic frequency, followed by diastolic spectral broadening.

Ultrasound examination is an important investigation in the management of the renal transplant recipient. Early graft dysfunction must be investigated to exclude a technical problem, with either the renal artery or vein, or a urinary leak. Colour Doppler scanning also provides valuable information about the vascular supply of the graft and the presence of arteriovenous fistulae following renal biopsy. Fluid collections appear as echo-free or echo-poor areas. Acute rejection, acute ischaemic tubular necrosis, and immunophyllin toxicity all cause an increase in intrarenal pressure and reduced dialytic blood flow (physiological dialysis).

Ultrasound guidance is used to drain perinephric collections and occasionally aspirate native renal cysts to relieve symptoms and for diagnostic purposes.

CT scanning

Ultrafast CT scanning, without contrast, is frequently used to image ureteric renal stones and the site of ureteric obstruction. In addition, CT provides vital information in determining the cause of ureteric obstruction by imaging the ureter, retroperitoneal space, and pelvis. Spiral or helical CT scans allow a three-dimensional reconstruction of the images and overcomes respiratory artefacts. These imaging techniques can be enhanced by contrast, for example, simple renal cysts do not change density following contrast. CT scanning is also used to investigate renal masses. Renal cell carcinomas vary in appearance, with some showing calcification both within and surrounding the tumour on non-enhanced scans, some are solid, and others are cystic or have necrotic centres. The majority of tumours are vascular and readily enhance with contrast; however, those with heavy calcification may not enhance.

Renal tract imaging in patients with acute pyelonephritis is usually requested to exclude obstruction or when there has been an inadequate response to treatment. CT scanning identifies the extent of disease and detects abscesses and/or obstruction. Whereas focal acute bacterial pyelonephritis should respond to antibiotics, renal abscesses may require drainage.

In renal trauma, contrast-enhanced CT scans provide information about renal anatomy and function, and perirenal collections, differentiating blood from urine. In addition, CT scanning provides valuable information about trauma to other intra-abdominal structures.

Magnetic resonance imaging

MRI has some advantages over CT. Tissues surrounded by fat, such as enlarged lymph nodes, or tumour extension into the renal vein are better demonstrated on MRI than CT. Thus, MRI is useful in staging renal cell carcinoma and is able to differentiate simple cysts complicated by haemorrhage from malignant cysts. The whole of the urinary tract can be visualized, in a manner similar to an IVU, by using a heavily weighted T_2 fast spin echo sequence. This rapid acquisition scan can be used to assess potential live donors for renal transplantation by demonstrating the renal vasculature, renal anatomy, and urinary drainage with one investigation.

Angiogram/DSA

Renal angiography remains the gold standard technique for assessing renovascular disease and for renal angioplasty and/or stenting. The side effects of renal angiography include an arterial puncture, the use of potentially nephrotoxic contrast agents, and the risk of dislodging aortic and renal artery plaques with cholesterol embolization.

Renal arteriography can be indicated in the investigation of renal ischaemia due to renal artery thrombosis or dissection, aortic dissection with extension into the renal arteries, or trauma to the renal artery. Renal and coeliac arteriography can establish a diagnosis of classical macroscopic polyarteritis nodosa.

Digital subtraction angiography (DSA) uses a venous injection of contrast and computer-derived images to view the major renal arteries. High doses of contrast media may be required to visualize the renal arteries and intrarenal vessels. DSA is a good screening test but may need to be followed by formal angiography.

Static nuclear imaging

Technetium-labelled dimercaptosuccinic acid (DMSA) binds to renal proximal tubular cells, and DMSA scans provide information about the relative function of each kidney and show areas of scarring due to renal stone disease, infection, and vascular disease.

DMSA scans are used to identify a non-functioning or absent kidney and detect ectopic kidneys and other congenital malformations, e.g. horseshoe kidney.

Dynamic imaging

Technetium-labelled mercaptoacetyltriglycine (^{99}Tc^{m}MAG3) is filtered by the glomerulus and then rapidly excreted by the kidney, providing three imaging phases: vascular, accumulation within the kidney, and then excretion. Renal artery stenosis and acute tubular necrosis can reduce uptake, flattening the second and third phases of the renogram.

Dynamic scans are used to assess urological obstruction. Occasionally, patients with polycystic kidney disease present with severe pain due to obstruction from a cyst, which can be detected by dynamic testing. In patients with dilated collecting systems, it is important to differentiate congenital megaureter from an obstructed system. Excretion may be slow due to pooling in a dilated system, but obstruction is unlikely if there is a brisk washout, following the administration of IV furosemide.

Following renal transplantation, isotope scans can be used to monitor graft function. In cases of major arterial or venous thrombosis and hyperacute rejection, the graft appears to have absent perfusion and may also show perirenal and urinary leaks before they are clinically manifest.

A MAG3 scan may detect patients with renal artery stenosis since they have a delay in uptake time, the time taken from injection to peak activity, and an increased intensity and duration of the accumulation or parenchymal phase on scanning.

Single-kidney GFR can be calculated, using the combination of EDTA and MAG3, so that the serial assessment of renal function can be determined over time, monitoring the rate of change in renal function in patients with renovascular disease.

PET CT scanning

Positron emission scanning, using fluoride-labelled deoxyglucose, combined with CT scanning, localizes areas of inflammation and, as such, has been shown to be helpful in imaging large-vessel vasculitis in cases of Takayasu's arteritis, infected cysts in patients with polycystic kidney disease, and active inflammation in retroperitoneal fibrosis.

Acute kidney injury

The clinical approach to patients with acute kidney injury (AKI)

The term acute kidney injury (AKI) was introduced to make clinicians aware of developing renal injury and, therefore, potentially allow interventions designed to prevent the development of renal failure requiring dialysis. AKI is associated with a rapid reduction in renal function, characterized by a fall in glomerular filtration rate (GFR), with corresponding increases in serum urea and creatinine.

AKI is defined as an 'abrupt (1–7 days) and sustained (>24 hours) decrease in glomerular filtration, urine output, or both'. AKI is divided into three levels of risk, injury, and failure and is defined 'acute' as changes in creatinine or urine output occur within a 48-hour time period (see Table 11.4). In both staging systems, renal dialysis is scored as failure or AKIN-3.

Incidence

The annual incidence of AKI in the UK is reported to be 500 per million, with some 200 per million requiring dialysis. The

Table 11.4 Acute kidney injury grading

Stage	Serum creatinine	Urine output
1	1.5–1.9 × baseline Or ≥ 0.3mg/dL (≥ 26.5µmol/L) increase	<0.5mL/kg/h for 6–12 hours
2	2.0–2.9 × baseline	<0.5mL/kg/h for ≥ 12 hours
3	3.0 × baseline Or Increase in serum creatinine to ≥ 4.0mg/dL (≥ 353.6µmol/L) Or Initiation of RRT Or In patients <18 years, decrease in eGFR to <35mL/min per 1.73m^2	<0.3mL/kg/h for ≥ 24 hours Or Anuria for ≥ 12 hours

Kidney Disease: Improving Global Outcomes (KDIGO) Acute Kidney Injury Work Group. KDIGO 2012 Clinical Practice Guideline for Acute Kidney Injury. *Kidney International*, Suppl. 2013; 3: 1–150, reproduced with permission.

risk of developing AKI increases with age (more than doubling in patients aged >85 years, compared to those <65), male sex, and ethnicity, being more common in African Americans than other racial groups in the USA.

Risk factors and causes

Following the introduction of the modified MDRD equation, it is now generally recognized that many patients who develop AKI do so on a background of pre-existing chronic kidney disease. Traditionally, the causes of AKI are divided into pre-renal, intrinsic, and post-renal aetiologies (see Figure 11.1). In hospitals, ~40–70% of cases of AKI are due to pre-renal causes, 10–50% intrinsic, with obstruction accounting for ~10%, whereas obstruction is a more common cause of AKI in the community (see Figure 11.2). The mortality in AKI is much higher in high TNF-alpha, low IL-10 producer phenotypes.

The clinical history is vital in helping to differentiate intrinsic AKI from obstruction and pre-renal (volume-responsive) causes and also the time course of AKI, compared to chronic kidney disease (see Figure 11.3). Pre-renal AKI is due to a reduction in renal perfusion, either in terms of renal artery blood flow and/or renal perfusion pressure or due to intrarenal ischaemia (see Table 11.5). Similarly, the history may reveal causes of intrinsic renal disease, such as drug-induced toxic or interstitial renal injury, pyelonephritis, and/or underlying vasculitis (see Table 11.6). Total anuria and loin pain may be suggestive of obstructive causes of renal failure (see Table 11.7). Although obstruction can cause AKI, typically, it causes acute-on-chronic kidney damage.

Clinical assessment

Thorough physical examination is required, not only to assess volume status (see next paragraph), but also to look for signs of small-vessel vasculitis and/or systemic disorders (nailfold infarcts, skin vasculitis, arthritis, oral ulceration, retinopathy), atrial fibrillation, hypo- and/or hypertension, the presence of cardiac murmurs, haemoptysis, abdominal distension, organomegaly, and/or ascites. A pelvic examination is mandatory to exclude an enlarged bladder, abnormal prostate, and/or gynaecological malignancy. Bedside urine dipstick testing may detect haematuria (due to excess red blood cells, haemolysis, and/or myoglobin), protein (glomerular, tubular, or overflow), leucocytes, and nitrites.

Volume assessment

In the early stages of AKI due to pre-renal aetiologies, appropriate fluid resuscitation may well prevent progression

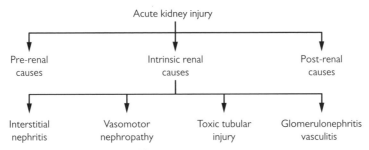

Figure 11.1 Broad categories of acute kidney injury.

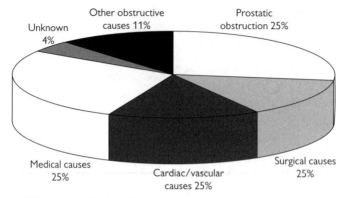

Figure 11.2 Causes of AKI in a community-based survey.

to established acute renal failure and, similarly, minimize AKI in cases of myeloma/light chain disease, rhabdomyloysis, and post-tumour lysis syndrome. However, in cases of established AKI, rapid fluid administration may cause pulmonary oedema. Review the clinical fluid balance charts and daily weights. Typically, hypovolaemic patients have cool peripheries, but patients with septic shock, liver failure, and carbon dioxide retention may well have warm peripheries despite renal hypoperfusion. A delayed capillary refill test >2 s after release of pressure is suggestive of hypovolaemia.

In hypovolaemic states, the jugular venous pulse (JVP) is low, and patients may need to be tilted head down before the JVP becomes visible. Fluid resuscitation should be designed to maintain tissue wellness (see Table 11.8) and restore tissue perfusion. In clinical practice, it can be very difficult to assess the adequacy of the circulating volume, as this depends upon both vasomotor tone and cardiac performance.

In a previously normotensive patient, tissue organ flow, including renal perfusion, should be maintained by ensuring a mean blood pressure ≥65 mmHg with fluid and/or vasopressors. If patients are preload (volume) responsive (see Table 11.5), then fluid resuscitation will be beneficial by increasing cardiac output and renal perfusion, whereas, if they are not, then vasopressors should be tried, as additional fluids may well be detrimental (for treatment algorithm, see Figure 11.4). In the non-ventilated patients, preload responsiveness can be assessed by monitoring the dynamic CVP during spontaneous respiration and also by assessing the change in pulse wave variability of the finger oxygen saturation probe (if the change in CVP is >1 mmHg), or change in pulse oxygen probe >10% suggests that the patient will be preload-responsive). Volume loading in patients with a CVP >12 mmHg is unlikely to increase cardiac output.

Investigations
Ultrasound is the key investigation, providing valuable information on renal size and intrarenal echogenicity. Small kidneys suggest pre-existing CKD, and obstruction is excluded by detecting bladder, prostate, and pelvic pathology, and hydronephrosis.

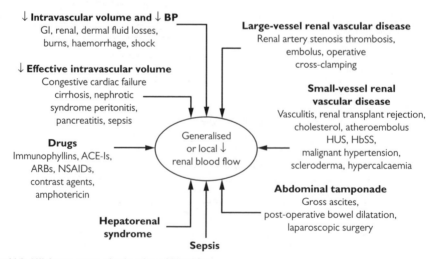

Figure 11.3 AKI due to causes of reduced renal blood flow.

Table 11.5 Causes of pre-renal AKI

Causes of reduced renal perfusion	
Volume loss	Haemorrhage
	Gastrointestinal fluid losses
	Burns
	Overdiuresis
Renal arterial obstruction	Renal artery thrombosis or embolus
	Renal artery stenosis
	Aortic aneurysm
Intrarenal ischaemia	Cardiogenic shock
	Systemic sepsis
	Hepatorenal syndrome
	Anaphylactic shock
	Nephrotic syndrome
	Abdominal compartment syndrome
	PAGE kidney
	Renal vein thombosis
	Right-sided heart failure
	Carbon dioxide retention
	Drugs, e.g. NSAIDs, ACE-Is, and ARBs and calcineurin inhibitors

Table 11.6 Causes of intrinsic AKI

Small-vessel vascular disease	
Occlusive	Cholesterol emboli, cryoglobulinaemia, HUS/TTP, DIC, malaria, sickle cell crisis, eclampsia, viral haemorrhagic fever
Vasculitic	Microscopic polyangiitis, polyarteritis nodosa, SLE, Henoch–Schönlein purpura (HSP), renal transplant rejection
Hypertensive	Malignant hypertension, scleroderma
Acute GN	Anti-GBM disease, post-infectious GN, idiopathic
Interstitial nephritis	
Drug-associated	Antibiotics, NSAIDs, aminoglycosides, tenofovir, indinavir
Post-infective	Leptospirosis, Epstein–Barr virus
Toxins	Radiocontrast media, myoglobin, haemolysis, myeloma/light chains, ethylene glycol, snake or spider venom
Heavy metals	Cisplatinum, lead, mercury
Crystals	Urate or oxalate
Infiltrative	Sarcoid or lymphoma
Infection	
Acute pyelonephritis	Bacterial infection
Immunological	
Renal transplant	Cellular rejection

All patients should have urine stick testing performed to detect blood, protein, glucose, and nitrites. Depending upon the history and physical examination, other investigations may be required (see Table 11.9). Urinary electrolytes may be helpful in determining those patients with potentially reversible pre-renal AKI; however, urinary sodium (U_{Na})

Table 11.7 Causes of post-renal (obstructive) AKI

Intraluminal	Calculus
	Blood clot
	Sloughed papilla
Intramural	Ureteric malignancy
	Ureteric stricture
	Post-irradiation fibrosis
	Bladder cancer
	Prostatic hypertrophy
Extramural	Retroperitoneal fibrosis
	Pelvic malignancy
	Ureteric ligation

excretion can be affected by pre-existing CKD and prior treatment with diuretics.

In those patients with pre-renal AKI, the fractional excretion of sodium (FE_{Na}) is <1%, and the fractional excretion of urea (FE_{Urea}) <35%. The normal FE_{Na} is >1%, and FE_{Urea} is >45%. However, FE_{Na} can be <1% in cases of cardiac failure, contrast nephropathy hepatorenal failure, or haem pigment nephropathy. The FE_{Urea} is a better discriminant of pre-renal AKI than FE_{Na}, as, even when patients have been given diuretics, the FE_{Urea} will be <35%, whereas the FE_{Na} is often >2%. In established AKI, both are elevated. In the

Table 11.8 Assessment of tissue 'well-being'

Variable	Desired range
Mean arterial blood pressure	>65 mmHg
S_VO_2 mixed venous oxygenation	>70% sat 4–6 kPa
$S_{CV}O_2$ central venous oxygenation	>65% sat
Arterial/venous lactate	<2.0 or <2.5 mmol/L
Base excess	±2 mmol/L
Capillary refill time	<2 s
Heart rate	<100 beats/min

Table 11.9 Investigations in the patient with AKI

Haematuria	Renal or urinary tract inflammation Myoglobinuria
Proteinuria	Glomerular or renal tubular disease
Urine nitrite	Urinary infection
Urine culture	Urinary infection
Urine microscopy	Red cell casts in glomerulonephritis/vasculitis, malignant cells, oxalate/indinavir/uric acid crystals/stones, eosinophils in interstitial nephritis
Urea and electrolytes	Increased creatinine, hyperkalaemia, and metabolic acidosis in AKI
CRP	Elevated in inflammation and sepsis
Calcium	Hypo- or hypercalcaemia in rhabdomyolysis, hypercalcaemia in myeloma, sarcoid, malignancy
Hypoalbuminaemia	Nephrotic syndrome, cirrhosis
Bilirubin	Raised in liver disease, leptospirosis, haemolysis
LDH and uric acid	Marked elevation in malignancy and haemolysis
CPK	Rhabdomyloysis, sickle cell crisis
Paraprotein or light chains or BJP	Myeloma Bence–Jones protein in urine in myeloma
Cryoglobulin	Hepatitis C/SLE/lymphoma
Haptoglobins	Reduced in haemolytic uraemic syndrome
Serum ACE	Raised in sarcoid
Eosinophilia	Vasculitis, cholesterol emboli
Thrombocytopenia	HUS or liver disease
Blood film	Red cell fragments in HUS, malarial parasites
Coagulation studies	DIC: sepsis, burns, fat emboli, heat stroke, eclampsia, amniotic fluid embolism, liver failure, and cancer
	Lupus anticoagulant
Autoantibodies	ANA, dsDNA anti-C1q, ENA in SLE
	RhF in cryoglobulimaemia
	ANCA in vasculitis, Wegener's granulomatosis, microscopic polyangiitis
	Proteinase 3 or myeloperoxidase (MPO) in Wegener's granulomatosis, microscopic polyangiitis
	Anti-GBM: Goodpasture's
	ENA in Sjögren's and scleroderma
	Antiphospholipid antibodies
Complement	Low C3 and/or C4 in SLE
	Low C4 in cryoglobulinaemia
Low serum complement activity	Acute post-streptococcal glomerulonephritis (GN), type II membranoproliferative glomerulonephritis (MPGN), subacute bacterial endocarditis, cryoglobulinaemia, 'shunt' nephritis
Blood cultures	To diagnose bacteraemia
Specific infections	Leptospirosis, *Legionella*, viral haemorrhagic fevers, malaria
Virology	HIV—FSGS/increased risk pre-renal AKI in patients taking HAART
	Hepatitis B and C—cryoglobulinaemia or GN, and risk of transmission on haemodialysis

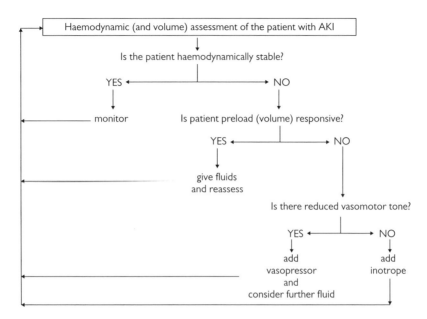

Figure 11.4 Clinical approach to volume and vasopressor management in the patient with AKI. After each step, reassess the patient. A typical vasopressor would be noradrenaline and a typical inotrope dobutamine. Vasomotor tone would normally be assessed invasively as systemic vascular resistance (SVR).

hepatorenal syndrome, the FE_{Urea} is low, and the urinary sodium concentration is often <10 mmol/L.

FE_{Na} = (urinary sodium concentration × plasma creatinine concentration × 100) / (plasma sodium × urinary creatinine).

Indications for renal biopsy
Renal biopsy should only be performed when the history, examination, or laboratory tests suggest the possibility of an underlying systemic disorder, amenable to specific treatment causing AKI. In addition, renal biopsy should be considered in those cases where there is doubt as to the cause of AKI, with no convincing history or documentation of vasomotor renal injury, and also when renal recovery has been delayed and a possible second pathology, such as a drug-induced interstitial nephritis may be involved.

Specific treatments to reverse AKI
Few specific drug treatments have been proven to prevent or shorten AKI, and thus loop diuretics and dopamine should not be routinely administered. Patients with pre-renal AKI should be appropriately resuscitated with fluids and/or vasopressors, as outlined previously. Renal obstruction and abdominal tamponade should be relieved. Specific drugs are appropriate in special circumstances to prevent or reduce AKI, including terlipressin in hepatorenal syndrome, rasburicase in tumour lysis syndrome, leukovorin to prevent methotrexate toxicity, and fomepizole in ethylene glycol poisoning. There are data to suggest that sodium bicarbonate or paracetamol may be useful in the management of rhabdomyolysis, but there are few or no data in man.

Recent studies suggest that blood glucose control can reduce the incidence of AKI. Otherwise, potential nephrotoxins, such as aminoglycosides, should be avoided and iodine-based contrast studies minimized and, if necessary, by using the smallest volume of hypo-osmolar contrast required for the study, with sodium bicarbonate prophylaxis. The current data are unclear as to whether N-acetylcysteine has an effect at preventing contrast-induced nephropathy.

Nutrition
Nutritional support for patients with AKI must take into account not only the specific metabolic disturbances associated with AKI, but also the underlying disease process. Enteral nutrition is preferred, and, as a general rule, patients with AKI should receive 20–35 kcal/kg/day, with up to a maximum of 1.7 g amino acids/kg/day if catabolic and receiving continuous renal replacement therapy. The majority of enteral and parenteral supplements designed for patients with AKI are low in sodium. Electrolytes should be closely monitored to avoid hyper- and hypokalaemia and hypophosphataemia. Trace elements and water-soluble vitamins should be supplemented.

Treatment of complications
Hyperkalaemia
Hyperkalaemia in AKI may lead to cardiac arrest. The ECG changes, which herald potential cardiac arrhythmias, include 'tenting' of the T waves and shortening of the QT interval. These are said to occur when the plasma potassium concentration increases to >5.5 mmol/L. More severe hyperkalaemia causes widening of the QRS

complex, with suppression of the P wave and lengthening of the PR interval.

Administration of 10 mL of 10% calcium gluconate over 2 minutes is the standard medical management of hyperkalaemia in patients with significant ECG changes (i.e not simply tenting of T waves). This should be repeated until the ECG changes reverse. Calcium ensures cardiac stability but does not affect the serum potassium concentration. To decrease serum potassium levels, the immediate treatments used are:

1. Salbutamol (10 mg via nebulizer).
2. Intravenous insulin and glucose (10 units insulin + 50 mL 50% glucose).
3. Isotonic sodium bicarbonate (volume depending upon patient volume assessment) for patients who are acidaemic (arterial pH <7.2).
4. Cation exchange resins (sodium or calcium polystyrene sulfonate 15 g by mouth 6-hourly or 15–30 g per rectum 6-hourly, with lactulose 20 mL qds) have a delayed effect, but it may be useful to start these sooner, rather than later.
5. Acute dialysis if no response.

Pulmonary oedema
Salt and water overload in AKI leads to pulmonary oedema, and, regrettably, many cases are iatrogenic. Patients should be treated with:

1. Supplemental oxygen (± CPAP +5 to +10 mmHg).
2. Intravenous diamorphine.
3. Intravenous GTN (glyceryl trinitrate) infusion.
4. Intravenous furosemide (furosemide infusion 5–10 mg/h).
5. Dialysis may be required in patients with oligo-anuric AKI.

Acute pericarditis
Pericarditis may develop as part of a systemic condition, such as SLE, causing AKI or due to uraemia per se. Typically, patients complain of anterior chest pain, worse on inspiration, with a postural component. The JVP may be elevated, with Kussmaul's sign (if there is an effusion to cause tamponade) and an audible friction rub detected. Urgent echocardiogram assessment is required to exclude a pericardial effusion. If there is an effusion with right atrial collapse, then aspiration should be considered, otherwise, urgent anticoagulant-free haemodialysis started.

Initiation of renal dialysis
The decision to start renal replacement therapy depends on the clinical assessment of the individual patient. General guidelines are set out in Table 11.10.

Survival and renal recovery following AKI
For hospital inpatients, an increase in serum creatinine is associated with stepwise increased risk of mortality, the relative risk of mortality increasing fourfold for a 0.3 mg/dL (27 micromoles/L) rise in creatinine, up to a fourteen fold increase for a 2.0 mg/dL (180 micromoles/L) increase. The overall survival of both patients with AKI and those requiring dialysis has improved over time, increasing from ~60% in 1988 to ~75% by 2002.

Renal recovery following severe AKI with acute tubular injury generally occurs within 21 days, although this is very variable, depending on the severity of the original insult, pre-existing kidney disease, and subsequent clinical course. As more patients are now surviving AKI, it is now becoming clear that renal recovery is often only partial, with reports

Table 11.10 Indications for renal replacement therapy in standard clinical practice in patients with AKI

Biochemical indications

Refractory hyperkalaemia >6.5 mmol/L

Serum urea >30 mmol/L

Refractory metabolic acidosis pH ≤7.1

Severe refractory electrolyte abnormalities: hypo- or hypernatraemia and hypercalcaemia

Tumour lysis syndrome with hyperuricaemia and hyperphosphataemia

Urea cycle defects and organic acidurias, resulting in hyperammonaemia, methylmalonic acidaemia

Clinical indications

Urine output <0.3 mL/kg for 24 h or absolute anuria for 12 h

AKI with multiple organ failure

Refractory volume overload

End-organ damage: pericarditis, encephalopathy, neuropathy, myopathy, uraemic bleeding

Create intravascular space for plasma and other blood product infusions and nutrition

Severe poisoning or drug overdose

Severe hypothermia or hyperthermia

suggesting 7% of survivors become dialysis-dependent within 3 years of the AKI event and 28% for those patients with pre-existing chronic kidney disease.

Following relief of renal obstruction, and also in the polyuric phase of recovering AKI, fluid balance may be problematic due to loss of water and electrolytes. In addition to sodium and potassium losses, patients may develop tetany and/or fitting due to profound hypocalcaemia/hypomagnesaemia. Careful monitoring of daily weights and electrolytes is mandatory to determine appropriate replacement.

Summary
The incidence of AKI is increasing and is more common with increasing age, male sex, and pre-existing chronic kidney disease. The majority of cases result from multiple insults; dehydration, drugs in conjunction with inflammation, and/or sepsis. Patients should be appropriately resuscitated to achieve a mean arterial blood pressure >65 mmHg and fluids given to maximize cardiac preload responsiveness without overloading the patient. Depending upon the individual history and examination, obstruction may need to be excluded by renal imaging and other investigations obtained to establish the cause of AKI.

Special cases of AKI
Hepatorenal syndrome (HRS)
HRS is defined as a sudden deterioration in renal function, occurring in patients with advanced liver disease. Most commonly, HRS occurs in patients with cirrhosis who have acute-on-chronic liver injury. HRS may also occur in patients

with acute liver failure (see 'Acute liver failure') or following surgical resection of the liver (small for size).

Classification of HRS

Since liver disease may be associated with glomerulonephritis and patients are prone to other causes of AKI, the diagnosis of HRS is based on exclusion of other causes. At present, the diagnostic criteria for HRS lag behind those of AKI and will need to be redefined, as, currently, HRS is diagnosed at a relatively late stage of AKI (stage 2 or 3).

- Cirrhosis with ascites or acute liver failure.
- Serum creatinine >1.5mg/dL (133 micromoles/L).
- Absence of shock.
- Absence of hypovolaemia, as defined by no sustained improvement of renal function (creatinine decreasing to <133 micromoles/L), following at least 2 days of diuretic withdrawal (if on diuretics), and volume expansion with albumin at 1 g/kg per day up to a maximum of 100 g/day.
- No current or recent treatment with nephrotoxic drugs.
- Absence of parenchymal renal disease, as defined by proteinuria <0.5 g/day, no microhaematuria (<50 red cells/high-powered field), and normal renal ultrasonography.

Standard laboratory creatinine measurements may be affected by bilirubin and other compounds in liver failure. HRS is further subdivided into HRS type I, in which the deterioration in renal function is relatively acute (within 2 weeks), with a doubling of, or an absolute increase in, serum creatinine to >2.5 mg/dL (220 micromoles/L), and type II, in which the deterioration in renal function is slower or does not meet the criteria for type I. Median survival is 1 month for type I HRS and 6 months for type II.

Pathogenesis of HRS

There are four factors involved in the pathogenesis of HRS. These are:

1. Development of splanchnic vasodilatation which causes a reduction in effective arterial blood volume and a decrease in mean arterial pressure.
2. Activation of the sympathetic nervous system and the renin-angiotensin-aldosterone system which causes renal vasoconstriction and makes renal blood flow much more sensitive to changes in mean arterial pressure.
3. Impairment of cardiac function due to the development of cirrhotic cardiomyopathy, which impairs the compensatory increase in cardiac output secondary to vasodilatation.
4. Increased synthesis of vasoactive mediators which decrease renal blood flow or glomerular microcirculatory haemodynamics, such as cysteinyl leukotrienes and endothelin-1. However, the role of these in the pathogenesis of HRS is unknown.

Risk factors for development of HRS

The probability of developing HRS in patients presenting with cirrhosis and ascites is 18% in the first year and approximately 40% at 5 years. Risk factors originally identified in 'stable' patients for the development of HRS include the presence of hyponatraemia, decreased solute-free water clearance, poor nutritional status, absence of hepatomegaly, arterial hypotension, and elevated plasma renin activity or norepinephrine concentrations. However, recent studies have shown that the development of sepsis is the most important risk factor.

Treatment of HRS

The most important steps in the management of a patient with advanced liver disease who has a rising serum creatinine are:

1. Screen for other causes of AKI (as previously described).
2. Give a volume challenge (e.g. 1 L crystalloid).
3. Stop all diuretics.
4. Stop all nephrotoxic drugs.
5. Screen urine, blood, and ascitic samples, and the chest for sepsis, and start broad-spectrum antibiotics.

If there is no response to these measures, then start treatment with terlipressin, together with albumin therapy for patients presenting with type 1 HRS. Patients should have a baseline ECG, and this should be repeated, if clinically indicated. Contraindications to terlipressin therapy include patients with known ischaemic heart disease or peripheral vascular disease. Terlipressin is started as a bolus injection of 0.5–1 mg every 4–6 hours. Albumin is given at an initial dose of 1 g/kg on day 1, followed by 40 g/day. The efficacy of therapy should be assessed by changes in serum creatinine. If serum creatinine does not decrease during therapy, the dose of terlipressin should be increased in a stepwise manner up to a maximum dose of 2 mg every 4 hours. The aim of therapy is to improve renal function sufficiently to decrease serum creatinine to <133 micromoles/L. For patients with a partial or no response, treatment should be discontinued within 14 days but earlier if there are significant side effects. Patients on terlipressin therapy should be carefully monitored for signs of cardiac arrhythmias or ischaemia, splanchnic or digital ischaemia, and fluid overload, with treatment modified or stopped accordingly. In patients with recurrence of HRS, therapy with terlipressin should be repeated and is frequently successful.

Alternative therapies to terlipressin include *Noradrenaline or midodrine plus octreotide*, both in association with albumin, but there is very limited information with respect to the use of these drugs in patients with type 1 HRS. *Transjugular intrahepatic portosystemic shunting* (TIPSS) can be used to treat HRS in cases refractory to standard medical therapy. TIPSS reduces portal pressures and increases renal plasma flow, with reduced intrarenal endothelin production. However, renal function may initially worsen, as does encephalopathy.

Patients with HRS may be considered for *liver transplantation*. However, unless they fulfil urgent criteria, most have to be managed conservatively. Liver transplantation offers between 65 and 90% survival. However, for patients with irreversible liver disease who are not suitable for transplantation, then a more palliative approach should be considered.

Many centres now consider combined liver and kidney transplantation if patients with HRS have been dialysis-dependent for more than 6 weeks.

Acute ischaemic AKI

Renal arterial occlusion leads to acute ischaemic AKI, and renal venous thrombus causes renal infarction. Renal artery or vein occlusion may be secondary to an underlying prothrombotic tendency (see haematology section). Nephrotic syndrome also leads to a prothrombotic state, with an annual risk of venous and arterial thrombosis of 1% and 1.5% per year, respectively, with a much higher incidence in the first 6 months after presentation. The underlying cause of the hypercoagulable state in patients with nephrotic syndrome is not well understood.

Causes of renal arterial or renal venous thrombosis

1. **Hypercoagulable** states—antiphospholipid syndrome, protein S or C deficiency, factor V Leiden mutation, nephrotic syndrome, malignancy.
2. **Vasculitis**.
3. **Arterial dissection** (trauma, post-surgery or angioplasty/stenting, Marfan's or Ehlers–Danlos syndromes).
4. **Embolic disease** (L > R) from atrial fibrillation, renal artery interventions.
5. Acute renal transplant **vascular rejection** may cause renal venous thrombosis or, rarely, intrarenal arteriolar thrombosis.
6. Renal vein thrombosis may also follow acute **pancreatitis** and IVC thrombosis.
7. Small-vessel ischaemia typically occurs with the **microangiopathic** diseases (see sections on HUS and scleroderma) and may be seen with intrarenal sickling (HbSS).

Renal cholesterol emboli syndrome
Cholesterol emboli to the kidney usually arise spontaneously from a ruptured arterial plaque. Emboli are more likely to enter the left renal artery. In addition to direct renal artery interventions, aortic atheroma can be dislodged during other radiological procedures.

Presentation of renal cholesterol emboli syndrome
Typical patients are male Caucasoids >40 years old or diabetics with hypertension and peripheral vascular disease. Acute presentations are associated with flank, abdominal, or back pain, and there may be signs of cholesterol embolization elsewhere, with livedo reticularis, peripheral digital ischaemia, gastrointestinal haemorrhage, and cholesterol emboli seen on fundoscopy (Hollenhorst plaques). Patients may be systemically unwell, with pyrexia. Laboratory investigations may show blood and protein on urinary dipstick, eosinophilia, with a raised LDH, AST, CRP, amylase. Less commonly, cholesterol embolization syndrome presents as an insidious illness, with pyrexia, malaise, weight loss, and non-specific symptoms.

Imaging in renal cholesterol emboli syndrome
In acute ischaemic AKI, dynamic scanning with DMSA or MAG3 (see dynamic imaging above) may demonstrate complete arterial obstruction by showing no renal perfusion in a kidney, which is known to be present on ultrasound scanning.

Treatment of renal cholesterol emboli syndrome
Urgent MRA is required to detect major acute arterial occlusion, as surgical or interventional radiology (thrombectomy, direct tPA lysis, and/or angioplasty) may be required to restore blood flow. Whereas conservative management is appropriate for cases of aortic dissection or cholesterol emboli, it is important to discontinue angiotensin-converting enzyme inhibitors or angiotensin receptor blockers, and statins may help to stabilize plaques. Renal support with haemodialysis may be required.

Anticoagulation is required for prothrombotic conditions to prevent additional thrombus formation, but there are reports of heparin therapy causing deterioration in patients with cholesterol emboli syndrome; thus, prostacyclin is preferred for patients with digital ischaemia.

Cholesteroli emboli syndrome usually occurs in patients with generalized atheroma and, therefore, these patients have a high risk for cardiovascular disease. Approximately 50–70% who require dialysis for AKI recover residual renal function, but the majority—if they survive—have CKD and subsequently progress to CKD stage 5 over time.

Rhabdomyolysis
Acute muscle injury leads to the release of myoglobin and myoglobinuria. Myoglobin causes AKI due to the generation of free radicals mediated through the ferryl radical of myoglobin. Thus, treatments which stabilize the ferryl myoglobin radical (e.g. alkali) or cause reduction of the radical (e.g. paracetamol) may be beneficial in treatment. At present, however, there are no controlled clinical trials for the treatment of rhabdomyolysis.

Aetiology of rhabdomyolysis
The causes of rhabdomyolysis are shown in Table 11.11.

Diagnosis of rhabdomyolysis
Myoglobinuria often has a brown smoky discoloration and gives a positive urine dipstick reaction for blood and protein, whereas, on urine microscopy, red blood cells are typically absent. The serum CPK is raised, and patients often have a metabolic acidosis, with hypocalcaemia, hyperphosphataemia, and AKI.

Isotope bone scans can be used to image affected muscle groups. In cases of compartment syndrome, direct tonometry may be required to assess pressure, and EMG is useful in assessing patients with myositis and/or dermatomyositis. Renal biopsy shows acute tubular injury, with myoglobin cast nephropathy.

Table 11.11 Causes of rhabdomyloysis

Muscle injury	Trauma, crush injury
	Compartment syndrome
	Immobilization, burns
	Electrocution, seizures
	Heat stroke
	Acute vascular ischaemia
	Sickle cell crisis
	Polymyositis
	Excessive exertion
	Status asthmaticus
Drugs	Statins, fibrates
	Antimalarials
	Ecstasy, cocaine
	Amphetamines
	Heroin, alcohol
Toxins	Snake venom
	Insect venom
	Fish venom
	Mercury
Bacterial infections	*Legionella, Leptospira*
	Salmonella, staphylococci, streptococci
Viral infections	Coxsackie, HIV, influenza
Inherited diseases	Malignant hyperthermia
	Neuroleptic malignant syndrome
	McArdle's syndrome
	Carnitine palmitoyltransferase deficiency
	Mitochondrial cytopathy
Endocrine	Hypothroidism
	Diabetic ketoacidosis

Management of rhabdomyolysis

In crush injuries, patients require active resuscitation prior to hospital transfer to minimize the risk of rhabdomyolysis. Initially give 0.9% Hartmann's solution 10–15 mL/kg/h or isotonic sodium bicarbonate solution (1.26%), as muscle injury leads to marked fluid losses into the injured area and hyperkalaemia. Hartmann's is preferable to normal saline, as the latter may cause a hyperchloraemic acidosis when infused at large volumes, and this may worsen renal injury in rhabdomyolysis. This is because slightly acidic conditions markedly enhance tissue injury by the ferryl myoglobin radical formed during rhabdomyolysis.

Concurrent injuries should be managed as appropriate. Fluid balance should be assessed (see AKI section). If the patient is passing urine, then intravenous crystalloid fluids are required to ensure a high urine ouput, aiming for >200 mL/h. If the patient is anuric, then it is important not to fluid-overload the patient and precipitate pulmonary oedema.

Hyperkalaemia may require emergency treatment (see hyperkalaemia section). For those with hypocalcaemia, calcium is only replaced if patients have a low ionized calcium with associated clinical consequences or ECG changes, as administration may exacerbate muscle injury by metastatic calcification in those patients who survive. Renal support should be instituted, if appropriate.

For malignant hyperthermia and/or neuroleptic malignant syndrome, treatment with sodium dantrolene, starting at 1 mg/kg IV up to a maximum dose of 10 mg/kg, may be required. For sickle crisis, exchange blood transfusion may be necessary. Patients with acute arterial occlusion or a compartment syndrome (>30 mmHg or clinical signs of hypoperfusion and/or sensory changes) require urgent surgical review for restoration of blood flow and to assess whether to perform a fasciotomy. During recovery, hypercalcaemia may develop.

Acute intravascular haemolysis

Acute intravascular haemolysis will result in the release of free haemoglobin, and this may cause AKI, complicated by hyperkalaemia, similar to rhabdomyoloysis. This may follow major or minor blood group-incompatible transfusions, autoimmune haemolytic anaemia, drug-induced haemolysis (penicillin, chloroquine), infections with malaria or mycoplasma, sickle cell crisis, glucose-6-phosphate dehydrogenase deficiency, toxins from snake bites, insect and jellyfish stings, and poisons, including arsenic. Contamination of dialysis water with copper, chloramines, or nitrites may cause haemolysis. Similarly, ill-fitting dialysis lines and misaligned blood pumps can cause massive mechanical-induced haemolysis during haemodialysis or coronary artery bypass grafting. Priming extracorporeal circuits with 5% dextrose can also cause acute haemolysis due to osmolar changes.

Multiple myeloma and monoclonal immunoglobulin deposition disease (MIDD)

There are five renal syndromes caused by plasma cell dyscrasias. These are:

1. Acute kidney injury.
2. Myeloma kidney (cast nephropathy).
3. Light chain AL amyloid.
4. Cryoglobulinaemia .
5. MIDD or immunoactoid glomerulopathy.

Causes of kidney injury

Waldenström's macroglobulinaemia, with increased IgM typically causes renal ischaemia due to hyperviscosity and predisposes to AKI.

AKI is common in multiple myeloma since patients become intravascularly volume-depleted due to hypercalcaemia and infections. In addition, binding of light chains in the renal tubule, typically Tamm–Horsfall protein in the distal tubule, causes tubular injury and obstruction (cast nephropathy). Approximately 50% of patients with multiple myeloma presenting with AKI will have pre-renal AKI and 50% cast nephropathy.

Cryoglobulinaemia may also cause kidney injury due to the deposition of IgM autoantibodies bound to IgG.

Deposition of monoclonal immunoglobulin (MIDD) or fragments may lead to proteinuria and CKD.

Management

Investigation should be as for myeloma (see 'Myeloma'), including free serum and urinary light chains, serum electrophoresis, Bence–Jones protein, and cryoglobulins.

Patients presenting with AKI should be volume-resuscitated, sepsis treated, and nephrotoxic drugs withdrawn, as, once dialysis is instituted, few patients recover residual renal function.

Thereafter, specific treatment is required to suppress the underlying B cell dyscrasis (see 'Myeloma'). There have been recent encouraging reports of recovery of renal function in cases of cast nephropathy-induced AKI, using the combination of bortezomib, a proteasome inhibitor with a superflux dialysis membrane, capable of removing free plasma light chains. Patients have an increased risk of infection, and mortality is typically twice that of a standard haemodialysis patient.

Haemolytic uraemic syndrome (HUS)

HUS is one of the thrombotic microangiopathies (see Table 11.12), characterized by a microangiopathic haemolytic anaemia, thrombocytopenia, and acute kidney injury. All of the thrombotic microangiopathies are characterized by endothelial cell activation, which consists of five core changes: loss of vascular integrity, expression of leucocyte adhesion molecules, cytokine production, upregulation of HLA molecules, and a change in phenotype from an anticoagulant to a procoagulant state. It is the latter that predisposes to the development of a *thrombotic microangiopathy*.

In childhood, the commonest association is following infection with the verocytotoxin-producing *E. coli* O157:H7 serotype, particularly in the under 5s. Other bacteria can also produce this shiga toxin (see Table 11.12), with a reported HUS incidence of two cases per 10^5. However, there have been an increasing number of childhood cases reported, following *S. pneumoniae* infection, which produces neuraminidase, causing red cell agglutination.

There are a number of familial forms of HUS, which are associated with deficiency of complement proteins or phenotypic alterations, which lead to the inability to switch off complement once activated. These include deficiencies or polymorphisms of complement inhibitory proteins factor H and I, complement protein 3, and membrane complement protein-1 (MCP-1).

Thrombotic thrombocytopenia (TTP) is typically due to reduced caspase activity such that large multimers of von Willebrand factor cannot be readily cleaved. This may be genetic but is often acquired due to antibody formation precipitated by infection, pregnancy, and drugs.

Table 11.12 Classification of thrombotic microangiopathies

Haemolytic uraemic syndrome

Diarrhoea-associated (90%)

E. coli O157:H7 (75%)

Other: Shigella dysenteriae serotype 1, Salmonella, Yersinia, Campylobacter

Non-diarrhoea-associated

Idiopathic (5–10%)

Familial: complement factors H and I, C3 deficiency, membrane complement protein-1

Drug-induced HUS: ciclosporin, tacrolimus, quinine, sirolimus, interferon alfa, crack cocaine, clopidogrel, ticlopidine

Cancer chemotherapy HUS: gemcitabine, cisplatinum, mitomycin, bleomycin, fluorouracil, radiotherapy

HIV-1-related HUS: occurs in 1%. Associated with CMV infection

Pregnancy-related: post-partum HUS

Malignancy-associated HUS: gastric, breast, colon, small cell lung cancer

Infection-related HUS: S. pneumoniae or Clostridia

Systemic disease-related: systemic lupus erythematosus, primary antiphospholipid syndrome, and cobalamin C disease

Other thrombotic microangiopathies

Pregnancy-related: pre-eclampsia, HELLP syndrome

Thrombotic thrombocytopenia, TTP: ADAMTS13 deficiency, post-infection, drug-related

Bone marrow transplantation: graft vs host disease, irradiation

Hypertension-related: malignant hypertension

Miscellaneous: HCV cryoglobulinaemia, polymyositis, dermatomyositis, glomerulonephritis, and POEMS syndrome (polyneuropathy, organomegaly, endocrinopathy, monoclonal gammopathy, and skin changes)

Reprinted by permission of Macmillan Publishers Ltd: Kidney International, Besbas N et al., 'A classification of hemolytic uremic syndrome and thrombotic thrombocytopenic purpura and related disorders', 70, 3, pp. 423–431, Copyright 2006.

Clinical presentation

HUS may present with diarrhoea, which may be bloody, fever, hypertension, fluid retention, abdominal pain (mesenteric ischaemia and pancreatitis), heart failure and ischaemic heart disease (coronary artery occlusion), and AKI. Cerebral presentations with confusion and/or localized cortical involvement are more common in TTP but can occur in HUS.

In women presenting in the third trimester, differentiation from severe forms of pre-eclampsia, such as the HELLP syndrome (haemolysis, elevated liver enzymes, and low platelets) may be difficult. Pre-eclamptic syndromes tend to be associated with less severe forms of haemolytic anaemia, the presence of hepatocellular necrosis, and rapid improvement following delivery. Features of pregnancy-related HUS include severe hypertension, neurological symptoms, fever, and renal failure requiring renal replacement therapy. Although plasma exchange increases survival rates, maternal mortality remains between 5 and 20%, and preterm delivery and intrauterine fetal death (approximately 30%) are frequent complications. Long-term follow-up is important because of the later development of renal failure and hypertension. About 50% of patients will have a recurrence.

Investigations

In diarrhoea-associated HUS, urine dipstick testing is strongly positive for blood and proteinuria, due to glomerular thrombosis and infarction, with positive testing for bilirubinuria. Full blood count may show a mild to moderate reduction in red blood cell count, an increased reticulocyte count, neutrophilia, and thrombocytopenia. Red cell fragments are usually visible on a blood film. Typically, standard laboratory clotting tests are normal or only marginally deranged, differentiating HUS from DIC. However, circulating prothrombin fragments and thrombin-antithrombin complexes are increased. Other key investigations include serum haptoglobins which should be markedly lowered, in association with an elevated lactate dehydrogenase, and bilirubin due to intravascular haemolysis. Persistently low C3 should suggest an underlying complement disorder. Neuraminidase-associated red cell agglutination is usually noted during attempts to cross-match blood.

An appropriate microbacteriology screen is required, including stool in diarrhoea-associated HUS and consideration of HIV and other precipitating infections. ADAMTS13 can now be assessed and is typically low in TTP (<5% of standard activity). Similarly, in familial cases, screening of factors H, I, and MCP-1 should be undertaken.

Treatment

All patients should receive supportive management, and platelet transfusions should be avoided, unless haemorrhage develops with a peripheral platelet count of <20 × 10^9/L. Treatment depends upon the underlying aetiology, including withdrawal of precipitating drugs and delivery in pregnancy-associated TTP.

- **Diarrhoea-positive HUS in childhood:** conservative management. No evidence for plasma exchange.
- **Diarrhoea-negative HUS:** fresh frozen plasma is a source of both von Willebrand proteases and complement inhibitory proteins. Solvent-treated plasma removes the large multimers of von Willebrand factor and is the preferable treatment. In most cases, plasma exchange is required, starting at 30 mL/kg/day, then reducing to 20 mL/kg/day, and continued until lactate dehydrogenase levels fall and platelet count increases.

Familial, genetic HUS/TTP may recur, requiring further plasma exchange, and potentially other therapies including eculizumab, intravenous immunoglobulin, rituximab, splenectomy, and vincristine.

Outcome

Childhood diarrhoea-associated HUS has an initial good outcome, with a reported mortality of <3%, but 40% subsequently develop hypertension and/or progressive CKD. However, HUS without diarrhoea has a more severe outcome, with many patients developing CKD requiring long-term dialysis. In these patients, it is important to define underlying genetic predispositions, as HUS is likely to return (50%), following transplantation in patients with complement factor H and I deficiencies, but <10% with MCP-1 abnormalities. Combined liver and renal transplantation has been used for factor H-deficient HUS.

Renal vasculitis

The kidney is frequently involved in systemic diseases which affect the endothelium. These include local endothelial thrombosis, haemolytic uraemic syndrome, and diseases causing small-vessel vasculitis, such as microscopic polyangiitis, systemic lupus erythematosus, Wegener's granulomatosis, and medium to large vessel vasculitis.

Renal vasculitis typically occurs in the setting of a systemic vasculitis, but occasionally the kidney is the only organ involved. Vasculitis may be primary (see Table 11.13); or secondary to infections (infective endocarditis, TB, leprosy, arboviruses, parvovirus), drugs (penicillamine, propylthiouracil, hydralazine, ciprofloxacin, 'crack' cocaine, amphetamines), post-vaccination (pneumococcus, influenza virus, hepatitis A and B, tetanus toxoid), and both solid organ tumours and haematological malignancies.

Renal vasculitis, microscopic polyangiitis (MPA), and Wegener's granulomatosis (WG) typically occur in middle-aged Caucasoids and peak between 65 and 74 years, with a slight male preponderance and an estimated incidence of 60 per 10^6/year.

Small-artery vasculitis

Presentation

Wegener's granulomatosis is a granulomatous vasculitis, whereas microscopic polyangiitis is a necrotizing vasculitis, and, although all the clinical features of microscopic polyangiitis may occur in cases of Wegener's granulomatosis, the converse is not true. Wegener's granulomatosis differs from microscopic polyangiitis, and patients may have nasal and sinus symptoms and also involvement of both middle ear and auditory nerve, with conductive and neurological hearing loss. In addition, Wegener's granulomatosis can affect the cartilage not only in the nose, but also the larynx, trachea, and large bronchi. Typically, Wegener's granulomatosis also affects the lower respiratory tract with granulomas, which may cavitate and become secondarily infected.

Although both microscopic polyangiitis and Wegener's granulomatosis may only affect the kidney, they generally present with the systemic manifestations of a generalized vasculitis, with a history of myalgia, arthralgia, weight loss, lethargy, night sweats, associated with a vasculitic skin rash, conjunctivitis, scleritis, and arthritis.

Investigations

Patients with a systemic vasculitis usually have non-specific abnormal laboratory investigations, including normochromic normocytic anaemia, with a neutrophilia and thrombocytosis. ESR and CRP are typically raised, with a reduced albumin. Urea and creatinine are raised in cases of renal involvement, as is often alkaline phosphatase.

Urine dipstick testing is usually strongly positive for blood and protein, and urine microscopy may confirm glomerular haematuria with red cell casts (nephritic presentation).

The majority of patients will have an elevated IgG, with positive immune complexes, and mildly elevated rheumatoid factor. However, the diagnosis is helped by a positive indirect antineutrophil cytoplasmic antibody test (ANCA). In the laboratory, there are two patterns of staining: perinuclear (pANCA) and cytoplasmic (cANCA). Specific ELISA tests are now available, and most pANCA results are due to anti-myeloperoxidase antibodies (anti-MPO) and cANCA due to proteinase 3 antibodies (PR3). Although PR3 antibodies are more common in cases of Wegener's granulomatosis and MPO in microscopic polyangiitis, there is major overlap between the antibody specificities and clinical disease. The standard tests are for IgG specificities, and, sometimes in the acute stage of the disease, antibodies may be of the IgM isotype or IgA. In some cases, other autoantibodies, such as anti-glomerular basement membrane antibodies may be present. Anti-endothelial cell antibodies have been reported in microscopic polyangiitis and Wegener's granulomatosis, as well as in the large-vessel vasculitides (see Table 11.13). However, the pathogenic role of these antibodies remains unclear.

Renal biopsy typically shows a necrotizing vasculitis, with glomerular capillary rupture and fibrin deposition within the glomerulus. Initially, this is segmental, causing limited damage within the glomerulus, with reactive proliferation of the parietal and visceral epithelial cells (podocytes). However, as the lesion expands and more fibrin is deposited within the glomerulus, with an associated inflammatory cell infiltrate, a crescent forms, compressing the remainder of the glomerular tuft, so shutting down the glomerulus, potentially resulting in a very aggressive disease with AKI.

Table 11.13 Classification of primary vasculitides

Vessel affected	Vasculitic condition
Aorta	Giant cell arteritis
	Takayasu's arteritis
Large to medium arteries	Polyarteritis nodosa
	Kawasaki disease
Small arteries	Microscopic angiitis
	Wegener's granulomatosis
	Churg–Strauss syndrome
Arterioles	Microscopic angiitis
	Wegener's granulomatosis
	Churg–Strauss syndrome
	Henoch–Schönlein purpura
	Cryoglobulinaemic vasculitis
Capillary	Microscopic polyangiitis
	Wegener's granulomatosis
	Churg–Strauss syndrome
	Henoch–Schönlein purpura
	Cryoglobulinaemic vasculitis
	Behçet's syndrome
	Leukocytoclastic vasculitis
Venules	Microscopic angiitis
	Wegener's granulomatosis
	Churg–Strauss syndrome
	Henoch–Schönlein purpura
	Cryoglobulinaemic vasculitis
	Behçet's syndrome
	Leukocytoclastic vasculitis
Veins	Wegener's granulomatosis
	Churg–Strauss syndrome
	Behçet's syndrome

Data from Jennette JC, et al., 'Nomenclature of Systemic Vasculitides', *Arthritis and Rheumatism*, 1994, published by Wiley.

Management

In patients with limited renal disease treatment depends upon the serum creatinine at presentation. For patients with a serum creatinine <500 micromoles/L, induction therapy designed to achieve remission should include oral cyclophosphamide 2.5–3.0 mg/kg/day (reduced to 2 mg/kg/day if the patient is aged >65 years old) and oral prednisolone, starting at 60 mg/day and then reducing in a stepwise fashion over time. Intravenous pulsed cyclophosphamide (10–15 mg/kg, given on average monthly) is equally effective as oral therapy but should be covered with mesna (2-**m**ercapto**e**thane **s**ulfonate **Na**) to minimize bladder toxicity. Rituximab and steroids may also be used as induction therapy, with reduced need for cyclophosphamide. This is a potent immunosuppressive regime, and patients are advised to take a bisphosphonate to reduce osteoporosis, low-dose septrin to prevent infection (*Pneumocystis carinii* and staphylococcal nasal carriage), oral nystatin, and proton pump inhibitors for gastric protection. In young patients, sperm and oocyte collection should be considered prior to cytotoxic therapy or ovarian protection with gonadotrophin antagonsim. If remission has been achieved, then after 3 months, cyclophosphamide can be replaced by azathioprine (2 mg/kg/day) or mycophenolate mofetil (2 g/day), as the risks of cyclophosphamide therapy, in terms of sterility, bladder cancer, and other haematological malignancies, are related to cumulative dosage. In the remission phase, immunosuppression should be progressively reduced to 5 mg/day of prednisolone and 1 mg/kg azathioprine. Generally, 18 months of remission are required before considering withdrawal of immunosuppression, although longer treatment may be required for PR3-associated vasculitic disease.

For patients presenting with a serum creatinine >500 micromoles/L, plasma exchange (60 mL/kg up to a maximum of 4 L), in addition to standard induction therapy, improves short-term renal outcomes. In addition, plasma exchange is recommended for all patients with pulmonary haemorrhage due to vasculitis, irrespective of serum creatinine.

Relapses may well occur during follow-up, particularly in those patients in whom there is no fall in anti-MPO or PR3 ELISA titres. In other patients, a rise in ELISA titre may herald disease relapse; however, bacterial infection can also cause an increase in ANCA titre, particularly if IgG is suppressed. Relapses should be treated by returning to induction therapy.

Outcome

Twenty-five years ago, Wegener's granulomatosis and microscopic polyangiitis were life-threatening diseases, whereas today the majority of patients survive their initial presentation, and more than 50%, initially requiring renal dialysis, become dialysis-independent. Even in those who remain dialysis-dependent, renal transplantation is feasible, but it is advisable to wait until the disease has been in remission for 12–18 months before embarking on transplantation.

Churg–Strauss syndrome

Patients with Churg–Strauss syndrome (CSS) typically have predominant extrarenal manifestations. Patients may have microscopic haematuria and proteinuria on dipstick testing. ANCA antibodies (typically anti-MPO) are present in more than 60% of patients referred with renal involvement.

Although peripheral eosinophilia is common in CSS, eosinophils are not always present in the renal biopsy. Biopsy appearances range from minor glomerular changes to focal segmental glomerulosclerosis and segmental necrotizing vasculitis with crescents.

Management is similar to that of microscopic polyangiitis/Wegener's granulomatosis. Patients with very high peripheral eosinophil counts who require dialysis may be at risk of eosinophil degranulation during extracorporeal treatment and encephalopathy due to the sudden release of eosinophil basic protein. As with PAN, patient survival depends on extrarenal disease, particularly cardiac involvement.

Polyarteritis nodosa (PAN)

PAN is a necrotizing vasculitis of medium-sized arteries, and patients typically present with fever, malaise, myalgia, gastrointestinal symptoms, hypertension, and renal involvement, which can include haematuria and renal infarction. Middle-aged white males (peak 40–50 years) are predominantly affected. PAN is a disease of larger pre-glomerular vessels, and renal biopsy shows glomerular ischaemia and infarction, rather than glomerulonephritis.

The majority of patients are ANCA-negative, and the diagnosis is established by mesenteric or renal angiography showing characteristic microaneurysms. Renal biopsy has an increased risk of bleeding and developing arteriovenous fistulae. Muscle biopsy may be helpful in showing vascular fibrinoid necrosis.

Treatment is the same as for microscopic polyangiitis and Wegener's granulomatosis, and the outcome has now improved, with 80% of patients surviving >5 years. Mortality is due to severe intestinal or cerebral vasculitis, and gel foam or coil ablation of aneurysms may be lifesaving in cases of haemorrhage.

Henoch–Schönlein purpura (HSP)

HSP is the most common vasculitis to affect children, with an incidence of 14 per 10^5, predominantly affecting boys, with a median age of 4 years. As with IgA nephropathy, HSP is more common in Northern Europe and Japan.

Aetiology

The aetiology remains unknown, although there are numerous reports of HSP following bacterial and viral infections, vaccinations, drugs, malignancy, and trauma. As yet, no genetic predisposition has been identified.

Presentation

The non-renal manifestations of HSP are more common in children than adults. Children typically develop palpable, non-blanching purpuric macules over the buttocks and symmetrically over the extensor surfaces of the lower limbs (particularly around the ankle) and forearms. The purpura may spread to other areas and typically appears as 'crops' of new lesions and may recur. Children often have recurrent abdominal pains and transient arthralgias. Occasionally, other organs, including the brain, can be affected, with chorea and pulmonary haemorrhage reported.

Isolated haematuria is the commonest finding in paediatric series; however, if haematuria persists, then proteinuria often supervenes and then hypertension as a marker of CKD. Fifty per cent of patients have a nephritic urinary sediment on presentation (glomerular haematuria with red cell casts). Heavy proteinuria is unusual in children but common in adults. Renal function is usually normal on presentation in children but often abnormal in adults.

Total serum IgA is usually increased at presentation due to an increase in polymeric IgA1. IgA immune complexes are often detected, including IgA-associated ANCA and RhF, which may develop due to aberrant glycosylation of

IgA1. In addition, antiphospholipid antibodies have been reported in some cases.

Although complement turnover is increased with reduced CH_{50} and properdin levels, complement proteins C3 and C4 are usually normal. Despite marked purpura, laboratory clotting times and peripheral platelet counts are normal.

Renal biopsy

Renal histology is variable, with six basic classes described, with a number of subclasses ranging from minimal glomerular damage to extensive crescent formation with fibrin deposition and diffuse endocapillary glomerulonephritis. The key finding is diffuse IgA deposition, often in combination with C3 and C5b–C9. Dense deposits can be located, with electron microscopy, in the mesangium.

Risk factors for progression and outcome

Renal function at the time of presentation is the most important factor in determining renal outcome, followed by hypertension, crescents on renal biopsy, and proteinuria. Approximately 30% of those who undergo renal biopsy develop progressive renal dysfunction over 10-year follow-up. Following renal transplantation, although IgA may be deposited in the transplant, HSP does not tend to recur in the graft.

Treatment of HSP

Steroids and other immunosuppressants have not been shown to affect outcome in mild cases of HSP. However, steroids and cyclophosphamide reduce the risk of progression to CKD in children with >50% crescents on renal biopsy. Typically, adults with vasculitic changes and/or crescents are treated similarly to microscopic polyangiitis/Wegener's granulomatosis.

Behçet's syndrome

Behçet's syndrome is a systemic vasculitis. Primary renal vasculitic involvement is relatively unusual. The kidney can be affected secondarily to renal vein thrombosis and amyloidosis. However, ciclosporin and tacrolimus are often used to treat Behçet's syndrome and the most common cause of renal impairment, and renal biopsy findings today is one of immunophilin nephrotoxicity.

Rheumatological diseases and glomerular disease

Rheumatoid arthritis can cause a low-grade focal glomerulonephritis and, rarely, a vasculitic crescentic nephritis. AA amyloid deposition may occur in patients with long-standing rheumatoid. The commonest cause of renal involvement in rheumatoid disease is drug nephrotoxicity.

Mixed connective tissue disease, dermatomyositis, and Sjögren's syndrome may all be associated with a low-grade focal glomerulonephritis and occasional membranous glomerulonephritis (MGN) and mesangiocapillary glomerulonephritis (MCGN). Sjögren's typically causes tubulointerstitial renal disease.

Systemic lupus erythematosus (SLE)

SLE is an autoimmune disease with multisystem involvement (see Chapter 16). Patients with SLE and/or the antiphospholipid syndrome may develop renal involvement. SLE can cause a myriad of renal syndromes, ranging from little or no involvement with normal urine dipstick testing, through to a rapidly progressive crescentic glomerulonephritis with AKI requiring dialysis. In addition, SLE with biopsy-proven glomerular disease can evolve with time. SLE can also cause interstitial renal disease, minimal change-like nephropathy, thrombotic microangiopathy, arteritis, and even renal artery stenosis.

Classes III and IV are subdivided into: (a) active, (c) chronic, or mixed (a/c). Class IV is also subdivided into segmental or global. Mixed membranous and proliferative glomerulonephritis is now termed class III + V or IV + V, previously termed membranoproliferative glomerulonephritis. Immune complexes typically stain for C1q, C3, and IgG.

Clinical presentation of lupus nephritis

Patients with SLE may have normal urinary dip stick testing or present with nephrotic syndrome or with a nephritic presentation and rapidly progressive AKI. Similarly, patients may present with renal involvement alone or as a multisystem disease with renal involvement. When patients present with rapidly progressive renal disease and hypertension, then cerebral involvement, particularly with seizures, due to a posterior leukoencephalopathy syndrome is a more frequent presentation.

Investigations may show complement abnormalities, with low C3, C4, and positive antiC1q, double-stranded DNA, and ENA (Ro, La, Jo, Sm, RNP) antibodies. In addition, the patient may have antiphospholipid antibodies and/or beta2 glycoprotein 1 antibodies. Coagulation tests may detect a lupus anticoagulant.

Treatment of lupus nephritis

There is significant risk of progression to CKD in lupus nephritis, and, as such, treatment is required for most patients, and responses may be complete or partial.

Typically, classes I and II are treated with steroids alone, whereas classes III, IV, and V require steroids and additional immunosuppressives including cyclophosphamide and rituximab.

There are two steroid regimes used to induce remissions, either starting with oral prednisolone 1 mg/kg/day and reducing in stepwise manner, according to clinical response, or an initial IV methylprednisolone 500 mg for 3 days, followed by 0.5 mg/kg/day, again then reducing the dose in a stepwise fashion.

Traditionally, cyclophosphamide has been given by intravenous pulses, and two commonly used regimens are: 500 mg every 2 weeks for six doses or 0.75 g/m^2/month for six doses, adjusted to maintain a peripheral neutrophil count >3–4 x 10^9/L (NIH). Mesna and IV fluids should be given to cover each pulse of cyclophosphamide, and additional precautions should be considered (listed under treatment of vasculitis). More recently, oral mycophenolate mofetil (MMF) has been proposed as being as effective as cyclophosphamide.

Calcineurin inhibitors and mycophenolate have been used to treat class V membranous lupus nephritis.

Approximately 20% of patients are intolerant of cyclophosphamide and/or MMF, and some 20% will fail to achieve remission. If this fails, then consider rituximab therapy, and continue with azathioprine 1.5–2.0 mg/kg/day.

If patients fail to achieve remission, consider a further course of intravenous methylprednisolone, followed by rituximab, or plasma exchange.

Risk factors for renal progression (e.g. hypertension) should receive standard management (see 'Chronic kidney disease').

In cases of relapse, which may be induced by reduction in immunosuppression and in those patients with persistently positive anti-dsDNA and/or low complement proteins or infection, consider repeating the renal biopsy, as the histological class may have changed. Reinstitute and/or increase immunosuppression in these cases, and consider rituximab and/or intravenous immunoglobulin therapy.

In those patients who progress to end-stage renal failure, renal transplantation is a viable option, although patients with lupus anticoagulant or antiphospholipid syndrome are more prone to thrombosis in the early post-transplant period.

Antiphospholipid syndrome (APS)

APS is defined as a positive anticardiolipin antibody and/or lupus anticoagulant on two separate occasions, with a history of arterial and/or venous thrombosis. APS may be primary when it occurs in the absence of any other disease, or secondary when associated with SLE or other autoimmune diseases.

Antiphospholipid syndrome may cause renal thrombotic microangiopathy, renal artery thrombosis, and increased risk of renal biopsy haemorrhage. In SLE-associated antiphospholipid syndrome without thrombosis, patients should be treated as for SLE, but with additional aspirin. However, after the first thrombotic event, formal lifelong anticoagulation with warfarin or an oral direct thrombin inhibitor must be considered.

Anti-glomerular basement membrane disease (anti-GBM)

Goodpasture's syndrome is an autoimmune disease characterized by antibodies to the carboxy terminal NC1 domain of the alpha 3 chain of type IV collagen, found in the glomerular, alveolar, choroid plexus, and retinal basement membranes.

Aetiology

Most patients with anti-GBM disease inherit the B1*1501 allele of the DR2 region of the HLA class II molecule, with weaker associations for DRB1*04 and DRB1*03. Although minor outbreaks have been reported, no specific environmental trigger factor has been positively identified.

Clinical presentation

Anti-GBM disease is typically characterized by a rapidly progressive glomerulonephritis, associated with pulmonary haemorrhage, the combination termed Goodpasture's syndrome. However, some patients can present decades later after episodes of haemoptysis, and, similarly, the deterioration in renal function can occur over months.

Most patients have a systemic illness with associated malaise, but weight loss and arthralgia are less common, compared to patients with systemic vasculitis. Pulmonary haemorrhage is reported to occur in 50% of patients, but can vary from minor haemoptysis to life-threatening pulmonary haemorrhage, which often remits and relapses spontaneously. Pulmonary haemorrhage can be precipitated by volume overload and respiratory infections.

Anti-GBM disease is rare, estimated at 1 per 10^6, and is not the only cause of a pulmonary renal syndrome (see Table 11.14). Anti-GBM antibodies have been reported in cases of ANCA-associated small vessel vasculitis and also, very rarely, in association with membranous glomerulonephritis, diabetes mellitus, viral infections (HIV and HCV), solid organ malignancy and lymphomas, and, exceptionally, following lithotripsy.

Typically, Caucasoid males in their 50s and 60s are most susceptible to anti-GBM disease, although this condition may occur in all age groups. Pulmonary haemorrhage is more common in younger patients and is more likely in smokers and those exposed to hydrocarbon fumes.

Investigations

Patients with anti-GBM disease may have a microcytic anaemia due to repeated blood loss from alveolar haemorrhage. Typically, there is peripheral leucocytosis and thrombocytosis, with raised ESR and CRP. The alkaline phosphatase may also be increased.

Table 11.14 Conditions causing rapidly progressive glomerulonephritis and pulmonary haemorrhage

Goodpasture's	Anti-GBM disease
ANCA-associated vasculitis	Microscopic polyangiitis
	Wegener's granulomatosis
	Hydralazine
	Penicillamine
Other vasculitides	SLE
	HSP
	Behçet's disease
	Mixed essential cryoglobulinaemia
	Rheumatoid vasculitis

Patients will have a positive indirect immunofluorescence test for anti-GBM antibodies, which can be confirmed by a specific ELISA. Renal biopsy shows a typical rapidly progressive glomerulonephritis with crescents. In particular, there is linear staining of the glomerular basement membrane on indirect immunostaining and absence of immune deposits.

Urine dipstick is usually strongly positive for blood and protein, with a nephritic sediment on microscopy.

Pulmonary haemorrhage is suggested by a sudden fall in haemoglobin and diffuse alveolar interstitial shadowing on CXR. Respiratory function tests showing an increased KCO are suggestive of pulmonary haemorrhage, and bronchoscopy may obtain haemosiderin-laden macrophages.

Treatment

Anti-GBM disease should be treated in the same way as microscopic polyangiitis or Wegener's granulomatosis. Plasma exchange should be instituted for those with pulmonary haemorrhage and/or presentation serum creatinine >500 micromoles/L (5.5 mg/dL), and continued according to antibody response.

However, renal outcome strongly depends on renal function at presentation, with only 8% of patients who were initially dialysis-dependent subsequently becoming dialysis-independent.

In those patients who remain dialysis-dependent, transplantation can be performed after a 6-month period with undetectable antibodies.

Interstitial renal disease

Interstitial renal disease is associated with inflammation and damage to the renal tubules and interstitium. This may be acute or chronic.

Acute tubulointerstitial nephropathy (ATIN)

ATIN is associated with an acute inflammatory interstitial infiltrate, including lymphocytes, macrophages, and sometimes granulomas and/or eosinophilias, with interstitial oedema, and may cause AKI.

ATIN may develop due to direct hypersensitivity reactions to drugs (antibiotics, NSAIDs, anticonvulsants, etc.) or cell-mediated tubulointerstitial disease (NSAIDs, cimetidine, CMV, sarcoid, Wegener's granulomatosis, tubulointerstitial nephritis and uveitis syndrome (TINU)). Other

Table 11.15 Non-drug causes of acute tubulointerstitial nephropathy

Bacterial
Streptococci, *Diphtheria*, pneumococci, brucellosis, *Legionella*, tuberculosis, typhoid, *Yersinia pseudotuberculosis*, Enterobacteriaceae, *Chlamydia*, mycoplasma, syphilis, leptospirosis

Viral
HIV, CMV, EBV, hanta virus, puumala virus, Crimean haemorrhagic fever, measles, echo virus, Coxsackie virus, adenovirus, mumps, influenza, herpes simplex, hepatitis A, hepatitis B, polyomavirus (BK virus)

Rickettsia
Rocky mountain spotted fever, Mediterranean spotted fever, Lyme disease

Parasitic
Toxoplasma, *Leishmania*, dengue fever

Systemic diseases
Sarcoidosis, Sjögren's syndrome, systemic lupus erythematosus

Idiopathic
Isolated or associated with unilateral or bilateral uveitis (TINU syndrome)

Table 11.16 Drug causes of acute tubulointerstitial nephropathy

Antibiotics: cephalosporins, macrolides (e.g. erythromycin), penicillins (e.g. amoxicillin), quinolones (e.g. ciprofloxacin), anti-tuberculous drugs (e.g. ethambutol, isoniazid, rifampicin), aminoglycosides (e.g. gentamicin), tetracyclines, or sulfonamides. *Miscellaneous*: nitrofurantoin, minocycline, colistin, co-trimoxazole, polmyxin, vancomycin, teicoplanin

Antivirals: adefovir, tenofovir, indinavir, foscarnet, aciclovir, atazanavir

Anticonvulsants: e.g. carbamazepine, phenytoin, valproic acid, lamotrigine, clozapine

NSAIDs: e.g. indometacin, ibuprofen, aspirin, naproxen, paracetamol, flurbiprofen, diclofenac, meloxicam, rofecoxib, sulindac, piroxicam

Diuretics: e.g. furosemide, bumetanide, ethacrynic acid, hydrochlorothiazide, indapamide

Contrast agents for radiology

Proton pump inhibitors: e.g. omeprazole, pantoprazole

ACE inhibitors: e.g. captopril

Anti-inflammatory bowel disease drugs: e.g. mesalazine, sulfasalazine

Miscellaneous: mefenamic acid, quinine, allopurinol, probenecid, diazepam, phenindione, azathioprine, bismuth salts, ciclosporin, interferon alfa, griseofulvin, clofibrate, fenofibrate, mercury salts, amphetamines, methyldopa, propranolol, warfarin, triamterene, cytosine arabinoside, some herbal medicines, streptokinase

Anti-arthritic drugs: penicillamine, gold salts, NSAIDs

H2 antagonists: e.g. ranitidine

Phenothiazines

Antithyroid drugs: e.g. carbimazole, propylthiouracil

causes include immune complex-mediated disease (SLE, Sjögren's syndrome) and antitubular basement membrane disease (MGN and drugs—meticillin cefalotin, allopurinol, phenytoin, SLE).

ATIN may be idiopathic, related to drug sensitivity (see Table 11.16), or follow infection (see Table 11.15). In addition, it may be associated with malignancy (lymphoma, T cell leukaemia, myeloma cast nephropathy (see 'Myeloma')) and immune-mediated diseases, including SLE, sarcoidosis, Sjögren's syndrome, tubulointerstitial nephritis and uveitis syndrome, with antitubular basement membrane antibodies, and renal allograft transplant rejection.

Presentation
ATIN may present as part of a systemic illness or with fever, skin rash, and arthralgia, following the introduction of a new drug, or illness. Urine dipstick testing may be positive for blood and protein, usually <100 mg/mmol creatinine (and tubular in origin—ratio of retinol-binding protein/creatinine > albumin/creatinine), with leucocytes and eosinophiluria and FE_{Na} usually >1. There may be a peripheral eosinophilia, thrombocytopenia, with autoimmune haemolysis and abnormal liver function tests.

Treatment
Management depends upon the underlying aetiology. In cases of suspected drug-associated ATIN the drug should be stopped. However, if renal function does not improve or the patient is dialysis-dependent, then prednisolone, starting at 1 mg/kg/day (up to a maximum of 60 mg), should be considered. The steroid is then weaned over 4 weeks, according to response. If renal function deteriorates after steroid withdrawal, then recommence prednisolone at 30 mg/day, with mycophenolate 2 g/day, and reduce dose over time.

Tubulointerstitial nephritis and uveitis syndrome (TINU)
TINU is a distinct syndrome, predominantly affecting women, and may be associated with NSAIDs or systemic conditions, such as SLE and Sjögren's syndrome. Infection with EBV and *Chlamydia* has also been reported. Patients present with painful red eyes due to bilateral uveitis, which may pre- or post-date the onset of acute tubulointerstitial nephropathy. Treatment is with either topical steroids to the eyes or systemic steroids, depending upon the severity of disease.

Drug-induced acute kidney injury
Both pharmaceutical drugs and herbal medicines can lead to a number of renal diseases. See Table 11.17. Some drugs affect creatinine secretion by the renal tubule and, therefore, cause an 'increase' in the serum creatinine, without necessarily altering renal function (amiloride, cimetidine, creatinine, fibrates, intravenous immunoglobulin, probenecid, spironolactone, triamterene, and trimethoprim), whereas other drugs interfere with the colour change of the standard Jaffe reaction used to measure creatinine (ascorbic acid, cephalosporins, flucytosine, levodopa, and methyldopa).

Drugs may cause kidney injury due to idiosyncratic reactions or toxicity, which may be due to dosage or altered pharmacokinetics in CKD, as many drugs are metabolized and/or excreted by the kidney. For example, extended-spectrum

Table 11.17 Drug-induced acute kidney injury (AKI)

Pre-renal AKI	Diuretics, NSAIDs, ACE-Is/ARBs, ciclosporin, tacrolimus, contrast media, interleukins, vasodilators (minoxidil, CCBs, hydralazine, diazoxide), tolvaptan
Thrombotic microangiopathy	Ciclosporin, tacrolimus, sirolimus, mitomycin, oral contraceptives, quinine, fluorouracil, ticlopidine, clopidogrel, interferon, valaciclovir, cisplatinum, gemcitabine, bleomycin
Cholesterol emboli	Streptokinase, warfarin, heparin
Tubular toxicity	Aminoglycosides, NSAIDs, paracetamol (acetaminophen), iodine and gadolinium radiocontrast media, cefaloridine, cefalotin, amphotericin, rifampicin, pentamidine, vancomycin, cisplatin, nedaplatin, methoxyflurane, streptozocin, mithramycin, foscarnet, intravenous immunoglobulin, interferon, mannitol, high molecular weight starches and dextrans, zoledronate, fosfamide, quinolones, cidofovir, adefovir, tenofovir, herbal remedies
Rhabdomyolysis	Statins, fibrates, ethanol, codeine, barbiturates, diazepam, cocaine, ectasy
Haemolysis	Quinine, quinidine, sulfonamides, hydralazine, dapsone, primaquine, triamterene, nitrofurantoin, phenytoin
Glomerular disease	Gold, pencillamine, NSAIDs, interferon-alpha, captopril, lithium, mefenamate, mercury, pamidronate, tolmetin, foscarnet, ciprofloxacin
Intratubular obstruction	Aciclovir, indinavir, phosphate-based bowel purgatives and enemas, triamterene, ganciclovir, foscarnet, sulfanilamide, methotrexate

penicillins and third-generation cephalosporins can accumulate in CKD stage 5 patients, causing encephalopathy and fitting. Thus, drug dosages should be checked prior to prescribing in patients with AKI or CKD.

Some drugs predispose to AKI by either reducing renal blood supply or causing intrarenal ischaemia (pre-renal AKI), or by predisposing the renal tubular cells to AKI due to the anti-mitochondrial effects of HAART. Some drugs cause glomerular or tubular injury, which may be a direct toxic action or due to interstitial nephritis (see ATIN section). NSAIDs, gold, penicillamine, and interferon beta have all been reported to cause nephrotic syndrome.

Some drugs primarily cause proximal tubular defects (acetazolamide) or distal tubular defects. For example, amphotericin typically affects the distal tubule, causing renal tubular acidosis and magnesium wasting. Cisplatinum also characteristically leads to renal tubular magnesium wasting and hypomagnesaemia. Drugs affecting the distal tubule can lead to nephrogenic diabetes insipidus, with increased water loss and hypernatraemia (lithium, demeclocycline, amphotericin, cidofir, didanosine, and foscarnet).

Cholinergic drugs and herbal remedies containing atropine may affect the bladder leading to urinary retention.

Scleroderma renal crisis

Develops in some 15% of cases of diffuse scleroderma and 2% of limited scleroderma (see Chapter 16), and it is more common in those with anti-RNA polymerase III antibody.

Patients typically present with a rapidly progressive illness or a subacute presentation in association with the new onset of scleroderma or active skin disease. Characteristic clinical features include new onset hypertension, AKI, pulmonary oedema, myocarditis with pericardial effusion, encephalopathy, and even seizures.

Management
Careful control of blood pressure is mandatory, aiming to reduce blood pressure slowly and avoid hypotensive episodes. Intravenous prostanoids (epoprostenol 0.2–2.0 ng/kg/min) are often used in combination with short-acting angiotensin-converting enzyme inhibitors (ACE-Is) and then converting patients to longer-acting ACE-Is and angiotensin receptor blockers (ARBs) in the longer term. Dialysis may be required in the short term, but around 50% of patients recover residual renal function on follow-up. Renal biopsy characteristically shows onion ring appearance of the renal arterioles and pinhole occlusion, with a microangiopathic appearance in the glomerular capillaries. In some patients, an MCGN appearance may be present, particularly in those with an SLE overlap syndrome. Scleroderma has not been reported to recur post-renal transplantation.

Malignant hypertension
Malignant hypertension, with microangiopathic haemolytic anaemia (see Chapter 4), can develop as an accelerated form of hypertension in patients with underlying chronic glomerulonephritis, more commonly in African/Afro-Caribbean patients and those with IgA nephropathy, critical renal artery stenosis (RAS), and those with acute scleroderma and/or SLE.

Further reading

Ashley C and Currie A, eds. (2004). *The renal drug handbook*, 2nd edn. Radcliffe Medical Press, Oxford.

Epocrates (for dosing, side effects, complications of drugs) <http://www.epocrates.com>.

European Vasculitis trial group. <http://www.vasculitis.org>.

Keeling D, Mackie I, Moore GW, Greer IA, Greaves M, British Committee for Standards in Haematology (2012). Guidelines on the investigation and management of antiphospholipid syndrome. *British Journal of Haematology*, **157**, 47–58. <http://www.guideline.gov/content.aspx?id=36927>.

Kidney Disease: Improving Global Outcomes (KDIGO) (2012). Acute Kidney Injury Work Group. KDIGO clinical practice guideline for acute kidney injury. *Kidney International*, (Suppl) **2**, 1–138.

National Institute for Health and Clinical Excellence (2013). Acute kidney injury: Prevention, detection and management of acute kidney injury up to the point of renal replacement therapy. NICE clinical guideline 169. <https://www.nice.org.uk/guidance/cg169/resources/guidance-acute-kidney-injury-pdf>.

Royal Infirmary of Edinburgh Renal Unit. <http://renux.dmed.ed.ac.uk/edren/EdRenINFOhome.html>.

Thomsen HS (2006). Guidelines for contrast media from the European Society of Urogenital Radiology. *European Journal of Radiology*, **60**, 307–13. <http://www.esur.org/guidelines/>.

Wadei HM, Mai ML, Ahsan N, et al. (2006). Hepatorenal syndrome: pathophysiology and management. *Clinical Journal of the American Society of Nephrology*, **1**, 1066–72.

Walters G, Willis NS, Craig JC (2008). Interventions for renal vasculitis in adults. *Cochrane Database of Systematic Reviews*, **16**, CD003232.

Haematuria and proteinuria

Glomerulonephritis

All forms of glomerulonephritis can present with either haematuria or proteinuria or acute kidney injury. The majority of patients present with haematuria.

The glomerulus is a highly specialized structure. The afferent arteriole divides into a capillary tuft of specialized capillaries with a fenestrated endothelium, giving direct contact between blood and the capillary basement membrane. Blood exits via the efferent arteriole. The capillary network is contained within Bowman's capsule, in which the visceral epithelium follows the basement membrane, with a series of foot processes from highly branched podocytes. As the glomerular capillaries have no muscular wall, increased capillary flow or pressure causes capillary dilatation, and one key role of the podocytes is to mechanically regulate the diameter of the capillaries. Within Bowman's capsule and adjacent to the basement membrane is the mesangium, comprising mesangial cells, extracellular matrix, and trafficking macrophages/monocytes. The mesangial cells can change phenotype into myofibroblasts and regulate the capillary surface area.

Glomerulonephritis describes several conditions which primarily affect the glomerulus. Damage or inflammation within the glomerulus will typically lead to proteinuria and/or glomerular haematuria. In the days before renal histology was available, patients with glomerular kidney disease were classified, according to clinical presentation, as nephrotic syndrome, typically with heavy proteinuria, peripheral oedema, normal or minimal hypertension, often with preserved renal function, and nephritic syndrome with glomerular haematuria, hypertension, and impaired renal function.

Patients with glomerulonephritis may present with *nephrotic syndrome, acute kidney injury* (AKI) or *haematuria*.

Presentation with nephrotic syndrome

Nephrotic syndrome may present acutely with a triad of heavy proteinuria (>3.5 g/day in adults or urine protein/Cr >350 mg/mmol), hypoalbuminaemia (<25 g/L), and peripheral oedema. The only difference between nephrotic syndrome and nephritic syndrome with heavy proteinuria is that the patient has decompensated in the former and developed peripheral oedema. Many patients lose >3.5 g protein per day in their urine without clinically evident oedema.

Clinical presentation of nephrotic syndrome

Depending upon the aetiology (see Table 11.18), the history of peripheral oedema can be abrupt, in cases of minimal change nephropathy, or develop insidiously over weeks with amyloid. Patients typically awake with periorbital oedema. In severe cases, extensive peripheral oedema develops, with scrotal oedema, ascites, pleural, and even pericardial, effusions. The renal interstitium becomes oedematous and increases intrarenal pressure, stretching the renal capsule, causing discomfort and backache, particularly over the renal angles.

If nephrotic syndrome persists, then xanthelasmata may develop due to hyperlipidaemia and nail changes secondary to chronic hypoalbuminaemia.

Aetiology of proteinuria

The filtration of proteins is restricted by the negative charge and anatomical structure of the glomerular basement membrane. Proteins that cross this filtration barrier are further restricted by the slit pores between the podocyte foot processes and proteins trafficked through the mesangium back to the renal hilum. The majority of proteins which manage to pass through the slit pore are then actively taken up by proximal tubular cells and degraded so that, normally, only a small amount of protein is excreted in the urine, around 150 mg/day.

Thus, damage to the glomerular basement membrane or the slit pore can lead to major proteinuria, overwhelming the reabsorption capacity of the proximal tubule.

Investigation of nephrotic syndrome

Urine dipstick testing should confirm heavy proteinuria. Blood on dipstick testing could be non-glomerular, in the case of renal vein thombosis, or glomerular, depending upon the cause of nephrotic syndrome. In minimal change glomerulonephritis, proteinuria tends to be selective, with a urinary albumin/IgG ratio or IgG/transferrin ratio <0.10 or preferably <0.05.

Total serum proteins are often <50 g/L, with an albumin of <20 g/L. Serum electrophoresis typically shows increased alpha 2 globulins and, to a lesser extent, beta 2 globulins, with decreased IgG. There may be a non-specific increase in some tumour markers due to increased hepatic protein synthesis.

The combination of hypoalbuminaemia and low total proteins can lead to hyponatraemia due to non-osmotic

Table 11.18 Changing aetiology of nephrotic syndrome with age

	Children	Young adult	Older adult
Minimal change	77%	23%	18%
Focal segmental sclerosis	8%	18%	15%
Mesangiocapillary glomerulonephritis	7%	13%	5%
Membranous glomerulonephritis	2%	10%	34%
Other proliferative glomerulonephritis	6%	30%	15%
Amyloid	<1%	2%	16%

hypersecretion of ADH. Serum calcium may be reduced due to hypoalbuminaemia, and ionized calcium may be low due to urinary loss of vitamin D binding protein.

Increased interstitial pressure can lead to a type IV renal tubular acidosis with hyperkalaemia due to tubular ischaemia, but, occasionally, proximal tubular ischaemia leads to phosphaturia and mild glycosuria.

Complement and autoantibody levels may help to determine the underlying aetiology. C3 levels may be low with membranoproliferative GN and post-infective GN, but normal in idiopathic nephrotic syndrome.

Hyperlipidaemia is typical, with increased total cholesterol, VLDL, IDL, and LDL cholesterol, due to a combination of increased hepatic synthesis and reduced catabolism by endothelial lipoprotein lipase. Urinary losses of HDL (HDL-3) and reduced activity of lecithin cholesterol acyltransferase also lead to a reduction in HDL-2. Thus, patients with nephrotic syndrome have a very atherogenic lipid profile.

Patients with nephrotic syndrome are procoagulant due to urinary losses of the natural anticoagulants antithrombin, proteins S and C, with increased hepatic synthesis of fibrinogen, factors V and VII, and von Willebrand factor.

Summary of findings in nephrotic syndrome
1. Heavy proteinuria (3.5 g/day).
2. Mild haematuria (glomerular or non-glomerular).
3. Low serum protein and albumin.
4. Hyperlipidaemia.
5. Procoagulant state.
6. Hypocalcaemia.
7. Hyponatraemia.
8. Complement levels may be low or normal, depending on aetiology.
9. Renal tubular acidosis.

Renal biopsy is required to help to define the underlying pathology, as specific management depends on the underlying condition.

Complications of nephrotic syndrome
Acute kidney injury
Although patients with nephrotic syndrome have peripheral oedema, it can be difficult to assess the effective plasma volume. Apart from careful clinical examination, a spot urinary sodium of <10 mmol/L (mEq/L) is suggestive of intravascular volume depletion. Increased renal interstitial pressure due to interstitial oedema increases renal tubuloglomerular feedback, causing glomerular shutdown and AKI. This reduction in effective renal perfusion can be exacerbated by drugs used to manage nephrotic syndrome: diuretics, ACE-Is, ARBs, and NSAIDs.

Occasionally, a secondary interstitial nephritis due to a reaction to drugs supervenes or the underlying glomerulonephritis transforms to a crescentic disease, e.g. with idiopathic membranous change and/or SLE.

Venous thrombosis
Patient mobility is limited in severe nephrotic syndrome. Bed rest, with foot elevation, is part of the management, so patients are at risk of DVT and pulmonary emboli. This is compounded by the underlying prothrombotic state.

AKI may develop due to renal vein thrombosis. This typically occurs in children but can also occur in adults, particularly those with membranous glomerulonephritis, and underlying malignancy.

Risk of infection
IgG, C3, and other opsonins can be lost in the urine in nephrotic syndrome, which increases the risk of infection from encapsulated bacteria. Severe oedema increases the risk of infection from skin commensals, which gain access to the subcutaneous tissues following minor trauma, causing cellulitis.

Cardiovascular risk
Studies have shown that, in cases of persistent nephrotic syndrome, there is an increased risk of atheromatous cardiac disease on long-term follow-up. Hyperlipidaemia should, therefore, be treated aggressively.

Nutritional losses
Continued protein loss results in significant skeletal muscle wasting, which is exacerbated by lack of exercise, due to lethargy, and steroid therapy. Appetite may be depressed due to intestinal oedema, but high-protein diets increase renal glomerular blood flow and may exacerbate glomerular damage and increase proteinuria.

Risk of chronic kidney disease (CKD)
Persistent nephrotic syndrome is a major risk factor for progression of renal disease. Heavy proteinuria results in increased renal proximal tubular protein reabsorption, which leads to tubular damage with increased interstitial inflammation and interstitial fibrosis.

Management of nephrotic syndrome
Depending on the underlying aetiology, specific therapy may be required. Otherwise, patients should receive conservative management, aimed at reducing proteinuria and other risk factors for progression of renal disease and cardiovascular risk.

General management should be designed to reduce and control peripheral oedema. The key initial assessment is to determine whether the patient is intravascularly depleted since administration of diuretics may precipitate AKI. If they are intravascularly volume-depleted, then the patient should be nursed in bed, with the foot of the bed elevated, and the administration of 100 mL 20% albumin is recommended. This should be followed by reassessment of volume status.

Once fluid resuscitation is complete or if there are signs of fluid overload, then patients should be salt-restricted (80–100 mmol sodium/day), which entails a no-added salt diet, and started on loop diuretics. Infusions of loop diuretics (eg furosemide 5–10 mg/h) are more effective than oral administration. When loop diuretics increase distal sodium delivery, there may be a secondary increase in distal tubular sodium reabsorption, thus minimizing the effect of the loop diuretic. Thus, combinations of furosemide with amiloride are much more effective. Patients should be weighed daily to monitor fluid losses and the response to therapy. Oral fluids should be limited to around 1.0 L daily. Initially, an optimum weight loss of 1.0 kg/day should be achieved. Occasionally, in severe cases, typically with very high renal interstitial pressure, ultrafiltration using haemofiltration or haemodialysis machines, is required. Once fluid has been removed, the renal interstitial pressure falls and the kidney becomes diuretic-responsive.

Provided the patient is not hypovolaemic, then ACE-Is should be used to reduce proteinuria and carefully increased, aiming for a blood pressure of <120/80 mmHg. The combination of an ACE-I and ARB is the most potent to reduce proteinuria, but combination therapy is not without complications.

Other drugs that can be used to reduce proteinuria include ciclosporin, tacrolimus, and NSAIDs. However, these drugs may predispose to AKI in the short term and chronic kidney damage in the longer term.

To prevent infection, patients with nephrotic syndrome should be given prophylactic oral phenoxymethylpenicillin (INN), provided there is no penicillin allergy, and they have been vaccinated against pneumococcus, meningoccocus, and/or *Haemophilus influenzae*, etc.

To reduce the risk of thrombosis, patients with a serum albumin of <25 g/L are typically given subcutaneous low molecular weight heparin acutely. Although heparins may not be as effective as in normal subjects, due to antithrombin deficiency (<60%), low molecular weight heparins cause less osteoporosis and are more reliable anticoagulants than unfractionated heparin.

If the nephrotic syndrome continues, then the choice of anticoagulation as an outpatient is dictated by local practice, as there are no evidence-based guidelines. The options include continuing with low molecular weight heparin, switching to warfarin, using oral antiplatelet therapy, and possibly using oral direct thrombin inhibitors.

Hypercholesterolaemia should be treated with a statin and hypertriglyceridaemia with omega-3 fish oils due to the increased risk of cardiovascular disease.

Nutritional supplements may be required, as patients with nephrotic syndrome can lose zinc, selenium, and other trace elements. Otherwise, patients are recommended to adhere to their low-salt diet, with a normal protein intake of 1.0–1.2 g/kg/day.

In refractory cases of nephrotic syndrome, e.g. associated with amyloid, continued nutritional losses lead to severe protein malnutrition. In these cases, a difficult decision has to be made with the patient that, despite apparently normal or good renal function, bilateral nephrectomy (surgical or medical embolization) and institution of haemodialysis are required to halt protein losses and allow adequate nutrition.

Minimal change glomerulonephritis (MCN)

MCN is the commonest cause of nephrotic syndrome in children (90%), 50% of teenagers, and 10–15% of adults. It is more common in boys.

Most cases are idiopathic, although there is an association with HLA-DR7, allergies (fungi, poison ivy, ragweed, timothy grass pollen, house dust, medusa stings, bee stings, cat fur, cow's milk protein, egg), drugs (NSAIDs, sulfasalazine, mesalazine, penicillamine, lithium, rifampicin, gold, mercury, trimethadione, pamidronate), viral infections and haematological malignancy (Hodgkin's disease, mycosis fungoides, chronic lymphocytic leukaemia, and chronic graft vs host disease post-bone marrow transplantation), and other diseases causing glomerulonephritis (SLE and IgAN).

Diagnosis is by renal biopsy which typically appears normal under light microscopy with negative immunofluorescence, and podocyte foot process effacement on electron microscopy

Natural history of MCN

Early spontaneous remission occurs in 5% of cases, and up to 50% and 70% may remit after 18 and 36 months, respectively. However, MCN is typically a relapsing condition, with 66% of children having at least one relapse. Less than 5% of children continue to relapse as adults. Typically, patients with MCN do not develop CKD.

Twenty-two per cent of patients aged >60 years old who present with MCN have an underlying malignancy. Thus, older patients should be screened for lymphoma, lung, breast, stomach, large bowel, and renal cancers.

Treatment of MCN

In addition to general supportive care (as previously described), specific treatment is required to induce remission and prevent relapse. Typically, when in remission, urine dipstick testing should be negative for protein.

Prednisolone is used as induction therapy in MCN, starting at 40–60 mg/day in adults, or pulsed methylprednisolone intravenously. About 50% of adults will remit within 4 weeks, and 50–75% of adults will relapse within 12 months. Ten to 25% will have frequent relapses.

Relapses are treated with increased oral prednisolone doses which are rapidly tapered to response and remission. Other drugs which have been used include: oral levamisole, ciclosporin, and tacrolimus. Cytotoxic therapy (e.g. cyclophosphamide and chlorambucil) has also been used to treat MCN, with 67% of adults achieving sustained remission after an 8–12-week course. More recently rituximab has been used for relapsing MCN.

Focal segmental glomerulosclerosis (FSGS)

FSGS is not a singular entity but a number of separate conditions, which lead to damage of the glomerular podocytes and proteinuria. FSGS accounts for some 30–50% of adult nephrotic syndrome.

Primary or idiopathic FSGS is due to a circulating factor which increases glomerular permeability and results in proteinuria. Patients with the variant of the apolipoprotein L1 gene are predisposed to FSGS. Any condition which increases the flow or pressure within the glomerular capillary network will cause FSGS, as the increased pressure/flow causes a response from the visceral epithelial cells (podocytes) and, ultimately, cell death of podocytes. Healing occurs with fibrosis, resulting in glomerular damage, initially starting at the glomerular hilum and then progressing outwards. Under normal conditions, not all nephron units work equally. Those at the juxtaglomerular junction function all day, whereas cortical nephrons tend to switch on according to need. Thus, FSGS tends to affect the juxtaglomerular nephrons first. As such, early in the disease, a renal biopsy may miss these glomeruli, and the biopsy may be reported as MCN. FSGS is a condition primarily affecting the podocytes, and there are a myriad of causes of FSGS (see Table 11.19), including hyperfiltration injury, which may be an adaptive response to reduced nephron numbers.

Clinical presentation of FSGS

FSGS typically presents with proteinuria, which can range from asymptomatic proteinuria through to nephrotic syndrome. At presentation, 30–50% of patients will have hypertension, 25–75% dipstick-positive haematuria, and 20–30% will have reduced renal function.

Renal pathology in FSGS

This presents a number of distinct histological variants. **Classic FSGS** reveals segmental sclerosis, involving part of the glomerular tuft in some, but not all, glomeruli (focal). Glomerular capillaries may be occluded by hyaline deposits (proteins in the capillary wall) and foam cells (lipid-laden macrophages). Immune complexes are absent on immunochemistry, but scattered deposits of IgM, C3, and C1 may be present in areas of sclerosis. Electron microscopy shows diffuse

Table 11.19 Secondary causes of FSGS

Genetic	Alpha actinin 4 (AD)
	Podocin (AR)
	TRPC6 (AD)
	CD2-AP
Infection	HIV-1
	Parvovirus B19
	SV40 virus
Drugs	Pamidronate
	Interferon alfa
	Lithium
	Heroin
Tumours	Lymphoma
	Burkitt's lymphoma
Hyperfiltration with reduced renal mass	Post-nephrectomy
	Chronic allograft nephropathy
	Reflux nephropathy
	Renal dysplasia
	Oligomeganephronia
	Cholesterol emboli
	Unilateral agenesis
	Intrauterine growth retardation
Hyperfiltration with normal renal mass	Hypertension
	Obesity
	Sickle cell anaemia
	Cyanotic heart disease
	Pre-eclampsia

AD, autosomal dominant; AR, autosomal recessive.

Table 11.20 Secondary causes of membranous glomerulonephritis

Immunological		
SLE		
Mixed connective tissue disease		
Rheumatoid arthritis		
Antiphospholipid syndrome		
Sjögren's syndrome		
Autoimmune hepatitis		
Autoimmune thyroiditis		
Anti-GBM disease		
Graft vs host disease	HLA antibody	
Renal transplant	Neutral endopeptidase	
Maternal antibody transfer		
Malignancy		
Solid organs	Lung	
	Breast	
	GI tract	
	Kidney	
	Prostate	
Haematological	Lymphoma	
	Hodgkin's	
Infection		
Parasite	Malaria	
	Schistosomiasis	
	Filariasis	
Bacterial	Leprosy	
	Syphilis	
Viral	Hepatitis B	
	Hepatitis C	
	HIV	
Drugs	penicillamine	
	Gold	
	Captopril	
	Probenecid	
	NSAIDs	
	Bucillamine	
Other	Diabetes	
	Sickle cell disease	
	Mercury	

podocyte foot process effacement. There is also an FSGS perihilar variant, in which there is >50% perihilar hyalinosis and sclerosis in those sclerotic glomeruli (typically seen in cases of hyperfiltration injury). Other variants include FSGS cellular variant, FSGS collapsing (typically reported with HIV and pamidronate), and an FSGS tip variant.

Medical management of FSGS

Patients with subnephrotic proteinuria are usually managed conservatively, aiming for strict blood pressure control, using ACE-Is and/or ARBs, and minimizing cardiovascular risk factors (see 'Chronic kidney disease').

FSGS presenting with nephrotic syndrome should initially be managed conservatively (as described previously). Patients with secondary FSGS may benefit from specific treatments, such as HAART for those due to HIV, potential precipitating drugs discontinued, and underlying malignancies treated. Otherwise, immunosuppression can be considered in cases of idiopathic FSGS, provided that eGFR >30 mL/min.

There is no agreed protocol treatment; however, most centres start with a trial of steroids, followed by combination therapies with immunosuppressive agents, similar to those used to treat MCN. The tip variant is more likely to respond to immunosuppressive treatment.

Membranous glomerulonephritis (MGN)

MGN occurs in 11 per million people and is the commonest cause of nephrotic syndrome in adults. It is twice as common in males. About 25% of cases are secondary to an underlying condition (see Table 11.20), including malignancy.

Aetiology of MGN

The majority of patients (70%) with idiopathic membranous nephropathy have IgG4 antibodies against a conformation-dependent epitope in the M type phospholipase A2 receptor present in the podocyte. About 5% have antibodies to thrombospondin type-1 domain-containing 7A (THSD7A) Idiopathic MGN is more common in adults than children (75% vs 25%). Although the association with malignancy increases with age (22% in those >60 years), there is also an association with HLA-DQA1.

Some cases of human MGN are associated with immune complex deposition in the GBM and are specific to the underlying disease (e.g. HBeAg and HBeAb in HBV).

Clinical outcome of MGN

Approximately one-third of patients undergo complete remission; one-third undergo a remitting and relapsing course and have an excellent renal prognosis. However, 30% never remit and progress to CKD.

Clinical assessment and investigation of MGN

It is important to obtain a full history and detailed examination of the patient to help to differentiate idiopathic from secondary causes of MGN. As with any renal condition, assessment of fluid volume status and renal function is mandatory. Urinary dipstick testing, with appropriate microscopy and quantification of proteinuria, is required.

Renal histology in MGN

Early in the course of MGN, the light microscopic findings may be normal, but then the GBM thickens, with basement membrane spikes appearing, typically demonstrated with silver staining. Characteristically, immunofluorescence detects IgG (predominantly IgG4), C3, and C5-9 in the GBM. IgA or IgM staining within the mesangium is more often associated with secondary causes of MGN. Occasionally, MGN can transform into a crescentic disease with anti-GBM antibodies. Dense deposits are apparent on electron microscopy, initially in the subepithelial space and which become surrounded by GBM. The position of these dense deposits has been used to stage MGN: **stage I:** subepithelial deposit; **stage II:** GBM projection between the deposits; **stage III:** new GBM surrounds the deposits; **stage IV:** highly thickened GBM, with loss of spikes. Podocyte foot process effacement is lost, as in any proteinuric state.

Risk of developing CKD in MGN

Older male patients are more likely to develop progressive CKD. The other main risk factors for progression are persistent nephrotic syndrome, impaired renal function at presentation, renal biopsy showing interstitial fibrosis and tubular atrophy.

Treatment of MGN

All patients should receive general supportive management to minimize proteinuria and reduce cardiovascular risk (see section on the management of nephrotic syndrome). In cases of secondary MGN, treatment of the underlying cause may sometimes lead to spontaneous remission of MGN.

Several treatments have been suggested to induce remission of nephrotic syndrome in patients with progressive MGN. These include: chlorambucil and steroids—methylprednisolone, 1 g IV for 3 days, followed by oral prednisolone 30–40 mg/day for 1 month, alternating with chlorambucil 0.1–0.2 mg/kg/day for 6 months, has been reported to decrease proteinuria and progression to CKD. An alternative regime uses cyclophosphamide 2.5 mg/day, instead of chlorambucil (modified Ponticelli regimen).

Another possibility is ciclosporin which has been reported to have higher rates of partial and complete remission. The results of a UK MRC trial investigating the effect of ciclosporin A and conservative management for progressive MGN is awaited.

Renal amyloidosis

Renal amyloidosis develops due to the deposition of amyloid fibrils within the glomerulus. Typically, these are monoclonal light chains (AL amyloid) or serum amyloid A protein (SAA or AA amyloid), and occasionally other proteins—fibrinogen A-alpha chain, transthyretin, lysozyme, apolipoprotein AI or AII, and gesolin. Typically, these amyloid deposits usually stain with Congo red and are birefringent under polarized light.

Aetiology of renal amyloidosis

The fibrils in AL amyloid are derived from monoclonal immunoglobulins. These are typically low-grade B cell dyscrasias and often very difficult to detect. Whereas AA amyloid results from persistent inflammation, with increased production of SAA1 and SSA2, which are broken down to amyloidogenic peptides which form the fibrils. In addition to chronic infections, chronic inflammatory diseases (typically arthritides and inflammatory bowel disease), and malignancy, there are a number of hereditary inflammatory conditions which predispose to AA amyloid, including familial Mediterranean fever, Muckle–Wells syndrome, and disorders of the TNF receptor (TRAPS).

Presentation

Renal amyloidosis, fibrillary glomerulopathy, and immunoactoid glomerulopathy usually present with nephrotic syndrome or proteinuria. Microscopic haematuria may also be present.

Renal biopsy appearance of renal amyloidosis

There is an increased risk of bleeding post-renal biopsy in cases of amyloid. Typically, on light microscopy, there is positive mesangial staining for Congo red and change in red to green colour of the deposits under polarized light. Fibrillary glomerulopathy and immunoactoid glomerulopathy often have a mesangiocapillary or atypical membranous appearance. Immunofluorecence and electron microscopy can be helpful in characterizing the deposits. In AL amyloid and immunoactoid glomerulopathy, the deposits are clonal, whereas, in fibrillary glomerulopathy, IgG is polyclonal but of κ4 isotype. In addition to glomerular deposition, AA amyloid is often found within in the interstitium.

Additional investigations in renal amyloidosis

Apart from the usual screening investigations for patients with nephrotic syndrome and additional standard serum and urine electrophoresis, immunofixation, and cryoglobulin measurement, a search for free λ and κ light chains should be made to look for an underlying B cell dyscrasia.

Treatment of renal amyloidosis

Medical management should be instituted to limit proteinuria (see section on the management of nephrotic syndrome). Specific treatment targeted at the B cells producing the amyloidogenic proteins is required in cases of AL amyloid, immunoactoid glomerulopathy, and fibrillary glomerulopathy (see section on multiple myeloma). Unfortunately, immunoactoid glomerulopathy tends to be refractory to treatment, and patients typically progress to CKD. Similarly, in cases of AA amyloid, specific treatment should be directed to the underlying cause. Familial Mediterranean fever may respond to colchicine therapy.

Mesangiocapillary glomerulonephritis (MCGN)

MCGN is synonymous with membranoproliferative glomerulonephritis and is an unusual cause of nephrotic syndrome (<10%) in Europe, with an incidence of 0.9 per 10^6. In Europe, MCGN may occur due to hepatitis C, typically in middle-aged and older men.

Aetiology of MCGN

MCGN arises due to glomerular damage from either chronic complement activation in the plasma or due to deposition of immune complexes and complement activation within the basement membrane.

MCGN is classified into **type I**, in which there are persistent circulating immune complexes or cryoglobulins (see Table 11.21) which activate complement. **Type II** results from persistent activation of the alternative complement pathway, typically due to C3 nephritic factor, an

Table 11.21 Classification of cryoglobulinaemias

Type	Constituent	Underlying pathology
I	Monoclonal IgG, IgM, or IgA	Myeloma Lymphoma Waldenström's
II	Monoclonal IgM rheumatoid factor and polyclonal IgG	'Essential' Hepatitis C Lymphoma Sjögren's syndrome
III	Polyclonal IgM rheumatoid factor and polyclonal IgG	SLE Rheumatoid arthritis Chronic infections Hepatitis C Hepatitis B Idiopathic

Reprinted from Elsevier, 57, 5, J-C Brouet et al., 'Biologic and clinical significance of cryoglobulins: a report of 86 cases', pp. 775–788, Copyright 1974, with permission from Elsevier.

Table 11.22 Secondary causes of MCGN

Cryoglobulinaemia	Type II or III
Viral	Chronic viral hepatitis B and C, HIV-1
Bacterial or fungal	SBE, abscess, shunt nephritis, bronchiectasis, TB, leprosy, Candida
Parasitic	Malaria or schistosomiasis
Autoimmune	SLE, Sjögren's, Castleman's disease, systemic sclerosis, mixed cryoglobulinaemia
Complement deficiency	Hereditary or acquired
Liver disease	Cirrhosis and alpha-1-antitrypsin deficiency
Miscellaneous	Sickle cell disease, cyanotic heart disease, sarcoid
Malignancy	CL, lymphoma, myeloma, light chain nephropathy, hydatidiform mole, ovarian dysgerminoma
C3 nephritic factor	Partial lipodystrophy
Factors H/I deficiency	Hereditary or acquired

autoantibody which activates C3 convertase. Rarely, type II is associated with defects of factor H or factor I, which prevent inhibition of the alternative complement pathway once activated. **Type III** has the same associations as type I, but plasma complement proteins C1q and C4 are usually normal.

Clinical presentation of MCGN

Patients typically present with a nephritic pattern, rather than nephrotic syndrome. Vasculitic rashes and joint involvement may suggest an underlying cryoglobulinaemia (see Table 11.22).

Renal biopsy appearance in MCGN

In all three types of MCGN, the light microscopy findings are similar with thickening of the GBM, mesangial expansion, and cellular proliferation, with an inflammatory cell infiltrate. Electron microscopy defines the subtypes; in type I, the immune deposits are subendothelial and occasionally mesangial and subepithelial, whereas, in type II, they are present in the central part of the GBM, known as the lamina densa, so have been named 'dense deposits'. In type III MCGN, the deposits are both subendothelial and subepithelial, so giving the GBM a layered appearance, and also in the mesangium.

Investigation of MCGN

Patients should be investigated for underlying causes. In particular, complement proteins should be measured, as C3 will be low in 50% of cases, and both classical pathway complement proteins (C2, C4, C1q) and terminal complement proteins (C5b-C9) will also be reduced in type I. Nephritic factor may be present. In MCGN type II, ~75% of patients will have a low C3 and nC3 nephritic factor; other classical complement proteins are typically normal, and the terminal complement proteins normal or low. Patients with MCGN type III usually have similar findings to type I patients, but the classical pathway complement proteins (C2, C4, and C1q) are typically normal.

Treatment of MCGN

As with other forms of glomerulonephritis, patients should be treated conservatively to control blood pressure, minimize proteinuria (see section on the management of nephrotic syndrome), and reduce cardiovascular risks.

Treatment should be targeted to the underlying disease. For example, HCV-induced MCGN type 1 may respond to peginterferon alfa therapy with ribavarin, with the disappearance of cryoglobulinaemic skin rash and remission of proteinuria. Recent small series have suggested that rituximab is effective in treating HCV-induced MCGN type I.

The prognosis depends upon the underlying aetiology. Progression to CKD is more likely in older male patients, who are hypertensive and have nephrotic syndrome and renal impairment at presentation. Therapy with aspirin and dipyridamole has also been reported to improve outcome in adults and children.

Essential or idiopathic MCGN type II does not respond to steroids or ciclosporin. High-volume plasma exchange (60 mL/kg) with fresh frozen plasma may have a role in terms of supplying factor H or factor I in those rare cases of factor H or I deficiency. Preliminary reports have suggested a role for rituximab in cases of C3 nephritic factor-induced MCGN type II.

Presentations with nephritic syndrome

Acute endocapillary glomerulonephritis (AEGN)

AEGN is the archetypical cause of nephritic syndrome, presenting with a nephritic urinary sediment, sometimes with macroscopic haematuria, hypertension, oliguria, peripheral oedema, and impaired renal function.

Traditionally, this develops 10–14 days following a Lancefield group A beta-haemolytic streptococcal infection, either a respiratory tract infection with serotypes 12, 1, 2, and 4 or skin infection with serotypes 49, 47, 55, and 57.

Aetiology

AEGN typically occurs post–infection, with antigen deposition in the glomerular basement membrane (see Table 11.23), which are then bound by circulating host antibody, so immune complexes form within the GBM. It most commonly occurs in children but may occur in adults.

IgA nephropathy (IgAN)

Berger's disease is defined as the deposition of IgA1 in the glomerular mesangium. It is the most common cause of glomerulonephritis in the developed world.

Aetiology of IgAN

IgAN typically affects young males aged 10–30 years old. Changes in glycosylation around the hinge region of the IgA1 molecule expose novel epitopes, allowing cross-reacting antibody formation, leading to circulating immune complexes which deposit within the renal mesangium, leading to local inflammation and injury. IgAN should be differentiated from secondary causes of intraglomerular IgA deposition, which are usually due to failure of the liver and/or spleen to remove IgA immune complexes (cirrhosis—particularly alcoholic, and coeliac disease) or elevated serum IgA (HIV-1 and AIDS), and/or IgA-associated vasculitis (Henoch–Schönlein purpura; see section on Henoch–Schönlein purpura). In addition, IgA may be deposited in other conditions, such as SLE, and has also been reported in post-infectious glomerulonephritis, particularly with *Staphylococcus aureus*.

Table 11.23 Infections associated with acute endocapillary glomerulonephritis

Bacteria	Streptococci
	Staphylococci
	Mycobacteria
	Meningococci
	Salmonella
Viruses	Hepatitis B
	Epstein–Barr virus
	Cytomegalovirus
	Rubella
	Mumps
Fungi	*Candida*
	Coccidioides
	Histoplasma
Parasites	Malaria
	Schistosomiasis
	Toxoplasmosis
	Filariasis

Clinical presentation of IgAN

Most patients are asymptomatic and are detected on urinary dipstick testing with microscopic haematuria although some patients develop frank macroscopic haematuria, or bleeding, following an upper respiratory tract infection, and may even develop AKI. Nephrotic syndrome develops in <5% of patients.

Natural history of IgAN

Approximately 30% of patients will develop slowly progressive CKD, requiring dialysis over 15–30 years, with a small proportion developing a rapidly progressive form leading to end-stage failure within 4 years. The majority of patients have stable renal function.

Risk factors for progression of IgAN

As with other forms of glomerulonephritis, older age, hypertension, increasing proteinuria, impaired renal function at presentation, and renal interstitial fibrosis with tubular atrophy on renal biopsy are all associated with progressive CKD.

Although around 30% of patients will have an increased serum IgA1 and increased λ to κ light chain ratio and other circulating autoantibodies, including IgA rheumatoid factor, these do not correlate with clinical outcome.

Treatment of IgAN

As with other forms of glomerulonephritis, strict blood pressure control, designed to minimize proteinuria, and reduction in cardiovascular risk factors is required (see 'Chronic kidney disease'). There is no firm evidence for any disease-modifying treatment at present.

In cases of crescentic IgA associated with a rapid decline in renal function, a trial of steroids and cyclophosphamide should be considered (see section on vasculitis treatment).

Diabetic nephropathy

It is important to be aware of diabetic nephropathy since this is the commonest cause of CKD stage 5, and many patients present acutely with complications of their disease. It occurs more frequently in some racial groups, such as West Indians, black Americans, and South Asians.

Management of diabetic nephropathy

If diabetic patients only have proteinuria, then diabetic nephropathy is most likely, particularly if they have diabetic retinopathy. However, diabetic patients may have alternative renal pathology, such as renal artery stenosis, autonomic bladder dysfunction, or recurrent UTIs. Patients presenting with sudden-onset proteinuria, and those with haematuria should be investigated accordingly.

Improve glycaemic control and lower blood pressure

For patients with diabetic nephropathy, progressive CKD can be slowed by a combination of tight glycaemic control (HbA1c <7.0 %), with strict blood pressure control (≤130/80 mmHg: but not too low a systolic pressure (>110 mmHg)), and minimizing proteinuria, coupled with reduction in cardiovascular risk factors. The combination of ACE-Is and ARBs is the most potent regimen for reducing proteinuria but can lead to hyperkalaemia, potentially preventing or restricting their use. Diabetes also causes renal tubular ischaemia, with type IV renal tubular acidosis, so patients are more prone to hyperkalaemia. Diuretics, initially thiazide and then loop diuretics, are important in preventing sodium retention and treating hypertension. If blood pressure remains elevated, beta-blockers, and then calcium channel blockers, should be added.

Renovascular hypertension

Narrowing of the main renal artery or arteries and renal artery stenosis (RAS) can lead to hypertension and CKD. In Western Europe, more than 90% of cases are due to atheroma (ARAS) and the remainder are generally due to fibromuscular disease (FMD). However, in Japan, RAS may be secondary to Takayasu's arteritis. Other causes include Castleman's disease, middle aortic arch and antiphospholipid syndromes. Occasionally, RAS develops in neurofibromatosis type 1.

Fibromuscular disease (FMD)

FMD leads to medial hyperplasia, with collagen deposition leading to areas of vessel wall thinning and thickening. It is more commonly found in middle-aged women but is thought to occur in around 5% of the population. It accounts for <1% of all hypertensive patients. In patients with hypertension and >50% narrowing of the renal artery, angioplasty with stenting is likely to cure the hypertension in 30% of patients.

Atheromatous renal artery stenosis

Most patients with atheromatous renal artery stenosis have hypertension, small-vessel renal disease, and CKD, which has been termed atherosclerotic renovascular disease. The prevalence of atheromatous renal artery stenosis increases with age, with some reports suggesting that >40% of patients are aged >75 years old. In addition, atheromatous renal artery stenosis is increased in patients with other vascular disease, including 30–50% of patients with peripheral vascular disease, 10–30% with coronary artery disease, and 30% of patients with aortic aneurysms. Apart from age, other risk factors include smoking, hyperlipidaemia, type 2 diabetes, and CKD.

Clinical presentation

Patients with atheromatous renal artery stenosis are usually diagnosed with CKD and hypertension but may present with AKI secondary to volume depletion, institution of ACE-Is/ARBs, post-radiocontrast imaging, cholesterol emboli syndrome (and/or sudden arterial occlusion), malignant phase hypertension, and cardiac failure.

RAS typically develops at, or within, 1 cm of the renal artery origin (ostium) from the aorta, probably due to shear stress. Vascular calcification is common, particularly in patients with CKD. Progression occurs over time such that, at diagnosis, around 30% of patients have bilateral disease. CKD develops due to a combination of small-vessel (intrarenal) disease, hypertension, ischaemia, and cholesterol embolization.

MRA is the diagnostic screening test of choice (see 'Investigation of the renal tract'). Although MRA will always overestimate the degree of stenosis, dynamic MAG3 captopril studies may be helpful in assessing the functional effect of RAS.

Management

Patients require appropriate blood pressure control and cardiovascular risk factor management (see 'Chronic kidney disease'). Once renal size has shrunk to <8 cm, then active treatment of the stenosis is usually futile. Treatment of the stenosis with angioplasty and/or stenting remains controversial, since only 30% of patients with >75% stenosis have an improvement of renal function post-angioplasty or stenting. However, most centres would treat RAS in cases of 'flash' pulmonary oedema, acute AKI secondary to RAS (due to acute occlusion), malignant phase hypertension, and severe difficult to control hypertension (four or more agents), provided the renal size was ≥8 cm.

Although ACE-Is and ARBs may potentially trigger AKI in patients with RAS, many patients benefit from these agents in helping to reduce intrarenal vascular disease progression. This may be a consideration in deciding whether to treat the stenosis, prior to commencing ACE-Is/ARBs.

Chronic tubulointerstitial nephropathy (CTIN)

Chronic tubulointerstitial nephritis is usually asymptomatic and presents with slowly progressive renal impairment. Urinalysis may be normal or show low-grade proteinuria (<1.5 g/day) and/or pyuria. Diagnosis depends on renal biopsy, which reveals variable cellular infiltration of the interstitium, tubular atrophy, and fibrosis. There are many causes, including sarcoidosis, drugs, irradiation, toxins, and metabolic disorders.

Diseases which cause acute tubulointerstitial nephropathy may evolve into chronic interstitial disease. By affecting the renal tubules and interstitium, these may lead to damage to the proximal tubule or the distal tubule, or both. Thus, conditions which cause tubulointerstitial nephropathy can lead to renal tubular acidosis, with systemic acidosis and consequent metabolic bone disease.

Renal tubular acidosis

Conditions which primarily affect the proximal tubule may cause a Fanconi-like syndrome, with associated proximal tubule defects, including renal glycosuria, bicarbonate losses (type 2 proximal renal tubular acidosis), phosphate wasting, aminoaciduria, and losses of small molecular weight proteins, such as vitamin D-binding protein.

Conditions which predominantly affect the distal renal tubule cause distal renal tubular acidosis (type 1), as the kidney cannot excrete an acid urine, and typically the minimum urine pH is >5.5. These patients have a normal anion gap but are prone to nephrocalcinosis and osteomalacia.

These conditions can be inherited diseases or acquired due to autoimmune diseases (SLE, Sjögren's syndrome, rheumatoid arthritis, primary biliary cirrhosis, chronic active hepatitis, Hashimoto's thyroiditis, cryoglobulinaemia), hypergammaglobulinaemia, upper urinary tract obstruction, nephrocalcinosis (medullary sponge kidney, hyperparathyroidism, milk alkali syndrome, Fabry's disease, Wilson's disease), renal transplantation—immediately post-operatively, sickle cell/HbSC disease, malaria, leprosy, and toxins (drugs—lithium, amphotericin, ifosfamide, vanadate, cyclamate, trimethoprim; toxins—toluene, benzene, glue sniffing).

Conditions which affect both proximal and distal tubules can cause type IV renal tubular acidosis, resulting in hypoaldosteronism and hyperkalaemia. These include pseudohypoaldosteronism (types 1 and 2), primary adrenal insufficiency, congenital hyperplasia, aldosterone synthase deficiency, drugs (potassium-sparing diuretics, heparins, ACE-Is >> ARBs, NSAIDs, ciclosporin, tacrolimus), diabetic nephropathy, HIV infection, SLE, severe nephrotic syndrome, and tubulointerstitial disease.

Specific types of CTIN
Sarcoidosis
Although sarcoidosis can be associated with glomerulonephritis, it is one of the classic forms of non-caseating granulomatous interstitial nephritis. Presentation is varied, ranging from AKI to CKD, Fanconi-like syndrome to distal renal tubular acidosis, with nephrocalcinosis, and calcium oxalate calculi. Treatment is with prednisolone 1–1.5 mg/kg/day (max 60 mg), but renal recovery may only be partial, dependent upon the amount of chronic damage. Sarcoid granuloma may recur post-transplantation.

Radiation nephritis
External irradiaton of >10 Gy in a single dose or >20 Gy in fractions over 4 weeks can lead to radiation nephritis. Symptoms and signs typically take 3 months or more to appear, with hypertension and fluid retention. ACE-Is and ARBs may help to reduce progression. Occasionally, an HUS-like syndrome can occur within weeks of irradiation (see section on HUS).

Sickle cell nephropathy
Sickle cell and HbSC disease may lead to repeated episodes of intrarenal sickling, leading to ischaemic chronic tubulointerstitial nephritis (CTIN) and papillary necrosis. This is less common now that management of sickling crisis has improved, and sickle cell patients typically develop CKD due to hyperfiltration FSGS.

Chinese herbal nephropathy
CTIN may be due to Chinese herbal medicines which contain aristocholic acid, a nephrotoxin from the Aristolachia species. Balkan nephropathy may be caused by a fungal toxin and also carries an increased risk for uroepithelial tumour.

Patients usually present with end-stage renal failure, with bilateral small kidneys, tubular proteinuria, and renal biopsy showing severe interstitial fibrosis. There is a marked increase in risk of uroepithelial tumour such that some centres advocate native ureteronephrectomy, prior to transplantation, with regular screening cystoscopy.

South Asian subcontinent nephropathy
After diabetes, the next most common cause of CKD in the South Asian subcontinent population, both in India and the UK, is a chronic interstitial nephropathy, which typically presents with CKD, hypertension, minor proteinuria (100–200 mg/mmol), with increased retinol binding/albumin ratio, and bilateral small kidneys. Renal biopsy shows

chronic tubulointerstitial nephritis. The aetiology is unknown. There is no specific treatment, and it does not recur post-transplantation

Central America and Sri Lanka also have an excess of interstitial nephritis.

Heavy metal-induced CTIN
This is secondary to lead, cadmium, arsenic, or mercury toxicity. Acute lead toxicity can cause a Fanconi-like syndrome, but chronic lead toxicity leads to hypertension and saturnine gout. Although chelation therapy (calcium edentate or dimercaprol) can successfully treat acute lead toxicity, it does not reverse the chronic fibrotic changes associated with chronic lead nephrotoxicty. Blood lead reflects recent exposure, and high levels (>3.9 micromoles/L or 80 mcg/dL in adults, and 2.3 micromoles/L or 45 mcg/dL in children) should prompt chelation therapy.

Cadmium exposure can also cause CTIN, with Fanconi syndrome. Arsenic poisoning typically causes jaundice and AKI, but CTIN often develops with chronic exposure or following acute poisoning in the survivors.

Mercury, uranium, and polonium typically cause AKI with acute tubular toxicity, but chronic low-dose exposure can lead to CTIN.

Analgesic nephropathy
CTIN due to phenacetin was widely reported, particularly in women, in the USA, Sweden, and Australia. Since then, it has been recognized that NSAIDs and other analgesics (paracetamol, in combination with aspirin, caffeine, and codeine) can cause a slowly progressive CTIN, which may present with acute pain due to papillary necrosis, and there is an increased risk of uroepithelial carcinoma.

Further reading
Angioplasty and Stent for Renal Artery Lesions trial (ASTRAL). <http://www.astral.bham.ac.uk>.

Birkeland SA and Storm HH (2003). Glomerulonephritis and malignancy: a population based study. *Kidney International*, **63**, 716–21.

Choudry D and Ahmed Z (2006). Drug-associated renal dysfunction and injury. *Nature Clinical Practice*, **2**, 80–91.

Davison AM, Camero JS, Grunfeld JP, et al., eds. (2006). *Oxford textbook of clinical nephrology*, 3rd edn. Oxford University Press, Oxford.

Floege J and Feehally J (2007). Introduction to glomerular disease: clinical presentations. In J Feehally, J Floege, E Johnson, eds. *Comprehensive clinical nephrology*, pp. 193–207. Mosby, St Louis.

Lai ASH (2006). Viral nephropathy. *Nature Clinical Practice*, **2**, 254–62.

Laing CM and Unwin RJ (2006). Renal tubular acidosis. *Journal of Nephrology*, **19** (Suppl 9), S46–52.

Naicker S, Fabian J, Naidoo S, Wadee S, Paget G, Goetsch S (2007). Infection and glomerulonephritis. *Seminars in Immunopathology*, **9**, 397–414.

National Kidney Federation. Information on renal biopsy. <http://www.kidney.org.uk/help/medical-information-from-the-nkf-/kidney-disease-biopsy/>.

Sclari F, Ravani P, Piola A, et al. (2003). Predictors of renal and patient outcomes in atheroembolic renal disease: a prospective study. *Journal of the American Society of Nephrology*, **14**, 1584–90.

The Internationsl IgA Nephropathy Network. <http://www.iganworld.org>.

Tryggvason K and Patrakka J (2006). Thin basement membrane nephropathy in adults with persistent haematuria. *Journal of the American Society of Nephrology*, **17**, 813–22.

US Food and Drug Administration. For gadolinium-based contrast agents and risk of NSF. <http://www.fda.gov/Safety/MedWatch/SafetyInformation/SafetyAlertsforHumanMedicalProducts/ucm225375.htm>.

Waldeman M, Crew RJ, Valeria A, et al. (2007). Adult minimal change disease. Clinical characteristics, treatment and outcomes. *Clinical Journal of the American Society of Nephrology*, **2**, 445–53.

Urinary tract infection (UTI)

Definitions
Asymptomatic bacteruria is a single isolate of $\geq 10^5$ colony-forming units/mL (CFU) in appropriately collected urine in asymptomatic patients. In comparison, lower UTI urine also contains leucocytes and the patient has symptoms of dysuria, suprapubic pain, frequency, urgency, and strangury. Acute pyelonephritis is an infection of the upper urinary tract, characterized by fever, loin pain, and dysuria. Reinfection is a separate infection after clearance of UTI, whereas a relapse is a recurrent UTI with the same organism which had not been successfully eradicated. Complicated infections are those occurring in an abnormal (congenital or acquired) upper or lower urinary tract.

Epidemiology
UTI is more common in women, with 50–60% suffering at least one UTI. Incidence is increased in young, sexually active, and post-menopausal women. Infection is more common in atonic bladders (spina bifida, MS, diabetic neuropathy) and following renal transplantation.

Microbiology
E. coli and coagulase-negative staphylococci (CNS) are the commonest bacteria causing UTI, although, in complicated infections, Pseudomonas and enterococci are increased. The bacterial spectum for lower and upper tract UTIs is similar, as most upper tract infections develop from ascending lower UTIs.

Pathogenesis
Host factors include short urethra and proximity to the anus in women, sexual intercourse, non-secretion of ABO blood group antigens, and P1 blood group phenotype (recognized by bacterial adhesins). Bacterial factors include fimbriae or other adhesion mechanisms. It is now recognized that bacteria may be taken up by the vesical mucosa, exist intracellularly, and then later undergo replication and release, so accounting for clinical relapses and reinfection.

When to treat asymptomatic bacteruria
Asymptomatic bacteruria increases with age in both sexes (20% of women >80, and 15% of men >75 years old). As patients are asymptomatic without pyuria, treatment is not warranted, except for pregnant women (increased risk of pyelonephritis, premature labour, and IUGR), patients due for urological intervention (increased risk of bacteraemia), and renal transplant recipients (risk of allograft pyelonephritis).
Treatment is antimicrobial therapy for 3–7 days.

What defines a urinary tract infection as significant?
Many patients will have symptoms of lower UTI but without a pure growth of $\geq 10^5$ CFU/mL. Contamination of urine samples is the main problem in trying to determine whether patients have UTI. Urine dipstick testing for leucocyte esterase is more predictable for detecting UTI than nitrites. Urine microscopy showing leucocytes (pyuria) is supportive of UTI (but can also be increased in interstitial nephritis and cystitis, renal calculi, tumours, infections with Chlamydia, TB, and ureaplasma). Urine cytology is helpful in demonstrating free bacteria but may also show intracellular bacteria. In a clean-catch (midstream) urine sample, a bacterial count of $\geq 10^2$ CFU/mL (or any bacteria in a suprapubic catheter specimen from infants <1 year), with pyuria and symptoms, is almost always a significant UTI.

Lower urinary tract infection
Lower UTI needs to be differentiated from urethritis (Chlamydia, Neisseria, herpes simplex), vaginitis (Candida, Trichomonas), pelvic inflammatory disease, and prostatis in men. Acute prostatitis requires ≥ 4 weeks' treatment with fluoroquinolones to prevent chronic infection.
Diagnosis (as described previously) is traditionally based on $\geq 10^5$ CFU/mL with pyuria and symptoms, although lower counts are acceptable.
Treatment is a 3-day course of trimethoprim, co-trimoxazole, or fluoroquinolones, or a single dose of amoxicillin (3g) or fosfomycin, or longer courses (7–10 days) of nitrofurantoin (if renal function is normal). Longer courses of antibiotics are required for complicated lower UTIs.
Patients with indwelling catheters are at increased risk of infection, and UTIs should be treated with broad-spectrum antibiotics for 7–10 days and the catheter changed, as bacteria can adhere in a biofilm to the catheter. Intermittent self-catheterization is associated with reduced risk of UTI.
Cranberry and/or blueberry juice (reduce bacterial adhesion) and avoidance of spermicidal creams may have benefit in preventing further UTIs. Frequent and double voiding may be helpful in complicated UTI due to vesicoureteric reflux (VUR: see section on VUR). Circumcision may reduce the risk of UTI in male infants with malformation of the lower urinary tract. Breastfeeding also reduces the risk of UTI in infants.
In cases of recurrent infections, continuous prophylactic antibiotics (trimethoprim or nitrofurantoin in adults) should be tried and only changed if resistance develops. Optimal duration of therapy has yet to be established.

Acute pyelonephritis (upper urinary tract infection)
Acute pyelonephritis may present with symptoms more in keeping with a lower UTI and mild flank pain, rather than fever, nausea, vomiting, and systemic sepsis. Incidence is $2/10^3$, and more common in women. Occasionally, it can cause AKI, particularly when associated with urinary tract obstruction.
Urine stick testing is typically positive for leucocyte esterase, nitrate, blood, and protein, with pyuria and $\geq 10^4$ CFU/mL on microscopy and culture. However, in cases of obstruction or perinephric abscess, the urine may be bland. Blood cultures may be positive.
Depending on the presentation, other conditions may need to be excluded (pneumonia, cholecystitis, pancreatitis, acute GN, renal vein thrombosis), and an USS may show increased intrarenal pressure with damped diastolic blood flow on colour Doppler, or a renal calculus. CT scanning may reveal stranding in the perirenal fat due to the inflammatory reaction and is useful in detecting complicated UTI.
Management depends on illness severity, ranging from oral antibiotics (fluoroquinolones) to hospital admission with intravenous fluids, and parenteral antibiotics (aminoglycosides, third-generation cephalosporins, extended-spectrum penicillins).
Perinephric abscesses should be treated with prolonged antibiotic courses (6–8 weeks), and percutaneous drainage may be required. Similarly, infected cysts in adult polycystic kidney disease (APKD) typically require antibiotics for ≥ 4 weeks and occasionally require drainage.

Emphysematous pyelonephritis

Diagnosis is made by KUB (kidney, ureter, and bladder) or CT scanning showing gas within the kidney due to gas-forming enterobacteriaceae. Typically found in diabetic patients with severe pyelonephritis. Due to high mortality (up to 60%), it has been traditionally treated by nephrectomy and broad-spectrum antibiotics.

Papillary necrosis due to pyelonephritis

Papillary necrosis may occur in cases of pyelonephritis, usually associated with ischaemia and typically in diabetics and those with HbSS/SC disease.

Urine infections in patients with ileal conduits or uterosigmoidostomy

Artificial bladders, historically uterosigmoidostomy, and then ileal loop conduits or bladder extensions have been formed for children with bladder atresia or other congenital development abnormalities and in adults post-cystectomy.

Most patients have a mild hyperchloraemic acidosis due to chloride-bicarbonate exchange by the bowel segment. During episodes of infection, reflux may occur and patients often become systemically unwell. Dehydration leads to severe metabolic acidosis, with Kussmaul respiration, as the longer urinary transit time in the bowel segment leads to increased bicarbonate losses. In addition, particularly in cases of uterosigmoidostomy, urease-producing bacteria may also lead to hyperammonaemia with encephalopathy.

Treatment is with appropriate antibiotics, aggressive rehydration with isotonic bicarbonate (may require potassium and calcium supplementation), and laxatives for cases of uterosigmoidostomy.

Tuberculous infections of the urinary tract

Renal tuberculosis accounts for 15–20% of extrapulmonary TB and is spread by haematogenous spread. It is more common in males, pre-existing renal tract abnormalities, and immunocompromised hosts. Renal transplant recipients with a past history of TB, or from countries with high endemic rates, should be offered isoniazid prophylaxis.

Renal TB may cause a chronic granulomatous interstitial nephritis, parenchymal calcification, papillary necrosis, pyonephrosis, and/or secondary AA amyloid. TB can also lead to ureteric strictures and stones, and a chronic interstitial cystitis with contracted small-volume bladder. Envionmental TB strains may cause chronic skin infection in renal transplant patients.

For diagnosis and treatment, see Chapter 5. In patients with renal impairment, there is increased risk of drug toxicity (streptomycin—nephrotoxicity; ethambutol—optic neuritis; and rifamipicin increases the metabolism of prednisolone and immunophyllins in renal ransplant recipients (rifabutin has less effect on cytochrome P450 metabolism)). In granulomatous TB, the addition of steroids to standard quadruple therapy increases renal recovery and, similarly, in TB peritonitis in peritoneal dialysis patients, reduces intraperitoneal adhesions.

Fungal infections in the urinary tract

Fungal infections may not only cause lower UTIs, but also upper tract infections, causing multiple renal abscesses, emphysematous pyelonephritis, papillary necrosis, and fungal balls. Fungal infections are more common in the immunocompromised and diabetics.

Treatment depends upon cultures and antimicrobial sensitivity. Fungi typically adhere to non-biological surfaces, so

treatment also requires removal of nephrostomy tubes, stents, and catheters.

Schistosomiasis

Schistosomiasis is a parasitic illness due to *S. haematobium* (Africa), *S. japonicum* (Far East), and *S. mansoni* (Africa, Central and South America, and parts of Asia), all of which can cause glomerulonephritis. However, *S. haematobium* can also cause bladder infestation, leading to a chronic interstitial cystitis, calcified small-volume bladder, bladder cancer, and obstruction, leading to upper tract dilatation and interstitial fibrosis.

Treatment should be directed to the parasite (praziquantel 40 mg/kg, although larger doses are required for *S. japonicum*) and then managing the obstruction, if required (see 'Urinary tract obstruction').

Vesicoureteric reflux (VUR) and reflux nephropathy

In cases of VUR, urine passes retrogradely from the bladder back towards the kidney. Primary VUR (1–2%) is thought to be due to abnormal ureteric insertion into the bladder, with loss of natural sphincter function, whereas secondary VUR follows obstruction, bladder dysfunction, and post-surgical re-implantation of the ureter (post-renal transplant).

Reflux nephropathy is the renal disease associated with VUR, which may be due to renal dysplasia associated with primary VUR, focal scarring secondary to urosepsis, and secondary FSGS due to hyperfiltration.

VUR is staged, according to the severity of calyceal dilatation and hydronephrosis (I to V), and divided into active (reflux occurs during micturition) and passive (no reflux on micturition). By definition, VUR is diagnosed on micturating cystourethrogram, but USS is the screening test of choice.

Secondary causes of VUR should be excluded and managed, as appropriate. In cases of primary VUR, treatment is designed to reduce frequency and promptly treat urosepsis to prevent further scarring. This includes adequate fluid intake, regular voiding, and double voiding with active VUR, avoiding constipation and maintaining perineal hygiene.

There is debate over the role of surgical treatment (laparoscopic infiltration of Teflon around the bladder ureteric orifice or re-implantation of the ureters), and most centres prescribe prophylactic antibiotics for 2 years. Rather than rotating antibiotics, a single agent, such as trimethoprim 1–2 mg/kg/day is prescribed and only changed when bacterial resistance occurs. VUR tends to regress with time, so antibiotics should be discontinued in cases with no infections and no new scars on DMSA scanning. Patients who develop proteinuria and hypertension should receive standard management (see 'Chronic kidney disease'). Reflux nephropathy accounts for 15% of end-stage kidney disease in adolescents.

Prune belly syndrome (Eagle–Barrett syndrome)

This comprises a triad of megacystis-megaureter, cryptorchidism, with deficient anterior wall musculature. The latter causes wrinkling of the anterior abdominal wall (prune belly) in infants. Patients (1 in 30,000) have large-volume bladder, with poor contraction, and high-grade VUR. Despite urological input, many develop progressive CKD due to additional renal dysplasia

Horseshoe kidney

In this developmental abnormality, the two lower poles of the kidney remain fused by an isthmus. The horseshoe kidney may be in the pelvis in 20% of cases. Complications include hypertension, VUR, pelviureteric obstruction, renal stones, malignancy, and progressive CKD.

Duplex ureter

Renal ureteric duplication (1%) is often familial, and the two ureters either fuse or enter the bladder separately, but occasionally into the urethra or vagina. The upper ureter typically enters the bladder inferomedially and predisposes to VUR. USS should detect duplex systems and also confirm dilatation and/or associated ureteroceles.

Further reading

Cochrane renal group. <http://www.cochrane-renal.org/>.

Crino PB, Nathanson KL, Henske EP (2006). The tuberous sclerosis complex. *New England Journal of Medicine*, **355**, 1345–56.

Hildebrandt F and Zhou W (2007). Nephronophthisis associated ciliopathies. *Journal of the American Society of Nephrology*, **18**, 1855–71.

National Institute for Health and Clinical Excellence (2007). Urinary tract infection: diagnosis, treatment and long-term management of urinary tract infection in children. <http://www.nice.org.uk/cg54>.

National Organization for Rare Disorders. <http://www.rarediseases.org/>.

Orphanet. Database of rare diseases. <http://www.orpha.net/>.

World Health Organization. International Programme on Chemical Safety. <http://www.who.int/ipcs/>.

World Health Organization. Schistosomiasis. <http://www.who.int/schistosomiasis/strategy/en/>.

Urinary tract obstruction

Urinary tract obstruction can follow congenital or development abnormalities, or acquired.

Congenital causes of urinary tract obstruction

Congenital urinary tract obstruction is more common in males and includes posterior urethral valves, meatal strictures, ureterocele, and pelviureteric junction (PUJ) obstruction, which may be bilateral in 20% of cases.

Acquired causes of urinary tract obstruction

The commonest cause of intrarenal obstruction is renal calculus disease, although sloughed papillae (see Box 11.3), fungal balls, and papillary cell carcinoma can also cause upper tract obstruction.

Renal calculus disease

In addition to obstruction by renal calculi, tubular obstruction can develop and cause AKI due to sudden microcrystal deposition, including uric acid following tumour lysis syndrome, or genetic defects of purine metabolism/renal tubular uric acid transport, calcium phosphate deposition secondary to high phosphate cathartics used for bowel preparation, and drug crystals (indinavir, aciclovir).

Renal calculi

The incidence of renal calculi increases with dietary sodium and meat intake and is more common in men and countries with hot climates. In North America and Europe, the incidence is around 1 per 10^3, with a prevalence of 10%. Renal stones recur in 30% and 70% of those with two previous stones. Renal calculi are increased in cases of structural abnormality of the renal tract (calyx diverticulum, caliectasis, medullary sponge kidney, PUJ obstruction, horseshoe kidney, pelvic kidney, malrotated kidney, VUR, megaureter, ureteric stricture, and ureterocele).

If possible, stones should be sent for biochemical analysis (80% calcium oxalate—may also contain calcium phosphate, 6–14% struvite, 5–10% uric acid, 5% calcium phosphate, 1–2% cystine). Otherwise, 24-hour urine collections for calcium, magnesium, oxalate, urate, phosphate, and citrate are required, with corresponding serum measurements, and additional serum chloride, bicarbonate, vitamin D, and PTH levels. Spot urine samples should be analysed for pH, specific gravity, and dibasic amino acids.

In cases of renal colic, many stones will pass spontaneously, and, provided there is no sepsis, a conservative approach may be initially adopted, aiming for pain relief, typically with NSAIDs and alpha-blockers, which have been reported to increase stone passage. If ureteric stones do not pass spontaneously, then extracorporeal shock wave lithotripsy (ESWL) may be successful, particularly for upper ureteric stones, although ureteric stents should be inserted for stones >2 cm.

Urate stones

Urate stones predominantly occur in men, are radiolucent, occur with high urinary uric acid (>4 mmol/day or a uric acid/creatinine ratio of >0.7 mmol/L or >1 mg/dL) and/or low pH (inherited disorders of purine metabolism, gout, leukaemias, psoriasis, uricosuric agents (probenecid), tumour lysis, ileostomy loop bladder). Treatment includes high fluid intake, avoiding high purine foods, urinary alkalinization (sodium or potassium citrate solution 50–60 mEq/day,

urocit-K wax tablets 20–40 mmol/day), and either allopurinol or febuxostat (for tumour lysis).

Stones secondary to urine infection

Magnesium ammonium phosphate (struvite) and calcium hydrogen phosphate stones develop in alkaline urine, created by urease-producing bacteria (produce ammonia), which include *Proteus*, particularly when associated with urinary stasis. This may result in staghorn calculi, which may need percutaneous nephrolithotomy, if refractory to ESWL.

Cystine stone disease

Cystinuria is a recessive genetic defect (4 per 1,000), leading to increased urinary excretion of dibasic amino acids (cystine, ornithine, lysine, and arginine). Cystine is more soluble in alkaline urine. Cystine stones are characteristically radiolucent.

Treatment includes high fluid intake, low sodium diet, urinary alkalinization, and treatment with either D-penicillamine (starting at 500 mg and titrating upwards to 2 g, according to response) or tiopronin (10–40 mg/kg/day), aiming for a urinary cystine <1,000 micromoles/L. Cystine stones are typically resistant to ESWL and often require percutaneous nephrolithotomy.

Calcium oxalate stone disease

Calcium oxalate stone disease occurs with hypercalciuria. Hypercalciuria may be related to increased intestinal calcium absorption due to increased dietary calcium, milk alkali syndrome, or increased $1,25(OH)_2$ vitamin D3 activity (secondary to sarcoidosis, hyperparathyroidism, and lithium). Distal renal tubular acidosis predisposes to calcium-based stones by causing a metablic acidosis, with alkaline urine, hypercalciuria, and hypocitraturia. Other renal conditions leading to hypercalciuria include Dent's disease and familial idiopathic hypercalciuria.

Whereas the concentration of most compounds in the urine are well below their solubility level, urinary oxalate is very close to its solubility limit, and thus calcium oxalate stones are common. Most oxalate is derived from endogenous hepatic metabolism and is raised in cases of primary hyperoxaluria (see section on hyperoxaluria). Oxalate is normally bound to calcium in the gut and the majority passed in the faeces. However, oxalate absorption can be increased by a low calcium diet, following gastric bypass surgery, small bowel Crohn's disease, pancreatic insufficiency, and treatment with orlistat. Oxalate in the gut can be broken down by *Oxalobacter formigenes*, and some stone formers lack these bacteria.

Treatment comprises high fluid intake, with adequate dietary calcium with low oxalate intake (avoid spinach, rhubarb, black tea, nuts, and vitamin C) and a trial of pyridoxine.

Box 11.3 Causes of papillary necrosis

Diabetes mellitus
Sickle cell or HbSC disease
Analgesic nephropathy
Renal amyloidosis
Acute pyelonephritis

Calcium phosphate disease

Pure calcium phosphate stones are relatively rare. They occur in alkaline urine, with hypercalciuria and hypocitrataemia, and are increased by distal renal tubular acidosis or hyperparathyroidism.

General management of calcium stone disease

High fluid intake and low sodium diet are the cornerstone of medical magement of renal calculus disease. Hypercalciuria can be reduced by thiazide diuretics. Hypocitraturia can be supplemented by sodium or potassium citrate solution 50–60 mEq/day or urocit-K wax tablets 20–40 mmol/day.

Ureteric obstruction

May be secondary to a renal calculus or blood clot (transitional cell and papillary carcinomas, renal arteriovenous malformations, renal trauma, polycystic kidney disease, endometriosis, and IgA nephropathy), and fungal balls. Following renal transplantation, a high ureteric stricture may develop, either as part of transplant rejection or ureteric ischaemia due to damage to the lower pole renal artery or ureteric blood supply. The ureter may become obstructed during its passage through the bladder wall, often in cases of cerebral palsy due to increased bladder wall thickening or stricture post-ureteric implantation (renal transplantation, ureteric-bowel anastomoses). Other causes of ureteric stricture include renal transitional cell carcinoma, radiotherapy, infection with *Schistosoma haematobium* and TB, and Wegener's granulomatosis. The ureters may also become obstructed by external compression due to retroperitoneal fibrosis, bladder, cervical, or prostate cancer, other retroperitoneal masses and/or tumours, pelvic inflammatory disease, uterine or bladder prolapse, gravid uterus, blood vessels (horseshoe kidney, retrocaval ureter), and surgical ligation.

Obstruction at the level of the bladder

Prostatic hypertrophy is the commonest cause of obstruction and accounts for 3–5% of CKD stage 5 in patients >65 years. Obstruction can also develop in patients with neuropathic bladders (spina bifida, multiple sclerosis, diabetes mellitus, spinal cord trauma), either secondary to a contracted, spastic, or atonic flaccid bladder. Schistosomal infection and chronic interstitial cystitis may lead to a contracted bladder and bladder neck. Strictures may also cause obstruction.

Urethral obstruction

Urethral strictures are much more common in men and may follow instrumentation, gonorrhoea, and other sexually transmitted infections but can occur following female circumcision.

Clinical presentation

Clinical presentation will depend upon the age of the patient, site, and duration of the obstruction. For example, obstruction due to urethral valves may be detected by fetal USS, and neonates may present with failure to thrive, vomiting, and a distended bladder. Older patients may be relatively asymptomatic or suffer mild flank discomfort, whereas renal colic is typically an abrupt presentation, with severe colicky pain radiating into the groin. Other presentations include urosepsis, haematuria, difficulty with micturition, and even anuria.

Clinical signs

Occasionally, hydronephrotic kidneys are palpable and may be tender. The bladder may be distended. Pelvic and rectal examination may detect prostatic hypertrophy, cancer, or other pelvic malignancy.

Investigations

Urine dipstick testing often detects blood and protein. Microbiology may be positive, and cytology detects malignant cells and schistosomal ova. Biochemical testing may show CKD or a distal renal tubular acidosis (hyperchloraemia with hyperkalaemia). Urine biochemistry may be helpful in investigating renal calculus disease (see section on renal calculi).

Imaging is vitally important to determine the level and help to define the cause of the obstruction. USS usually detects hydronephrosis (unless acute; see Investigation of the renal tract), and CT-KUB is now the standard investigation for renal calculus. In cases of ileal conduit, additional investigations will be required, such as ileal loopogram for investigation of obstruction, for example, in cases of artificial bladder reconstruction and ante- or retrograde studies to investigate intrinsic ureteric obstruction.

Dynamic nuclear medicine scanning, particularly with furosemide, is helpful in assessing potential obstruction when anatomical scans show dilatation, for example, in cases of PUJ dilatation, megaureters, and bladder dysfunction. Sometimes, direct pressure measurements are required to investigate compression of the transvesical ureter.

Management of obstruction

Management is designed to relieve pain and the obstruction, treat infection, and then the underlying cause. If patients present with AKI or end-stage CKD, then they may have to be dialysed and stabilized prior to relieving the obstruction. Depending upon the level of obstruction, simple bladder catheter or suprapubic catheterization may be appropriate. Obstructing ureteric calculi may require surgical removal. In cases of upper tract obstruction, a temporary nephrostomy tube may be required, and then, when inflammation has settled, the nephrostomy should be replaced with either an antegrade or a retrograde stent, depending upon the cause and site of the obstruction. Patients may become profoundly hypotensive post-nephrostomy, particularly when infection complicates obstruction, and, therefore, patients should be adequately resuscitated and, if sepsis suspected, antibiotics started prior to the relief of the obstruction. Strictures in the ureter and urethra may require direct visualization with biopsy or brushings for cytology.

Following relief of obstruction, there may be a post-obstructive diuresis, which needs appropriate fluid replacement. Hypokalaemia, hypocalcaemia, and hypomagnesaemia may develop if the diuresis is excessive, and replacement of these electrolytes is required.

Specific management may be required, depending upon the underlying cause of the obstruction. For example, in cases of idiopathic retroperitoneal fibrosis, medical therapy (prednisolone 30 mg/day, and then reducing prednisolone, according to CRP response and disease activity shown on PET CT scanning) and surgical ureterolysis may be required. Bladder outflow obstruction due to prostatic hypertrophy should be treated by either transurethral resection or medical therapy with alpha-blockers and finasteride.

Retroperitoneal fibrosis

Retroperitoneal fibrosis is typically an autoimmune periaortitis, characterized by IgG4 autoantibodies, although it may be secondary to other causes of fibrosis in the retroperitoneal area. It is three times more prevalent in men, with a peak incidence in the 6th and 7th decades of life. Although patients may present with acute kidney injury, the majority present with flank pain, hypertension, venous thrombosis, and raised serum creatinine. Some patients may have systemic symptoms. The incidence is increased in patients taking specific antihypertensive drugs (practolol (no longer available), methyldopa, hydralazine, atenolol), ergot-containing drugs, and dexamfetamine (INN).

Diagnosis is made with CT scanning which shows encasement of the ureter. Management typically involves ureterolysis and steroids with tamoxifen.

Further reading

Kermani TA, Crowson CS, Achenbach SJ, Luthra HS (2011). Idiopathic retroperitoneal fibrosis: a retrospective review of clinical presentation, treatment, and outcomes. *Mayo Clinic Proceedings*, **86**, 297–303.

Tumours of the renal tract

Renal cell carcinoma

The incidence of renal cell carcinoma is increasing, now accounting for 2–3% of all cancers. They typically occur in men aged 60–70 years old. Potential risk factors include cigarette smoking, hypertension, and obesity.

These adenocarcinomas are subdivided, according to appearance: clear cell (75%), papillary type 1 (5%), papillary type 2 (10%), chromophobe (5%), oncocytoma (5%), collecting duct (<1%), and medullary carcinoma (rare).

Only a minority of patients present with the classic triad of flank pain, palpable mass, and haematuria. Many renal cell carcinomas are incidentally detected on USS and CT scans. Renal cell carcinomas may cause paraneoplastic disease and/or present as a consequence of secondary spread.

Patients with suspected renal cell carcinoma should be investigated by CT scanning of the chest and abdomen and isotope bone scanning to qualify the anatomical size of the tumour and assess metastatic spread. PET-CT scanning may replace CT scanning for tumour staging. There is a risk of seeding tumour in a biopsy needle track, and, therefore, only occasionally, in atypical cases, is fine needle biopsy performed for diagnostic purposes.

In cases of localized renal cell carcinoma, radiofrequency ablation or cryotherapy may be used for small-sized tumours (<4 cm), rather than partial nephrectomy, and total nephrectomy is reserved for larger-sized tumours. Metastatic disease can be treated with interferon alfa, and some newer angiogenesis inhibitors including sorafenib, sunitinib, bevacizumab, and the mTor inhibitor temsirolimus, offer additional survival benefit. Prognosis is better for renal cell tumours limited to the kidney, and chromophobe type > papillary > clear cell. There is a risk of recurrence in the contralateral kidney.

Wilm's tumour

Wilm's tumour (8 per 10^6) is the commonest malignancy of the renal tract in childhood and accounts for 8% of childhood malignancies. Children typically present with a mass, detected by a parent, or loin pain, haematuria, or symptoms and signs from secondary spread. Even in cases with no metastases, preoperative chemotherapy (for 6 weeks—the duration and intensity depending upon tumour staging and biopsy appearance) is recommended before nephrectomy. Five-year survival for favourable histological types with no metastases is around 100%.

Transitional cell carcinoma

Transitional cell carcinoma (TCC) can arise from the lining of the upper renal tract from the renal calyces down to the urethra. Unlike other tumours, additional synchronous primary tumours may occur.

Predisposing factors include smoking and exposure to aniline dyes, beta-naphthylamine, benzadine, phenacetin (analgesic nephropathy), cyclophosphamide, Balkan nephropathy, Chinese herbal nephropathy, coffee, and some hereditary conditions, such as Lynch syndrome.

Typical presentations include haematuria, clot colic, and loin pain. Investigations include urine cytology, CT-IVU, with ureteroscopy and/or retrograde studies, and cystoscopy to exclude urethral or bladder tumour.

Nephroureterectomy remains the standard treatment, with a 60–90% 5-year survival for carcinoma in situ or non-invasive papillary tumour. Survival is very poor for high-grade tumours or more extensive disease. Follow-up is required due to the risk of other tumours developing.

Bladder tumours

Bladder cancer is the second commonest tumour of the renal tract and the fifth commonest cancer in the UK. It is more common in elderly Caucasoid men.

Transitional cell carcinoma is the commonest histological type (90%), with the same risk factors as for TCC of the upper tract, but with exposure to irradiation, prolonged immunosuppression (renal transplant recipients), chronic cystitis, bladder calculi, indwelling urinary catheter, bilharzias, and industrial exposure (aniline dyes and rubber) as additional risk factors.

Most patients present with haematuria or urinary frequency, urgency, and dysuria.

Cystoscopy allows visualization and tumour biopsy (papillary, sessile, or carcinoma in situ). All patients should be screened with CT-IVU to exclude upper tract tumours. In more extensive cancers, metastatic spread should be excluded with isotope bone scans and CXR/chest CT.

Cancers which have not invaded the muscle layer are treated by transurethral resection, followed by intravesical chemotherapy (mitomycin or epirubicin or doxorubicin), and patients followed up, as recurrence is common (60–70%). Patients with higher-grade tumour are given prophylactic intravesical chemotherapy or BCG (may cause fever, arthralgia, hepatitis, and pneumonitis), and recurrence may prompt more aggressive therapy. If the muscle layer has been breached, then radical cystectomy with urinary diversion should be offered or radiotherapy for those unfit for major surgery, both combined with chemotherapy (such as gemcitabine and cisplatin (INN)). Other tumour types, adenocarcinoma, and squamous cell cancers should also be treated by radical cystectomy.

Prostate tumours

Prostatic adenocarcinoma is the commonest cancer in men in the Western World, with an incidence of 98 per 10^5. The incidence is increasing, which may reflect PSA screening. Risk factors, apart from age, include race (Afro-Caribbeans > Caucasoids > South Asian subcontinent) and a positive family history.

Most patients are asymptomatic at presentation but may have lower urinary tract symptoms, and develop bladder or upper tract obstruction. Some present with metastatic disease, in particular bone pain.

Most prostate cancers develop posteriorly and may be palpable on rectal examination. PSA, particularly a free/bound ratio <0.23, is suggestive of prostate cancer, but histological diagnosis is required by transrectal US-guided biopsy.

Adenocarcinoma is, by far, the commonest histological type, although other tumour types may occur. Cancers are histologically graded by the Gleason staging system, which correlates with staging and prognosis (Gleason stage 6, good prognosis; 7, intermediate; and 8–10, poor prognosis).

Bladder outflow obstruction should be treated by transurethral resection. For localized low-grade disease, patients may be offered watchful waiting, with active treatment if the disease progresses, or active treatment. This includes radical prostatectomy, external radiotherapy, and brachytherapy (insertion of radioactive seeds into the prostate), as all treatments currently appear to offer similar survival. When the cancer is locally advanced, then treatment options include external radiotherapy, radical prostatectomy, and hormone therapy. Hormone modulation (surgical orchidectomy, LHRH agonist, antiandrogens, or oestrogens) is the only treatment option for metastatic disease. Metastatic disease should be treated with appropriate palliative therapy.

Further reading

European Association of Urology. <http://www.uroweb.org>.

Chronic kidney disease (CKD)

The key management strategy for patients with CKD is to prevent and/or slow down the rate of progression of underlying renal disease. In cases of microscopic polyangiitis, SLE, or diabetes, specific treatment aimed at the underlying disease is appropriate

For the staging system of CKD, see Table 11.24. Although some 5% of the general population have CKD 3, the majority have relatively stable renal function, and only a minority progress to stage 5 CKD (estimated at 0.1% of the population), with a far larger number of patients dying of cardiovascular disease. Thus, the second strand of treating CKD patients is to minimize cardiovascular risk factors.

Hypertension and proteinuria are the two major risk factors for progression of CKD. Renal biopsy assessment of the amount of interstitial fibrosis and scarring, is associated with progression; the greater the degree of tubular loss, the greater risk of progressive CKD.

Hypertension in chronic kidney disease (CKD)

The prevalence of hypertension increases as patients progress from CKD stage 3 to 5 such that the majority of patients starting dialysis have left ventricular hypertrophy. Hypertension is partially due to increased centrally driven sympathetic nervous system activity and sodium retention. As renal function declines, the ability of the kidney to excrete sodium falls, leading to sodium retention. Traditionally, sodium retention was thought to result in expansion of the extracellular fluid volume, as sodium is osmotically active and so retains water. Expansion of the extracellular volume leads to increased cardiac filling pressures and cardiac volume, so leading to natriuretic peptide release and a corresponding natriuresis. However, if this

compensatory response is inadequate, patients develop signs of extracellular fluid overload, such as peripheral oedema. It is now recognized that sodium gain can also be non-osmotic, with sodium exchanging for intracellular potassium, particularly in muscle, and also as sodium is positively charged associating with negatively charged proteoglycans in tissue matrix. As patients progress from CKD 3 to 5, cardiotonic steroids increase and, by inhibiting sodium-potassium ATPase, increase sodium retention. Sodium retention in blood vessel walls increases arterial stiffness, which can be detected by increased pulse wave velocity. It has been suggested that statins may help to reduce the progression of CKD, and the mechanism may be by reducing these cardiotonic steroids.

Thus, the management of hypertension in CKD patients should aim to increase sodium excretion with loop diuretics, as traditional thiazide diuretics are ineffective in CKD 4/5 patients, in addition to antihypertensive agents which reduce visceral sympathetic activity (ACE-Is, ARBs, and beta-blockers).

Blood pressure targets depend on the individual patient and rate of underlying progression but should be <140/90 mmHg, and <130/80 mmHg in those with progressive disease. Even lower targets (125/75 mmHg) are recommended for those with proteinuria (PCR >100 mg/mmol) and/or type 1 diabetes. Patients should be advised to monitor their blood pressure at home.

Management of proteinuria in CKD

The greater the urinary protein leak, the greater the risk of progression of CKD. In part, proteinuria is dependent on blood pressure control, and, therefore, a lower systolic blood pressure target is required. ACE-Is appear to have an additional beneficial effect in terms of lowering proteinuria, and this can be increased when combined with ARBs. However, this combination may increase the risk of hyperkalaemia, particularly in diabetics who may be predisposed to hyperkalaemia due to type IV (combined proximal and distal) renal tubular acidosis.

Cardiovascular risk factor modification

Patients should be advised to alter lifestyle, to stop smoking, take regular exercise, reduce weight if appropriate, and eat a healthy low-salt diet. Potential nephrotoxin drugs should be avoided (e.g. NSAIDs).

Aspirin and statins should be prescribed. Homocysteine accumulates as CKD progresses, and this can be partially reversed by folate. Uric acid is a risk factor for both cardiovascular disease and renal progression. Allopurinol accumulates as renal function declines, and, therefore, dose modification is required.

Specific treatments for patients with CKD

As patients progress towards CKD 5, anaemia develops due to both a reduction in erythropoietin and also iron deficiency. Patients with CKD absorb less iron than normal, and they should be treated with iron to maintain an iron saturation >25%, and erythropoietin to maintain a haemoglobin 10–12 g/dL.

Vitamin D deficiency becomes more common, as patients progressing from CKD 3 not only have reduced $1,25(OH)_2D_3$ (1,25-dihydroxyvitamin D_3, 1,25-dihydroxycholecalciferol) due to reduced renal 1 hydroxylation but also reduced $25OHD_3$ (25-hydroxyvitamin D).

Table 11.24 The CKD staging system. The suffix (p) is used to denote the presence of proteinuria, as defined by an albumin/creatinine ratio of ≥30 mg/mmol, which is equivalent to a protein/creatinine ratio of ≥50 mg/mmol (≥0.5 g/24 h)

GFR category	GFR (ml/min/1.73m^2)	Terms
G1	≥90	Normal or high
G2	60–89	Mildly decreased*
G3a	45–59	Mildly to moderately decreased
G3b	30–44	Moderately to severely decreased
G4	15–29	Severely decreased
G5	<15	Kidney failure

Abbreviations: CKD, chronic kidney disease; GFR, glomerular filtration rate.

*Relative to young adult level

In the absence of evidence of kidney damage, neither GFR category G1 nor G2 fulfill the criteria for CKD.

Kidney Disease: Improving Global Outcomes (KDIGO) Acute Kidney Injury Work Group. KDIGO Clinical Practice Guideline for Acute Kidney Injury. *Kidney International* Suppl. 2012; 2: 1–138, reproduced with permission.

Phosphate retention occurs as renal function declines. Hyperphosphataemia leads to hyperparathyroidism and should be treated when phosphate levels are >1.5 mmol/L (4.5 mg/dL), typically with calcium-based phosphate binders taken prior to eating.

As renal function declines, patients may become acidotic and require bicarbonate supplementation. However, if this is given as sodium bicarbonate, then the additional sodium load must be considered.

CKD patients may also develop hyperplastic gastric polyps due to increased gastrin. Other hormonal abnormalities include hyperprolactinaemia, which reduces female fertility and may lead to male gynaecomastia.

Patients with CKD are advised to have annual flu vaccinations and also to be vaccinated against hepatitis B and pneumoccocus.

Haemodialysis

Haemodialysis is the commonest treatment provided for end-stage kidney disease worldwide. Typically, most patients dialyse thrice weekly, and small solutes pass by diffusion from the patient's blood across the dialyser membrane into the dialysate. Additional ultrafiltration is used to remove fluid and sodium which have accumulated in the interdialytic interval. The actual dose delivered is probably equivalent to an eGFR of 12–15 mL/min. Thus, patients continue to develop metabolic bone disease, soft tissue vascular calcification, and require erythropoietin to prevent anaemia. Mortality remains high, with 5-year mortality in the USA approximately equivalent to patients with Duke's B carcinoma of the colon. Sepsis and cardiovascular mortality are the commonest modes of death, followed by treatment withdrawal. The commonest cause of infection relates to central venous access catheters. These disseminate infection, causing bacterial endocarditis, cerebral abscesses, intervertebral discitis, and osteomyelitis, with some 300–400 UK haemodialysis patients dying annually from infections. Central venous access catheters predispose to venous thrombosis and superior vena cava stenosis and also intra-atrial thrombus formation. These patients can present with facial and periorbital oedema, widened neck, and fixed jugular veins. In addition, pulmonary, or even cerebral, emboli may occur through a patent foramen ovale.

Although cardiovascular risk is increased in dialysis patients, sudden cardiac death due to arrhythmias is more common than that due to myocardial ischaemia. Hypertension remains prevalent with arteriosclerosis, and patients are at increased risk of stroke.

Occasionally, patients will collapse shortly after starting a haemodialysis treatment. This can be due to an air embolus, due to a fault in priming of the dialysis circuit, or an acute reaction to heparin, either as an allergic reaction or due to heparin-induced thrombocytopenia (HIT). The HIT can cause a pulmonary embolus, or more likely an acute pulmonary leak syndrome (acute respiratory distress syndrome), or bradykinin production due to a reaction between the patient's blood and the dialyser circuit, made worse by co-prescription of ACE-Is.

Very occasionally, massive haemolysis occurs during dialysis due to contamination of the water supply (peroxide, chloramines) or due to a mechanical fault with the blood pump.

Intradialytic hypotension, requiring intervention, occurs in around one in six haemodialysis sessions, as the rate of ultrafiltration exceeds the rate of plasma refilling from the extravascular space. The fall in plasma osmolality during

dialysis can also lead to brain oedema due to the gradient which develops between plasma urea and brain urea; this can cause headache, restlessness, and confusion and is made worse by an underlying structural brain abnormality.

Haemodialysis does not readily remove middle-sized toxins, so beta-2 microglobulin accumulates, causing carpal tunnel median nerve compression in patients dialysing for 12–15 years or more. In longer-term patients, it can be deposited in the shoulder, lower cervical and lumbar spine, causing a destructive arthropathy.

Peritoneal dialysis

Peritoneal dialysis is one of the main modalities for treating patients with CKD stage 5. Patients either perform 3–4 manual exchanges of peritoneal dialysis fluid per day (chronic ambulatory peritoneal dialysis; CAPD) or use an overnight cycling machine (APD), with or without daytime exchanges. The major complications of peritoneal dialysis are infections, typically peritonitis and volume overload, usually secondary to ultrafiltration failure.

Peritonitis typically presents with sudden onset of generalized abdominal pain. Patients may be febrile, with clinical signs of guarding with rebound peritonism and hypotension. The differential diagnosis is that of an acute surgical abdomen. In peritoneal dialysis peritonitis, the peritoneal dialysis effluent will be cloudy, with an increased total WBC >100/mm³, with >50% polymorphonuclear leucocytes (4-hour dwell of dialysate). Usual causes are Gram-positive skin organisms, and, once blood and peritoneal effluent cultures have been sent, empirical intraperitoneal antibiotics should be commenced and patients treated by CAPD (e.g. gentamicin loading dose 8 mg/L, followed by 4 mg/L, cephradine loading dose 250 mg/L, maintenance dose 125 mg/L), with increased dose for patients with residual renal function, until directed by microbacteriology results. If patients fail to respond within 72 hours, catheter removal should be considered.

Patients on peritoneal dialysis can develop volume overload due to leaks, including scrotal and pleural collections, or due to loss of peritoneal membrane function. In patients with symptomatic volume overloaded, changing the peritoneal dialysis prescription to one using higher glucose concentration fluids (2.27% glucose) and reducing the dwell time to two hours, should improve ultrafiltration in the short term. If this is not effective then ultrafiltration with haemodialysis should be considered.

Patients who have been treated for >4 years on peritoneal dialysis may be at increased risk of encapsulating peritoneal sclerosis (EPS). In this condition, the small bowel becomes encapsulated in a fibrous sheath, causing small bowel obstruction and malnutrition. Patients may present with signs of small bowel obstruction, malnutrition, and recurrent ascites which may not present until after the patient has transferred to haemodialysis and/or even transplantation.

Further reading

Feehally J, Griffith KE, Lamb EJ, O'Donoghue DJ, Tomson CRV (2008). Early detection of chronic kidney disease. *BMJ*, **337**, 845–7.

K/DOQI (2007). Clinical practice guidelines and clinical practice recommendations for diabetes and chronic kidney disease. *American Journal of Kidney Diseases*, **49**, S1–179.

National Kidney Foundation (2002). K/DOQI clinical practice guidelines for chronic kidney disease: evaluation, classification, and stratification. *American Journal of Kidney Disease* 39 (Suppl 1): S1–266.

NDT-Educational, for European best practice guidelines. <http://www.ndt-educational.org/>.

National Institute for Health and Clinical Excellence (2014). Chronic kidney disease: early identification and management of chronic kidney disease in adults in primary and secondary care. NICE clinical guideline 182. <https://www.nice.org.uk/guidance/cg182/resources/guidance-chronic-kidney-disease-pdf>.

Taal M and Tomson C (2007). UK Renal Association clinical practice guidelines for the care of patients with chronic kidney disease. <http://www.renal.org/Libraries/Old_Guidelines/Module_1_-_Chronic_Kidney_Disease_CKD_-_4th_Edition.sflb.ashx>.

Renal transplant patients

Acute complications post-renal transplantation

During the first 3 months following renal transplantation, patients are exposed to high levels of immunosuppression and are more susceptible to both atypical infections and renal allograft rejection.

Following the introduction of induction therapy to prevent IL-2 activation of lymphocytes, the incidence of acute rejection in the first 3 months following transplantation has fallen from ~50% to 20%. In comparison, AKI post-transplantation, due in part to ischaemia-reperfusion injury, occurs in around 50% of renal transplants. However, it is unusual following live related transplantation but is more common when donors after cardiac death are used.

Although dynamic nuclear medicine scans and ultrasound are used to monitor renal allografts (see 'Investigation of the renal tract'), these cannot differentiate AKI from rejection, and, therefore, renal biopsy remains the standard test for excluding rejection. Rejection is classified as vascular when lymphocytes invade the endothelium, and cellular when collections of lymphocytes are detected in >25% of the interstitium. The degree of transplant rejection is graded by the Banff criteria.

Oral immunosuppressive regimes typically use tacrolimus and, occasionally, ciclosporin. These drugs increase the risk of glucose intolerance, hypertension, gout, and have a narrow therapeutic index, with high levels causing nephrotoxicity. Drug interactions that increase tacrolimus and ciclosporin levels, risking toxicity, occur with diltiazem, fluconazole, ketoconazole, and macrolides (apart from azithromycin). Drugs which reduce effective plasma levels include rifampicin, phenytoin, and carbimazole.

Cellular rejection is usually treated with three daily doses of methylprednisolone (500 mg), followed by an increase in background oral immunosuppression. If this fails to control rejection, then a 10–14-day course of antithymocyte globulin (ATG; or occasionally, OKT3 monoclonal antibody) is used. If patients have developed cytotoxic antibodies to the allograft, then rituximab, or plasma exchange with/without intravenous immunoglobulin, is used.

Infection may be transferred from the donor, or by infected organ transport medium.

Atypical infections are relatively common (see Table 11.25). To prevent infections, most patients are given prophylactic co-trimoxazole and valganciclovir (if CMV-naive) for the first 3 months post-transplantation.

In addition, viral reactivation may lead to tumours, including EBV-associated post-transplant lymphoproliferative disease, HHV-8-induced Kaposi's sarcoma, and HPV-induced squamous cell carcinoma (skin, anus, vulva, and cervix). In addition, patients may develop dementia due to infection with JC virus (progressive multifocal leukoencephalopathy) and either tropical spastic paraparesis or T cell leukaemia/lymphoma with HTLV-1.

Post-transplant lymphoproliferative disease occurs in 1–2% of transplant recipients. Patients often present with lymphadenopathy, or graft dysfunction, and, in many cases, the lymphoma is driven by EBV.

Table 11.25 Infections in the immunocompromised host

Days post-transplant		Organism
7–30 days	Viral	Herpes simplex
		VZV primary
		CMV primary
		EBV primary
		CMV reactivation
	Bacterial	*Clostridium difficile*
	Fungal	*Candida*
30–180 days	Viral	CMV primary
		CMV reactivation
		EBV primary
		EBV secondary
	Bacterial	*Legionella*
		Listeria
		Mycobacteria
	Fungal	*Pneumocystis*
		Nocardia
		Cryptococcus
	Parasite	*Toxoplasma*
		Strongyloidosis
>180 days	Viral	Influenza
		VZV reactivation
	Bacterial	*Pneumococcus*
		Listeria
		Mycobacteria
		Psittacosis
	Fungal	*Pneumocystis*
		Nocardia
		Cryptococcus

Renal transplant artery stenosis

Stenosis may develop at the site of the surgical anastomosis. Angioplasty and/or stenting are the treatments of choice.

Further reading

American Society of Transplantation. <http://www.a-s-t.org/>.
American Society of Transplant Surgeons. <http://www.asts.org/>.

![Chapter 12]

Anticoagulation and transfusion

The coagulation cascade and coagulation tests

The dual need for blood to remain fluid in an intact circulation, but to coagulate where the vascular endothelium has been breached, has resulted in the development of a highly sophisticated mechanism of blood coagulation, a major component of haemostasis (the cessation of blood loss from a damaged vessel). This coagulation mechanism comprises two components which occur together, more or less immediately, when the endothelium is damaged: primary haemostasis, in which platelets are activated at the site of endothelial injury to form a platelet plug, and secondary haemostasis, whereby a series of coagulation proteins become activated in a complex cascade to produce fibrin strands which strengthen the platelet plug.

Primary haemostasis

Immediately after the vessel endothelium is damaged, platelets bind to the subendothelial collagen via their glycoprotein GP Ia/IIa collagen receptors. The binding is enhanced by the presence of von Willebrand factor (vWf), an essential adhesive substrate that mediates the formation of a platelet thrombus. The vWf acts as a bridge between the collagen and the platelets, via the platelet surface glycoprotein receptors GP Ib and GP IIb/IIIa (see Figure 12.1). This process activates the platelets, resulting in a physical shape change and the release of compounds from the platelet granules (ADP, serotonin, vWf, platelet factor 4, thromboxane A2), which stimulate further binding of additional platelets to collagen and fibrinogen to form the primary haemostatic plug at the site of vascular injury.

Secondary haemostasis

Consists of a series of serine proteases activated sequentially (see Figure 12.2). Once activated, each protease catalyses the reaction on its substrate protease, ultimately resulting in the formation of a fibrin clot.

This cascade has two components:
- Tissue factor pathway (previously the extrinsic pathway).
- Contact activation (intrinsic) pathway.

The tissue factor pathway is the more important, but both activate the final common pathway, whereby thrombin is generated which then converts soluble fibrinogen to insoluble fibrin.

The tissue factor pathway is activated when endothelial damage results in the release of tissue factor (TF) into the circulation. This binds to and activates FVII to form TF-VIIa, which, in turn, activates FIX (part of the intrinsic pathway) and FX by a factor of about 30,000-fold. Together with FVa, FXa forms the prothrombinase complex which acts to convert prothrombin to thrombin in the presence of calcium ions and phospholipids, provided by activated platelets. This prothrombinase complex activates prothrombin at a rate 300,000 times greater than that of FXa and calcium alone. Thrombin, in turn, converts fibrinogen to fibrin, the basis of the haemostatic plug. There are numerous other positive and negative feedback control loops. Thus, FVII is also activated by thrombin, FXII, FXIa, FXa, and plasmin, whilst the activation of FX by TF-FVIIa is inhibited by the tissue factor pathway inhibitor. Thrombin activates both FV and FVIII and releases FVIII from being bound to vWf. FVIIIa has 50 times the coagulant activity of its inactive precursor FVIII and acts as the co-factor for FIXa (forming the 'tenase' complex) that activates FX. This activation of FVIII to FVIIIa, and consequent generation of the intrinsic 'tenase' complex, is a key step in the amplification of the coagulation cascade.

The contact activation pathway is initiated by the activation of FXII, high molecular weight kininogen (HMWK), and prekallikrein. FXIIa converts FXI to FXIa, which, in turn, activates FIX to FIXa. Together with FVIIIa, FIXa forms the tenase complex which activates FX to FXa. Activation of the contact activation pathway by this route plays only a minor role in coagulation, and indeed individuals with severe deficiencies of HMWK, prekallikrein, and FXII do not have a clinical bleeding disorder.

Final common pathway: thrombin plays a central role in the coagulation cascade. Its primary function is the conversion of soluble fibrinogen to insoluble fibrin, but, in addition, it activates FVIII and FV. Thrombin also activates FXIII, and FXIIIa forms covalent bonds between fibrin monomers, thereby polymerizing, and thus strengthening, the fibrin clot.

Thrombin, in the presence of thrombomodulin, also activates protein C, a major anticoagulant. Together with protein S and phospholipid, protein C inhibits the coagulation sequence by inactivating FVa and FVIIIa. Co-factors are required for the correct functioning of this coagulation cascade. These are:
- Calcium is necessary for the binding of FXa and FIXa via the terminal gamma carboxyl groups onto phospholipid

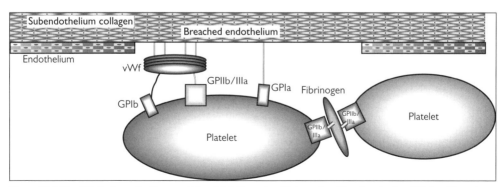

Figure 12.1 Simplified schematic diagram of the platelet/vessel wall interaction. Note the role of von Willebrand factor in acting as a bridge between the platelet and the vessel wall via the GPIb and GPIIb/IIIa receptors. GPIb can bind directly to subendothelial collagen, whilst GPIIb/IIIa receptors enhance platelet-platelet aggregation, mediated by fibrinogen and von Willebrand factor (not shown).

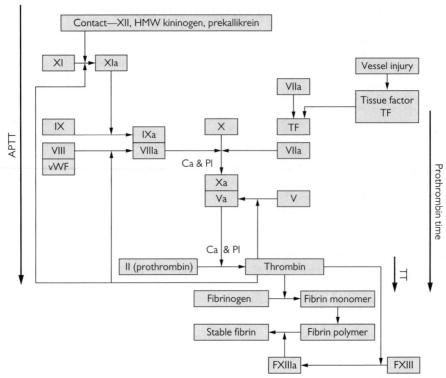

Figure 12.2 The coagulation cascade. Bold arrows emphasize the central role of thrombin in the blood coagulation pathway: cleaving of fibrinogen to fibrin and activation of factors V, VIII, XI, and XIII. Activation of antithrombin, protein C, and protein S are not included. Ca, calcium; Pl, platelet membrane phospholipid.

surfaces (principally supplied by platelet), which allows the tenase and prothrombinase complexes to function.

• Vitamin K, a fat-soluble vitamin, is required for the production of carboxyl groups on the glutamic acid residues of factors II (prothrombin), VII, IX, and X. The interaction of these coagulation factors with their substrates requires the presence of these carboxyl groups to bind to calcium ions. Vitamin K is also necessary for the production of the anticoagulants protein C, protein S, and protein Z.

Regulation of the coagulation system: if left unopposed, the activated coagulation system would rapidly result in widespread thrombosis, as the catalytic nature of coagulation reactions allows tremendous amplification of the initial stimulus. The presence of regulators in the system serves to prevent this. The chief regulators are:

• Protein C: a vitamin K-dependent serine protease enzyme activated by thrombin in the presence of thrombomodulin on cell surface membranes. Together with protein S and calcium ions, activated protein C cleaves activated FVa and FVIIIa, thereby inactivating them. The structurally altered factor V Leiden is relatively resistant to the action of activated protein C, and hence possession of this variant leads to a predisposition to thrombosis (activated protein C resistance).

• Antithrombin (previously antithrombin III) is a serine protease inhibitor. It inactivates thrombin, FXa, FIXa, FXIa,

and FXIIa by binding to, and blocking, the active site of these proteases, making them inaccessible to their usual substrate. Antithrombin activity is greatly enhanced by the presence of heparin, which accelerates the rate of thrombin inactivation by 3,000-fold and inactivation of FXa up to 1,000-fold. Antithrombin deficiency predisposes to thrombosis and can occur due to an absolute reduction in synthesis (type I deficiency) or due to the presence of a structurally abnormal antithrombin which cannot bind to substrates or to heparin, thereby reducing its enzymatic activity (type II deficiency).

Fibrinolysis: is the process by which the blood clot is resorbed and is dependent upon the enzyme plasmin, which is subject to a range of activators and inhibitors. The inactive form plasminogen is trapped within the thrombus and is converted to the active plasmin by urokinase and tissue plasminogen activator (tPA), which is released by damaged endothelium. tPA is inhibited by plasminogen activator inhibitors, and plasmin is inactivated by alpha-2 antiplasmin and alpha-2 macroglobulin in the plasma.

Coagulation tests

Full blood count and blood film

This is important, especially to assess thrombocytopenia. The finding of a low platelet count should be confirmed by examination of the blood film so that artefactual clumping of the platelets (a common EDTA-dependent phenomenon) is excluded. Additional associated features may be noted, e.g. the presence of abnormal white cells denoting bone marrow infiltration or replacement, fragmented red cells (seen in microangiopathic haemolysis, thrombotic thrombocytopenia (TTP), and disseminated intravascular coagulation (DIC)), or the presence of an otherwise normal blood count and film (characteristic of autoimmune thrombocytopenia— idiopathic thrombocytopenia (ITP)).

Prothrombin time (PT)
This is a screening test of the tissue factor (extrinsic) pathway. It measures the coagulation system from FVII through FX, FV, prothrombin, and fibrinogen. Tissue thromboplastin (derived from brain) and calcium are used to activate the pathway in vitro. As the procoagulant activity of tissue thromboplastins differs, the results may be expressed as an international normalized ratio (INR), a calibration against a primary World Health Organization standard thromboplastin. The normal range is 10–14 seconds (INR 0.8–1.2). The PT is most sensitive to the level of FVII, which has the shortest half-life of all the coagulation factors (3–6 hours) and which falls first when production of vitamin K-dependent coagulation factors is compromised. The PT is, therefore, sensitive to the coagulation effects of warfarin therapy, liver disease, and DIC.

Activated partial thromboplastin time (APTT)
This screening test measures the contact activation (intrinsic) pathway. It is sensitive to deficiencies of FVIII, IX, XI, and XII, in addition to the components of the final common pathway FX, FV, prothrombin, and fibrinogen. The technique involves the addition of a surface activator (e.g. kaolin), phospholipids, and calcium to a citrated sample of plasma to initiate clot formation. The normal range varies, according to the particulars of the technique used by the laboratory, but is usually 30–40 seconds. The APTT may be abnormal in haemophilia A and B, deficiencies of FXII (not normally associated with bleeding disorders), FXI (haemophilia C), and disorders of the final common pathway as well as multiple factor deficiencies. It is sensitive to the presence of inhibitors, especially lupus anticoagulants and heparin, although its sensitivity to these inhibitors can vary. Furthermore, the presence of raised levels of FVIII, which may occur in reaction to stress (including surgery), can reduce the sensitivity of the APTT. The reduced sensitivity of the APTT in this setting should be remembered when monitoring unfractionated heparin therapy in the postoperative period, as undue reliance on the APTT may lead to dangerous errors in the adjustment of heparin doses.

Thrombin time (TT)
This measures the conversion of fibrinogen to fibrin in citrated plasma by the addition of bovine thrombin. It is sensitive to deficiencies of fibrinogen, structural abnormalities of fibrinogen (dysfibrinogenaemia), and thrombin inhibitors. The reference range is in the order of 14–16 seconds, depending on the particular laboratory methodology used.

Collection of blood for coagulation tests
An important practical aspect of coagulation tests is the need to ensure the blood sample is obtained correctly. Ideally, the first tube in a case where multiple specimens are drawn should never be used for coagulation assays because tissue thromboplastin from the initial venepuncture may affect coagulation test results. In addition, the tube(s) for coagulation testing should be filled before any tubes containing EDTA. If coagulation tests are the only studies ordered, a discard tube should be drawn before filling the citrate tube used for the tests. The anticoagulant of choice for coagulation testing is sodium citrate, which reversibly chelates calcium (a prerequisite for a number of reactions on the coagulation cascade). Commercially available evacuated tubes (blue topped in the Vacutainer system) are manufactured to draw nine parts of whole blood to one part of liquid sodium citrate already present in the tube. Thus, when using an evacuated system, blood must be allowed to flow into the tube until it stops automatically. This provides for the 90% fill ratio required for coagulation testing. Underfilling of the tube results in artefactually long coagulation test times. The plasma specimen should be tested within 4 hours of collection, and, if not, then the samples should be frozen until testing.

Inhibitor screening and specific assays of coagulation factors
If the screening tests (PT, APTT, TT) are abnormal, then an inhibitor screen is appropriate. The addition of normal plasma to the patient's test plasma, usually in a 50:50 ratio (often referred to as a '50:50' mix), will correct any coagulation factor deficiencies in the test plasma, resulting in a normalization of the screening test. By contrast, the presence of an inhibitor in the patient's plasma will be much less affected by the added normal plasma, and hence the coagulation test will fail to correct to a normal or near normal result. The inhibitor screen can be further refined by incubation of the patient's test plasma with normal plasma to detect a time-dependent inhibitor, e.g. factor VIII inhibitors. If correction occurs with the addition of normal plasma, then the patient's plasma is depleted of one or more coagulation factors.

Specific assays for these coagulation factors can be performed on citrated plasma. The choice of which specific factor assays to undertake is based on which screening test is abnormal and the clinical circumstances of the patient. For example, in a male patient with a normal PT, but a prolonged APTT, who is bleeding, then assays for inhibitors of FVIII, FXI, and FXI may be performed initially. By contrast, the isolated finding of a prolonged APTT in an individual who has no bleeding history may be investigated first by an assay for FXII and lupus anticoagulant.

Platelet function tests
The use of the bleeding time, which was subject to considerable observer error and occasionally left a scar, has now largely been replaced by the platelet function analysis-100 (PFA-100) as a screening test for platelet function defects. In this test, citrated blood is drawn through a membrane coated with platelet activators (collagen, ADP, adrenaline/epinephrine). Aggregation of the platelets in the presence of these activators is measured by the time taken for the apertures in the membrane to occlude and for the blood flow to stop (the 'closure' time). The PFA-100 test is dependent on platelet function, the plasma vWf level, platelet number, and (to some extent) the haematocrit. It is particularly sensitive to von Willebrand's disease and the effects of aspirin.

Platelet aggregometry is the 'gold standard' of platelet function tests and measures the aggregation of platelets by light absorption in response to ADP, collagen, ristocetin, arachidonic acid, and adrenaline (epinephrine). Different patterns of aggregation are associated with different platelet disorders.

Additional tests are available in specialist centres to measure platelet glycoproteins and platelet alpha and dense granules.

Hypercoagulable disorders

Over 100 years ago, Virchow described the pathological basis for the risk factors for thrombosis being alterations in:
- The flow of blood.
- The blood vessel wall.
- The coagulability of blood.

The term thrombophilia refers to a predisposition to thrombosis, which can be both inherited and acquired. It is not a disease in itself, and most people with thrombophilia never experience symptomatic thrombosis. When thrombotic episodes occur, they are usually venous in nature and multifactorial in origin, resulting from the interplay of environmental factors with the individual's thrombotic predisposition.

The recognized risk factors for venous and arterial thrombosis differ, reflecting the differing pathophysiology of the two processes (see Table 12.1).

The inherited or familial disorders that predispose to thrombosis include:
- Antithrombin deficiency.
- Protein C deficiency.
- Protein S deficiency.
- Activated protein C resistance.
- Factor V Leiden.
- Prothrombin G20210A.
- Hyperhomocysteinaemia.
- Elevated plasma levels of:
  - Fibrinogen or factors II, VIII, IX, XI.
- Dysfibrinogenaemia.

The causes of acquired deficiencies of the naturally occurring anticoagulants antithrombin, protein C, and protein S are shown in Table 12.2. The prevalence and incidence of thrombosis associated with the more common inherited thrombophilia conditions are available in Heit 2007 (see Further reading).

To evaluate a patient with a history of venous thromboembolism (VTE), consideration must be given to both the possible acquired and inherited contributing factors. A detailed history must include possible immediate high-risk events (e.g. surgery, trauma), drugs (particularly the oral contraceptive in women), symptoms that might suggest a systemic disease (e.g. SLE) or underlying malignancy as well as the presence of any past personal or family history of VTE. The occurrence of a thrombosis without a clear provoking cause or in an unusual location (e.g. upper arm, cerebral vein, portal vein, etc.) should prompt consideration of an occult malignancy. Whilst there is no clear consensus on the cost benefit of widespread screening for malignancy in the setting of unprovoked VTE, it is reasonable to investigate individual patients, based upon the results of the history, examination (including rectal examination and pelvic examination in women), and routine laboratory investigations (blood count, renal and liver function, bone biochemistry, PSA in men over 50 years of age, urinalysis, and a chest X-ray).

Who to test

Most patients with VTE should not be routinely tested for inherited thrombophilia. Consideration should be given in the following circumstances:
- Thrombosis at a young age (<40 years).
- Thrombosis in unusual sites (e.g. cerebral, portal circulation, upper limb, etc.).

Table 12.1 Acquired risk factors for thrombosis

Venous thrombosis

Immobilization: 10-fold increased risk with bed rest >3 days, plaster cast, paralysis

Immobility during travel: 2 to 3-fold increased risk

Trauma

Post-operative state

Pregnancy: 10-fold increased risk compared to non-pregnant

Puerperium: 25-fold increased risk compared to non-pregnant/non-puerperal

Malignancy

Pelvic obstruction

Age: (<40 years old, annual incidence 1/10,000, 60–69 years old annual incidence 1/1000, >80 years old annual incidence 1/100

Oestrogen therapy: 2.5-fold increased risk, raloxifene and tamoxifen 2 to 3-fold increased risk

Combined oral contraceptives: 3 to 6-fold increased risk

Varicose veins: 1.5 to 2.5-fold risk after major general/orthopaedic surgery

Family history of VTE

Hospitalization: 10-fold increased risk

Anaesthesia: 2 to 3-fold increased risk of postoperative VTE in general anaesthesia compared to spinal/epidural

Central venous catheters: femoral route 11.5-fold increased risk compared with subclavian access

Obesity: 2 to 3-fold risk if BMI >30 kg/m^2

Hyperviscosity

Congestive cardiac failure

Inflammatory bowel disease

Nephrotic syndrome

Antiphospholipid syndrome (lupus anticoagulant)

Myeloproliferative diseases

Thrombotic thrombocytopenic purpura

Heparin-induced thrombocytopenia

Paroxysmal nocturnal haemoglobinuria

Arterial thrombosis

Family history

Male gender

Hyperlipidaemia

Hypertension

Diabetes mellitus

Antiphospholipid syndrome (lupus anticoagulant)

Myeloproliferative diseases

Hyperhomocysteinaemia

Smoking

Collagen vascular diseases

Elevated fibrinogen

Elevated factor VIII

Part derived from the Scottish Intercollegiate Guidelines Network (SIGN), Guideline 122 (2010). Prevention and management of venous thromboembolism. <http://www.sign.ac.uk/pdf/qrg122.pdf>.

- Unprovoked (idiopathic) recurrent venous thromboembolism.
- Family history of VTE, especially if a first-degree relative has had a VTE event at a young age.
- Neonatal thrombosis and purpura fulminans.
- Warfarin-induced skin necrosis.

Table 12.2 Some causes of acquired deficiencies of antithrombin, protein C, and protein S

	Antithrombin	Protein C	Protein S
Neonate	X	X	X
Pregnancy	X		X
Liver disease	X	X	X
Acute thrombosis	X	X	
Sepsis	X	X	X
DIC	X	X	X
Nephrotic syndrome	X		X
Drugs			
Heparin	X		
Warfarin		X	X
L-asparaginase	X	X	X
Oestrogens	X		X

X indicates an acquired deficiency of the indicated factor may occur.
Source: Thrombophilia: Common Questions on Laboratory Assessment and Management. John A Heit. *Haematology* 2007: 127-135 (American Society of Haematology Education Programme Handbook 2007. <http://asheducationbook.hematologylibrary.org/cgi/reprint/2007/1/127>).

- Recurrent miscarriages (>3) without fetal chromosomal abnormality.

There is no recommendation to screen women without a family history of venous thromboembolic disease prior to oral contraception. To prevent one death from pulmonary embolism (assuming a 1% case fatality rate for all VTE events), then over 2 million women would need to be screened prior to starting the oral contraceptive, and a large number of women who were heterozygote carriers would be denied the use of the oral contraceptive, and some would suffer thrombotic complications from the additional pregnancies that would arise if this strategy was adopted.

There is little evidence to support testing for inherited thrombophilia defects in the setting of arterial thrombosis (e.g. myocardial infarction, stroke). There is some evidence that factor V Leiden and the prothrombin gene mutation may contribute to the risk of these arterial events, in conjunction with other known risk factors (e.g. smoking, hypertension), whilst data on antithrombin, protein C and protein S are conflicting.

Principles for thrombophilia testing

- Testing should only be undertaken when the result is likely to influence management. There are no good data to support indefinite anticoagulation after a single venous thromboembolic event, even in the presence of a defined thrombophilia defect, save perhaps in the event of a massive/life-threatening thrombosis (especially if unprovoked). An exception might be where an individual has more than one inherited thrombophilic defect. The intensity of anticoagulation in an affected individual is the usual recommended INR of 2.5, irrespective of the presence or absence of a thrombophilic defect. Thus, thrombophilia (TPH) testing in an individual who has had a single VTE episode should rarely be undertaken.
- A negative thrombophilia screen does not imply that the patient has no risk of a recurrent VTE event.

- As thrombophilia testing involves genetic testing, patients should be carefully counselled about this in advance of the test. Considerable anxiety may be generated from the results, especially if they are not interpreted within the circumstances of the testing procedure. Furthermore, such tests might have an impact on life insurance issues.

When to test

- As a rule, the tests should not be performed during the acute phase of a VTE event nor if the patient is on a vitamin K antagonist (VKA: e.g. warfarin), as this reduces the levels of protein C and protein S. These tests should be undertaken after the patient has been off the VKA for at least 2 weeks, and preferably 4 weeks, to avoid obtaining a falsely low protein C or S result.
- Testing for inherited thrombophilia in children is not generally recommended.

Testing asymptomatic individuals

Most people who have inherited thrombophilia will never suffer a thromboembolic event. Therefore, a positive thrombophilia result in an asymptomatic individual (e.g. a family member of an affected person) does not constitute grounds to recommended long-term prophylactic anticoagulation, as the cumulative risk of bleeding would outweigh the risk of thrombosis in these individuals. It follows that testing of asymptomatic family members should be done only after careful consideration of the potential benefits. For example, the results of testing may help to identify risk factors for thrombosis, which might encourage a change in lifestyle or the use of prophylactic anticoagulation for high-risk situations (e.g. surgery). In pregnancy, the finding of the commonest defect, factor V Leiden, in a woman without a personal history of thrombosis is not generally considered sufficient grounds for antenatal prophylactic anticoagulation, although post-partum prophylaxis may be considered advisable.

Box 12.1 Thrombophilia screening—laboratory tests
Full blood count
ESR
Coagulation screen (PT and APTT)
Antithrombin
Protein C
Protein S
Activated protein C resistance
Factor V Leiden
Prothrombin gene mutation
Plasma homocysteine
Fibrinogen assay
Lupus anticoagulant
Anticardiolipin antibodies
Beta-2 glycoprotein 1 antibody

What to test for

Laboratory screening tests for thrombophilia are outlined in Box 12.1. The likelihood of a positive test result is partly related to the nature of the thrombotic event. Where the thrombosis is in an unusual location (cerebral, retinal, portal vein), then an acquired condition is often implicated as the underlying predisposing factor (e.g. myeloproliferative disease, oral contraceptive, recent surgery, or trauma). In addition, of the inherited thrombophilia defects, it is more likely, in these circumstances, that factor V Leiden or prothrombin G20120A will be implicated, rather than the rarer deficiencies of antithrombin, protein C, or protein S.

By contrast, where an individual has suffered a VTE before the age of 40 years old or has a first-degree family history of such or has a history of recurrent VTE, then the diagnostic yield of deficiencies of antithrombin, protein C, and protein S may reach 20–30%, especially if more than one of these risk factors is present. Similarly, factor V Leiden has been found in up to 50% in selected individuals who have suffered a VTE.

Prediction of recurrent thrombosis

Following VTE, there is evidence that the inheritance of more than one thrombophilia defect increases the risk of a recurrence. However, there is conflicting evidence that the inheritance of one thrombophilia defect on its own increases the risk of recurrent thrombosis, compared to the individual without a defined thrombotic defect. Thus, predicting the likelihood of a recurrent VTE event is not necessarily served by the finding of a single inherited thrombophilia defect; indeed, in 40–50% of families with a history of VTE, no laboratory abnormality can be identified.

An exception may be the inheritance of type 1 antithrombin deficiency, which is associated with a particularly high rate of thrombosis in pregnancy.

The circumstance of the first thrombosis is important in predicting the recurrence rate. A first thrombosis that occurs in association with temporary predisposing factors (trauma, surgery, pregnancy, etc.) is less likely to predict a recurrence than one that is spontaneous, where the recurrence rate is approximately 10% per year once the individual is off warfarin. This risk of recurrence appears to be highest in the first 2 years which has implications for the duration of anticoagulant therapy in these circumstances. This is an area of considerable ongoing research.

Air travel

Debate exists as to how to advise individuals with a past history of VTE or who are known to have an inherited TPH defect on the risks of air travel. Overall, the risks of fatal VTE are low—in the order of 1 in 1 million for transatlantic air flights. In this context, 'long' air flights are those of more than 4–6 hours. The risk of VTE appears to relate mostly to the period of inactivity and hence is a potential factor in all forms of long-distance travel. Standard advice comprises avoidance of excess alcohol, the regular flexion of the ankles to effect calf compression, and the wearing of compression travel socks, although the efficacy of this advice has been questioned. There are no data to support 'routine' thromboprophylaxis with stockings or heparin, but these may be considered in individuals with additional risk factors for VTE. There is no convincing evidence to support the use of aspirin.

Further reading

British Committee for Standards in Haematology (2005). Risk of venous thrombosis and long distance travel (including air flights) Information for travellers. BCSH Approved Document (2005). <http://www.bcshguidelines.com/documents/venousthromb_travel_bcsh__23052005.pdf>.

Chee YL and Watson HG (2005). Air travel and thrombosis. *British Journal of Haematology*, **130**, 671–80.

Heit, JA (2007). Thrombophilia: Common Questions on Laboratory Assessment and Management. *Haematology*, 127–35 (American Society of Haematology Education Programme Handbook, 2007, <http://asheducationbook.hematologylibrary.org/content/2007/1/127.long>).

Janssen H, Meinardi J, Vleggaar F, et al. (2000). Factor V Leiden mutation, prothrombin gene mutation, and deficiencies in coagulation inhibitors associated with Budd-Chiari syndrome and portal vein thrombosis: results of a case-controlled study. *Blood*, **96**, 2364–8.

Margaglione M, D'Andrea G, Colaizzo D, et al. (1999). Coexistence of Factor V Leiden and Factor II A20210 mutations and recurrent venous thromboembolism. *Thrombosis and Haemostasis*, **82**, 1583–7.

Mateo J, Oliver A, Borrell M, et al. (1997). Laboratory evaluation and clinical characteristics of 2,132 consecutive unselected patients with venous thromboembolism—results of the Spanish multicentre study on thrombophilia (EMET Study). *Thrombosis and Haemostasis*, **77**, 444–51.

Pradoni P, Lensing AWA, Cogo A, et al. (1996). The long term clinical course of acute deep venous thrombosis. *Annals of Internal Medicine*, **125**, 1–7.

National Institute for Health and Clinical Excellence (2010). Venous thromboembolism: reducing the risk. Reducing the risk of venous thromboembolism (deep vein thrombosis and pulmonary embolism) in patients admitted to hospital. NICE clinical guideline 92. <http://www.nice.org.uk/guidance/cg92/resources/guidance-venous-thromboembolism-reducing-the-risk-pdf>.

Rosendaal FR (1996). Oral contraceptives and screening for factor V Leiden. *Thrombosis and Haemostasis*, **75**, 524–5.

Schreijer AJ, Cannegieter SC, Doggen CJ, Rosendaal FR (2009). The effect of flight-related behaviour on the risk of venous thrombosis after air travel. *British Journal of Haematology*, **144**, 425–9.

Schulman S, Granqvist S, Homstrom M, et al. (1997). The duration of oral anticoagulation after a second episode of venous thromboembolism. *New England Journal of Medicine*, **336**, 393–8.

Scottish Intercollegiate Guidelines Network (SIGN) (2010). Prevention and management of venous thromboembolism. Guideline 122. <http://www.sign.ac.uk/pdf/qrg122.pdf>.

van den Belt AGM, Sanson B-J, Simioni P, et al. (1997). Recurrence of venous thromboembolism in patients with familial thrombophilia. *Archives of Internal Medicine*, **157**, 2227–32.

Walker ID (1997). Congenital thrombophilia. *Baillière's Clinical Obstetrics and Gynaecology*, **11**, 431–45.

Walker ID, Greaves M, Preston FE, on behalf of the Haemostasis and Thrombosis Task Force, British Committee for Standards in Haematology (2001). Guideline—investigation and management of heritable thrombophilia. *British Journal of Haematology*, **114**, 512–28.

Watson HG and Baglin TP. BJH Guideline (2010). Guidelines on travel-related venous thrombosis. *British Journal of Haematology*, **152**, 31–34.

Anticoagulation

Anticoagulant drugs

Heparin

Mechanism and pharmacology
Unfractionated heparin (UFH: molecular weight 15,000–18,000) is a mucopolysaccharide obtained from lung and gut tissue of pigs and cattle. It must be given parenterally, is protein-bound in the plasma, inactivated in the liver, excreted in the urine, and has a variable plasma half-life depending on dose, generally in the order of 1 hour. The anticoagulant effect of heparin is dependent on the presence of functioning antithrombin to which it binds, thereby accelerating the irreversible inactivation of thrombin, FX, FIX, and FXI. Given intravenously, the anticoagulant effect of heparin is effectively instant. Subcutaneous unfractionated heparin may be only 50% bioavailable or less, and peak plasma levels occur after 30–60 minutes.

Low molecular weight heparins (LMWH) (molecular weight 2,000–10,000) are produced by depolymerization of heparin. They are more bioavailable, with a longer plasma half-life than unfractionated heparin (3–5 hours), allowing once daily subcutaneous administration. They bind to antithrombin, but their small molecular weight results in the heparin-antithrombin complex having its greatest effect on the inactivation of FXa, with little effect on thrombin. Their anticoagulant effect is more predictable than unfractionated heparin and laboratory monitoring is not generally required.

Therapeutic doses of unfractionated heparin are usually given by continuous IV infusion, and laboratory monitoring is required to ensure adequate anticoagulation whilst minimizing the risks of bleeding. The therapeutic target for activated partial thromboplastin time (APTT) is 1.5–2.5 times the mean normal reference range for the laboratory (as different laboratories use different techniques, it is the ratio that is important, not the absolute clotting time). Alternatively, the anti-Xa assay can be used, especially where the APTT may be difficult to interpret (e.g. in the presence of a lupus anticoagulant), with the target therapeutic range being 0.3–0.7 U/mL. In some circumstances, 'heparin resistance' can occur, in which the impact of even high doses of heparin on the APTT is minimal. This can be due to antithrombin deficiency but, more commonly occurs in the setting of acute phase reactions, perhaps due to elevated FVIII levels. This explains why, following surgery, apparently high (and dangerous) levels of heparin may be seemingly required to provide a therapeutic anticoagulant effect when monitored by the APTT. In this situation, the use of unfractionated heparin should be monitored, using the anti-Xa assay.

Low molecular weight heparins are given subcutaneously and are the treatment of choice for the prophylaxis and management of deep vein thrombosis and pulmonary embolism as well as being used in the treatment of acute coronary syndromes. The outpatient management of patients with DVT has become routine, as patients can be taught to self-inject their LMWH. Laboratory monitoring is not required, as the anticoagulant effect is predictable. However, when monitoring is deemed necessary, e.g. when LMWH accumulates in renal failure (creatinine clearance <30 mL/min), potentially resulting in excessive anticoagulation, or when LMWH is used in pregnancy, then the anti-Xa assay must be used to assess the heparin dose. Blood sampling for anti-Xa levels should be done 4 hours after the last subcutaneous dose. The therapeutic range of heparin, using the chromogenic anti-Xa assay, is usually 0.3–0.7 U/mL, although the predictive value of the anti-Xa result is poor in terms of antithrombotic efficiency and bleeding risk.

Heparin-induced thrombocytopenia (HIT)

Mild thrombocytopenia induced by heparin use within the first 24 hours is relatively common (HIT, type 1). It is due to platelet clumping and not clinically relevant.

The more severe HIT type 2 typically occurs after 5–10 days of heparin exposure on first time use (it may occur earlier if there has been previous exposure to heparin) and is due to immune-mediated consumption, caused by an antibody against a complex of heparin and platelet factor 4. It can present with both arterial and venous thrombosis, the platelet count usually falling to around 50% of the pre-treatment levels, and only falling to $<20 \times 10^9$/L in 10% of patients. This type 2 phenomenon occurs in about 3–5% of patients on first exposure to unfractionated heparin for more than 4 days. It is less frequent with LMWH, in the order of 0.2%.

All patients receiving heparins should have a baseline pre-treatment platelet count performed and repeated at 24 hours if they have been exposed to heparin within the last 100 days. In cases of first exposure, a platelet count should be performed on alternate days (unfractionated heparin) and every 2 to 4 days (LMWH) from days 4 to 14. Obstetric patients receiving treatment doses of LMWH should have platelet counts performed every 2–4 days from days 4 to 14 but do not need platelet monitoring if using prophylactic doses. If the platelet count falls by 50% or more and/or the patient develops new thrombosis or skin allergy between days 4 and 14 of heparin administration, then HIT should be considered. Unless there are significant contraindications, then heparin should be stopped and an alternative anticoagulant started in full dosage whilst laboratory tests are performed. Alternative anticoagulants (see below) include the heparinoid danaparoid (IV infusion for VTE therapy and SC route for thromboprophylaxis) and lepirudin, a hirudin given by IV infusion.

Alternatives to heparin for use in HIT

Danaparoid is a mixture of heparin sulphate, chondroitin sulphate, and dermatan sulphate and is described as a heparinoid. It is used subcutaneously for thromboprophylaxis in orthopaedic and general surgery and may also be used intravenously as an alternative to heparin in the context of HIT. Cross-reactivity with heparin may occur. The major adverse effect is bleeding, and it must be used with caution in hepatic or renal impairment. Monitoring is with the anti-Xa assay. It is not available in the USA.

Lepirudin is a direct thrombin inhibitor biosynthetically derived from the saliva of the medicinal leech *Hirudo medicinalis*. It is licensed as an alternative to heparin in HIT, as it does not cross-react with HIT antibodies. It is given intravenously as a bolus of 0.4 mg/kg, followed by a continuous infusion of 0.15 mg/kg/hour. Both the bolus and infusion dose must be reduced in renal insufficiency. It is monitored with the APTT 4 hours after the first dose, then daily (target APTT ratio is 1.5–2.5 mean of the control). There is no antidote. If bleeding occurs, the drug should be withdrawn, the APTT monitored, and red cell transfusions given as necessary. The half-life is 1–3 hours in normal volunteers but may be up to 2 days in dialysis-dependent patients.

Heparin-associated osteopenia

Long-term heparin use is associated with bone density loss in up to 15% of patients receiving UFH for 3 months or more, with symptomatic vertebral fractures occurring in 2% of cases. The risk is lower with LMWH, and it is now used in preference to UFH, if long-term heparin use is planned.

Reversal of heparin

The short IV half-life of UFH results in rapid diminution of the anticoagulant effect once stopped, and, in most cases, this is all that is needed. However, protamine sulfate can be used for the urgent reversal of UFH. It is given by slow intravenous infusion at a dose of 1 mg per 100 units of heparin to be reversed. The dose should not normally exceed 50 mg over 10 minutes. Monitor its effect with the APTT, because rebound anticoagulation can occur as the half-life of protamine is brief. If given in excess, protamine has anticoagulant properties (e.g. it can interfere with the conversion of fibrin by thrombin), so the required dose must be calculated with care. Protamine is less effective in reversing the effect of LMWH and may need to be given repeatedly, as heparin enters the circulation from the subcutaneous depot.

Protamine is ineffective at reversing fondaparinux.

There are anecdotal reports of the use of recombinant factor VIIa being used to reverse life-threatening bleeding associated with LMWH and fondaparinux (see section on newer anticoagulants), although clinical experience is limited.

Oral anticoagulants

Oral anticoagulants are usually derived from coumarins or indandione. Warfarin, a coumarin, is most commonly used. It blocks the hepatic carboxylation of the glutamic acid residues of the vitamin K-dependent coagulation factors II, VII, IX, and X and interferes with the production of the anticoagulants protein C and protein S. Importantly, within the first 24 hours of use, the fall in plasma protein C occurs to a greater extent than the coagulation factors, which may result in a temporary prothrombotic state. In the setting of venous thromboembolism (VTE), the patient must receive heparin to cover the first few days of warfarin anticoagulation to prevent untoward thrombosis, which may present with severe skin necrosis.

The full anticoagulant effect of warfarin may take up to 4 days to develop, reflecting the different rates at which the vitamin K-dependent coagulation factors fall. FVII has the shortest half-life (3–6 hours), with levels falling within 24 hours of warfarin administration. This is reflected in the prolongation of the prothrombin time, which is most sensitive to FVII levels. However, the full anticoagulation effect of warfarin is not fully established until the other vitamin K-dependent coagulation factors have fallen, which, for prothrombin (factor II), may take up to 3 days.

For this reason, heparin therapy for acute VTE should not be stopped immediately the patient achieves a therapeutic INR but should be continued for at least 2 further days.

Where rapid induction of warfarin therapy is required, e.g. in the context of acute thrombosis, then a loading dose regimen is used, typically using daily doses of warfarin of 10 mg, 5 mg, and 5 mg on days 1, 2, and 3, respectively. Guided regimes, using Fennerty charts or similar algorithms, are commonly used. An initial dose of 5 mg should be used in those patients who are likely to be sensitive to warfarin (e.g. the elderly, cardiac failure or liver disease, or those at high risk of bleeding). The INR should be measured daily to permit dose adjustments. In most cases, a rapid induction is not essential, in which case a slow induction regimen is safer (e.g. 2 mg daily for 2 weeks) and can be done on an outpatient basis. This is the preferred induction regimen wherever possible.

Coumarin therapy is monitored using the international normalized ratio (INR). This is the prothrombin time adjusted to take into account the sensitivity of the thromboplastin reagent, calibrated against a WHO standard. It allows direct comparison of prothrombin time results, using any thromboplastin reagent. The range of INR in a normal unanticoagulated individual is 0.8 to 1.2, and the target INR in most indications for oral anticoagulation is 2.5 (range 2.0 to 3.0). Exceptionally, the target INR is higher (e.g. prosthetic mitral valve—target INR 3.0–3.5). Indications for oral anticoagulation and recommended target INRs have been recently published by the British Committee on Standards in Haematology.

Warfarin is highly protein-bound, and its pharmacokinetics are, in part, affected by two important genetic polymorphisms (VKORC1 and CYP2C9). These partially account for the range of dosing requirements between different individuals and different races (higher doses are required for African Americans and lower doses for Asians). Many drugs interfere with warfarin protein binding and metabolism, and most of these increase the anticoagulant effect of warfarin (see Table 12.3). Antibiotic therapy is a particularly common cause of increased warfarin effect, and anticoagulated patients should have their INR checked if on oral antibiotics for more than 5 days. If a drug is prescribed which is known to potentiate warfarin, then a simultaneous minor reduction of the warfarin dose should be considered.

Reversal of warfarin

The risk of bleeding associated with warfarin therapy is related to the INR and increases rapidly once the INR is greater than 5.0. The management of a high INR due to excess oral anticoagulation is based on the value of the INR (which relates to the risk of bleeding) and whether the patient is actively bleeding or not. Guidelines have been published by the British Committee on Standards in Haematology, updated in 2005 (see Further reading). A summary is shown in Table 12.4. If the INR is greater than 4.5 and the patient is not bleeding, it is often sufficient to omit one or two daily doses of warfarin. Where the INR is very high (>8), then it may be prudent to administer a small dose of vitamin K (0.5 to 2.0 mg), which can be given intravenously or orally (the IV preparation can be given orally). Vitamin K only partially reverses the warfarin effect until about 6 hours, full reversal taking up to 24 hours. In the event of life- or limb-threatening bleeding, a higher dose of 5–10 mg IV of vitamin K may be required. This may render the patient warfarin-resistant for up to 3 weeks.

For the immediate reversal of oral anticoagulation, the use of prothrombin complex concentrate (PCC) is preferred to fresh frozen plasma, as it more efficiently reverses the INR and can be given in lower volumes more quickly. The dose of IV PCC is 15 IU/kg–50 IU/kg, depending on the INR. If FFP is used, the dosage is 15 mL/kg, which may be an excessively large volume to completely reverse a dangerous INR (>8). In either case, the use of either PCC or FFP should be combined with vitamin K, and the INR checked within 30 minutes of the administration of the coagulation product and 4–6-hourly for 24 hours thereafter, to ensure adequate and sustained reversal. It may be necessary to administer a second dose of PCC or FFP, as rebound

Table 12.3 Some interactions with coumarin oral anticoagulants

Drugs that enhance anticoagulant effect		Drugs that reduce the anticoagulant effect	
Reduced albumin binding	Sulfonamides		
Inhibition of hepatic metabolism of warfarin	Allopurinol Amiodarone Cimetidine Clarithromycin Erythromycin Metronidazole Omeprazole Phenytoin Sulfonamides Tricyclic antidepressants	Increased hepatic metabolism of warfarin	Barbiturates Rifampicin
Alteration of hepatic receptor site for warfarin	Thyroxine Quinidine		
Reduced synthesis of vitamin K	Aspirin (in high doses) Some cephalosporin antibiotics	Increased synthesis of clotting factors	Oral contraceptives Dietary supplements (containing vitamin K)
Liver disease	Reduced synthesis of vitamin K-dependent clotting factors	Hereditary resistance to coumarin oral anticoagulants	
Reduced absorption of vitamin K	Antibiotic therapy (many) Laxatives Malabsorption	Pregnancy (warfarin and other coumarin oral anticoagulants should generally be avoided in pregnancy)	
Other	NSAIDs		

anticoagulation can occur. Management of the patient should be in close collaboration with the haematology department.

Management of perioperative anticoagulation
The management of a patient undergoing surgery and on oral anticoagulation is based on:

- The perceived risk of bleeding, based on the nature of the surgery (major or minor surgery).

Table 12.4 Management of bleeding and excessive anticoagulation

INR	Action
INR >8.0, no bleeding or minor bleeding; no other risk factors for bleeding	• Stop warfarin, and recheck INR daily. • If there are other risk factors for bleeding (e.g. age >70, thrombocytopenia, previous bleeding episodes, recent surgery, concomitant aspirin), then give 0.5–1 mg of vitamin K (use IV preparation orally or give dose IV). • When INR <5, review need for anticoagulation. • Restart warfarin, if appropriate, at reduced dose.

Major bleeding (irrespective of INR)*	• Stop warfarin, and give 5 mg vitamin K IV.
	• In severe bleeding, consider using prothrombin complex concentrate (PCC):
	  – 15 U/kg where INR >5.
	  – 30 U/kg where INR <5.
	  – 50 U/kg if there is intracerebral bleeding.
	• The alternative to PCC is FFP 15 mL/kg.
	• Check INR immediately following the administration of PCC (i.e. after 30 minutes) and again 4–6 hours later and then daily.
	• PCC (or FFP) and vitamin K may need to be repeated if bleeding continues/INR rises/or complete reversal of warfarin is required.
	• When INR <5, review need for anticoagulation.
	• Restart warfarin, if appropriate, at reduced dose.

* Complete reversal of warfarin in patients with mechanical heart valves may cause prolonged anticoagulant resistance and the possibility of valve thrombosis and emboli—degree of reversal will depend on type of valve; consult cardiology.

Source: Thrombophilia: Common Questions on Laboratory Assessment and Management. John A Heit. *Haematology* 2007: 127-135 (American Society of Haematology Education Programme Handbook 2007. <http://asheducationbook.hematologylibrary.org/cgi/reprint/2007/1/127>).

- The perceived risk of thrombosis if anticoagulation is withdrawn.

If the risk of bleeding during surgery is low, then oral anticoagulation can be continued, provided the INR is within the therapeutic range and less than 3.0 (e.g in dental surgery, cataract surgery, upper and lower endoscopy with or without a biopsy). In other instances, it may be sufficient to reduce the dose of warfarin 4 days prior to surgery to bring the INR down to a lower value of 1.5–2.0. If the perioperative bleeding risk is high, then warfarin is stopped 4 days before the surgery and consideration given to bridging therapy with LMWH in prophylactic or weight-adjusted doses. This should be continued until oral anticoagulation has been resumed and a therapeutic INR achieved. Bridging therapy with a continuous intravenous infusion of unfractionated heparin is generally not advised, as it is associated with a higher risk of perioperative bleeding, not least because the APTT is often relatively insensitive to its effect in the immediate post-operative period, as previously discussed.

Pregnancy

Warfarin crosses the placenta, whereas heparin does not. In the first trimester of pregnancy, warfarin is potentially teratogenic whilst, later in pregnancy, its anticoagulant effect on the fetus can result in intrauterine fetal bleeding. If either prophylactic or therapeutic anticoagulation is required during pregnancy, then LMWH heparin is the preferred anticoagulant.

Venous thromboembolism is the leading cause of maternal death in the UK. Prophylactic anticoagulation may be considered in women at increased risk of VTE. This includes those with:

- A previous history of unprovoked thrombosis.
- A thrombotic event and an inherited thrombophilia genotype, or family history of thrombosis.
- No personal history of thrombosis but a high-risk inherited thrombophilia genotype (homozygous factor V Leiden or prothrombin gene mutation, protein C deficiency, combined defects).

Prophylactic LMWH heparin should be started early in pregnancy and continued until 6 weeks post-partum. A switch to oral warfarin can be made in the post-natal period, if convenient. The usual prophylactic once-daily dose of LMWH (e.g. 40 mg of enoxaparin, 5,000 units of dalteparin) may be modified in patients at especially high risk of VTE. As heparin is cleared from the circulation more quickly later in pregnancy, it may be administered twice daily. Monitoring anti-Xa level is generally not required, unless high doses of heparin are used.

Treatment of an established venous thromboembolic event during pregnancy is based on therapeutic doses of LMWH, monitored by the anti-Xa assay, and continued throughout the pregnancy and for at least 6–12 weeks postpartum. The total duration of therapeutic anticoagulation should be at least 6 months.

The management of labour in women who are on LMWH requires coordination between the obstetrician, the anaesthetist, and the haematologist. Because of the risk of spinal haematoma during epidural catheter insertion and removal, the timings of epidural anaesthesia and previous LMWH administration need to be coordinated. As a guide, at least 12 hours should have elapsed from the last dose of prophylactic LMWH and 24 hours from the last therapeutic dose before an epidural is performed. LMWH should not be given for at least 4 hours after the epidural catheter has been inserted or removed, and the cannula should not be removed within 10–12 hours of the most recent injection. Obstetric units must have agreed protocols for the management of women in labour who are receiving anticoagulants.

In the post-partum period, both heparin and warfarin can be used. Heparin is not secreted into breast milk whilst the quantity of warfarin that gets into breast milk is minimal, and so breastfeeding is considered safe for both anticoagulants.

Self-testing of warfarin

A growing number of people on long-term warfarin are now testing their own INR readings on portable handheld devices, and some undertake self-dosing on the basis of the INR results. In all cases, they should be encouraged to do this after discussion with the appropriate clinical staff and suitable training, with regular quality control checks of the accuracy of the results obtained on the handheld machines and their dosing decisions.

Newer anticoagulants

Dabigatran and rivaroxaban are licensed for short-term prophylactic use in joint surgery, for the prevention of stroke in patients with non-valvular atrial fibrillation, and (in the case of rivaroxaban) for the treatment of deep vein thrombosis and the prevention of recurrent venous thromboembolism (i.e. DVT and PE). They are orally active, fixed-dose, direct inhibitor anticoagulants that do not require monitoring and have a rapid onset of action. Drug and food interactions are minimal. There is no antidote available to reverse their anticoagulant effect, but this is short-lived, as plasma half-lives are in the order of 12–16 hours. There are anecdotal reports of the beneficial reversal effect of prothrombin complex concentrate (PCC) and recombinant factor VII (rVIIa) in the setting of major bleeding, although the use of these clotting agents is off licence in this setting.

Dabigatran is an orally administered direct thrombin inhibitor and approved for the prophylaxis of VTE in hip and knee surgery. In this context, it has been shown to be as effective as enoxaparin 40 mg daily. It is also approved for the prevention of stroke in patients with non-valvular atrial fibrillation who meet appropriate criteria.

Rivaroxaban is an orally active direct inhibitor of FXa, licensed in Europe for the prevention of VTE in adults undergoing elective hip and knee replacements. It is given at a fixed dose once daily, and onset of action occurs 3 hours after oral dosing. In a phase III study, a 10 mg dose of rivaroxaban was found to be significantly more effective for extended thromboprophylaxis than once-daily 40 mg subcutaneous dose of enoxaparin in patients undergoing elective total hip arthroplasty. Both drugs had similar safety profiles. It has now been approved for the prevention of stroke in patients with non-valvular atrial fibrillation and also for the treatment of deep vein thrombosis and prevention of recurrent venous thromboembolism.

Apixaban is a new direct inhibitor of FXa, being investigated as a prophylactic anticoagulant in orthopaedic surgery.

Fondaparinux is a synthethic polysaccharide that inhibits FXa in the presence of antithrombin. It is administered subcutaneously once daily and has a lower incidence of associated thrombocytopenia than unfractionated heparin and LMWH. It is licensed for the prophylaxis of VTE in orthopaedic and abdominal surgery and the treatment of VTE and acute coronary syndromes. It is renally excreted and should not be used in renal failure. There is no specific antidote.

Antiplatelet agents

(See 'Transfusion and management of bleeding'.)

Aspirin irreversibly inhibits platelet cyclo-oxygenase (COX), thereby inhibiting thromboxane A2 production. The result is a reduced aggregation response to collagen, ADP, low concentrations of thrombin, and TXA2. Aspirin is effective at inhibiting platelet aggregation (a COX 1 activity) at lower doses than required for its anti-inflammatory effects (a COX 2-dependent activity). Platelet inhibition persists for the life of the platelet (8–10 days), but, as 10% of platelets are replaced every 24 hours, overall platelet activity returns to >50% within 5–6 days of the last dose. Aspirin is widely used in the prevention of thrombotic events in patients with vascular disease.

Clopidogrel, a thienopyridine, irreversibly inhibits platelet function through a variety of mechanisms, not all of which are fully understood. It has no direct effect on cyclo-oxygenase, thromboxane synthesis, phosphodiesterase, or adenosine uptake. Its major action appears to be by inhibiting platelet ADP receptor sites which blocks activation of the glycoprotein IIb/IIIa pathway. This is pivotal in platelet activation and the cross-linking of platelets by fibrin. It is used for the prevention of vascular ischaemic events in patients with symptomatic atherosclerosis, acute coronary syndromes, and, in combination with aspirin, as prophylaxis against thrombosis following coronary artery stenting. Adverse effects include haemorrhage (more frequently in combination with aspirin), neutropenia (rare), and thrombotic thrombocytopenic purpura (very rare).

Other antiplatelet agents include the platelet glycoprotein IIb/IIIa receptor antagonists, used in acute coronary syndromes (abciximab, tirofiban, eptifibatide), and dipyridamole, an inhibitor of thromboxane synthesis and phosphodiesterase. See also Chapter 4 on cardiac diseases and shock for further information.

Further reading

Baglin T, Barrowcliffe TW, Cohen A, Greaves M for the British Committee for Standards in Haematology (2006). Guidelines on the use and monitoring of heparin. *British Journal of Haematology*, **133**, 19–34.

Baglin TP, Keeling DM, Watson HG for the British Committee for Standards in Haematology (2005). Guidelines on oral anticoagulation (warfarin): third edition–2005 update. *British Journal of Haematology*, **132**, 277–85.

Baglin T, Gray E, Greaves M, *et al.* (2010). Clinical guidelines for testing for heritable thrombophilia. *British Journal of Haematology*, **149**, 209–220.

Eriksson BI, Borris LC, Friedman RJ, *et al.* (2008). Rivaroxaban versus enoxaparin for thromboprophylaxis after hip arthroplasty. *New England Journal of Medicine*, **358**, 2765–775.

Eriksson BI, Dahl OE, Rosencher N, *et al.* (2007). Dabigatran etexilate versus enoxaparin for prevention of venous thromboembolism after total hip replacement: a randomized, double-blind, non-inferiority trial. *Lancet*, **370**, 949–56.

Haemostasis and Thrombosis Task Force, British Committee for Standards in Haematology (2001). Investigation and management of inheritable thrombophilia. *British Journal of Haematology*, **114**, 512–28.

Keeling D, Baglin T, Tait C; British Committee for Standards in Haematology. Guidelines for oral anticoagulation with warfarin—fourth edition. <http://www.bcshguidelines.com/documents/warfarin_4th_ed.pdf>.

Levine M, Hirsh J, Gent M, *et al.* (1994). A randomized trial comparing activated thromboplastin time with heparin assay in patients with acute venous thromboembolism requiring large daily doses of heparin. *Archives of Internal Medicine*, **154**, 49–56.

Martel N, Lee J, Wells PS (2005). Risk for heparin-induced thrombocytopenia with unfractionated and low-molecular-weight heparin thromboprophylaxis: a meta-analysis. *Blood*, **106**, 2710–5.

National Institute for Health and Clinical Excellence (2012). Dabigatran etexilate for the prevention of stroke and systemic embolism in atrial fibrillation. <http://www.nice.org.uk/TA249>.

National Institute for Health and Clinical Excellence (2012). Rivaroxaban for the prevention of stroke and systemic embolism in people with atrial fibrillation. <http://www.nice.org.uk/TA256>.

National Institute for Health and Clinical Excellence (2012). Rivaroxaban for the treatment of deep vein thrombosis and prevention of recurrent deep vein thrombosis and pulmonary embolism. <http://www.nice.org.uk/TA261>.

National Patient Safety Agency. Managing patients who are taking warfarin and undergoing dental treatment. <http://www.nrls.npsa.nhs.uk/EasySiteWeb/getresource.axd?AssetID=60028&>.

No authors listed (1998). Guidelines on oral anticoagulation: third edition. *British Journal of Haematology*, **101**, 374–87.

Royal College of Obstetricians and Gynaecologists Guidelines (2015). Thrombosis and embolism during pregnancy and the puerperium, reducing the risk. Green top guideline 37a. <http://www.neonatalformulary.com/pdfs/uk_guidelines/ENOXAPARIN-thromboprophylaxis_in_pregnancy_guideline.pdf>.

Warkentin TE (1998). Clinical presentation of heparin-induced thrombocytopenia. *Seminars in Haematology*, **35** (Suppl 5), 9–16.

Watson H, Davidson S, Keeling D (2012). Guideline on the diagnosis and management of heparin-induced thrombocytopenia: second edition. *British Journal of Haematology*, **159**, 528–540.

Factors contributing to coagulation failure and DIC

The primary function of the coagulation system is to maintain vascular integrity without compromising vascular patency. Despite the presence of a vast excess of coagulation proteins and platelets, blood remains fluid in its basal state. This is enabled by a number of adaptive measures that suppress the coagulation mechanisms:

- Coagulation factors circulate in an inactive form and only promote blood clotting if activated.
- Endothelium lining blood vessels is devoid of thrombogenic tissue factor and collagen, and this prevents the activation of platelets and the coagulation cascade, unless the endothelium is breached.
- Blood flow through the vessels ensures that activated coagulation proteins are inactivated in the liver.
- Circulating anticoagulants in the blood and their activation by feedback mechanisms integral to the coagulation cascade serve to keep the procoagulant activity of blood in check.

Failure of the coagulation system occurs when the balance between procoagulant and anticoagulant activity is pathologically disturbed, resulting in bleeding or thrombosis. A paradigm for coagulation failure is the widespread inappropriate intravascular deposition of fibrin that occurs with the consumption of coagulation factors in disseminated intravascular coagulation (DIC).

DIC comprises the following components:

- Exposure of blood to procoagulants.
- Formation of fibrin in the circulation.
- Fibrinolysis.
- Depletion of clotting factors.
- End-organ damage.

Central to this process is the uncontrolled and excessive production of thrombin, the central regulator of the coagulation cascade. This, in turn, results in the widespread intravascular deposition of fibrin, leading to systemic microvascular thrombosis and consumption of coagulation proteins. The normal regulatory mechanisms that keep the balance between procoagulant and anticoagulant activity of blood is greatly disturbed, resulting in overwhelming failure of the coagulation system. Regardless of the initiating trigger, the pathophysiology of DIC is essentially similar in all conditions.

Activation of haemostasis

The primary event leading to the excessive inappropriate production of thrombin is the release or expression of tissue factor in the circulation. This occurs with damage to the vascular endothelium and exposure of transmembrane glycoprotein tissue factor, or its release into the circulation from tissues rich in tissue factor (e.g. brain, lung, placenta) or the upregulation and increased expression of tissue factor by circulating monocytes in response to endotoxin and other cytokines, as occurs in severe sepsis. The increased expression of tissue factor binds to FVIIa to form the extrinsic factor Xase complex, activating both factors IX and X, overwhelming the antithrombotic regulatory mechanisms that keep this process in check (antithrombin and tissue factor pathway inhibitor). This, in turn, results in the production of the prothrombinase complex (FX, FV, phospholipids, and calcium ions), leading to the explosive generation of thrombin which acts on fibrinogen to form the fibrin clot.

With the widespread production of fibrin, there follows extensive fibrinolysis, largely mediated by the release of tissue plasminogen activator (tPA) from damaged endothelium, converting thrombus-bound plasminogen to plasmin. Fibrinolysis is further enhanced by the destruction of plasma inhibitors of tPA by activated protein C, produced by the action of thrombin on protein C via thrombomodulin. Plasmin digests fibrin, fibrinogen, factors V and VIII and produces a variety of split products from fibrin and fibrinogen by cleavage of peptide bonds. These fibrin degradation products (FDPs) inhibit thrombin and fibrin polymerization, leading to further coagulation defects.

The combined action of thrombin and plasmin results in the depletion of fibrinogen and all coagulation factors, whilst the systemic deposition of thrombi in the vasculature results in platelet aggregation and deposition in vessels. This platelet deposition contributes to thrombotic process and to thrombocytopenia, leading to enhanced bleeding.

Clinical features

In acute DIC, the consumption of clotting factors resulting from the extensive activation of the coagulation cascade, together with the systemic activation of fibrinolysis, leads to a clinical state dominated by profound generalized bleeding. Blood oozes from venepuncture sites, intravenous catheters, and wound sites. There may be bleeding into the deeper tissues, including the gastrointestinal tract, the lungs, the oropharynx, and, in obstetric cases, from the vagina. Less commonly, microthrombi in the circulation may lead to skin lesions, renal failure, ischaemia and ultimately gangrene of the extremities (fingers and toes), and cerebral infarcts.

Occasionally, activation of the coagulation mechanisms occurs more slowly, and the liver is able to compensate for the consumption of clotting factors, and the bone marrow can maintain adequate platelet numbers. In these patients, a state of compensated chronic DIC exists, in which the primary manifestation is widespread arterial and venous thrombosis, rather than bleeding. In this situation, some of the laboratory coagulation tests remain normal because the coagulation factors are not depleted. An example is the hypercoagulable state associated with malignancy, particularly with mucin-secreting adenocarcinomas (Trousseau syndrome).

Aetiology

The major causes of DIC are:

Infection

DIC was originally described as a complication of meningococcal septicaemia. However, DIC can occur in a variety of Gram-positive and Gram-negative infections as well as viral infections (hepatitis, varicella, cytomegalovirus, HIV) and falciparum malaria. It is common in Gram-negative sepsis and may occur in 30 to 50% of such cases. In severe sepsis, tissue factor is released due to endothelial damage and its expression is increased by circulating monocytes and macrophages. Furthermore, endotoxin activates both the tissue factor (extrinsic) pathway directly and the intrinsic pathway by acting on FXII, which, in turn, stimulates kinin production, leading to increased vascular permeability, vasodilatation, and shock.

Major surgery and trauma

DIC is a complication of major surgery and extensive trauma where severe tissue damage results in tissue factor and phospholipid release into the circulation. Together with the sustained systemic inflammatory response syndrome (SIRS), the severity of the DIC in these situations can be a predictor of adverse outcome. DIC is especially common after head injury, occurring within a few hours of trauma, and associated with a higher mortality.

Malignancy
The third most common cause of DIC, after infection and trauma, is malignancy. Hypercoagulable states with chronic DIC are common. Laboratory tests of haemostasis are variable, depending on the degree to which the liver and bone marrow can compensate for the consumption of clotting factors and platelets. Whilst thrombosis is the predominant manifestation in chronic DIC induced by many disseminated malignancies, extensive and life-threatening haemorrhage is the principal complication of the acute DIC associated with acute promyelocytic leukaemia. This may occur at presentation or after the start of chemotherapy treatment. In these cases, the induction of leukaemia tumour cell differentiation with retinoic acid, plus appropriate supportive therapy, can lead to improvement in the coagulopathy.

Obstetric complications
DIC can occur with amniotic fluid embolism, abruptio placentae, eclampsia and severe pre-eclampsia, the HELLP syndrome, and retained dead fetus and septic abortion. Release of procoagulants into the maternal circulation from the placenta or fetus is the likely cause of the DIC in obstetric cases.

Other conditions associated with DIC
These include:
- Giant haemangioma (Kasabach–Merritt syndrome).
- Acute haemolytic transfusion reaction (usually ABO incompatibility and, most commonly, a clerical error).
- Insertion of a peritoneovenous shunt, with entry of procoagulants (endotoxin, etc.) from the ascitic fluid into the circulation.
- Snake bites—especially from the venom of vipers.
- Hepatic failure and cirrhosis—reduced synthesis of coagulation proteins and absorbed endotoxin from the gut contribute to the DIC.
- Heat stroke and burns result in tissue factor release from widespread tissue damage.
- Purpura fulminans, usually associated with homozygous protein C deficiency in the neonatal period, can lead to widespread skin necrosis and DIC.
- Catastrophic antiphospholipid syndrome.
- Paroxysmal nocturnal haemoglobinuria can cause venous thrombosis, occasionally, with DIC.

Laboratory tests
The major laboratory findings of DIC are:
- Thrombocytopenia—in >95% of cases.
- Reduced fibrinogen levels.
- Prolonged thrombin time (TT)—in 70–80% of cases.
- High levels of fibrin degradation products (FDPs) and D-dimers in blood and urine. If both are present and clinical suspicion of DIC is high, then almost all cases will be confirmed to have DIC.

- Prolongation of the APTT and PT in 50–75% of cases. Blood film examination—in about 50% of cases, the blood film will show red cell fragments due to damage sustained by the erythrocytes as they shear through the fibrin strands in the microcirculation. When fragments are present in high numbers on the film, then other causes of red cell fragmentation should be considered (e.g. TTP, microangiopathic haemolytic anaemia).
- The degree to which the clotting times (TT, APTT, PT) are prolonged relate to the overall reduction in the level of circulating coagulation factors; they may be normal in chronic DIC but are characteristically prolonged in acute DIC. Similarly, levels of FV and FVIII are reduced in the acute setting but are normal in chronic DIC.

DIC is primarily a clinical diagnosis, supported by the laboratory findings. Since this clinical condition is dynamic and changes rapidly, the results of laboratory tests may already be 'out of date' by the time they become available. This potential inability for laboratory assays to reflect the state of the coagulation system in real time should always be recognized when interpreting the results of the tests.

Treatment of DIC
This has recently been summarized by the British Committee on Standards in Haematology. The treatment of DIC is based on the following principles:
- The primary goal is to treat the underlying condition which has initiated DIC and 'switch off' the stimulus that maintains it. Thus, treatment of sepsis, shock, trauma, and obstetric complications is vital.
- Transfusion of platelets is reserved for patients who are actively bleeding or at high risk of doing so, e.g. about to undergo an invasive procedure. In this situation a platelet count of 50×10^9/L should be the target.
- FFP and cryoprecipitate should be considered in patients with prolonged coagulation times (PT and APTT) who are bleeding. Concentrates (e.g. prothrombin complex concentrate) can be used to correct the coagulopathy if the patient is fluid-overloaded and cannot safely be given FFP, although such concentrates will not replace all of the coagulation proteins. In non-bleeding patients, clotting products to correct laboratory abnormalities is inappropriate.
- The judicious use of therapeutic doses of heparin should be considered in cases where thrombosis predominates, e.g. in severe purpura fulminans. If concomitant bleeding is present, then continuous infusion of unfractionated heparin at the weight-adjusted dose of 10 U/kg/h may be appropriate. In this circumstance, APTT monitoring is not required and is difficult, as the underlying DIC may complicate interpretation. Clinical observation for signs of bleeding is important. Prophylactic doses of heparin (usually low molecular weight heparin) should be given to critically ill patients who are not bleeding but are at high risk of venous thrombosis.
- There are insufficient data to support the use of antithrombin concentrate.
- Antifibrinolytic agents are not generally recommended in DIC. However, tranexamic acid (1 g tds) may be used in patients with severe primary hyperfibrinolytic states (e.g. in acute promyelocytic leukaemia and prostrate cancer) and significant bleeding.

Blood and blood components

The *Handbook of Transfusion Medicine United Kingdom Blood Services* (2013) is an excellent text on the practical aspects of blood transfusion medicine. This contains essential information on blood components and their use.

Blood comprises cellular components (predominantly red cells and platelets) and plasma, from which a variety of other components are derived (coagulation products and immunoglobulins). In the western world, whole blood is now seldom used for routine blood transfusion, as there is a need to fractionate plasma. The need to produce factor VIII for the care of haemophiliac patients in the 1980s led to the development of blood component therapy, whereby patients were transfused with the specific component of blood they required (red cells, platelets, fresh frozen plasma, and cryoprecipitate).

All blood donations are tested for the following and only released if negative for:

- HIV antibody.
- HTLV antibody.
- Hepatitis B surface antigen.
- Hepatitis C antibody and RNA.
- Syphilis antibody.

Depending on the history of the donor and the need for specific blood products, other tests may be undertaken, including cytomegalovirus antibody, malaria antibodies, *T. cruzi* antibodies, and West Nile virus RNA.

The estimated risks of transfusion-transmitted viral disease for 2007 are:

- HIV—0.25 per million donations.
- Hepatitis B—1.62 per million donations.
- Hepatitis C—0.02 per million donations.
- HTLV—0.10 per million donations.

Indications for the transfusion of blood components

Prior to undertaking blood product transfusion, and in line with Patient Blood Management (2012), consideration should be given to the possible use of blood conservation strategies.

Red cells

Transfusion of red cells is undertaken to improve the oxygen-carrying capacity of the blood where such a reduction causes a clinically significant problem and where correction is considered likely to benefit the patient. It is an important part of the management of significant blood loss. Thus, red cell transfusion is the mainstay of treatment of inherited disorders of haemoglobin production (e.g. haemoglobinopathies—thalassaemias and sickle cell disease) as well as acquired marrow conditions resulting in anaemia (e.g. myelodysplasias, leukaemias, bone marrow metastases). However, transfusion may not be required in haematinic insufficiency (deficiencies of iron, vitamin B12, or folic acid) if the underlying deficiencies are corrected, unless the anaemia is especially symptomatic. Red cells are supplied with minimal plasma (about 20 mL in each unit), the remainder of the fluid being saline with added adenine, glucose, and mannitol (SAGM or optimal additive solution (OAS)). The mean volume of a unit of red cells is 282 mL, with a haematocrit of 57% (equivalent to 55 g of Hb per pack). The shelf life of a unit is 35 days, stored between +2°C and +6°C. Red cells need to be compatible with the recipient's ABO (and usually rhesus D) blood group, and the infusion of each unit should be completed within 4 hours of leaving the blood bank fridge.

Platelets

Platelet transfusions are indicated to prevent or treat untoward bleeding in thrombocytopenic patients or in significant platelet functional defects. A single adult pooled dose of platelets (volume approximately 310 mL) is derived from four donors (apheresed platelets come from a single donor). The mean number of platelets per adult dose is about 300×10^9 and, for a 70 kg adult, can be expected to immediately raise the platelet count by $20–40 \times 10^9/L$, provided there is no excessive consumption of platelets, either by immunological mechanisms or by splenic pooling in an enlarged spleen. Ideally, they should be ABO- and rhesus D-compatible with the recipient and be administered through a standard blood administration set or a platelet infusion set. An adult dose of platelets can be infused in 30 minutes.

Fresh frozen plasma

Fresh frozen plasma (FFP) is indicated in the treatment of bleeding from coagulation deficiencies where specific virally inactivated coagulation factor replacement is not available (e.g. DIC, liver disease, massive transfusion, and occasionally to reverse warfarin). It is also used in the management of thrombotic thrombocytopenic purpura. It is not indicated as a method of blood volume replacement. It has been widely used without clear indication or good evidence of efficacy and is as likely to transmit viral infections as whole blood or red cells. Its inappropriate use constitutes the largest avoidable risk to patients of transfusion-transmitted infection worldwide. In the UK, it may be subject to pathogen-reducing processes to reduce this risk. All children under the age of 16 who require FFP should receive methylene blue-treated FFP. One donor pack contains 220 mL of plasma (with anticoagulant, the total volume is 270 mL), an estimated 20–50 mg of fibrinogen, >0.7 IU/mL of FVIII, and a variable amount of other coagulation factors. Once defrosted, the unit should be transfused within 24 hours (but sooner if not kept at +2°C to +6°C in the interim). The rate of infusion is, in part, dependent on the cardiovascular state of the patient, as infusion of multiple units of FFP may lead to circulatory overload. FFP should be ABO-compatible with the patient to avoid haemolysis but does not need to be rhesus D-matched.

Cryoprecipitate

This is produced by controlled thawing of FFP to produce a precipitate that is rich in fibrinogen, von Willebrand factor (vWf), and factor VIII:C (FVIII:C). A single donation of 20–50 mL contains 80–300 units of FVIII:C and vWf and 300–600 mg of fibrinogen. Cryoprecipitate is used to correct low fibrinogen levels (e.g. in massive transfusions where FFP is inadequate). In the past, it was used to treat haemophilia A and von Willebrand's disease, although this has now been superseded by the advent of virally inactivated factor concentrates. The usual adult dose is two, five donor pools (five donor pools can be supplied by the regional transfusion centre), or ten, single donor units. This adult dose contains 3–6 g of fibrinogen in 200–500 mL and would be expected to raise the fibrinogen concentration in an adult by 1 g/L.

Plasma derivatives

Products which are derived from plasma include:

- Albumin—supplied as 4.5% and 20% concentrations, in various volumes. Both concentrations contain approximately 140 mmol/L of sodium chloride. The volume required to provide any given amount of albumin is about one-quarter when using the 20% concentration, compared to the 4.5% concentration. However, it is hyperoncotic and may result in volume overload. Albumin is licensed for the restoration and maintenance of circulating blood volume. The 20% solution is primarily used in patients with liver failure or nephritic syndrome.

- Human immunoglobulin—this may be supplied as an intramuscular preparation (usually for passive immunization against hepatitis A or to prevent rhesus D sensitization in RhD-negative pregnant woman). Intravenous preparations are used in the replacement of IgG in immunodeficiency syndromes or as immunomodulatory treatment in immune-mediated disorders (e.g. idiopathic thrombocytopenic purpura). In some circumstances specific anti-D immunoglobulin can be administered via the IV route to prevent RhD sensitization in pregnant women who have had a large feto-maternal bleed.

- Clotting factor concentrates—those derived from plasma are virally inactivated and include:
  - Factor VIII (some preparations contain von Willebrand factor). Used in haemophilia A and some cases of von Willebrand's disease.
  - Factor IX. Used in haemophilia B.
  - Prothrombin complex concentrate (containing factors II, VII, IX, and X). Used in the management of bleeding in which multiple factor deficiencies have been implicated and in the reversal of coumarin (e.g. warfarin) overdose.
  - Others: protein C concentrate, FEIBA (factor eight inhibitor bypassing activity), antithrombin, fibrinogen, von Willebrand concentrate, C1 esterase inhibitor.

Recombinant clotting factors

Recombinant clotting factors are expensive but do not carry any risk of viral transmission. They are:

- Factor VIII—most haemophilia A patients in the UK are treated with recombinant FVIII.
- Factor IX—for haemophilia B patients.
- Factor VIIa—licensed for use in haemophilia A patients with inhibitors, those with Glanzmann's thrombocythaemia, and for the rare patient with congenital FVII deficiency. It has been used 'off label' in the management of massive haemorrhage, but, as its mechanism of action is dependent upon the presence of sufficient platelets and coagulation factors, it should only be employed after sufficient replacement of these blood products. It is extremely expensive and should only be used within the context of a protocol that has been agreed with the haematologists, in the management of massive transfusion.

Special requirements of blood products

Gamma irradiation

This is recommended for cellular blood products where there could be a risk of transfusion-associated graft versus host disease (TA-GVHD; Table 12.5). This occurs when immunocompetent transfused donor lymphocytes mount an immunological response against an immunocompro-

Table 12.5 Special requirements

Indications for gamma irradiation of cellular blood products

Intrauterine and exchange transfusions

Transfusion from family members (first- and second-degree)

HLA-matched platelets

Autologous haemopoietic stem cell recipients:
 All transfusions given 7 days or less prior to stem cell harvesting
 All transfusions given from the start of conditioning therapy to 3 months post-transplant (6 months post-transplant if total body irradiation has been used)

Allogeneic haemopoietic stem cell recipients:
 All transfusions from the start of conditioning until graft vs host disease prophylaxis has been stopped

Patients who have received purine analogue chemotherapy (e.g. fludarabine, cladribine, pentostatin (INN)). Irradiated blood products required indefinitely

Hodgkin's lymphoma—all stages of disease. Irradiated blood products required indefinitely

Congenital immunodeficiencies affecting T cells (e.g. SCID, Di George's syndrome, Wiskott–Aldrich syndrome, etc.)

Any granulocyte transfusion for any recipient

Note: whilst not considered mandatory, some units irradiate blood products for HIV patients.

Irradiation may be recommended in the future for patients receiving forthcoming immunomodulatory monoclonal antibody drugs and other chemotherapy agents.

CMV antibody-negative components

CMV antibody-negative allogeneic stem cell recipients

CMV antibody-negative pregnant women

Intrauterine transfusion

HIV patients

---

mised transfused recipient. Leucocyte depletion of blood products does not provide sufficient protection against TA-GVHD. Gamma irradiation is not required for FFP, cryoprecipitate, or fractionated plasma products.

CMV-negative blood products

This should be used in CMV antibody-negative patients at risk of CMV infection due to their immunocompromised state (see Table 12.5). Leucocyte depletion of blood products (routine in the UK) may confer equivalent protection against transfusion-transmitted CMV infection in these patients as with the use of CMV-negative blood products, although, as yet, there is no consensus.

Competency assessment in blood transfusion

Following the National Patient Safety Agency Safer Practice Notice 14 in November 2006, it is now a requirement in England that all persons involved in the process of blood transfusion undergo a competency assessment every 3 years, with respect to the particular aspect of the transfusion process that they practise (e.g. the obtaining of a blood sample for transfusion cross-match, the administration of blood components). This reflects the recognition that blood transfusion carries significant risks, is a complex process, and needs strict checks in place at each stage of the process.

Further reading

Department of Health (2007). Health Service Circular. Better blood transfusion—safe and appropriate use of blood. <http://www.transfusionguidelines.org.uk/docs/pdfs/nbtc_bbt_hsc_07.pdf>.

Norfolk D (2013). Handbook of transfusion medicine. United Kingdom Blood Services. 5th Edition. <http://www.transfusionguidelines.org.uk/transfusion-handbook>.

National Blood Transfusion Committee (2014). Patient Blood Management. <http://www.transfusionguidelines.org.uk/uk-transfusion-committees/national-blood-transfusion-committee/patient-blood-management>.

National Patient Safety Agency (2006). Safer practice notice 14. Right patient, right blood, pp. 2–6. <http://www.transfusion-guidelines.org.uk/docs/pdfs/bbt-02_npsa-notice-14.pdf>.

SHOT (2008). SHOT Annual Report 2007. Summary, p. 106. <http://www.shotuk.org/wp-content/uploads/2010/03/SHOT-Report-2007.pdf>.

Bleeding disorders

Inherited coagulation disorders

Inherited disorders of all coagulation factors have been described. Haemophilia A (FVIII:C deficiency), haemophilia B (FIX deficiency), and von Willebrand's disease are the most common.

Haemophilia A

Haemophilia A is an inherited deficiency of functioning FVIII and occurs in 1 in 5,000–10,000 live male births. Factor VIII is coded by a large gene carried on the long arm of the X chromosome. A number of defects in this gene result in haemophilia A, although spontaneous mutations occur in one-third of cases with no family history. Males are affected whilst females born to affected males are obligate carriers. Occasionally, females may have symptomatic haemophilia A, most commonly due to excessive lyonization of FVIII (or IX in haemophilia B) alleles in obligate carriers. Lyonization (also known as X-inactivation) is the process by which one X 'shuts-down' or does not express itself. In a female, if the X chromosome with the Haemophilia gene is the 'active' chromosome then she will have lower levels of FVIII (or IX) and symptomatic disease.

Prenatal diagnosis can be undertaken. The fetus can be tested, using chorionic villous sampling at 8–10 weeks' gestation, to provide DNA for analysis, or at 16 weeks by amniocentesis. The latter is associated with a 0.5–1.0% miscarriage rate. At 16–20 weeks, fetal FVIII level can be assayed in umbilical cord blood, but this carries a 1–6% fetal loss rate.

The hallmark of haemophila is spontaneous bleeding into the muscles and joints (haemarthrosis). The knee is most commonly affected, but bleeding can occur in the elbows, ankles, shoulders, and wrists. Recurrent bleeding into the joint causes degeneration of the cartilage and destruction of the joint space, with reactive synovial hypertrophy. The synovium becomes fragile and hence more prone to bleeding, resulting in further spontaneous bleeding, and a 'vicious' cycle is established that results in potential progressive joint destruction. Bleeding episodes do not usually start until the child starts walking, usually at about 1 year old. Prior to this, the child may present with bleeding after circumcision or a scalp haematoma immediately following a difficult birth, e.g. forceps delivery.

Bleeding into muscles is the second most common manifestation of haemophilia. The presentation depends on the location of the bleed, the muscles involved, and whether there are features of compression secondary to a compartment syndrome. Bleeding into a fascial compartment can cause ischaemia, necrosis, contraction, and nerve damage, whilst bleeding into a large muscle group not confined by fascial planes is more likely to resolve without complications. Retroperitoneal or psoas bleeding can cause referred groin pain and reduced ipsilateral hip movement. If the femoral nerve is compressed, then permanent disability may result. Diagnosis is confirmed on ultrasound, CT, or MRI scanning.

Intracranial haemorrhage is the most common cause of death from bleeding and can occur spontaneously, or with minimal trauma and may present with headache, nausea and vomiting, or seizures. Following even apparently trivial head trauma, the patient should receive immediate factor concentrate to raise the levels to 100% of normal, even before CT/MRI. Other bleeding manifestations include spontaneous haematuria, which is usually painless, unless ureteric clot forms, gastrointestinal and oropharyngeal bleeding (retropharyngeal bleeding is particularly dangerous, as airway obstruction can occur).

Laboratory diagnosis

Outside of prenatal diagnosis (as described previously), the possibility of haemophilia should be considered in those presenting with a compatible bleeding history and a prolonged APTT but normal PT, thrombin time, and platelet function tests. The addition of normal plasma to the patient's plasma, usually in a 1:1 proportion (the 50:50 mix), will correct the prolonged APTT, thereby ruling out the presence of an inhibitor (lupus anticoagulant, FVIII inhibitor, heparin). Specific factor assays will isolate the deficient factor. A FVIII level <1% (<0.01 U/mL) indicates severe haemophilia, between 1 and 5% (1 U/mL–5 U/mL) is moderate, and mild haemophilia when the FVIII level is >5% (5 U/mL).

Development of antibodies (inhibitors) to FVIII occurs in about 10% of haemophilia A patients. These inhibitors neutralize administered FVIII, resulting in an ineffective rise in factor VIII levels, following administration. The diagnosis should be considered if a rise is not demonstrated by factor assay after giving concentrate and requires a formal screen and assay to quantify the level of inhibitor (Bethesda units).

Treatment of haemophilia

Patients with haemophilia should be treated in specialist haemophilia centres, which comprise multidisciplinary teams, including haematologists, specialist nurses, rheumatologists, orthopaedic surgeons, hepatologists, physiotherapists, dentists, and obstetricians.

The cornerstone of haemophilia care is the use of factor concentrate for the treatment or prevention of bleeding episodes. Both factor VIII and factor IX concentrates are administered intravenously and are available as recombinant or virucidally treated plasma products of different degrees of purity. The dose is determined by the activity of the concentrate (IU/mg), the degree to which the patient's deficient factor needs to be raised, and the specific factor involved (where 100 IU/dL = 100% of mean normal level). Thus, bleeding is usually controlled in haemophilia A by raising the FVIII level, but this may need to be to 100% for severe bleeds. Factor VIII concentrates raise the patient's plasma FVIII level by 2 U/dL per unit infused per kilogram. Thus, the dose of factor VIII concentrate to be infused in units is:

$$\frac{\left(\text{weight in kg} \times \text{increment of FVIII required in U/dL}\right)}{2}$$

Typically, minor, moderate, and major bleeds require FVIII levels of 20–40, 30–60 and 60–100 IU/dL (or % of normal) respectively, with repeat infusion every 8–24 hours until resolution. Minor and major surgical procedures require 30–60 or 60–100 IU/dL (or % of normal) respectively with repeat infusion every 8–24 hours until haemostasis (or wound healing). Concentrate should be administered rapidly at the onset of bleeding without waiting for investigations. Haemophilia centres frequently arrange home supplies of concentrate after teaching patients or carers to administer concentrates during bleeding episodes. Regular prophylactic factor concentrate administration may be given to prevent the development of a target joint.

Desmopressin may be used to raise the FVIII level for short periods in mild or moderate haemophilia A, for example, in advance of dental or minor surgical procedures or to control a bleeding event. When given intravenously at a dose of 0.3 mcg/kg, the FVIII levels will increase 2–4-fold within 45–60 minutes, as FVIII is released from endothelial cells. Repeated use of IV desmopressin in a short period will exhaust these stores and become ineffective (tachyphylaxis). It is often combined with tranexamic acid (1 g tds for 7–10 days—initially IV, then orally) to counteract the fibrinolysis, which desmopressin stimulates. Desmopressin is a synthetic analogue of the antidiuretic vasopressin and may result in excessive water retention, and patients should restrict their fluid intake to 2 L for 24 hours after use. It can be given subcutaneously or intranasally. It should be used with caution in the elderly because of thrombotic complications (e.g. myocardial infarction).

As discussed, inhibitors (anti-FVIII alloantibodies) develop in about 10% of haemophilia A patients, especially in children with severe disease, and neutralize the infused FVIII. If present in low titre, they can be overcome by higher doses of concentrate, but, at higher titres, it may be necessary to use bypassing agents (e.g. prothrombin complex concentrates, FEIBA) or recombinant FVIIa until bleeding is controlled. In the longer term, strategies to induce immune tolerance may be employed, e.g. daily administration of factor concentrate, to suppress the production of antibody by the immune system.

Haemophilia B

Like haemophilia A, haemophilia B (Christmas disease) is a sex-linked disease, affecting males with deficient FIX production. The incidence is about one-fifth of haemophilia A, at 1 in 30,000 live male births. Clinical presentation is identical to haemophilia A and only distinguished by the specific FIX assay. Again, APTT is prolonged, but the PT is normal. Treatment is with FIX concentrates which have a longer half-life than FVIII and do not need to be administered so frequently. As a guide, the dose can be estimated by:

$$\frac{(\text{weight in kg} \times \text{increment of FIX required in U} / \text{dL})}{1}$$

Desmopressin has no activity in haemophilia B.

von Willebrand's disease

von Willebrand's disease is the commonest inherited bleeding disorder, occurring in up to 1% of the population. Usually inherited in an autosomal dominant fashion, it presents in either sex, with bruising and mucosal bleeding of variable intensity (epistaxis, menorrhagia, gum bleeding, bleeding from dental and operative procedures). It may be due to an overall reduction in von Willebrand factor (vWf: type 1—70% of cases) or to a qualitative abnormality of the vWf protein (type 2), resulting in a functional deficit. Rarely, there is complete absence of the vWf protein (type 3) when the disease may present with haemarthroses and muscle bleeds, which are otherwise rare.

Laboratory diagnosis

vWf has two functions: firstly, it acts as a bridge between the subendothelial collagen and platelets, without which the primary haemostatic platelet plug cannot form effectively. Secondly it functions as a carrier for FVIII, without which FVIII is degraded more quickly, resulting in a reduced plasma FVIII level. Routine coagulation screening tests may, therefore, show a prolonged APTT by virtue of the reduced plasma FVIII, but they do not detect the vWF protein, as it does not directly take part in the coagulation cascade. However, because platelet function is affected, the PFA-100 test may be abnormal, and the diagnosis can be confirmed by demonstrating reduced platelet aggregation in the presence of ristocetin (vWf:RiCoF) and collagen (vWf:CB). Quantitative assays of the vWf, together with analysis of the structure of the protein, allow determination of the type of the disease.

Treatment

This is based on local measures and antifibrinolytics:

- Tranexamic acid (1 g tds) is used as an adjunct to other treatments. It can be administered as a mouthwash for oral or dental bleeding (IV preparation diluted in water or orange juice).
- Desmopressin (0.3 mcg/kg IV, subcutaneously or intranasally) will raise the vWf in type 1 disease by release from the endothelial stores. It may be given 1–2 hours before any operative procedure, repeated 8–12 hours later, and then again daily for 2–3 days, if necessary. Tachyphylaxis can occur. Intravenous infusion may cause hypo- or hypertension and headache, which resolve on slowing the infusion. Hyponatraemia can result from water retention, and water consumption should be restricted for 24 hours. Occasionally, it has been associated with thrombosis.

  Tranexamic acid is often given, along with desmopressin, to inhibit fibrinolysis.

  Desmopressin has no activity in type 2 or type 3 disease and may cause thrombocytopenia in type 2B disease.

- von Willebrand factor concentrates are available for patients with very low vWf levels.

Pregnancy

vWf levels rise 2–3-fold in pregnancy, and women with type 1 disease seldom need treatment antenatally or during labour. However, vWf may fall quickly in the post-natal period when treatment with desmopressin may be required intermittently for a few weeks after childbirth if bleeding is problematic. It may be given intranasally (300 mcg dose for patients >50 kg, 150 mcg dose for patients <50 kg). For women with low levels of vWf during pregnancy, and especially during labour, then IV desmopressin or vWf concentrates are used.

Less common inherited coagulation disorders

Inherited disorders of all the coagulation factors are described and present with variable bleeding manifestations. They are rare and are generally inherited in a recessive autosomal fashion. The effect of the specific deficiency on the screening tests can be predicted from the coagulation cascade.

Deficiencies of FXII (which is not associated with bleeding) and FXI can be detected by a prolonged APTT.

FVII deficiency presents with an isolated prolonged PT.

The rare deficiencies of FX, FV, and prothrombin result in prolongation of APTT and PT.

Hypofibrinogenaemia or dysfibrinogenaemia is associated with prolongation of the APTT, PT, and the thrombin time. Usually, these prolonged coagulation screening tests will correct with the addition of normal plasma (50:50 mix), differentiating them from the presence of inhibitors.

Inherited vascular disorders

Vascular disorders can be inherited or acquired and result in bleeding from small vessels, often the skin and mucous membranes. Standard coagulation screening tests and platelet function tests are normal.

Hereditary haemorrhagic telangiectasia (Osler–Weber–Rendu syndrome)—autosomal dominant inheritance
This disease presents with telangiectasia, developing from childhood onwards in the skin, mucous membranes, and internal organs. Arteriovenous malformations occasionally form in the lungs and brain, whilst gastrointestinal haemorrhage and recurrent epistaxes are common. Iron deficiency anaemia is common. Treatments include laser therapy, embolization, tranexamic acid, oestrogens, and supplementary iron.

Connective tissue disorders
Rare inherited metabolic disorders of connective tissue present with extreme joint laxity, skin stretching, and defective platelet aggregation with resultant purpura and ecchymoses. They include Ehlers–Danlos syndrome, pseudoxanthoma elasticum, osteogenesis imperfecta (also presents with multiple bone fractures), and Marfan's syndrome (tall stature, lens dislocation, and a predisposition to aortic aneurysm).

Inherited disorders of platelet function
These rare autosomal recessive disorders comprise defects in platelet adhesion to von Willebrand factor (Bernard–Soulier syndrome, a disorder of the GP1b-IX-V complex), defective platelet aggregation (Glanzmann's thrombocythaemia, a disorder of the GPIIb-IIIa complex), and disorders of platelet secretion and signal transduction (e.g. storage pool diseases). They present with mucocutaneous bleeding and excessive haemorrhage, following surgery or trauma.

Inherited thrombocytopenias
These are rare but can occur due to the inheritance of mutations in the non-muscle myosin heavy chain gene (*MYH-9* gene). Examples include May–Hegglin anomaly, Epstein syndrome, and Fechtner syndrome.

Acquired bleeding disorders
Acquired vascular disorders
- Henoch–Schönlein purpura—usually an IgA-mediated vasculitis, seen most commonly in children after upper respiratory tract infections. It presents with purpura on the buttocks and extensor surfaces (legs and elbows), and occasionally abdominal pain and haematuria. Renal failure may occur but it is usually self-limiting. For further information, see Chapter 11.
- Infections—vascular damage or immune complex formation may cause purpura as a complication of a wide range of bacterial, viral, and rickettsial infections (measles, dengue fever, meningococcal infections).
- Senile ('actinic' or 'atrophic') purpura—a manifestation of age-related atrophy of the supporting tissues of cutaneous blood vessels.
- Scurvy—results from poor collagen formation from vitamin C deficiency, with perifollicular haemorrhage and mucocutaneous bleeding.
- Steroid therapy—long-term steroid therapy (or uncontrolled Cushing's syndrome) results in defective vascular supporting tissue due to reduced collagen synthesis.
- Amyloid—inherited or an acquired disorder, e.g. a manifestation of an underlying plasma cell dyscrasia. Purpura are common, mostly due to increased capillary fragility, as the abnormal protein is deposited between the endothelium and basement membrane. The purpura are often around the periorbital or pressure areas.

- Simple easy bruising—occurs commonly in women of childbearing age. It is not a pathological entity.

Acquired platelet function disorders
- Antiplatelet drugs—aspirin inhibits thromboxane A2 production, resulting in defective aggregation to ADP and adrenaline, whilst clopidogrel inhibits the binding of ADP to its platelet receptor. In both cases, the platelet is affected for its lifespan of 8–10 days. The anti-GPIIb/IIIa receptor antibodies abciximab, eptifibatide, and tirofiban are used in patients undergoing percutaneous coronary intervention, usually in combination with heparin and/or aspirin. Normalizing of platelet function occurs within 12–48 hours of infusion. If untoward bleeding occurs, this can be partially corrected by platelet transfusions, which may also be required if severe thrombocytopenia complicates the use of these platelet receptor inhibitors.
- Uraemia—impairment of renal function per se does not affect platelet numbers but inhibits platelet function and platelet-vessel wall interactions. Anaemia of renal failure also contributes to the bleeding tendency, which is usually mucocutaneous. Treatment includes correction of the anaemia with red cell transfusions or erythropoietin, dialysis, DDAVP, cryoprecipitate infusions, conjugated oestrogens, and platelet transfusions.
- Acute leukaemias, myelodysplastic and myeloproliferative diseases, dysproteinaemias (myeloma, macroglobulinaemia)—in addition to thrombocytopenia, these disorders may adversely affect platelet function through a variety of mechanisms. Treatment is directed at the underlying disorder, although platelet transfusions may be needed in the short term.

Acquired thrombocytopenia
Thrombocytopenia occurs due to failure of bone marrow production, increased consumption or destruction of platelets in the circulation, or increased splenic pooling (see Table 12.6).

Idiopathic thrombocytopenic purpura (ITP)
ITP (also known as autoimmune thrombocytopenia) results from the immune destruction of the patient's platelets by the macrophages of the reticuloendothelial system, predominantly in the spleen. The production of the antiplatelet antibody is often idiopathic but may be a secondary event in other diseases (SLE, HIV, EBV, lymphomas, and CLL.). Immune destruction of platelets is also recognized as a side effect of a number of drugs (see Table 12.7).

In adults, ITP is usually chronic, whilst in children, the disease is usually self-limiting and frequently precipitated by a viral infection or vaccination. Chronic ITP may present with isolated thrombocytopenia, with platelet counts as low as $5-10 \times 10^9/L$, but an otherwise normal blood count. The blood film may show giant platelets and have features of any associated disease (e.g. atypical lymphocytes in infectious mononucleosis) but is often otherwise unremarkable. Bleeding manifestations are very variable, as platelet turnover in ITP is substantially increased and the circulating platelets are highly metabolically active. In part, depending on the degree of thrombocytopenia, the patient may present with widespread bruising, purpura (often more severe on the legs), epistaxis, and mucous membrane bleeding. Intracranial bleeding is a rare, but dangerous complication. Alternatively, there may be few, or no, bleeding manifestations, and the thrombocytopenia is an incidental finding.

Table 12.6 Causes of thrombocytopenia

Reduced production	Congenital	Thrombocytopenia-absent radii (TAR) syndrome Fanconi anaemia Wiskott–Aldrich syndrome
	Acquired	Aplastic anaemia Myelofibrosis Leukaemia and lymphoma Myelodysplasia Marrow infiltration (metastatic malignancy) Myeloma Megaloblastic anaemia HIV infection Myelosuppressive drugs Ionizing radiation Paroxysmal nocturnal haemoglobinuria (PNH)
Increased destruction	Immune	Idiopathic thrombocytopenia purpura (ITP) Drugs Post-transfusion purpura (PTP) Autoimmune diseases (SLE, Evans' syndrome, Graves's disease) Viral infections (HIV, hepatitis C, EBV) Heparin-induced thrombocytopenia (HIT) Neonatal alloimmune thrombocytopenia (NAIT) Neonatal autoimmune thrombocytopenia (ITP)
	Non-immune	Sepsis Thrombotic thrombocytopenic purpura (TTP) Haemolytic uraemic syndrome (HUS) Haemolysis, elevated liver enzymes, low platelets (HELLP)/eclampsia Disseminated intravascular coagulation (DIC) Burns Aortic valve dysfunction (natural or replacement) Fat embolism Type IIB von Willebrand's disease Snakebites Giant cavernous haemangioma (Kasabach–Merritt syndrome)
Increased sequestration	Splenomegaly	Various

Diagnosis of ITP is based on history and examination, the blood count and film, the finding of a normal coagulation screen, and occasionally a bone marrow examination if there are atypical features or if the patient is older than 60 years old (to exclude myelodysplasia). There is no reliable specific test for ITP and hence is a diagnosis of exclusion of the other causes of thrombocytopenia.

Management of this disorder is primarily directed to controlling the bleeding manifestations, if present, rather than raising the platelet count for its own sake. Treatment should take into account the chronicity of the disorder, recognizing that control is more often achieved than cure. The toxicity of long-term treatment (especially steroids) can be substantial, especially if given solely to control the platelet count, irrespective of bleeding.

Table 12.7 Drugs implicated in thrombocytopenia

Reduced production	Dose-related marrow suppression	Cytotoxic drugs Ethanol Others—chloramphenicol, co-trimoxazole
	Idiosyncratic marrow suppression	Chloramphenicol Co-trimoxazole Penicillamine
Increased destruction	Immune	Analgesics Antimicrobials—penicillin, sulfonamides Anticonvulsants—sodium valproate, carbamazepine, diazepam Diuretics—thiazides, furosemide, acetazolamide Oral hypoglycaemics—chlorpropamide, tolbutamide Others—heparin, methyldopa, quinine, quinidine
Platelet aggregation		Heparin

As a guide, acceptable platelet counts in ITP are:
- Dentistry—10×10^9/L.
- Dental extractions—30×10^9/L.
- Regional dental block—30×10^9/L.
- Minor surgery—50×10^9/L.
- Major surgery—80×10^9/L.
- Epidural anaesthesia—80×10^9/L.

The main treatment options are:
- Steroids—prednisolone 1 mg/kg for 2–3 weeks, or pulsed dexamethasone 20–40 mg daily for 4 days. Steroids raise the platelet count in about 75% of cases.
- Intravenous immunoglobulin (IVIG)—0.4 g/kg/day for 5 days or 1 g/kg for 2 days. Approximately 80% of patients respond to IVIG, but the response is often short-lived (3 weeks).
- Intravenous anti-D—may be used in rhesus D-positive patients with a functioning spleen. The response rate is about 80% and can last for 3 months. It frequently causes a fall in the haemoglobin of ~1 g/dL due to haemolysis and should be used with caution in patients who have a positive direct antiglobulin test.
- Rituximab—this anti-CD20 antibody, licensed for the treatment of non-Hodgkin's lymphomas and CLL, has proved successful in refractory ITP. It may result in reactivation of hepatitis B, so testing for the presence of hepatitis B should be done prior to use.
- Splenectomy—the spleen is usually the chief site of platelet destruction in ITP, and splenectomy will result in a sustained rise in the platelet count in 80% of patients. Splenic scanning with radiolabelled platelets can predict the likely outcome of splenectomy in advance of the operation. Preoperative vaccination with Pneumovax®, Hib (*Haemophilus influenzae* type b), and Meningovax® is essential, as is postoperative prophylactic use of phenoxymethylpenicillin (erythromycin if penicillin-allergic).
- Immunosuppression can be achieved with a variety of steroid-sparing agents in those refractory cases not responding to acceptable doses of steroids. Drugs include azathioprine, mycophenolate mofetil, cyclophosphamide, ciclosporin, and vincristine.
- Eltrombopag and AMG 531—these recently developed agents stimulate platelet production and have been shown to have activity in relapsed or refractory ITP.

Post-transfusion purpura
Thrombocytopenia occurring 7–10 days following a blood transfusion, is thought to result from the development of antibodies directed at the donor's platelet antigens (usually HPA-1a antigen). It is more common in women, who may have become immunized to the platelet antigen in previous pregnancies. Treatment is with steroids and IV immunoglobulin.

Heparin-induced thrombocytopenia (HIT)
Usually occurs 5–10 days after starting heparin treatment and is more common with unfractionated heparin than low molecular weight heparins. For further details, see section on heparin in Anticoagulation.

Thrombotic thrombocytopenic purpura (TTP) and haemolytic uraemic syndrome (HUS)
Both disorders result when platelet aggregation occurs *in vivo*, resulting in widespread platelet thrombosis and embolization within the microvasculature. The red cells undergo shearing and fragmentation as they pass through these thrombi.

The cause of TTP and HUS is the presence of ultralarge von Willebrand factor multimers (ULVWF), which stimulate platelet aggregation via GP1a receptors. In health, these multimers are normally broken down by a metalloprotease (ADAMTS13). This becomes depleted in TTP and HUS due to inherited or acquired factors. Reduced production may be due to genetic mutations in the familial forms, or in acquired forms, due to the production of IgG autoantibodies secondary to infections (e.g. HIV, *E. coli* infections), some drugs (clopidogrel, ticlopidine, ciclosporin, mitomycin C), autoimmune or connective tissue disorders, and pregnancy.

The classical five presenting features are:
- Thrombocytopenia.
- Microangiopathic haemolytic anaemia with red cell fragmentation.
- Neurological complications (especially in TTP).
- Renal failure (more so in HUS).
- Fever.

Not all five features may be present in one case, especially in the early stages of the disease. In addition to the anaemia and thrombocytopenia, laboratory investigations show red cell fragments on the blood film, a normal coagulation screen, raised unconjugated bilirubin and reticulocytosis (features of haemolysis), biochemical markers of renal failure, and a raised LDH. LDH and platelet count can be used to monitor disease progress.

Immediate treatment is with plasma replacement, most commonly plasma exchange with FFP, and high-dose steroids. Longer-term control may be gained with the use of immunosuppressive agents (steroids, vincristine, azathioprine, cyclophosphamide, IV immunoglobulins, and rituximab).

Acquired inhibitors of coagulation
The development of autoantibodies directed against coagulation factors can occur spontaneously or with other conditions.

The lupus anticoagulant
This inhibitor is directed against phospholipid-dependent coagulation reactions and classically occurs in SLE. However, it may be present in other autoimmune diseases or develop spontaneously. It may prolong the APTT, which does not adequately correct with the addition of normal plasma (50:50 mix). Specific and sensitive tests are available, e.g. dilute Russell's viper venom time—DRVVT. It is frequently found in association with anti-cardiolipin antibodies, also directed against lipid antigens. Despite its name and the *in vitro* effect of prolonging the APTT, it is not associated with bleeding but is an acquired risk factor for venous and arterial thrombosis and recurrent miscarriage.

Autoantibodies directed against specific coagulation factors
This rarely but can be associated with severe bleeding disorders. Acquired haemophilia is due to autoantibodies to FVIII and occurs in both sexes. It can occur post-partum, in association with autoimmune disease (e.g. rheumatoid arthritis), and in cancer. Most commonly, there is no identifiable underlying cause, other than old age. The APTT is prolonged and is not corrected in a 50:50 mix with normal plasma. Immediate treatment is with high doses of FVIII concentrate or with recombinant FVIIa or activated prothrombin complex concentrate. Immunosuppressive regimens are usually required.

Autoantibodies to von Willebrand factor are found in many diseases, most commonly lymphoproliferative and myeloproliferative disease, as well as autoimmune diseases. Acquired von Willebrand's disease is recognized in hypothyroidism and may resolve with appropriate thyroid replacement therapy.

Autoantibodies have been described to virtually all the other specific coagulation factors but are rare.

Liver disease

In liver disease, coagulation can be severely affected due to:
- Reduced absorption of fat-soluble vitamin K in biliary obstruction, with reduced synthesis of factors II, VII, IX, and X (vitamin K-dependent).
- Reduced synthesis of clotting factors (II, VII, IX, X, V, and fibrinogen).
- Synthesis of structurally abnormal fibrinogen (dysfibrinogenaemia), with reduced function.
- Reduced synthesis of the anticoagulants antithrombin and protein C.
- Impaired clearing of activated clotting products from the circulation.
- Hypersplenism from portal hypertension, with reduction in the circulating platelet count.

Laboratory tests of coagulation in liver failure typically show varying degrees of prolongation of the prothrombin time (the most sensitive test), the APTT, and the thrombin time, with correction on the addition of normal plasma (50:50 mix). D-dimers and fibrin degradation products, normally cleared by the liver, may be raised. The platelet count is often reduced. The degree of hypersplenism correlates poorly with the physical size of the spleen. The bleeding tendency in liver disease may be exacerbated by acquired functional disorders of platelets and reduced thrombopoietin levels.

Treatment of the coagulopathy of liver disease is based on the replacement of clotting products, predominantly with FFP and cryoprecipitate if fibrinogen is low. Platelet transfusions may be required to temporarily raise the platelet count. These strategies have only temporary effects on the haemostasis and should be reserved for acute bleeding or prior to interventional procedures. There is a poor correlation between the bleeding risk of liver biopsy and the prolongation of the laboratory coagulation tests. The traditional practice of infusing FFP prior to a liver biopsy if the PT is 3 seconds above normal has little proven evidence base. If the risk is significant, then a transjugular biopsy of the liver should be performed. Post-biopsy bleeding is more common in cirrhotic livers; however, the most reliable indicator of biopsy-related bleeding is the presence of hepatic malignancy.

Vitamin K deficiency

Vitamin K is stored in the liver and is essential for the hepatic synthesis of coagulation factors II, VII, IX, and X, as well as the anticoagulants protein C and protein S. Deficiency of this vitamin occurs due to:
- Diet—deficiency of vitamin K is rare in healthy adults but can occur in intensive care.
- Malabsorption—vitamin K is absorbed in the ileum and requires the formation of mixed micelles of bile salts and broken down fats from the action of pancreatic lipases. Poor absorption occurs in biliary obstruction and pancreatic insufficiency.
- Haemorrhagic disease of the newborn—neonates are born with low levels of vitamin K and the associated

dependent clotting factors. This deficiency can be exacerbated by breastfeeding, the immaturity of the liver, and reduced bacterial synthesis of the vitamin in the gut. Haemorrhage can occur within the first week of life and, occasionally, during the first 2 months. Vitamin K is now given at birth.
- Warfarin and other vitamin K antagonists—interfere with the reduction of vitamin K epoxide, required in the gamma carboxylation pathway of the vitamin K-dependent clotting factors. Without gamma carboxylation, these clotting factors cannot bind calcium ions on phospholipid membranes, an essential component of the coagulation cascade. A state of acquired vitamin K deficiency is, therefore, induced.

Laboratory tests in vitamin K deficiency show prolongation of the PT and APTT that correct with the addition of normal plasma. Thrombin time and fibrinogen assays are normal.

Treatment of vitamin K deficiency
- Prophylaxis—neonates receive prophylactic vitamin K.
- Treatment of deficiency—can be oral (usually 5 mg daily) or parenteral (10 mg IV, given slowly).
- Reversal of warfarin overdose—small doses (0.5–2 mg) are usually sufficient to reverse an excessively high INR and may be given IV or orally (the IV route is more rapid). In the case of life-threatening bleeding, factor concentrate should be given and a higher dose of vitamin K (5–10 mg). This may result in resistance to the effect of warfarin for up to 3 weeks.

Further reading

Afdhal N, McHutchison J, Brown R, et al. (2008). Thrombocytopenia associated with chronic liver disease. Journal of Hepatology, 48, 1000–7.

Allford S, Hunt BJ, Rose P, Machin SJ, on behalf of the Haemostasis and Thrombosis Task Force of the British Committee for Standards in Haematology (2003). Guidelines on the diagnosis and management of the thrombotic microangiopathic haemolytic anaemias. British Journal of Haematology, 120, 556–73.

Baglin TP, Keeling DM, Watson HG for the British Committee for Standards in Haematology (2005). Guidelines on oral anticoagulation (warfarin): third edition—2005 update. British Journal of Haematology, 132, 277–85.

Chee YL, Crawford JC, Watson HG, Greaves M (2008). Guidelines on the assessment of bleeding risk prior to surgery or invasive procedures. Guideline for the British Committee for Standards in Haematology. British Journal of Haematology, 140, 496–504.

Davies JM, Lewis MPN, Wimperis J, et al, on behalf of the British Committee for Standards in Haematology (2011). Review of guidelines for the prevention and treatment of infection in patients with an absent or dysfunctional spleen. British Journal of Haematology, 155, 308–317.

Goulis J, Chau TN, Jordan S, et al. (1999). Thrombopoietin concentrations are low in patients with cirrhosis and thrombocytopenia and are restored after orthotopic liver transplantation. Gut, 44, 754–8.

Keeling D, Tait C, Makris M (2008). Guideline on the selection and use of therapeutic products to treat haemophilia and other hereditary bleeding disorders. A United Kingdom Haemophilia Center Doctors' Organization (UKHCDO) Guideline—approved by the British Committee for Standards in Haematology. Haemophilia, 14, 671–84.

Provan D, Newland A, Bolton-Maggs P, et al. (2003). Guidelines for the investigation and management of idiopathic thrombocytopenic purpura in adults, children and in pregnancy. British Journal of Haematology, 120, 574–96.

Transfusion and management of bleeding

The *Handbook of Transfusion Medicine United Kingdom Blood Services* 5th Edition (2013) is a comprehensive text on the practical aspects of blood transfusion medicine. Much of the guidance in this section is drawn from this reference, and the reader is also referred to <http://www.transfusionguidelines.org.uk/>.

Blood is an expensive resource and carries risks associated with transfusion. There is now widespread recognition of the need to minimize its use where possible. Strategies to conserve blood include:

- Correction of haematinic deficiencies contributing to anaemia.
- Stopping drugs that interfere with blood coagulation (e.g. aspirin, warfarin).
- Use of erythropoietin in appropriate cases to raise the patient's haemoglobin concentration.
- Minimize intraoperative blood loss:
  - With appropriate surgical techniques.
  - Intraoperative cell salvage.
- Use of drugs to promote haemostasis (e.g. fibrin sealants, tranexamic acid).
- Implementation of maximum blood ordering schedules (MSBOS).
- Implement critical use of blood transfusion triggers.

Blood transfusion threshold triggers

The decision to transfuse blood should not be taken solely on the basis of an arbitrary haemoglobin value but should take account of the wider circumstances of the patient. Such factors include:

- The haemoglobin value.
- The severity of symptoms and signs relating to anaemia.
- Age.
- Comorbidity, including:
  - Likelihood of bleeding (type of surgery, haemostatic results).
  - Ischaemic heart disease/cardiomyopathy/heart failure.
  - Chronic lung disease.
  - Pre-existing bone marrow failure.
  - High tissue oxygen demand (sepsis, pyrexia, inflammation).

In the surgical or critically ill patient who is not actively bleeding (and in whom the replacement of blood volume is not an issue), the following thresholds for transfusion have been found to be helpful:

- No cardiovascular disease and younger patients—maintain haemoglobin between 7 and 9 g/dL.
- Known cardiovascular disease—maintain haemoglobin between 9 and 10 g/dL.

Anaemias due to chronic medical conditions require a different approach with consideration of:

- The severity of bone marrow failure.
- Contributing correctable factors (e.g. iron deficiency due to chronic bleeding, B12 or folate deficiency, coagulopathies, haemolysis).
- Other potential strategies to correct the anaemia (e.g. use of erythropoietin, haematinic replacement).

No single haemoglobin value can be advised as a transfusion trigger in medical patients with chronic anaemia, as individual tolerance to degrees of anaemia varies considerably. As a general rule, it is reasonable to transfuse chronically anaemic normovolaemic patients up to a haemoglobin value of 8 g/dL if symptomatic, unless they have significant ischaemic heart disease, in which case a value of 9–10 g/dL is recommended.

Management of bleeding in the surgical patient

Why do surgical patients bleed?

Surgical technique and changes in the haemostatic mechanisms play a part in the propensity for bleeding in surgical patients. Good surgical technique is clearly vital in this regard, as, without it, the likelihood of bleeding from an undisclosed damaged vessel is high. This, in turn, may result in an increased need for transfusion and changes in the haemostatic mechanism, which exacerbate the bleeding.

Identification of patients preoperatively at risk of bleeding

Consideration should be given to the following:

- **The history.** A previous personal or family history of excessive bleeding may point to an underlying familial haemorrhagic disorder, of which von Willebrand's disease is the most common (autosomal dominant). Its incidence may be as high as 1:100 to 1:1,000. Specific questions should be asked about bleeding following previous surgery (including dental surgery), menstrual bleeding, and family history. The history is especially important, as standard coagulation screening tests (PT, APTT, and thrombin time) will not pick up some mild abnormalities of coagulation or reliably detect certain specific inherited coagulation disorders, including von Willebrand's disease and some platelet disorders.

- **The type of surgery planned**. The more extensive the surgery, the greater the risk of bleeding. In addition, certain tissues are rich sources of activators of plasminogen (prostate, meninges, brain), the release of which can lead to fibrinolytic activation and excessive bleeding. A history of previous similar surgery may also be a predictor of bleeding (e.g. repeat total hip operation).

- **The use of antithrombotic drugs:**
  - **Aspirin**. The antiplatelet action of cyclo-oxygenase inhibition is prolonged, and patients on aspirin should ideally cease taking it about 10 days prior to surgery to allow for the production of new platelets. This is especially so where perioperative bleeding might prove catastrophic (e.g. during neurosurgery). However, low-dose aspirin (75 mg daily) should not be stopped before operations with a high risk of vascular complications and where the risk of uncontrolled bleeding is minimal (e.g. coronary artery surgery). It need not be stopped prior to cataract surgery.
  - **Clopidogrel**. This antiplatelet drug is frequently used, in combination with aspirin, as prophylaxis against thrombosis following coronary artery stenting and in acute coronary syndromes. Elective surgery should ideally be postponed until the minimal recommended period of clopidogrel therapy has elapsed (5–7 days). If this is not possible, then the balance between the risks of coronary artery thrombosis versus perioperative bleeding needs to be considered, often in consultation with a cardiologist. It may be considered

permissible to keep the patient on low-dose aspirin during the perioperative period.

Warfarin (and other coumarin oral anticoagulants)

The management of patients established on warfarin who are to undergo elective procedures is based on the appreciation of thrombotic risk if not anticoagulated, in comparison to the haemorrhagic risk of the operation exacerbated by anticoagulation.

Low thrombotic risk patients

This category includes most patients taking warfarin and includes those in atrial fibrillation on warfarin for prophylaxis against cerebral embolism. These patients do not require any additional thromboprophylaxis to that recommended for the type of surgery or interventional procedure being undertaken. They can stop their warfarin 4 days prior to the date of the operation, by which time the INR should be less than 1.5. The use of prophylactic doses of low molecular weight heparin during the perioperative period should be governed by the thrombotic risk of the surgery being undertaken.

High thrombotic risk patients

These include patients on long-term warfarin for a strong personal history of recurrent thrombosis and those with prosthetic heart valves. These patients require thromboprophylaxis during the surgical period. The options are to use full-dose intravenous unfractionated heparin to achieve an APTT of between 1.5 and 2.5 or low molecular weight heparin (LMWH) by subcutaneous injection at doses determined by the thrombotic risk to the patients. Intravenous heparin is inconvenient, but, as its half-life is short (in the order of 1 hour), its dose can be titrated against the APTT at frequent intervals. It can be rapidly reversed, should the need arise, with protamine, although ceasing the infusion is often sufficient. It is the method of choice in managing patients with high-risk artificial heart valves but must be monitored meticulously, especially in the immediate postoperative setting when the APTT may not be as sensitive to its effects, partly due to raised levels of FVIII:C. In this postoperative setting, use of the anti-Xa assay may more accurately reflect the heparin levels. Subcutaneous LMWH has the advantage of being easy to administer and the patient can be taught to self-administer at home the day after stopping the warfarin prior to admission. The anti-Xa assay is the method of choice for monitoring LMWH. LMWH is more difficult to reverse than unfractionated heparin, being less affected by protamine and having a longer systemic half-life. However, its convenience has led to its use in most high thrombotic risk patients, other than those with high-risk artificial heart valves.

Transfusion of red cells in the surgical patient

Transfusing red cells to achieve a haemoglobin (Hb) concentration of 10 g/dL, irrespective of circumstances, is no longer appropriate. Current evidence suggests that, in critically ill patients, a Hb of 7 g/dL is as effective, and possibly more so, than a Hb of 10 g/dL, except for patients with cardiorespiratory disease. The transfusion trigger should be tailored to the individual patient needs.

Transfusion in acute blood loss

This section covers the management of patients who are actively bleeding to the extent that they are at risk of becoming significantly hypovolaemic. It applies equally to the management of surgical and medical patients (especially those with gastrointestinal haemorrhage), as well as trauma patients.

The objective is to prevent tissue hypoxia by maintaining adequate red cell volume. Treatment and prevention of shock is important, as, once shock has become established, then complications increase, either directly as a result of the persistent hypotension or due to the complications of massive blood transfusion. Massive transfusion is arbitrarily defined as the replacement of the whole blood volume in less than 24 hours (the blood volume is 7% of ideal body weight in an adult) or 50% of blood volume in 3 hours. Complications from large-volume transfusion include:

1. **Dilutional coagulopathy**. Coagulation factors fall at variable rates with blood volume replacement, dependent on their distribution between intravascular and extravascular space and on the body's ability to replace the falling levels. In general:
   - Fibrinogen level will fall <1 g/dL after a 12 unit transfusion (1.5 x blood volume).
   - Prothrombin time ratio (test result/control) will increase to >1.5 when coagulation factors have fallen to 50% of normal after 8–12 units of red cells transfused (1–1.5 x blood volume) and reach >1.8 when twice the blood volume has been replaced.
   - Platelet count halves with every replacement of the blood volume and will fall to $50-100 \times 10^9/L$ after a two-volume transfusion (15 units), or less if the starting platelet count was lower.

2. **Disseminated intravascular coagulation**. Arises when there is activation of the coagulation system with consumption of clotting proteins and platelets, leading to widespread microvascular bleeding, with or without thrombosis (see 'Factors contributing to coagulation failure and DIC' earlier in this chapter). It occurs, most commonly, in sepsis, obstetrics, and in trauma cases. The trigger for activation of the coagulation system is tissue damage. This may be due to direct trauma or secondary to systemic hypotension, hypothermia, sepsis, or obstetric complications, with the release of large amounts of tissue thromboplastin. Venomous snakes (particularly vipers, including rattlesnakes) can be a common cause of DIC.

3. **Acid-base disturbances**. Lactic acidosis, and consequent metabolic acidosis resulting from poor tissue perfusion, combined with oliguria from shock, can exacerbate bleeding.

4. **Hypocalcaemia.** If large volumes of citrated anticoagulated blood are transfused, as in multiple transfusions of red cells or plasma, this may cause hypocalcaemia. This can reduce myocardial contractility and promote vasodilatation, thus exacerbating shock and microvascular bleeding. To counteract this, IV calcium chloride (10 mL of 10% given slowly +/- ECG monitoring as there is a risk of arrhythmias with rapid IV administration) can be given in large-volume transfusions, repeating the calcium assay immediately afterwards (on a blood gas analyser, if necessary).

5. **Hyperkalaemia**. This can complicate massive blood transfusion, due to the high extracellular potassium content of stored red cells, and is aggravated by the acidosis and renal impairment associated with shock. Hyperkalaemia should be treated in standard fashion with insulin and glucose and, if necessary, renal support.

6. **Hypothermia**. As red cells are stored at 4–6°C and if large volumes are transfused, then this can contribute directly to hypothermia, which can reduce oxygen delivery to the tissues.

Management of massive transfusion

The management of massive transfusion requires a coordinated approach between the clinicians, the hospital laboratories, blood bank, and the regional transfusion centre. Good communication is essential, as blood products may need to be ordered in advance of their immediate need, and time is usually required for their delivery from the transfusion centre. Special requirements may need to be considered, e.g. irradiated or CMV-negative blood, although, in life-threatening bleeding, it may not be possible to accommodate these requirements. All hospitals should have a massive transfusion protocol that involves all the parties and is practised regularly. After a massive transfusion incident, feedback and analysis of how it was conducted is valuable in refining the hospital protocol.

Communication

Communication between the surgical theatres and blood bank is essential. A single individual should be delegated to be the communication coordinator and liaise early with blood bank, so blood stocks can be checked, work prioritized, and staff deployed effectively. ITU should be informed, and senior surgical and anaesthetic staff should attend to ensure maximum chances of arresting surgical bleeding as quickly as possible.

The consultant haematologist should provide advice on the use of blood product components and communicate between the clinical team and the regional transfusion centre, as necessary.

Investigations

Samples for the following should be sent to the laboratory urgently:

- Full blood count.
- Coagulation screen.
- Cross-match sample.
- Biochemistry sample.

Repeated sampling at regular intervals is necessary during the course of the massive transfusion as is the need for blood component therapy. There is an inevitable delay between the blood sampling and test results being available. This has led to the use of near patient testing in some hospitals, particularly thromboelastography (TEG), a technique that examines whole blood clotting and subsequent clot lysis. TEG requires experienced analysis and regular use to maintain skills to ensure consistent results. Its use is not yet widespread in the UK.

Accurate patient identification—this is essential. All patients receiving a blood transfusion must wear an identification wristband with the unique hospital number (possibly to be replaced by their NHS number in the future). The hospital must have a tried and tested method of identifying unconscious patients, as it is crucial to avoid misidentification between multiple patients.

Blood component therapy in massive transfusion

There is a paucity of randomized controlled trials to support the recommendations for blood component therapy in massive blood transfusion, as there are practical difficulties in conducting trials in this area. The following recommendations comply with the British Committee on Standards in Haematology guidelines on the management of massive blood loss.

Red cells

Red cells provide oxygen-carrying capacity to the tissue, enhance platelet margination and function, and contribute to the maintenance of haemostasis. Transfusion of red cells needs to take into account multiple factors—blood volume indicators (blood pressure, pulse, CVP, wedge pressure, etc.), the rate of bleeding, comorbidity (age, cardiovascular and respiratory disease), and the haemoglobin concentration. The haemoglobin and haematocrit may significantly underestimate the degree of tissue underperfusion and should not be the sole guide for red cell transfusion, although, if the Hb is less than 6 g/dL, then red cells are almost certainly indicated.

In the face of massive bleeding, the immediate aim is to restore the blood pressure. Initially, crystalloids (or occasionally colloids) are used as volume expanders. Currently there is no evidence that colloid infusions are associated with a lower mortality rate than crystalloids. If crystalloids are used, then a slightly greater volume may be needed. In the emergency situation, uncross-matched group O, rhesus D-negative ('flying squad') blood can be given, but, within 5 minutes of receiving an EDTA sample for 'group and screen', the blood bank can issue uncross-matched red cells compatible with the patient's blood group. A full cross-match takes about 40 minutes, and cross-matched red cells, or red cells released by electronic issue, should be used as soon as possible. In the event that there is a shortage of red cells which are the same ABO group as the patient, then group-compatible cells may be used (see Table 12.8).

Cryoprecipitate

A rich source of fibrinogen, FVIII:C, and von Willebrand factor that should be given if fibrinogen is less than 1 g/dL. The adult dose is two pools (equivalent to ten single donor units), which should increase fibrinogen levels by 1 g/dL.

Platelets

Can be expected to fall to $50 \times 10^9/L$ once there has been a 1.5 or 2.5 blood volume replacement. Patients undergoing massive transfusion should not have their platelet count fall below this critical level, and it should be maintained at higher levels in the event of there being multiple injuries or central nervous system (CNS) damage. In practice, a platelet transfusion trigger of $75 \times 10^9/L$ in the setting of massive transfusion is advised, with a higher value of $100 \times 10^9/L$ being recommended for patients with CNS injury.

There is often a delay in obtaining platelets, which are not routinely stored on site in hospital blood banks, as they are ordered from the regional transfusion centre. One adult dose of platelets (either apheresed from a single donor or pooled from four separate donations) can be expected to raise the patient's platelet count by $20–40 \times 10^9/L$, although this may be less in the face of ongoing haemorrhage, circulating volume replacement, or DIC. The platelets can be transfused through a standard blood administration set or a platelet giving set, with a fresh giving set for each administration of platelets.

The platelet count must be monitored closely with full blood counts (or with TEG, if available) in massive transfu-

Table 12.8 Group-compatible red cells

Patient group	1st choice	2nd choice
A	A	O
B	B	O
AB	AB	A or B
O	O	None

sion, and it may be necessary to request platelets from the blood bank pre-emptively once it is clear that the count is falling and especially if the haemorrhage is continuing.

Recombinant FVIIa

rFVIIa has been used, with increasing frequency, 'off label' in massive transfusion, although there are no randomized controlled data to define clear indications for patients with intracranial haemorrhage. It is costly, and guidelines should be drawn up locally, with the haematologist to oversee its use. The usual dose is 90 mcg/kg, repeated after 2 hours, if necessary. It is potentially thrombogenic and is relatively contraindicated in patients with a history of venous thromboembolism, myocardial infarction, cerebrovascular disease, or metastatic carcinoma.

The pre-emptive use of coagulation products in massive transfusion

Where massive transfusion is expected, e.g. in major trauma or obstetric haemorrhage, there may be a case for the early use of coagulation components (predominantly FFP and platelets), transfused as a pre-defined ratio of the number of red cell units transfused. This approach is to try to prevent a coagulopathy developing, as, once it has occurred, it can be difficult to correct. It also recognizes that monitoring of blood coagulation involves an inevitable delay between the blood sample collection and the result being available. Such an approach (e.g. the issue of one unit of FFP for every two units of red cells, and one unit of platelets for six units of red cells) should be agreed in advance, a protocol drawn up and be subject to audit. It should be recognized that its adoption does not abolish the need for repeated monitoring of the coagulation and platelets.

Further reading

Department of Health (2007). Health Service Circular. Better blood transfusion—safe and appropriate use of blood. <http://www.transfusionguidelines.org.uk/docs/pdfs/nbtc_bbt_hsc_07.pdf>.

Herbert PC, Wells G, Blackman MA, et al. (1999). A multicentre, randomised controlled clinical trial of transfusion requirements in critical care. New England Journal of Medicine, **340**, 409–17.

National Blood Transfusion Committee (2014). Patient Blood Management. <http://www.transfusionguidelines.org.uk/uk-transfusion-committees/national-blood-transfusion-committee/patient-blood-management>.

National Patient Safety Agency (2006). Safer practice notice 14. Right patient, right blood, pp 2–6. <http://www.npsa.nhs.uk/nrls/alerts-and-directives/notices/blood-transfusions/>.

Perel P and Roberts IG (2007). Colloids versus crystalloids for fluid resuscitation in critically ill patients. Cochrane Database of Systematic Reviews, **4**, CD000567.

Stainsby D, MacLennan S, Thomas D, et al., on behalf of British Committee for Standards in Haematology (2006). Guidelines on the management of massive blood loss (BJH Guideline). British Journal of Haematology, **135**, 634–41.

Immunocompromised patients, including HIV-positive patients

HIV and other causes of immunodeficiency

HIV infection

There are approximately 35 million people infected with HIV around the world. Despite the increasing and wider coverage of highly active combination antiretroviral therapies (cART), infections secondary to HIV-associated immune suppression accounted for most of the 2 million deaths associated with HIV in 2008. Opportunistic infections occur with pathogens that would not normally cause disease in the immune-competent host. In the developed world, opportunistic infections still account for up to a quarter of all deaths in HIV-infected adults, since many patients remain unaware of their diagnosis and present with an opportunistic infection as the initial indicator of their HIV.

In the UK, there are approximately 87,000 people living with HIV, of whom approximately 25,000 are unaware of their diagnosis. A national audit of death amongst HIV-infected patients in 2005 identified infections as a cause of mortality in almost 25% and that, in a quarter of these patients, the diagnosis was too late to prevent mortality. A small minority of patients succumb to serious infections because of persisting immune deficiency as a result of non-adherence to cART or as a result of multiple cART-resistant HIV.

HIV testing

Testing for HIV can be carried out by any trained healthcare worker who can competently obtain voluntary informed consent from the patient. There is no need for HIV testing to be the domain of specialist nurses, health advisors, or doctors.

Where possible, laboratories should offer fourth-generation HIV tests (combination of antigen and antibody testing) which reduces the 'window' period between infection to a positive test to 4 weeks. Positive tests should be confirmed by further testing, as per local/national laboratory guidelines. HIV RNA quantitative (HIV viral load) tests should not be used for the diagnosis of HIV infection.

Point of care testing for HIV is increasingly used for rapid turnaround results, with either finger-prick blood or mouth swabs. These tests are particularly useful where testing is carried out in community settings or where rapid results are imperative in clinical decision-making (e.g. testing a source patient to make a decision regarding post-exposure prophylaxis). It should be noted that these tests have slightly reduced sensitivities and specificities, compared to fourth-generation antigen/antibody tests.

An urgent referral to the local HIV specialist service should be offered to all patients testing HIV-positive. Arrangements should be in place to provide appropriate counselling for post-test risk reduction strategies. This can be arranged by onward referral to the local sexual health service or voluntary sector organizations.

Patients testing HIV-negative in the 'window' period, in other words, within 12 weeks of a risk activity, should be offered follow-up repeat testing.

Who to test

In the UK, 'opt out' HIV testing has been successfully implemented in the antenatal setting and has had a major impact on reducing mother-to-child HIV transmission.

The UK HIV testing guidelines (2008) recommend the following HIV testing strategies.

Universal HIV testing in the following settings

- GUM or sexual health clinics.
- Antenatal services.
- Termination of pregnancy services.
- Drug dependency programmes.
- Healthcare services for those diagnosed with TB, HBV, HCV, and lymphoma.

Where local prevalence exceeds >2 in 1,000 population

- All patients registering at a general practice.
- All general medical admissions to hospital.

HIV testing should be routinely offered to the following

- All patients where HIV enters the differential diagnosis of disease.
- All patients with a diagnosed STD.
- All sexual partners of HIV-infected patients.
- All men who have sex with men.
- All female partners of men who have sex with men.
- All patients reporting a history of IV drug use.
- All patients from a high HIV-prevalent country (>1%).
- All patients who report sexual contact with individuals from a country with a high HIV prevalence (>1%).

Clinical indicator diseases where HIV testing should be considered

- **Respiratory**—bacterial pneumonia, aspergillosis.
- **Neurology**—aseptic meningitis/encephalitis, space-occupying lesions (SOL) of unknown cause, Guillian–Barré syndrome, transverse myelitis, peripheral neuropathy, dementia, leukoencephalopathy.
- **Dermatology**—severe/recalcitrant seborrhoeic dermatitis, severe/recalcitrant psoriasis, multi-dermatomal or recurrent herpes zoster.
- **Gastroenterology**—oral candidiasis, oral hairy leukoplakia, chronic diarrhoea of unknown cause, weight loss of unknown cause, *Salmonella*, *Shigella* or *Campylobacter* enteritis, HBV or HCV infection.
- **Oncology**—anal cancer or intraepithelial dysplasia, lung cancer, seminoma, head or neck cancers, Hodgkin's lymphoma, Castleman's disease.
- **Gynaecology**—vaginal intraepithelial neoplasia, cervical intraepithelial neoplasia grade 2 or above.
- **Haematology**—unexplained cytopenias.
- **ENT**—lymphadenopathy of unknown cause, chronic parotitis, lymphoepithelial parotid cysts.
- **Ophthalmology**—infective retinal diseases, including herpes viruses and toxoplasma, any unexplained retinopathy.
- **Other**—mononucleosis-like syndrome (primary HIV infection), pyrexia of unknown origin, any lymphadenopathy of unknown cause, any sexually transmitted infection. Anyone with elevated immunoglobulin G.

General principles in the management of HIV-infected patients

The care of patients with HIV infection should be managed by physicians specializing in HIV medicine. In the UK, this is usually within GU medicine or infectious diseases services with a specialist interest in managing patients with HIV infection.

Because of the many potential drug-drug interactions for patients on cART and a natural history that may be very different, co-infections (TB, viral hepatitis) and other conditions (end-stage renal disease, lymphoma, etc.) that require other specialist input should always be co-managed with HIV physicians, and many units have models of multidisciplinary joint specialist care for such patients.

The main framework of HIV care revolves around:

- Prevention of opportunistic infections.
- Managing combination antiretroviral therapy (cART).
- Monitoring for, and managing, complications associated with cART.
- Managing co-infections and other HIV-associated conditions.
- Provision of socio-psychological support.

Antiretroviral therapy

Highly active cART has revolutionized HIV care. Morbidity and mortality from AIDS has reduced drastically in the last decade, and there is even a suggestion that patients who achieve CD4 count rises over 500 cells/microlitre in the developed world can expect a normal life expectancy.

There are a number of different drugs from five different classes of agents that are currently licensed for the treatment of HIV infection.

- Nucleos(t)ide analogues (NAs): zidovudine (AZT), didanosine (DDI), stavudine (D4T), lamivudine (3TC), abacavir, tenofovir, and emtricitabine (FTC).
- Non-nucleoside reverse transcriptase inhibitors (NNRTIs): nevaripine, efavirenz, etravirine, rilpivirine (licensed 2014/2015).
- Protease inhibitors (PIs): ritonavir, saquinavir, indinavir, lopinavir, atazanavir, fosamprenavir, darunavir.
- Integrase inhibitors: raltegravir, elvitegravir (boosted with cobicistat), dolutegravir (licensed 2014/2015).
- Entry inhibitors: enfuvirtide (INN), maraviroc.

By virtue of the fact that HIV multiplies at a very high rate (1 billion new virus particles produced every day), together with the fact that replication lacks proofreading, means that resistance to antiviral therapy can develop very rapidly. This can be overcome by using a combination of antiretroviral therapies from different classes that rapidly suppresses viral replication. This led to the concept of highly active combination antiretroviral therapy.

It should be noted that most cART agents are associated with short- and long-term side effects. Agents within the NNRTI and PI classes are cytochrome P450 isoenzyme subclass metabolized, and many are inducers or inhibitors of these enzymes. There is, therefore, the need to carefully consider risk versus benefit of cART and to monitor for, and manage, side effects. Healthcare workers managing HIV-infected patients on cART need to be aware of the potential for drug interactions, often with serious consequences.

When to start cART

The ultimate aim of cART is to promote immune reconstitution by suppressing viral replication, thereby preventing HIV-related mortality and morbidity. A secondary aim is to reduce HIV viral load in blood, semen, and vaginal fluid and, therefore, preventing HIV transmission.

Peripheral blood CD4 counts, HIV-associated symptoms, the presence of an opportunistic infection or other AIDS-defining diagnoses, and the presence of HIV-associated comorbidities are central to the decision regarding when to start cART.

Most national and international guidelines suggest starting cART for the following groups of patients:

- Patients with an opportunistic infection or another AIDS-defining illness (lymphoma, Kaposi's sarcoma, cervical carcinoma, etc.), regardless of CD4 count.
- Patients with symptomatic HIV infection.
- Patients with a CD4 count <350 cells/microlitre (in the UK); other guidelines suggest treatment at CD4 <500 cells/microlitre.
- Patients with HIV-associated comorbidities—HBV co-infection, HCV co-infection, HIV-associated nephropathy, older patients.
- Patients with primary HIV infection, especially where there is neurological involvement, any AIDS-defining illness, or confirmed CD4 <350 cells/microlitre.
- For patients where treatment may prevent onward transmission (in sero-discordant couples for example).

These guidelines are evolving, and, as new-generation antiretroviral therapies with fewer short- and long-term side effects become available, there will be a move towards earlier initiation of cART.

Further reading

British HIV Association, British Association of Sexual Health and HIV, British Infection Society (2008). UK National Guidelines for HIV testing 2008. <http://www.bhiva.org/documents/Guidelines/Testing/GlinesHIVTest08.pdf>.

Infections in the HIV-infected patient

The predisposition to infection in the HIV-infected patient is attributable to a number of immune defects associated with HIV, including:

- T lymphocyte defects, including reduced CD4 lymphocyte numbers and a defect in T regulatory cells, with a resultant defect in cell-mediated immunity.
- Defective antibody production.
- Defective mucosal immunity.
- Neutropenia.
- Deficiency in complement activation.

Moreover, lifestyle and nosocomial practices, including intravenous drug use, sexual practices, and the increasing use of indwelling catheters in hospitals, contribute to the pattern and incidence of infections.

This chapter will concentrate on the recognition, management, and prevention of common opportunistic infections associated with HIV-related immunodeficiency.

Peripheral blood CD4 lymphocyte counts

Predisposition to opportunistic infections and their prevention

The association between groups of infections at different thresholds of peripheral blood CD4 cell counts has been well documented (see Table 13.1).

This has led to a number of recommendations for the use of antimicrobials as primary prophylaxis against a number of specific opportunistic infections. It also endorses the widely accepted recommendation of starting cART at a CD4 threshold of 350 cells/microlitre to prevent immune deterioration and the risk of serious opportunistic infections. Specific prophylactic regimens and thresholds will be discussed for each of the opportunistic infections in detail in the following sections.

Pneumocystis pneumonia (PCP)

PCP is caused by a ubiquitous fungal organism *Pneumocystis jirovecii* that shares many properties with protozoa. Whether PCP occurs as a result of reactivation of previously acquired infection or as a result of a new infection in the immune compromised host remains controversial. Before the advent of cART and primary preventative therapy, PCP was the commonest pulmonary opportunistic infection in the western world. The vast majority of cases occur in patients with a CD4 count <200 cells/microlitre. Patients with a low CD4 % (<14%), recurrent bacterial pneumonia, oropharyngeal candidiasis, unintentional weight loss, and high HIV plasma viral loads should also be considered at risk of PCP.

Clinical manifestations

Dry cough and progressive exertional dyspnoea over a period of weeks, often associated with fever and pleuritic chest pain, is the most common presentation of PCP. Atypical presentations include rapidly progressive dyspnoea associated with haemoptysis and pleuritic chest pain.

Diagnosis

In the early stages of the disease the chest radiograph (CXR) may be normal. The typical finding of perihilar alveolar shadowing sparing the lung bases may be a relatively late finding. High-resolution CT scan of the thorax may reveal the characteristic alveolar inflammation of PCP early in the disease. Likewise, exercise-induced oxygen desaturation is often an early feature and, in the correct clinical context, should prompt a search for evidence of PCP infection. A raised serum LDH, associated with typical pulmonary symptoms, should also raise the index of suspicion of PCP.

The definitive diagnosis is established by demonstrating *Pneumocystis jirovecii* organisms in appropriate respiratory specimens by histochemical or immunofluorescent stains. Sensitivity for positive tests vary from clinic to clinic but are generally lower for induced sputums (50–90%), compared to a bronchoalveolar lavage (>90%).

Treatment

Treatment should not be delayed whilst awaiting confirmation of diagnosis. Organisms are often present in respiratory specimens for up to 10 days after starting therapy.

- **Co-trimoxazole.** 120 mg/kg per day IV is the treatment of choice. The dose may be reduced to 90 mg/kg per day after the first 3 days, if the initial clinical response is satisfactory, to complete a 21-day course. For mild to moderate disease, oral co-trimoxazole at a dose of 1,920 mg three times a day for 21 days may be used.
- **Corticosteroids.** Patients with moderate to severe disease (defined as patients with PaO_2 <9.3 kPa or O_2 saturations <92%) should receive corticosteroids within 72 hours of starting PCP treatment. This should normally be oral

Table 13.1 Infections associated with falling CD4 counts

CD4 count (cells/microlitre)	Infectious complications
>500	Pulmonary tuberculosis, acute retroviral syndrome
200–500	Pneumococcal and other bacterial pneumonias Pulmonary tuberculosis Oropharyngeal candidiasis Cryptosporidiosis (self-limited) Oral hairy leukoplakia Herpes simplex (oral/genital) Kaposi's sarcoma (cutaneous) Herpes zoster
<200	*Pneumocystis jirovecii* pneumonia (PCP) Miliary/extrapulmonary tuberculosis Disseminated histoplasmosis and coccidioidomycosis Progressive multifocal leukoencephalopathy (PML)
<100	Disseminated herpes simplex virus Toxoplasmosis Cryptococcosis Chronic cryptosporidiosis Microsporidiosis Candidal oesophagitis Visceral or pulmonary Kaposi's sarcoma
<50	Disseminated cytomegalovirus (CMV) Disseminated *Mycobacterium avium* complex (MAC)

prednisolone (or an equivalent dose of IV methylprednisolone) at a starting dose of 40 mg bd, tapered over 21 days.

Alternative agents to co-trimoxazole
In patients intolerant of/allergic to co-trimoxazole, the following antimicrobials may be used as alternatives. Check for G6PD deficiency before prescribing primaquine, dapsone, or atovaquone.

- **Clindamycin/primaquine**—the preferred alternative in moderate to severe disease. The usual dose is clindamycin 600–900 mg tds IV plus oral primaquine 15 mg/day.
- **Pentamidine** IV—4 mg/kg/day. This requires monitoring for infusion-associated hypotension and hypoglycaemia. It may also cause significant nephrotoxicity and acute pancreatitis.
- **Dapsone/trimethoprim**—oral dapsone 100 mg od plus trimethoprim 20 mg/kg/day is an alternative for mild to moderate disease.
- **Atovaquone** 750 mg bd is also an alternative for mild disease.

Primary prophylaxis for PCP
Co-trimaxozole at a dose of 960 mg/day or 960 mg three times a week or 480 mg/day are equally as efficacious for preventing PCP in HIV-infected patients with CD4 <200 cells/microlitre.
In patients intolerant of co-trimaxozaole, the following are alternatives:

- Nebulized pentamidine—300 mg once a month. Please note this requires a high-particulate nebulizer.
- Oral dapsone 50–100 mg od.
- Atovaquone 750 mg bd.

Secondary prophylaxis for PCP
All patients with PCP should be treated with secondary prophylaxis (as described previously) until sufficient immune restitution following cART has been achieved.
Prophylaxis may be stopped once patients have achieved CD4 >200 cells/microlitre (at least two readings 3 months apart), with undetectable HIV RNA following successful cART.

Pneumococcal pneumonia and bacteraemia

Infections with *Streptococcus pneumoniae* are commoner in HIV-infected patients and may be encountered at any CD4 counts. Rates of bacteraemia associated with pneumonia are higher than in the general population.

Diagnosis and management
Diagnosis and management is similar to non-HIV-infected patients and should include a CXR, blood cultures, and a urine test for pneumococcal antigens. Antibiotic therapy should be guided by local guidelines for the management of community-acquired pneumonia and bacteraemia. Intravenous amoxicillin or co-amoxiclav remains the treatment of choice. In the UK, most strains remain sensitive to penicillin, but antimicrobial sensitivity testing is essential.

Prevention
The 23-valent polysaccharide pneumococcal vaccine is recommended for all HIV-positive patients. The vaccine response may be poor in patients with low CD4 counts, and vaccination may be repeated following cART-associated immune reconstitution.

Central nervous system infections and diseases

CNS disorders are common in the context of HIV infection. They can manifest in a variety of ways, including meningoencephalitis, encephalopathy, radiculitis, transverse myelitis, and space-occupying intracerebral infections involving a number of pathogens, including HIV per se.

HIV-associated encephalopathy
This is a common manifestation of HIV infection and may be seen during acute HIV seroconversion. A more progressive form characterized by cognitive behavioural changes and motor manifestations may be encountered as disease progresses. AIDS dementia complex (ADC) or HIV-associated dementia syndrome (HADS) is often seen in HIV-infected adults with CD4 <200 cells/microlitre and is characterized by cognitive, motor, and behavioural changes.
Diagnosis is by exclusion of other disorders that may cause similar manifestations, particularly CNS infections with the herpes group of viruses, syphilis, and vitamin B12 deficiency. MRI scan of the brain often shows cerebral atrophy with associated hyperintense bilateral periventricular white matter changes. CSF examination may show slightly raised protein (usually <1 g/dL) associated with a normal CSF glucose. The CSF is normally acellular, and the presence of a pleocytosis should prompt a search for alternative pathogens. CSF HIV RNA levels are often quite high.
The cornerstone of management is cART therapy with agents that penetrate into the CSF.

Progressive multifocal leukoencephalopathy (PML)
PML is a debilitating demyelinating CNS disease caused by JC virus, a member of the polyoma group of viruses. The infection is usually acquired in childhood and the associated CNS manifestations progress as the CD4 counts decline. The virus is thought to infect oligodendrocytes in the brain.

Clinical manifestations
PML presents as progressive multifocal neurological deficits in HIV patients with CD4 counts <50 cells/microlitre. Systemic manifestations are virtually always absent. Seizures may be rarely associated with PML. Multiple focal motor and sensory deficits distinguish this from HIV-associated encephalopathy.

Diagnosis and management
MRI scan of the brain shows the characteristic multifocal bilateral T2 hyperintense lesions, without enhancement or oedema. Detection of JC virus in the CSF, using PCR-based nucleic acid detection tests, clinches the diagnosis. Rarely, a brain biopsy may be required. cART is the only therapy shown to be beneficial in PML, with stabilization of CNS and arrest of demyelination.

Cryptococcal meningitis
Cryptococcosis is caused by subtypes of the encapsulated yeast *Cryptococcus neoformans*. Although meningitis is the commonest clinical infection, these organisms can cause pneumonia, skin infections, and biliary tract infections in immunocompromised hosts. In HIV-infected patients, cryptococcal meningitis is rarely seen in patients with CD4 >100 cells/microlitre.

Clinical manifestations
The commonest symptoms associated with cryptococcal meningitis are fevers and headaches ± meningism. In some cases, signs and symptoms of meningism may be completely absent. There is often an associated increase in intracranial

pressure which may manifest as isolated VIth nerve palsy and reduced conscious levels. Seizures are rarely seen but may indicate the presence of intracerebral cryptococcomas in association with meningitis.

Diagnosis

CT and MRI imaging of the brain may be normal or may show evidence of a communicating hydrocephalus. CSF examination characteristically shows a high opening pressure, with moderately increased CSF protein (often 1–1.5 g/dL) and a low CSF glucose. CSF pleocytosis may be absent. India ink stains reveal the characteristic budding yeasts, and CSF cryptococcal antigen testing by latex agglutination test is positive. Serum cryptococcal antigen tests are highly sensitive and specific tests, and a positive test should prompt a search for cryptococcal disease. In patients with a high burden of cryptococcosis, CSF and, occasionally, blood will be culture-positive. A high opening pressure, associated with a low CSF glucose and an absence of pleocytosis, positive blood cultures, and a CSF CrAg >1:1024 are bad prognostic markers in CSF meningitis.

Treatment

- Induction therapy with liposomal amphotericin (3–5 mg/kg/day), together with flucytosine 100 mg/kg/day, is the initial treatment of choice.
- Fluconazole (400 mg/day IV), together with flucytosine, may be preferred when monitoring of renal function and serum electrolytes is not possible.
- Itraconazole, voriconazole, and posiconazole should be reserved for those who are intolerant of the above regimens and for when there is availability for adequate sensitivity testing. Caspofungin has no activity against *Cryptococcus neoformans*.
- Lumbar punctures should be repeated daily and CSF pressure reduced to <20 cmH$_2$O. Placement of lumbar CSF drains or VP shunts may be considered for patients with resistant raised CSF pressures.
- Two weeks of induction therapy is followed by 10 weeks of fluconazole 400 mg/day.
- All patients should then receive fluconazole 200 mg/day as secondary prophylaxis until CD4 >200 on cART.

Toxoplasma encephalitis

Cerebral toxoplasmosis is caused by the protozoa *Toxoplasma gondii* and is the commonest cause of an intracerebral space-occupying lesions in HIV-infected patients. Most infections are due to reactivation of previously acquired infections, and it is, therefore, useful to document evidence of baseline anti-toxoplasma antibodies in newly diagnosed HIV-positive patients.

Clinical manifestations

The clinical features are those of a space-occupying CNS lesion, with focal neurological deficits, often associated with seizures evolving over days to weeks. Some patients may present with diffuse encephalitis and a reduced conscious level, associated with raised intracranial pressure. Unusual presentations include transverse myelitis, cauda equina syndromes, and personality changes.

Diagnosis

Diagnosis is based on the presence of ring-enhancing lesions with associated oedema, often best appreciated on MRI scans. Toxoplasmosis can manifest as a single space-occupying lesion. It is often difficult to differentiate CNS toxoplasmosis from cerebral pyogenic abscesses, cerebral tuberculomas, and primary CNS lymphoma on clinical and radiological grounds. The presence of anti-toxoplasma antibodies in blood is almost universal in HIV-positive patients and does not help with the diagnosis. The absence of serum anti-toxoplasma IgG may be helpful in ruling out toxoplasmosis since most infections are reactivation and patients with advanced immune suppression may lose antibodies. Nucleic acid testing for *Toxoplasma gondii* by PCR in CSF is highly specific but has low sensitivity, and CSF testing is often unsafe in patients with space-occupying lesions with a mass effect.

Diagnosis is often only confirmed by characteristic signs, symptoms, radiological changes, and a radiological response to empirical therapy after an appropriate interval (usually 2–4 weeks). In the absence of appropriate response or where there is a high index of suspicion for an alternative diagnosis (for example, with a negative toxoplasma IgG), a brain biopsy may be required.

Treatment

- Pyrimethamine (loading dose of 200 mg, followed by 50–75 mg/day), together with sulfadiazine (15 mg/kg qds) plus folinic acid (15 mg/day), is the preferred first-line treatment.
- Clindamycin (600 mg qds IV) may be used as an alternative to sulfadiazine in sulfa-allergic patients.
- Alternative regimens, including co-trimoxazole or azithromycin, clarithromycin, dapsone, or atovaquone plus pyrimethemaine and folinic acid have lower efficacies.
- Treatment should be continued for 6–8 weeks and radiological response documented by repeated CNS imaging. Completion of treatment should be followed by secondary prophylaxis (using the same drugs but at lower doses) until CD4 count >200 cells/microlitre following cART.
- Corticosteroids may be required when patients have significant mass effect from pre-lesional oedema.
- Anticonvulsant therapy should be offered to patients with seizures or high risk of seizure activity.

Primary prophylaxis

HIV patients with a CD4 count of <200 cells/microlitre should be offered primary prophylaxis with either co-trimoxazole (480 mg or 960 mg od) or dapsone (50 mg od), together with weekly pyrimethamine (50 mg).

Diarrhoeal disease in HIV-infected patients

Diarrhoea, in the context of HIV infection, has a number of different causes, ranging from associations with cART agents to opportunistic infections. Here, we will consider two important causes in patients with advanced immune suppression.

Cryptosporidiosis

This is a disease caused by a species of the protozoan parasite *Cryptosporidium* which mainly infects the small bowel. The organism is ubiquitous in the environment. Outbreaks have been associated with faecal contamination of recreational water facilities, and person-to-person transmission has been described amongst men who have sex with men.

Clinical manifestations

The most common presentation is of profuse, non-bloody, watery diarrhoea, often accompanied by fever. In patients with low CD4 counts, prolonged illness may present with cholangitis.

Diagnosis

The oocysts can be visualized in stool specimens or tissue, using acid-fast stains. In cases where stool specimens fail to make a diagnosis, small intestine biopsy is often invaluable. The organism is easily identified with H&E stains, either as a single organism or in clusters on the mucosal brush border.

Treatment

Management is largely supportive with fluid and electrolyte replacement. Early cART to restore CD4 counts is the only definitive therapy. Antiparasitic agents like nitazoxanide and paramomycin have no role on their own but may be used as an adjunct to cART. Treatment with antimotility agents may be used for symptom control.

Microsporidiosis

Microsporidiosis is an infection caused by a number of species of ubiquitous organisms related to fungi. *Encephalitozoon* spp., *Trachipleistophora* spp., and *Pleistosphora* spp. are amongst the many microsporidia that cause human disease. Clinical disease is rarely seen in patients with CD4 counts >100 cells/microlitre.

Clinical manifestations

Diarrhoeal illness with malabsorption is the commonest manifestation, although encephalitis, myositis, and disseminated multiorgan involvement have also been described. *Trachipleistophora* spp. have been associated with encephalitis and disseminated disease.

Diagnosis

The spores may be visualized in stool specimens by direct microscopy, although this may be difficult because of their small size. Definitive diagnosis is often by examination of small bowel biopsy specimens. Small bowel biopsies should be obtained in all patients with HIV and low CD4 counts with unexplained diarrhoea.

Treatment

cART is the only definitive therapy for diarrhoeal disease caused by microsporidia. Fluid and electrolyte replacement, together with nutritional support and antimotility agents, may be useful.

Itraconazole and albendazole, in combination, may be used in disseminated disease caused by *Trachipleistophora* spp.

Mycobacterial disease in HIV-infected patients

Mycobacterium tuberculosis (mTB) complex

On a worldwide basis, tuberculosis is the commonest opportunistic infection encountered in HIV-infected patients and accounts for 15% of all AIDS-related deaths globally.

Patients with latent TB and HIV infection have an 8–10% annual risk of TB reactivation, compared to a 2% lifetime risk of reactivation in HIV uninfected patients. Unlike other opportunistic infections, the relationship between absolute CD4 counts and the risk of TB reactivation or primary infection with progression to active disease is not well established. In other words, patients with HIV infection may present with active tuberculosis at any CD4 count.

Clinical manifestations

The classical presentation of pulmonary infiltrates with upper zone cavitation is also seen in HIV-positive patients with good CD4 counts. However, with advancing immune suppression, presentation is often less classical, with more involvement of lower and middle lobes, hilar and paratracheal lymphadenopathy, pericarditis and less evidence of cavitation. Extrapulmonary disease is also more common in the context of HIV co-infection. Multiorgan involvement, TB lymphadenitis, and CNS tuberculosis are also more often seen in HIV-positive patients, regardless of CD4 counts. The association of advanced HIV immune suppression with high mycobacterial loads may manifest with a sepsis syndrome and multiorgan failure.

In patients with subclinical TB, the initiation of cART may result in an 'unmasking' phenomenon. Similarly, paradoxical fevers, worsening clinical signs and symptoms may also occur in patients on TB treatment shortly after starting cART. This is termed 'immune restitution inflammatory syndrome' (IRIS).

Diagnosis of tuberculosis

Active TB

The definitive diagnosis of TB is based on a positive culture of appropriate specimens. Even with the use of liquid culture media, it generally takes 2–4 weeks to get positive TB cultures. In patients with low CD4 counts and high mycobacterial loads, it may be possible to get positive blood cultures.

The demonstration of acid and alcohol fast bacilli (AAFBs) by Ziehl–Neelsen or auramine stains in acquired specimens is helpful. The use of nucleic acid amplification techniques (e.g. mTB-PCR) is useful in identifying AAFBs as mTB, since other mycobacteria can cause disease in HIV-positive patients.

Sensitivity testing is mandatory in HIV-positive patients because of their increased risk of acquiring drug-resistant mTB. Molecular analysis for mutations associated with rifampicin and isoniazid resistance is a quick and sensitive method for the early identification of drug-resistant TB but is only available in specialist laboratories.

For many patients, anti-tuberculous therapy is commenced on the basis of a high index of clinical suspicion. This is not unreasonable as long as specimens have been submitted for TB culture prior to commencement of anti-TB therapy.

Latent TB

TB skin testing using PPD may be useful in identifying patients with latent TB, but false negative tests may be seen in patients with low CD4 counts.

The interferon-gamma release assays (TB-IGRAs) may perform better in HIV-positive patients, both in terms of fewer false negatives and in that they have no cross-reactivity with BCG or common environmental mycobacteria. Please note that currently a positive result does not distinguish between active and latent disease.

Treatment of active TB

For general principles for treatment of active TB, see Box 13.1, and for TB treatment regimens in drug-susceptible mTB, see Box 13.2.

When to start cART in antiretroviral naive HIV/TB patients

There is a need to find the optimum time to start cART in the treatment of naive HIV-positive patients with a new diagnosis of TB. This needs to take into consideration the risk of further opportunistic infections that can be averted by early cART, versus the risk of IRIS early in the course of cART, and also the risk of drug-drug interactions that may potentially jeopardize both treatments. Furthermore, cART, in addition to anti-TB therapy, may impose a high pill burden that may not be acceptable to many patients.

Box 13.1 General principles for treatment of active TB

a) Wherever possible, tuberculosis treatment for HIV co-infected patients should be supervised by multidisciplinary teams with expertise in managing such patients.

b) Treatment regimens should be guided by the availability of sensitivity testing results.

c) There are a number of clinically relevant interactions between rifamycins and boosted protease inhibitors (PIs) and non-nucleoside reverse transcriptase inhibitors (NNRTIs).

d) Judicious use of therapeutic drug monitoring is recommended both for rifamycins and components of cART when used together to guide appropriate drug dosing.

e) Directly observed therapy should be carried out whenever possible.

f) Administration of once or twice weekly long-acting rifamycins should be avoided in HIV-positive patients because of the risk of drug-drug interactions and the possibility of variable absorption.

g) HIV-positive patients are at higher risk of drug-induced hepatotoxicity from anti-TB therapy. This risk is increased further by co-infection with HBV/HCV. All HIV-positive patients should have regular monitoring for hepatotoxicity.

Box 13.2 TB treatment regimens in drug-susceptible mTB

1. 6 months of therapy should be sufficient for all extra-CNS tuberculosis and 12 months for CNS disease.

2. The induction phase should consist of four drugs, including isoniazid, rifampicin, pyrazinamide, and ethambutol. Moxifloxacin or streptomycin can be used as alternatives where ethambutol use is contraindicated (e.g. patients with renal failure).

3. Rifabutin, at a dose of 150 mg three times a week, should replace rifampicin when boosted PIs are used as part of cART.

4. The dose of efavirenz should be increased to 800 mg/day when used as a component of cART during standard quadruple anti-TB treatment.

5. The continuation phase, consisting of isoniazid and rifampicin or rifabutin, may need to be prolonged in patients in whom pyrazinamide is not used in the induction phase or in patients with cavitatory lung disease in whom sputum culture results are still positive after 2 months of therapy.

6. Pyridoxine at a dose of 25 mg/day should be used in all patients for the duration of isoniazid therapy to prevent occurrence of peripheral neuropathy.

- All patients with TB and a CD4 count <500 cells/microlitre should start cART as soon as possible
- In patients with CD4 counts between 350 and 500, physicians may want to wait until the end of the induction phase of anti-TB treatment (2 months) before commencing cART.
- In patients with CD4 <350 cells/microlitre, cART should be started as soon as possible. Some physicians prefer to wait for 2 weeks after commencement of anti-TB treatment.

TB immune restitution inflammatory syndrome (IRIS)

This is an inflammatory response seen typically between 2 and 12 weeks after starting cART in patients on anti-TB treatment. It represents, in very simplistic terms, an immune response to residual mycobacterial antigens by cART-reconstituted cellular responses and is seen in about 20% of individuals. It is associated with a number of factors, including disseminated TB, initiation of cART within 2 months of anti-TB treatment, low CD4 counts, and a rapid fall in HIV viral load.

Clinical manifestation

Clinical presentation is wide and varied but is characterized by high fevers, often in association with new or worsening lymphadenopathy, pulmonary infiltrates, pleural and/or pericardial effusions, enlarging CNS tuberculomas, or worsening meningeal inflammation. The presentation may be with inflammation at a site distant from the area of the original involvement with TB. It is important to note that IRIS is a diagnosis of exclusion, and, in particular, drug-resistant TB, new opportunistic or secondary infections, and drug reactions need to be carefully excluded.

Management of TB-IRIS

Once the diagnosis is certain, oral corticosteroids are the treatment of choice.

- Prednisolone, at a dose of 20–40 mg for 4–8 weeks, is the most widely used regimen and is sufficient for most patients.
- If the diagnosis is certain, there is never a need to stop or interrupt cART.
- Some patients may require prolonged and repeated courses of corticosteroids.
- Leukotriene inhibitors may be used in patients refractory to, or intolerant of, corticosteroids.
- Be vigilant for secondary infections in patients with low CD4 counts on prolonged corticosteroid therapy, especially with regard to fungal infections (aspergillosis, cryptococcosis) and CMV reactivation.

Management of latent TB in the HIV-infected host

In view of the high risk of TB reactivation with advancing immune suppression, there is intense debate amongst the HIV community regarding the role of chemoprophylaxis for latent TB infection. With the advent of early cART and the achievement of effective immune restitution, much of this risk is abrogated, and early cART remains the mainstay of TB prevention. Furthermore, as highlighted previously, there are difficulties in establishing the diagnosis of latent TB in this group of patients. The use of short courses of combination therapy with rifampicin and pyrazinamide are associated with unacceptable risk of severe hepatotoxicity. Studies using short courses of isoniazid chemoprophylaxis have shown short-term mortality benefits but only in patients with positive PPD skin tests.

Mycobacterium avium intracellulare complex (MAC)

Disseminated MAC is predominantly seen in patients with advanced immune suppression (CD4 <50 cells/microlitre) and is rare in the era of cART. The disease is caused by environmental mycobacteria. Person-to-person transmission does not occur.

Clinical presentation

Disseminated MAC typically presents with unexplained fevers, often associated with hepatosplenomegaly and lymphadenopathy. It is characterized by pancytopenia, as a result of bone marrow infiltration, and hypersplenism. Patients may also report weight loss, anorexia, and night sweats. Unusual focal manifestations may include oral ulceration, osteomyelitis, septic arthritis, myocarditis, and pericarditis.

Diagnosis

The definitive diagnosis of disseminated MAC is established by positive blood or bone marrow aspirate culture or culture from a normally sterile site. A single positive culture from stool, sputum, or bronchoalveolar lavage, in the absence of clinical symptoms or radiological changes, should not prompt treatment.

Because of the high mycobacterial loads characteristic of disseminated MAC infections, the organisms may be visualized as AAFB-positive in appropriate histological or cytological specimens. Disseminated MAC infections are rarely associated with granuloma formation.

Treatment

Treatment usually comprises a combination anti-mycobacterial therapy for at least 12 months. Unlike mTB, sensitivity testing is rarely helpful and, apart from macrolides, does not correlate to clinical response *in vivo*. cART should be commenced (or modified if the patient is already on treatment) to ensure early and effective immune replenishment.

- First-line therapy is with a macrolide (clarithromycin 500 mg bd or azithromycin 500 mg od), together with ethambutol (15 mg/kg/day).
- Rifabutin (300 mg/day) may be added if there are concerns about macrolide sensitivity in patients with CD4 <25 cells/microlitre and/or in patients with features of severe illness. Note: if a boosted PI is used for cART, the dose of rifabutin is 150 mg three times weekly or 450 mg od with efavirenz.
- Fluoroquinolones and aminoglycosides may be used for patients in whom treatment failure, following first-line therapy, is suspected. In these cases, at least two new agents should be commenced.
- Treatment should be for at least 12 months and should continue for a minimum of 3 months after adequate immune response to cART is evident (undetectable HIV viral load and CD4 >100 cells/microlitre)

MAC prophylaxis

Primary prophylaxis may be considered for patients with a CD4 count <50 cells/microlitre whilst cART is initiated and immune restoration achieved.

- Azithromycin, 1,250 mg on a weekly basis, is the commonest regimen used.
- Alternatives are clarithromycin 500 mg bd, or rifabutin od (dose adjustments may be required for interactions with cART components).

Further reading

Kaplan JE, Benson C, Holmes KH, et al. (2009). Guidelines for the prevention and treatment of opportunistic infections in HIV infected adults and adolescents. *MMWR Recommendations and Reports*, **58** (RR-4), 1–207.

British HIV Association Guidelines for the treatment of HIV-1-positive adults with antiretroviral therapy 2012 (updated November 2013). <http://www.bhiva.org/documents/Guidelines/Treatment/2012/hiv_v15_is1_Rev.pdf>.

European AIDS Clinical Society Guidelines v 7.1 November 2014. <http://www.eacsociety.org/files/guidelines_english_71_141204.pdf>.

Post-exposure prophylaxis (PEP) for prevention of HIV infection

Studies of primary HIV infection and animal models of HIV infection have demonstrated that there is a 'window' period from exposure to HIV to the establishment of systemic disseminated viral infection. It is estimated that once HIV crosses a mucosal barrier, it may take up to 48–72 hours before HIV can be detected in regional lymph nodes and up to 5 days before HIV is detected in the blood. This represents a window of opportunity to prevent infection with the timely use of antiretroviral therapy.

A case control study in 1997 by the CDC, of the administration of zidovudine prophylaxis to healthcare workers exposed to HIV was associated with an 80% reduction in HIV seroconversion. This established the principles of modern occupational PEP to prevent HIV infection.

PEP has not only successfully prevented HIV infection following occupational exposure, but is commonly used to prevent vertical HIV transmission. This is achieved by the administration of antiretroviral therapy to the at risk neonate for 4–6 weeks within 48 hours of birth.

More recently, studies in macaques have also suggested that PEP may be effective in preventing infection, following vaginal or rectal exposure to HIV. This established the phenomenon of PEP following sexual exposure (PEPSE).

In order to make an appropriate risk assessment for the administration of PEP, it is important to be able to appraise the risk of infection following an exposure. The risk of HIV infection is proportional to the risk of the exposure, the likelihood of the source being HIV-positive, and having infective virus present in the fluid exposed to.

The following are the risks of HIV transmission (per exposure), based on exposure from a known HIV-positive source (2006 British Association for Sexual Health and HIV (BASHH) guidelines for post-exposure prophylaxis (PEP) after sexual exposure (PEPSE) to HIV):

- Blood transfusion (1 unit): 90–100%.
- Receptive anal intercourse: 0.1–3.0%.
- Receptive vaginal exposure: 0.1–0.2%.
- Insertive vaginal intercourse: 0.03 –0.09%.
- Insertive anal intercourse: 0.06%.
- Oral intercourse: 0–0.04%.
- Needle-stick injury: 0.3%.
- Sharing injecting equipment: 0.67%.
- Mucous membrane exposure: 0.09%.

The risks from an unknown source will clearly depend on the likelihood of HIV infection (HIV prevalence) in subgroups in the general population. In the context of occupational exposure in a healthcare setting, this can be established by HIV-testing the source. It should be noted that, in the UK, informed consent is required before HIV testing of the source case is carried out, even in the healthcare setting.

PEP regimens

Since the advent of combination therapies for the treatment of established HIV infection, PEP regimens have also evolved to consist of triple therapies to ensure effectiveness of therapy. However, the efficacy of PEP wanes with increasing time to administration following exposure. Furthermore, it should be borne in mind that antiretroviral regimens are associated with significant side effects. Fulminant hepatic failure has been reported in patients exposed to nevirapine as part of PEP regimens. Moreover, failure to take PEP properly because of side effects may result in HIV infection with drug-resistant strains. As more patients commence early cART, and with increasing antiretroviral resistance, both in patients with chronic HIV infection and in primary infections, it is important that the correct PEP regimen is chosen.

- Following possible exposure to HIV, an appropriate risk assessment must be carried out immediately by healthcare professionals experienced in HIV PEP administration.
- If benefits outweigh risks, PEP should be administered immediately, and within 72 hours of exposure, for maximum efficacy.
- The specific PEP regimen should be constructed, based on the likelihood of drug sensitivity in the index case
- In the case of an unknown or untested source, the standard regimen is tenofovir, emtricitabine (as a fixed-dose combination tablet, Truvada® once a day), and ritonavir boosted lopinavir (a fixed-dose combination, Kaletra® two tablets bd).
- A baseline sample should be stored for retrospective testing in case of subsequent HIV seroconversion.
- Testing for, and vaccination against, HBV should be carried out as appropriate.
- In the case of sexual exposure, appropriate screening, treatment and counselling for other sexually transmitted infections should be offered.
- Standard anti-nausea and antimotility agents for diarrhoea should be part of PEP packs.
- Recipients of PEP should have weekly monitoring of full blood counts, renal function, and liver function.
- PEP should be administered for 4 weeks for maximum efficacy.

HIV testing following completion of PEP

Recipients of PEP should be closely monitored for signs and symptoms of HIV seroconversion and offered early HIV testing if seroconversion is suspected.

A negative fourth-generation combined antigen/antibody HIV test 12 weeks after completion of PEP is fairly definitive evidence of lack of HIV infection, and further testing after that time is not recommended.

Further reading

Fisher M, Benn P, Evans B, et al. (2006). UK guideline for the use of post-exposure prophylaxis for HIV following sexual exposure. International Journal of STD & AIDS, **17**, 81–92.

Nandwani R, on behalf of the Clinical Effectiveness Group of the British Association for Sexual Health and HIV (BASHH) (2006). 2006 United Kingdom national guideline on the sexual health of people with HIV: sexually transmitted infections. <http://www.bashh.org/documents/60/60.pdf>.

Non-HIV causes of immunodeficiency

Immunodeficiency may be caused by failure of any component of the immune system and results in increased susceptibility to infections.

Patients may be aware that they have an immunodeficiency state or it may be unrecognized. Suspect immunodeficiency if there are recurrent, serious, persistent, or unusual infections and if there is a known family history of immunodeficiency.

Secondary causes of immunodeficiency are common in a variety of disorders, including lymphoproliferative disease, liver disease, malnutrition, multiple myeloma, malignancy, as well as bacterial or viral infections, such as HIV (see 'Infections in the HIV-infected patient'), or following splenectomy.

The causes of immunodeficiency are shown in Box 13.3.

Antibody deficiency

Antibody deficiency occurs in children and adults. Most antibody deficiencies are acquired and >90% present at >10 years old. Patients present with recurrent chest or ENT infections (see Figure 13.1) (adapted from Hermaszewski and Webster 1993). This may lead to chronic otitis media, deafness, sinusitis, bronchiectasis (IgA deficiency), or pulmonary fibrosis. Often there is involvement of another system, such as skin (boils, abscesses), gut infections, or meningitis. Diarrhoea ± malabsorption may be caused by *Giardia lamblia*, bacterial overgrowth, *Cryptosporidium*, *Campylobacter*, or viral infections. Some patients present with a pernicious anaemia-like syndrome but lack antibodies to gastric parietal cells or intrinsic factor. Bacterial infections are often due

> **Box 13.3** Causes and presentations of immunodeficiency
>
> **Antibody deficiency.** Recurrent severe or persistent sinopulmonary infections, chronic diarrhoea, malabsorption.
>
> **Phagocyte dysfunction or deficiency.** Recurrent pyogenic skin sepsis, invasive fungal infection, recurrent oromucocutaneous ulceration, granulomatous inflammation.
>
> **Defective cell-mediated immunity.** Patients with more than one of the following infections: virus, e.g. CMV; intracellular bacteria (e.g. mycobacteria); fungal infections; protozoal infections; and certain malignancies, e.g. Kaposi's sarcoma or EBV-driven lymphoma (see 'Infections in the HIV-infected patient').
>
> **Complement deficiency.** Encapsulated bacterial sepsis, e.g. meningitis, lupus-like syndrome, vasculitis, haemolytic uraemic syndrome. neisserial infection.
>
> **Hyposplenism.** Severe recurrent encapsulated bacterial sepsis, e.g. meningitis, severe malaria, *Babesia* infection, cellulitis by *Capnocytophaga*.

to common organisms, such as *Streptococcus pneumoniae* or *Haemophilus influenzae*.

There may be non-infectious manifestations, including autoimmune phenomona (15%), thyroid disease, haemolytic anaemia, immune thrombocytopenic purpura, or arthropathy (12%). Septic arthritis may be caused by mycoplasma. Some patients present with failure to make specific antibodies, following vaccination. Diagnosis is made by measurement of immunoglobulins. Management is by monthly infusion of immunoglobulins to prevent further infections.

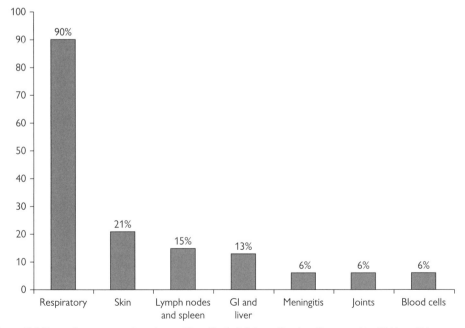

Figure 13.1 Presenting symptoms in patients with antibody deficiency. Data from Hermaszewski and Webster, 'Primary hypogammaglobulinaemia: a survey of clinical manifestations and complications', *Quarterly Journal of Medicine*, 1993; **86**: 31–42.

Phagocyte dysfunction or deficiency

The major role of neutrophils is to kill bacteria and fungi. Neutrophil dysfunction may be due to neutropenia (lack of neutrophils) or due to abnormal neutrophil function. Mild neutropenia is often asymptomatic and may be racial (e.g. Africans). Life-threatening infections tend to occur when the neutrophil count falls below 0.5×10^9/L.

Patients present with recurrent prolonged bacterial infections, often with few signs or symptoms, despite severe infection. The commonest organism is *Staphylococcus aureus* which tends to be poorly responsive to antibiotics and involve skin and mucous membranes. Pneumonia is associated with high mortality.

Impaired neutrophil function may be due to abnormal adhesion (e.g. leucocyte adhesion deficiency), poor migration of neutrophils towards a source of infection, impaired chemotaxis (i.e. decreased in infections or burns), abnormal phagocytosis (impaired opsonization; e.g. C3 deficiency or severe immunoglobulin deficiency), or reduced respiratory burst (e.g. primary in chronic granulomatous disease, or secondary in infection, malnutrition, liver disease, or burns (see Table 13.2)). Chronic granulomatous disease is a group of inherited disorders caused by failure to exert a respiratory burst. These classically present in childhood.

Complement deficiency

Complement deficiency is usually secondary to diseases which consume complement, e.g. SLE or some forms of glomerulonephritis, but may be inherited (usually autosomal recessive).

Patients present with recurrent pyogenic infections, with increased susceptibility to neisserial infection or associated immune complex disorders (e.g. SLE). Patients with C1, C2, or C4 deficiency may present with SLE-like symptoms with arthralgia and glomerulonephritis. Recurrent bacterial infections may also occur with encapsulated organisms due to impaired opsonization.

Patients with C3 deficiency present with a variety of life-threatening infections, such as meningitis, septicaemia, pneumonia. Deficiency of C5-8 (components of the membrane attack complex) is associated with severe neisserial infection.

General principles

Clinical approach

Immunosuppression can cause infections to be more frequent, more severe, or with organisms that are not normally pathogenic (opportunistic infections). Where infections are more frequent without increased severity, the major consideration is the prevention of future episodes. Increased severity of infection, for example in febrile neutropenia, means the clinician must have a low threshold for rapidly administering broad-spectrum antibiotics. Opportunistic infections broaden the causes of any infective syndrome and may require specific antibiotics to

be used, in addition to the usual choices, for example, the addition of co-trimoxazole for PCP in lower respiratory tract infection.

Opportunistic infections by site

- **Respiratory:** PCP, *Aspergillus*, *Nocardia*, *Cryptococcus*, respiratory syncytial virus.
- **Gastrointestinal:** *Candida*, CMV, HSV, atypical mycobacteria.
- **Nervous system:** *Toxoplasma*, *Cryptococcus*, *Listeria*, *Nocardia*, CMV.
- **Skin:** *Pseudomonas*, CMV.
- **Undifferentiated fever:** fungaemia, CMV, EBV, atypical mycobacteria.

There are few specific guidelines regarding the management of immunosuppressed patients, so the usual principles of management of infections apply, but with a greater emphasis on completing each stage rapidly. The patient should be assessed clinically and the cause and degree of immunosuppression considered. History is important, considering occupational, sexual, travel, and nosocomial exposures.

The nature of the immunosuppression will inform the likely pathogens and, therefore, the antimicrobials required (see relevant sections for details). The clinical features associated with infection, including fever, pain, and examination findings may be reduced in immunosuppression, and subtle abnormalities should be pursued. Infection may occur in unusual sites as well as with unusual organisms. The clinician should consider syndromes, such as sinusitis, pyomyositis, and psoas abscess. Also remember that bacteraemia or fungaemia may cause endocarditis or seeding to distant sites (e.g. right-sided endocarditis and septic emboli to the lungs).

Supportive management should be commenced with intravenous fluids and oxygen. Consider the need for higher level care early. Comorbidities, such as diabetes, should be managed appropriately, and patients admitted unwell on oral steroids should receive intravenous doses. It is vital that sufficient material for culture is taken quickly from blood and other sites before antibiotics are commenced. However, collection of these samples should not be allowed to significantly delay the administration of empirical antibiotics. For example, antibiotics should be commenced before procedures, such as lumbar puncture, which may be time-consuming and initially unsuccessful.

Empirical antibiotic cover should be broad and tailored to cover both common community-acquired pathogens and those pathogens to which the patient is susceptible. This may require the advice of a microbiologist. Isolation should be considered, either to protect the patient from nosocomial infection (e.g. in febrile neutropenia) or to isolate the source of infection (e.g. in MRSA). The patient should be reassessed frequently for response and to ensure that other infections are not developing.

Radiological investigation is often helpful if the diagnosis remains unclear. CT scanning with contrast is first line; consider HRCT of the chest if fungal infection is suspected or CT PET in fever of unknown origin. If an infective site is identified, specific diagnosis with biopsy, aspiration, or bronchoalveolar lavage should be pursued. Some infections may require surgical intervention, particularly intra-abdominal or soft tissue collections or osteomyelitis.

Table 13.2 Causes of neutropenia

1. **Decreased marrow production**
   a. *Primary*, e.g. cyclical neutropenia, chronic benign neutropenia, or familial neutropenias
   b. *Secondary*, e.g. cytotoxic drugs, aplastic leukaemia, leukaemia, infections, drug reactions
2. **Increased destruction by bone marrow**
   For example, hypersplenia, immune-mediated neutropenia

The management of infections, once a microbiological diagnosis has been made, is similar in immunocompetent and immunosuppressed individuals. Antibiotic therapy is guided by the sensitivities of the organism and dosing is usually unchanged. Narrowing the spectrum of administered antimicrobials reduces side effects and reduces the likelihood of secondary infection with hospital-acquired organisms, such as *Clostridium difficile*.

There is relatively little evidence about the use of antimicrobials in immunosuppression outside of HIV and febrile neutropenia. In some settings, it is appropriate to extend the course of antibiotics, compared with immunocompetent hosts, and, in some specific cases, long-term prophylaxis is indicated. In complex cases, the advice of an experienced microbiologist is helpful. The decision to stop antibiotics is usually made on clinical grounds and informed by markers, such as CRP. Even in expert hands and after prolonged courses, infection may recur. Patients should be informed that this is a possibility and to re-present early if there are any signs of recurrence.

General principles

- Rapid clinical assessment to identify clinical syndrome, level of care required, and the nature and degree of immunosuppression.
- Take cultures early from appropriate sites.
- Commence broad-spectrum antimicrobials whilst culture results are awaited; in many cases, it is possible to do this within 1 hour.
- Reassess frequently for response, complications, and as results are available.
- Seek a specific radiological or microbiological diagnosis which may allow rationalization of antibiotics.
- When the patient improves, consider measures to reduce the likelihood of future infections with the same or different organisms.
- A microbiologist or infectious disease physician can help to guide management at each stage.

Asplenia or splenectomy

Asplenia may be due to surgical splenectomy, congenital absence of the spleen or functional asplenia, characterized by the presence of Howell–Jolly bodies on the peripheral blood film and seen in a range of haematological disorders, such as sickle cell disease, thalassaemia major, and a range of lymphoproliferative disorders, in addition to SLE, portal hypertension, and graft versus host disease (GVHD). In all cases, the absence of the spleen leads to increased susceptibility to infection by a variety of organisms, as the splenic macrophages responsible for the phagocytosis of opsonized intravascular organisms are lost (see Box 13.4). In particular, these patients are susceptible to infection by the encapsulated bacterium *Streptococcus pneumoniae* which accounts for 50–90% of bacteraemias post-splenectomy.

Diagnosis

Hyposplenism or asplenia may be diagnosed by the presence of increased numbers of erythrocyte Howell–Jolly bodies, absence of spleen on ultrasound or computed tomography scanning, and failure of splenic uptake of technetium-99-tagged meta-stable sulphur colloid. The measurement of specific antibodies to pneumococcal polysaccharides and its responses after test vaccination with the 23-valent pneumococcal polysaccharide vaccine may demonstrate impaired specific antibody responses to polysaccharide antigens.

Management

Elective splenectomy should be postponed after infancy. If the patient has not been immunized, immunization should be given several weeks before elective splenectomy. Following splenic injury, repair or partial splenectomy, instead of complete splenectomy, is performed whenever possible. Splenic autotransplantation done at the time of surgery will preserve the antibody responses to vaccines.

Vaccination

- *H. influenzae*, pneumococcal, and meningococcal vaccines are required for all splenic-deficient patients.
- Children <2 years: conjugated *H. influenzae* and 7-valent pneumococcal vaccine.
- Children >2 years: pneumococcal polysaccharide and quadrivalent meningococcal vaccines.
- Booster vaccinations are given every 5 years.

Overwhelming post-splenectomy infection

Overwhelming post-splenectomy infection (OPSI) is the syndrome of rapidly progressive sepsis in asplenic patients. The presentation is typically of fevers with rigors, pharyngitis, myalgia, and sometimes vomiting and/or diarrhoea. It has a lifetime incidence of 5% and carries a mortality of 50%. It can occur at any time following splenectomy, although the majority of cases are within the first few years. It is a medical emergency and requires the rapid administration of appropriate intravenous antibiotics and intensive care. *Neisseria meningitidis* infection is no more common or serious than in normal individuals.

Key points in the history

- Use of prophylactic antibiotics (most commonly, phenoxymethylpenicillin or erythromycin in penicillin allergy).
- Up-to-date vaccinations against pneumococcus, *Haemophilus influenzae* b, and meningococcus.
- Recent travel and potential exposure to resistant *Streptococcus pneumoniae* or malaria.
- Tick bites or potential exposure to ticks that may transmit the organisms responsible for human ehrlichiosis or babesiosis. Concurrent infections are possible due to bites from dually infected ticks.
- Other recent trauma or wounds that may represent a port of entry, particularly bites.

Investigation and management of overwhelming post-splenectomy infection

Rapid assessment of the patient and aggressive fluid resuscitation is required. Blood cultures should be taken as soon as possible and are positive in 95% of cases. Empiric antibiotic therapy with an intravenous beta-lactam antibiotic at

---

Box 13.4 Common infections in patients without a spleen

Streptococcus pneumoniae
Haemophilus influenzae type b
Staphylococcus aureus
Salmonella species
Escherichia coli
Klebsiella species
Capnocytophaga canimorsus
Babesia and *Ehrlichiosis* species
Malaria

high dose should be commenced immediately. Third-generation cephalosporins, such as ceftriaxone, are recommended, particularly in patients who have been taking prophylactic oral phenoxymethylpenicillin. For patients who may have penicillin-resistant streptococcal infection, which is prevalent in Spain and the USA, a glycopeptide, such as vancomycin or teicoplanin should be added. In beta-lactam allergy, a glycopeptide may substitute for ceftriaxone, but this requires the addition of a second agent to cover the Gram-negative organisms, such as a quinolone. Ideally, one with some activity against Gram-positive organisms, such as moxifloxacin, should be used.

Where the patient may have been exposed to the intra-cellular parasites causing malaria or babesiosis, thick and thin blood films should be examined urgently. These organisms are difficult to distinguish on microscopy, and findings should be correlated with the history. Widely available malaria antigen tests may be helpful to distinguish these infections where the cause remains unclear. Intensive care assessment and transfer should be sought rapidly where appropriate.

Empiric antibiotics in OPSI
- First line: ceftriaxone.
- Alternatives (e.g. allergy): vancomycin or teicoplanin and moxifloxacin or alternative quinolone.
- Resistant streptococci suspected: ceftriaxone and vancomycin/teicoplanin.

Ongoing management
Antibiotic therapy can be modified in the light of blood cultures. If Gram-negative bacilli are seen, consider broadening the antibiotics to cover *Pseudomonas aeruginosa* while identification and sensitivities are awaited. Duration of antibiotic therapy should be based on clinical and biochemical response as there are currently no trials available for guidance. We would recommend at least 14 days antibiotic therapy in patients with bacteraemia.

Some sources recommend the administration of intravenous immunoglobulin 0.4 g/kg daily for 3 days. There are no human trials to support this practice, but one study showed benefits in splenectomized rats with post-splenectomy pneumococcal sepsis.

Prevention of future episodes
All patients with splenic dysfunction or post-splenectomy should take lifelong prophylactic phenoxymethylpenicillin (or erythromycin in the case of beta-lactam allergy). Hyposplenic patients should be offered polyvalent pneumococcal vaccine every 5 years and *Haemophilus influenzae* b and meningococcus C conjugate vaccines if not previously vaccinated. Yearly influenza vaccination should also be offered.

Some sources recommend that patients keep a supply of stand-by antibiotics to be used in case of febrile illness and that patients be instructed to contact a doctor immediately if any are used. Co-amoxiclav at a dose of 625 mg tds would be first line, with moxifloxacin or linezolid as alternatives in severe beta-lactam allergy.

Malaria, babesia, and ehrlichia

The advice of a specialist infectious disease physician should be sought if these infections are suspected. Babesiosis and ehrlichiosis are particularly rare and difficult to diagnose. We recommend treating with antibacterials whilst investigating the patient.

Malaria
Asplenic patients travelling to malarious areas should take meticulous care to avoid mosquito bites, with the use of insect repellent and mosquito nets, and should take appropriate malarial prophylaxis for the area. Malaria infection in hyposplenic patients should be treated, as per severe *Plasmodium falciparum* infection (see 'Malaria' in Chapter 6). There should be a low threshold for the use of empiric antibacterial agents in these patients.

Babesiosis
This zoonosis of rodents and other mammals causes severe human disease almost exclusively in hyposplenic patients. It is caused by a number of related protozoan species of the genus *Babesia* transmitted by the bite of infected *Ixodes* ticks. The distribution is limited to areas of the north-west USA and small pockets in south-east Europe. Quinine and clindamycin, either intravenously or at high dose orally, are first line. Alternatively, atovaquone and azithromycin have a similar efficacy and may be better tolerated.

Ehrlichiosis
Ehrlichiosis is caused by a number of species of intracellular spirochetes of the genuses *Ehrlichia* and *Anaplasma* which are transmitted by *Ixodes* ticks across Europe and North America. It presents with fever, chills, and commonly headache, with or without nausea and vomiting. Infection in hyposplenic patients is reportedly more severe than in normal individuals. The diagnosis is usually based on serology, and doxycycline 100 mg bd for 14–21 days is the mainstay of treatment. Where dual infection is suspected, separate treatment for babesiosis and ehrlichiosis must be given.

Further reading

Bach O, Baier M, Pullwitt A, et al. (2005). Falciparum malaria after splenectomy: a prospective controlled study of 33 previously splenectomized Malawian adults. *Transactions of the Royal Society of Tropical Medicine and Hygiene*, **99**, 861–7.

Cadili A (2010). Encapsulated bacterial infections following splenectomy. *Reviews in Medical Microbiology*, **21**, 7–10.

Davidson RN and Wall RA (2001). Prevention and management of infections in patients without a spleen. *Clinical Microbiology and Infection*, **7**, 657–60.

Davies JM, Barnes R, Milligan D (2002). Update of guidelines for the prevention and treatment of infection in patients with an absent or dysfunctional spleen. *Clinical Medicine*, **2**, 440–3.

Goldblatt F, Chambers S, Rahman A, Isenberg DA (2009). Serious infections in British patients with systemic lupus erythematosus: hospitalizations and mortality. *Lupus*, **18**, 682–9.

Lynch AM and Kapila R (1996). Overwhelming post-splenectomy infection. *Infectious Disease Clinics of North America*, **10**, 693–707.

Secondary immunodeficiency in malignancy or post-chemotherapy

Most cancer chemotherapy produces a dose-dependent pancytopenia which is immunosuppressive because it frequently causes neutropenia. However, cancer chemotherapy may lead to profound suppression of cellular and humoral immunity. Newly acquired delayed-type hypersensitivity (DTH) and primary humoral responses appear to be more susceptible to drug-induced immunosuppression than secondary memory immune responses. Neutropenia can occur transiently, typically 7–14 days following a chemotherapy cycle, and may be profound. Febrile neutropenia (FN) or neutropenic sepsis can progress rapidly and carries a mortality of 10%. Multiple international bodies have published guidelines on the management of febrile neutropenia (including NICE clinical guideline 151 (CG151) 2012). We summarize the various guidelines below.

Cancer chemotherapy often damages mucosal surfaces, increasing the risk of oropharyngeal, respiratory, gastrointestinal, urinary, and bacteraemic infections. Chemotherapeutic drugs that cause mucositis include chlorambucil, cisplatin, cytarabine (Ara-C), doxorubicin, fluorouracil (5-FU), and methotrexate. Damage to the ciliary function of the respiratory tract increases the risk of pneumonia. Methotrexate and vincristine inhibit phagocytosis and the killing ability of granulocytes, producing qualitative impairment of host defence mechanisms. Cytotoxic agents produce suppression of cellular immunity. Impaired cellular immunity may also occur after prolonged corticosteroid therapy (e.g. in patients with CNS tumours) and may lead to opportunistic infections (e.g. PCP, mycobacterial, fungal).

Malignancy in itself can predispose to infection, either due to local effects or due to bone marrow suppression (particularly leukaemia and non-Hodgkin's lymphoma). Local effects need to be considered on a case-by-case basis. For example, bronchial carcinoma, causing distal lung collapse, may lead to recurrent lower respiratory tract infection due to the inability to expel secretions on coughing. Extended courses of antibiotics may be required, and prophylactic antibiotics should be considered. Ideally, the local effect should be removed. In this case, stenting or ablation of the tumour may be possible. Another common local predisposing effect is tumour necrosis. This produces a region that is difficult for both antibiotics and the immune system to penetrate. Excision may be considered, but often this is contraindicated by the functional status of the patient. Again, extended courses of antibiotics may be required. Fungating tumours with superinfection may be amenable to topical antibiotics, such as metronidazole.

Febrile neutropenia

Commonly, fever is the only sign of severe infection in neutropenic patients, as neutropenia prohibits the local inflammation that is responsible for clinical signs. Case definitions vary slightly; most authors would agree that a patient with a single temperature measurement of 38.5°C or two measurements of 38.0°C, 1 hour apart, and a neutrophil count of <0.5 x 10^9/L, following chemotherapy, would have FN. Some guidelines permit a slightly lower fever or a neutrophil count up to 1.0 x 10^9/L if it is expected to fall. Such patients should be managed by the oncology or haematology service administering the chemotherapy or by medical professionals with experience in FN.

Common aetiological agents by site

- **Unknown:** coagulase-negative staphylococci, *Escherichia coli*, *Enterococcus* species.
- **Lung:** *Pseudomonas aeruginosa*, pneumococci, alpha-haemolytic streptococci, *Acinetobacter* species.
- **Abdomen:** *E. coli*, *Pseudomonas aeruginosa*, *Clostridium* species, *Enterococcus* species, *Klebsiella* species.
- **Urogenital:** *E. coli*, *Klebsiella* species, *P. aeruginosa*.
- **Soft tissues:** *Staphylococcus aureus*, alpha-haemolytic streptococci.
- **Central lines:** coagulase-negative staphylococci, *Corynebacteriae*, *Propionibacterium* species, *Candida albicans*, *Candida tropicalis*.

Assessment and investigation

Rapid assessment and administration of appropriate antibiotics is essential. Key points in the history include the chemotherapy administered, any recent surgery, any antibiotic prophylaxis, and any prior infections. Available microbiological information, particularly with reference to resistant organisms is essential. Multiple sets of blood cultures should be taken, at a minimum either two peripheral or one peripheral and one from every lumen of any indwelling line. In addition throat swabs and cultures from any sites that may represent an infective focus, such as wound or line sites or urine and stool, should be obtained. Do not perform digital rectal examination, as this can cause bacteraemia. A chest radiograph should be performed routinely. Consider nasopharyngeal swabs for respiratory virus PCR, particularly during influenza season. Aggressive fluid resuscitation may be required; hypotension disproportionate to fever may be suggestive of Gram-negative bacteraemia. The Multinational Association for Supportive Care in Cancer index (MASCC index) has been used for risk stratification and can be used before the neutrophil count is available and without access to specific information about the disease or therapeutic status of the patient. Available in J Klastersky *et al.* (2000).

Antibiotics in febrile neutropenia

Despite appropriate cultures being taken, no causative organism is identified in most cases of febrile neutropenia. A clinical diagnosis of a source of infection is apparent in 10–20% of cases, and bacteraemia is identified in 15–25%. As a result, antimicrobial use in febrile neutropenia is largely protocol-driven. There is ongoing discussion about the most appropriate antibiotics for empiric therapy, and most hospitals have local guidelines, which should ensure easy and rapid access to the required agents. These should also take into account the local prevalence of antibiotic-resistant organisms. Antibiotics should be administered within 1 hour of the arrival of the patient in the emergency department. Neutropenia is largely predictable, and there is little reason to wait for the FBC before commencing antibiotics.

In patients with low-risk MASCC scores who do not have pneumonia, indwelling catheter infections, or severe soft tissue infection, oral antibiotics can be considered. Some units consider patients for outpatient oral therapy; this should only be used for patients who will be discharged to a safe environment with rapid (less than 1 hour) access to an inpatient unit with 24-hour cover, and they must be reviewed daily. In 20% of cases, readmission is required. This management option is not recommended for non-specialists. Oral quinolone plus co-amoxiclav (clindamycin may substitute in penicillin allergy) is recommended in patients who have not taken quinolone prophylaxis.

Empiric intravenous antibiotics remain the mainstay of treatment and should be administered to all other patients. Recommended regimens include meropenem, imipenem, piperacillin/tazobactam, or ceftazidime monotherapy or dual therapy with either aminoglycoside plus piperacillin/tazobactam, piperacillin/tazobactam plus ciprofloxacin, or aminoglycoside plus ceftazidime. Monotherapy regimes are associated with fewer adverse events and similar survival when compared to regimens containing aminoglycosides. A macrolide should be added in the case of community-acquired pneumonia. Vancomycin should be added empirically if there is an indwelling venous catheter or soft tissue infection is suspected clinically or if the patient is known to be colonized by MRSA. It should be considered in patients who have taken ciprofloxacin or co-trimoxazole prophylaxis or in whom septic shock develops. It should also be added into the existing regime if Gram-positive organisms are identified on blood cultures, pending identification and sensitivities. Add metronidazole if *Clostridium difficile* is suspected, and consider including it, if intra-abdominal sepsis is among the differential diagnoses and where the patient is not already receiving piperacillin/tazobactam or meropenem (which have good anaerobic cover).

Ongoing management
The patient should receive frequent reassessment initially, particularly where fluid resuscitation has been required. Granulocyte colony-stimulating factor (G-CSF) may be administered in pneumonia or severe infection or in prolonged neutropenia. At 48 hours, if the fever continues, the patient should be reassessed and, if deteriorating, should be investigated for resistant bacterial or fungal infection. Such patients should be managed by physicians with experience in febrile neutropenia, with microbiology input. CT of the chest and abdomen should be considered to look for evidence of fungal infection. Empiric antibiotics can be broadened, according to protocol or microbiological advice. If VRE are suspected, consider linezolid or daptomycin; carbapenem-resistant *Pseudomonas aeruginosa* may be sensitive to piperacillin/tazobactam or aminoglycoside; if carbapenem-resistant Gram-negative bacilli are suspected, consider colistin or tigecyclin. *Pneumocystis jirovecii* pneumonia should be suspected in patients with diffuse lung infiltrates and exertional hypoxia and is treated with high-dose co-trimoxazole.

Once fever and neutropenia have resolved, consider switching to oral antibiotics. Low-risk patients can be transferred to oral therapy and considered for early discharge. High-risk patients should continue IV antibiotics until clinically well. Some guidelines recommend stopping aminoglycosides at this point to reduce associated complications.

Intravenous catheter infection
Evidence on the recommended management of IV catheter infections is conflicting. Ideally, the line should be removed, if possible. Depending on the causative organism, it may be possible to preserve the line, for example, using teicoplanin as a line lock in *Staphylococcus aureus* IV catheter infection. However, treatment failure is common, and the convenience of retaining the line must be balanced against the possibility of peripheral seeding of bacteria. In *Candida* IV catheter infection, the line must be removed.

Antifungal agents
If fever continues after 4–7 days, empirical antifungal agents are commonly recommended. Liposomal amphotericin or an echinocandin, such as caspofungin, are suitable agents. Fluconazole can be used in patients at low risk of *Aspergillus* infection and who have not received azole prophylaxis. Once begun, antifungal agents should be continued until the patient is no longer neutropenic or for a minimum of 14 days in proven fungal infection.

Further reading
Aapro MS, Bohlius J, Cameron DA, et al. (2011). 2010 update of EORTC guidelines for the use of granulocyte-colony stimulating factor to reduce the incidence of chemotherapy-induced febrile neutropenia in adult patients with lymphoproliferative disorders and solid tumours. *European Journal of Cancer*, **47**, 8–32.

de Naurois J, Novitzky-Basso I, Gill MJ, Marti FM, Cullen MH, Roila F (2010). Management of febrile neutropenia: ESMO Clinical Practice Guidelines. *Annals of Oncology*, **21** (Suppl 5), v252–6.

Freifeld AG, Bow EJ, Sepkowitz KA, et al. (2011). Clinical practice guideline for the use of antimicrobial agents in neutropenic patients with cancer: 2010 update by the infectious diseases societies of America. *Clinical Infectious Diseases*, **52**, e56–93.

Innes H, Lim SL, Hall A, et al. (2008). Management of febrile neutropenia in solid tumours and lymphomas using the Multinational Association for Supportive Care in Cancer (MASCC) risk index: feasibility and safety in routine clinical practice. *Supportive Care in Cancer*, **16**, 485–91.

Klatersky J et al. (2000). The Multinational Association for Supportive Care in the Cancer Risk Index: A Multinational Scoring System for Identifying Low-Risk Febrile Neutropenic Cancer Patients. *Journal of Clinical Oncology*, **18**, 16, 3038–51.

Klatersky J and Paesmans M (2013). The Multinational Association for Supportive Care in Cancer (MASCC) risk index score: 10 years of use for identifying low-risk febrile neutropenic cancer patients. *Supportive Care in Cancer*, **21**(5), 1487–95.

National Comprehensive Cancer Network (NCCN) (2009). Prevention and treatment of cancer-related infections v2. <http://www.nccn.org/professionals/physician_gls/f_guidelines.asp#supportive>.

National Institute of Health and Care Excellence (2012). Neutropenic sepsis: prevention and management of neutropenic sepsis in cancer patients. NICE clinical guideline 151. <https://www.nice.org.uk/cg151>.

Immune dysfunction and systemic illness

A variety of chronic diseases can cause low level immuno-suppression, leaving the patient susceptible to infection. This immune dysfunction is caused by a range of mechanisms from anatomical defects to direct effector cell dysfunction. In the following sections, we discuss a number of common diseases that have immune dysfunction as a feature.

Diabetes mellitus

The prevalence of type 2 diabetes mellitus continues to rise and predisposes to infection in a number of ways. Elevated glucose in blood and tissues not only provides nutrition for bacteria, but also impairs lymphocyte function, leading to the so-called 'lazy lymphocyte' syndrome. This leads to a recently identified 2-fold increase in susceptibility to tuberculosis. In addition, neuropathy and arteriopathy combine to cause ulcers, and skin breakdown acts as a portal of infection. Glycosuria predisposes to urinary tract infection. Both fungal and bacterial infections are more prevalent in diabetes and may act synergistically, particularly in the leg where dermatophyte infections of the foot provide an entry point for Gram-positive bacteria to cause cellulitis. In poorly controlled diabetics, inflammation is impaired, and clinical signs may be slight when compared with the bacterial burden. This is particularly the case with soft tissue infections in adipose tissue of obese patients where extensive tissue necrosis can occur without obvious skin change. Diabetic patients also respond to sepsis differently to non-diabetics, with an increased incidence of acute kidney injury but less ARDS.

Common pathogens in diabetes mellitus
- *Staphylococcus aureus*.
- Group B *Streptococcus*.
- *Escherichia coli*.
- *Candida albicans*.
- *Pseudomonas aeruginosa*.

Clinical approach
Diabetic patients with sepsis may have one of a wide range of pathogens or may have polymicrobial infection. Bacteria often behave differently in a high-glucose environment, for example, *Staphylococcus aureus* infections can be gas-forming. In addition, diabetic patients have frequently had previous antibiotic exposure which predisposes to resistant organisms. It is important to establish the presence or absence of MRSA carriage early to guide management. Cultures should be taken from blood and any potential focus of infection, and antibiotics should be commenced which are broad enough to cover the likely pathogens. In most cases, these will be the same as for non-diabetic patients. Meticulous glucose control with sliding scale insulin improves outcomes, and metformin should be stopped, as it can cause metabolic acidosis. Infected fluid collections should be managed in conjunction with the appropriate surgical team. Extended courses of antibiotics may be required. For soft tissue infections, antibiotics with good tissue penetration, such as clindamycin or linezolid, may be preferred, although there is little trial evidence of superiority over traditional beta-lactam antibiotics.

Connective tissue diseases

Diseases, such as systemic lupus erythematosus (SLE) commonly cause immune dysfunction. In the case of SLE, this dysfunction affects both innate and adaptive immunity. Patients may be functionally hyposplenic and have disorders of complement function. Early complement disorders impair opsonization of encapsulated organisms; late disorders increase susceptibility to *Neisseria* species. Pneumonia is the most common clinical presentation.

Infection accounts for 25% of deaths in SLE. Most organisms identified from SLE patients are normal pathogenic bacteria, such as *Streptococcus pneumoniae* or *Haemophilus influenzae*. Oral prednisolone is a particular risk factor, with each 10 mg per day increasing the risk of infection 11-fold. The majority of deaths are in patients with serologically active disease and receiving high dose prednisolone and at least one other immunosuppressive agent. It is important to recognize the possibility of rapid progression in these patients. A significant proportion of *Haemophilus* isolates are resistant to amoxicillin, so co-amoxiclav or a cephalosporin, such as cefuroxime, are recommended, in addition to a macrolide, in community-acquired pneumonia.

In other connective tissue diseases, a range of local factors predispose to particular infections. Lung fibrosis increases the risk of pneumonia, and oesophageal dysfunction (e.g. in systemic sclerosis) can lead to aspiration pneumonia. Soft tissue infections, particularly with *Staphylococcus aureus*, are common in patients with calcinosis, severe Raynaud's, and digital infarcts. Group G *Streptococcus* pyomyositis may develop in patients treated with chlorambucil. *M. avium intracellulare* may be a cause of septic arthritis. In patients with scleroderma *Nocardia* may cause ocular infections. Oesophageal fungal infections may also occur in patients with or without oesophageal involvement.

Chronic liver disease

Cirrhosis is associated with a 2–3-fold increase in hospital admissions for sepsis and death from sepsis, and up to 25% of patients admitted with cirrhosis develop a bacterial infection during hospitalization. In addition, ongoing chronic excessive alcohol intake is associated with impaired cell-mediated immunity and susceptibility to bacterial and mycobacterial infection. Patients are at risk from both Gram-positive and Gram-negative infections. The gut is a major source of infecting bacteria, and pneumonia caused by Gram-negative organisms is more common in cirrhotic patients. In addition, sepsis is associated with an increased risk of acute kidney injury, and this is an independent risk factor for death in these patients. Careful fluid balance is, therefore, a priority, and clinicians should have a low threshold for invasive monitoring and management on an intensive care unit with the input of specialist hepatologists.

Spontaneous bacterial peritonitis (SBP) may develop in any patient with cirrhosis, portal hypertension, and ascites. Clinical features are often absent (25%), and SBP may be present in 15% of patients admitted with ascites, so it is essential that all patients with ascites have an ascitic tap to assess the presence of SBP on admission. Symptoms may include malaise, encephalopathy, fever, and abdominal pain (60%). Rigors are rare. An ascitic fluid polymorphonuclear leucocyte count of >250/mm^3 is diagnostic of SBP. *E. coli*, staphylococci, and pneumococci may be isolated from ascitic fluid cultures. Anaerobes are rarely isolated. Secondary bacterial peritonitis from gut perforation or punctured bowel post-paracentesis may yield multiple organisms. The antibiotic of choice is cefotaxime or another third-generation cephalosporin. Second-line antibiotics include co-amoxiclav and ciprofloxacin in patients who are not on quinolone prophylaxis. Aminoglycosides frequently cause renal failure in this context and should be avoided. Patients who develop SBP need long-term prophylaxis and specific management, including supplementation with albumin (see Chapter 8).

Down's syndrome

Trisomy 21 leads to a wide range of immunological dysfunction with disordered T and B cells and reduced responses to a range of vaccines, including pneumococcal, influenza, polio, tetanus, and pertussis. Much of the pathology in Down's syndrome is thought to be due to premature ageing. B cell function appears to deteriorate after 6 years, with increased class 1 and 3 IgG at the expense of classes 2 and 4 with decreased IgM. However, recent studies suggest this is an oversimplification and that multiple immune disorders are intrinsic to Down's syndrome. In childhood, recurrent ENT infections are common. Macroglossia and altered airway anatomy are likely contributors to the primary immune dysfunction. In adulthood, pneumonia is a more common infection. Autoimmune and lymphoproliferative disorders are also prevalent. In general terms, management is as for normal adults, but the physician should be aware that the patient may respond poorly to treatment. In addition, patients with learning difficulties may not cooperate with treatment, and early sedation and ventilation should be considered.

Renal impairment and dialysis

Renal impairment leads to chronic inflammation, with activation of Toll-like receptor pathways. Uraemia leads to reduced synthesis of nitric oxide by macrophages and impaired apoptosis of neutrophils. Furthermore, haemodialysis may provoke further inflammation due to the bioincompatibility of the materials used and low-level contamination of dialysis fluid by bacterial wall components. Peritoneal dialysis fluid has a low pH, high glucose and lactate, and contains glucose degradation products, all of which have been shown *in vitro* to produce chronic immune activation. Both haemodialysis and peritoneal dialysis breach the skin which normally acts as a major barrier to infection. As a result, the pathogens involved in these cases tend to be staphylococci, either *S. aureus* or coagulase-negative staphylococci. In renal dialysis patients, infection is the leading cause of death after cardiovascular events.

Haemodialysis fistula and vascath infection

- Take blood cultures from peripheral sites and intravenous catheters. *S. aureus* is the commonest pathogen.

- Vancomycin is recommended for patients with extended hospital exposure or who have ever had MRSA colonization or infection. In dialysis patients, a single dose is sufficient until the next dialysis.
- In critically ill patients, consider additional Gram-negative and *Candida* cover. Fluconazole can be used in patients without recent azole exposure; otherwise, consider an echinocandin, such as caspofungin.
- Intravenous catheters should be removed if infected with *S. aureus*, *P. aeruginosa*, mycobacteria, or fungi. With other organisms, salvage therapy can be considered with antibiotic line locks, e.g. teicoplanin for coagulase-negative staphylococci.

Peritoneal dialysis peritonitis

- *S. aureus* and *P. aeruginosa* are the most common, and most serious infections.
- Exit site infections may be treated with oral antibiotics to cover *S. aureus*.
- Exit site infections may progress to peritonitis.
- Peritonitis typically presents with cloudy fluid and abdominal pain; however, in some cases, the fluid remains clear.
- Diagnosis is by increased WCC in aspirated dialysis fluid; the exact level is dependent on the 'dwell time' of the fluid; >100 cells/microlitre after 2 hours is positive.
- Empirical antibiotics are either vancomycin or a cephalosporin for Gram-positive organisms and a third-generation cephalosporin or aminoglycoside for Gram-negative organisms.
- Intraperitoneal antibiotics are superior to intravenous.
- In all, except coagulase-negative staphylococcal infections, the catheter must be removed rapidly, rather than subject the patient to ongoing peritonitis.

Further reading

Esper AM, Moss M, Martin GS (2009). The effect of diabetes mellitus on organ dysfunction with sepsis: an epidemiological study. *Critical Care*, **13**, R18.

Foreman MG, Mannino DM, Moss M (2003). Cirrhosis as a risk factor for sepsis and death analysis of the National Hospital Discharge Survey. *Chest*, **124**, 1016–20.

Li PK, Szeto CC, Piraino B, *et al.* (2010). Peritoneal dialysis-related infections recommendations: 2010 update. *Peritoneal Dialysis International*, **30**, 393–423.

Mermel LA, Allon M, Bouza E, *et al.* (2009). Clinical practice guidelines for the diagnosis and management of intravascular catheter-related infection: 2009 Update by the Infectious Diseases Society of America. *Clinical Infectious Diseases*, **49**, 1–45.

Solid organ transplant

Recipients of solid organ transplants receive relatively high doses of immunosuppressive drugs for a few months following transplantation, followed by maintenance at the lowest effective immunosuppressive dose. Transplant recipients are susceptible to bacterial, viral, and fungal infection, and post-transplant infection now exceeds acute rejection as the main cause of hospitalization post-transplant. Fungal infection is also associated with reduced graft survival. Acute infection in transplant recipients, particularly during the first 6 months post-transplant or for any infection other than simple bacterial infections, should be managed by, or in conjunction with, a specialist transplantation unit, as modifications of immunosuppressive therapy may be required. In this regard, acute infection is a risk factor for graft rejection, so immunosuppression should not be reduced acutely, except on the advice of experienced transplant clinicians.

Infections can be grouped according to the time post-transplant and epidemiologically by source, either donor-derived, recipient-derived, nosocomial, or community-acquired.

It is difficult to assess the level of immunosuppression of the patient, as this is a function of medication, tolerance of the graft, and individual variation. In addition, susceptibility to infection is influenced by vaccination and prophylaxis.

High risk factors
- Anti-T cell antibodies (alemtuzumab) in induction.
- Pulsed corticosteroids.
- Plasmapheresis.
- Early graft rejection.
- Graft dysfunction.
- High risk of rejection (e.g. due to poor HLA match).
- Surgical complications.

Early period (0–1 months)
Patients in the initial post-transplant period are rarely seen in acute medicine, as they tend to remain under the direct care of the transplantation service. Infections in these patients tend to be recipient-derived infections, including *Aspergillus* and *Pseudomonas* or, most commonly, nosocomial. Likely nosocomial pathogens depend on the post-operative course but include MRSA, VRE, resistant *Candida* species, *Clostridium difficile*, and intra-abdominal Gram-negative rods in the event of anastomotic leaks, other surgical complications, or catheter-associated infections. In particular, renal transplant recipients are at risk of Gram-negative bacteraemia. Uncommonly, infections are donor-derived, including HSV and lymphocytic choriomeningitis virus (LCMV).

Intermediate period (1–6 months)
In this period, tolerance to the graft is established. Most febrile episodes are due either to viral infections or acute rejection. Historically, *Pneumocystis jirovecii* and CMV were important pathogens, but most patients now receive co-trimoxazole and antiviral prophylaxis with an agent, such as valganciclovir. Co-trimoxazole is effective prophylaxis against PCP, *Toxoplasma gondii*, *Listeria monocytogenes*, most urinary tract infections, and some *Nocardia* strains. As a result, other infections are prominent, such as BK polyoma-virus which causes nephritis in renal transplant recipients and has become an increasingly well-recognized cause of

graft failure over the past decade. Patients are commonly asymptomatic and present with worsening renal function. Diagnosis is by PCR for BK virus DNA in blood or urine, and treatment requires a reduction in immunosuppression, with or without antiviral medication, such as cidofovir or leflunomide. Untreated graft failure rates are between 30% and 60%.

Other common intermediate period infections include *Clostridium difficile*, adenovirus, influenza, and *Mycobacterium tuberculosis*.

Late period (>6 months)
After the first 6 months, post-transplantation immunosuppression is reduced, so risk of infection falls. The risk period for reactivation of latent donor and recipient-derived infections has passed, and patients have less healthcare exposure, so most infections are community-acquired. Community-acquired pneumonia and urinary tract infections are common (and rates of resistance to antibiotics in this context are increasing), as are *Aspergillus* and other fungal infections and opportunistic bacterial infections with *Listeria* or *Nocardia*. Treatment is with the usual antimicrobials used for these infections, but prolonged courses should be considered, following discussion with microbiology or infectious diseases physicians. Late-stage viral infections include CMV (commonly presenting with colitis or retinitis), HSV, HBV, HCV, EBV causing post-transplant lymphoproliferative disease (PTLD), and JC polyomavirus causing progressive multifocal leukoencephalopathy.

CMV post-transplant
In immunocompetent hosts, primary infection is either asymptomatic or causes an EBV-like glandular fever. CMV in transplant recipients causes both direct and immunological effects. Direct effects of CMV infection include viraemic symptoms of fever, malaise, arthralgia, and end-organ damage causing retinitis, nephritis, hepatitis, colitis, carditis, and pneumonitis. CMV reactivation may occur due to increases in immunosuppression or acute infection, causing lymphocyte activation. Serology can help to assess susceptibility but is unhelpful in acute infection when CMV viraemia measurement by PCR of serum is used. Intravenous ganciclovir is the recommended therapy; oral valganciclovir is an alternative but is not recommended in GI disease. Relapse is common with inadequate therapy and risks the development of resistant CMV, which is treated with more toxic agents, such as cidofovir or foscarnet.

CMV reactivation also causes immune activation and cytokine-mediated effects which can cause allograft rejection or failure and be a risk factor for opportunistic infection and for EBV-associated PTLD.

Post-transplant lymphoproliferative disease
PTLD is a term encompassing a range of lymphoproliferative disorders and occurs in up to 10% of transplant recipients, with a mortality of 50%.

Presentations of PTLD
- Fever or mononucleosis-like illness.
- Abdominal mass.
- Allograft infiltration.
- Hepatic or pancreatic dysfunction.
- CNS disease.

EBV viral load testing and EBV staining on histology may guide diagnosis. Treatment is by reduction of immunosuppression, and, for progressive disease, chemotherapy or radiotherapy may be required.

Further reading

Al-Hasan MN (2009). Incidence rate and outcome of Gram-negative bloodstream infection in solid organ transplant recipients. *American Journal of Transplantation*, **9**, 835–43.

Dall A and Hariharan S (2008). BK virus nephritis after renal transplantation. *Clinical Journal of the American Society of Nephrology*, **3**, S68–75.

Dharnidharka VR, Stablein DM, Harmon WE (2004). Post-transplant infections now exceed acute rejection as cause for hospitalization: a report of the NAPRTCS. *American Journal of Transplantation*, **4**, 384–9.

Fishman JA (2007). Infection in solid-organ transplant. *New England Journal of Medicine*, **357**, 2601–14.

Immunosuppressive therapy

Management of infections in the context of immunosuppressive therapy is challenging. This is because manifestations of infection and exacerbations of the underlying rheumatological disease may be identical, immunosuppression may mask clinical signs, and a wide range of organisms may be implicated. In addition, the underlying disorder commonly predisposes to infection, so the contribution of the therapeutic agent may be unclear.

Predominant pathogens by site

1. Respiratory tract: *Streptococcus pneumoniae*, *Haemophilus influenzae*, *Staphylococcus aureus*, *Legionella* spp. and enteric Gram-negative rods are the most frequent cause of pneumonia. *Pneumocystis carinii* is the most common opportunistic pulmonary infection in rheumatology patients. Other pathogens include fungi (*Aspergillus* spp. *Cryptococcus neoformans*, *Coccidiodes immitis*, *Histoplasma capsulatum*), mycobacteria, *Nocardia* spp., and cytomegalovirus (CMV) (rare).
2. Urinary tract: enteric Gram-negative organisms and *Enterococcus* spp.
3. CNS: the most common pathogens include *C. neoformans*, *Listeria monocytogenes*, *S. pneumoniae*, *H. influenzae*, *N. meningitidis*, and *Nocardia* spp. Less common pathogens include *Mycobacterium tuberculosis*, *C. immitis*, *Strongyloides stercoralis*, *Toxoplasma gondii*, *Aspergillus* spp., and JC virus (PML).
4. Bone and joint: *S. aureus* (most common), Gram-negative rods.
5. Bacteraemia without an obvious source: *S. aureus*, enteric Gram-negative rods.

Corticosteroids

Daily oral corticosteroids are used in a wide variety of diseases. Their actions are wide-ranging, with reduced B, T, and antigen-presenting cell activity, impaired NO and cytokine synthesis by macrophages, and reduced neutrophil and eosinophil function. It is unusual for short courses to lead to infection, but regular use, particularly at high doses, predisposes to a wide range of infections, including both Gram-positive and Gram-negative bacteria, *Candida* spp., and herpesviruses, including HSV and VZV. At doses above the equivalent of prednisolone 1 mg/kg/day, opportunistic infections, e.g. with PCP, *Cryptococcus* and *Listeria monocytogenes* become increasingly common.

Tacrolimus and sirolimus

These agents impair T cell function and proliferation and thereby cause a secondary impairment of B cell antibody production due to reduced T helper cell function. They predispose to a similar range of infectious agents as cyclophosphamide, although infectious complications appear to be less frequent. Conflicting data exist regarding HSV reactivation with topical tacrolimus, with some studies showing increased reactivation and others no change.

Methotrexate

Methotrexate inhibits T cell cytokine production and induces T cell apoptosis. Once weekly methotrexate remains a mainstay of treatment in rheumatoid arthritis. This low-dose therapy is associated with no increased susceptibility to infection. This is believed to be due to the improved inflammatory and immunological function on methotrexate.

Methotrexate may be continued through very mild viral infections but, in severe infections requiring hospital admission, methotrexate should be withheld until antibiotics are complete and the patient is clinically well. Methotrexate can be continued through uncomplicated shingles if oral aciclovir is commenced. In more severe VZV infection (e.g. multidermatomal shingles or primary chickenpox), IV aciclovir should be used and methotrexate discontinued for 5–10 days until resolution.

Azathioprine

Azathioprine therapy has been shown not to be an independent risk factor for infection in a case series of 223 patients with SLE; however, azathioprine-induced bone marrow suppression does cause significant immunosuppression. This may be because azathioprine use is associated with reduced requirement for corticosteroids, which have been shown to predispose to infection in a dose-dependent manner. Pneumonia, in the context of azathioprine use, is associated with poorer outcome.

Ciclosporin

Ciclosporin down regulates IL-2 production and inhibits T cell proliferation and activation. *In vitro*, it causes mild inhibition of replication of certain fungal, helminthic, and protozoal organisms, but these are of no clinical significance. In high doses, the drug causes marked immunosuppression and renders the patient susceptible to infection by a wide range of viruses, bacteria, and fungi. In a non-transplantation setting, there is little evidence of increased infection. In one series on patients with myasthenia gravis, the number of infections requiring antibiotics was greater in the placebo arm. In 1,000 patients treated with low-dose ciclosporin, one patient developed *Legionella* pneumonia, and three cases of aseptic meningitis were reported. Aseptic meningitis was reported in other early studies with ciclosporin. Ciclosporin is known to increase susceptibility to herpesvirus infection, and it is likely that some of these episodes represent reactivations of HSV. Many antibiotics interact with ciclosporin metabolism, and levels should be monitored carefully while infection is treated. Levels are increased by amphotericin, erythromycin, itraconazole, and ketoconazole. Levels are reduced by rifampicin, isoniazid, co-trimoxazole, and imipenem. Cefuroxime, cefotaxime, co-trimoxazole, ketoconazole, amphotericin, and aciclovir can cause additive nephrotoxicity when co-administered with ciclosporin, and, if possible, ciclosporin should be withdrawn whilst the patient is on antibiotics. In the context of transplantation, this is rarely possible (see 'Solid organ transplant').

Mycophenolate mofetil

Mycophenolate mofetil is a newer immunosuppressive agent that is replacing cyclophosphamide for indications, such as lupus nephritis. It suppresses lymphocyte proliferation, antibody production, and NK cell activity. As a result, it predisposes to infection with herpesviruses; in one trial with 11 clinically significant infections, eight were with herpesviruses: four VZV (shingles), two HSV, and two CMV. In these cases, we recommend withdrawing the mycophenolate while the infection is treated. Progressive multifocal leukoencephalopathy has also been reported with mycophenolate. Withdrawal of the drug and supportive care are the only treatments.

Cyclophosphamide

Cyclophosphamide impairs both T and B cell function and, in one series of patients with rheumatoid arthritis, was associated with a 6-fold increased risk of infection requiring hospitalization. Infection does not correlate well with dose, duration, or leucopenia and is most common in males over 60 years of age. Infections may be caused by standard bacteria as well as by herpesviruses, respiratory viruses, and opportunistic infections, such as tuberculosis, *Cryptococcus*, *Pneumocystis jirovecii*, *Listeria*, *Nocardia*, and a variety of fungal infections.

Anti-TNF agents

Compared to other disease-modifying anti-rheumatic drugs (DMARDs) the anti-tumour necrosis factor (anti-TNF) agents infliximab, adalimumab, and etanercept do not increase the overall incidence or severity of infection when adjusted for age, sex, and disease severity. They are, however, associated with a 4-fold increased risk of serious skin and soft tissue infections, as well as an increased risk of infections with intracellular bacteria. In the British Biologics Register report (2006), there were 19 intracellular bacteria infections in the anti-TNF group and 0 in the control group. Ten were caused by *Mycobacterium tuberculosis*; the rest were *Listeria monocytogenes*, *Salmonella* species, *Legionella pneumophila*, and one case of *Mycobacterium fortuitum*. The sites of these infections were unusual; seven of the ten tuberculosis cases were extrapulmonary and two of the *Listeria* and two of the *Salmonella* infections involved the joints. There were no significant differences between the three agents, although case numbers were small. Other sources suggest that infliximab is the most immunosuppressant of the three agents and may predispose to tuberculosis most strongly.

Anti-TNF agents and tuberculosis

All patients commenced on anti-TNF agents are screened by chest radiograph (CXR) and interferon-gamma release assay (IGRA) before the drug is commenced and treated for latent tuberculosis if this is detected. IGRA has high sensitivity for tuberculosis exposure in normal individuals, but the sensitivity in patients with connective tissue disease is unclear, particularly in patients taking regular DMARDs or corticosteroids. The CXR may contribute to the disproportionately low number of cases of pulmonary TB seen. Tuberculosis infection is most common in the first 3 months after initiation of therapy and, in these cases, represents reactivation of latent disease. There is, however, a low overall incidence of TB infection, even in prolonged use, which is thought to represent new infection. Tuberculosis in these patients may present acutely with pneumonia, lymphadenopathy, or meningitis. Diagnostic methods are unchanged and based on identifying acid-fast bacilli in the relevant tissue or fluid, either by direct microscopy or TB culture. The burden of mycobacteria may be higher in these patients, aiding rapid diagnosis. Treatment for tuberculosis is as normal; anti-TNF agents should be withdrawn during treatment but may be reintroduced once treatment is completed. There are theoretical reasons to believe that treatment could be reintroduced more rapidly in drug-sensitive disease, as the bulk of mycobacterial burden is cleared in the first 2 weeks, and anti-TNF agents have been used in paradoxical reaction (an effect opposite to that which would normally be expected) with success, but no trial data exist to support this practice.

Primary immunodeficiency disease

Primary immunodeficiencies are rare inherited disorders, often with recessive or X-linked recessive inheritance (see Table 13.3). Patients present in childhood with recurrent

Table 13.3 Primary immunodeficiency diseases and associated pathogens

Disorder	Functional deficiency	Predominant pathogens
B cell defects		
X-linked agammaglobulinaemia (XLA)	Absent B cells; sinopulmonary infections, enterovirus meningoencephalitis	Pneumococci, *Haemophilus*, mycoplasma, *Giardia*, poliovirus, echovirus, Coxsackie virus
X-linked hyper-IgM syndrome (XHIM)	Low IgA, low IgG, elevated IgM, T cell defect, neutropenia, interstitial pneumonia	As above and *Pneumocystis jirovecii*
Activation-induced cytidine deaminase deficiency (AID)	Autosomal recessive hyper-IgM syndrome, antibody deficiency	As above for XLA
NFkB essential modulator deficiency (NEMO)	Autosomal recessive hyper-IgM syndrome, antibody deficiency, reduced NK cytotoxic activity, hyperhidrotic ectodermal dysplasia	As above for XLA
Common variable immunodeficiency (CVID)	B and T cell defect, hypogammaglobulinaemia; poor vaccine antibody response, autoimmune cytopenia, alopecia areata, vitiligo, rheumatoid arthritis, SLE, sprue-like syndrome, malignancy	Encapsulated bacteria, *Giardia* spp., *Yersinia spp.*, *H. pylori*, *H. jejuni*
Good's syndrome	CVID with thymoma, aplastic anaemia, agranulocytosis, thrombocytopenia	As above for CVID
IgG subclass deficiency	IgG2 and IgA deficiency with recurrent infections; IgG2 and IgG4 with chronic mucocutaneous candidiasis and bronchiectasis; IgG1 with pyogenic lung infections; IgG3 with respiratory and gut infections; IgG2 with poor polysaccharide responses	*Streptococcus pneumoniae*, *Candida* spp.

Table 13.3 Primary immunodeficiency diseases and associated pathogens (continued)

Disorder	Functional deficiency	Predominant pathogens
Specific antibody deficiency	Poor antibody responses to polysaccharide vaccine	*Streptococcus pneumoniae*
Selective IgA deficiency	Allergy, autoimmunity, malignancy, infections of respiratory/urinary tract, sprue-like syndrome	Encapsulated bacteria
Selective IgM deficiency	Septicaemia, meningitis, pneumonia, otitis, pyogenic skin infection	*Meningococcus*, Gram-negative organisms, *Pneumococcus*
Transient hypogammaglobulinaemia of infancy	Prolonged low IgG for first 2 years, no specific antibody deficiency	Unknown
T cell defects		
X-linked severe combined immunodeficiency (SCID)	Absent T cells, present B cells, absent NK cells; T– B+ NK–	*Candida* spp., *Cryptococcus*, *Histoplasma*, *Nocardia*, *P. carinii*, *Toxoplasma*, *cryptosporidium*, herpes simplex, varicella zoster, cytomegalovirus, adenovirus, parainfluenza, respiratory syncytial virus, *M. tuberculosis*, *M. avium complex*, *Listeria monocytogenes*
JAK3 deficiency	Absent T cells, present B cells, absent NK cells; T– B+ NK–	As above for X-linked SCID
Recombinase activating gene (RAG), Omenn's syndrome	T– B– NK+	As above for X-linked SCID
IL-7 receptor deficiency	T– B+ NK+	As above for X-linked SCID
Adenine deaminase deficiency (ADA)	T– B– NK–	As above for X-linked SCID
Purine nucleoside phosphorylase deficiency (PNP)	T– B+ NK+	As above for X-linked SCID
CD3 T cell receptor defects	T– B+ NK+	As above for X-linked SCID
MHC class I defects	T– B+ NK+, absent CD4	As above for X-linked SCID
MHC class II defects	T- B+ NK+, absent CD8	As above for X-linked SCID
ZAP70 defects	T+ B+ , absent CD8	As above for X-linked SCID
Idiopathic CD4 lymphopenia (Nezelof syndrome)	Reduced CD4, autoimmune cytopenia, lymphoma	Chronic mucocutaneous candidiasis, herpesviruses, Gram-negative sepsis
Thymic hypoplasia (DiGeorge syndrome)	Low T cell numbers, poor vaccination responses, congenital heart disease, hypocalcaemia	*Pneumocystis jirovecii*, *C. albicans*
Wiskott-Aldrich syndrome (WAS)	T cell defect, poor vaccination antibody responses, eczema, thrombocytopenia, malignancy, arthritis, haemolytic anaemia, vasculitis	*Streptococcus pneumoniae, H. influenza, Varicella, P. carinii*
Chronic mucocutaneous candidiasis (CMC)	Variable response to *Candida*, defects of mannan processing	Chronic *Candida* infections of skin, nails, and mucous membranes, pyogenic infections of skin, sinopulmonary tract and urinary tract, *Histoplasma capsulatum*
Hyper-IgE syndrome	Elevated IgE, impaired antibody response to polysaccharides, IgE antibodies to *S. aureus*	*S. aureus, C. albicans, Aspergillus* spp.
Ataxia telangiectasia	Variable T and B cell defects, malignancy, defective DNA repair, oculocutaneous telangiectasia, progressive cerebellar ataxia	Opportunistic infections, aspiration pneumonia
X-linked lymphoproliferative disease (XLP)	Inability of T cells to control Epstein–Barr virus, malignancy	Fulminant infectious mononucleosis
Cartilage hair hypoplasia	Moderate to severe T and B cell defect, short limb dwarfism, malignancy	*Varicella, Vaccinia*, oral candidiasis

Table 13.3 Primary immunodeficiency diseases and associated pathogens (continued)

Disorder	Functional deficiency	Predominant pathogens
Complement and cytokine disorders and abnormal neutrophils		
Complement C1q	Classical pathway, SLE, glomerulonephritis	Pyogenic infections, including meningitis, *Streptococcus*, *Staphylococcus*
Complement C1r/C1s	Classical pathway, SLE	As above for Complement C1q
Complement C4	Classical and Lectin pathways, SLE	As above for Complement C1q
Complement C2	Classical and Lectin pathways, SLE, juvenile rheumatoid arthritis	Pyogenic infections, e.g. pneumonia, meningitis, pyogenic arthritis with *Streptococcus pneumoniae*
Complement C3	SLE, glomerulonephritis	Pyogenic infections
Factor B	Alternative pathway	Neisseria infections, e.g. meningitis, sepsis, pyogenic arthritis; brucellosis, toxoplasmosis
Factor D	Alternative pathway	Neisseria infections
Properdin	Alternative pathway	Neisseria infections, rarely pyogenic infections
Mannose-binding lectin	Lectin pathway, SLE	Recurrent infections
Complement C6-C9	Membrane attack complex	Neisseria infections
Factor I	Haemolytic uraemic syndrome	*Streptococcus pneumoniae, Neisseria meningitidis*
Factor H	Glomerulonephritis	Neisseria infections
C1 inhibitor	Hereditary angioedema	Nil
Congenital neutropenia	Neutrophil <100/microlitre	Pyogenic infections including *Staphylococcus* and *Streptococcus* spp., fungal infections including *Aspergillus*
Shwachman's syndrome	Neutropenia and pancreatic insufficiency	*Staphylococcus aureus, Haemophilus influenzae, Streptococcus pneumoniae*, Gram-negative bacilli including *Pseudomonas* spp.
Chediak–Higashi syndrome	Neutrophil motility disorder, oculocutaneous albinism, giant lysosomal granules, absent NK cell activity	Recurrent pyogenic infections
Chronic granulomatous disease	Granulomatous lesions of GI tract, urinary tract, osteomyelitis, liver abscess, skin abscess, defect of NADPH oxidase complex	Catalase-positive *Staphylococcus aureus, Escherichia coli, Serratia marcescens, Salmonella, Chromobacterium, Candida albicans, Aspergillus*, and catalase-negative *Streptococcus pneumoniae*
Leucocyte adhesion deficiency 1	Defect of LFA-1 (CR3, CR4, CD11a, b , c), Absent CD18, absent NK cell activity	<0.5% activity fatal; 3–10% activity presents with recurrent mucous membrane ulcers, severe periodontal disease, recurrent skin abscesses
Leucocyte adhesion deficiency 2	Absence of Sialyl Lewis^X due to defect of fucose transporter, mental retardation, short stature, Bombay (hh) blood phenotype	Recurrent bacterial infections—pneumonia, periodontitis, otitis media, cellulitis
Interferon-gamma receptor 1 or 2 deficiency	Fever, wasting, lymphadenopathy, chronic anaemia, elevated inflammatory markers, asthma, glomerulonephritis, vasculitis	Disseminated BCG, disseminated mycobacterial infection
Interleukin-12/IL-12R deficiency	Th1 deficiency, decreased IFN gamma production by T and NK cells	*Staphylococcus aureus, Streptococcus pneumoniae, Haemophilus influenzae*, disseminated infections with BCG, *M. avium* complex, non-tuberculous mycobacteria, *Salmonella, Nocardia asteroides*

severe infections. They are best managed in conjunction with experienced specialist immunologists.

In the acute setting, general principles apply; there is little evidence available to guide practice. Thorough clinical assessment is important, and patients should be thoroughly reassessed on a regular basis for evidence of deterioration, complications, and superadded infections. Multiple cultures should be taken of blood, urine, wounds, and other potential infective foci.

Empirical antibiotics should be selected to cover common pathogens for the clinical syndrome and for the pathogens to which the patient is particularly susceptible. The microbiological history of the patient is important, particularly the resistance profile of any organisms previously identified. Microbiological advice may be instructive. Normal antibiotic doses are usually sufficient. GM-CSF is of benefit in the primary neutrophil disorders.

Radiological investigation, particularly CT scanning of the chest and MRI of the brain, can identify characteristic appearances of certain infectious agents, such as *Aspergillus* or PML, as well as identifying infectious foci where clinical signs are masked.

As these patients can deteriorate rapidly, clinicians should have a low threshold for escalation of care to HDU/ICU.

Further reading

Bradley JD, Brandt KD, Katz BP (1989). Infectious complications of cyclophosphamide treatment for vasculitis. *Arthritis & Rheumatism*, **32**, 45–53.

Dixon WG, Watson K, Lunt M, Hyrich KL, Silman AJ, Symmons DP (2006). Rates of serious infection, including site-specific and bacterial intracellular infection, in rheumatoid arthritis patients receiving anti–tumor necrosis factor therapy: results from the British Society for Rheumatology Biologics Register. *Arthritis & Rheumatism*, **54**, 2368–76.

Houssiau FA, D'Cruz D, Sangle S, et al. (2010). Azathioprine versus mycophenolate mofetil for long-term immunosuppression in lupus nephritis: results from the MAINTAIN Nephritis Trial. *Annals of the Rheumatic Diseases*, **69**, 2083–9.

McLean-Tooke A (2009). Methotrexate, rheumatoid arthritis and infection risk—what is the evidence? *Rheumatology*, **48**, 867–71.

Chapter 14

Psychiatric diseases and emergencies

Acute psychiatric emergencies

Patients with psychiatric illness (including deliberate self-harm and alcohol/drug abuse) account for ~5–10% of acute hospital admissions. Their care may be compromised, as they are often complex cases and frequently exhibit disturbed or aggressive behaviour. In addition, assessment may be difficult, as the environment is often inappropriate (e.g. emergency room, hospital ward) and/or due to associated alcohol and drug intoxication. It is important to bear in mind that:

- Most aggressive, abusive, or bizarre behaviour is due to alcohol intoxication, drugs, and medical, rather than psychiatric illness.
- Alcohol withdrawal is a medical emergency and requires medical, not psychiatric referral.
- Significant illness can be missed (e.g. myocardial ischaemia, subdural haematoma) in the intoxicated, abusive, or aggressive patient. A period of observation may be required.
- Acute confusion and delirium are nearly always due to organic, rather than psychiatric causes.

The psychiatric history

A careful systematic approach to the patient presenting with suspected psychiatric illness usually results in an accurate diagnosis. Ideally, the interview should be conducted in a quiet and relatively private area. However, the need for privacy must not compromise safety, and support staff must be immediately available, if necessary. Relatives, GPs, paper and electronic hospital records, and community mental health teams may be able to provide additional important information and corroboration of the patient's history.

The key features of the psychiatric history are:

Presenting complaint
Examine the individual complaints, and determine the course, severity, and effect of each on the person's life and work. Assess when they were last well and what factors have caused the patient to be referred or to present on this occasion. Assess mental state (see section on mental state examination) and the patient's personality. Determine what the patient wants (e.g. advice, treatment, or admission) and whether these requests are appropriate.

Current mood
Assess the patient's mood and how they feel about themselves and other people. Do they enjoy themselves? Are they sad or depressed?

Past psychiatric history
Assess previous psychiatric and/or physical illness, outpatient contact (keyworker, community mental health team), and hospital admissions (especially if compulsory). Accurately record psychiatric and other medications.

Family history
Family history should include specific enquiry about psychiatric disorders among close blood relatives.

Personal history
Childhood circumstances, education (± academic achievements), bereavements, parental and family relationships (e.g. domestic violence, adoption, single-parent family), and friends.

Work history
Determine whether the patient is employed and the effect of current and previous employment on mental state. Assess whether previous psychiatric or other illness has affected employment.

Marital/relationship history
Enquire about personal relationships, which may provide information about the patient's personality. Recent separations (or sexual abuse) may be a major factor in the presenting complaint.

Social circumstances
Assess where the patient is staying, whether they are sharing, and the type of accommodation. Ask if the patient has any dependants. Income, debt, social support, and financial circumstances should be reviewed.

Substance misuse
Try to estimate alcohol, tobacco, and drug misuse. Patients do not always underestimate use.

Criminal/forensic history
Determine whether the patient has any impending criminal charges or court appearances due. Record previous criminal charges or convictions.

The mental state examination

Following a thorough history, assess the patient's mental state. If a background history cannot be collected (e.g. aggression, violence), the observations collected when assessing mental state are even more crucial to diagnosis. The key components of mental state examination are:

Appearance and behaviour
Determine whether the patient is clean, tidy, and appropriately dressed or neglected. Is their behaviour consistent or labile and unpredictable? Assess whether the patient's facial expression, posture, and movement suggest anxiety, depression, withdrawal, low mood, fear, or aggression. Examine for abnormal, inappropriate, or dystonic movements and grimaces. Does the patient respond appropriately and maintain eye contact or are they easily distracted? Is there any suggestion that they are hallucinating or responding to no obvious stimuli?

Speech
Record the rate, volume, spontaneity and intonation of speech, and associated dysarthria and dysphasia. Is there any suggestion of perseveration, garbled speech, or flight of ideas (i.e. sudden switching to new themes) or vagueness? Has the patient invented new words (neologisms) or used unusual phrases?

Mood
On the basis of the patient's appearance and behaviour, assess the patient's mood (e.g. sad, depressed), opinion of themselves, and view of the future. Ask about suicidal thoughts. Also enquire about irritability, loss of memory (especially short-term memory), appetite, libido, sleep, concentration, and fluctuations in mood.

Thought abnormalities and insight
These include thought blocking and flight of ideas. Concrete thinking (i.e. impairment of abstract or symbolic thinking) can be assessed by asking the patient to interpret a simple proverb. Ideas of reference (i.e. a feeling that others are talking about, or looking at the patient for some reason, but with preserved insight, unlike delusions), persecutory delusions (i.e. a firm, usually false, belief, unshakeable by logical argument or contrary experiences and out of context with the patient's cultural norms), and passivity (i.e. an experience of being under external control; often associated with schizophrenia) may require direct enquiry to

become evident (e.g. by asking about neighbours or electrical equipment). Does the patient believe they are ill and would they accept treatment?

Hallucinations

Record the nature and specific content of hallucinations. Be aware that visual, tactile, and olfactory or gustatory hallucinations may be associated with organic disease.

Cognitive function

This is determined by formally evaluating higher mental function. It is an essential part of the assessment and prevents organic neurological disease being inappropriately labelled as psychiatric or 'functional' illness and leading to the wrong treatment. Cognitive assessment should include level of consciousness, orientation, attention and concentration, registration of new information, short- and long-term memory, and the ability to interpret instructions and carry out tasks. It is usually assessed using the mini-mental state examination.

The mini-mental state examination and score

The mini-mental state examination (MMSE) is a screening tool for the assessment of cognitive function and was originally designed for use in the elderly but has been adapted for general adult use, as reported in Box 14.1.

The maximum score for the mini-mental test is 30 points. A score of 23 is the cut-off point for significant impairment. The abbreviated mental test score is illustrated in Box 14.1.

Physical examination

This specifically looks for physical illnesses that can be associated with psychiatric disturbance (e.g. substance withdrawal, thyroid disease, epilepsy, cerebrovascular disease, and head trauma). Examination and investigation of violent or aggressive patients can be difficult, but, if possible, exclude focal neurological signs, meningism, intoxication, head injury, and organic confusional states. Record pulse, blood pressure, respiratory rate, oxygen saturation, temperature, blood glucose, urinalysis. Arrange routine blood tests, thyroid function tests, toxicology screens (urine or blood), chest X-ray, and clinically relevant CT scans. Occasionally, electroencephalography is necessary.

Assessing and managing the potentially violent patient

Violent and abusive behaviour is relatively rare and most commonly associated with intoxication (e.g. alcohol, drugs) or organic acute confusional states (e.g. sepsis, hypoglycaemia), rather than mental illness. It is often associated with personality disorders, a previous history of violence,

dementia, frontal lobe brain damage, schizophrenia or other psychoses (e.g. mania), and post-ictal states.

The interview

During the interview, it is essential to ensure the safety of both the patient and the interviewer. Before the interview, ensure staff know where the interview is taking place and what to do in an emergency. There must be an appropriate means of summoning help (e.g. a panic button), and the response must be immediate. Obtain as much information as possible beforehand (i.e. relatives, GP, social workers).

The interview should be in a quiet, comfortable, and preferably non-clinical area. Ideally, the interviewer should be accompanied (e.g. by a nurse). The door of the interview room should open outwards, and the interviewer should sit between the patient and the door to facilitate rapid exit. Avoid directly facing the patient during the interview, as this can appear confrontational (i.e. sit at an angle). Never turn your back on the patient, especially when leaving.

Conduct the interview calmly, maintaining a reassuring and non-judgemental attitude. Speak slowly and clearly, and avoid excessive eye contact. Allow the patient time to air their immediate grievance or complaint with the minimum of interruption.

Managing violent behaviour

Initially, exclude an organic cause for abusive or violent behaviour. Remember that hypoglycaemia, hypoxaemia, sepsis, post-ictal confusion, or a distended bladder in an intoxicated patient can all present, and are often missed, as causes of aggressive behaviour.

Drug and alcohol intoxication is a common cause of aggressive behaviour, but, in most cases, a calm, courteous manner avoids the need for further intervention. Similarly, patients with drug-induced psychosis can often be 'talked down' without the need for tranquillization. However, stimulant drugs (e.g. amphetamines, ecstasy) and hallucinogens (e.g. LSD) that cause violent, agitated behaviour may require restraint and sedation to avoid harm to the patient and staff.

Restraint

If restraint is required, ensure adequate support is available, including nursing and/or security staff. Ideally, three staff trained in 'control and restraint' or 4–6 untrained staff will be required. Police may be available to help. During restraint, ensure that the airway and breathing are not compromised at any time. Only release restraint when the risk of violence has abated (e.g. after sedation). Never try to remove a weapon from a patient. Summon police assistance, and try to persuade them to put the weapon down, and move away from that area (i.e. do not try to retrieve the weapon).

Box 14.1 Abbreviated mental test score	
Question	**Score**
What is your age?	1 for exact age
What is your date of birth?	1 for date and month (not year)
What year is it?	1 for current year only
What time of day is it?	1 for nearest hour
Where are we (place/address)?	1 for exact name/address of hospital
Register three line address and recall at the end of the test	1 if correctly registered and recalled at the end of the test
Who is the Queen?	1 for the current monarch
What year was World War 1?	1 for either first or last year
Count back from 20 to 1	1 if no mistakes
Identify 2 people (names/job)	1 if both recognized
Total score 10; less than 7 abnormal.	

Reproduced from Hodkinson HM, 'Evaluation of a mental test score for assessment of mental impairment in the elderly', *Age and Ageing*, 1972, 1, 4, pp. 233–238, by permission of Oxford University Press and The British Geriatrics Society.

Emergency sedation/tranquillization

Emergency sedation should only ever be used as a last resort when violent or aggressive patients cannot be 'talked down' and/or remain a danger to themselves and/or other people. Throughout sedation, 'de-escalation' techniques should continue to be employed, including reassurance and treatment in an appropriate environment. All sedative/tranquillizer drugs have side effects, especially in the emergency setting, and respiratory depression must be anticipated. Facilities for resuscitation should be available, and it is important to monitor vital signs, including oxygen saturation and respiratory rate. Emergency sedation/tranquillization may be given as oral, intramuscular, or intravenous preparations, depending on the urgency.

- **Oral (PO) sedation** is preferred from a safety point of view. In non-psychotic patients, give lorazepam 1–2 mg PO. In psychotic patients, use lorazepam 1–2 mg PO and an antipsychotic drug such as olanzapine 5–10 mg PO. Allow sufficient time for the drugs to work before giving a second dose.
- **Intramuscular (IM) sedation** is given if oral therapy is refused or inappropriate (i.e. a more rapid onset of action is required). In non-psychotic patients, give lorazepam 1–2 mg IM. In psychotic patients, give lorazepam 1–2 mg IM or promethazine 50 mg IM. Haloperidol is no longer considered a safe option, as it requires a pre-treatment ECG and risks acute dystonic reactions. Intramuscular diazepam and chlorpromazine are best avoided.
- **Intravenous sedation** provides an immediate response and is only required in exceptional circumstances (ideally with appropriate consultation, although this may not be possible in an emergency). Consider use of intravenous diazepam, 10 mg over at least 5 minutes. Try to avoid barbiturates and clomethiazole, as they are more likely to cause respiratory depression.

Ongoing management

Liaise with the psychiatric team about current and ongoing management. Arranging a psychiatric nurse to aid nursing on a medical ward is often an excellent option, providing support and reassurance for the patient, nursing and medical staff.

Legal issues in acute psychiatry

The Mental Health Act, UK 1983

In the UK, the rights and procedures for managing patients with mental illness are addressed in the Mental Health Act. Although slightly different rules apply in Scotland, the principles are the same. In other jurisdictions, local regulations should be reviewed.

The Mental Health Act allows for the compulsory detention and treatment of a patient with mental illness and/or mental impairment of a nature and/or degree that requires inpatient treatment against their wishes. Patients who need to be in hospital, because of a risk to their health and safety, or for the protection of others, may be detained or brought into hospital if the appropriate people agree that this is necessary.

Section 2

Section 2 allows a period of assessment and/or treatment for up to 28 days. It is usually applied to patients presenting for the first time or known patients with a new problem.

Section 3

Section 3 may follow Section 2 and allows detention for treatment for up to 6 months. Both Sections 2 and 3 require opinions from two appropriately qualified doctors and an approved mental health professional/social worker (AMHP). Patients may appeal against both Sections 2 and 3.

Section 4

Section 4 allows patients to be brought into hospital for up to 72 hours with only one medical opinion (not necessarily a psychiatrist) and that of an AMHP. It is only used in emergencies.

Section 5

Section 5 allows for hospital inpatients to be detained by a single doctor under Section 5(2) or a nurse under Section 5(4) whilst awaiting assessment (see further text). In the accident and emergency department, they must be detained under common law (see further text).

Section 136

Section 136 allows the police to bring a patient to a place of safety (e.g. accident and emergency) for assessment by a doctor and AMHP who may then arrange a Section 2 or 3, if necessary.

A patient may be sectioned either in the community or in hospital. They may be detained and nursed on a medical ward if they require medical treatment.

Common law

Common law allows:

- A medical practitioner to act in the patient's best interest in an emergency when they are unable to give consent (e.g. unconscious or if conscious but lack capacity).
- Detention of a patient, pending assessment, or treatment against their will if deemed necessary, in an emergency.
- Treatment given in the best interest of the patient if it is carried out to save life or to ensure improvement or prevent deterioration of physical or mental health.

Always document that you are giving treatment in the best interest of the patient under common law. However, as a rule of thumb, common law only supports emergency acts to save life and limb over a timescale of minutes. For more sustained interventions, over several hours or days, doctors should rely on the Mental Capacity Act (2005).

Consent and capacity

Lack of capacity to consent to, or refuse medical interventions is surprisingly common (over 20% of general hospital inpatients). It is often assumed that mental illness is the most frequent cause, although substance abuse and organic illness with loss of capacity is probably more common. The key issue when deciding if a patient has the competence to accept or refuse treatment is whether or not they have 'capacity'. Emergency treatment may be given against a patient's will if they lack capacity under common law or, if time allows, under the Mental Capacity Act (MCA, 2005).

To have capacity, they must be able to take in and retain the information necessary to make the decision and understand the consequences of refusal. They must believe the information and assess it in order to arrive at a decision. The patient should be assisted to communicate, if possible. Capacity may fluctuate over time in an individual. In addition, the patient may have capacity to make some decisions but not others.

Although mental illness and cognitive impairment may impair capacity, this is not always the case (and has been tested in law). It must be remembered that disagreeing with medical advice does not constitute incapacity.

Once incapacity is evident with regard to a specific proposed medical or surgical intervention, the MCA describes a number of steps that should be taken to establish 'the best interests' for that individual. The doctor's best judgement in isolation is no longer sufficient when determining the treatment of incapacitous patients. These steps should be pursued and documented if time allows:

- What would this patient have wanted for themselves in this circumstance when they did have capacity? This usually involves consulting those close to the patient and checking whether any advance directive, either written or verbal, exists. If there are no close relatives/others, an independent mental capacity advocate should be appointed.
- The intervention must be necessary and the least restrictive option chosen.

In UK law, a third party cannot consent on behalf of an adult patient (i.e. proxy consent). The situation in children is different, and appropriate senior advice should be obtained. Most medical defence organizations offer 24 hour helplines.

The Mental Health Act does not allow doctors to treat mentally ill patients for physical problems against their will. Such treatment is illegal, even if the physical problem is due to the mental problem (e.g. liver failure after paracetamol overdose). The only exception to this rule is if the physical condition is the cause of the mental condition (e.g. detention and treatment of confusion due to organic illness). Treating a patient who has the capacity to refuse is potentially a criminal offence. However, treatment in an emergency, when the issue of capacity is unclear, is unlikely to be criticized.

Compulsory detention of patients

In an emergency, a patient can be detained under common law if it is in the best interests of the patient. In this situation, security staff should be asked to detain the patient until a psychiatric opinion can be obtained. It should be documented that this is being done under common law.

Patients who do not wish to stay in hospital can sometimes be persuaded to stay. However, if this proves impossible and there is concern for the patient's safety if they leave the ward, then it may be necessary to use physical restraint to prevent them from leaving whilst awaiting psychiatric assessment of their capacity to decide to leave.

If there is no psychiatric team on site, Section 5(2) and Section 5(4) of the Mental Health Act make provision for detention of these patients whilst awaiting assessment

Section 5(2)

Section 5(2) allows any inpatient on a ward to be prevented from leaving for a maximum of 72 hours. Form H1, which should be available on the wards, should be completed and the duty psychiatry team and mental health duty social worker informed. It is a holding measure, pending full assessment by appropriately qualified doctors and an AMHP. Section 5(2) does not allow medical treatment of any kind to be enforced. This would have to be given under common law if against the patient's wishes.

Any medical practitioner may use Section 5(2), but it must be applied on behalf of the patient's consultant or their nominated deputy (i.e. a member of the team who is covering their patients out of hours). Section 5(2) expires when the patient has been reviewed by an appropriately qualified doctor and has been converted to a Section 2 or 3 or cancelled.

Section 5(4)

Section 5(4) entitles a qualified nurse to detain a patient for up to 6 hours whilst awaiting a doctor (i.e. if the doctor is not on site) to assess the patient for Section 5(2). If the doctor subsequently detains the patient under Section 5(2), the 72-hour duration is deemed to have started when the nurse imposed Section 5(4).

Patients in accident and emergency departments or outpatient departments should be detained under common law, pending psychiatric assessment, as Section 5(2) and Section 5(4) are only applicable to inpatients.

The mentally ill patient in hospital

Patients with chronic mental illness, including schizophrenia and depression, are more susceptible to organic ill health and may require admission to hospital and treatment of non-psychiatric disease. They are already at a significant disadvantage due to the stigma associated with mental illness, and these patients often need additional reassurance and support to help them cope with what is often perceived as a potentially threatening hospital environment.

Occasionally, psychiatric ward patients, sectioned under the Mental Health Act, become medically unwell and require transfer to a medical ward. This is acceptable, but it is important to ensure ongoing psychiatric support, as these patients often have serious mental illness and may become disturbed. They can be nursed on open wards, but sectioned patients should be supervised by a registered mental health nurse at all times. If a patient is very disturbed, they may need more than one nurse. Most psychiatric wards do not have the trained staff or equipment for even basic medical interventions (e.g. intravenous drips), and patients must be medically stable and relatively independent before they can return to a psychiatric ward. Good communication with the psychiatric team aids transfer back to the psychiatric ward and ongoing medical care.

Important guidelines for the care of mentally ill patients whilst in hospital include:

- Continue regular psychiatric drugs. Suddenly stopping some medications like serotonin reuptake inhibitors and lithium can precipitate psychiatric crises. Ensure depot injections (slow release medications) are administered at the appropriate time.

- Before stopping a psychiatric drug for a medical reason, consult a psychiatrist for advice.

- If you are concerned about a patient's mental state during their hospital admission, contact the psychiatric team and, if necessary, ask them to review the patient.

- Remember that new onset of confusion is organic, until proved otherwise, and should be investigated and treated as in a non-psychiatric patient.

- Liaise with the patient's mental health and psychiatric teams who may be able to provide valuable support whilst in hospital. Community mental health social workers may be able to help with complex discharge planning.

Acute clinical psychiatric problems

Acute confusion, delirium, or organic brain syndrome

Acute confusional states or 'delirium' are relatively common, particularly in elderly care, trauma, and orthopaedic patients. It affects up to 10% of acute medical admissions and >30% of elderly patients during their hospital stay and is more common in patients with dementia.

Clinical features

The hallmarks of an acute confusional state (delirium) are disorientation in time and place, disturbed consciousness and impaired short-term memory. It has a rapid onset (hours, days) that fluctuates over time and is worse at night ('sundowning'). The disturbed global consciousness may cause excitement and overactivity or drowsiness and stupor. Cognitive function is impaired with reduced short- and long-term memory, disorientation, incoherent speech, and reduced attention. There may be perceptual disturbances, especially in visual and tactile modalities, which include visual distortions, illusions (which may be frightening), and hallucinations. Mood is often labile, with apathy, depression, irritability, and perplexity. Motor activity is often increased but is usually purposeless. Many show autonomic overactivity, with tachycardia, sweating, and dilated pupils. About 10% of cases exhibit aggressive behaviour. The sleep-wake cycle is often disturbed. The features of the underlying cause are often detectable (see next section).

Causes

These include:

- Metabolic derangements (e.g. hypoglycaemia, hyponatraemia, renal or liver failure, acidosis, hypercalcaemia).
- Hypoxaemia, hypercapnia, or tissue hypoxia (e.g. carbon monoxide poisoning).
- Pain or discomfort (e.g. constipation, distended bladder).
- Endocrine derangement (e.g. thyrotoxicosis, hypothyroidism, diabetes mellitus, Addison's disease).
- Infection, either localized or systemic.
- Neurological disease (e.g. post-ictal states, meningitis, subdural haematoma, etc.).
- Cardiac disease (e.g. heart failure, myocardial ischaemia, endocarditis).
- Alcohol or drug withdrawal.
- Related to prescription drugs (e.g. opiates, sedatives, steroids, digoxin, cimetidine, analgesics, diuretics, anticholinergics, anti-parkinsonian, etc.) and recreational drugs (e.g. ecstasy, amphetamines, LSD).

Diagnosis

A careful physical and mental state examination is required in all acutely confused patients. Review the notes, and obtain a history from friends and relatives, focusing primarily on premorbid functioning, onset and course of the confusion, and previous use and abuse of alcohol and drugs. The mini-mental state and abbreviated mental state examinations give a rapid estimate of key cognitive functions.

The main priority is to identify treatable or life-threatening conditions. Look carefully for evidence of alcohol or drug intoxication or withdrawal. Vivid hallucinations, in the absence of a previous history of mental illness, may indicate alcohol withdrawal. Review the drug chart for potential precipitants (e.g. steroids, opiates). Exclude hypoglycaemia, head injury, liver failure, cardiac, respiratory, abdominal, and neurological abnormalities, including acute urinary retention, sepsis, and focal neurological signs. Carbon monoxide poisoning and endocarditis are rare but easily missed. Document vital signs and Glasgow coma scale in all cases.

Mandatory investigations include routine blood tests, including liver and renal function, blood glucose, calcium, arterial blood gases (and carbon monoxide levels), saturation, blood cultures, C-reactive protein, urinalysis, electrocardiogram, and chest radiographs. Further tests should be based on clinical suspicion, including toxicology screen, cardiac enzymes, thyroid function tests, B_{12} and folate, syphilis (and, very rarely, Lyme disease) serology, porphyrins, amylase, lumbar puncture, electroencephalography, and brain CT scans.

Unfortunately, acute confusional state is often misdiagnosed as a functional psychosis (e.g. mania, depression, and late-onset schizophrenia) or dementia. Dementia is defined as an acquired progressive decline in intellect, personality, and behaviour. It is irreversible and, importantly, is typically associated with a normal level of consciousness. Box 14.2 demonstrates how dementia and delirium can be differentiated.

Management

Treat the cause

Always consider the possibility of alcohol withdrawal. It is often possible to treat the acute confusional state conservatively whilst awaiting the response to therapy directed at the precipitating cause.

Orientation

Nurse the patient in a quiet, well-lit room on a general medical ward, with familiar nursing staff and, if possible, with a family member in attendance to aid orientation. Ensure glasses and hearing aids are available. Clocks and family photographs may help. Patients are often very anxious and may need repeated explanations and reassurance.

Dehydration and electrolyte imbalance

These are common, irrespective of the underlying cause, and should be corrected.

Sedation

Sedation may be required for aggressive or undesirable behaviour. It is best given in small incremental oral doses, using a treatment protocol. Offer liquid preparations if tablets are refused. Parenteral medication may be needed in more severely disturbed patients. Treatment regimes use either antipsychotic drugs or benzodiazepines.

- **Antipsychotic drugs** are preferred, although there is some concern that these may increase stroke and mortality in older patients. Oral haloperidol is still considered first-line therapy but should be avoided in patients with

Box 14.2 Differentiation between delirium and dementia

Delirium	vs	Dementia
Rapid <---------------------	Onset ------------------>	Gradual
Fluctuating <--------------	Course ----------->	Slowly progressive
Clouded <-----------	Conscious level -------------->	Alert
Incoherent /++ <--	Thought content ------->	Impoverished/--
Common <------------	Perceptual ---------->	Auditory (30%)
especially Visual	Abnormalities	Visual

Parkinson's disease, as they are very sensitive to neuro-leptics and may develop extrapyramidal side effects. It should also be avoided in patients at risk of arrythmias due to prolonged QTc syndromes and those who have taken ecstasy, amphetamines, cocaine, or GHB.

Haloperidol is best given orally as small incremental doses: 1–2.5 mg 1–2-hourly (max dose 20 mg daily) in patients <65 years old or 0.5–1 mg 1–2-hourly (max dose 5 mg daily) in the elderly (i.e. >65–75 years old). Intramuscular doses are 1–3 mg, 1–2-hourly (max dose 15 mg) in patients <65 years old and 0.5–1 mg 1–2-hourly (max 5 mg daily) in the elderly.

Atypical antipsychotics, such as olanzapine (2.5–5 mg) and risperidone (1–2 mg), are preferred by some authorities.

- **Benzodiazepines** should only be used in patients with Parkinson's disease, parkinsonism, Lewy body-type dementia, during alcohol withdrawal, and in patients with drug toxicity, including ecstasy, cocaine, amphetamines, and GHB. It is best given orally or intramuscularly in small incremental doses (e.g. lorazepam 1 mg 1–2-hourly in patients <65 years old or 0.5 mg 1–2-hourly in the elderly, i.e. >65–75 years old). The maximum daily dose is 4 mg. These drugs may exacerbate the confusion, precipitate hypotension, and potentiate the risk of falls. Longer-acting benzodiazepines are used in alcohol withdrawal (e.g. chlordiazepoxide).

Reassess the patient after 20–30 minutes to determine the effect of the sedation, and supplement with further small doses, as required. If parenteral medication is required, lorazepam and haloperidol are probably the best combination. If repeated doses of these are required, monitor vital signs in view of the risk of respiratory depression and perform an ECG to exclude QTc prolongation (i.e. a prelude to life-threatening tachyarrhythmias).

Patients with ongoing acute confusion may require regular sedation (e.g. haloperidol 0.5 mg tds, risperidone 0.25 mg bd). Regular use of benzodiazepines may induce tolerance and dependence.

Prognosis

Acute confusion is associated with increased mortality, may increase hospital stay by up to 10 days, and can produce residual cognitive impairment. Duration depends on the speed of diagnosis and the underlying cause. If the cause is reversible, recovery is rapid, with return to premorbid functional level. Delirium may occur on a background of dementia, lasting for days or even weeks, and often has a poor outcome.

Alcohol abuse and alcohol withdrawal

Excessive alcohol consumption is associated with significant health and social problems. In the UK, heavy drinking, defined as >8 units/day for men and >6 units/day for women, affects 23% of men and 9% of women. Alcohol dependence occurs in 6% of men and 2% of women; it is increasing in women and young people. Alcohol is a factor in 20% of work-related fatalities, 30% of road traffic fatalities, drowning, and suicides, 50% of homicides and most assaults.

Aetiology

Aetiology is multifactorial. Social factors include occupation (e.g. doctors, sales people), peer group (e.g. Scots), and the cost of alcoholic drinks. Genetic factors have been identified, with increased incidence in some families and racial groups (e.g. indigenous Americans) due to differences in alcohol metabolism. Behavioural factors include the association with pleasure and social reinforcement.

Alcohol abuse

Alcohol abuse describes regular or binge consumption, sufficient to cause physical, neuropsychiatric, and social damage. The conventional safe drinking limits are 21 units per week for men and 14 units per week for women, with 2 drink-free days each week, where 8 g or 10 mL of alcohol is 1 unit and represents half a pint of beer or a small glass of wine. In the UK, safe limits have been changed to <4 units/day for men and <3 units/day for women.

Alcohol intoxication

Alcohol intoxication is characterized by slurred speech, impaired coordination and judgement, flushing, labile affect, unsteady gait, and nystagmus. Alcohol intoxication is frequently associated with abusive or violent behaviour and should be managed as described previously. Hypoglycaemia may occur both during intoxication and in the following 24 hours in those who present with alcoholic ketoacidosis (e.g. chronic alcoholics, children, binge drinkers). If severe, it can cause coma, a medical emergency requiring airway protection and exclusion of other potential causes (e.g. hypoglycaemia, head injury). Differential diagnosis includes other causes of acute confusion, especially head injury.

Alcohol dependence

Alcohol dependence is a syndrome associated with the compulsion to drink, preoccupation with alcohol, loss of the ability to regulate alcohol intake, fixed drinking patterns, withdrawal phenomena, and altered tolerance to the intoxicant effects of alcohol (i.e. initially increased but dramatically reduced later in the syndrome).

Detection and assessment of alcohol-related problems

Alcohol abuse and dependence are not always clinically obvious. Hospital staff must have a high index of suspicion, as early detection is vital to avoid long-term health problems and withdrawal.

Physical examination may reveal alcoholic stigmata, including those of liver disease (e.g. spider naevi, gynaecomastia, jaundice), peripheral neuropathy, bruising due to coagulopathy, ataxia, and other cerebellar signs. Macrocytosis, elevated INR, raised gamma glutamyl transferase or other liver function tests, and a raised blood alcohol level on investigation suggests excessive alcohol intake.

The CAGE questionnaire is a useful, and commonly used, screening tool for the detection of problem drinking. A single positive answer is significant, and >1 is probably diagnostic of chronic alcohol dependence.

Alcohol withdrawal
Simple alcohol withdrawal

Simple alcohol withdrawal occurs within 24–48 hours of abstinence and is often uneventful. In some cases, it can be managed as an outpatient. Initial symptoms include anxiety, agitation, irritability, tremor, tachycardia, hypertension, sweating, hyperactivity, nausea, vomiting, diarrhoea, insomnia, delirium, hallucinations, and mild pyrexia. These symptoms peak at 12–24 hours and usually subside by 48 hours.

Generalized, self-limiting tonic-clonic seizures can occur during this early period, especially in those with known epilepsy, but status epilepticus is rare. The fits can be precipitated by photic stimulation and flickering lights but do not show the EEG characteristics of epilepsy.

Severe withdrawal or delirium tremens

Severe withdrawal or delirium tremens ('DTs') occurs in 5% of cases of alcohol withdrawal, usually 3–4 days after cessation of alcohol. It is a medical emergency, with an untreated mortality of ~15%. In addition to the symptoms of withdrawal, there may be confusion and disorientation, hallucinations (visual or tactile), irritability, labile mood, and sinister fleeting delusions which can be very frightening. Rarely, lactic acidosis, ketoacidosis, or high fever can occur. Deaths tend to be due to arrhythmias, precipitated by electrolyte disturbances, acidosis, or alcohol-related cardiomyopathy, infection, or cardiovascular collapse. Exclude hepatic encephalopathy, hypoglycaemia, subdural haematoma due to head trauma, and Wernicke–Korsakoff syndrome (see following paragraph) in these patients.

Wernicke–Korsakoff syndrome

Wernicke–Korsakoff syndrome is a complication of acute thiamine deficiency which may occur in chronic alcoholism. Wernicke's encephalopathy comprises the triad of acute confusion, ataxia (cerebellar type), and ophthalmoplegia with nystagmus and VI nerve palsy. Peripheral neuropathy may also occur, but not all the symptoms may be present.

If Wernicke's encephalopathy is untreated, most patients will develop Korsakoff's syndrome (amnesic syndrome) with severe confusion, impaired long-term memory, and confabulation. There may be overt psychosis.

Alcoholic ketoacidosis

Alcoholic ketoacidosis is uncommon but occurs when an alcoholic stops drinking, vomits repeatedly, and does not eat. It is due to fatty acid breakdown, complicated by dehydration from vomiting. Investigation reveals a high anion gap metabolic acidosis, a reduced bicarbonate, and low $PaCO_2$. The pH is very variable, as the metabolic acidosis may be buffered by a metabolic alkalosis due to vomiting and/or respiratory alkalosis. Differential diagnosis includes salicylate, methanol, and ethylene glycol poisoning. Consider ICU/HDU admission.

Management of alcohol withdrawal

General measures

- Simple alcohol withdrawal can often be treated as an outpatient. However, patients with a history of seizures or delirium tremens or features suggestive of delirium tremens should be treated on a medical ward.
- Prevent disorientation by nursing the patient in a well-lit room. Exclude or treat hypoglycaemia. Treat intercurrent infections (e.g. pneumonia, cellulitis).
- Consider rehydration, with intravenous fluids if necessary, and monitor urine output. Avoid normal saline in known chronic liver disease. In alcoholic ketoacidosis, consider sodium bicarbonate (in addition to intravenous fluids), and monitor electrolytes and blood sugar closely.
- B complex vitamins are required to prevent Wernicke–Korsakoff syndrome. Initial parenteral therapy as Pabrinex® (1–2 pairs of ampoules daily for 3 days, with each pair of ampoules being given intravenously over 8 hours whilst observing for anaphylaxis) is followed by oral therapy for a week, with thiamine 100 mg orally twice daily or vitamin B tablets (compound strong) two tablets three times daily. Wernicke's encephalopathy requires a longer period of intravenous Pabrinex® (at least 5 days).
- Severe hypophosphataemia may complicate alcohol withdrawal and should be corrected with intravenous phosphate if the serum phosphate is <0.6 mmol/L. Magnesium deficiency should also be corrected.

Sedation

- Long-acting benzodiazepines are required for the treatment of alcohol withdrawal. The drug of choice is chlordiazepoxide (Librium®), but diazepam may be used, especially if an intravenous agent is required. Lorazepam, which is not metabolized in the liver, is a better choice in chronic liver disease.
- A typical management algorithm for alcohol withdrawal syndrome is shown in Box 14.3. Initially, give a single oral dose of chlordiazepoxide, based on the severity of the patient's symptoms. This is followed by chlordiazepoxide (0, 25, or 50 mg every 2 hours for a further 24 hours, depending on the symptom score derived from the clinical institute withdrawal assessment of alcohol scale-revised (CIWA-Ar) score (see Box 14.4). If the CIWA-Ar score is 0–9 or the patient is asleep, no treatment is required; if the score is 10–14, give 25 mg or if the score is >15, give 50 mg chlordiazepoxide. The total dose of chlordiazepoxide given in the first 24 hours is calculated, and a reducing regime should be prescribed, based on this baseline (see Box 14.3)).
- Haloperidol (2.5–5 mg) may be useful in severe agitation. Oral clomethiazole (INN), although used in the past, is no longer recommended, as it is addictive and dangerous if combined with alcohol. Although previously recommended, carbamazepine is probably ineffective, even in those with a history of withdrawal seizures.

Seizure therapy

- Withdrawal seizures are usually self-limiting but may be treated with intravenous diazepam (10 mg given over 5 minutes).
- Phenytoin is less effective but should be added if there is a history of epilepsy or recurrent seizures.

Follow-up and support

- Arrange referral to an alcohol dependence clinic and self-help groups like Alcoholics Anonymous (AA).
- Abstinence is the most realistic long–term aim, rather than controlled drinking. Psychotherapy, relapse prevention strategies, and development of social routines not dependent on alcohol are all useful.
- Treat coexistent depression and anxiety.
- Acamprosate, which reduces craving, and disulfiram, which induces nausea if the patient drinks alcohol, can be considered by addiction specialists.

Prognosis

Alcohol dependence is associated with remission and relapse and premature death in 40% of patients (15% due to

---

Box 14.3 Management algorithm for alcohol withdrawal

1. **Stat dose of chlordiazepoxide** based on symptom severity.
2. **Prescribe chlordiazepoxide 0, 25, or 50 mg 2-hourly for 24 h**, depending on the CIWA-Ar score (score 0–9 = 0 mg; score 10–14 = 25 mg; score >15 = 50 mg).
3. **Total dose of chlordiazepoxide on day 1 (stat + prn) is calculated and determines the 5-day reducing regime.**

Day 1	Day 2	Day 3	Day 4	Day 5
300 mg severe	60 mg × 4	50 mg × 4	30 mg × 4	20 mg × 4
250 mg	50 mg × 4	40 mg × 4	25 mg × 4	15 mg × 4
200 mg moderate	40 mg × 4	30 mg × 4	20 mg × 4	10 mg × 4
150 mg	30 mg × 4	20 mg × 4	15 mg × 4	7.5 mg × 4
100 mg mild	20 mg × 4	15 mg × 4	10 mg × 4	5 mg × 4

If on day 5 the patient is taking chlordiazepoxide >40 mg daily, consider a longer reducing dose.

Box 14.4 Clinical institute withdrawal assessment of alcohol scale, revised (CIWA-Ar)

10-point questionnaire: add up total score for each question. If score 10–14, give 25 mg; and if >15, give 50 mg of chlordiazepoxide.

1. *Nausea and vomiting.* Ask 'Do you feel sick?', 'Have you vomited?' Scale 0–7: 0 = nil, 1 = mild nausea, 4 = intermittent nausea, 7 = constant nausea and vomiting.
2. *Tremor.* Observation: arms extended and finger spread. Scale 0–7: 0 = no tremor, 4 = moderate with arms extended, 7 = severe, even at rest.
3. *Sweats.* Observation; scale 0–7: 0 = no sweats, 4 = beads of sweat on forehead, 7 = drenching sweats.
4. *Anxiety.* Ask 'Do you feel nervous?'. Scale 0–7: 0 = at ease, 4 = moderate anxiety or 'guarded', 7 – acute panic, severe anxiety as in delirium.
5. *Agitation.* Observation; scale 0–7: 0 = normal, 4 = restless, fidgety, 7 = paces back and forth, very restless.
6. *Tactile disturbances.* Ask 'Have you any itching, pins and needles, burning, bugs crawling under you skin?' Scale 0–7: 0 = none, 4 = moderate hallucinations, 7 = severe hallucinations.
7. *Auditory disturbances*: Ask 'Are you more aware of sounds around you?' 'Are you hearing anything that disturbs you?', 'Are you hearing things you know are not there?' Scale 0–7: 0 = none, 4 = moderate hallucinations, 7 = continuous hallucinations
8. *Visual disturbances.* Ask 'Does the light appear too bright?', 'Are you seeing anything that disturbs you?', 'Are you seeing things you know are not there?' Scale 0–7: 0 = none, 4 = moderate hallucinations, 7 = continuous hallucinations.
9. *Headache.* Ask 'Does your head feel different?', 'Do you have a band round your head?' Scale 0–7: 0 = no, 4 = moderate, 7 = very severe.
10. *Orientation.* Ask 'What day is this?', 'Where are you?', 'Who am I?' Scale 0–4: 0 = orientated, 2 = disorientated for date, <2 days, 4 = disorientated for place and person.

Reproduced with permission from Sullivan JS *et al.*, 'Assessment of alcohol withdrawal the revised clinical institute withdrawal assessment for alcohol scale (CIWA-Ar)', *Addiction*, 84, 11, pp. 1353–1357. © 2006 John Wiley and Sons.

suicide). They have increased rates of physical injury (especially head injury), heart disease, malignancy, and stroke.

Deliberate self-harm and suicide

Deliberate self-harm

In the UK, deliberate self-harm accounts for 10% of acute medical admissions and has an annual incidence of 2–3/1,000 people. Associated psychiatric illness is not always present, affecting perhaps 50% of cases, most of whom have depression. Self-poisoning accounts for 90% of cases of self-harm, and the remainder are physical self-injury. Unlike suicide, deliberate self-harm is more common in young, mainly female, low social class, and single (or divorced) patients. As in suicide, deliberate self-harm is associated with psychiatric illness, especially depression, and personality disorder

Most episodes are impulsive and associated with alcohol consumption. However, 1–2% of these patients commit suicide within a year, which is 100 times greater than in the general population. About 50% of successful suicide cases have a previous history of deliberate self-harm, and in the presence of depression this is the single best predictor of successful suicide. About 20% of cases will repeat the self-harm within a year.

Assessment

Assessment is important to detect those at risk of future self-harm and to identify those with genuine suicidal intent or significant mental illness who require referral for psychiatric review and treatment and to arrange aftercare in the community. Box 15.5 summarizes the factors associated with an increased risk of suicide in deliberate self-harm patients.

Key areas of assessment which may identify increased risk of psychiatric illness or subsequent suicide and the need for psychiatric referral include:

- Demographic and personal factors. Suicide risk is higher in older men, who are single or divorced, recently separated, unemployed with physical illness, and living in social isolation.
- The events and circumstances leading up to the self-harm.
- Previous psychiatric illness (e.g. depression, personality disorder) and episodes of self-harm.
- Premeditation (i.e. saving of pills, choosing a time when least likely to be detected), preparation for (e.g. preparation of a will, organizing finances), true intent (i.e. a sustained wish to die, not wishing to seek help after the self-harm event), and the level of concealment (i.e. arranged secretly) of the deliberate self-harm event.
- The outcome of the event (i.e. was the discovery accidental?).
- Associated alcohol and substance abuse or dependence.

The acronym SAD PERSONS may be a useful aide-memoire for the risk factors for suicide: **S**ex, **A**ge, **D**epression, **P**revious attempts, **E**thanol abuse, **R**ational thinking loss (especially psychosis), **S**ocial support lacking, **O**rganized plan, **N**o pastimes, and **S**ickness.

Management

Management of repeated deliberate self-harm can be difficult, as these patients often have personality disorders. Always try to maintain an empathic and professional approach to these patients, and avoid and discourage the negative attitude adopted by many staff. Multidisciplinary (e.g. emergency room, community psychiatric and nursing team) management plans may successfully discourage habitual self-harmers.

Not all adult self-harm patients need psychiatric referral, and outpatient management may be an option. However, when in doubt, refer. If a patient at high risk of suicide refuses to stay for further assessment, it may be necessary to detain them under common law, pending urgent psychiatric review. If you are satisfied that the risk of suicide is relatively low and does not merit detention, then allow the patient to be discharged, but ensure the GP is informed.

Risk of further non-fatal self-harm is most likely if there have been repeated previous episodes (e.g. recurrent

Box 14.5 Risk of suicide

Male
Elderly (especially in women)
Separated, widowed, or divorced
Living alone
Unemployed or retired
Psychiatric illness (especially depression/schizophrenia)
Alcoholism, alcohol abuse
Personality disorder (i.e. sociopathic)
Violent deliberate self-harm (e.g. shooting, hanging)
Physical illness (e.g. terminal, painful)

overdoses), if aged under 35 years old, being female, single, separated, unemployed, or from a lower social class. Substance and alcohol abuse, personality disorder, previous psychiatric illness, and a criminal history are also associated with recurrence.

Specific therapy involves treatment of underlying psychiatric illnesses, psychotherapy, behavioural therapy, and intensive follow-up with social support. Ensure the GP is informed.

Suicide

Suicide is defined as intentional self-inflicted death. It is most common in Eastern European states and Russia. There are about 5,000 suicides annually in the UK (~1% of all deaths), and it is more common in men. In the UK, the suicide rate is about three times higher in men than in women. Recently, in developed countries, there has been a sharp rise in the rate of suicide in young men, but the highest rates are still in older men (>65 years old).

Aetiological causes of suicide

These may be:

- **Social.** In Emile Durkheim's social model, suicide is classified as:
  - **Egoistic.** This describes the effect of separation of an individual from an established social group. It occurs following bereavement, house moves, in people living alone, immigrant, and divorced or single people. Mental illness (e.g. depression, schizophrenia) is a significant cause of social isolation.
  - **Anomic.** This reflects the effect of society's disintegration and loss of common values. It is illustrated by the association between suicide and unemployment/homicide rates, the increased urban suicide rate, compared to rural societies, and the decrease during wartime (i.e. social cohesion in adversity). The relationship of suicide to job loss or unemployment is also found at an individual level in men and the mentally ill who are at greater risk of unemployment.
  - **Altruistic.** This is suicide undertaken for a cause or movement (e.g. religious suicide bombers).
- **Biological.** Serotonergic underactivity has been demonstrated in the CSF and brains (i.e. low 5-HT levels and receptors) of both successful and attempted suicide patients. A positive family history of suicide is also associated with increased risk.
- **Psychiatric.** There is strong association between suicide and psychiatric illness, and, retrospectively, a psychiatric diagnosis can be made in most successful suicides. The lifetime risk of suicide is increased in depression (15%), schizophrenia (10%), alcoholism (~4%) and, less consistently, substance misuse, personality disorders, and anorexia nervosa. In older patients, there is a strong association with depression and chronic painful illness, whereas, in young men, substance misuse and personality disorders are more common.

Suicide prevention

Suicide prevention requires early detection of both psychiatric illness and/or actively suicidal patients. Careful assessment of risk and urgent admission for safety (with compulsory detention under the Mental Health Act, if required), with intensive psycho- and pharmacological therapy may be necessary. At the population level, reducing unemployment and decreasing access to methods of self-harm may also reduce suicide rates. For example, access to firearms has been associated with suicide rates in the USA. In the UK, public health initiatives include reducing the availability and size of paracetamol and aspirin packs.

Substance abuse and misuse

Drug abuse is common. In the UK, ~10% of the population have used cannabis in the last year, and half a million people take ecstasy each weekend. The main causes are availability and peer pressure. It is more common in the young (12–24 years old), males, and socio-economically deprived groups. Iatrogenic factors may be involved (e.g. prescribed benzodiazepines), and there is an association with psychiatric illness, especially personality disorders.

Most drugs are obtained illicitly, but some may be obtained legally from pharmacies (e.g. codeine), over the shop counter (e.g. solvents), or as therapeutic prescription drugs (e.g. benzodiazepines).

Classification

Classification of substance abuse is by:

The type of drug used

- **Opiates** (e.g. heroin, morphine, methadone). These can be smoked ('chasing the dragon'), sniffed, taken orally, intravenously ('mainlining'), intramuscularly, or subcutaneously ('skin popping'). Opiates produce an initial pleasurable rush with histamine release (itchy eyes), followed by a sense of peace or detachment, and finally central nervous depression. Tolerance and withdrawal develop rapidly. Accidental overdose is characterized by miosis and respiratory depression, and chronic abuse by tremor, constipation, malnutrition, and apathy. About 10% of users become dependent, and 2–3% die annually. Early (24–48 hours) withdrawal symptoms include flu-like symptoms, craving, and sweating. Later features (7–10 days) include agitation, restlessness, tachycardia, mydriasis, and diarrhoea/abdominal cramps. Opiate dependence is treated with methadone (opioid agonist) or buprenorphine (partial agonist).
- **Stimulants** (e.g. amphetamines, cocaine). Oral or intravenous amphetamines cause euphoria, mydriasis, and tachycardia, followed by depression, headache, and fatigue. Occasionally, acute use causes psychosis. 'Crystal meth' is a long-acting methamphetamine which can be taken orally, smoked, or sniffed. It is more potent, long-acting, and potentially more harmful. 'Khat' contains an amphetamine-like stimulant that causes euphoria and excitement. It is smoked or chewed by Somali communities and until recently was not a controlled substance in the UK. It has recently been reclassified as a Class C controlled drug.
  Cocaine is sniffed, chewed, or taken intravenously. It increases energy, and intoxication resembles hypomania with restlessness and anorexia. Hallucinations, including formication (i.e. insects crawling under the skin), and paranoid psychoses may occur. Profound depression and insomnia ('the crash') precede withdrawal. 'Crack' is a purified, highly addictive type of cocaine which is smoked. A brief 'high' is followed by withdrawal and associated persecutory delusions.
- **Hallucinogens** (e.g. LSD, ecstasy, 'magic mushrooms') increase perception, produce physical effects (e.g. mydriasis, vasoconstriction), and may occasionally result in psychoses. However, they do not cause dependence. Overdose may cause seizures. Ecstasy (an amphetamine analogue) has mixed stimulant and hallucinogenic effects. It may cause hyperactivity, hyperpyrexia, and dehydration with severe thirst. Subsequent hyponatraemia is due to excessive water intake.

- **Benzodiazepines** cause respiratory depression in overdose, dependence, withdrawal, including seizures and tolerance. Dependence may be iatrogenic, following medical prescription.
- **Cannabis** (e.g. skunk, marijuana, or 'pot'/'grass') produces a sense of euphoria, well-being, and hallucinations. It increases appetite and reduces temperature. Psychological, rather than physical, dependence occurs. Use of cannabis (especially skunk, which has a high THC content) is associated with an increased incidence of schizophrenia, and this effect seems particularly marked in users under 17 years of age. Adverse responses include transient psychoses, flashbacks, apathy, conjunctival irritation, and reduced spermatogenesis.
- **Solvents** are usually sniffed. They are often used by young boys and may cause a rash around the mouth and/or nose. Drowsiness follows initial euphoria, and chronic use is associated with weight loss, cognitive impairment, nausea, and peripheral neuropathy. Adverse effects can be fatal and include bronchospasm, cerebral and/or hepatorenal damage, arrhythmias, and aplastic anaemia. Psychological dependence is common, but physical dependence rare.
- **Phencyclidine** (e.g. PCP, 'angel dust') is usually smoked. It produces euphoria and analgesia, but toxic effects include impaired consciousness and psychoses requiring antipsychotic agents.
- **Club drugs** (e.g. gamma hydroxybutyrate (GHB), rohypnol, ketamine, ecstasy (MDMA; see above), methamphetamine (see above)) are a pharmacologically heterogeneous group of psychoactive drugs that tend to be abused by teens and young adults at nightclubs, concerts, and parties. GHB is a central nervous system depressant that produces euphoria, increased sexual drive, and tranquility but also negative effects including coma, amnesia, and hallucinations. Rohypnol is a benzodiazepine. Both drugs can be obtained as colourless and odorless forms that can be combined with alcohol and used to commit sexual assualts ('date-rapes') due to their ability to sedate victims.

The disorder it produces

- Intoxication (i.e. impaired consciousness, behaviour, affect, cognitive perception).
- Dependence (i.e. physical, psychological, tolerance).
- Withdrawal (i.e. time-limited physical and psychological symptoms, following withdrawal of a drug after prolonged use). Depends on the substance and previous dose.
- Harmful use (i.e. health, social damage, vascular complications).
- Psychotic disorder (e.g. hallucinations, persecutory delusions, psychomotor disturbances).
- Amnesic effects, with impairment of memory and cognitive function (e.g. alcohol).
- Residual or later psychotic disorders (e.g. cannabis).

Drugs may also be classified by the harm they cause. The most harm is caused by class A drugs (e.g. opiates, cocaine), then class B drugs (e.g. ecstasy, cannabis), and finally class C.

Complications

Most dependent drug users present at times of crisis (e.g. overdose, withdrawal) or with medical complications. Less than 10% actively seek help.

Overdose

Overdose is usually inadvertent. Initially, protect the airway, and exclude hypoglycaemia or serious head/other injury. Opiate overdose is usually due to taking an unexpectedly pure drug or as a result of reduced tolerance after a period of abstinence. It presents with reduced consciousness, respiratory depression, and pinpoint pupils, although hypoxia can cause pupillary dilatation. Hypothermia, pulmonary oedema, and rhabdomyolysis may need to be excluded. Treatment is with naloxone (0.4–0.8 mg intravenously, repeated as necessary). The patient should not be discharged until 6 hours after the last dose of naloxone.

Intoxication

Intoxication requires little intervention in mild cases. Having excluded serious problems, observation until ambulant and orientated is usually all that is required.

Mild benzodiazepine and depressant drug intoxication is similar to that seen with alcohol. Severe intoxication causes hypotonia, diplopia, nystagmus, and mydriasis.

Solvent intoxication is associated with agitation, euphoria, drowsiness, slurred speech, and unsteady gait. There may be a perioral rash.

Stimulants (e.g. cocaine, ecstasy) cause restlessness, pyrexia, and sympathomimetic effects. Severe cases may develop seizures, paranoia, or violent behaviour. Ecstasy may cause an idiosyncratic reaction, similar to malignant hyperthermia. Occasionally, cocaine can cause chest pain, arrhythmias, and even myocardial infarction, due to coronary artery spasm, with ischaemia.

Drug withdrawal

Drug withdrawal can sometimes be difficult to differentiate from intoxication, alcohol withdrawal, drug-related effects (e.g. stimulant-induced psychosis), and organic disease. Careful observation and symptomatic treatment with small doses of benzodiazepines may be required.

Vascular complications

Vascular complications due to intravenous injections include phlebitis, endocarditis, and deep venous thrombosis. Accidental arterial injection may result in fistulae, major bleeding, false aneurysms, and peripheral embolization which may cause significant limb or cerebral ischaemia, with rhabdomyolysis, renal failure, and limb loss.

Septic arthritis

Septic arthritis should be suspected in intravenous drug users who present with acutely painful joints (especially the hip). Antibiotics, joint aspiration, and repeated surgical irrigation may be required.

Skin infections

Skin infections, including cellulitis, abscesses (which may be deep or interconnected with false aneurysms), and extensive skin necrosis may follow subcutaneous drug injections. Treatment includes antibiotic therapy and, in many cases, surgical review and/or debridement.

Management

Management should ideally be multidisciplinary, particularly if there is coexistent psychiatric illness (dual diagnosis).

General

Treatment may be in the community, hospital, or residential settings. It should aim to minimize the risk of self-harm. For example, needle exchanges aim to reduce the risk of HIV infection and hepatitis. Minor painful complaints should be managed with simple analgesics (e.g. paracetamol) which are as effective as in non-drug users. However, these patients are at risk of all the normal medical complaints (e.g. renal stones), and opiate analgesics must not be withheld, if needed.

Underlying psychiatric illness must be detected and treated. Local drug addiction and rehabilitation centres are essential.

Specific
Psychological approaches, including cognitive behavioural therapy, and self-help groups like Narcotics Anonymous are effective.

Pharmacological therapy is used as an antidote to overdoses (e.g. naloxone), prevention or alleviation of withdrawal (e.g. benzodiazepines), or substance replacement (or maintenance) therapies (e.g. methadone) to avoid the need for intravenous opiates.

Maintenance prescriptions are carefully managed by the addiction services and pharmacists, and hospital physicians should not prescribe or supply outpatient controlled drugs to dependent drug users without consulting the patient's GP or these services. Relapse prevention with naltrexone or acamprosate may be considered.

Depression

The lifetime risk of significant depression is about 10% for men and 20% for women. The population prevalence is about 4–5%. It usually presents in the third decade of life and is more common in women from lower socio-economic classes, middle or old age, and in urban, rather than rural, areas. About 15% of patients with severe, recurrent depression eventually commit suicide, and suicidal ideation, or even minor self-harm, in a depressed patient is significant.

Aetiology
Aetiology is complex and includes genetic, environmental, social, and neurobiological factors.

Neurochemical/hormonal
Neurochemical/hormonal mechanisms include the 'monoamine theory' which is largely based on the efficacy of antidepressant medications. Some studies have shown serotonin and noradrenaline metabolites to be reduced in the cerebrospinal fluid and urine of depressed patients. Another theory implicates hypothalamic-pituitary-adrenal axis dysfunction, based on the hypercortisolaemia and disrupted diurnal secretion of cortisol seen in depressed individuals, along with failure to suppress on the dexamethasone suppression test. However, to date, there are no reliable diagnostic biomarkers of depression. The sleep EEG also shows characteristic changes in depression.

Genetic factors
Genetic factors appear to predispose to depression and have been demonstrated in twin and adoption studies. Mood disorders are more common in the relatives of depressed patients.

Psychosocial factors
Life events associated with loss (e.g. bereavement, separation, divorce, loss of status, ill health) increase the rate of depression by sixfold (compared with a normal population) in the following 6 months. Previous childhood abuse, early maternal loss, adverse social circumstances, lack of a confiding relationship, unemployment, domestic unhappiness, or more than three children <14 years old at home can increase susceptibility.

Physical illnesses
Physical illnesses, including hypothyroidism, other endocrine disorders, some viral infections and malignancy, certain medications (e.g. steroids), and recent childbirth are associated with depression. Coexisting psychiatric illness can make diagnosis difficult.

Clinical presentation
Clinical presentation includes the three core symptoms of persistent low mood (usually worse in the morning), loss of enjoyment and interest in activities that were previously pleasurable (termed anhedonia), and decreased energy.

Additional features include reduced concentration and attention, decreased self-esteem and confidence, memory disturbances (especially short-term), ideas of guilt and worthlessness, pessimism regarding the future, and ideas of self-harm. Somatic features include sleep disturbance with early morning waking, decreased appetite, weight loss, constipation, reduced libido, and amenorrhoea.

The patient may exhibit self-neglect and psychomotor retardation. Low mood may be masked by anxiety, with agitation, irritability, and hypochondrial preoccupations. Cognition is often impaired, with reduced attention and decisiveness, but improves with effort. Psychotic features may occur in severe cases, with hallucinations and delusions which are usually mood-congruent. Thus, hallucinations are usually auditory, in the second person, and accusing, abusive, or persecutory (e.g. encouraging suicide). Likewise, delusions are nihilistic, with ideas of poverty (i.e. no clothes), absence of body parts (e.g. no bowel), ill health, or death.

Atypical depression often occurs in adolescence and results in reversal of somatic symptoms, with increased appetite and weight, anxiety-related insomnia with subsequent oversleeping, and reversed diurnal mood variation.

Treatment
Treatment of mild or moderate depression is usually undertaken in the community. Detection of depression should be an important priority for all healthcare workers. Unfortunately, many cases fail to be detected or are missed when presenting with other medical conditions, with potentially serious consequences. Initial management requires assessment of the risk of suicide or self-neglect. Psychiatric referral is advised if suicide risk is high or symptoms are severe or fail to respond to initial treatment. Coexisting physical and substance abuse should be treated.

Pharmacological therapy
Selective serotonin reuptake inhibitors (SSRI) are the commonest drug therapy for depression and are effective in about two-thirds of cases. They may fail due to non-compliance or inadequate dose. Citalopram and sertraline are most often used in patients with comorbid medical problems, as they generally have least interactions with other medications. Combination drug therapies, including antipsychotic agents, may be required in severe cases. Ongoing antidepressant therapy for at least 6 months substantially reduces the risk of relapse, and prophylactic therapy may be essential in severe disease with recurrent relapses (see section on prognosis). When discontinuing antidepressant medication, taper slowly to avoid withdrawal symptoms.

Electroconvulsive therapy
Electroconvulsive therapy is very effective and may be life-saving in severe depression, particularly when associated with stupor or psychosis.

Cognitive behavioural therapy
Cognitive behavioural therapy and other types of psychotherapy are as effective as drug treatments in non-psychotic depression. It can be first-line therapy in mild depression and used in combination with pharmacological therapy in more severe disease.

Prognosis
A single episode of depression usually lasts 3–6 months, but 20% of patients may remain depressed for 2 or more years. About 50% of cases relapse, increasing to 80% in severe disease. Recurrent episodes become increasingly severe, with shorter depression-free periods. Predictors of poor outcome are initial severity, early age of onset, and associated psychiatric or medical comorbidity. In these cases, prophylactic

therapy is particularly important. Lifetime risk of suicide is 15% in severe depression, but successful therapy can reduce this and overall morbidity.

Psychotic illness

Psychosis is best defined as a severe mental disturbance with loss of insight, characterized by loss of contact with reality and in which delusions, hallucinations, and disorganised thinking are often present. Clinically significant psychosis affects about 3% of the general population; the most common conditions are schizophrenia and bipolar affective disorders (i.e. manic-depressive illness). Other psychotic illnesses include drug-induced psychoses, brief psychotic episodes (i.e. lasting less than the duration required to diagnose schizophrenia), schizoaffective disorders (i.e. combined affective and schizophrenic symptoms), and isolated delusional disorders (in which other areas of mental function are well preserved).

Schizophrenia

Schizophrenia means split mind and is characterized by splitting of normal links between mood, perception, thinking, behaviour, and contact with reality. It affects all areas of personal function, including perception, mood, thought content and process, speech, motivation, and behaviour. Schizophrenia differs from bipolar affective disorder, in which normal function is regained between episodes.

The lifetime risk of developing schizophrenia is 1%, affecting men and women equally. Incidence is 2/1,000 individuals per year, and peak incidence is in the late teens and early adulthood.

Aetiology

Aetiology includes genetic, socio-economic, and neurobiological factors.

- **Genetic.** There is a strong genetic link, with the risk of developing schizophrenia estimated at ~50% in a monozygotic twin whose other twin has schizophrenia, ~12% in children of schizophrenics, and 2.5% in a second-degree relative of a schizophrenic, compared with a risk of 1% in the general population.
- **Socio-economic factors** include an increased risk in those born in urban areas, Afro-Caribbean populations, and those with shy, suspicious, and overcompliant personalities. Relapse is higher in families with high levels of expressed emotions. Schizophrenics tend to drift to lower social classes.
- **Neurobiological.** Excess dopamine with overactivity in the mesolimbic system is associated with the development of schizophrenia. Stimulant drugs like amphetamines release dopamine and can precipitate psychosis. Similarly, antipsychotic drugs which block dopamine receptors are effective therapies. Chronic schizophrenia is associated with reduced brain size and enlarged lateral ventricles, and neurodevelopmental abnormalities (e.g. low birthweight babies, perinatal injuries) have been implicated as potential causes for schizophrenia.

Clinical features

Clinical features are initially non-diagnostic. No single symptom is pathognomonic, and hallucinations or delusions only confirm psychosis. Classifications of schizophrenia are based on the presence of previous or current psychosis for >1 month and the absence of predominantly affective symptoms. Mental state examination helps exclude organic and affective disorders, as non-auditory hallucinations are more common in organic disease, and delusions in depression and mania are mood-congruent.

The commonest pattern of illness is of acute exacerbations, with increasing residual impairment between episodes. About a third of patients who have a first episode never have another. Another third develop chronic illness, requiring repeated admissions and long-term care.

Schneider's first rank symptoms for the diagnosis of schizophrenia may, confusingly, also occur in mania and other conditions. They include auditory hallucinations, in which two or more voices discuss or make a running commentary about the patient; thought echo, in which voices repeat the subject's thoughts out loud or anticipate thoughts, and thought withdrawal, insertion, or broadcasting. There may be somatic passivity in which emotions and actions are externally controlled or imposed; and delusional perceptions, in which a delusional meaning is imposed on a real perception (i.e. I saw a bird in the sky, and I knew the police wanted to kill me).

Second rank symptoms are less specific and include secondary delusions and catatonic behaviour. Thought disorders with neologisms (i.e. new words), concrete thinking, and 'word salad' (jumbled nonsense) can also occur.

Symptoms are often divided into positive (e.g. hallucinations, delusions), negative (i.e. flat affect, poverty of speech, poor motivation), and cognitive (e.g. poor attention/memory).

Classifications

Classifications include:

- Type 1 with acute onset, positive symptoms (e.g. hallucinations), normal brain ventricular size, which responds to neuroleptics and has a good prognosis, and Type 2 with chronic negative symptoms, enlarged ventricles, which responds poorly to neuroleptics and has a poor prognosis.
- Differentiation into subtypes of schizophrenia, including: paranoid schizophrenia which is common and associated with delusions and auditory hallucinations; catatonic schizophrenia which is rare; hebephrenic (disorganized) schizophrenia which has an early onset, poor prognosis, and unpredictable behaviour; and residual (chronic) schizophrenia in which negative symptoms predominate.

Management

Management of first-episode schizophrenia requires prompt referral to the psychiatric team for two reasons. First, the duration of untreated psychosis affects the long-term prognosis and, secondly, the risk of suicide in schizophrenia is high during a first episode (when the patient is perplexed or terrified by the novel psychotic phenomena and responds unpredictably). Classical antipsychotic drugs alleviate hallucinations and delusions but do not control negative symptoms, although the newer atypical antipsychotic drugs are helpful in this respect. The antipsychotic effects may take 10–14 days to develop. Cognitive therapy may help to control distressing auditory hallucinations.

In known schizophrenics, close liaison with the psychiatric multidisciplinary team (including the community psychiatric nurse and psychiatrist) is essential to decide whether the patient should be admitted or treated in the community and what treatment should be given. All patients receiving secondary psychiatric services are managed through the Care Programme Approach, in which they are assigned a care coordinator who will provide support, monitor their mental state, and ensure treatment compliance. Social support, including accommodation and community rehabilitation services, are vital to maximize patient independence and, if possible, return to work.

Prognosis

After a first psychotic episode, 90% will be well within 12 months, but 70–80% will relapse within 5 years. In addition to taking medication, avoiding illicit drug use (e.g. cannabis) and excessive stress reduces the risk of relapse. Ten years after the diagnosis of schizophrenia, about 50% of patients continue to have relapses, with no or minimal disability between relapses; 25% have chronic disease with significant disability. Lifetime risk of suicide in schizophrenics is ~10%.

Mania and hypomania

Mania and hypomania are less common than depression but often require compulsory hospital admission. Onset may be acute or gradual, with pathologically elevated mood, hyperactivity, poor judgement, and lack of insight. These episodes may be associated with depression (bipolar affective disorder or manic-depressive syndrome), may follow severe stress, physical illness, or childbirth, or may occur spontaneously. Mania can be precipitated by medications (e.g. antidepressants, steroids, substance abuse with amphetamines), lithium withdrawal, or electroconvulsive therapy. Relationships, employment and finances can be severely affected.

Manic patients tend to be overactive, cheerful, and have a decreased requirement for sleep. They are easily distracted and demonstrate flight of ideas, delusions (often grandiose), hallucinations, and promiscuity. They tend to be impetuous, irresponsible. Irritability can be the dominant symptom and may be expressed in terms of the interviewer's shortcomings, anger, and occasionally violence. Hypomanic patients do not exhibit delusions, hallucinations, or complete disruption of normal activity.

Overt mania is best treated in hospital, but, as insight is often lacking, compulsory admission may be required. Antipsychotic drugs like olanzapine are used to treat the acute episode, and electroconvulsive therapy can be effective in severe cases. Prophylactic lithium therapy for recurrent mania is effective in about 60% of cases. Alternative agents include sodium valproate, carbamazepine, and depot medications.

Munchausen's syndrome

A disorder characterized by recurrent hospital admissions, with factitious symptoms and signs of physical illness and a morbid attraction to the sick role. It is usually more common in men, with onset aged 30–40 years old. Psychiatric illness is rare, but there may be an underlying personality disorder. The cause is unknown. It may take many years before the cause of the patient's repeated admissions to hospital is known, and, during this time, they may undergo multiple investigations and operations.

Suspicion should be raised in patients a long way from home, with incomplete and inconsistent disclosure of personal details, in those with excellent knowledge of their previous treatment, dramatic recent illness (e.g. surgery), multiple scars or laparotomies, multiple allergies, and unusual demands.

Management

It is important to exclude physical disease, and admission for observation may be necessary. If suspicious, discreetly contact the general practitioner or other hospitals involved with previous admissions to corroborate the history. Record details of the admission carefully, and offer the patient help to manage the syndrome. However, once discovered, most patients simply self-discharge.

The detection of factitious disorder in healthcare workers has serious consequences, as the Clothier report (1994) advises that patients with severe personality disorder should be prevented from working in health-related disciplines.

Further reading

AA in the United States. <http://www.aa.org/subpage.cfm?page=26>.

Alcoholics Anonymous (Great Britain). <http://www.alcoholics-anonymous.org.uk>. UK national helpline: 0845 769 7555. World service: <http://www.aa.org>.

Depression Alliance. <http://www.depressionalliance.org>. Tel: 08451 232 320.

Friedman RA (2006). Violence and mental illness—how strong is the link? *New England Journal of Medicine*, **355**, 2064–6.

General Medical Council. <http://www.gmc-uk.org>. Tel: 0161 923 6602.

Inouye SK (2006). Delirium in older persons. *New England Journal of Medicine*, **354**, 1157–65.

Jones R (2014). *Mental Health Act Manual*, 17th edn. Sweet & Maxwell, London.

Langlands RL, Jorm AF, Kelly CM, Kitchener BA (2008). First aid for depression: a Delphi consensus study with consumers, carers and clinicians. *Journal of Affective Disorders*, **105**, 157–65.

Luty J (2006). What works in alcohol use disorders? *Advances in Psychiatric Treatment*, **12**, 13–22.

Maj M (2005). 'Psychiatric comorbidity': an artefact of current diagnostic systems? *British Journal of Psychiatry*, **186**, 182–4.

Medical Defence Union. <http://www.the-mdu.com>. 24 h helpline: 0800 716 646.

Medical Protection Society. Email: info@mps.org.uk or querydoc@mps.org.uk. Tel: 0845 605 4000.

Mind (the UK leading mental health charity and support group). <http://www.mind.org.uk>. Tel: 0300 123 3393.

Morgan JF (2007). 'Giving up the culture of blame': risk assessment and risk management in psychiatric practice. Briefing document for Royal College of Psychiatrists. Royal College of Psychiatrists: London. <http://www.rcpsych.ac.uk/pdf/Risk%20Assessment%20Paper%20-%20Giving%20up%20the%20Culture%20of%20Blame.pdf>.

Mueser KT and McGurk SR (2004). Schizophrenia. *Lancet*, **19**, 2063–72.

Narcotics Anonymous UK. <http://www.ukna.org>. Tel: 0207 730 0009. UK national helpline: 0300 999 1212.

National Institute for Health and Clinical Excellence (2004). NICE guidelines on self-harm. Clinical guideline 16. <http://www.nice.org.uk/guidance/cg16>.

National Institute for Health and Clinical Excellence (2009). NICE guidelines on schizophrenia. Clinical guideline 92. <http://www.nice.org.uk/guidance/cg82>.

National Institute for Health and Clinical Excellence (2009). NICE guidelines on depression. Clinical guideline 90. <http://www.nice.org.uk/guidance/cg90.>.

Public Health England (2007). Drug misuse and dependence—UK guidelines on clinical management. HMSO, London. <http://www.nta.nhs.uk/uploads/clinical_guidelines_2007.pdf>.

Scottish Intercollegiate Guidelines Network. The management of harmful drinking and alcohol dependence in primary care annex 4. The one minute Paddington Alcohol Test (PAT). <http://www.sign.ac.uk/guidelines/fulltext/74/annex4.html>.

Royal College of Psychiatrists, Royal College of Physicians (2003). *The psychological care of medical patients, a practical guide*. 2nd edn. Royal College of Psychiatrists and Royal College of Physicians, London.

The national confidential enquiry (NCI) into suicide and homicide by people with mental illness. Health Quality Improvement Partnership. Annual Report: England, Northern Ireland, Scotland and Wales 2015. <http://www.bbmh.manchester.ac.uk/cmhs/research/centreforsuicideprevention/nci/reports/NCISHReport2015bookmarked.pdf>.

The Samaritans. <http://www.samaritans.org>. Tel: 08457 909 090; Republic of Ireland Tel: 1850 609 090. Outside the UK: <http://www.befrienders.org>.

World Health Organization. The ICD-10 classification of mental and behavioural disorders. World Health Organization, Geneva. <http://www.who.int/classifications/icd/en/bluebook.pdf>.

Haematological emergencies

Introduction

This chapter describes the common haematological emergencies that are encountered in acute medicine. Throughout this chapter, we will use case studies to illustrate various points. However, since terminology in haematology can be confusing, an understanding of the origin of haematopoiesis may help to categorize diseases.

Early in the process of differentiation, haematopoietic stem cells divide into lymphoid and myeloid cells.

- Lymphoid precursors develop into B cells, T cells, and natural killer cells.
- Myeloid precursors divide into red cell, platelet, and granulocyte precursors (eventually neutrophils, monocytes, eosinophils, and basophils).

Most coagulation factors are synthesized in the liver. Diseases are categorized as those that affect red or white cells, haemostasis and thrombosis, transfusion, and malignant or non-malignant processes.

Red cell disorders include:

- Abnormalities in the haemoglobin molecule: sickle cell anaemia and thalassaemia.
- Reduced enzymes within the red cell: G6PD and pyruvate kinase deficiency.
- Structural abnormalities of the red cell: hereditary spherocytosis and elliptocytosis.
- Other causes of peripheral destruction of red cells: autoimmune haemolytic anaemia, microangiopathic haemolytic anaemia.
- Reduced production of red cells: haematinic deficiencies, anaemia of chronic disease, red cell aplasia, aplastic anaemia.
- Iron overload from transfusion and genetic abnormalities: primary and secondary haemochromatosis.

White cell disorders include:

- Leukaemias: malignancy of the haematopoietic precursors in the bone marrow and blood. These can be acute or chronic, and lymphoid or myeloid. Abnormalities in myeloid precursors can manifest themselves as overproduction (myeloproliferative disorders) or under-/inefficient production (myelodysplasia).
- Myeloproliferative disorders: polycythaemia rubra vera, essential thrombocythaemia, and myelofibrosis.
- Myelodysplasia: refractory anaemia (RA), refractory cytopenia with multilineage dysplasia (RCMD), refractory anaemia with excess of blasts (RAEB).

Blood transfusion

Blood transfusion and reactions to transfusion encompasses not only transfusion of red cells, but also platelets, coagulation factors, and intravenous immunoglobulin.

Haemostasis and thrombosis

Haemostasis is achieved by a combination of platelets, coagulation factors, coagulation inhibitors, fibrinolysis, and blood vessels. Abnormalities in any of these elements can lead to:

1. Bleeding disorders: inherited (haemophilia, von Willebrand's disease (vWD)), acquired (vitamin K deficiency, liver disease), and platelet disorders (qualitative and quantitative).
2. Clotting disorders—arterial and venous (see acute thrombosis later in this chapter and Chapter 12).

This chapter complies with the British Committee for Standards in Haematology guidelines which can be accessed via <http://www.bcshguidelines.com/4_HAEMATOLOGY_GUIDELINES.html>.

Acute leukaemias

Case study

A 22-year-old student nurse was taken to hospital by ambulance, unconscious. She was accompanied by a friend who reported that she had been tired and unwell for the last month and had initially presented to her GP with a sore throat and fever, for which she had been treated with co-amoxiclav. A week earlier, she had presented to the accident and emergency (A&E) department with epistaxis, requiring nasal packs. Thrombocytopenia was noted. She was discharged, and review by her GP was arranged for the following morning. Over the course of the day prior to her second presentation, she complained of increasing headache and, that evening, was found unconscious in her room. On examination, she was obtunded, with a reduced Glasgow coma score (GCS) of 8/15, oral candidiasis, petechiae on her arms and legs, and fundoscopy revealed bilateral papilloedema. A full blood count reported a haemoglobin of 9.5 g/dL, WCC 8.2×10^{-9}/L, platelets 23×10^{-9}/L, and clotting profile PT 35.0, APTT 51.5, and fibrinogen 0.5 g/L Following further deterioration of her conscious level, she was intubated and mechanically ventilated. The subsequent CT head scan demonstrated a large intracerebral haemorrhage. Blood film examination was consistent with acute promyelocytic leukaemia. She was initially treated with clotting factors, and plans were made to do a bone marrow aspiration and commence treatment with ATRA (all trans-retinoic acid). However, her GCS continued to deteriorate, and her pupils became fixed and dilated. A repeat CT head scan showed herniation of the cerebellar tonsils through the foramen magnum, and she was eventually pronounced dead on ITU.

Background

Acute leukaemias are divided into acute lymphoblastic leukaemias (ALL) and acute myeloid leukaemias (AML). Acute promyelocytic leukaemia (APML) is a subtype of AML and is a particularly important diagnosis to make in haematology. It can be associated with early life-threatening bleeding and disseminated intravascular coagulation (DIC), yet the long-term outcome for such patients, with prompt treatment, is excellent.

ALL has a bimodal incidence; the first peak is in children (aged 2–10 years old) and is associated with high remission rates and excellent long-term survival with modern chemotherapy regimens. The second peak is in adults and appears to be a biologically different disease with much poorer outcomes.

Acute myeloid leukaemia is the most common leukaemia in adults. AML may occur de novo or be secondary to myelodysplasia, myeloproliferative disorders, previous cytotoxic chemotherapy, ionizing radiation, and constitutional chromosomal abnormalities (e.g. Down's syndrome).

Presentation of acute leukaemia

Acute leukaemias are aggressive diseases that present with bone marrow failure and organ infiltration. A high index of suspicion is needed to diagnose bone marrow failure, as symptoms can easily be ascribed to other causes (see Box 15.1, Table 15.1).

Organ infiltration may lead to hepatosplenomegaly, lymphadenopathy, gum hypertrophy, mediastinal masses, and testicular swelling.

Box 15.1 Signs and symptoms of bone marrow failure

- Anaemia—tiredness, shortness of breath, pallor
- Neutropenia—fever, sore throat, oral *Candida*, cellulitis, respiratory infection, etc.
- Thrombocytopenia—bruising, petechiae, epistaxis, menorrhagia

Table 15.1 Initial assessment of a patient with suspected acute leukaemia

History of any symptoms of bone marrow failure, previous haematological disease, previous chemotherapy treatment

Examination for signs of bone marrow failure (e.g. pallor, infection, petechiae) and organ infiltration (hepatosplenomegaly, lymphadenopathy, gum hypertrophy, testicular enlargement in males)

FBC with film: to detect pancytopenia and circulating blasts

Clotting profile, including fibrinogen: to rule out DIC

Urea and electrolytes: to assess renal function as may need imminent chemotherapy

Liver function: to assess baseline function prior to chemotherapy (may be deranged with infiltration/sepsis)

CRP: signs of infection are common at presentation

CXR: for signs of pneumonia and to rule out mediastinal masses

Bone marrow aspirate and trephine, with cytogenetics, immunophenotyping and possibly molecular studies (organized by haematology services)

Management of acute leukaemia

The management of acute leukaemias can be divided into general supportive measures and treatment of specific types of leukaemia.

General supportive measures

1. **Blood product support.** Frequent blood and platelet transfusions are required due to bone marrow failure and chemotherapy-induced myelosuppression. Current guidelines for blood transfusion are a haemoglobin (Hb) <8 g/dL, but a higher threshold may be required if a patient has comorbidity, such as cardiovascular disease. Platelets are transfused if $<10 \times 10^{-9}$ in an otherwise well patient, and $<20 \times 10^{-9}$ if septic, and should be discussed with the haematology team in a patient with active bleeding or if the patient is about to undergo an intervention (e.g. central line, surgery). CMV-negative blood should be given until the CMV status is known by checking serology, as reactivation of this virus can cause serious morbidity if the patient were to undergo a bone marrow transplant in the future. In patients with clotting abnormalities, replacement factors may be required in the form of FFP, prothrombin complex concentrate, cryoprecipitate, or fibrinogen concentrate. Of particular note, ALL patients receiving asparaginase therapy may have low fibrinogen levels due to drug-induced reductions in antithrombin III

levels. Discussion with the local haematology department is required before giving factor replacement, as there may be variations in local protocols.

2. **Treatment and prophylaxis of infection.** It is common for patients with a new diagnosis of leukaemia and in those already on treatment to present with fever. Local treatment protocols for neutropenic/non-neutropenic fever should be followed. The use of antibiotic prophylaxis during neutropenia (e.g. ciprofloxacin) varies between units and also for particular patients (e.g. recurrent Gram-negative sepsis). Viral prophylaxis (e.g. aciclovir) is often given to prevent herpes reactivation. Patients with prolonged neutropenia are at risk of yeast infection (e.g. *Candida*; usually pharyngitis or oesophagitis) and invasive fungal infection (e.g. *Aspergillus* with invasive lung infection). After 96 hours of antibiotic therapy, patients with prolonged fever are usually investigated with a serum *Aspergillus* galactomannan, antifungal agent level, and high-resolution CT scan, looking for typical fungal features in the chest.

Fungal prophylaxis may be with itraconazole (oral), fluconazole (oral), or liposomal amphotericin (IV). It should be noted that fluconazole gives protection against *Candida* but not *Aspergillus*. However, itraconazole may not be co-prescribed with vinca-alkaloids (usually a component of ALL therapy) or gemtuzumab (a part of some AML regimes).

- Proven or suspected *Candida* infection is usually treated with fluconazole or itraconazole.
- Proven or suspected *Aspergillus* infection is usually treated with liposomal amphotericin or caspofungin.
- Patients with ALL are at high risk of *Pneumocystis jirovecii* pneumonia (PCP) and are given co-trimoxazole prophylaxis (see also Chapters 6 and 13), possibly with folic acid rescue (as co-trimoxazole may cause folate deficiency).

3. **Progesterones** are usually given to premenopausal women to prevent menstruation when undergoing intensive chemotherapy.

4. **Prevention of tumour lysis syndrome** (see section on 'Chemotherapy-related complications', later in this chapter).

5. **Fertility**. Sperm cryopreservation should be offered to all men wishing to preserve their reproductive potential before commencing intensive chemotherapy. Women are at risk of reduced fertility and premature menopause. However, it is often impractical and dangerous to delay for IVF treatment, and embryo storage is often arranged in women.

6. **Insertion of a central venous catheter.** This is usually in the form of a tunnelled Hickman line. It provides easy access for blood tests, chemotherapy, and blood product support. The tunnel site can be a frequent focus for infection and, if this occurs, should be treated, according to local protocols (usually with MRSA cover after line cultures and swabs).

7. **Viral screen.** Patients are usually screened for HIV and hepatitis B and C infection before commencing chemotherapy. Patients receiving high-dose chemotherapy, particularly with corticosteroids, are at risk of hepatitis B reactivation and fulminant liver failure. Those with past hepatitis B infection should be given lamivudine prophylaxis during treatment.

Specific treatments
The treatment of acute leukaemia is divided into the categories of APML, AML, and ALL. Patients are frequently enrolled onto current clinical trials.

Acute promyelocytic leukaemia (APML)
Treatment for APML is different from treatment of other forms of AML. Current standard treatment is four blocks of chemotherapy, including ATRA (all-trans retinoic acid, the acid form of Vitamin A). ATRA induces differentiation of leukaemic promyelocytes, into 'mature, differentiated' malignant cells that initially undergo spontaneous apoptosis. Consequently ATRA may induce remission but it is short-lived without 'traditional' chemotherapy. Arsenic trioxide has been the standard concurrent chemotherapy since 2013 as it has a better side-effect profile than previous therapy with low-dose anthracycline (e.g. daunorubicin, mitoxantrone) and is followed by 2 years of maintenance treatment (e.g. methotrexate and ATRA). Initial remission rates are about 90% and prolonged survival is achieved in >60%. A complication of treatment is development of the ATRA syndrome which may be caused by neutrophilia, secondary to promyelocyte differentiation. Symptoms include fever, weight gain, acute respiratory distress, and pleural/pericardial effusions. Patients may require steroid treatment, with or without temporary discontinuation of ATRA.

Acute myeloid leukaemia (AML)
All other subtypes of acute myeloid leukaemia are treated in broadly the same way. Decisions about the type of treatment a patient receives is determined by the patient's fitness for intensive treatment, their age, their risk (defined by cytogenetics and response in the bone marrow after treatment), and availability of a sibling donor. Treatment options include 3–4 courses of intensive chemotherapy; two courses of intensive therapy, followed by a standard allograft; three courses of chemotherapy, followed by a 'mini' allograft; or non-intensive chemotherapy. It may be more suitable to give non-intensive treatment in the elderly or those with comorbidity, in the form of low-dose subcutaneous chemotherapy. The intention of low-dose treatment is palliation.

Acute lymphocytic leukaemia (ALL)
Around 85% of children with ALL are now cured. The treatment involves alternating intensive inpatient and less intensive outpatient blocks of therapy. After the last intensive block, girls go on to have a 2-year outpatient maintenance treatment and boys for 3 years (due to the worse prognosis for males).

ALL in adults has a much poorer prognosis than that in children, and survival rates have not improved significantly in the last two decades. Five-year survival for patients under 60 is approximately 30–40%, less than 15% for patients over 60 years, and less than 5% for patients older than 70 years.

Young adults with ALL are now treated on paediatric protocols, and UKALL 2003 accepts young adults up to the age of 25 years. Treatment for adults involves remission induction, which can be via a number of protocols. It usually involves steroids, vincristine, anthracyclines, asparaginase, cyclophosphamide, and cytarabine therapy. The remission induction phase can take many weeks. High-risk patients and those with an HLA-matched sibling may be offered an allogeneic bone marrow transplant. Other options include imatinib maintenance for those who have the Philadelphia chromosome; a low-intensity approach to remission induction in those over 60 years old to preserve quality of life as far as possible; and intensification chemotherapy post-remission induction for those not suited to a transplant.

Hyperleucocytosis
Case study
A 26-year-old man with no previous medical history was admitted to the emergency department with a 1-day history

of confusion and a 1-week history of shortness of breath on exertion. The patient had presented to a community-based practice 3 days earlier, at which time examination of the lungs and a chest X-ray (CXR) were normal. In the 24 hours before admission, the patient's family had noted that he was confused and that he was complaining of a headache.

Physical examination revealed diffuse, bilateral retinal haemorrhages and a fine petechial rash below the knees. Pulse oximetry demonstrated arterial hypoxaemia, and a CXR identified bilateral, fine interstitial and alveolar space shadowing. A full blood examination revealed a white cell count of 300×10^9/L, haemoglobin 7.5 g/dL, and a platelet count of 13×10^9/L. Examination of the peripheral blood film demonstrated leukaemic blasts which were immunophenotyped, using flow cytometry, and confirmed the diagnosis as acute myeloid leukaemia.

The patient was initially treated with intravenous fluids, without blood transfusion, and tumour lysis syndrome prophylaxis. He subsequently underwent leukapheresis with a single plasma volume exchange. Chemotherapy was commenced shortly afterwards. The following day, his white cell count was 160×10^9/L, and his confusion had resolved completely. His breathlessness improved gradually over the next 48 hours.

Background

Most patients with acute leukaemia or with aggressive lymphomas in leukaemic phase, present with non-specific constitutional symptoms, features of bone marrow failure, or are referred, following the detection of an abnormal blood count. A small proportion of patients present acutely with hyperleucocytosis. This is defined as a white cell count in excess of 100×10^9/L. Such patients are often extremely unwell, with multiple organ dysfunction, and require prompt intervention. Patients frequently require specific intervention, in addition to chemotherapy, for the underlying malignancy.

Pathophysiology

Patients with hyperleucocytosis present with a constellation of symptoms and signs that are primarily due to leukostasis. This refers to the impaired passage of circulating tumour cells in the microcirculation of the tissues and organs of the body. Leukostasis can occasionally be encountered at white cell counts of $<100 \times 10^9$/L. Conversely, some patients with haematological malignancies may present with counts in excess of 100×10^9/L and may not have any features of hyperleucocytosis. Clearly, cell surface adhesion molecules and their interaction with the endothelium are important in determining which patients develop this clinicopathologic syndrome, in addition to the absolute white cell count. Clinical manifestations of this syndrome are protean; most patients present with neurological or pulmonary manifestations. Early deaths are most frequently due to intracranial haemorrhage or respiratory failure.

When the pulmonary microvasculature is affected, patients usually present with shortness of breath. Importantly, the CXR may be discordant with the patient's symptoms. Confusion may occur in patients without evidence of haemorrhage due to leukostasis in the microvasculature of the central nervous system. Focal neurological deficits usually herald the onset of intracranial haemorrhage. Small-vessel occlusion may account for retinal vein thrombosis, myocardial infarction, or other life-threatening ischaemia.

Laboratory evaluation

A full blood count will confirm the presence of leucocytosis. A blood film examination is essential for further characterization of the tumour cells. There is frequently anaemia and thrombocytopenia. Disseminated intravascular coagulation may occur, especially in patients with acute myeloid or acute lymphoblastic leukaemia. A bone marrow examination is often required to completely characterize the cause.

Prevention and management

There are a number of therapeutic interventions that are required, in addition to the identification and treatment of the underlying cause. In the acute setting, aggressive fluid administration, with appropriate monitoring of the extracellular fluid volume status, is required. Blood transfusion should be avoided, unless there is evidence of critical tissue hypoxaemia, as this may aggravate the sludging of cells in the microcirculation. Prompt attention should be given to the assessment for, and prevention of, tumour lysis syndrome (see 'Chemotherapy-related complications', later in this chapter).

The platelet count and coagulation profile must be carefully monitored, as disseminated intravascular coagulation may develop. This is especially important in this patient group who may require insertion of large-diameter central venous access lines for the administration of chemotherapy.

To abrogate the symptoms of hyperleucocytosis, the number of circulating tumour cells must be reduced. This is achieved either with chemotherapy designed to cause cell death and reduce the overall tumour burden or through leukapheresis, which simply removes the fraction of whole blood which is most concentrated with the tumour cell population. Chemotherapy should be regarded as the central element of treatment and should begin as soon as the diagnosis of the tumour subtype is confirmed.

Leukapheresis requires suitable vascular access and an apheresis machine to remove the malignant population and to re-infuse plasma. This technique should be considered in all patients with symptoms and in those patients with a leucocyte count above 100×10^9/L. Although the evidence base is poor, many clinicians proceed directly to chemotherapy without leukapheresis in patients with blast counts $100-200 \times 10^9$/L but in the absence of symptoms. Leukapheresis offers a prompt reduction in the circulating white cell count. However, without chemotherapy, the white cell count will subsequently climb, as more tumour cells are mobilized from the extravascular compartment. The technique can be repeated during the first 24–48 hours until chemotherapy takes full effect. Its main disadvantage is the requirement for central venous access and the need for specialized training and equipment which is not available in all centres.

Summary

Hyperleucocytosis is a medical emergency. It requires rapid identification, treatment directed at the underlying cause, and consideration of other methods to improve blood circulation in the microvasculature. Early identification and treatment are essential, as this syndrome has a high mortality, but prompt therapy rapidly alleviates potential complications.

Further reading

Inaba H, Greaves M, Mullighan CG (2013). Acute lymphoblastic leukaemia. *Lancet*, **381**, 1943–55.

Lo-Coco F, Avvisati G, Vignetti M, *et al*. (2013). Retinoic acid and arsenic trioxide for acute promyelocytic leukemia. *New England Journal of Medicine*, **369**, 111–121.

Rowe JM and Goldstone AH (2007). How I treat acute lymphocytic leukemia in adults. *Blood*, **110**, 2268–75.

Yanada M (2015). Time to tune the treatment of Ph+ ALL. *Blood*, **125**, 3674–5

Haemolytic anaemias

Case study

A 34-year-old Caucasian accountant presented to A&E with increasing lethargy. He was accompanied by his wife who had noticed his eyes were slightly yellow. Of note, his previous medical history included idiopathic thrombocytopenic purpura (ITP), which was currently in remission, and there had been no recent bruising or bleeding. He had received no recent blood transfusions, there had been no recent travel, and he did not take any regular medication. He had no personal or family history of G6PD deficiency. On examination, he was jaundiced and looked pale. He had a palpable spleen that extended 3 cm below the costal margin. Initial tests in A&E showed a Hb 5.5 g/dL, WCC 9 × 10^9/L, neutrophils 8.0×10^9/L, and platelets 180×10^9/L. His bilirubin was 50 micromoles/L, but otherwise his liver function was normal. After liaison with haematology, further tests were undertaken. A blood film showed polychromasia and spherocytes. The reticulocyte count was 250×10^9/L, and serum lactate dehydrogenase (LDH) was raised at 2,500 IU/L. Serum haptoglobin was undetectable, and a direct antiglobulin test (DAT, previously known as the direct Coomb's test), was positive for complement and IgG, which is a warm-reacting antibody. He was diagnosed with warm autoimmune haemolytic anaemia (and Evans' syndrome, as he already had a diagnosis of ITP). He was treated with prednisolone 1 mg/kg/day by the haematology team. There was a good recovery in his haemoglobin level, and he was discharged after 4 days and followed up in the outpatient department.

Background

Normal red cell lifespan is 120 days after which cells are removed by the reticuloendothelial system (i.e. bone marrow, spleen, and liver). Haemoglobin is broken down to haem and globin. The globin is broken down to amino acids which are then re-utilized for protein synthesis. The haem is broken down to iron and protoporphyrin which is converted to unconjugated bilirubin. Conjugation occurs in the liver. This is then excreted from the gut as stercobilinogen, and after reabsorption, from the kidney as urobilinogen.

There are many conditions that may lead to a shortening of red cell survival. The bone marrow has a huge ability to expand red cell production, but, if the rate of destruction outstrips marrow production, anaemia will result.

Biochemical markers of accelerated red cell destruction are apparent in haemolytic anaemia; the reticulocyte count (i.e. immature red cells) will be raised due to hyperplastic erythropoiesis in the marrow. Bilirubin will increase due to increased haem breakdown. The LDH will be high, as there is increased cell turnover. Haptoglobins are plasma proteins capable of binding haemoglobin. Consequently, when free haemoglobin is raised, haptoglobulin levels will be low. In addition, the spleen enlarges due to expansion of the reticuloendothelial system.

Increased red cell destruction can be caused by a number of abnormalities (see Table 15.2). If red cells are destroyed within the circulation, this is termed intravascular haemolysis, whereas destruction within the reticuloendothelial system is extravascular haemolysis.

A blood film is often essential for diagnosis in haemolytic anaemia. It may be difficult to establish a differential based on history and examination alone, and blood film findings may trigger the differential diagnosis and prompt further history taking and investigations. Table 15.3 illustrates the typical clinical approach to a patient with suspected haemolytic anaemia.

Table 15.2 Causes of haemolytic anaemia

Acquired

1. Immune: **alloimmune** (HDN, haemolytic transfusion reaction, bone marrow allograft); **autoimmune** (warm, cold)
2. Red cell fragmentation syndromes (MAHA): TTP/HUS/DIC/prosthetic heart valves
3. Infections (sepsis, malaria)
4. Paroxysmal nocturnal haemoglobinuria

Inherited

1. Membrane disorders (hereditary spherocytosis, elliptocytosis)
2. Enzyme disorders (G6PD and PK deficiency)
3. Haemoglobinopathies (sickle cell anaemia, thalassaemias)

MAHA, microangiopathic haemolytic anaemia; TTP, thrombotic thrombocytopenic purpura; DIC, disseminated intravascular coagulation; HUS, haemolytic uraemic syndrome; PK, pyruvate kinase; G6PD, glucose-6-phosphate dehydrogenase.

Table 15.3 Approach to a patient with suspected haemolytic anaemia

1. History: any known personal or family history of haemoglobin, red cell or enzyme abnormality. Any recent blood transfusion, travel (malaria), drug history, B symptoms (fever, night sweats, weight loss; often associated with lymphoma)
2. Examine: for jaundice and splenomegaly
3. FBC with film (see Table 15.1)
4. Tests for evidence of haemolysis: reticulocyte count, serum LDH, bilirubin, haptoglobin, urinary haemosiderin (in chronic intravascular haemolysis), urobilinogen, urinary haemoglobin
6. Consider G6PD testing (although may be falsely normal in an acute haemolytic episode), DAT (? with determination of warm or cold antibody if positive; three thick and thin films for malaria; consider haemoglobin electrophoresis (but haemoglobinopathies are usually diagnosed in childhood)

LDH, lactate dehydrogenase; DAT, direct antiglobulin test or direct Coomb's test.

The direct antiglobulin test (DAT), previously known as the direct Coomb's test, helps determine the cause of haemolytic anaemia. Circulating IgG autoantibodies bind to antigens on the red blood cell (RBC) surface membrane, and this leads to complement binding to the bound IgG. These bound autoantibodies can be detected by the DAT test (or direct Coomb's test); the RBCs are washed (removing the patient's own plasma) and then incubated with antihuman globulin (also known as 'Coomb's reagent'). If this produces agglutination of RBCs, the direct Coomb's test (DAT) is positive, a visual indication that antibodies are present.

Management of haemolytic anaemias

Warm autoimmune haemolytic anaemia

This is caused by the production of antibodies against red cell antigens (usually of the Rh group). The antibodies are most commonly IgG and react more strongly at 37°C than 4°C. Hence, they are termed warm antibodies. Initially monocytes and macrophages (usually in the spleen) remove part (i.e. 'take a bite out of') of the red cell membrane and the cells change shape from biconcave discs to spheres as they lose membrane (i.e. microspherocytes). Then, the whole cell is sequestered by the reticuloendothelial system (i.e. extravascular haemolysis). Patients often have splenomegaly.

The disease runs a remitting and relapsing course, and if associated with ITP, is known as Evans' syndrome. The condition is usually idiopathic but may be secondary to lymphoproliferative disorders, such as chronic lymphocytic leukaemia (CLL) or autoimmune disorders, such as systemic lupus erythematosus (SLE).

Treatment is usually commenced with prednisolone 1 mg/kg/day, and then the dose is gradually tapered down. Other methods of immunomodulation may be required, such as azathioprine, cyclophosphamide, and rituximab. Intravenous immunoglobulin (IVIG) is sometimes helpful in refractory cases. Patients are usually commenced on folic acid maintenance, as they are at risk of deficiency due to high cell turnover. Occasionally, when haemolysis is severe, blood transfusion is required. Cross-matching in this case is difficult, and the least incompatible blood is selected. Difficult cases may be treated with splenectomy.

Many drugs can cause warm autoimmune haemolytic anaemias. This usually involves one of three mechanisms:

1. True autoimmune haemolytic anaemia (e.g. methyldopa).
2. The drug may attach to the red cell membrane and acts as an antigen, inducing an antibody reaction (e.g. penicillins, cephalosporins).
3. Drug-antibody complexes attach to the red cell, causing deposition of complement. This results in red cell removal by the reticuloendothelial system (e.g. quinine).

Drug-induced haemolytic anaemia usually resolves with discontinuation of the drug. Transfusion may be required in severe cases.

Cold autoimmune haemolytic anaemia

This is caused by antibodies that react most strongly with red cells at colder temperatures (e.g. <32°C). The antibody is usually an IgM. Red cells in the peripheral circulation become coated with antibody where the temperature is cooler. As IgM can fix complement, there may be intravascular, as well as extravascular, haemolysis.

Causes include lymphoproliferative disorders, mycoplasma pneumonia, and infectious mononucleosis. Patients may have mild jaundice and splenomegaly. The blood film classically shows red cell agglutinates.

Management includes keeping the patient warm and treating the underlying cause. Steroids are generally ineffective. If the cause is not apparent, it may be appropriate to actively search for a lymphoproliferative disorder (e.g. CT scan, bone marrow biopsy). In some cases, chlorambucil or cyclophosphamide are used.

Haemolytic disease of the newborn – See Section on 'Obstetric Issues' later in this chapter.

Haemolytic transfusion reactions – See Section on 'Haemostasis and transfusion-related emergencies' later in this chapter and Chapter 12.

Red cell fragmentation syndromes

In these syndromes, there is intravascular haemolysis due to mechanical destruction of red cells. This may be caused by cells passing through abnormal endothelium due to fibrin deposition in disseminated intravascular coagulation (DIC), vasculitis-induced inflammation, or platelet adherence in thrombotic thrombocytopenic purpura (TTP). Mechanical heart valves or transjugular intrahepatic portosystemic (TIPS) shunts can also cause physical damage to red cells when they pass through. The blood film will show red cell fragmentation and irregularly contracted cells. There may be accompanying thrombocytopenia in the case of DIC and TTP. Of note, untreated TTP has a very high mortality, and, if this condition is suspected, rapid treatment with plasma exchange must ensue (see Chapter 12, section on 'Bleeding disorders').

Infections

Haemolysis may be precipitated by DIC or oxidative stress in those who are glucose-6-phosphate dehydrogenase (G6PD) deficient. In the case of malaria, there may be extravascular haemolysis of parasitized cells or intravascular haemolysis (i.e. blackwater fever).

Paroxysmal nocturnal haemoglobinuria

This is a clonal disorder of stem cells that results in a structural abnormality at the cell surface. This leads to chronic intravascular haemolysis. Patients are also at risk of thrombosis and iron deficiency from chronic urinary haemosiderinuria. The diagnosis is made by immunophenotyping, which shows loss of the regulatory proteins CD55 and CD59. Haemolysis can be reduced by treatment with the antibody eculizumab. Long-term anticoagulation may be required.

Membrane disorders (e.g. hereditary spherocytosis, elliptocytosis)

Hereditary abnormalities in the red cell cytoskeleton can lead to changes in the shape of the cell. Less surface area can lead to early destruction in the reticuloendothelial system. Symptoms are highly variable, with fluctuating jaundice and splenomegaly in most patients. There is usually a chronic compensated haemolysis, but parvovirus infection may precipitate an aplastic crisis. A blood film will show spherocytosis, and the DAT will be negative. There will be increased osmotic fragility (i.e. increased rupture of cells when incubated with saline of various concentrations, when compared with normal cells). Splenectomy is an effective therapy to reduce haemolysis but should be delayed as long as possible. Folic acid prophylaxis may be given.

Hereditary elliptocytosis is a similar condition with an elliptical appearance of red cells. Phenotypically, it is usually a milder disorder.

Glucose-6-phosphate dehydrogenase (G6PD) deficiency

G6PD is a metabolic enzyme involved in the pentose phosphate pathway. Deficiency of the enzyme leads to decreased levels of the membrane-bound enzyme complex, nicotinamide adenine dinucleotide phosphate-oxidase (NADPH), which maintains the levels of reduced glutathione. This is critical to the defence of red blood cells against oxidative stress. Glucose-6-phosphate dehydrogenase deficiency is an X-linked recessive disorder, which is more prevalent in Africa, the Mediterranean, the Middle East, and South East Asia. People with G6PD deficiency are asymptomatic; however, various precipitants of oxidative stress may lead to intravascular haemolysis (see Box 15.2). There may be abdominal and back pain and dark urine from

---

Box 15.2 Causes of haemolytic anaemia in G6PD deficiency

Acute infections
Fava beans
Antimalarials: primaquine, chloroquine
Antibiotics: co-trimoxazole, nitrofurantoin, ciprofloxacin, dapsone, sulfonamides
Analgesics: high-dose aspirin
Diabetic ketoacidosis

haemoglobinuria. Young red cells have normal levels of G6PD; therefore, levels may be artificially raised during a haemolytic crisis. These episodes are usually self-limiting. It may be a cause of neonatal jaundice and a congenital non-spherocytic anaemia.

A blood film may show irregularly contracted and 'blister' cells. Supravital dyes will show Heinz bodies. Management involves stopping any precipitating agents and blood transfusion may be required in severe or symptomatic anaemia. Intravenous fluid is given to maintain a good urine output. Neonatal jaundice is sometimes treated with an exchange transfusion.

Haemoglobinopathies
See Section on 'The haemoglobinopathies and acute presentations' later in this chapter.

Plasma cell myeloma

Case study

A 59-year-old teacher is admitted to the emergency department by ambulance with a fractured shaft of femur, following a fall down a few stairs at work. The orthopaedic team arranges for an open reduction and internal fixation of the fracture. He is a type 2 diabetic on metformin 500 mg three times daily (tds), and he has mild chronic kidney disease. He is anaemic with an Hb of 9.2 g/dL and an MCV of 85 fL. His white cell count and platelet counts are normal. His creatinine is 450 micromoles/L, and the corrected calcium is raised at 2.89 mmol/L; albumin is 20 g/L, and CRP is 65 mg/L (INR <5). The medical registrar is asked to review him in view of his significant renal impairment. Further investigations are conducted. The blood film shows marked rouleaux formation; the ESR is 95 mm/h; immunoglobulin analysis demonstrates immune-paresis, and serum protein electrophoresis reveals an IgG kappa paraprotein of 25 g/L. Urinary Bence–Jones proteins are detected. The haematology team reviews the patient, as plasma cell myeloma is suspected. A bone marrow biopsy shows 15% plasma cells, with kappa light chain restriction. A skeletal survey reveals numerous lytic lesions, and the orthopaedic team feels his right humerus is at risk of fracture and needs prophylactic pinning. His blood beta-2 microglobulin is raised. He is treated with intravenous fluids to try and improve his renal function, and pamidronate (60 mg) to treat his hypercalcaemia. He is commenced on pulsed daily dexamethasone 40 mg for 4 days. Plasma exchange is also considered. The femur is fixed as an emergency, with no complications. His renal function improves, and the creatinine falls to 150 micromoles/L. He is commenced on regular cyclophosphamide and thalidomide, and his humerus is pinned 2 weeks later. He requires intensive input from occupational therapy and physiotherapy. Three weeks later, he is discharged, with follow-up in the haematology outpatient department.

Background

Plasma cells are terminally differentiated B lymphocytes that secrete immunoglobulin. The class that they secrete (IgG, IgA, IgM, IgD, IgE) depends on cell signalling during their maturation. Plasma cell myeloma is caused by a malignant clone of plasma cells. These cells may secrete a clone of immunoglobulin or light chains (called M-protein). The criteria for diagnosing plasma cell myeloma are described in Table 15.4, and the recommended clinical assessment of a patient with suspected plasma cell myeloma is shown in Table 15.5. If the M-protein and bone marrow clonal plasma cells are lower than the stated levels for asymptomatic myeloma, with no related organ involvement or other B cell lymphoproliferative disorder, a condition called monoclonal gammopathy of undetermined significance (MGUS) may be diagnosed. MGUS requires no specific treatment, but there is a 1% risk of progression annually, so surveillance is required. Plasma cell myeloma can be divided into asymptomatic (smouldering) or symptomatic (see Table 15.4). The main complications of symptomatic plasma cell myeloma are:

1. Hypercalcaemia: plasma cells produce cytokines that stimulate osteoclastic activity. This leads to bone resorption and release of calcium into the serum, with associated complications.

2. Acute kidney injury (AKI) is commonly due to tubular damage from light chain deposition (i.e. Bence–Jones proteins). It can also be a complication of hypercalcaemia and hyperuricaemia.

Table 15.4 Diagnostic criteria for plasma cell myeloma

Symptomatic plasma cell myeloma

M-protein in serum or urine*

Bone marrow clonal plasma cells or plasmacytoma°

Related organ or tissue impairment^ (CRAB: hyper**C**alcaemia, **R**enal impairment, **A**naemia, **B**one lesions)

Asymptomatic (smouldering) myeloma

M-protein in serum at myeloma levels >30 g/L

± 10% or more clonal plasma cells in bone marrow

No related organ or tissue impairment (end-organ damage or bone lesions (CRAB: hypercalcaemia, renal insufficiency, anaemia, bone lesions)) or myeloma-related symptoms^

---

* No level of serum or urine M-protein is included. M-protein in most cases is >30 g/L of IgG or >25 g/L of IgA or >1 g/2 h of urine light chain, but some patients with symptomatic myeloma have levels lower than these.

° Monoclonal plasma cells usually exceed 10% of nucleated cells in the marrow, but no minimal level is designated because about 5% of patients with symptomatic myeloma have <10% marrow plasma cells.

^ The most important criteria for symptomatic myeloma are manifestations of end-organ damage, including anaemia, hypercalcaemia, lytic bone lesions, renal insufficiency, hyperviscosity amyloidosis, or recurrent infections.

Reproduced with permission from The International Myeloma Working Group, 'Criteria for the classification of monoclonal gammopathies, multiple myeloma and related disorders: a report of the International Myeloma Working Group', *British Journal of Haematology*, 121, 5, pp. 749–757, © 2003, John Wiley and Sons and British Society for Haematology.

Table 15.5 Clinical approach to a patient with suspected plasma cell myeloma

1) History: ask about bone pain, urine output, symptoms of hypercalcaemia (e.g. polyuria, polydipsia, abdominal pain, constipation, mental disturbance), recurrent infections, symptoms of hyperviscosity (see section on 'Hyperviscosity syndrome' below and the section on 'Hyperleukocytosis' above), and symptoms of cord compression

2) Examination: exclude cord compression; look for any evidence of infection or amyloid (e.g. facial purpura, peripheral neuropathy, carpal tunnel syndrome, and organomegaly)

3) Full blood count (looking for anaemia, thrombocytopenia, leucopenia)

4) Clotting screen: may be bleeding tendency from M-protein interference with clotting factors; patient may be on warfarin

5) Group & save: in case anaemia requires transfusion

6) ESR: raised

7) Renal function: may be impaired

8) Liver function: prior to chemotherapy

9) Bone profile: hypercalcaemia is a common complication

10) Serum and urine protein electrophoresis and immunofixation: to detect an M-protein (i.e. 'paraprotein' in blood or 'Bence–Jones protein' in urine)

11) Serum immunoglobulins: to detect immune-paresis

12) Uric acid: may be raised

13) LDH: as a marker of cell turnover

14) X-ray any sites of bone pain, looking for lytic lesions

15) Consider MRI if suspicion of cord compression

16) Diagnostic tests to be organized by haematology team: bone marrow biopsy, skeletal survey ± serum free light chains (if non-secretory myeloma is suspected)

17) Prognostic markers: beta-2 microglobulin, albumin, and cytogenetics

3. Anaemia: this may be due to bone marrow failure from the replacement of normal haematopoiesis with plasma cells or due to decreased erythropoietin levels from renal failure.

4. Bone lesions: osteoclastic activity leads to lytic lesions in the bones. As well as causing pain, this can lead to pathological fractures. Vertebral fractures and plasmacytomas (i.e. localized tumour of plasma cells) near the spinal cord can cause spinal cord compression.

5. Infections: there may be a decrease in normal polyclonal immunoglobulins, and hence patients may be at increased risk of infection.

6. Amyloidosis: deposition of abnormal immunoglobulin or light chains in organs can lead to amyloid deposition. This may present with purpura, organomegaly, macroglossia, peripheral neuropathy, or carpal tunnel syndrome.

7. Hyperviscosity—see Section on 'Hyperviscosity syndrome' below and the Section on 'Hyperleukocytosis' above.

Management

The management of plasma cell myeloma can be divided into the management of complications and the management of the underlying disease.

Management of complications

1. Hypercalcaemia: initial management involves rehydration with intravenous fluid and treatment with a bisphosphonate. Pamidronate 90 mg is given by IV infusion over 90 minutes and may be repeated after 72 hours if hypercalcaemia persists. Reduced doses may be required in renal failure, and the patient should be managed in conjunction with the renal team.

2. Acute kidney injury (see also Chapter 11): requires rehydration with treatment of any underlying cause (i.e. hypercalcaemia and hyperuricaemia) and avoidance of nephrotoxic drugs. Liaison between the renal and haematology teams is essential for the management of acute kidney injury. Plasma exchange may be used to try to reduce the light chain load on the kidneys, and pulsed high-dose steroid is required for definitive treatment of the myeloma.

3. Anaemia: may require transfusion or may be supported with erythropoietin if there is renal insufficiency. Always exclude haematinic deficiency and abnormal thyroid function as causes of anaemia.

4. Bone lesions and cord compression: any bony lesion at risk of fracture needs to be discussed with the orthopaedic team, as they may require prophylactic fixation. Impending or actual cord compression requires urgent MRI and discussion with radiotherapy and neurosurgical teams about definitive management. Steroids (e.g. dexamethasone 4 mg qds) should be started immediately. Patients with myeloma are maintained on regular bisphosphonates.

5. Hyperviscosity: see Section on 'Hyperviscosity syndrome' below and the Section on 'Hyperleukocytosis' above.

6. Infections: rapid treatment of any infection is essential.

Specific treatments

Specific therapies depend on the age and fitness of the patient and whether the disease is responsive. Asymptomatic (smouldering) myeloma, is not treated, but monitored closely, until symptoms occur. The only potentially curative treatment for symptomatic plasma cell myeloma is a stem cell transplant which may be carried out in the fittest patients. However, most patients with myeloma are older and have significant comorbidities, and the choice is usually between intensive treatment, followed by an autologous stem cell transplant, or non-intensive treatment. Examples of intensive chemotherapy combinations include Z-Dex (i.e. idarubicin and dexamethasone) and CDT (i.e. cyclophosphamide, dexamethasone, and thalidomide). This is usually followed by a melphalan-conditioned autograft. Non-intensive regimes include MPT (i.e. melphalan, prednisolone, and thalidomide) and CDT (with reduced-dose dexamethasone). Treatment for relapsing disease includes bortezomib and lenolidamide. Of note, thalidomide and lenolidamide are associated with an increased risk of veno-occlusive disease, and these patients are normally maintained on warfarin thromboprophylaxis.

Prognosis

Plasma cell myeloma is usually an incurable disease, with a median survival in the range of 3–4 years. Plasma cell myeloma can be staged, using the international staging system, which has stages I–III. A raised beta-2 microglobulin and low serum albumin are associated with a shorter median survival.

Hyperviscosity syndrome (HVS)

As serum proteins or cellular components increase, the blood becomes more viscous causing vascular stasis and hypoperfusion (see also section on 'Hyperleukocytosis' above). HVS refers to the symptoms triggered by this increase in blood viscosity. The characteristic triad of clinical symptoms includes spontaneous bleeding from mucous membranes, visual disturbances due to retinopathy, and neurologic symptoms ranging from headache, confusion, and vertigo to seizures and coma. Constitutional symptoms and cardiorespiratory symptoms such as shortness of breath, hypoxaemia, acute respiratory failure, and hypotension may also result from 'sludging' of blood within the microvascular circulation. Clinical sequelae of HVS can include congestive heart failure, ischaemic acute tubular necrosis, pulmonary oedema with multiorgan failure, and death if treatment is not promptly initiated.

Increased serum viscosity is usually due to raised circulating serum immunoglobulins, as in multiple myeloma (particularly IgA and IgG3) and the monoclonal gammopathies (e.g. Waldenström macroglobulinaemia, which accounts for ~85% of HVS due to the large size of its associated IgM paraproteins). It can also result from increased cellular blood components (typically white or red blood cells or platelets) in hyperproliferative states such as the leukaemias (may occur with a white blood cell count >10^6; see also Section on 'Hyperleukocytosis' above), polycythaemia, myeloproliferative disorders, essential thrombocytosis, sickle cell anaemia, and sepsis. The underlying pathology determines the clinical features. Serum hyperviscosity due to excess immunoglobulins causes neurologic or ocular disorders, whereas raised blood cell counts (e.g. polycythaemia) and reduced deformability of red blood cells (e.g. sickle cell anaemia) result in reduced capillary perfusion ('sludging') and increased organ congestion.

The diagnosis of HVS is confirmed by measurement of elevated serum viscosity in a patient with characteristic clinical manifestations of HVS. Normal plasma viscosity is between 1.4 and 1.8 centipoises (where 1.0 centipoise equates to the viscosity of water) while symptoms of HVS typically occur at >4-5 centipoise (i.e. ~4-5 times more viscous than water) although no exact diagnostic cut-off exists. If hyperviscosity is suspected, treatment may need to start prior to obtaining the laboratory viscosity level. Patients will also have laboratory (and clinical) evidence of their underlying disorder. Those with myeloma will typically display rouleaux formation on a peripheral smear and a large globulin gap, indicative of a significant paraprotein load.

Plasmapheresis is the treatment of choice to decrease viscosity in the initial management and stabilization of HVS from elevated immunoglobulin levels (e.g. in myeloma), whereas leukapheresis or phlebotomy may be employed in a leukaemic or polycythaemic crisis, respectively. Pheresis (especially leukapheresis) may precipitate tumour lysis syndrome which requires appropriate therapy. Blood transfusions should be used with caution as they can increase serum viscosity. Hydration and phlebotomy are useful temporizing measures whilst preparing pheresis. The underlying disease (e.g. multiple myeloma, blood dyscrasias) requires definitive treatment with the appropriate oncologic therapy (e.g. chemotherapy, steroids), or the HVS will recur within a few weeks, requiring further pheresis.

Further reading

National Comprehensive Cancer Network (NCCN); Clinical Practice Guidelines in Oncology. Version 2 (2014). Multiple Myeloma. <www.nccn.org/professionals/physician_gls/PDF/myeloma.pdf> and <http://williams.medicine.wisc.edu/myeloma.pdf>.

Swerdlow SH, Campo E, Harris NL, *et al.*, eds. (2008). *World Health Organization classification of tumours of haematopoietic and lymphoid tissues*, 4th edn, Vol 2. IARC Press, Lyon.

Haemostasis and transfusion-related emergencies

Fundamentals of haemostasis

Normal haemostasis depends on a delicate balance between maintaining circulating blood in a liquid state and clot formation at sites of injury, followed by clot dissolution. The five major factors essential for haemostasis and examples of abnormalities that can occur in each group are listed as follows:

1. Platelets: thrombocytopenia and thrombocytosis (see Chapter 12 and section on 'Bleeding disorders'), hereditary platelet function disorder, antiplatelet medication, von Willebrand's disease.
2. Coagulation factors: anticoagulant medication, haemophilia, DIC, liver failure, vitamin K deficiency.
3. Coagulation inhibitors: these may develop in treated haemophilia patients.
4. Fibrinolysis system: rare hereditary deficiencies.
5. Blood vessels: Henoch–Schönlein purpura, hereditary haemorrhagic telangiectasia (HHT), vasculitis, steroids.

Introduction to coagulation testing

Coagulation screening tests are increasingly a part of routine blood testing, and it is important to have a basic understanding of the coagulation cascade and an algorithm for managing an abnormal result. The activated partial thromboplastin time (APTT) is used to test the intrinsic pathway, and the prothrombin time (PT) is used to test the extrinsic pathway. The thrombin time and fibrinogen assay are both sensitive to fibrinogen levels. It should be noted that these tests have a limited relationship to coagulation *in vivo*. Although it is beyond the scope of this chapter to discuss these complexities, the basic principles are outlined. It is important to remember that patients may have a bleeding disorder with normal coagulation testing and, conversely, no bleeding disorder with abnormal coagulation testing. The coagulation tests were designed to screen for factor deficiencies in clinically suspicious cases. These results may be invaluable for management decisions in relevant patients (e.g. the bleeding patient, sepsis and DIC, APML) but may cause confusion when done indiscriminately in otherwise well patients. A review of the bleeding history is, therefore, important if an assessment of bleeding risk is needed. Recent BCSH guidelines on the assessment of bleeding risk prior to surgery or invasive procedures have made the following recommendations:

1. Indiscriminate coagulation screening prior to surgery or other invasive procedures to predict post-operative bleeding in unselected patients is not recommended (grade B, level III).
2. A bleeding history, including details of family history, previous excessive post-traumatic or post-surgical bleeding, and use of antithrombotic drugs, should be taken in all patients preoperatively and prior to invasive procedures (grade C, level IV).
3. If the bleeding history is negative, no further coagulation testing is indicated (grade C, level IV).
4. If the bleeding history is positive or there is a clear clinical indication (e.g. liver disease), a comprehensive assessment, guided by the clinical features, is required (grade C, level IV).

Table 15.6 shows an approach to further assessment of an abnormal coagulation result. Results can be abnormal due to underfilling of the coagulation tube, increased cuff

Table 15.6 Approach to abnormal coagulation results

1. *Isolated prolongation of the APTT*
   i) Repeat the test if the first occasion.
   ii) Perform an APTT 50:50 mix (see text).
   iii) If there is no correction, send samples for the investigation of a lupus anticoagulant.
   iv) If there is correction, consider congenital deficiencies (factors VIII, IX, XI, XII or mild II, V, X), von Willebrand's disease, heparin (consider reptilase time, see text). Discuss investigation of these disorders with haematology.

2. *Isolated prolongation of the PT*
   i) Repeat the test if the first occasion (is patient on oral anticoagulants?).
   ii) Perform a PT 50:50 mix (see text).
   iii) If no correction, send samples for investigation of lupus anticoagulant.
   iv) If correction occurs, consider vitamin K deficiency (risk factors include parenteral feeding, malabsoption, and long-term antibiotics) and a trial of vitamin K if suspicion remains.
   v) If correction occurs, also consider factor VII deficiency, liver disease and portal vein thrombosis, and mild factor II, V, and X deficiencies. Discuss with haematology if the cause is not obvious and further investigation is required.

3. *Prolonged APTT and PT, with normal fibrinogen and platelet count*
   i) Repeat the test if the first occasion, and check the history in relation to liver disease, vitamin K deficiency, sepsis, anticoagulant drugs, and massive transfusion.
   ii) Consider a possible trial of vitamin K if the history is suggestive (usually PT more prolonged than APTT).
   iii) Discuss with haematology if the cause is not obvious (may be rare combined deficiency).

4. *Prolonged PT, APTT, low fibrinogen, and low platelet count*—DIC (see later in this chapter, and Chapter 12, section on 'Factors contributing to coagulation failure and DIC'.).

pressure during venepuncture, and delayed assay. Therefore, if the initial results are unexpected, repeat the test. A useful test is an APTT or PT 50:50 mix, in which the patient's plasma is mixed with normal plasma. If the coagulation defect does not correct, it suggests an inhibitor is present, e.g. lupus anticoagulant. If it does correct, it is suggestive of a factor deficiency. It is important to note that a prolonged clotting result may not be associated with a bleeding tendency. For example, a prolonged APTT may be caused by a lupus anticoagulant which can be associated with a thrombotic state or a factor XII deficiency which is of no clinical significance. In contrast, factor XIII deficiency is associated with severe bleeding, but APTT and PT are normal, which reinforces the importance of taking a bleeding history. Of note, a reptilase time is referred to in Table 15.6. This is a test that can be done if prolonged coagulation results are thought to be due to heparin. It produces normal clotting results in the presence of heparin but is prolonged in the presence of low fibrinogen or albumin levels.

Management of over-anticoagulation

Recommendations for management of bleeding and excessive anticoagulation with warfarin have been made by the British Committee for Standards in Haematology (1998, 2005, 2011).

For those patients taking warfarin, the risk of reversing anticoagulation should always be weighed against the risk of continued bleeding without reversal. In general, active bleeding is more life-threatening than any of the conditions whose risk is enhanced by reversal of anticoagulation. See Table 15.7.

The annual risk of embolization in non-anticoagulated patients with prosthetic heart valves is 4% for aortic and 8% for mitral valves overall, with greater risk associated with caged ball valves, especially the Starr–Edwards type.

The annual risk of stroke in non-anticoagulated patients with AF is 3–5% (relative risk 2.5 to 3) but is much lower in those <75 years without comorbidity.

If a patient who is anticoagulated with intravenous unfractionated heparin (UFH) is bleeding, the infusion should be stopped. This is an effective intervention, as UFH has a short half-life. In addition, UFH is rapidly reversed with protamine sulfate, and 1 mg will neutralize 80–100 units UFH when administered within 15 minutes of the heparin dose, and less is required if there has been a longer period since UFH administration. Low molecular weight heparin is incompletely reversed by protamine, and we would recommend discussion with the local haematology services in both of the above situations. Fresh frozen plasma (FFP) is ineffective for reversal of heparin and should not be used for this purpose.

Disseminated intravascular coagulation (DIC)

DIC is a syndrome caused by the introduction of procoagulant material into the circulation or widespread endothelial damage (see Table 15.8). This leads to the consumption of coagulation factors and deposition of fibrin in the microcirculation. The course is usually acute, although some cases may be chronic. Most cases are associated with a haemorrhagic syndrome, although some patients have thrombotic complications.

The diagnosis of DIC needs to take into account the clinical condition of the patient and laboratory tests. The platelet count is likely to be low or falling, although other causes, such as sepsis alone, may account for thrombocytopenia. The PT and APTT may be normal or prolonged. The fibrinogen level may be normal or low. Fibrin degradation products and D-dimers are raised. A blood film may show red cell fragmentation.

The management of DIC should primarily be aimed at treating the underlying cause. Beyond that, treatment depends on the clinical state of the patient. The following is a summary of some of the main recommendations from recent BCSH guidelines.

1. It is important to repeat tests since DIC is a dynamic process.
2. Transfusion of platelets and plasma (components) should not be primarily based on laboratory results but reserved for patients who are bleeding or at high risk of bleeding.
3. Where thrombosis predominates, therapeutic doses of heparin should be considered. If unfractionated heparin is used (due to short half-life and reversibility), monitoring of the APTT may be complicated and clinical observation for signs of bleeding are important.
4. In critically ill, non-bleeding patients, prophylaxis for venous thromboembolism with prophylactic doses of heparin or low molecular weight heparin is recommended.
5. Recombinant human activated protein C (rAPC) has been withdrawn from the market worldwide (2012) due to increasing uncertainty about its efficacy and the risk of bleeding. An amendment has been made to the BCSH

Table 15.7 Management of bleeding and excessive anticoagulation with warfarin

3.0 < INR < 6.0 (target INR 2.5) 4.0 < INR < 6.0 (target INR 3.5)	1. Reduce warfarin dose or stop 2. Restart warfarin when INR <5.0
6.0 < INR < 8.0 No bleeding or minor bleeding	1. Stop warfarin 2. Restart when INR <5.0
INR >8.0 No bleeding or minor bleeding	1. Stop warfarin 2. Restart when INR <5.0 3. If other risk factors for bleeding, give 0.5–2.5 mg vitamin K (oral)
Major bleeding	1. Stop warfarin 2. If available, give prothrombin complex concentrate (50 U/kg), in preference to FFP (15 U/kg) 3. Give 5–10 mg vitamin K IV

Table 15.8 Conditions associated with DIC

Trauma
Organ destruction, e.g. pancreatitis
Malignancy Solid tumours Leukaemia
Obstetric Amniotic fluid embolism Placental abruption Pre-eclampsia
Vascular abnormalities Large haemangiomata Vascular aneurysm
Severe liver failure
Toxic and immunological insults
Snakebites
Recreational drugs
ABO transfusion incompatibility
Transplant rejection

Data from British Committee for Standards in Haematology (2009) – Guidelines for the diagnosis and management of disseminated intravascular coagulation. M Levi, CH Toh, J Thachil, HC Watson. <http://www.bcshguidelines.com/pdf/DICFinal_230109.pdf>.

guidelines and it is no longer recommended for use in patients with severe sepsis and DIC.

6. In general, patients with DIC should not be treated with anti-fibrinolytic agents. However, in DIC characterized by a primary hyperfibrinolytic state, there may be a role for tranexamic acid.

An introduction to blood component therapy

There has been a move over recent years to make blood transfusion safer and avoid unnecessary blood transfusion. There is still morbidity and mortality associated with blood transfusion, and this is collated on a yearly basis in the UK's independent SHOT (Serious Hazards of Transfusion) report. The 2007 SHOT report found one transfusion-related death (probably due to TRALI (transfusion-associated lung injury)). Morbidity included 332 episodes of an incorrect blood component being transfused, 115 acute transfusion reactions, and 25 transfusion-transmitted infections.

Red cells

Some recommendations in the 2001 BCSH guideline (currently under revision) for the clinical use of red cell transfusions include:

- In acute blood loss, transfuse when Hb <7 g/dL or <8 g/dL in those who would tolerate anaemia poorly (e.g. age >65 years, cardiovascular or respiratory disease).
- In chronic anaemia, the cause should be established, and treatment with red cell transfusions should not be given where effective alternatives exist (e.g. treatment of iron deficiency anaemia, megaloblastic anaemia, autoimmune haemolytic anaemia).

Platelets

- BCSH guidelines for the use of platelet transfusions (2003) recommend prophylactic platelet transfusions for bone marrow failure (e.g. due to disease, cytotoxic therapy, or irradiation). During acute blood loss there is also consensus that the platelet count should not be allowed to fall below 50×10^9/L (see also section on 'Massive transfusion' later in this chapter). A higher target level of 100×10^9/L has been recommended for those with multiple trauma or central nervous system injury. As noted above transfuse when Hb <7 g/dL or <8 g/dL in those who would tolerate anaemia poorly (e.g. age >65 years, cardiovascular or respiratory disease). Note that a platelet count of around 50×10^9/L is expected when red cell concentrates equivalent to approximately two blood volumes have been transfused.
- In thrombocytopenia, not due to bleeding, with or without chronic anaemia, the cause should be established. Prophylactic platelet transfusions may be indicated when reductions are due to cytotoxic therapy, irradiation, and some diseases associated with marrow failure (e.g. acute promyelocytic leukaemia). As discussed above, in chronic anaemia, treatment with red cell transfusions should not be given where effective alternatives exist (e.g. treatment of iron deficiency anaemia, megaloblastic anaemia, autoimmune haemolytic anaemia). The indications (i.e. to prevent spontaneous haemorrhage) and thresholds for platelet use in thrombocytopenia, not related to acute bleeding, have recently been reviewed. In general, the thresholds have been reduced and the current recommendations are:
  - 10×10^9/L, with no additional risk factors (sepsis, use of antibiotics, and other abnormalities of haemostasis).
  - For patients without risk factors, a threshold of 5×10^9/L may be appropriate if there are concerns regarding alloimmunization, but there may be difficulties in establishing an accurate platelet count <10×10^9/L.
  - A specific platelet threshold may not be appropriate for patients with chronic stable thrombocytopenia.

In the case of surgical prophylaxis, the following thresholds have been recommended:

- For lumbar puncture, epidural anaesthesia, gastroscopy and biopsy, insertion of indwelling lines, transbronchial biopsy, liver biopsy, laparotomy or similar procedures, the platelet count should be raised to at least 50×10^9/L.

- For operations to critical sites, such as the brain or eyes, the platelet count should be raised to 100×10^9/L.

The 2004 BCSH guidelines (currently under review) for the use of fresh frozen plasma, cryoprecipitate, and cryosupernatant, recommend the following clinical indications:

Fresh frozen plasma (FFP)

- For a single (e.g. inherited) factor deficiency where no virus-safe, fractionated product is available.
- Multiple coagulation factor deficiencies (e.g. DIC, see Section above and Chapter 12; Section 'Factors contributing to coagulation failure and DIC').
- Thrombotic thrombocytopenic purpura (TTP) for daily plasma exchange.
- Reversal of warfarin in severe bleeding where prothrombin complex concentrate is not available.
- Surgical bleeding and massive transfusion.
- Note that children born after 1st January 1996 should only receive pathogen-reduced FFP (PRFFP). This PRFFP is from countries with a low bovine spongiform encephalopathy incidence as recommended by the Department of Health.

Cryoprecipitate

The most common use is to enhance fibrinogen levels in dysfibrinogenaemia and the acquired hypofibrinogenaemia seen in massive transfusion and DIC. It is usually given if the fibrinogen level is less than 1 g/L, although there is no absolute threshold.

Red cell antibodies

Hundreds of red cell antigens have been described. They can be clinically significant when a person lacks an antigen and makes an antibody. In the case of a blood transfusion, this can lead to a haemolytic transfusion reaction, and in pregnancy, haemolytic disease of the newborn. For what happens when a sample is cross-matched, see Table 15.9.

The ABO blood group system consists of four groups A, B, AB, and O. There are naturally occurring IgM antibodies in the serum of the absent antigen.

The Rhesus blood group system consists of five main antigens including C, D, E, c and e. The significance of the Rh group is the association of anti-D and anti-c with haemolytic disease of the newborn. Women who are RhD-negative are given antenatal anti-D prophylaxis at 28 and 34 weeks to prevent immunization. All sensitizing events should be treated with anti-D. If women have already developed antibodies, these should be monitored, with referral of moderate- and high-risk cases to a fetal medicine centre.

Other blood groups—other antibodies that are routinely screened for include MNS, P, Lu, Kell, Kp, Le, Fy, and Jk.

Table 15.9 What happens to the cross-matched sample?

1) The sample is ABO and RhD-typed.
2) An antibody screen is done to look for circulating antibodies in the recipient.
3) If the antibody screen is positive, the antibody is identified, using an antibody panel.
4) If a clinically significant antibody is identified, blood negative for that antigen must be selected.
5) Cross-match is done either serologically or electronically, depending on clinical scenario.
6) Patients with sickle cell anaemia and thalassaemia are also matched for Rh antigens (C, D, E, c, e) and Kell.

Transfusion reactions

Transfusion reactions may be acute or delayed.

Acute transfusion reactions

Acute haemolytic transfusion reactions
This is usually caused by transfusion of ABO-incompatible blood due to clerical errors. Complement-mediated intra-vascular haemolysis of transfused cells occurs, leading to DIC and acute kidney injury. Mortality is approximately 10%. Signs and symptoms usually occur within minutes of starting the transfusion. Patients may present with agitation, nausea, back pain, pain at venepuncture sites, and shock. They may develop haemoglobinaemia and haemoglobinuria. Table 15.10 summarizes the approach to the management of a patient with an acute transfusion reaction.

Anaphylaxis
Rarely, IgA-deficient patients develop an anaphylactic reaction to IgA in transfused blood. This may be a life-threatening complication, presenting with urticaria, bronchospasm, and hypotension. Treatment is as for other causes of anaphylaxis, with adrenaline, hydrocortisone, and chlorpheniramine.

Febrile non-haemolytic reactions
These have become much less common since the introduction of universal leucodepletion of blood. They are caused by anti-HLA or leucocyte antibodies in the recipient against donated cells. Pyrexia usually occurs later in the transfusion. It can be managed by slowing down the transfusion and treatment with antipyretics.

Transfusion-associated circulatory overload
This can be a problem, particularly in the elderly or those with a history of cardiac failure. Management is with diuretic therapy.

Bacterial contamination
This occurs most frequently with platelet transfusions and has a high mortality. Treatment involves stopping the transfusion and management of septic shock.

Transfusion-associated lung injury (TRALI)
This is caused by antibodies in the donor to patient leuco-cytes. It is usually associated with transfusions of FFP. As antibodies occur more frequently in multiparous women, FFP is solely extracted from male donations. Patients present with a respiratory reaction, including cough, fever, and breathlessness. There are pulmonary infiltrates on chest X-ray. Management involves respiratory support.

Table 15.10 Approach to transfusion reaction

1) Check airway and breathing.
2) Ensure adequate access.
3) Replace IV giving set, and give fluid resuscitation (if compromise is not caused by fluid overload).
4) Check patient identity with donor pack.
5) Take a blood sample for cross-match. Send to the laboratory with a donor pack for a pre- and post-transfusion cross-match and post-transfusion DAT.
6) If bacterial contamination is suspected, the transfusion laboratory should organize blood cultures from the donated pack; take blood cultures from patient, and initiate broad-spectrum antibiotics.
7) If an anaphylactic reaction is suspected, consider hydrocortisone, adrenaline, and chlorpheniramine.
8) Monitor urine output, and consider a CVP line.
9) Consult senior medical staff with regards to the need for further circulatory/ventilatory support.

Delayed transfusion reactions

Delayed haemolytic transfusion reactions
These are usually caused by IgG antibodies that are un-detectable on initial cross-match. It may present with a drop in haemoglobin 5–10 days after transfusion.

Transfusion-associated graft versus host disease (TA-GVHD)
This is a universally fatal condition, caused by donor T lymphocyte attack against an immunosuppressed recipient. Therefore, patients at risk (e.g. bone marrow transplant patients, Hodgkin's disease patients, those who have received purine analogues, and fetuses receiving intrauterine transfusion) receive irradiated blood products. The incidence of TA-GVHD has decreased significantly since universal leucodepletion of blood was introduced.

Post-transfusion purpura
This usually presents 5–10 days after a transfusion with thrombocytopenia. The recipient has platelet-specific antibodies that cause destruction of their own and transfused platelets. It is normally self-limiting but may need treatment with intravenous immunoglobulin (IVIG) or plasma exchange.

Iron overload
This is mainly a problem for those on regular transfusion programmes (e.g. sickle cell anaemia, thalassaemia). Treatment requires iron chelation therapy.

Non-bacterial infections
UK blood donations are currently screened for hepatitis B, hepatitis C, HIV, syphilis, HTLV, malaria, and CMV (although CMV-negative blood products are only issued to those with special requirements). The current risks for viral transmission from blood products in the UK include:

- Hepatitis B—1 in 850,000.
- HIV—1 in 4,850,000.
- Hepatitis C—1 in 50,670,000.

In addition, there have been no reported cases of transmission of nvCJD from blood transfusion since 1999.

Approach to a patient with an acute transfusion reaction
If a patient presents with a fever >40°C at the start of a transfusion or any signs of shock or hypoxia at any point, stop the transfusion immediately.

Massive transfusion

There are various definitions of massive blood loss. The total blood volume in adults is defined as 7% of ideal body weight. Therefore, in a 70 kg man, this would be nearly 5 L. In the acute setting, a useful definition is 50% loss of blood volume in 3 hours or 150 mL/min. The recent BSCH guideline for the haematological management of major haemorrhage (2015) suggests an alternative definition, of bleeding which leads to a heart rate >110 beats/min and/or systolic blood pressure <90 mmHg, in the acute situation.

The management aims in a patient requiring a massive transfusion are:

1. Maintaining tissue perfusion and oxygenation.
2. Arrest of bleeding by treating the cause.
3. Judicious use of blood component therapy to correct coagulopathy. In this regard, the 2015 BCSH guideline recommends serial haemostatic tests (i.e. PT, APTT, fibrinogen) every 30-60 minutes depending on the severity of the haemorrhage to ensure appropriate use of haemostatic blood components.

Table 15.11 summarizes the approach to a patient with massive blood loss.

Table 15.11 Approach to a patient with massive blood loss

1) Check airway and breathing.
2) Insert 2 large-bore peripheral cannulae.
3) Ensure accurate patient identification (especially in the unconscious patient).
4) Bloods for full blood count, clotting screen, fibrinogen, group and cross-match, urea and electrolytes, liver function, blood gas.
5) Administer pre-warmed crystalloid fluids, as required, to avoid hypotension or a urine output <0.5 mL/kg/h.
6) Contact the clinician in charge, consultant anaesthetist, transfusion biomedical scientist, and haematologist.
7) Early surgical/obstetric/radiological intervention.
8) Transfusion of blood products—see below.
9) Documentation—a legal requirement for traceability of blood components.
10) Maintain ionized calcium >1.13 with calcium chloride.
11) Arrange ITU bed.

Red cell transfusion
The urgency of the need for transfusion must be assessed clinically. In extreme emergencies, group O RhD-negative blood may be required. It is acceptable to transfuse RhD-positive blood to males or post-menopausal females of unknown blood group. Once a patient's blood group has been identified, group-specific blood should be issued. This should be fully compatible, if time permits. After one blood volume has been replaced, serological cross-match of blood is no longer required. The haemoglobin should be maintained between 70–80 g/L, although it should be noted that the haemoglobin is often a poor indicator of blood loss in the acute setting.

Platelet transfusion
Current BCSH guidelines (2015) recommend maintaining a platelet count greater than 50×10^9/L. If a patient has multiple trauma, CNS trauma, or platelet function abnormality (secondary to cardiopulmonary bypass, uraemia, or antiplatelet agents), it is recommended that the platelet count is maintained above 100×10^9/L.

Fresh frozen plasma (FFP)
FFP is the component of choice to manage the coagulopathy of bleeding, although the supporting data is limited. The previous 2006 BCSH massive transfusion guidelines recommended that the need for FFP should be anticipated after 1–1.5 × blood volume replacement. However, the most recent BCSH guidelines for major haemorrhage (2015) recommend that FFP is given in the initial resuscitation process in a ratio of 1:2 of FFP:red blood cells until the results of coagulation tests (e.g. PT, APTT, etc) are available to guide ongoing therapy. In traumatic bleeding an initial ratio of 1:1 is recommended. Once bleeding is under control, further FFP should be guided by abnormalities in coagulation tests with an FFP transfusion trigger of PT and/or APTT of >1.5 times normal. Use of FFP should not delay fibrinogen supplementation if it is required. FFP is normally given at a dose of 12–15 mL/kg. Thirty-minute thawing time has to be allowed for.

Cryoprecipitate
Hypofibrinogenaemia is common during major haemorrhage, and fibrinogen is the first factor to fall to critical levels. Fibrinogen levels <1 g/L are likely after 1–1.5 times blood volume replacement. It is currently recommended

(BCSH 2015) that the fibrinogen level should be maintained at >1.5 g/L. FFP alone may be sufficient to maintain fibrinogen levels at >1.5g/L, unless there is DIC. However, if levels are <1.5 g/L, fibrinogen should be replaced in the form of cryoprecipitate. Two, five donor, pools of cryoprecipitate contain 3–6 g of fibrinogen, in a volume of 200–500 mls, and would typically raise the plasma fibrinogen level by ~1 g/L. Alternatively, if the concentration of fibrinogen in cryoprecipitate is inadequate, fibrinogen concentrate can be given as per local protocols.

Prothrombin complex concentrate
This should only be used in bleeding associated with anticoagulant overdose and is not recommended in major haemorrhage unless part of a clinical trial.

Recombinant activated factor VIIa
This is licensed for use in haemophiliacs and has been used off licence in massive transfusion with anecdotal reports of success. Sound evidence from controlled trials is not yet available. The current BCSH guidelines (2015) do not recommend its use in the management of major haemorrhage, unless as part of a clinical trial.

Tranexamic acid
The BCSH guidelines (2015) recommend that adult trauma patients with, or at risk of major haemorrhage, in whom antifibrinolytics are not contraindicated, should be given tranexamic acid as soon as possible after injury, at a dose of 1 g intravenously over 10 minutes followed by a maintenance infusion of 1 g over 8 hours. Its use should also be considered in non-traumatic major bleeding.

Risks of massive transfusion
The most serious risk is giving the wrong blood to the wrong patient. It is especially important in an emergency situation with an unconscious patient, to make sure there is adherence to policies on blood labelling. There is also a risk of ionized hypocalcaemia from citrate toxicity, particularly with deranged liver function. This should be corrected with calcium chloride (not gluconate, as it requires liver metabolism). There is also a risk of hyperkalaemia due to the extracellular potassium in red cells. All risks associated with blood product transfusion apply.

Haemophilia emergencies
Haemophilia A (factor VIII deficiency) and haemophilia B (factor IX deficiency) are sex-linked recessive disorders. Symptoms depend on factor levels and can be classed as mild (>5% factor level), moderate (1–5% factor level), or severe (<1% factor level). Diagnosis is made in childhood, often after post-circumcision bleeding or with bleeding out of proportion to the injury. Patients with mild haemophilia A or B can be treated with tranexamic acid for cuts or dental extraction. Mild haemophilia A can sometimes be treated with DDAVP for the same indications. Spontaneous bleeding (e.g. soft tissue bleeds, haemarthroses) is treated with recombinant factor concentrate. Major surgery and post-traumatic bleeding also need cover with factor concentrates. Prophylactic treatment has dramatically changed the outlook for severe haemophilia. Patients may also have treatment 'on demand' at the first sign of a bleed. Patients with haemophilia attend specialized centres with multidisciplinary management. They usually carry a card with details of their diagnosis. If a patient presents with a bleeding emergency or requires any intervention, this should always be discussed with haematology services.

Further reading

Baglin TP, Barrowcliffe TW, Cohen A, Greaves M; British Committee for Standards in Haematology (2006). Guidelines on the use and monitoring of heparin. *British Journal of Haematology*, **133**, 19–34.

Baglin TP, Keeling DM, Watson HG; British Committee for Standards in Haematology (2005). Guidelines on oral anticoagulation: third edition 2005 update. *British Journal of Haematology*, **132**, 277–85.

British Committee for Standards in Haematology (2011). Guidelines on oral anticoagulation with warfarin: fourth edition. *British Journal of Haematology*, **134**, 311–324.

British Committee for Standards in Haematology (2003). Guidelines for the use of platelet transfusions. *British Journal of Haematology*, **122**, 10–23.

Cannegieter SC, Rosendaal FR, Briet E (1994). Thromboembolic and bleeding complications in patients with mechanical heart valve prostheses. *Circulation*, **89**, 635–41.

Chee YL, Crawford JC, Watson HG, Greaves M; British Committee for Standards in Haematology (2008). Guidelines on the assessment of bleeding risk prior to surgery or invasive procedures. *British Journal of Haematology*, **140**, 496–504.

Department of Health (1998, 2002, 2007). Better Blood Transfusion—Department of Health Circular. <http://www.transfusionguidelines.org.uk/index.aspx?Publication=BBT>.

Fakhry SM and Sheldon GF (1994). Massive transfusion in the surgical patient. In LC Jeffries, ME Brecher, eds. *Massive transfusion*. American Association of Blood Banks, Bethesda.

Hunt BJ, Allard S, Keeling D, *et al.*; British Committee for Standards in Haematology (2015). A practical guideline for the management of those with, or at risk of major haemorrhage. *British Journal of Haematology*, doi: 10.1111/bjh.13580 or <http://www.bcshguidelines.com/documents/Major_Haemorrhage.pdf>.

Levi M, Toh CH, Thachil J, Watson HC; British Committee for Standards in Haematology (2009). Guidelines for the diagnosis and management of disseminated intravascular coagulation. *British Journal of Haematology*, **145**, 24–33.

Murphy MF, Wallington TB, Kelsey P, *et al.*; British Committee for Standards in Haematology (2001). Guideline for the clinical use of red cell transfusions. *British Journal of Haematology*, **113**, 24–31.

National Blood Transfusion Committee (2014). Patient Blood Management. <http://www.transfusionguidelines.org.uk/uk-transfusion-committees/national-blood-transfusion-committee/patient-blood-management>.

NHS Blood and Transplant and Health Protection Agency (Centre for Infections) (2008). Infection surveillance annual report 2007. NHSBT/HPA annual report (2007). <http://www.hpa.org.uk/web/HPAwebFile/HPAweb_C/1227255714122>.

O' Shaughnessy, C Atterby, P Bolton Maggs, M Murphy, D Thomas, S Yates, LM Williamson (2004); British Committee for Standards in Haematology. Guidelines for the use of fresh-frozen plasma, cryoprecipitate and cryosupernatant. *British Journal of Haematology*, **126**, 11–28. Amendments 2005, 2007.

SHOT (Serious Hazards of Transfusion) report (2007). <http://www.shotuk.org>.

Stainsby D, MacLennon S, Thomas D, Izaac J, Hamilton PJ; British Committee for Standards in Haematology (2006). Guidelines on the management of massive blood loss. *British Journal of Haematology*, **135**, 634–41. Updated 2015, see Hunt BJ, *et al.*, above.

Acute thrombosis

Case study

A 63-year-old man presents to accident and emergency with a painful and swollen left leg. He has noticed worsening symptoms for the last 2 days. He has no chest pain or breathlessness. On examination, he has unilateral swelling of the left leg that is measured to be 4 cm greater than the right. There is tenderness along the deep venous system, with superficial collateral veins seen. Respiratory examination is normal, as are an ECG and chest X-ray. His full blood count shows a Hb 9.2 g/dL, WCC 5.8 × 10^9/L, neutrophils 3.2 × 10^9/L, and platelet count 1,067 × 10^9/L. His biochemistry is normal, and urine dipstix is unremarkable. He is given a dose of low molecular weight heparin, as a deep vein thrombosis is suspected and sent for a Doppler ultrasound. This is confirmed, and he is referred to the haematology services for further investigation and the anticoagulant team for warfarinization. Iron deficiency is excluded as a cause of thrombocytosis, and further investigations are carried out. He is found to have a JAK2-positive myeloproliferative disorder. He is commenced on hydroxyurea therapy to reduce his platelet count, with regular follow-up.

Background

It is important, when assessing thrombosis, to have a different approach for arterial and venous thrombosis (see Boxes 15.3, 15.4; see also Chapter 4, section 'Thromboembolic disease'). Arterial thrombosis is generally associated with underlying atherosclerosis. Therefore, history taking should be focused on cardiovascular risk factors. It is only in unusual cases (see Box 15.4) that investigation for a thrombophilia needs to be carried out. This should be done in liaison with haematology.

Most episodes of venous thrombosis are precipitated. Therefore, careful history and examination are required (see Tables 15.12 and 15.13) to determine the underlying cause. Some people have a tendency to thrombosis (thrombophilia). There are a number of heritable conditions that are associated with an increased risk of thrombosis. However, many individuals with these conditions are asymptomatic. Also, many individuals presenting with thrombosis will have no laboratory abnormalities. Therefore, care must be taken not to overassess the risk in a patient with a positive thrombophilia screen and likewise to give false reassurance to a person with a negative screen.

Heritable thrombophilias

Laboratory testing can be carried out for the following genetic variants associated with thrombosis:

- Antithrombin deficiency.
- Protein C deficiency.
- Protein S deficiency.
- Activated protein C (APC) resistance and factor V Leiden.
- Prothrombin G20210A mutation.
- Dysfibrinogenaemia.
- Elevated factor VIII levels.
- Hyperhomocysteinaemia.

The acute thrombotic state and anticoagulation can affect some thrombophilia assays; therefore, it is recommended that testing is done at least 1 month after completion of a course of anticoagulation.

Box 15.3 Risk factors for venous thromboembolism

Surgery or trauma
Obesity
Dehydration
Sepsis
Immobility
Pelvic obstruction
Malignancy (including myeloproliferative disorders)
Nephrotic syndrome
Pregnancy and the combined contraceptive pill
Heparin-induced thrombocytopenia
Paroxysmal nocturnal haemoglobinuria
Behçet's disease
Heritable thrombophilias (see text)

Box 15.4 Risk factors for arterial thrombosis

Smoking
Hypertension
Diabetes
Hypercholesterolaemia
Family history of ischaemic heart disease
Hyperhomocysteinaemia
Lupus anticoagulant
Occasionally heritable thrombophilias

Table 15.12 Approach to a patient with suspected venous thrombosis

1. History—how old is the patient? Is there any history of recent surgery or trauma? Is there any malignancy or systemic disorder? Has there been a previous thrombosis? Could they be pregnant or on the oral contraceptive pill? Has there been a history of miscarriage? Is the thrombosis at an unusual site? Is there a family history of thrombosis?

2. Examination—examine site of suspected thrombosis: is there tenderness along deep veins, size difference between limbs or visible superficial collateral veins. Are the arterial pulses normal?

3. Urine dipstix—to rule out nephrotic syndrome

4. Blood tests—full blood count and biochemistry profile

5. Other investigations—CXR (looking for malignancy); consider faecal occult blood test

6. Referral for investigation of thrombophilia—tests above; normal, with unprecipitated venous thromboembolism in a young adult with a strong family history; or thrombosis at an unusual site; or recurrent thromboembolism

Antiphospholipid syndrome

This is a syndrome of thrombosis associated with recurrent miscarriage and laboratory evidence of an antiphospholipid antibody. There may also be thrombocytopenia and skin changes (e.g. livedo reticularis). Thrombosis may be venous or arterial. The antiphospholipid antibody may be the lupus anticoagulant or other antibodies, such as anti-cardiolipin or anti-beta-2 glycoprotein.

The following recommendations comply with the 2001 BCSH guidelines for investigation and management of heritable thrombophilia.

Table 15.13 Approach to a patient with suspected arterial thrombosis

1) History—are there risk factors for atherosclerosis (i.e. smoking, hypertension, diabetes, hypercholesterolaemia, family history of ischaemic heart disease)? Is there a history of miscarriage?
2) Examination—examine for pulses at area of thrombosis, any cardiac murmurs, xanthelasma, signs of peripheral vascular disease.
3) Investigations—full blood count, urea and electrolytes, liver function, fasting lipids and glucose; consider ECHO and carotid artery Doppler for embolic sources.
4) Consider—angiography by vascular surgeons/interventional radiology.
5) If normal angiography or patient less than 50 years old, consider investigating for lupus anticoagulant, anti-cardiolipin antibody, protein S deficiency, and homocysteine levels.

Management of acute venous thrombosis

- DVT or PE; give low molecular weight heparin for a minimum of 5 days, followed by oral anticoagulation for a minimum of 6 months, aiming for a target INR of 2.5.
- A shorter period (e.g. 3 months) may be acceptable when the thrombus is confined to distal veins or there is evidence of a temporary risk factor that is no longer present.
- If there is a persisting thrombotic risk factor (e.g. cancer or high-risk thrombophilic defect), consideration should be given to extending the period of anticoagulation.

- If there is recurrent thrombosis on treatment, a higher target INR is recommended.
- If there is a recurrent event when the patient was not anticoagulated, it is sufficient to reintroduce coumarin at a target INR of 2.5 after initial treatment with low molecular weight heparin.
- Patients who have had two or more apparently spontaneous venous thrombotic events require consideration for indefinite anticoagulation.

Prevention of thrombosis

- All patients with a past history of venous thromboembolism (with or without a heritable thrombophilia) should be considered for short-term anticoagulation for periods of increased risk (e.g. surgery).
- Similarly, affected (with an identifiable thrombophilia), but asymptomatic, relatives of those who have had a thrombosis should be considered for thromboprophylaxis for similar high risk periods.

Further reading

Haemostasis and Thrombosis Task Force, British Committee for Standards in Haematology (2001). Investigation and management of heritable thrombophilia. *British Journal of Haematology*, **114**, 512–28.

Laffan MA and Manning RA (2012). Investigation of a thrombotic tendency. In BJ Bain, I Bates, Laffan MA, Lewis SM, eds. *Dacie and Lewis's Practical Haematology*, 11th edn, pp. 447–67. Churchill Livingstone, Philadelphia.

Obstetric issues

Haemolytic disease of the newborn (and fetus)

Case study

A 24-year-old clinically obese lady was admitted to the labour ward, with regular contractions at 38 weeks' gestation. She was ABO blood group O and RhD-negative and had received 500 IU of anti-D immunoglobulin as routine antenatal anti-D prophylaxis (RAADP) at 28 and 34 weeks. A cardiotocograph (CTG) showed fetal distress, and the baby was delivered by emergency Caesarean section. The baby's blood group on cord blood was ARhD-positive; Hb was 5.3 g/dL, and bilirubin was 100 micromoles/L. An acid elution test (modified Kleihauer-Betke) test was done to screen for fetomaternal haemorrhage and gave a result of 50 mL. Flow cytometry was carried out to quantify the bleed, and a result of 85 mL was obtained. A diagnosis of haemolytic disease of the newborn (HDN) was made, and the baby was given a top-up transfusion and phototherapy for jaundice. The mother had already been given 500 IU of anti-D IM post-delivery. Following discussion with the local transfusion centre, she was given a further 8,000 IU of anti-D intravenously. A sample taken 72 hours later showed anti-D was still present. Four days post-partum, she developed chest pain, breathlessness, and her haemoglobin oxygen saturation was measured at 91% on room air. The medical registrar was called. A V/Q scan revealed a large left pulmonary embolus. She was therapeutically anticoagulated, and made a good recovery. She was discharged home with her baby 5 days later. She had a repeat antibody screen 6 months later, which did not detect anti-D, but she was counselled about the risk of HDN in relation to future pregnancies.

Background

Haemolytic disease of the newborn and fetus leads to a shortened fetal red cell lifespan. This is due to fetal cells leaking into the maternal circulation and IgG antibodies that are able to cross the placenta, causing destruction of fetal red cells. The most common cause is anti-D antibodies produced by an RhD-negative mother against an RhD-positive fetus. Hence, there is a national routine antenatal anti-D prophylaxis (RAADP) programme to prevent immunization. The other antibodies that may be significant are anti-c, anti-Kell, and rarely ABO. If a mother is found to have antibodies at routine screening, these need to be discussed with the transfusion laboratory to determine their clinical significance and to assess if any further action is required.

In the UK, approximately 85% of the population is RhD-positive and 15% RhD-negative. As the majority of RhD-negative women will have an RhD-positive partner, there is a high likelihood that they will also have an RhD-positive child—61% in first pregnancy.

If a RhD-negative woman becomes immunized, subsequent pregnancies with an RhD-positive fetus may result in severe fetal anaemia. Before fetal medicine and monitoring were established, this often resulted in hydrops fetalis and death. The bilirubin produced by haemolysis is removed by the maternal liver but, after delivery, will accumulate due to immaturity of the neonatal liver. This can lead to cerebral toxicity (kernicterus) and may require phototherapy or even exchange transfusion.

Once a woman has developed immune anti-D antibodies, it is too late to give anti-D, as she is sensitized. The aim is to treat any sensitizing event (where fetal RhD-positive cells may leak into the maternal circulation) with anti-D to scavenge the D antigens on these cells so that the mother does not mount an immune response against them.

Management

Routine blood tests

As part of the routine booking blood tests in early pregnancy, a woman should be ABO and RhD-typed and an antibody screen performed. The antibody screen should be repeated at 28 weeks prior to the administration of anti-D prophylaxis. If antibodies are found on screening, antigen specificity needs to be typed to determine if this could be clinically significant and appropriate follow-up blood tests organized.

RAADP

Anti-D is a blood product, and women should be counselled prior to its administration and sign an informed consent form. Details of administration must also be recorded to ensure traceability of blood products. Anti-D must not be given to an RhD-positive mother.

There is debate about the exact dose of anti-D that should be given, but it is recommended that at least 500 IU is given at 28 and 34 weeks of pregnancy or, alternatively, 1,500 IU at 28 weeks.

Immune antibodies

Occasionally there is doubt as to whether anti-D detected in the mother is immune antibodies or passive antibodies from RAADP. If there is any doubt, anti-D should still be given whilst this is being established. If a woman has a level of anti-D greater than 4 IU/mL, a rising level, or a history of HDN, she should be referred to a fetal medicine unit. With an anti-c level greater than 7.5 IU/mL, she should be referred to a fetal medicine centre, and, with other antibodies, a titre greater than 1:32 is considered significant. If an antibody is detected at any time, it should be monitored at least monthly until 28 weeks and then every 2 weeks. It is now possible to monitor haemolytic disease in the fetus by middle cerebral artery Doppler, and an 'at-risk' fetus' can be supported with intrauterine transfusions.

Sensitizing events

The possible sensitizing events where anti-D should be considered are:

- Amniocentesis or cordocentesis and chorionic villus sampling.
- Other *in utero* therapeutic interventions/surgery (e.g. intrauterine transfusion, shunting).
- Antepartum haemorrhage (APH).
- Ectopic pregnancy.
- External cephalic version.
- Falls/abdominal trauma.
- Intrauterine death or miscarriage.
- Termination of pregnancy.

If a woman is RhD-negative, the following doses of anti-D should be given (see Table 15.14). At birth, if a RhD-positive child is born to a RhD-negative mother, 500 IU of anti-D should be given whilst awaiting results of fetomaternal haemorrhage (FMH) testing.

Fetomaternal haemorrhage (FMH) quantification

FMH should be quantified, following the birth of a RhD-positive baby to a RhD-negative mother, and also after any

Table 15.14 Recommended dose of anti-D in relation to gestation period

Gestation (confirmed by scan)	Dose of anti-D
<12 weeks miscarriage with no instrumentation	No anti-D required
<12 weeks therapeutic termination	250 IU anti-D
12–20 weeks	250 IU anti-D
>20 weeks and at birth	Quantify volume of FMH, and give appropriate anti-D

sensitizing event after 20 weeks of pregnancy. There are two methods of quantification.

- Firstly, the acid elution test (modified Kleihauer-Betke test), which is used as a screening tool. It works on the principle that fetal HbF is more resistant to alkali degradation and acid elution than adult HbA. Adult cells become ghost-like, whereas fetal cells can be stained.
- Secondly using a method of systematic counting, the volume of fetal haemorrhage can be calculated. It is, however, subject to more error than flow cytometry, and there can be false positives. Therefore, any bleed greater than 2 mL should be confirmed by flow cytometry.

The standard post-partum dose of 500 IU of anti-D covers a bleed up to 4 mL. If the bleed is larger than this, an additional dose is required. Anti-D is routinely given intramuscularly, and additional dosing above a 4 mL bleed

is calculated as 125 IU per 1 mL of fetal Rh-positive cells. If there is a very large bleed, it may be preferable to give anti-D intravenously. Dosing is different, and, in this scenario, there should be discussion with a transfusion consultant. A repeat FMH test and antibody screen should be done at 48–72 hours, and, if fetal cells are still present, the above process is repeated. If fetal cells are cleared, but there is no anti-D detected, a further standard dose is given.

Thrombosis in pregnancy
See Chapter 21; Section 'Medical emergencies in pregnancy'.

Further reading
Austin E, Bates S, de Silva M, *et al.*; British Committee for Standards in Haematology (2009). Guideline for the estimation of fetomaternal haemorrhage. <http://www.bcshguidelines.com/documents/BCSH_FMH_bcsh_sept2009.pdf>.

Gooch A, Parker J, Wray J, Qureshi H; British Committee for Standards in Haematology (2006). Guideline for blood grouping and antibody testing in pregnancy. <http://www.bcshguidelines.com/documents/antibody_testing_pregnancy_bcsh_07062006.pdf>.

National Institute for Health and Clinical Excellence (2008). Pregnancy—routine anti-D prophylaxis for rhesus negative women (review of TA41). <http://guidance.nice.org.uk/TA156/Guidance/pdf/English>.

Parker J, Wray J, Gooch A, Robson S, Qureshi H; British Committee for Standards in Haematology (2006). Guidelines for the use of prophylactic anti-D immunoglobulin. <http://www.bcshguidelines.com/documents/Anti-D_bcsh_07062006.pdf>.

Qureshi H, Massey E, Kirwan D, *et al*; British Committee for Standards in Haematology (2014). Guideline for the use of anti-D immunoglobulin for the prevention of haemolytic disease of the fetus and newborn. *Transfusion Medicine*, **24**, 8–20.

Acute problems in bone marrow transplant patients

Background

Bone marrow transplantation involves a conditioning process (i.e. chemotherapy ± radiotherapy), to remove a patient's haematopoietic system or to severely depress a host's immunity and the administration of exogenous stem cells. If these 'exogenous' cells are from the patient, it is termed an 'autologous' transplant, and, if the cells are from another person, it is an 'allogeneic' transplant. The donor in an allogeneic transplant could be an HLA-matched sibling or an HLA-matched unrelated donor (MUD). The mortality associated with sibling allografts is lower than MUD allografts. There is also variation in the conditioning regimes used, and older patients, or those with a worse performance status, are often considered for a reduced intensity conditioning (RIC) regime, rather than a fully myeloablative regimen. Stem cells may be harvested from the peripheral blood, the bone marrow, or cord blood.

Infections in bone marrow transplant and neutropenia

Infection is a significant cause of morbidity and mortality, following bone marrow transplantation. The risk of infection is higher after an allogeneic transplant, and the infections can be divided into three periods. Firstly, there is an aplastic phase until neutrophil engraftment. Patients are at risk of bacterial, fungal, and viral (particularly Herpes simplex virus (HSV)) infections. The second phase is from neutrophil engraftment until the third or fourth month and is characterized by a deficiency in cell-mediated immunity. Acute Graft Versus Host Disease (GVHD) is the main risk factor during this phase, and delayed recovery of the immune system is associated with infections. Viral infections are especially common during this time. The third phase is after the fourth month and is the late post-transplantation period. Chronic GVHD puts patients at risk of infection, and there may be associated immunoglobulin deficiency. In particular, there may be an increased risk of infection with encapsulated bacteria, e.g. *Haemophilus influenzae*, *Streptococcus pneumoniae*. There is a lower incidence of infection after autologous transplantation, and the risk of fungal infection is extremely low in the absence of other risk factors.

Neutropenic sepsis is a common cause of hospital admission in all haematology patients, not just following bone marrow transplantation. Neutropenia is usually defined as an absolute neutrophil count less than 2.0×10^9/L. However, patients are considered most vulnerable to infection when the absolute neutrophil count is $<0.5 \times 10^9$/L. Haematology patients are usually neutropenic from bone marrow failure (e.g. due to chemotherapy, marrow replacement with disease, haematinic deficiency, etc.). Other causes of neutropenia include drugs (e.g. chloramphenicol, clozapine), viral infections, cyclical neutropenia, and autoimmune neutropenia. The management of a patient with a bone marrow transplant and/or neutropenia and fever is summarized in Table 15.15.

Investigation and management of infections

Preventative measures

Neutropenic patients should be reverse barrier-nursed in a side room. Dietary advice should be given regarding safe food preparation and the avoidance of foods known to contain bacterial or fungal organisms. Regular mouthwashes and topical oral antifungal agents (e.g. amphotericin lozenges) are given routinely to prevent oral infections. All allograft patients are started on phenoxymethylpenicillin prophylaxis. Antifungal

Table 15.15 Approach to a patient with a bone marrow transplant or neutropenia and fever

1. ABC: airway, breathing and circulation.
2. History—are there any symptoms of infection? What is the underlying diagnosis and what chemotherapy has been given? If a BMT, are there any symptoms of GVHD (skin changes, diarrhoea, jaundice, any other new symptoms)? Establish the date of the transplant, type of transplant (autograft, allograft, MUD donor, sibling donor). Has there been acute or chronic GVHD? What is the CMV status of donor and recipient? What immunosuppression is the patient currently on? What infections have they had since the transplant? What anti-infective prophylaxis are they currently taking?
3. Examination—perform a full physical examination, looking for any signs of infection. Note particularly if there is tenderness around any tunnelled venous lines. Are there any skin changes (GVHD)? Are there signs of jaundice?
4. CXR—check for evidence of pneumonia.
5. FBC—is there neutropenia, thrombocytopenia, or anaemia?
6. U&E—look for acute kidney injury.
7. LFTs—raised bilirubin and ALP occur in GVHD; liver function may be deranged in sepsis.
8. Bone profile—diarrhoea may cause electrolyte derangement.
9. LDH—may be raised in haemolysis.
10. CRP—as an indicator of infection.
11. Septic screen—peripheral and central blood cultures, sputum culture, stool culture (for microscopy, culture and sensitivity, *Clostridium difficile* toxin, and electron microscopy), midstream urine, and urine for pneumococcal and *Legionella* antigen; consider nasopharyngeal aspirates if coryzal; swab indwelling catheter sites if any sign of infection; throat swabs if painful or injected fauces.
12. Fluid resuscitation and antibiotics as per local policy
13. Early liaison with haematology services.
14. Further investigations—immunosuppressant drug levels (trough ciclosporin or tacrolimus level); consider CMV, EBV, and adenovirus PCR,? HHV6 PCR, serum galactomannan (*Aspergillus* antigen), antifungal trough level.

prophylaxis (e.g. itraconazole) is given to all allograft patients and also to patients with acute leukaemia and those with prolonged steroid treatment. PCP prophylaxis is given to allogeneic transplant recipients, patients receiving purine analogues (fludarabine and cladrabine), alemtuzumab treatment (anti-CD52 monoclonal antibody), patients with ALL (acute lymphoblastic leukaemia), and those receiving prolonged high-dose steroid therapy. This is usually given as co-trimoxazole but can be substituted with nebulized pentamidine in allogeneic stem cell transplant when stem cells have been given but not yet engrafted. Aciclovir prophylaxis is usually recommended for those who are HSV-seropositive in allografts and autografts. Transplant patients who are CMV-seronegative with a CMV-seronegative donor, require CMV-negative blood products to prevent infection. Recommendations for antibacterial prophylaxis with quinolones (e.g. ciprofloxacin) are variable from centre to centre and depend on local resistance patterns.

Bacterial infections

In the immediate post-transplant period before neutrophil engraftment, bacterial infections are frequent. In many cases of neutropenic sepsis, there may be no organism grown on cultures. Commonly isolated organisms include Gram-positive organisms, such as coagulase-negative *Staphylococcus* and Gram-negatives, such as *E. coli* or *Pseudomonas* species. In the late transplant period, infections with encapsulated bacteria, as described previously, are more common. Local anti-infective guidelines should be followed when treating sepsis. In neutropenic sepsis, broad-spectrum antibiotics (e.g. beta-lactams, ceftazidine) should be given promptly. Centres vary in the use of aminoglycosides, which may be reserved for hypotensive shock after fluid resuscitation. A glycopeptide may be added if there is a suggestion of a line infection, soft tissue infection, or the detection of Gram-positive organisms in blood cultures. Antibiotics should be adjusted, according to sensitivities of isolates from cultures. *Clostridium difficile* stool infection should be treated with either metronidazole or vancomycin orally for 10–14 days. Atypical cover with a macrolide (e.g. clarithromycin) should be considered if atypical pneumonia is suspected.

Fungal infections
If there is no resolution of fever within 3–5 days of antibiotic treatment, then fungal infection should be considered. The most serious fungal infection is *Aspergillus*. Routine investigations of a suspected fungal infection in a transplant patient include the monitoring of serum galactomannans (*Aspergillus* antigen), checking that antifungal drug levels are therapeutic, and a high resolution CT scan. The CT scan may show the classic 'halo' sign or cavitation of *Aspergillus* infection. Treatments include caspofungin, liposomal amphotericin, and voriconazole. Local guidelines should be followed.

Viral infections
Herpes simplex virus (HSV) reactivation is common in seropositive patients and can result in mucosal ulceration. Treatment is with high-dose aciclovir. Routine screening for cytomegalovirus (CMV) viraemia now occurs in all allograft recipients, particularly in the early post-transplant period. Infection should also be considered in those receiving purine analogues and alemtuzumab treatment. Infection is associated with pneumonitis, oesophagitis, hepatitis, retinitis, and myelosuppression. A significant viral load is treated with either ganciclovir or foscarnet. The choice of antiviral agent may be influenced by comorbidities. For example ganciclovir may cause myelosuppression, and foscarnet renal impairment. Varicella zoster (VZV) infections are more common in the late transplant period, and treatment is with high-dose intravenous aciclovir or oral valaciclovir. HHV6 infection can be associated with pneumonitis, encephalitis, and delayed engraftment. Treatment is with ganciclovir. Epstein–Barr virus (EBV) infection is associated with post-transplant lymphoproliferative disorders (PTLD), more commonly seen in solid organ transplants than bone marrow transplants. Adenovirus is associated with a high mortality rate; and although there is limited evidence, current treatment approaches include cidofovir and ribavirin. Other viral infections include respiratory viruses, such as respiratory syncytial virus (RSV), influenza, parainfluenza, and rhinovirus. There is a very high mortality associated with these infections. Oseltamivir has been used for treatment of influenza. Nebulized ribavirin has been used in RSV infection, although evidence of benefit is limited.

Pneumocystis jirovecii pneumonia (PCP)
This causes pneumonia (e.g. amphotericin lozenges) infiltrates and hypoxia. Prophylaxis is given in the form of co-trimoxazole tablets or pentamidine nebulizers for at least 6

months. Treatment of infection is with high-dose co-trimoxazole and steroids (see also Chapter 13).

Cytopenias after bone marrow transplant
Graft failure
Neutrophil engraftment, following a bone marrow transplant, is normally defined when a neutrophil count of $>0.5 \times 10^9/L$ is achieved on the first of 3 days. Platelet counts are useful indicators if levels of $>20 \times 10^9/L$ and $>50 \times 10^9/L$ are achieved on the first of 3 consecutive days. Primary graft failure is when these values are never achieved after transplant, and secondary graft failure when they are achieved but then subsequently lost.

Graft failure is more common in conditions where there is previous alloimmunization from repeated transfusion, T cell-depleted transplants, reduced intensity conditioning regimes, unrelated donor transplants, and mismatched transplants.

In patients with suspected graft failure, myelosuppresive drugs should be changed to non-myelosuppressive alternatives (e.g. ganciclovir and co-trimoxazole). A virology screen (PCR) should also be sent, as viral infection is a significant cause of aplasia, hypoplasia, and haemophagocytosis (e.g. EBV, CMV, parvovirus, adenovirus, HHV6). Chimerism studies are also sent, as these assess the level of donor cells and recipient cells. The results may show all donor, all recipient, or mixed cells.

Approaches to the management of graft failure depend on the cause and include G-CSF administration, manipulation of immunosuppressive therapy, infusion of donor lymphocytes (DLI), and donor stem cells with or without conditioning.

ABO mismatch
A number of bone marrow transplants will have ABO mismatching between the donor and recipient. This is associated with an increased risk of delayed red cell engraftment, pure red cell aplasia, haemolysis, and increased red cell requirements.

ABO incompatibility is defined as major or minor. Major is when the recipient immune system can produce antibodies against the donor red cells (i.e. donor is group B, and the recipient is group O). Minor incompatibility is when the donor immune system can produce antibodies against the recipient red cells (i.e. group O donor and group A recipient). There can also be both major and minor incompatibility present, for example, if there is a group B donor and group A recipient. Close monitoring is required in the immediate post-transplant period to detect these complications.

As a patient's blood group may change during the transplant period, the recipient's group is used prior to the transplant and following the transplant, the following strategy is used.

- Major ABO mismatch—administer group O red cells until ABO antibodies are no longer detectable and the antiglobulin test is negative. Give platelets and plasma of the recipient's group until recipient red cells are no longer detected.
- Minor ABO mismatch—administer group O red cells until the ABO antibodies are no longer detectable and the antiglobulin test is negative. Again, give platelets and plasma of the recipient's group until recipient red cells are no longer detected.
- When both major and minor incompatibility are present, red cells should again be group O until ABO antibodies are no longer detected, but platelets and plasma should be group AB until recipient red cells are no longer detected.

Graft versus host disease (GVHD)

This can be divided into acute and chronic. Acute usually occurs within the first 100 days after an allogeneic transplant, and chronic occurs more than 100 days after but there can, however, be crossovers. Acute GVHD is thought to be a three-step process; conditioning, the effect of malignancy, and previous treatments lead to a huge release of chemokines and cytokines. This activates the immune system, in particular, the antigen-presenting cells of the host. Donated T cells interact with these antigen-presenting cells, leading to activation and expansion, and consequent immune-mediated organ damage. There are many risk factors for developing acute GVHD, including older donors and recipients, matched unrelated donor transplants rather than sibling, and alloimmunized donors (e.g. women who have had multiple pregnancies, or donors who have been transfused).

Acute GVHD is graded by involvement of skin, liver, and the gastrointestinal tract. Other characteristics include fever and involvement of other tissues and organs, such as the mucous membranes and bronchi. Skin involvement can vary from a maculopapular rash, involving the palms and soles, to a bullous desquamating condition. Liver involvement is typified by a cholestatic picture, with raised bilirubin and alkaline phosphatase, with relative sparing of the transaminases. Liver dysfunction can also be caused by drugs and infections, and it can be difficult to determine the aetiology. Gut involvement can lead to symptoms of nausea, vomiting, abdominal pain, and diarrhoea, which may be associated with massive fluid losses.

There are classic histological appearances associated with this entity. Skin or gastrointestinal biopsies should be taken to establish the diagnosis. CMV infection must be excluded in the case of a gastrointestinal biopsy, as this infection causes similar symptoms and histologically may be difficult to differentiate from early GVHD. Liver biopsy is only performed in complex cases.

Chronic GVHD: the manifestations of chronic GVHD are variable. Developing acute GVHD is the strongest risk factor for developing chronic GVHD. The clinical features may be similar to autoimmune disease, with scleroderma or Sjögren-like reactions, liver dysfunction, bronchiolitis obliterans, debility, weight loss, and severe immunosuppression.

Management

Patients with acute GVHD should be managed by a transplant haematologist. Preventative strategies include a calcineurin inhibitor (ciclosporin or tacrolimus), sometimes with another agent such as methotrexate or mycophenolate mofetil (MMF). Treatment of established acute GVHD involves supportive measures and steroid therapy. If this fails, secondary treatments (e.g. higher-dose steroids, tacrolimus, anti-thymocyte globulin monoclonal antibodies (ATG)) may be required, but the outlook for this group of patients is poor, and these decisions are made at a senior level.

Chronic GVHD is managed with supportive measures and specific treatments. Supportive measures include adequate nutrition and symptom control (e.g. artificial tears for dry eyes). As there is an increased risk of opportunistic infection, prophylactic, phenoxymethylpenicillin should be lifelong; antifungal therapy should be considered, and PCP prophylaxis given for 6 months after stopping immunosuppressive therapy. CMV surveillance is done routinely, as reactivation is common. Specific treatments include steroids and ciclosporin as first-line agents, along with various therapies for refractory cases, including psoralen with ultraviolet A (PUVA), MMF, thalidomide, tacrolimus, and rituximab.

Further reading

Cordonnier C (2008). Infections after HSCT. In E Apperley, E Carreras, E Gluckman, et al., eds. *Haematopoietic stem cell transplantation*, pp. 199–217. European School of Haematology (ESH-EBMT Handbook). <http://www.esh.org/online-training/handbook/>.

Devergie A (2008). Graft versus host disease. In E Apperley, E Carreras, E Gluckman, et al., eds. *Haematopoietic stem cell transplantation*, pp. 219–34. European School of Haematology.

Pamphilon DH (2008). Transfusion Policy. In E Apperley, E Carreras, E Gluckman, et al., eds. *Haematopoietic stem cell transplantation*, pp. 146–63. European School of Haematology.

Potter M (2009). Graft failure. In J Treleaven, AJ Barrett, eds. *Haematopoietic stem cell transplantation in clinical practice*, pp. 382–5. Churchill Livingstone Elsevier, Edinburgh.

Ruutu T. European Group for Blood and Marrow Transplantation (2011). Engraftment. <https://www.ebmt.org/Contents/Resources/Library/Slidebank/Documents/EBMT%202011%20SC%20Slide%20Bank/1439%20Ruutu.pdf>.

Chemotherapy-related complications

Tumour lysis syndrome

Case study

A 24-year-old healthcare assistant from Zimbabwe was an inpatient on the haematology ward. She had recently been diagnosed with HIV and Burkitt's lymphoma, with extensive abdominal disease. She started chemotherapy with R-CODOX-M (rituximab, cyclophosphamide, vincristine, methotrexate). The medical registrar had been called to review the patient the following evening, as her serum creatinine had increased from 45 to 200 micromoles/L. The potassium was 6.9 mmol/L, phosphate 3.5 mmol/L, corrected calcium 1.15 mmol/L, and uric acid 0.80 mmol/L. The patient had been given allopurinol prophylaxis and intravenous hydration to prevent tumour lysis syndrome. On examination, there was evidence of volume overload, with a 6 kg gain in weight over the preceding 36 hours. She was oliguric with a urine output of 10–15 mL per hour. ECG changes were consistent with hyperkalaemia. A diagnosis of tumour lysis syndrome was made. Treatment for her electrolyte disturbance was commenced, with insulin/glucose (INN) (20 units of short-acting insulin over 1 hour with 50 mL of 50% dextrose), 10 mL of 10% calcium gluconate, 15g four times daily (qds) of Calcium Resonium®, and a phosphate binder, e.g. sevelamer 2.4 g/day. She was also started on rasburicase rescue treatment. After an urgent renal ultrasound excluded obstruction, 80 mg of furosemide was given to try to initiate a diuresis. Despite all these measures, she remained hyperkalaemic, hyperphosphataemic, and oliguric, and the renal team transfered the patient to their unit for dialysis. After 5 days, there was a significant improvement in her renal function, and she was transferred back to the haematology ward.

Background

Tumour lysis syndrome causes metabolic disturbances due to rapid necrosis of tumour cells. A combination of hyperuricaemia, hyperkalaemia, hyperphosphataemia, secondary hypocalcaemia, and acute kidney injury is observed and usually occurs following initiation of chemotherapy. This syndrome is more common in malignancies with a high proliferation index (e.g. Burkitt's lymphoma and leukaemias with high white cell counts (AML, ALL, CML)) and a heavy burden of disease.

Pathophysiology

Hyperuricaemia

The breakdown of purine residues from tumour cells results in the production of hypoxanthine and xanthine and finally uric acid. The crystals can cause renal failure and arthropathy.

Hyperkalaemia

Rapid cell lysis results in the release of intracellular potassium into the extracellular compartment. Acute kidney injury exacerbates the hyperkalaemia, and this may cause arrhythmias.

Hyperphosphataemia and secondary hypocalcaemia

Large amounts of phosphate are released by tumour cell lysis. This binds with calcium, generating calcium phosphate crystals. These crystals also contribute to the development of acute kidney injury.

Table 15.16 Approach to a patient with suspected tumour lysis syndrome

1) History: What is the underlying malignancy? What is the tumour burden (i.e. pre-treatment white cell count, LDH)? When was chemotherapy started (i.e. is there a temporal relationship between the onset of the changes and the administration of chemotherapy)? Was appropriate tumour lysis prophylaxis given?
2) Examination: Is there evidence of intravascular or extracellular fluid volume expansion (e.g. pulmonary oedema, oliguria)?
3) Blood tests: Full blood count, urea and electrolytes, liver function, bone profile, LDH, uric acid, magnesium and CRP.
4) CXR: if breathless or signs of pulmonary oedema.
5) ECG: if any electrolyte disturbance.
6) Hyperkalaemia: 20 units of Actrapid® or other short-acting insulin over 1 hour in 50mL of 50% glucose (INN), 10mL of 10% calcium gluconate, and 15g qds of Calcium Resonium®
7) Hyperphosphataemia: phosphate binders such as aluminium hydroxide or sevelamer 2.4–4.8 g/day in divided doses.
8) Renal impairment: urgent renal ultrasound to rule out obstructive nephropathy.
9) Meticulous fluid balance.
10) Aggressive intravenous hydration with diuretics, if this can be tolerated, aiming for urine output 80–100 ml/m^2/hr.
11) Early liaison with renal services regarding the need for dialysis.
12) Early liason with haematology services regarding rasburicase or allopurinol treatment.

Prevention and management

Identification of patients at risk, and prevention of tumour lysis, are an important consideration during treatment of haematological malignancies (see Table 15.16).

Allopurinol inhibits the enzyme xanthine oxidase which catalyses the rate-limiting step in uric acid formation. Although less uric acid crystals are formed, hypoxanthine and xanthine can also form insoluble crystals, leading to nephropathy. It is given at a dose of 300 mg once a day with normal renal function, and 100 mg once daily in renal impairment. Caution is required when given with chemotherapeutic agents that are purine analogues (e.g. azathioprine, 6-mercaptopurine), as the metabolism of these agents can be impaired, resulting in significant toxicity to the patient.

Rasburicase is a recombinant form of urate oxidase that may be used to prevent or treat tumour lysis syndrome. It is contraindicated in G6PD deficiency. It is given at a dose of 200 mcg/kg/day for up to 7 days. There is local variation in guidance for the duration of treatment required.

Recommendations for the prevention of tumour lysis syndrome, according to risk

- Low risk—close monitoring of biochemistry and renal function.
- Intermediate risk—hydration and allopurinol.
- High risk—hydration and rasburicase. (see Table 15.17)

Central venous catheter-related issues

There are many types of indwelling central venous access devices, each with advantages and disadvantages.

Table 15.17 Patient stratification by risk

Type of Cancer	Patient Stratification by Risk		
	High	Intermediate	Low
NHL	Burkitt's, lymphoblastic, B-ALL	DLBCL	Indolent NHL
ALL	WBC ≥ 100	WBC 50–100	WBC ≤ 50
AML	WBC ≥ 50, monoblastic	WBC 10–50	WBC ≤ 10
CLL		WCC 10–100, tx with fludarabine	WBC ≤ 10
Other haematological malignancies (including CML and multiple myeloma) and solid tumours		Rapid proliferation with expected rapid response to therapy	Remainder of patients

NHL = non Hodgkin's lymphoma, ALL = acute lymphocytic leukaemia, AML = acute myeloid leukaemia, CLL = chronic lypmphocytic leukaemia, CML = chronic myeloid leukaemia, DLBCL = diffuse large B-cell lymphoma

A recent BCSH guideline has reviewed the indications and complications of central venous catheters.

Types of catheter

Non-tunnelled catheters
These are temporary lines that are inserted directly into a vein, such as the internal jugular, subclavian, or femoral vein.

Skin-tunnelled catheters (Hickman lines)
These offer a lower risk of infection than non-tunnelled lines but must be inserted by an interventional radiologist or surgeon, and removal may require blunt dissection if they have been *in situ* for more than a few weeks. They are suitable for long-term use and are ideal in many haematology patients who are having long regimes of chemotherapy and who require frequent blood product support.

Ports (Portacath)
The entry port is like a button under the skin. There is no external part to this catheter, and consequently it is more cosmetically acceptable. There is a lower risk of infection, but the port must be inserted and removed by a surgeon; accessing the device is more difficult and requires specialized training. It is, therefore, most useful for patients requiring long-term infrequent access, such as those with sickle cell anaemia or thalassaemia who have regular blood transfusions.

Apheresis non-tunnelled and tunnelled catheters (Vascath)
These are large-bore catheters that are used when high-flow rates are required, such as renal dialysis, plasmapheresis, and peripheral stem cell harvest. Tunnelled catheters are used if they are needed longer term. They require flushing with heparin to ensure patency.

PICC (peripherally inserted central catheter)
These are normally inserted via the antecubital fossa and are relatively easy to insert and remove. They are most suited to outpatient care. They have a higher risk of thrombosis and a shorter lifespan than centrally placed catheters.

Complications associated with catheters
The main complications of catheters are infection, malfunction, and thrombosis. The following is a summary of the 2007 BCSH guideline on management.

Catheter related infection
There are three types of catheter-related infection:

1. A catheter-associated bloodstream infection is defined as at least two positive blood cultures with the same organism, taken at different venepuncture sites at different times, and evidence of colonization of the line with the same organism.

2. An exit site infection—there is erythema, tenderness, and occasional discharge at the exit site.

3. A tunnel site infection—this is characterized by erythema and tenderness along the tunnel site.

If there is a suspicion of a catheter-related infection, peripheral and line cultures (including all line lumens with the culture bottles labelled accordingly) should be taken, as well as swabs of the exit site. Management requires:

- Removal of any infected catheter that is no longer required.
- Empirical treatment with a glycopeptide (e.g. teicoplanin).
- Adjustment of antibiotic therapy, according to isolates.
- Treatment for 10–14 days until the infection resolves.
- Remove the catheter if there is evidence of progression of the infection or bloodstream infection with *Staphylococcus aureus*, *Pseudomonas* species, mycobacterium species, or fungi.

Catheter malfunction
Catheter occlusion may be due to kinking of the catheter, being 'pinched off' between the clavicle and first rib, a fibrin sheath at the tip, intraluminal thrombus, or migration of the tip into a smaller vessel. Plain X-ray may help to make the diagnosis. Where intraluminal thrombus is thought to be the cause of occlusion, injection with Hepsal, urokinase, or tPA (alteplase) may help to unblock it. External damage to a catheter can be repaired with catheter repair kits by those experienced in doing so. Non-tunnelled lines can be replaced by re-inserting the guidewire, removing the line, and replacing it with a fresh line.

Catheter-related thrombosis
A high level of suspicion is needed to diagnose line-related thromboses. Any upper limb or facial swelling should be investigated with imaging. If a thrombosis is confirmed, the line must be removed. Anticoagulation should be discussed with haematology services. The level and duration of anticoagulation will depend on the platelet count, previous thrombosis, concurrent malignancy or treatment with thrombogenic drugs such as thalidomide, lenolidamide, and L-asparaginase.

Further reading

Bishop L, Dougherty L, Bodenham A, et al. (2007). Guidelines on the insertion and management of central venous access devices in adults. *International Journal of Laboratory Hematology*, **29**, 261–78.

Coiffier B, Altman A, Pui CH, Younes A, Cairo MS (2008). Guidelines for the management of pediatric and adult tumour lysis syndrome: an evidence-based review. *Journal of Clinical Oncology*, **26**, 2767–78.

Approach to the patient with peripheral blood cytopenias

Peripheral blood cytopenias in patients who present to the emergency department or in community practice are usually manifestations of systemic infection and/or inflammation, rather than evidence of a primary haematological disorder. Clinical presentation is almost always dominated by the underlying illness and its pathogenesis, rather than symptoms due directly to the cytopenias.

Nevertheless, a comprehensive approach to every patient who presents with anaemia, neutropenia, and/or thrombocytopenia is important to detect serious haematologic illness which may require prompt intervention and to address the sequelae of cytopenias in patients with systemic illness and associated secondary haematologic manifestations.

A general approach to the patient will be discussed in the first instance, and then specifics about each of the cytopenias will follow.

Case study

A phone call was received from a GP regarding an 86-year-old woman. She had symptoms of fever, fatigue, breathlessness, and a productive cough. Blood tests were performed, with a presumed diagnosis of a lower respiratory tract infection. Full blood count revealed Hb 103 g/L, MCV 83.2, WCC 1.79 × 10^9/L, neutrophils 0.81 × 10^9/L, lymphocytes 0.88 × 10^9/L, and platelets 32 × 10^9/L. A blood film revealed red cell anisocytosis, atypical lymphocytes, dysplastic neutrophils, and no platelet clumping evident. The morphology indicated an authentic pancytopenia.

Since the patient was febrile, she was admitted with neutropenic sepsis. Blood cultures were taken, and she was treated with intravenous broad-spectrum antibiotics. A chest X-ray showed right basal consolidation, in keeping with a right lower lobe pneumonia. Bone marrow examination went on to reveal myelodysplasia, with failure of normal haematopoiesis evident in all cell lines.

Pathophysiology

Anaemia

Defined as a haemoglobin of <13 g/dL in a man and <11.5 g/dL in a woman. Anaemia is common and can occur for a myriad of reasons. It is not a diagnosis in itself, and the reason for anaemia should always be considered. The mean cell volume (MCV) is useful to differentiate the various causes. Macrocytic anaemia (MCV >100 fL) is seen in liver disease, B12 or folate deficiency, haemolytic disease, and dysplastic bone marrow. Normocytic anaemia (MCV 78–98 fL) is seen in combined iron/haematinic deficiency, anaemia of chronic disease, and recent bleeding. Microcytic anaemia (MCV <76 fL) is seen in iron deficiency, haemoglobinopathy, and chronic disease. This classification emphasizes the importance of a thorough history (e.g. has the patient noticed recent bleeding or is there a family history of haemoglobinopathy?) and examination (e.g. jaundice in suspected haemolysis).

Leucopenia

Defined as a total white cell count of <4 × 10^9/L. It is usually more helpful to classify according to the neutrophil count, which has most impact on the total white cell count. Neutropenia is a neutrophil count of <2.0 × 10^9/L, and has a close bearing on the risk of infective complications. There is a significant risk of infection with neutrophil counts of <0.5 × 10^9/L. Causes include drugs (e.g.

cytotoxics, NSAIDs, antibiotics commonly), post-infection, immune-related, Felty's syndrome (seen with splenomegaly and rheumatoid arthritis), and haematological malignancies, including acute leukaemia and myelodysplasia. Lymphopenia is defined as a lymphocyte count of <1.5 × 10^9/L. It is seen in many medical conditions, including HIV, acute infection, lymphoma, carcinoma, tuberculosis, and cardiac failure.

Thrombocytopenia

Defined as a platelet count <150 × 10^9/L. It is difficult to predict at what count an individual is more susceptible to bleeding. The risk of spontaneous haemorrhage is significantly greater at counts < 5–10 × 10^9/L, and is of particular concern with regard to intracerebral bleeding. Presenting features include purpura, epistaxis, bleeding gums, or menorrhagia. Causes can be divided into increased consumption and decreased production. Increased consumption may be due to drugs, infection (including HIV), DIC, idiopathic thrombocytopenic purpura (ITP), transfusion post-massive haemorrhage, SLE, thrombotic thrombocytopenic purpura (TTP), chronic lymphatic leukaemia (CLL) and lymphoma, and hypersplenism. Decreased production occurs with drugs (including alcohol), chemicals, viral infection (including HIV), marrow infiltration, and leukaemia.

Laboratory evaluation

Anaemia

In addition to haemoglobin levels, anaemia can be further characterized by blood film examination (i.e. to inspect the appearance of erythrocytes), reticulocyte count, haemoglobin electrophoresis, haematinics, and full iron studies.

Leucopenia

As with the other cell lines, blood film microscopy is helpful to examine the appearance of the leucocytes, for example, dysplastic neutrophils in a post-infectious neutropenia. Bone marrow biopsy may be important if there is suspicion of haematological malignancy, particularly if there is reduction of other cell lines in a patient with lymphadenopathy or hepatosplenomegaly. Bone marrow aspirates may be sent for immunophenotyping, and cytogenetics can further distinguish a clonal disorder, such as an acute leukaemia or lymphoma.

Thrombocytopenia

A low platelet count should be confirmed by checking the sample for clots and the film for platelet aggregation, both of which would cause a spuriously low result by artefact.

Management

Anaemia

Correction of the haemoglobin must stem from addressing the cause. This may require further investigation, for example, the iron-deficient patient may require gastroscopy and/or colonoscopy to detect occult blood loss from a bowel malignancy. Bone marrow biopsy may be necessary to examine the erythroid line maturation. Transfusion should be reserved for patients who are compromised by their anaemia, and only after appropriate investigation, especially in the case of haemolysis, and usually after preliminary measures, such as iron replenishment have been undertaken.

Leucopenia

Treatment of patients with leucopenia is primarily aimed at reducing the risk of infection, for example, barrier nursing with or without isolation, use of prophylactic antibiotics, and consideration of potential fungal infection. Neutropenic sepsis remains a medical emergency, and inexplicable fevers in severely neutropenic patients should be treated urgently with intravenous broad-spectrum antibiotics. If leucopenia is persistent, granulocyte-colony stimulating factor (G-CSF) may be indicated to boost neutrophil production.

Thrombocytopenia

The underlying condition should be treated. Platelet transfusion is warranted in life-threatening haemorrhage in thrombocytopenic patients. This should be discussed with a haematologist, particularly if there is concern regarding TTP or heparin-induced thrombocytopenia (HIT).

Pancytopenia

This refers to a reduction in all cell lines. A haematology work-up is important to exclude causes, such as a severe B12 or folate deficiency. The paucity of all cell lines in the peripheral blood can relate to bone marrow failure. In turn, this may stem from a reduction in haemopoietic cells, as in aplastic anaemia; malignant replacement of marrow, as in leukaemia, lymphoma, or myeloma; or infiltration of abnormal tissue, as in myelofibrosis or amyloidosis. This will be evident from bone marrow examination.

Summary

Individual cytopenias result from many different causes, varying from infection to immune-related causes. Differential diagnosis, investigation, and management must be directed at the particular cytopenia. For example, anaemia due to iron deficiency, a common problem in the outpatient setting, may be due to a colonic cancer diagnosed as a result of gastroenterological investigation. In contrast, sepsis in a neutropenic patient may stem from bone marrow failure, which may be further delineated by bone marrow examination.

Further reading

Mehta A and Hoffbrand V (2009). *Haematology at a glance*, 3rd edn. Wiley-Blackwell, Oxford.

Provan D, Singer CRJ, Baglin T, Dokal I (2009). *Oxford handbook of clinical haematology*, 3rd edn. Oxford University Press, Oxford.

The haemoglobinopathies and acute presentations

Case study

A 22-year-old university student of Nigerian descent attends accident and emergency with chest pain, a productive cough, and shortness of breath. He is known to have sickle cell anaemia (HbSS), and has recently had an upper respiratory tract infection with a cough productive of green sputum. He has been taking prophylactic penicillin V, is up to date with his vaccinations, and is not on an exchange transfusion programme. On examination, there are crepitations in the left lung base, and his oxygen saturation is 82% on room air. There is evidence of left basal consolidation on chest X-ray. Full blood count demonstrates a Hb 6.2 g/dL, WCC 11.5 x 10^9/L, neutrophils 8.9 x 10^9/L, and platelets 105 x 10^9/L. His CRP is raised at 251, and other blood tests are unremarkable. He is commenced on oxygen therapy, opiate analgesia, and broad-spectrum antibiotics. He is diagnosed with an acute chest syndrome, so an exchange transfusion is performed manually, following which he starts to feel symptomatically much better. After 5 days of intravenous antibiotics, he is converted to oral antibiotics. He is discharged home 2 days later, with haematology clinic follow-up.

Introduction

Haemoglobinopathies are the result of either the synthesis of an abnormal haemoglobin (e.g. HbS resulting in sickle cell anaemia) or reduced alpha or beta chain production (thalassaemia).

Patients with thalassaemia syndromes have a variety of clinical manifestations, but these are usually of a chronic nature, e.g. transfusion dependence, leading to iron overload and subsequent hepatic, cardiac, and endocrine problems. Therefore, most problems are managed in the outpatient setting.

Most haemoglobinopathy emergencies involve patients with sickle cell anaemia. Homozygous sickle cell anaemia (HbSS) is the most severe haemoglobinopathy commonly encountered in the acute setting in the UK. Compound heterozygote disorders (HbSC, HbSbeta-thal) may also result in significant sickling. At low oxygen tensions, HbS forms insoluble crystals, leading to sickling of red cells and occlusion of the microcirculation. Vaso-occlusive crises can be precipitated by various insults, including cold weather, dehydration, infections, and exercise. People with sickle cell trait (HbAS) are usually asymptomatic, however, under intense stressful conditions e.g. exhaustion, severe hypoxia, and/or aggressive infection, sickling may occur.

General approach to a patient with sickle cell anaemia

An assessment of the patient should involve a search for evidence of dehydration, infection, severe anaemia, hypoxaemia, neurological signs, organomegaly, and priapism (see Table 15.18). The majority of admissions will be for an uncomplicated painful crisis. Initial management is aimed at prompt and effective pain control. National guidelines for opiate analgesia in this setting are summarized in Table 15.19 (see also NICE guideline CG143 2012).

Note that adjuvant non-opioid analgesia should be considered in all patients, e.g. paracetamol, ibuprofen. Laxatives, antiemetics, antipruritics, and prophylactic anticoagulation for patients likely to be bed-bound for more than 16 hours a day are other important elements of patient care.

Table 15.18 Approach to a patient with sickle cell anaemia attending A&E

1. Prompt medical assessment and delivery of analgesia, oxygen therapy, and fluid.
2. History—have there been any infective symptoms, shortness of breath, neurological symptoms, priapism? Do they carry a haemoglobinopathy card and do they have their own protocol for analgesia? Are they taking penicillin V and up to date with vaccinations?
3. Examination—oxygen saturations, observations, any chest signs, organomegaly, or neurology.
4. Blood tests—full blood count, urea and electrolytes, liver function, CRP, group and save.
5. CXR—if respiratory signs or symptoms.

Table 15.19 Outline of the management of acute pain in opioid-naive adults

1. Rapid clinical assessment.
2. If pain is severe and oral analgesia is not effective, give strong opioids. Morphine: 0.1 mg/kg IV/SC, repeated every 20 min until pain controlled. Then 0.05–0.1 mg/kg every 2 h IV/SC/PO—consider PCA or diamorphine: 0.1 mg/kg IV/SC, repeated every 20 min until pain controlled. Then 0.05–0.1 mg/kg every 2 h IV/SC—consider PCA.
3. Give adjuvant non-opioid analgesia: paracetamol, ibuprofen, diclofenac, keterolac.
4. Prescribe laxatives routinely and other adjuvants, as necessary. Laxatives: lactulose 10 mL bd, senna 2–4 tablets od, docusate 100 mg bd. Antipruritics: hydroxyzine 25 mg bd. Antiemetics: prochlorperazine 5–10 mg tds, cyclizine 50 mg tds. Anxiolytic: haloperidol 1–3 mg PO/IM bd.
5. Monitor pain, sedation, vital signs, respiratory rate, and oxygen saturations every 30 min until pain controlled and stable, and then every 2 h.
6. Give rescue doses of analgesia every 30 min for breakthrough pain: 50% of maintenance dose.
7. If the respiratory rate is less than 10/min, omit maintenance analgesia. If severe respiratory depression/sedation occurs, give 100 mcg naloxone IV, repeating every 2 min, as necessary.
8. Consider reducing analgesia after 2–3 days and replacing injections with an equivalent dose of an oral opiate.
9. Discharge patients when pain is controlled and improving without analgesia or on acceptable doses of oral analgesia.
10. Arrange any necessary home care and an outpatient follow-up appointment.

Reproduced with permission from DC Rees et al., 'Guidelines for the management of the acute painful crisis in sickle cell disease', British Journal of Haematology, 120, 5, pp. 744–752, © 2003, John Wiley and Sons and British Society for Haematology.

The use of pethidine in the UK for painful vaso-occlusive crises is the cause of much controversy. Its metabolite nor-pethidine is a cerebral irritant and has been reported to be associated with a risk of seizures. Therefore, the current NICE guideline CG143 (2012) states 'do not offer pethidine for treating pain in an acute painful sickle cell episode'.

Good oral fluid intake should be encouraged, however, if this is not possible consider replacement via intravenous or nasogastric routes.

Patients with sickle cell anaemia are rendered hyposplenic from vaso-occlusive crises, and it is recommended that they are suitably vaccinated and take oral penicillin prophylaxis from diagnosis. If patients are febrile (>38°C), they should be started on antibiotics, as per local protocols.

Blood transfusion may be required in the acute setting if there is an acute chest syndrome, neurological symptoms, priapism, multi-organ failure, a sequestration crisis, or severe anaemia for that patient (usually Hb <5 g/dL) but particularly if reticulocytopenic. Some situations may be managed with a 'top-up' transfusion. Exchange transfusion is necessary if there are severe clinical features or if there is no improvement despite initial simple transfusion. This may either be done on an apheresis machine or manually by removing and transfusing blood through a large-bore cannula or a central line. Decisions regarding this will need discussion with the local haematology service. Blood is matched for ABO, Rh C, D, E, and Kell due to the high frequency of antibody formation. It is, therefore, vitally important to provide the clinical information to the transfusion laboratory before requesting a cross-match.

Specific complications

Acute chest syndrome

This is a life-threatening complication and presents with fever, chest pain, shortness of breath, falling oxygen saturations, and new pulmonary infiltrates on chest X-ray. It requires prompt treatment with analgesia, oxygen, simple or exchange transfusion depending on progression, and ventilatory support, as necessary. There is often an infectious precipitant that should be treated appropriately.

Cerebral crisis

Cerebral sequestration occurs more commonly in children and those with HbSS. It may present as a CVA with hemiparesis, decreased conscious level, etc. It must be treated with an urgent exchange transfusion. Patients who have suffered a cerebral crisis are often maintained on an exchange transfusion programme. Transcranial Doppler studies in children can screen those children at risk.

Priapism

This is a urological emergency and requires prompt intervention. Symptoms may be relieved with analgesia and fluid but may require intracavernosal aspiration with or without full exchange transfusion. Early liaison with the haematology/urology services is recommended.

Visceral blood sequestration

This mainly occurs in children with sickling in organs, such as the liver and spleen, with pooling of large blood volumes. Patients may present with organomegaly and severe anaemia.

Aplastic crises

This may be caused by parvovirus infection and is characterized by marked anaemia with a low reticulocyte count.

Further reading

Howard J, Hart N, Roberts-Harewood M, et al., on behalf of the BCSH Committee (2015). Guideline on the management of acute chest syndrome in sickle cell disease. British Journal of Haematology, **169**, 492–505.

National Institute for Health and Care Excellence (2012). Sickle cell acute painful episode: management of an acute painful sickle cell episode in hospital. NICE clinical guideline 143. <https:www.nice.org.uk/guidance/cg143>.

Rees D, Olujohungbe A, Parker N, Stephens A, Telfer P, Wright J (2003). Guideline for the management of the acute painful crisis in sickle cell disease. British Journal of Haematology, **120**, 744–752.

Yardumian A (2007). Sickle cell disease: protocol for the management of adult patients, p. 27, North Middlesex Hospital.

Rheumatology

Arthritis

Arthritis is a term used to describe a wide variety of pathologies. By definition, it implies inflammation within a joint, and this may manifest as joint pain, swelling, and stiffness. In considering the differential diagnosis of a patient presenting with arthritis, it is helpful to consider six broad categories of disease types (see Table 16.1). Infection may cause a septic arthritis or may stimulate an immune response that leads to sterile inflammation of a joint known as reactive arthritis. Crystal deposition may stimulate an inflammatory reaction within joints. The aetiologies of rheumatoid arthritis, psoriatic arthritis, and spondyloarthritis are uncertain, but all three diseases are characterized by prominent inflammation and may be associated with joint destruction. The aetiology of osteoarthritis is likewise unclear, although cartilage degeneration, bone remodelling, and synovial inflammation may all play a role. Trauma may result in structural damage with consequent inflammation. Patients with a connective tissue disease or vasculitis often experience joint pain and stiffness, although overt joint swelling is less common, and these conditions are considered later in this chapter.

Whilst there is no absolute correlation between numbers of joints involved at presentation and disease type, the pattern of joint involvement can be helpful in making a diagnosis. In particular, an acute monoarthritis is usually due to septic arthritis, crystal arthritis, or reactive arthritis.

Septic arthritis and discitis
Septic arthritis
Septic arthritis is a medical emergency and should always be considered and excluded as a diagnosis in a patient with an acute monoarthritis. Factors that predispose to septic arthritis include dermatological conditions, such as psoriasis or eczema, skin trauma, cellulitis, diabetes, dental infections, intravenous drug use, and immunosuppression. *Staphylococcus aureus* accounts for most cases and is found in 60% of infected joints. Beta-haemolytic streptococcal infection occurs in 10% of cases. Gram-negative bacteria are less commonly found but may cause joint sepsis in more elderly individuals, particularly where there has been a urinary tract infection or recent abdominal surgery. *Mycobacterium tuberculosis* accounts for a smaller proportion of cases. Gonococcal septic arthritis should be suspected in a patient with high-risk sexual activity. Salmonella and fungi may cause infection in the immune-compromised patient.

Clinical features
Patients present with a painful, hot, and swollen joint. Knees are most commonly affected and account for 60% of cases; hips are involved in 10% of cases; other joints are much less commonly involved. Infection of multiple joints, rather than a single joint, occurs in 10% of cases. Gonococcal arthritis, in particular, may present with a polyarthritis, and there may be an associated pustular or vesicular rash and tenosynovitis. Tuberculous septic arthritis often has an insidious onset, even in the immunocompetent patient, presenting as a chronic joint effusion. Care needs to be taken with diabetic, elderly, and immunosuppressed patients, in whom symptoms are often atypical. An associated osteomyelitis should be suspected if patients are experiencing bone pain and tenderness.

Investigation
The diagnosis requires the involved joint to be aspirated and the sample of synovial fluid sent for urgent microscopy for organisms and for culture. Polarizing microscopy of the synovial fluid should also be carried out to exclude the differential diagnosis of gout or pseudogout. Aspiration for suspected septic arthritis of the hip should be carried out under ultrasound guidance. Microscopy and culture of the aspirates from gonococcal septic arthritis have a poor yield, and the patient should additionally be referred to a GU clinic for urethral swabs. Aspiration of prosthetic joints should not be carried out by physicians, and patients should be referred for urgent orthopaedic assessment. Needle aspiration of a joint is not contraindicated in patients taking warfarin, although due care must be taken.

In all cases, blood cultures should also be taken.

The white cell count, erythrocyte sedimentation rate, and C-reactive protein should be measured and renal and liver function assessed, both to detect organ damage and because the readings may influence antibiotic choice.

Plain X-rays will not be helpful in diagnosing septic arthritis. However, the presence of chondrocalcinosis may provide evidence in support of pseudogout as a differential diagnosis. Where there is an associated osteomyelitis, then the plain films may demonstrate a periosteal reaction. In this situation, an MRI is much more sensitive and will demonstrate marrow oedema adjacent to the infected joint.

Management
Empirical treatment with intravenous antibiotics should be started as soon as the joint has been aspirated. The current recommendation from the British Society of Rheumatology (BSR) is to initiate treatment with IV flucloxacillin. Local policies may suggest the addition of penicillin or gentamicin. If the patient is penicillin-allergic, then IV clindamycin is suggested. If Gram-negative infection is suspected, then patients should be treated with a second-or third-generation cephalosporin. Clearly, the initial Gram stain will influence antibiotic choice. The treatment may subsequently be amended, according to bacterial growth and reported sensitivities. In general, treatment is given intravenously for

Table 16.1 Broad categories of arthritis

Aetiology	Disease
Infection	Septic arthritis
	Discitis
Reactive to infection	Classical reactive arthritis
	Post-streptococcal
	Associated with a range of other infections
Crystal deposition	Gout
	Calcium pyrophosphate deposition disease
Unknown primary aetiology with prominent immunopathology	Rheumatoid arthritis
	Psoriatic arthritis
	Spondyloarthritis
Unknown primary aetiology with degenerative features	Osteoarthritis
Trauma	Structural damage to ligaments and cartilage

2 weeks and then orally for a further 4 weeks. The requirement for this length of treatment is not based on clear evidence, and shorter treatment regimens are now proposed. The joint should be aspirated to dryness on initial presentation and should be re-aspirated if there is a recurrent effusion. Arthroscopic washout may be required. Weight bearing through the infected joint should be avoided until signs of improvement are evident. Infected joints are very painful, and it is important to provide adequate analgesia. C-reactive protein (CRP) should be measured serially, as it is a good indicator of improvement in this condition.

Discitis

The term discitis refers to inflammation of an intervertebral disc. The condition is usually infective in aetiology, and, as in septic arthritis, the commonest organism found is *Staphylococcus aureus*. Discitis most likely arises from haematogenous spread of bacteria from another primary site of infection. There is often an associated osteomyelitis of the vertebral body.

Clinical features

Patients usually present with back pain and fever. In many cases, the onset is insidious, resulting in a delay in diagnosis. There will be tenderness over the affected disc and restriction of spinal movements. It is very important to undertake a neurological assessment to look for evidence of cord compression. Assessment of power is frequently difficult, as patients are in severe pain, but changes in sensation and abnormalities of tendon jerks may be more readily detected. Features of a cauda equina syndrome, such as urinary retention or poor anal tone, must be looked for.

Investigation

Plain radiographs of the spine may show loss of disc space and a periosteal reaction, but these abnormalities often take several weeks to develop. A soft tissue shadow adjacent to the spine suggests the presence of a paraspinal abscess. Plain abdominal radiographs may show loss of the psoas shadow, indicating a psoas abscess. CT scans are informative, but an MRI scan of the spine is the investigation of choice. Following this, a CT-guided needle biopsy/ aspirate of the possibly infected disc should be undertaken. As for investigation of septic arthritis, blood cultures should be taken, together with samples for haematology and biochemistry.

Management

Empirical treatment with IV antibiotics should be started as soon as a sample has been obtained for culture. Flucloxacillin with gentamicin is usually recommended initially, although the choice will depend on the initial Gram stain. An associated paraspinal abscess may need surgical drainage, and a spinal surgeon should be consulted urgently if neurological features develop. Depending on the extent of disease, patients may need to remain in bed for the first 2 weeks and may require a brace when they do start to mobilize. Antibiotics are given for 6–8 weeks, and the duration of IV antibiotics is usually longer than that for septic arthritis; it may extend for the full 6 weeks period. Patients should not switch from IV to oral antibiotics until the acute phase response has markedly improved (ESR less than half initial value) and the patient is pain-free and mobile.

Reactive arthritis

Reactive arthritis describes an inflammatory arthritis, occurring as part of the immune response to an infectious agent and with a sterile joint aspirate.

Classical reactive arthritis

The classical form of reactive arthritis is usually triggered by urethral infection with *Chlamydia trachomatis* or by gastrointestinal infection with *Salmonella*, *Shigella*, *Campylobacter*, or *Yersinia* spp. Males are much more commonly affected than females, and there is a strong association with the presence of the MHC class I allele HLA-B27. The role that this molecule may play in the pathogenesis of the condition remains unclear. It is presumed that bacteria stimulate an immune response that results in immunopathology.

Clinical features

Patients commonly present with a single hot and swollen large joint (typically a knee), and the clinical picture may be indistinguishable from that of septic arthritis or crystal arthritis. On occasions, more than one peripheral joint and/ or the sacroiliac joints may be involved. Patients may also develop conjunctivitis, circinate balanitis, and a scaly rash on the soles of the feet termed keratoderma blenorrhagica. Urethritis may be a feature and can be 'infectious', in association with *Chlamydia*, or sterile following gastrointestinal infection. The triad of arthritis, conjunctivitis, and urethritis has been referred to as Reiter's syndrome. As some patients present with only an inflamed joint whilst others present with more than these three features, the term is now best avoided. Systemic features of fever, malaise, and myalgias may be present.

Investigation

The affected joint should be aspirated and the fluid sent both for Gram staining and culture plus microscopy for crystals to exclude the differential diagnoses of septic or crystal arthritis. The diagnosis should then be made on clinical grounds. The presence of HLA-B27 increases the likelihood of reactive arthritis, but the test is not diagnostic, and individuals who are HLA-B27 –ve may still have the condition. The WCC and CRP may be significantly elevated. If urethritis is present or there is a relevant sexual history, then urethral swabs should be sent and may be informative, with respect to *Chlamydia*. If there is a history of diarrhoea, then a stool sample should be sent for culture; however, these rarely prove positive by the time the arthritis has developed. In the acute setting, radiographs are not usually helpful. However, in some cases, particularly where the arthritis persists, an MRI scan may be appropriate to exclude the differential diagnosis of mechanical derangement and to confirm the presence of synovitis.

Management

The arthritis will usually respond to intra-articular injection with corticosteroid. For larger joints 20–80 mg methylprednisolone or 10–40 mg triamcinolone are used. 10–25 mg hydrocortisone is more appropriate for small joints. Patients will also benefit from resting the joint and a regular NSAID. Urethral infection, if demonstrated, should be treated, although this may not affect the course of the arthritis. If the arthritis recurs, then the joint should be re-injected with corticosteroid. If the patient has not improved by 3 months, then consideration should be given to starting either sulfasalazine or methotrexate.

The outcome from classical reactive arthritis is very variable; it has been described as the disease of one-thirds; in one-third of cases, the condition is acute and self-limiting; in one-third of cases, it demonstrates a relapsing/remitting course but ultimately improves, and, in one-third of cases, it becomes chronic.

Streptococcus-associated arthritis

Group A beta haemolytic streptococci are a common cause of sore throats and cellulitis. They can also trigger autoinflammatory and autoimmune conditions, including glomerulonephritis, vasculitis, reactive arthritis, and rheumatic fever. The latter two conditions are characterized by joint involvement.

Post-streptococcal reactive arthritis

Patients experience pain and swelling, usually affecting a single large joint, 1–2 weeks after the acute streptococcal infection. In some individuals, more than a single joint is affected, although the condition is typically an oligoarthritis, rather than a polyarthritis. The pattern of arthritis and the lack of other features distinguish this condition from rheumatic fever. Cultures should be performed to identify the streptococcal infection; in most cases, the organism is identified from throat swabs. Serological tests may also provide information about recent streptococcal infection. The joint aspirate itself will be sterile. Treatment of the acute arthritis is as for classical reactive arthritis, with intra-articular corticosteroids and NSAIDs. The streptococcal infection should be treated with penicillin. Views are mixed as to whether long-term prophylaxis with penicillin is beneficial in adults with this form of reactive arthritis; in general, it is not given, following a single episode, but may be considered if recurrent episodes occur.

Rheumatic fever

The incidence of rheumatic fever has declined over the past century, although there has been a small increase in reported cases over the past two decades. The changing incidence relates to the introduction of antibiotics in the 1940s but may also reflect changes in the prevalent subtypes of streptococci. The condition usually affects children and is rarely seen in adults. It usually presents 2–6 weeks after the primary streptococcal infection, and the characteristic features are of a migratory polyarthritis that generally affects large, rather than small, joints, carditis, subcutaneous nodules, erythema marginatum, and chorea. The modified Jones criteria are used to aid diagnosis; in the presence of evidence of recent streptococcal infection, then the presence of two major or one major and two minor criteria are required to make a firm diagnosis (available in Jones TD, 1944, 'The diagnosis of rheumatic fever', JAMA, 126, 8, pp. 481-84).

The group A streptococcal infection should be treated with penicillin V for 10 days or with IM benzathine benzylpenicillin if compliance is likely to be a problem. Erythromycin is an alternative if the patient is allergic to penicillin. Following initial treatment, prophylaxis with phenoxymethylpenicillin PO bd or benzathine benzylpenicillin IM monthly should be continued for at least 5 years (and until the age of 18 in children). Longer-term prophylaxis may be considered in individuals with cardiac complications of the disease and in those who are recurrently exposed to streptoccoal infection. Salicylates are conventionally used for the management of arthritis, although other NSAIDs may be effective. Patients with severe carditis are often also given oral prednisolone. Cardiac failure and chorea should be managed in the usual way. Rheumatic fever is associated with the development of cardiac valvular abnormalities, and these may need longer-term medical and/or surgical management.

Acute sarcoidosis

Acute sarcoidosis is also known as Löfgren's syndrome; it tends to affect males more than females and has higher incidence during spring. The aetiopathogenesis of acute sarcoidosis is not understood. The observation that cases often present in the first few months of the year has suggested that it is triggered by an environmental, and possibly an infectious, agent. There is also some evidence to suggest it is more common in individuals after they have attended large gatherings, consistent with the idea that the disease represents a response to an infectious agent. The presentation and prognosis of acute sarcoidosis are different from those of chronic sarcoidosis, and every effort should be made to distinguish the two at presentation.

Clinical features

The three classical features of acute sarcoidosis comprise a periarthritis, generally of the ankles, erythema nodosum, and bilateral hilar lymphadenopathy. Patients usually experience severe unilateral or bilateral ankle pain and have difficulty weight bearing. The joints tend to be erythematous, with evidence of soft tissue swelling, although the range of movement is relatively well preserved. Imaging studies have shown that the inflammatory changes lie within the subcutaneous tissues, rather than within the joint itself. The appearances can resemble those of gout or of cellulitis. Erythema nodosum is a helpful sign if present but is often absent in men. Patients usually experience fevers and general malaise.

Investigation

Blood tests will show an elevated neutrophil count, with a high CRP. The serum ACE should be requested, although this can be within the normal range; a high serum ACE tends to correlate with poorer outcome in joint disease. The chest radiograph (CXR) will demonstrate enlargement of the hilar lymph nodes. The combination of periarthritis of the ankles and bilateral hilar lymphadenopathy has a very high specificity for the diagnosis of acute sarcoidosis. Where patients present with erythema nodosum and hilar lymphadenopathy without the classical periarthritis, then further investigations are warranted to exclude other conditions, such as TB and lymphoma.

Management

Acute sarcoidosis is almost always a self-limiting illness, with 95% of individuals recovering completely within 1–2 years. Most patients improve within the first 3–6 months. Only a very few individuals go on to develop a chronic form of the disease. There is no need for any specific treatment. However, the periarthritis does usually respond symptomatically to the use of regular NSAIDs, and these are first-line therapy. Where these are not effective or where there are significant systemic features, then prednisolone may be used at an initial dose of 15–20 mg od, tailing by 5 mg every month.

Virus-associated arthritis

Infection with many different viruses may be associated with the development of inflammatory arthritis (see Table 16.2). The pathophysiology of the arthritis is poorly understood in most cases but is likely to reflect the immunopathology, rather than the direct effects of the virus infection. In most cases, the arthritis is transient, polyarticular, and not associated with the development of joint destruction. The joint symptoms may be treated symptomatically with analgesics and non-steroidal anti-inflammatory drugs. Where arthritis becomes chronic, as in some patients with hepatitis C infection, then treatment with disease-modifying agents, such as methotrexate, can have a beneficial effect.

Table 16.2 Patterns of arthritis in viral infections

Virus	Arthritis
Parvovirus B19	Transient peripheral polyarthralgias or polyarthritis. More common in adults than children
Hepatitis B	Polyarthritis that commonly involves the hands and knees. Transient or persistent in those with chronic HBV viraemia
Hepatitis C virus (with or without cryoglobulinaemia)	Peripheral polyarthralgias or polyarthritis. May be persistent
Rubella	Transient polyarthritis
HIV	Transient polyarthritis associated with primary infection. Relatively high frequency of some other forms of arthritis (e.g. reactive arthritis) during persistent infection
Epstein–Barr virus	Transient polyarthritis or knee monoarthritis
Varicella zoster	Transient oligoarthritis
Mumps	Transient oligoarthritis
Adenovirus or Coxsackie viruses A9, B2, B3, B4, and B6	Recurrent polyarthritis

Crystal arthritis

Gout

Gout refers to a form of inflammatory arthritis caused by uric acid crystals. It affects men more commonly than women and is a further cause of an acute monoarthritis that may be clinically indistinguishable from a septic arthritis.

The degradation of the purine bases (AMP and GMP) involves their conversion to xanthine; this is then converted by xanthine oxidase to uric acid which is excreted in urine. Concentrations of uric acid may rise for several reasons, including high levels of purine consumption, abnormalities in purine metabolism, and failure to effectively excrete uric acid. Within synovial joints, high concentrations of uric acid result in the development of monosodium urate crystals which trigger an inflammatory response. At a clinical level, predisposing factors for the development of gout include a diet rich in purines, excess alcohol intake, myeloproliferative disorders, tumour lysis syndrome, dehydration, particularly following surgery, obesity, hypothyroidism, thiazide diuretics, and renal impairment. Where there is a strong family history, then inherited abnormalities of enzymes involved in purine metabolism or of a urate transporter within the kidney may be present.

Clinical features

Patients usually present with acute onset of severe pain and swelling, affecting a single joint. The first metatarsophalangeal (MTP) joint is most commonly affected, although any peripheral joint can be involved, and, on occasions, multiple joints are affected. There is classically very prominent sensitivity of the joint and surrounding skin such that the patient does not even like the sensation of a sheet over their joint in bed. The joint is usually warm and erythematous. Individuals may also present with acute bursitis, often involving the olecranon or prepatellar bursae. In cases of chronic hyperuricaemia, tophi may develop. These often form within the soft tissues of the fingers and toes or over the olecranon. Tophi may also form along the course of tendons or on the ear helix. Urate deposition may occur within the renal pelvis and ureters, resulting in renal calculi or in the renal medulla, resulting in 'urate nephropathy'. Whilst the initial presentation of gout is usually with monoarticular disease, over time, the condition may become polyarticular and resemble rheumatoid arthritis.

Investigation

Aspiration of the affected joint is required to formally confirm the diagnosis. Polarized light microscopy will demonstrate the presence of negatively birefringent, spindle-shaped crystals. The synovial fluid should also be Gram-stained and cultured to exclude septic arthritis. Whilst joint aspiration is ideal, this may not be possible, particularly where a small joint, such as the first MTP, is involved, and, in these cases, the diagnosis is based predominantly on the clinical picture. The serum urate can be a useful guide, although it may be normal, particularly in the context of an acute episode of gout. Repeat analysis, once the flare has settled, can be helpful. During the acute attack, the neutrophil count will usually be high, as will the CRP. Radiographs may demonstrate 'mouse bite' erosions, which classically occur at the joint margin, rather than the articular surface. Individuals with gout are at increased risk of hypertension, hyperlipidaemia, and type 2 diabetes; patients should be examined and investigated for these conditions. All individuals presenting with gout should have their renal function checked.

Management

Patients presenting with acute gout should be treated with an NSAID or colchicine and will usually require treatment for up to 4 weeks. If they are unable to tolerate either, then prednisolone can be used at a dose of 10–20 mg orally or depomedrone can be administered IM at a dose of 120 mg. Injection of an inflamed joint with 20–80 mg methylprednisolone or 10–40 mg triamcinolone is also usually effective. Patients should be advised to avoid foods high in purine, to moderate their alcohol intake, to ensure they remain well hydrated and, if appropriate, to lose weight. Where patients experience multiple attacks of gout, and particularly where the plasma urate is high, then treatment with allopurinol is recommended. This should not be commenced for at least 4 weeks after an acute flare but may then be introduced at an initial dose of 100 mg od, increasing by 100 mg od every 1–2 weeks until the plasma urate is <350 micromoles/L. Paradoxically, the introduction of allopurinol often precipitates flares of gout, and patients should be warned of this and given NSAID or colchicine prophylaxis for at least 6 weeks and ideally until they are established on a stable dose of allopurinol. A patient who is taking allopurinol and experiences an episode of acute gout should be treated with NSAIDs or colchicine as usual and allopurinol continued until the flare has settled.

Allopurinol has been associated with the development of toxic epidermal necrolysis and Stevens–Johnson syndrome, and patients should be warned to stop taking the drug if they develop a rash or mucosal ulceration. Allopurinol enhances the effects and increases the toxicity of azathioprine, and drug doses should be reduced accordingly.

Febuxostat is a newer xanthine oxidase inhibitor, prescribed at a dose of 80 mg daily, escalating to 120 mg daily, if required; it may be used where allopurinol is contraindicated or not tolerated. The uricosuric drugs sulfinpyrazone, probenecid, and benzbromarone are used much less commonly.

Calcium pyrophosphate deposition disease

Calcium pyrophosphate crystals may be deposited within cartilage and are associated with the development of acute calcium pyrophosphate crystal arthritis (previously termed pseudogout). Crystals may also be deposited in joints affected with osteoarthritis, and, occasionally, the recurrent inflammation in these joints may mimic rheumatoid arthritis (previously termed pseudorheumatoid arthritis).

The biochemical abnormalities that lead to deposition of calcium pyrophosphate crystals are poorly understood, although it is thought that increased breakdown of ATP may produce high levels of inorganic phosphate that can bind to calcium, with subsequent deposition of the crystals within cartilage. The condition affects women more than men, is rare in individuals <50 years, and is increasingly common with increasing age. It occurs more often in individuals with haemochromatosis, acromegaly, ochranosis, and hyperparathyroidism.

Clinical features

Many individuals with radiological evidence of calcium pyrophosphate deposition are asymptomatic. A proportion develops an acutely painful and swollen joint that clinically resembles gouty arthritis or septic arthritis. The wrist or knee is most commonly involved. Others develop calcium pyrophosphate crystal deposition in osteoarthritic joints, with involvement of large, and sometimes small, joints. These patients often present with acute-on-chronic joint swelling, and, where the metacarpophalangeal (MCP) joints are involved, the differential diagnosis may include seronegative rheumatoid arthritis.

Investigation

The diagnosis depends on the demonstration of calcium pyrophosphate crystals. In cases of acute calcium pyrophosphate crystal arthritis, the joint should be aspirated and examined under polarized light; rhomboid-shaped, positively birefringent crystals will be seen. The sample should also be Gram-stained and cultured to exclude septic arthritis. The white cell count (WCC) and CRP may be raised. In both acute and chronic presentations, radiographs may demonstrate chondrocalcinosis. This is particularly commonly seen in the triangular cartilage of the wrist and the menisci of the knees. It may also be seen within the acetabular labrum of the hips and the fibrocartilage of the symphysis pubis. Further laboratory tests should include calcium, phosphate, parathyroid hormone (PTH), and iron studies.

Management

Patients presenting with acute calcium pyrophosphate arthritis may be treated with an intra-articular injection of corticosteroid (20–80 mg methylprednisolone or 10–40 mg triamcinolone) or orally with an NSAID or, if these drugs are contraindicated, with colchicine and prednisolone at a dose of 10–20 mg od. Similarly to gout, the condition will also respond to an IM injection of 120 mg depomedrone. Patients who have more widespread, chronic inflammatory arthritis, associated with calcium pyrophosphate deposition, may show a symptomatic response to longer-term NSAIDs or low-dose prednisolone. Any underlying condition, such as haemochromatosis or hyperparathyroidism, should be actively managed.

Rheumatoid arthritis

Rheumatoid arthritis is a symmetrical polyarthritis that is common and affects females more often than males. It is a very significant cause of pain and disability, much of which can be prevented by early diagnosis and appropriate treatment.

The aetiology and pathogenesis of rheumatoid arthritis is poorly understood. There is a strong genetic influence on disease susceptibility, some of which relates to polymorphisms of the HLA class II DR beta chain and the protein tyrosine phosphatase non-receptor 22. This, together with the clinical observation that inhibition of T cell co-stimulation in vivo, using a CTLA4-Ig fusion protein, is an effective treatment for rheumatoid arthritis, suggests that T cells play a role in the pathogenesis of rheumatoid arthritis. However, there is also evidence for involvement of other components of the immune system. The finding of rheumatoid factor (antibodies directed against the Fc region of IgG) in individuals with rheumatoid arthritis has long suggested a failure of B cell regulation. The high specificity of antibodies directed against citrullinated self proteins for rheumatoid arthritis further implies an abnormality of B cell tolerance. The observation that B cell depletion is an effective form of therapy for rheumatoid arthritis supports the idea that this arm of the adaptive immune response is important in pathogenesis. In vitro cultures of synovial tissue have demonstrated that TNF-alpha and IL-1 are pivotal in triggering the cytokine cascade that promotes inflammation, and this lends support to the idea that production of these cytokines by monocyte-derived and other cell populations within the joint are an important downstream event in joint inflammation. The efficacy of TNF-alpha blockade in treatment is consistent with these in vitro observations. Further work has supported the idea that IL-6 also has an important role in disease pathogenesis and represents a therapeutic target. Whilst the ongoing research has led to valuable gains in terms of diagnostic tools and therapies, it has not, as yet, led to an understanding of what might actually trigger the disease in susceptible individuals.

Clinical features

The presentation of rheumatoid arthritis may be very acute, with symptoms developing overnight, or may be more gradual, with symptoms progressing over the course of a few weeks or months. In either case, patients will usually give a history of pain, stiffness, and swelling that particularly affect their small joints. Symptoms are often most severe in the mornings or after periods of inactivity and may improve, to some extent, with use of the joints. The arthritis classically involves the MCP and proximal interphalangeal (PIP) joints as well as the wrists and forefeet. However, involvement of all other peripheral joints, with the exception of the distal interphalangeal (DIP) joints, may occur. Examination may reveal swelling affecting the joints, consistent with synovitis and effusions. In early cases, swelling may not be clinically obvious, although the joints will usually be tender to pressure. A small proportion of individuals present atypically with large joint arthritis. Patients may also experience bursitis, usually affecting the olecranon or subacromial bursae and tenosynovitis, occasionally with associated tendinopathy and rupture. Joint inflammation may result in nerve entrapment, and compression of the median nerve (carpal tunnel syndrome) is particularly common. Systemic features, including lethargy, fevers, anorexia, and weight loss, may be present.

Untreated, patients develop cartilage damage, bony erosions, and soft tissue damage, with increasing joint destruction and deformity. The classical features are of swan necking and boutonnière deformities of the fingers, Z deformities of the thumbs, ulnar deviation at the MCP joints, subluxation of the carpus, fixed flexion deformity at the elbows, flattening of the longitudinal arch of the feet, with splaying of the forefeet and clawing of the toes. In the spine, atlantoaxial subluxation may occur, most commonly in the anterior plane; vertical subluxation is rare but even more serious, as it causes brainstem impingement.

The development of rheumatoid nodules, vasculitis, pulmonary effusions, or fibrosis is relatively rare early in the course of the disease but may occur with time. With current treatment regimens, amyloidosis is extremely unusual. Felty's syndrome describes a triad of RA, splenomegaly, and leucopenia; it is now also unusual. Large granular lymphocytic leukaemia, a syndrome of splenomegaly, neutropenia, and large granular lymphocytes, is felt to be a variant of Felty's syndrome and again is very rare.

In the longer term, patients with rheumatoid arthritis are at increased risk of cardiovascular disease and osteoporosis. They are also at increased risk of lymphoma, particularly if their rheumatoid arthritis is very active.

Investigation
The ESR and CRP are likely to be raised, consistent with an inflammatory process. Serial estimations of these markers are helpful in monitoring disease activity. The FBC, U&E, and LFTs should be checked; there may be anaemia of chronic disease, and the results of the tests may influence treatment choice and/or serve as baseline values in monitoring for treatment toxicity. Most laboratories will still test for rheumatoid factor; this will be present in approximately 60–70% cases. However, it is not highly specific and may also be positive in patients with Sjögren's syndrome, SLE, hepatitis C, infective endocarditis, and cryptogenic fibrosing alveolitis, as well as in a proportion of healthy adults. Many laboratories will test for anti-CCP (cyclic citrullinated peptide) antibodies. Although only present in approximately 60–70% of cases, they are much more specific than rheumatoid factor and identify a cohort of individuals likely to develop erosive disease. A smaller proportion of patients will be positive for antinuclear antibodies (ANA).

X-rays of the hands and feet are usually performed on presentation, although many patients will not have abnormalities at this time. Over time, the typical features of periarticular osteopenia, erosions of the articular surface, narrowing of the joint space, and joint subluxation can occur. Early radiographic changes often involve the feet, rather than the hands, but also include erosion of the ulnar styloid. X-rays should be repeated every 1–2 years to look for evidence of disease progression. Ultrasound scanning with the use of Doppler is a very useful tool early in the course of disease and can be used to identify active synovitis, tenosynovitis, and microerosions. MRI scans, particularly when performed with gadolinium enhancement, will likewise give detailed information about synovitis and erosive damage.

The classification criteria for rheumatoid arthritis were developed by the American College of Rheumatology (ACR) in 1987 and adapted by the European League Against Rheumatism (EULAR) in 2010 to aid earlier diagnosis (see Table 16.3).

Table 16.3 ACR-EULAR classification criteria for rheumatoid arthritis

A. Joint involvement:	
1 large joint	0
2–10 large joints	1
1–3 small joints	2
4–10 small joints	3
>10 joints (at least 1 small)	5
B. Serology:	
Low +ve RhF or anti-CCP	2
High +ve RhF or anti-CCP	3
C. Acute phase reactants:	
Raised CRP or ESR	1
D. Duration of symptoms >6 weeks	1

Patients may be classified as having rheumatoid arthritis if the total score is 6/10 or greater.

Reproduced with permission from D Aletaha et al., '2010 Rheumatoid arthritis classification criteria: an American College of Rheumatology/ European League Against Rheumatism collaborative initiative', *Arthritis & Rheumatism*, 62, 9, pp. 2569–2581, published by Wiley, © 2010 by the American College of Rheumatology.

In practice, anti-CCP antibodies and soft tissue ultrasound or MRI facilitate early diagnosis and allow prompt initiation of treatment, with consequent reduction in the risk of developing joint destruction and disability.

Management
The management of patients with rheumatoid arthritis requires a multidisciplinary team, with input from nurses, therapists, and doctors. The principal aims of medical management are to control symptoms and to minimize joint damage. Achievement of these aims will require consideration of the use of five broad categories of drugs for each patient (see Table 16.4). Care needs to be taken to minimize the considerable risks of side effects associated with the drugs used.

In Europe, the disease activity score using 28 points (DAS28) has become an integral part of the assessment and monitoring of rheumatoid arthritis. The DAS28 is a composite score (available online), derived from a tender joint score, swollen joint count, a visual analogue score of global health, and measurement of ESR. Ideally, drug therapy should be escalated until disease remission, defined as a DAS28 score of <2.6, is achieved.

Table 16.4 Drugs used in management of rheumatoid arthritis

Broad category	Examples
Analgesics	Paracetamol, codeine, tramadol
Non-steroidal anti-inflammatory drugs	Naproxen, diclofenac, ibuprofen, etoricoxib
Corticosteroids	Prednisolone, depomedrone, methylprednisolone
Classical disease-modifying anti-rheumatic drugs	Methotrexate, sulfasalazine, hydroxychloroquine, leflunomide
Biologic disease-modifying anti-rheumatic drugs	Adalimumab, etanercept, infliximab, golimumab, certolizumab, rituximab, tocilizumab, abatacept

Analgesics and non-steroidal anti-inflammatory drugs need to be considered in all patients. Many patients benefit from using paracetamol or a paracetamol/codeine combination on an as-needed basis, together with a regular long-acting NSAID, if required. Complications of NSAIDs include peptic ulceration and cardiovascular disease. Given the chronicity of the disease, then concomitant treatment with a gastroprotectant, such as a proton pump inhibitor, is appropriate in most individuals.

Corticosteroids are effective in the management of rheumatoid arthritis but are associated with high risks of complications. In the context of first presentation of disease, corticosteroids improve symptoms and may reduce early erosive damage. They may be administered intramuscularly, using a dose of 120–160 mg methylprednisolone, or given orally, usually at a dose of 10–15 mg od, although some studies have suggested a role for higher doses. IV steroid regimes are now rarely needed. In patients already on treatment with disease-modifying and biologic agents presenting with disease flares, IM, oral, or IV corticosteroids may likewise be used to suppress disease activity. However, the risk:benefit ratio is less convincing than for early disease, and they should be administered judiciously. It may also be appropriate to administer corticosteroids intra-articularly. This is a highly effective means of treating synovitis within a single joint and reduces the risks of systemic side effects. Smaller, more superficial joints are generally treated with up to 25 mg hydrocortisone whilst larger joints are treated with 20–80 mg methylprednisolone. The corticosteroid may be mixed with a small amount of lidocaine (INN) (0.2–2 mL of 1% or 2% lidocaine (INN) depending on the joint) in order to minimize discomfort felt from further distension of the joint capsule with fluid.

Classical disease-modifying anti-rheumatic drugs (DMARDs) should be considered in all patients with a diagnosis of rheumatoid arthritis. Before starting the drugs, all patients should be counselled about adverse effects, drug monitoring regimes, and given access to telephone helplines. Patients should be advised about the effects of the drugs on fertility and the risks of teratogenicity. Precise guidelines relating to each agent are available on the BSR website. UK guidance recommends the use of at least two classical DMARDs. For the majority of patients, methotrexate will be a first-choice, and the dose will be escalated to 20–25 mg weekly, as needed. Subcutaneous methotrexate is a good alternative to the tablets where gastrointestinal intolerance or poor responsiveness is a problem. A weekly dose of folic acid is usually also given in an effort to reduce methotrexate toxicity. Hydroxychloroquine and/or sulfasalazine will usually also be prescribed, particularly if disease control is not achieved with methotrexate. Leflunomide may be used for patients intolerant of methotrexate.

Where classical DMARDs fail to adequately control disease activity, then 'biologic' DMARD' therapies may be introduced. TNF-alpha antagonism (with infliximab, adalimumab, certolizumab, golimumab, etanercept), B cell depletion (with rituximab), IL-6 receptor blockade (with tocilizumab), and T cell co-stimulation blockade (with abatacept) are now all approved by the National Institute for Health and Care Excellence (NICE) for the treatment of rheumatoid arthritis (see Table 16.5).

NICE imposed constraints on the use of these drugs, and they may only be given following inefficacy of, or intolerance to, at least two classical DMARDs and only continued if the patient has a sustained clinical response. Where possible, the drugs are given in combination with

Table 16.5 NICE-approved 'biologic' disease-modifying anti-rheumatic drugs (DMARDs) for the management of rheumatoid arthritis

Drug	Description
Infliximab	Chimeric monoclonal antibody specific for TNF-alpha. Administered by infusion every 8 weeks
Adalimumab	Fully humanized monoclonal antibody specific for TNF-alpha. Administered fortnightly subcutaneously
Certolizumab	Recombinant humanized antibody Fab fragment specific for TNF-alpha conjugated to polyethylene glycol in order to extend the half-life of the compound. Administered fortnightly subcutaneously
Golimumab	Fully humanized monoclonal antibody specific for TNF-alpha. Administered every 4 weeks subcutaneously
Etanercept	Recombinant protein comprising part of the p75 TNF receptor linked to the Fc component of IgG. Binds to TNF-alpha and TNF-beta. Administered weekly by subcutaneous injection
Rituximab	Chimeric monoclonal antibody specific for CD20 expressed specifically by B cells. Rituximab given IV on two occasions 2 weeks apart results in B cell depletion. Plasma cells are not depleted, and Ig levels remain within the normal range. Treatment repeated after at least 6 months and following recovery of B cells and relapse of arthritis
Tocilizumab	Humanized monoclonal antibody specific for IL-6 receptor. Given by intravenous infusion every 4 weeks
Abatacept	Fusion protein comprising extracellular domain of CTLA4 and the Fc region of IgG1. Given by intravenous infusion every 4 weeks or by weekly subcutaneous injection

methotrexate to maximize response rates and reduce immunogenicity.

The use of TNF-alpha antagonists is associated with a reduction in capacity for protective immunity and hence an increase in risk of both acute and chronic infection. The most important risk relates to TB where reactivation or reinfection may occur, usually within 12 months of starting treatment. Patients should be assessed for risk, according to British Thoracic Society guidelines, and given prophylaxis or treatment drug regimens, as appropriate. Current policy is that TNF-alpha antagonists should be used with care in patients with HIV infection or prior hepatitis B infection and avoided in active hepatitis B or C infection. There have been concerns about the long-term risk of malignancy in patients treated with TNF-alpha antagonists. Available data are generally reassuring with respect to incidence of solid tumours, at least within the first 10 years of treatment. There may be a small increase in the risk of certain types of skin cancer, and patients should be counselled about sun exposure. Current guidelines suggest that TNF-alpha antagonists should be avoided for a minimum of 10 years, following treatment for a previous malignancy. The drugs should not be used in women who are pregnant or breastfeeding, in individuals with grade 3 or 4 congestive heart failure or with a history of demyelination. It is important that they are temporarily stopped in the context of acute infection.

The use of rituximab may be considered in patients with active rheumatoid arthritis who have failed to respond to classical DMARDs and TNF alpha antagonists. Again, it is usually given in combination with methotrexate. Patients may be retreated every 6 months or when B cell levels recover and disease relapses. There is no clear guidance as to how many times treatment can be repeated. Whilst TB infection is of less concern in patients receiving rituximab, hepatitis B reactivation is well documented. A rare association between progressive multifocal leukoencephalopathy (PML) and patients receiving rituximab, mainly in the context of lymphoproliferative disorders, has been observed. Rituximab may be used safely in individuals with a prior history of malignancy.

Tocilizumab is a humanized anti-IL-6 receptor antibody which blocks the interaction between the cytokine IL-6 and its receptors on a range of cells, including T cells, B cells, macrophages, and osteoclasts. It is most effective when given in combination with methotrexate. Infection risks are increased, and all patients should be screened for TB and hepatitis B and C infection prior to receiving tocilizumab.

Abatacept is a fusion protein of cytotoxic T lymphocyte associated antigen 4 (CTLA4) and IgG1; it serves to inhibit T cell co-stimulation. As with the other biologics, it is usually given in combination with methotrexate, and patients should be screened for, and counselled about, infection.

Early diagnosis, rapid conventional drug escalation regimes, and the use of the biologic agents have improved outcome from rheumatoid arthritis. In the long-term, patients remain at increased risk of both cardiovascular disease and osteoporosis. QRISK2 should be used to calculate cardiovascular risk, and the WHO FRAX calculator may be used to estimate fracture risk. Other risk factors for these conditions need to be identified and actively managed. Bone density scans should be performed, if required, and osteoporosis treated with bisphosphonates or an alternative agent, if appropriate.

Psoriatic arthritis

Psoriatic arthritis refers to a seronegative inflammatory joint disease found in approximately 5–8% patients with psoriasis. The aetiopathogenesis of the condition is not well understood. Genetic factors affect susceptibility, and associations with specific HLA class I and II alleles have been described, possibly suggesting a role for T cells or NK cells. Mononuclear cells infiltrate the synovium within joints. Similar to other forms of inflammatory arthritis, interactions between infiltrating and resident cells may occur, with increased cytokine expression, proliferation of the synovial lining, and the development of erosive damage.

Clinical features

A variety of clinical manifestations and several distinct patterns of disease have been described, although overlap between the patterns is common (see Table 16.6). The involvement of the DIP joints, early involvement of entheses (sites of tendon and ligament attachment to bone), and dactylitis (sausage finger, reflecting involvement of entheses and tendons as well as joints within the digits) are characteristic.

Asymmetric oligoarticular disease is the most common form of psoriatic arthritis, although a polyarticular 'rheumatoid-like' arthritis may also occur. A small proportion of patients present with arthritis that predominantly affects

Table 16.6 Clinical patterns of psoriatic arthritis

Type of arthritis	Frequency (%)
Asymmetrical oligoarthritis	50
'Rheumatoid-like' polyarthritis	15
DIP joint arthritis	10
Axial (sacroiliac) disease	20
Arthritis mutilans	5

the DIP joints. Involvement of the sacroiliac joints, often with an asymmetric pattern, is also well described. Rarely, a destructive form of psoriatic arthritis termed 'arthritis mutilans' develops. The psoriasis itself may be very mild, restricted to the nails, or, in some instances, may post-date the arthritis in terms of onset. The peak onset of arthritis occurs between 30 and 55 years.

Investigation

There are no specific diagnostic tests. Blood tests are often unhelpful, and ESR and CRP are normal in over 50% of patients. The rheumatoid factor, ANA, and anti-CCP antibodies will generally be negative, although the lack of specificity of the first two detracts from the significance of the results. Imaging studies can be contributory and may demonstrate erosions occurring particularly at the cartilaginous edge of the joint. MRI scans may demonstrate associated enthesopathy. In severe disease and in arthritis mutilans, osteolysis results in the typical 'pencil in cup' appearances. However, in many patients, the changes seen on imaging will not be diagnostic, and the differential may include rheumatoid arthritis, osteoarthritis, or gout. Overall, the diagnosis must be based on the clinical picture, with the most helpful clues being a history or family history of psoriasis, the presence of nail dystrophy, the presence of dactylitis, involvement of entheses, and arthritis involving the DIP joints.

Management

The approach to management of psoriatic arthritis is similar to that for rheumatoid arthritis. Analgesics and/or NSAIDs should be used for symptom control. Corticosteroids play a role, although the use of intermittent systemic corticosteroids may lead to an exacerbation of cutaneous disease. The evidence showing that DMARDs reduce joint destruction and disability is weaker in psoriatic arthritis than rheumatoid arthritis. However, they should be offered to patients who fail to respond adequately to NSAIDs or who are developing erosive disease. Most rheumatologists use methotrexate as the first-choice agent, and this drug will also have a beneficial effect on the skin. Leflunomide, sulfasalazine, and ciclosporin are alternatives.

TNF-alpha antagonists have been shown to be effective in the management of psoriatic arthritis. Infliximab, etanercept, adalimumab, and golimumab have all been approved by NICE for use where a patient has ongoing active disease with three or more tender and swollen joints and where treatment with at least two classical DMARDs has failed. Infliximab should be reserved for patients who are intolerant of the subcutaneous drugs or who would have major difficulties in administering them. Rituximab is not used in the management of psoriatic arthritis. Ustekinumab, used for the management of cutaneous psoriasis, also has proven benefit for the associated arthritis.

Spondyloarthritis

Ankylosing spondylitis

Ankylosing spondylitis describes an inflammatory arthritis that affects the sacroiliac joints and spine. Approximately 30% of patients will also develop a peripheral large joint oligoarthritis.

The association between specific subtypes of the class I allele HLA-B27 and ankylosing spondylitis is well known; within Caucasian populations, 92% of patients, compared with 8% of the general population, express an HLA-B27 gene. Studies suggest that other genes are also associated with disease development. At present, the mechanism by which HLA-B27 might predispose to ankylosing spondylitis remains unclear, and the predilection of the disease for the axial skeleton is not understood. The spectrum of disease severity and progression is very wide; the factors that influence this are largely unknown, although females tend to have more restricted disease than males.

Clinical features

Ankylosing spondylitis is more common in men than women, with a peak age of onset between the ages of 20 and 35 years. Patients present with lower back pain, with a prominent history of early morning stiffness. As the disease progresses, spinal pain may become a feature, with initial discomfort often occurring at the thoracolumbar junction. Over time, patients may develop loss of the lumbar lordosis and a stooped posture (sometimes referred to as a question mark posture). When examining a patient with suspected spondyloarthritis, each region of the spine and sacroiliac joints should be examined for pain and restriction of movement. The main clinical tests used to assess the axial skeleton in this condition are occiput-to-wall distances, chest wall expansion, Schoeber's test, and Patrick's test (see Table 16.7).

Pain and swelling of peripheral joints, particularly the hips and knees, may occur in an asymmetrical manner, and the arthritis may sometimes be destructive. Enthesitis is common and most characteristically involves the insertion of the Achilles tendon. Extra-articular manifestations of ankylosing spondylitis include anterior uveitis, apical pulmonary fibrosis, aortitis, aortic regurgitation, and cardiac conduction defects. Atlantoaxial subluxation and cauda equina syndrome can also occur. The inflammatory state predisposes to cardiovascular disease, osteoporosis, amyloidosis, and to anaemia of chronic disease.

Investigation

Radiographs of the sacroiliac joints should be requested and examined for irregularities, sclerosis, or fusion of the sacroiliac joints; changes can be graded from 1 to 4 (available in Dale K, 'Radiographic gradings of sacroiliitis in Bechterew's syndrome and allied disorders', *Scandinavian Journal of Rheumatology*, Suppl, 1979, 32, pp. 92–7).

Importantly, longitudinal studies have suggested that it takes a mean of 7 years for the inflammatory process to result in sacroiliac joint damage detectable on plain radiographs. During this time, abnormalities within the sacroiliac joints may be detected, using either a radionuclide bone scan or by MRI imaging, preferably performed with gadolinium enhancement.

In later disease, radiographs of the spine may demonstrate squaring of the vertebrae, enthesitis, and then erosion of vertebral borders (Romanus lesion), syndesmophyte

Table 16.7 Examination of the axial skeleton

Tests of cervical spine movement
Occiput-to-wall distance: horizontal distance between occiput and wall when patient stands, with heels and buttocks against wall, and attempts to place occiput to wall. This should normally be zero.
Tragus-to-wall distance: horizontal distance between right tragus (the small pointed eminence of the external ear) and wall when patient stands with heels and buttocks against wall without rotation. More useful for comparative measurements.

Test of thoracic spine movement
Chest expansion: normal thoracic spine movement is indicated by chest expansion of 5 cm or more between full expiration and inspiration measured at the fourth intercostal space.

Tests of lumbar spine movement
Schoeber's test: the L5 lumbar vertebra is identified by a horizontal line drawn through the dimples of Venus. The examiner measures 5 cm below and 10 cm above this line. An increase in this distance by 5 cm or more when the patient bends forward to touch their toes is considered normal.
Lumbar lateral flexion: distance travelled down the outer leg by the middle finger as the patient laterally flexes their spine, with both feet on the floor, knees extended, and without rotation. The mean of the right and left side measurements is taken and should be 10 cm or greater.
Finger-to-floor distance: distance between tip of middle finger and the floor, following maximal lumbar forward flexion with knees extended.

Tests of sacroiliac joint tenderness
Pelvic compression: compression of the pelvis, with the patient lying on one side, will elicit sacroiliac joint pain when this joint is inflamed.
Patrick's test: the knee is flexed and the heel placed on the opposite knee to achieve a position of flexion, external rotation, and abduction. Downward pressure on the flexed knee will cause pain in the contralateral sacroiliac joint if it is inflamed.

formation, and calcification of spinal ligaments to produce spinal fusion (bamboo spine).

Blood tests are rarely helpful, and the ESR and CRP may not be raised despite active disease.

Plain CXR should be carried out in patients with signs of fibrosis and ECG and ECHO requested in patients with bradycardia or murmurs.

The diagnosis of ankylosing spondylitis depends on fulfilment of the modified New York criteria (1984), and this involves demonstration of at least grade 2 sacroiliitis (see Table 16.8). Patients who do not fulfil New York criteria for the diagnosis of ankylosing spondylitis may fulfil the newer Assessment of Spondyloarthritis International Society (ASAS) 2009 criteria for diagnosis of an 'axial spondyloarthritis', in which MRI findings and HLA-B27 status are considered.

Several scoring systems have been developed to assess physical function and structural damage in patients with ankylosing spondylitis. The most commonly used is the Bath Ankylosing Spondylitis Disease Activity Index (BASDAI). This is a composite index that considers patients' responses to six questions relating to fatigue, axial pain, peripheral pain, enthesopathy, and stiffness, and a score of 4/10 or greater is considered to signify active disease.

Table 16.8 Modified New York diagnostic criteria for ankylosing spondylitis

Radiological criteria

1. Sacroiliitis: At least grade 2 bilaterally or grade 3 or 4 unilaterally

Clinical criteria

1. Low back pain and stiffness for more than 3 months that improves with exercise but is not relieved by rest
2. Limitation of motion of the lumbar spine
3. Limitation of chest expansion relative to normal correlated for age and sex

A diagnosis of ankylosing spondylitis requires the radiological and at least one clinical criterion to be satisfied.

Reproduced with permission from van der Linden S et al., 'Evaluation of diagnostic criteria for ankylosing spondylitis. A proposal for modification of the New York criteria', *Arthritis & Rheumatism*, 27, pp. 361–368, published by Wiley © 1984 American College of Rheumatology.

Management

NSAIDs and physiotherapy are essential for pain control and maintenance of mobility. Sulfasalazine may be effective in the management of an associated peripheral arthritis, and, as an alternative, some physicians may use methotrexate or leflunomide in this context. None of these DMARDs has a role in management of the axial disease. Likewise, corticosteroids do not have a role in the management of axial disease. NICE have approved the use of adalimumab and etanercept in ankylosing spondylitis in patients with evidence of ongoing disease activity with a BASDAI of ≥4 despite sequential trials of treatment with two different NSAIDs.

Miscellaneous spinal conditions

Several disorders can be confused with ankylosing spondylitis. These include osteitis condensans ilii, a benign disorder of multiparous women characterized by a triangular area of dense sclerotic bone on the iliac side of the sacroiliac joints.

Diffuse idiopathic skeletal hyperostosis (DISH or Forestier's disease) is a condition in which large bridging osteophytes extend between vertebral bodies. The sacroiliac joints are not involved. It usually occurs in males over the age of 50 years.

Patients with reactive arthritis, psoriatic and enteropathic arthritides may develop axial skeletal involvement with sacroiliitis but rarely develop significant spinal disease.

Connective tissue disease

Connective tissue diseases comprise multisystem inflammatory disorders. Whilst some features, such as arthralgias and Raynaud's phenomenon are common to many of these disorders, others are more disease-specific. These features, together with the profile of autoantibodies, enable classification to the major disease types described. It is important to remember that each diagnostic label covers a broad spectrum of disease severity. Some patients have features that are suggestive of a connective tissue disease but do not fulfil diagnostic criteria for any specific condition, and the term 'undifferentiated connective tissue disease' is sometimes used in this context.

Systemic lupus erythematosus

Systemic lupus erythematosus (SLE) is a chronic, multisystem, inflammatory connective tissue disorder of unknown aetiology. The age of onset is usually between 15 and 45 years; it is more common in females and in people of black African descent. Its pathogenesis is not well understood. There may be abnormalities of apoptosis, with the subsequent development of autoantibodies directed particularly against nuclear antigens and the formation of immune complexes.

Clinical features
Most patients have constitutional symptoms; fatigue is particularly common, but low-grade fevers and weight loss are also often present. Arthralgias affect the vast majority of patients, although joint swelling is rare. A malar or 'butterfly' rash that extends across the nasal bridge occurs in over 50% of patients, and more general cutaneous photosensitivity is also common. Diffuse hair fall, recurrent oral ulcers, lymphadenopathy, and Raynaud's phenomenon are often present. There may be involvement of the heart (pericarditis, myocarditis, or sterile endocarditis) and lung pleura (pleurisy and pleural effusions). Abdominal pain with vomiting and diarrhoea may suggest involvement of the gastrointestinal tract, and an autoimmune hepatitis may occur. Renal involvement, leading to the development of a nephritic or nephrotic syndrome, is a serious manifestation of disease. Neurological involvement may present in a variety of ways, with headaches, seizures, psychoses, or cranial and peripheral neuropathies.

The diagnosis of SLE is predominantly made on clinical grounds but is supported by the presence of antibodies specific for nuclear antigens. The Systemic Lupus International Collaborating Clinics (SLICC) have revised the ACR classification criteria for SLE (see Table 16.9). A patient must satisfy at least four criteria, including at least one clinical and one immunological criterion, or must have biopsy-proven lupus nephritis in the presence of antinuclear antibodies or anti-dsDNA antibodies.

Investigations
Investigations are to confirm the diagnosis, assess disease activity, and identify end-organ involvement or damage.

The SLICC classification criteria highlight the importance of testing for antinuclear antibody (ANA), anti-dsDNA, and anti-Sm antibodies. ANA have a high sensitivity for SLE, and their absence should raise concerns about the accuracy of this diagnosis and prompt investigation for other conditions. Lymphoma, chronic infections, or fibromyalgia are important differentials to consider. ANA have relatively low specificity for SLE, particularly where the titre is low. They may

Table 16.9 Outline of SLICC 2012 classification criteria for SLE

Clinical criteria	Immunologic criteria
1. Acute cutaneous lupus	1. ANA
2. Chronic cutaneous lupus	2. dsDNA
3. Oral or nasal ulcers	3. Anti-Sm
4. Non-scarring alopecia	4. Antiphospholipid Ab
5. Arthritis	5. Low complement (C3, C4)
6. Serositis	6. Direct Coomb's test (in absence of haemolytic anaemia)
7. Renal disease	
8. Neurologic disease	
9. Haemolytic anaemia	
10. Leucopenia	
11. Thrombocytopenia	

Reproduced with permission from M Petri *et al.*, 'Derivation and validation of the Systemic Lupus International Collaborating Clinics classification criteria for systemic lupus erythematosus', *Arthritis & Rheumatism*, 64, 8, pp. 2677–2686, published by Wiley, © 2012 by the American College of Rheumatology.

be found in a proportion of the normal population and are associated with other autoimmune diseases; the pattern of staining may be helpful in this respect (see Table 16.10).

Anti-dsDNA and anti-Sm antibodies have high specificity for the diagnosis of SLE. Some patients may have antibodies to other extractable nuclear antigens, including Ro, La, and RNP.

Disease activity is usually reflected in a high ESR and low complement (C). C4 tends to fall in mild/moderate disease whilst C3 will be low in more active disease. The level of anti-dsDNA binding can reflect disease activity in some patients. The CRP is less sensitive to SLE activity and is usually normal, although it may be elevated if the patient has synovitis or serositis. In general, an elevated CRP in SLE should signal the possibility of concomitant infection.

Blood tests, including FBC, U&E, and LFTs as well as urine dipstix, are essential preliminary tests to screen for the presence of haematological, renal, or hepatic manifestations of disease. Anaemia is common and may be multifactorial, but anaemia of chronic disease or haemolytic anaemia is well recognized. Further investigation of the latter should include a blood film, urinalysis, plasma bilirubin, Coomb's test, and reticulocyte count. Macrophage activation syndrome is a rare cause of anaemia in SLE and other connective tissue diseases. Leucopenia is also common but is rarely clinically important unless associated with drug tox-

Table 16.10 ANA staining patterns and their associations with connective tissue diseases

Pattern of ANA staining	Associated connective tissue disease
Diffuse	SLE
Nucleolar	Diffuse systemic sclerosis
Speckled	SLE, mixed connective tissue disease, Sjögren's syndrome
Centromere	Limited cutaneous systemic sclerosis

icity. A moderate thrombocytopenia may be seen, particularly where there is an associated antiphospholipid syndrome.

A positive urine dipstix for blood or protein suggests lupus nephritis. The urine should be microscoped to look for cellular casts, plasma albumin and protein excretion quantified. Request a renal ultrasound and make a referral to a nephrologist with a view to a renal biopsy. The association between nephrotic syndrome and high risk of vascular thrombosis should be borne in mind; abdominal pain in a patient with a nephrotic syndrome may reflect renal vein thrombosis and should be investigated with Doppler ultrasound.

Chest pain and breathlessness may reflect cardiac, pulmonary, or pleural disease. The possibility of pulmonary embolus should be considered, especially with an associated antiphospholipid syndrome. Appropriate investigations may include plain CXR, ECG, oximetry, and arterial blood gases. An ECHO should be carried out if pericardial disease is suspected, and a CT pulmonary angiogram should be performed if a PE is suspected.

Patients with muscle aches may have underlying myositis as part of SLE or an overlap syndrome. The CK should be measured, and, if raised, further investigations would include an EMG, an MRI to identify involved muscles, and a biopsy of the involved musculature.

Patients with neuropsychiatric symptoms should have an MRI of the brain to look for cerebral vasculitis. It may be hard to distinguish between this and atherosclerotic disease. An MRI may also show the rare reversible posterior leukoencephalopathy syndrome (RPLS), characterized by headaches, hypertension, visual loss, renal impairment, and fits. The importance of this diagnosis lies in the fact that it should not be treated with immunosuppressive medication, and management should focus on control of hypertension and seizures.

Management
SLE is a chronic disease, and patients will face many years of treatment. It is very important to balance the benefits and the side effects of treatment carefully.

The majority of patients should receive hydroxychloroquine which has been shown to reduce organ damage and mortality.

Patients with very mild disease may require no other specific treatment, although they should be advised to avoid sun exposure or use sunblock due to photosensitivity. Arthralgias may respond to occasional use of analgesics and NSAIDs. Mepacrine has been used to manage discoid lupus where hydroxychloroquine is ineffective. Topical corticosteroids may be helpful in the management of cutaneous disease.

Glucocorticoids have been a cornerstone of management but should always be used at the lowest possible dose.

Azathioprine is usually an effective steroid-sparing agent. All patients should have their thiopurine methyltransferase (TPMT) levels checked before starting azathioprine. If levels are within the normal range, then doses of up to 2.5 mg/kg are usually tolerated. If levels are consistent with heterozygous TPMT status, then half the normal dose of azathioprine may be used. Where TPMT levels are very low, azathioprine should be avoided. The FBC and LFTs must be monitored regularly; guidelines on an appropriate monitoring regime are provided by the British Society of Rheumatology (BSR). Low-dose weekly methotrexate or mycophenolate mofetil have been used as alternatives to azathioprine.

Table 16.11 Therapy for lupus nephritis

Class	Therapy
Minimal change	No immunosuppressive therapy
Mesangial	Prednisolone if proteinuria >1 g/day
Focal and diffuse proliferative nephritis	Prednisolone + Mycophenolate or low-dose intravenous cyclophosphamide. Azathioprine may be used for milder cases. Higher doses of cyclophosphamide may be required for severe cases. Rituximab may be considered, in addition to Mycophenolate, and may have a steroid-sparing role
Membranous	Prednisolone ± Mycophenolate

Management of renal disease will depend on the class of nephritis found on biopsy (see Table 16.11). Use of IV corticosteroids and cyclophosphamide may be warranted; the latter is usually given as intermittent IV pulses, rather than daily oral doses. More recently, Mycophenolate mofetil has shown encouraging results for the treatment of proliferative lupus nephritis. While case series have demonstrated rituximab to be an effective treatment, this has not been borne out in randomized trials, and the role of rituximab in lupus nephritis remains unclear. The use of both agents is associated with fewer side effects than conventional corticosteroid plus cyclophosphamide regimens.

Nephrotic patients with a significantly low albumin are at increased risk of vascular thrombosis, and prophylactic anticoagulants may be indicated.

Evidence relating to the efficacy of treatment of CNS lupus is limited. However, the European League Against Rheumatism guidelines 2012 reported benefit from the addition of cyclophosphamide to corticosteroids for patients with severe neuropsychiatric manifestations related to inflammation.

Pregnancy in individuals with SLE should be managed by a specialized obstetric unit. It is important to control SLE activity prior to, and during. Prednisolone, azathioprine, and hydroxychloroquine may be used. Cyclophosphamide, mycophenolate, and methotrexate must be avoided. Anti-Ro and anti-La antibodies may cross the placenta and may sometimes cause the transient condition of neonatal lupus. These antibodies can cross-react with fetal cardiac conduction tissue, resulting in cardiac conduction defects which may be permanent. Pregnant women with these antibodies should be monitored by a specialist unit with facilities for fetal cardiac ultrasound.

Antiphospholipid syndrome

Antiphospholipid syndrome is a condition characterized by vascular thrombosis or pregnancy morbidity, in association with the presence of antiphospholipid antibodies (see Table 16.12). It may occur in isolation or in association with another autoimmune condition.

Clinical features
Patients may present with thrombotic events that affect the arterial or, more frequently, the venous circulation. Pregnancy losses may occur in the first trimester, but more commonly in the second trimester. Given the frequency of early miscarriage in the general population, the specificity of

Table 16.12 Sydney criteria for diagnosis of antiphospholipid syndrome (2006)

Clinical criteria

1. Vascular thrombosis; may affect arteries, veins, or small vessels.
2. Pregnancy morbidity; one or more spontaneous abortions >10 weeks' gestation or three or more spontaneous abortions <10 weeks' gestation or one or more premature births <34 weeks due to eclampsia or severe placental insufficiency.

Laboratory criteria

1. Medium to high levels of IgG or IgM anti-cardiolipin antibodies.
2. Medium to high levels of IgG or IgM anti-beta-2-glycoprotein antibodies.
3. Presence of lupus anticoagulant.

Laboratory features must be confirmed on two occasions at least 12 weeks apart.

One clinical and one laboratory criteria are required to make the diagnosis.

Reproduced with permission from Miyakis S et al., 'International consensus statement on an update of the classification criteria for definite antiphospholipid syndrome (APS)', *Journal of Thrombosis and Haemostasis*, 4, pp. 295–306, © 2006, John Wiley and Sons and International Society on Thrombosis and Haemostasis.

this event is low. Antiphospholipid syndrome may also result in premature births associated with pre-eclampsia and placental insufficiency. Features of antiphospholipid syndrome not included in the formal diagnostic criteria, but which are relevant, include cardiac valve disease, livedo reticularis, nephropathy, headache, migraine, and neurological disease relating to microangiopathy. These features can be seen in the context of other connective tissue diseases and would normally prompt further investigation, even in the absence of a distinct thrombotic event.

Investigation
Three types of antibodies may be found in an antiphospholipid syndrome, and tests for all three should be performed in each patient. Anti-cardiolipin and anti-beta-2-glycoprotein antibodies may be tested for directly. The concept of a lupus anticoagulant is more complex. Reactivity of a lupus anticoagulant is targeted at plasma coagulation molecules; paradoxically, *in vitro*, this acts as an inhibitor of some assays, including the APTT, KCCT, or dRVVT so that clotting times appear prolonged. This abnormality is not corrected by the addition of normal plasma. Provided no specific clotting factor inhibitors are present, then the test confirms the presence of a lupus anticoagulant. Whilst the presence of each type of antibody within the diagnostic criteria does correlate with an increased risk of thrombosis, the presence of a lupus anticoagulant appears to be associated with the highest risk. Antiphospholipid antibodies are commonly found in patients with SLE, Sjögren's syndrome, and idiopathic thrombocytopenic purpura (ITP) and may be found in patients with HIV and hepatitis C. They may be found in patients taking chlorpromazine, phenytoin, hydralazine, and a number of other medications. They are also present in approximately 5–10% of the normal population. Notably, only a proportion of individuals with the relevant antibodies will experience a thrombotic episode and have a true antiphospholipid syndrome.

Other investigations indicated include FBC, as the antiphospholipid syndrome is often associated with a modest thrombocytopenia (50,000–100,000/microlitre), Imaging studies should be used to confirm a thrombotic event. ECHO will detect valvular abnormalities. Investigation of renal function will be appropriate if microangiopathic disease affecting the kidneys is suspected.

Management
The effectiveness of primary prevention of thrombosis in individuals with a positive antiphospholipid antibody test is unproven. Many clinicians will, however, prescribe low-dose aspirin for patients with SLE. Patients should be advised to reduce other risk factors for thrombosis, such as smoking and use of the oral contraceptive pill. Hypertension and hyperlipidaemia should be managed actively.

Approximately 50% of patients with antiphospholipid antibodies and a previous thrombotic event will go on to have further thrombotic events. Lifelong anticoagulation with warfarin is recommended for these individuals. The target INR should be 2–3 for patients with a previous single venous thrombosis, and 3–4 for patients with recurrent venous thrombosis or a previous arterial thrombosis.

Pregnant women with antiphospholipid antibodies and a history of thrombosis or previous miscarriage should receive low molecular weight heparin, in addition to low-dose aspirin, and be counselled about the risks of heparin-induced thrombocytopenia and osteoporosis.

Sjögren's syndrome

Sjögrens's syndrome is a chronic inflammatory condition characterized by lymphocytic infiltration of the exocrine glands.

Clinical features
Sjögren's syndrome usually presents between the age of 40 and 60 years and affects women much more often than men. It can be a primary disease or occur in association with other inflammatory conditions, such as rheumatoid arthritis or SLE.

Reduced tear secretion may result in damage to the corneal and conjunctival epithelium (keratoconjunctivitis sicca). Patients generally experience a sensation of grittiness and may notice redness of the eyes and sun sensitivity. Keratoconjunctivitis sicca is not diagnostic of Sjögren's syndrome.

Reduced salivary secretion will lead to dryness of the mouth (xerostomia), with difficulty in swallowing, speaking without breaks, and increased dental caries. Enlargement of the salivary glands may occur, either intermittently or persistently.

In addition, patients often experience very prominent fatigue and widespread arthralgias. The joint involvement is non-erosive. Other features include low-grade fevers, glandular enlargement, and dyspareunia. Involvement of the respiratory tract, with dryness of the trachea or lymphocytic infiltration of the lung interstitium, is common but rarely clinically significant. Lymphocytic infiltration of the gastrointestinal tract can also occur, resulting in abdominal pain and, occasionally, in malabsorption. Involvement of the liver is very well described. Furthermore, Sjögren's syndrome is often found in association with primary biliary cirrhosis. Lymphocytic infiltration of the kidneys may cause renal tubular acidosis. More rarely, membranoproliferative nephritis may occur, usually in association with the presence of cryoglobulins. A peripheral vasculitis, presenting as purpura, is seen in a small proportion of patients. A wide spectrum of CNS manifestations has been described.

Patients with primary Sjögren's syndrome are at increased risk of lymphoma, with some studies suggesting 4% of patients will develop a lymphoma in their lifetime. These are generally B cell in origin and should be suspected in all patients with lymphadenopathy, major organ enlargement, and persistent salivary gland enlargement.

Investigation
The American-European Consensus criteria may be used to facilitate the diagnosis of Sjögren's (see Table 16.13).

In general, patients will tend to satisfy criteria 1, 2, 3, and 6, and tests to demonstrate abnormal salivary flow or a lip biopsy are rarely performed. Newer classification criteria are being developed, requiring patients to be positive for two of three objective tests, including serology, ocular staining, and salivary gland biopsy. It is not always necessary to make a definitive diagnosis; treatment is symptomatic, in general, and an expectant approach can often be taken.

Schirmer's test is used to demonstrate dryness of the eyes. This involves measuring the wetness of a strip of filter paper placed under the lower eyelid. A measurement of less than 5 mm after 5 min indicates inadequate lacrimation. The total Ig levels are generally high, with an associated rise in the ESR. CRP is not usually raised. The ANA is often positive, with specificity for the Ro and La antigens. The RhF is positive in over 50% cases. The renal function, including bicarbonate, should be checked to investigate the possibility of development of renal tubular acidosis. Imaging studies are not helpful in making the diagnosis. CT or MR imaging may help if there is concern about the possible development of a lymphoma.

Management
Treatment is predominantly symptomatic. Artificial tears, such as hypromellose eye drops, should be applied frequently. More viscous preparations, such as those containing soft paraffin, may be beneficial if applied at night. Symptoms from a dry mouth are often best treated with frequent sips of water. Artifical saliva sprays or lozenges may provide temporary symptomatic relief. Sugar-free chewing gum or oral pilocarpine may increase saliva secretion in individuals with residual salivary gland function. Hydroxychloroquine may be helpful if there is prominent inflammatory disease and particularly where patients experience troublesome arthralgias. Prednisolone is rarely indicated but may be used in more severe disease.

Scleroderma
Scleroderma or systemic sclerosis describes a condition characterized by chronic inflammation, fibrosis, and vascular damage, with consequent ischaemia. It affects women more commonly than men. The disease is classified into four subtypes, depending on the extent of skin and major organ

Table 16.13 Revised international classification criteria for Sjögren's syndrome

I. Ocular symptoms: a positive response to at least one of the following questions:

    1. Have you had daily, persistent, troublesome dry eyes for more than 3 months?

    2. Do you have a recurrent sensation of sand or gravel in the eyes?

    3. Do you use tear substitutes more than 3 times a day?

II. Oral symptoms: a positive response to at least one of the following questions:

    1. Have you had a daily feeling of dry mouth for more than 3 months?

    2. Have you had recurrently or persistently swollen salivary glands as an adult?

    3. Do you frequently drink liquids to aid in swallowing dry food?

III. Ocular signs—that is, objective evidence of ocular involvement defined as a positive result for at least one of the following two tests:

    1. Schirmer's I test, performed without anaesthesia ($\leq$5 mm in 5 minutes)

    2. Rose bengal score or other ocular dye score ($\geq$4 according to van Bijsterveld's scoring system)

IV. Histopathology: In minor salivary glands (obtained through normal-appearing mucosa) focal lymphocytic sialoadenitis, evaluated by an expert histopathologist, with a focus score $\geq$1, defined as a number of lymphocytic foci which are adjacent to normal-appearing mucous acini and contain more than 50 lymphocytes per 4 mm^2 of glandular tissue

V. Salivary gland involvement: objective evidence of salivary gland involvement defined by a positive result for at least one of the following diagnostic tests:

    1. Unstimulated whole salivary flow ($\leq$1.5 ml in 15 minutes)

    2. Parotid sialography showing the presence of diffuse sialectasias (punctate, cavitary or destructive pattern), without evidence of obstruction in the major ducts

    3. Salivary scintigraphy showing delayed uptake, reduced concentration and/or delayed excretion of tracer

VI. Autoantibodies: presence in the serum of the following autoantibodies:

    1. Antibodies to Ro(SSA) or La(SSB) antigens, or both

Table 16.14 Subtypes of systemic sclerosis

Disease subtype	Major clinical features	Autoantibody
Pre-scleroderma	Raynaud's phenomenon with nail fold capillary changes	Anti-SCL70 Anti-centromere
Limited cutaneous scleroderma	Raynaud's phenomenon Skin involvement limited to hands and forearms, feet, and face Calcification, telangiectasia, upper GI tract involvement, isolated pulmonary hypertension	Anti-centromere
Diffuse cutaneous scleroderma	Raynaud's phenomenon Skin involvement that extends beyond forearms Interstitial lung disease, renal disease, diffuse GI tract involvement, myocardial disease, myositis, arthritis	Anti-SCL70
Scleroderma sine scleroderma	No skin involvement Typical pulmonary, GI tract, cardiac, or renal disease	Anti-SCL70 Anti-centromere

involvement (see Table 16.14). The clinical presentation correlates with the type of autoantibody found.

Clinical features

The vast majority of patients experience significant Raynaud's phenomenon as an early manifestation. Skin involvement may follow, initially with a feeling of 'puffiness' and subsequently a feeling of 'tightness' with the development of the classically 'leathery' skin texture. The extent of skin involvement distinguishes between the limited cutaneous and diffuse cutaneous forms of disease. The former was often previously referred to as CREST as an acronym for the major features of calcinosis, Raynaud's phenomenon, oesophageal involvement, sclerodactyly, and telangiectasia. The acronym does not, however, include one important manifestation of the disease; the isolated pulmonary hypertension that affects 10–15% of patients. Whilst patients with the diffuse form of the disease may also have many of these manifestations, they are at greater risk of developing myositis, arthritis, interstitial lung disease, more diffuse GI disease with dysmotility and bacterial overgrowth, and renal disease. The last is the most severe manifestation of systemic sclerosis and usually presents as a hypertensive renal crisis, with accelerated hypertension, oliguria, and the development of a microangiopathic haemolytic anaemia.

Investigations

Patients usually have a positive ANA, and the staining pattern may reveal an anti-centromere or anti-topoisomerase (SCL70) pattern. Recent studies show a proportion of patients, particularly those with the diffuse cutaneous form of disease, may have an anti-RNA polymerase antibody, rather than an anti-topoisomerase antibody, although testing for this is not yet routinely available.

Approximately 80% of patients with limited cutaneous disease will have an anti-centromere antibody whilst just over 50% of those with diffuse cutaneous disease will have anti-SCL70 or RNA polymerase reactivity. However, a proportion of patients are seronegative, and the diagnosis has to be made on clinical grounds. Inflammatory markers are not usually raised, and complement studies are normal. Further investigation will depend on the clinical presentation. CXR, pulmonary function tests, and a high-resolution CT scan may be required to investigate interstitial pulmonary disease. An ECG and echocardiogram, with monitoring of pulmonary artery pressures, will be useful in monitoring cardiac disease and pulmonary hypertension.

Cardiac catheterization should be considered in patients requiring further investigation for possible pulmonary hypertension. Barium or endoscopic studies will be required for investigation of GI disease. The presence of hypertension should lead to investigation for renal disease

Management

The management of systemic sclerosis is controversial. Treatments aimed at the immune response, the vasculature, and the fibrotic process have all been considered. There is no single management approach for this condition, and each manifestation of disease needs to be treated on merit.

Raynaud's phenomenon is a prominent symptom and may be severe, with consequent digital ulceration and infection. Simple advice about maintaining reasonable ambient temperature levels at home and the use of gloves and hand-warmers should be given. Patients should be advised to use copious amounts of hand cream to minimize cracking of dry, poorly perfused skin. Beta-blockers should be discontinued. Nifedipine may relieve the symptoms of Raynaud's phenomenon but is frequently associated with side effects. Losartan is a better tolerated alternative, and diltiazem, fluoxetine, and pentoxifylline have all been used. Where the condition is severe, then a course of 5 days of intravenous iloprost may provide some benefit that appears to last for a few weeks/months. Digital infection should be treated promptly with antibiotics and the presence of osteomyelitis considered where digital ulceration is deep or chronic.

Histopathological studies have confirmed inflammatory infiltrates during the early, oedematous phase of skin disease. Both corticosteroids and other immunosuppressive agents, such as mycophenolate, may have a role in the management of this phase. High doses of corticosteroid have been associated with an increased risk of hypertensive renal crisis and are to be avoided, if possible, particularly in those with anti-SCL70 or anti-RNA polymerase antibodies. Doses should be kept to <10–20 mg prednisolone daily.

Fibrosis of the GI tract leads to loss of peristalsis, gut dilation, and bacterial overgrowth, with consequent malabsorption. Upper GI symptoms often respond to a proton pump inhibitor (PPI). Prokinetic agents, such as metoclopramide, may be helpful. Diarrhoea is usually secondary to bacterial overgrowth and is treated with antibiotics. Dietary supplements should be given to patients with malabsorption. Parenteral nutrition may be required in very resistant cases.

Like other connective tissue diseases, the pattern of interstitial lung disease seen in systemic sclerosis is characteristically that of a non-specific interstitial pneumonitis (NSIP). Whilst corticosteroids are generally used to manage NSIP in the context of a connective tissue disease, they need to be used carefully in this patient group because of the risk of precipitating a renal crisis. Where HRCT suggests evidence of active alveolitis with a ground glass appearance, cyclophosphamide should be considered.

Pulmonary hypertension can arise due to primary pulmonary vascular disease or secondary to interstitial lung disease. Bosentan, sildenafil, epoprostenol, as well as anticoagulation have all been used to treat pulmonary hypertension in the context of systemic sclerosis. Patients with this complication should be managed by a specialist centre.

Scleroderma renal crisis is a medical emergency and reflects microangiopathy of renal vessels, resulting in malignant hypertension. Patients should be managed in a high dependency or intensive care environment. ACE inhibitors and IV epoprostenol (INN) infusions should be given, aiming for a gradual lowering of blood pressure. Prazosin and doxazosin can also be used. If seizures or severe left ventricular dysfunction complicate the condition, then more rapid reduction in blood pressure may be required. Plasma exchange should be considered in the presence of microangiopathy.

Idiopathic inflammatory myopathies

The idiopathic inflammatory myopathies include dermatomyositis, polymyositis, and inclusion body myositis. The last presents as an asymmetric distal weakness, usually in individuals older than 50 years. It has characteristic biopsy findings, and there is no clearly effective treatment. Dermatomyositis and polymyositis share many features and are considered next. They usually affect adults, with peak incidence between the ages of 40 and 50 years old. Dermatomyositis may also affect children.

Clinical features

Both dermatomyositis and polymyositis present with a proximal, symmetrical, progressive weakness. Patients report difficulty with standing from sitting, with climbing stairs, and with raising their hands above their heads. Involvement of the pharyngeal muscles may cause dysphagia and aspiration. Involvement of respiratory muscles may also be a feature leading to respiratory failure. Dermatomyositis is associated with a heliotrope rash that classically affects the eyelids and forehead but also commonly involves the extensor aspects of the fingers and knees. Skin involvement without muscle disease has been reported (dermatomyositis sine myositis). Gottron's papules (red, often scaly, bumps overlying the knuckles of the fingers), mechanic's hands (roughening and cracking of the skin of the tips and sides of the fingers, resulting in irregular,

dirty-appearing lines that resemble those of a manual labourer), subcutaneous calcification, Raynaud's syndrome, and arthralgias may also occur. Some patients may have systemic features, including low-grade fevers, malaise, and weight loss. Very importantly, there is an association between inflammatory myositis and malignancy, particularly cancers of the gut, lung, and ovary. Myositis may present up to 2–3 years before or after the presentation with malignancy.

Investigation

The creatinine kinase is usually significantly elevated. However, the myositis can be patchy, and it is possible for the creatinine kinase to be within the normal range despite significant disease. Electromyography (EMG) studies will reveal myopathic potentials characterized by increased spontaneous activity, with fibrillations, complex repetitive discharges, sharp waves and early recruitment, and short-duration, low-amplitude polyphasic units on voluntary activation. MRI scanning will show abnormalities of signal intensity within involved muscles. The site of abnormality should be used to guide muscle biopsy. Histopathology in polymyositis typically demonstrates endomysial infiltration with CD8+ T cells and muscle fibre necrosis and regeneration. In dermatomyositis, infiltration is in the perivascular and perifascicular regions, typically with CD4+ T cells and B cells. Many patients will have a positive ANA, although the fine specificity of the autoantibodies is varied. Anti-synthetase antibodies, including anti-Jo-1, OJ, EJ, KS, PL-7, and PL-12, may be seen, as may anti-Mi-2 and anti-SRP antibodies. Anti-RNP antibodies are seen in mixed connective tissue disease, and anti-Ku is associated with an overlap syndrome with sclerodermatous features.

Investigations should be done to look for an underlying malignancy. Most physicians will undertake a CT scan of the chest, abdomen, and pelvis and investigate suggestive symptoms carefully. Malignancy may present some time after the myositis.

Management

Myositis usually responds to high-dose corticosteroid, and initial treatment is commonly with IV methylprednisolone, followed by oral prednisolone. It is very common for the disease to relapse as corticosteroids are withdrawn, and patients often require low-dose methotrexate or azathioprine to facilitate reduction of corticosteroid doses. Ciclosporin may be effective in interstitial lung disease in patients with myositis. Courses of IV immunoglobulin (IVIG), repeated at monthly intervals, may also be effective. More recent reports suggest benefit from mycophenolate, rituximab, TNF-alpha blockers, and tocilizumab in some patients.

Vasculitis

Vasculitis describes an inflammatory disorder of the blood vessels. Patients present both with systemic features, such as malaise, fevers, and arthralgias, and with more specific, localized features that depend on the specific blood vessels involved. The vasculitides have been classified, according to the size of the vessels involved, following the Chapel Hill Consensus Conference on the nomenclature of systemic vasculitis (see Table 16.15).

A subset of the small-vessel vasculitides are associated with the presence of antineutrophil cytoplasmic antibodies (ANCA) (see Table 16.16). The vast majority of patients with microscopic polyangiitis, over half of patients with eosinophilic granulomatosis with polyangiitis, and a small minority of patients with granulomatosis with polyangiitis will have a p-ANCA antibody. In contrast, a c-ANCA is found in the majority of patients with granulomatosis with

Table 16.15 Classification of vasculitis

Large vessel	Giant cell arteritis
	Takayasu's arteritis
Medium vessel	Polyarteritis nodosa
	Kawasaki disease
Small vessel ANCA-associated	Microscopic polyangiitis
	Granulomatosis with polyangiitis
	Eosinophilic granulomatosis with polyangiitis
Small vessel immune complex	Anti-glomerulobasement membrane disease
	Cryoglobulinaemic vasculitis
	IgA vasculitis
	Hypocomplementaemic urticarial vasculitis
Variable vessel vasculitis	Behçet's disease
	Cogan's syndrome
Single-organ vasculitis	Cutaneous leukocytoclastic vasculitis
	Cutaneous arteritis
	Primary CNS vasculitis
	Isolated aortitis
	Others
Vasculitis associated with systemic disease	Lupus vasculitis
	Rheumatoid vasculitis
	Sarcoid vasculitis
	Others
Vasculitis associated with probable aetiology	Hepatitis C virus-associated cryoglobulinaemic vasculitis
	Hepatitis B virus-associated vasculitis
	Syphilis-associated aortitis
	Drug-associated immune complex vasculitis
	Drug-associated ANCA-associated vasculitis
	Cancer-associated vasculitis
	Others

Data from Jennette JC, et al., 'Overview of the 2012 revised International Chapel Hill Consensus Conference nomenclature of vasculitides', *Clinical and Experimental Nephrology*, 2013, published by Springer Verlag.

Table 16.16 Classification of ANCA-associated vasculitis

p-ANCA	Microscopic polyangiitis
Perinuclear pattern of staining Specificity for myeloperoxidase (MPO)	Eosinophilic granulomatosis with polyangiitis
	Granulomatosis with polyangiitis
c-ANCA	Granulomatosis with polyangiitis
Cytoplasmic pattern of staining Specificity for serine proteinase 3 (PR3)	Eosinophilic granulomatosis with polyangiitis

Reproduced from *Annals of the Rheumatic Diseases*, R Watts et al., 'Development and validation or a consensus methodology for the classification of the ANCA-associated vasculitides and polyarteritis nodosa for epidemiological studies', 66, 2, pp. 222–227, Copyright 2007, with permission from BMJ Publishing Group Ltd.

polyangiitis and a minority of patients with microscopic polyangiitis.

Many patients with vasculitis will require treatment with high-dose corticosteroids and other immunosuppressive drugs over prolonged periods of time. Protocols for regular monitoring for drug toxicity must be in place. Bone protection may be required in those receiving corticosteroids. Infection prophylaxis may be appropriate in those receiving cyclophosphamide and mycophenolate. Individuals must also be advised about possible long-term risks of malignancy as well as the effects of drugs on fertility and fetal development.

Giant cell arteritis and polymyalgia rheumatica

These conditions are often considered to form part of the same disease spectrum and usually present in individuals over the age of 55 years. Giant cell arteritis is sometimes termed temporal or cranial arteritis. It is a granulomatous form of vasculitis that typically involves the superficial temporal, posterior ciliary, and ophthalmic arteries. However, other vessels, including the retinal, extracranial, vertebral, internal, and external carotid as well as the subclavian and brachial arteries or the aortic arch itself, may be involved. The pathological basis for polymyalgia rheumatica is less well understood. However, approximately 15% of patients with polymyalgia rheumatica develop giant cell arteritis, and a proportion of those without symptoms of giant cell arteritis have been shown to have characteristic histopathological changes when biopsies have been performed.

Clinical features
Patients with polymyalgia rheumatica usually present with limb girdle pain and weakness. The onset is often fairly acute, with symptoms developing over a few days. They report difficulty standing from sitting, climbing stairs, and lifting their arms. The symptoms are most prominent in the mornings. There may be associated fatigue, malaise, and low-grade fever. The limb girdle musculature is often tender, and examination confirms weakness of shoulder and hip movements. Some patients have swelling of their hands with pitting oedema.

Patients with giant cell arteritis may have some polymyalgic features. However, they usually also experience temporal headaches, with jaw claudication and scalp tenderness. Visual symptoms are important and include blurring, double vision, and irreversible visual loss. The temporal artery may be tender and visibly inflamed or may be pulseless. Visual field testing may reveal abnormalities; an inferior altitudinal defect due to anterior ischaemic optic neuropathy is most characteristic. Fundoscopy may show optic disc oedema. Inflammation of the aorta and its branches may also occur, leading to carotidynia, atypical chest pain, and vascular bruits.

Investigation
In patients with polymyalgia rheumatica or giant cell arteritis, both the ESR and CRP are usually, but not invariably, elevated. Patients may have a normochromic, normocytic anaemia and a slightly elevated platelet count. ANA and ANCA are usually negative.

There is no specific diagnostic test for PMR. Whilst imaging studies are often not required for diagnosis, USS or MRI of the shoulders and hips may show evidence of bursitis, synovitis, and tenosynovitis.

A temporal artery biopsy should be performed if giant cell arteritis is suspected. The characteristic lesions tend to be patchy ('skip lesions'), so a negative result does not exclude the condition. The biopsy may be informative, even if treatment with corticosteroids has been initiated, although it should be performed as promptly as possible, and is much less likely to be diagnostic after 2 weeks of treatment. If more widespread vasculitic changes are suspected, then a PET scan or PET-CT scan can be helpful in identifying areas of active arteritis.

Management
Patients who present acutely with polymyalgia rheumatica and without evidence of giant cell arteritis should generally be treated with oral prednisolone at a dose of 15 mg daily. They usually show a clear response to treatment within a few days. The dose of prednisolone may then be gradually tapered over the course of approximately 18 months. Where symptomatic relapse occurs as the dose of prednisolone is reduced, care must be taken to exclude other causes of pain and stiffness or elevated acute phase markers. If there is difficulty in withdrawing corticosteroids, then the addition of low-dose methotrexate or azathioprine may facilitate this. Polymyalgia rheumatica is usually a self-limiting disease, and there is no good evidence that modest-dose corticosteroids alter the overall outcome or decrease the likelihood of development of giant cell arteritis. As such, there is no absolute requirement to treat patients with prednisolone. If steroid side effects are a problem, palliation of symptoms with analgesics is occasionally a reasonable alternative approach.

In contrast, patients with suspected giant cell arteritis are a medical emergency and must be treated with high-dose corticosteroids (prednisolone 40–60 mg/day). Many physicians will give IV methylprednisolone if there is concern about visual symptoms or disc oedema to minimize the risk of permanent visual loss. Low-dose aspirin and a proton pump inhibitor should also be prescribed. Once symptoms are controlled and the ESR and CRP have fallen, the dose of prednisolone may be gradually tapered. Treatment is usually continued for a minimum of 2 years. Relapses of the condition should be managed with an increase in the dose of prednisolone. There may be a case for the introduction of low-dose methotrexate or azathioprine as a second agent to facilitate steroid withdrawal.

Takayasu's arteritis

This form of large-vessel vasculitis affects the aorta and its branches. It is very rare but usually presents in young women; it is more frequent in those of Asian descent. Two phases are described: an acute inflammatory phase, characterized by a granulomatous inflammatory reaction with the vessel walls, and a later sclerotic phase, with fibrosis of vessel intima and adventitia and scarring of the media. This pathological progression may be reflected in the clinical features, an initial illness characterized by constitutional features, followed by later features of claudication. In many patients, the two phases coexist.

Clinical features
Patients often have systemic features of fevers, malaise, and weight loss. They may present with symptoms of claudication, usually involving the jaw or upper limbs. Neurological features include TIAs and CVAs as well as headaches and visual loss. Patients may develop aortic regurgitation, secondary to involvement of the aortic root, and may also development ischaemic heart disease. Involvement of the pulmonary vasculature may lead to pulmonary hypertension, which is often asymptomatic. Renovascular disease may present as hypertension, and mesenteric artery involvement may lead to abdominal symptoms. Examination may reveal bruits over involved arteries, asymmetric pulses, and differences in blood pressure between the arms.

Investigation
Patients usually have an elevated ESR and CRP, a normochromic normocytic anaemia, and an elevated platelet count, consistent with a significant inflammatory illness. Classical angiography or MR angiography (MRA) has been the standard tool for diagnosis and demonstration of the extent of the arterial lesions. As part of MRA, fast spin echo sequences may be helpful in demonstrating vessel wall oedema, suggestive of active disease. PET scanning has been shown to facilitate early diagnosis and provide information about disease activity. Tissue biopsy is rarely possible or appropriate.

Management
The condition responds to immunosuppression; initial treatment is with corticosteroids. Low-dose methotrexate, azathioprine, or mycophenolate have been used as additional agents to help suppress disease activity as prednisolone is withdrawn. Cyclophosphamide may be considered in cases of severe or unresponsive disease. Response to treatment should be monitored, using the ESR and CRP. Sequential PET scanning may also be informative. Critical stenosis may be treated with angioplasty or bypass grafts, if necessary, although outcome is variable. Surgery may be indicated for aortic aneurysms or for significant aortic regurgitation. Where possible, active disease should be controlled prior to surgical intervention.

Polyarteritis nodosa

Polyarteritis nodosa was previously used as a term to describe a spectrum of vasculitic illnesses. Following the Chapel Hill Consensus Conference in 1994, it is used in a more specific way to describe a rare medium-vessel arteritis that characteristically results in microaneurysm formation and thrombosis, leading to bleeding and infarction. Polyarteritis nodosa may be associated with viral infection, particularly hepatitis B infection. It should be distinguished from microscopic polyangiitis, which affects smaller vessels and is more common.

Clinical features
Polyarteritis nodosa affects men more than women and usually presents in late middle age. Patients experience constitutional symptoms of fevers, malaise, weight loss, and arthralgias. The arteritis itself tends to involve vessels supplying skin, peripheral nerves, the gut, and the kidneys. The manifestations of disease, therefore, include skin nodules, ulceration or gangrene, mononeuritis multiplex, bowel infarction, renovascular hypertension, or renal infarction. The lungs and kidney glomeruli are rarely affected. A limited form of disease that just affects the skin has been described.

Investigation
Patients will have an elevated ESR and CRP, anaemia of chronic disease, and thrombocytosis, consistent with an inflammatory process. Approximately 10% of patients are hepatitis B surface antigen-positive. ANA and ANCA are usually negative. The diagnosis should be based on histopathology, where possible; biopsies may be taken from involved skin, nerves, or kidneys and will demonstrate a focal necrotizing arteritis. Where this is not possible, visceral angiography or MRA may be helpful and demonstrate the typical aneurysms and arterial wall irregularities. These appearances are most often seen in the kidneys, liver, and mesenteric arteries and are a feature of late and severe, rather than early, disease.

Management
Treatment is with high-dose oral prednisolone, tapered over the course of 12–18 months. Where the disease is severe with evidence of end-organ damage, then IV methylprednisolone may be given at the start of treatment, and cyclophosphamide may be used to induce remission. Maintenance therapy with azathioprine should be introduced, following cyclophosphamide withdrawal. Patients with coexisting hepatitis B infection should not receive cyclophosphamide and should taper doses of prednisolone as quickly as possible. They should also be treated with lamivudine or interferon alfa.

Granulomatosis with polyangiitis
Granulomatosis with polyangiitis (previously known as Wegener's granulomatosis) is a form of systemic vasculitis involving small vessels that classically affects the upper and lower respiratory tract and the kidneys.

Clinical features
This is a very rare condition that may present in a wide variety of ways. Involvement of the upper airways may result in nasal discharge or obstruction, oral or nasal ulceration, perforation of the nasal septum, destruction of the nasal cartilage leading to a saddle deformity of the nose, middle ear congestion with poor hearing, and subglottic stenosis with hoarseness or stridor. Lower airway involvement with granulomatous infiltrates or alveolar capillaritis may result in breathlessness and pulmonary haemorrhage. The development of a glomerulonephritis causes a nephritic or, more rarely, a nephrotic syndrome. Involvement of the skin, with palpable purpura, joints with arthralgias or arthritis, and nerves with a mononeuritis multiplex may also occur. A retro-orbital inflammatory mass may cause proptosis and diplopia. Patients usually also have constitutional symptoms which include low-grade fevers, weight loss, and malaise.

Investigation
As with other forms of vasculitis, patients will have elevated inflammatory markers, normochromic normocytic anaemia, and thrombocytosis. They are also likely to have a positive ANCA, most commonly a c-type ANCA, with specificity for proteinase 3. The titre of ANCA often fluctuates with disease activity, with levels rising prior to disease flares. Urinalysis should be performed to detect microscopic haematuria and proteinuria, and the latter should be quantified. Plasma urea, creatinine, and electrolytes should be evaluated. CXR, lung function tests, and, if necessary, a high-resolution CT scan should be done to investigate possible pulmonary involvement.

Whilst the clinical picture and positive ANCA may be highly suggestive of granulomatosis with polyangiitis, the diagnosis is best made on the histopathology. Tissue may be obtained from the upper respiratory tract or from the kidneys. Occasionally, it proves necessary to perform a lung biopsy, although this should be avoided, if possible. The samples will demonstrate a small-vessel vasculitis, typically with granulomata. The characteristic renal lesion is a focal segmental glomerulonephritis which is pauci-immune, with crescents in severe cases.

Management
The outcome from Wegener's granulomatosis is very poor without treatment. As with other forms of vasculitis, high-dose oral prednisolone is given and tapered when disease activity is controlled. Where disease is severe, with evidence of end-organ damage, then IV methylprednisolone may be given at the start of treatment, and cyclophosphamide is also given for 3–6 months. This is followed with azathioprine or low-dose weekly methotrexate. Rituximab is an alternative to cyclophosphamide and is usually favoured in relapsing patients. There may be a role for plasmapheresis, mycophenolate, or IVIG, although the evidence for these treatments is more limited. In cases of limited Wegener's granulomatosis, then treatment with oral steroids and methotrexate may suffice. The disease tends to relapse, and there is some evidence to suggest that daily treatment with co-trimoxazole can reduce relapse rates.

Microscopic polyangiitis
Microscopic polyangiitis (previously known as microscopic polyarteritis) is a form of small-vessel vasculitis associated with the presence of p-ANCA antibodies. The involvement of arterioles, capillaries, and venules distinguishes this condition from polyarteritis nodosa, and the absence of granulomata or upper respiratory tract involvement distinguishes it from granulomatosis with polyangiitis.

Clinical features
The disease usually affects individuals in late middle age. Constitutional features include malaise, fevers, arthralgias, myalgias, and weight loss. Approximately 50% of individuals will have evidence of a vasculitic-type skin rash. Many will present with evidence of pulmonary or renal involvement. A mononeuritis multiplex is a frequent feature. Cardiac, ocular, and gastrointestinal involvement may occur.

Investigation
Blood tests will usually show a normochromic normocytic anaemia, thrombocytosis, and elevated ESR and CRP. Renal function may be abnormal, and urinalysis may show evidence of proteinuria and haematuria. ANCA is positive in 80% of cases, with specificity being more often for myeloperoxidase (p-ANCA) than for proteinase 3 (c-ANCA). CXR and pulmonary function tests are used to identify pulmonary involvement. Diagnosis is best based on histopathology, with biopsies taken from the skin, kidney, or a nerve,

depending on involvement. The biopsy may show a leukocytoclastic vasculitis, with or without segmental fibrinoid necrosis of the media. The renal tissue will usually show a pauci-immune focal segmental necrotizing glomerulonephritis.

Management
There is a spectrum of disease severity in patients with microscopic polyangiitis, and treatment choice should reflect this. Initial treatment is usually with high-dose prednisolone (1 mg/kg/day), tapered after 1 month. In severe disease, treatment with cyclophosphamide or rituximab is also given. Where disease is less severe, low-dose oral methotrexate may be used as an alternative. Once disease control has been achieved, then cyclophosphamide, if used, should be replaced by azathioprine or low-dose methotrexate. Low-dose prednisolone at a dose of approximately 10 mg daily should be continued. Treatment may usually be withdrawn after 18–24 months. Relapses should be treated in a similar way to the original presentation.

Eosinophilic granulomatosis with polyangiitis
Eosinophilic granulomatosis with polyangiitis (previously known as Churg–Strauss syndrome) is a small-vessel vasculitis characterized by the presence of eosinophils.

Clinical features
The disease usually develops over the course of 3–10 years. The early features are of allergic rhinitis and asthma. This is followed by the development of eosinophilic infiltrates and then by evidence of vasculitis with granulomatous inflammation. In these later phases of disease, patients will also likely experience constitutional symptoms. The peripheral nerves, skin, GI tract, lungs, and heart are commonly involved. Mononeuritis multiplex is a particularly prominent feature, occurring in >75% of patients. Purpuric skin lesions may be present in up to 50% of patients. Abdominal pain with diarrhoea and GI bleeding may occur. Haemoptysis secondary to pulmonary disease is a recognized feature. Cardiac involvement with the development of ischaemic heart disease, myocarditis, pericarditis, and cardiac failure is well recognized and a very important cause of mortality in this condition. Renal involvement is less common and usually less severe than that seen with many other forms of vasculitis.

Investigation
Blood tests show an elevated CRP and ESR and a peripheral eosinophilia (>10%). IgE levels are often elevated. The ANCA is positive in most patients, with a perinuclear staining pattern (p-ANCA) and specificity for myeloperoxidase. Biopsy is helpful in confirming the diagnosis, and samples may be taken from skin, nerves, muscle, or kidney. Histopathology will demonstrate necrotizing granulomata of small arteries and venules with an eosinophilic centre. Renal biopsy will show a pauci-immune focal segmental glomerulonephritis.

Management
Eosinophilic granulomatosis with polyangiitis is usually treated with oral prednisolone alone. Where disease is not responsive and important end-organ damage is occurring, then cyclophosphamide, rituximab, azathioprine, and mycophenolate have all been used.

IgA vasculitis
IgA vasculitis (previously known as Henoch–Schönlein purpura) is a small-vessel vasculitis characterized by the presence of a purpuric rash, arthritis, abdominal pain, and renal involvement. Approximately 50% of patients have a preceding upper respiratory tract illness, and ASO titres are raised in some individuals. Other infections or foods, drugs, and insect bites may act as triggers for the condition.

Clinical features
IgA vasculitis affects children much more commonly than adults. In most, it is a relatively benign self-limiting form of vasculitis, although the condition may last for several months and can relapse. The disease is generally less benign in adults, and outcomes can sometimes be poor.

The vast majority of patients have a palpable purpuric rash that particularly involves the buttocks and legs. Subcutaneous oedema of the hands and feet is often present. Arthralgias affecting the knees and ankles are common. Abdominal pain and tenderness is a classical feature; the small bowel is usually involved by the vasculitic process. Rarely, acute pancreatitis may be the presenting feature. Renal involvement is less frequent, but macroscopic haematuria may be a feature, and 2–5% of patients progress to renal failure, requiring dialysis. Vasculitis affecting cardiac, pulmonary, and neural tissues has been described, although it is uncommon.

Investigation
Blood tests may show evidence of an acute phase response and disturbance of renal function. Serum IgA levels may be elevated. ANA and ANCA will usually be negative. Proteinuria or haematuria will be evident on urinalysis in approximately 20% of cases. Histopathology with immunofluorescence testing is the most useful diagnostic test. Tissue is usually obtained from the skin, and the typical findings are of a leukocytoclastic vasculitis with perivascular IgA deposits. It is occasionally appropriate to obtain a renal biopsy. The usual findings are of mesangial proliferation (diffuse or focal segmental), with mesangial IgA deposition.

Management
In general, treatment is supportive, with full recovery expected within 3–6 months. No specific treatment is given for the rash. Treatment of the arthritis is conventionally with NSAIDs, although a short course of oral steroids may be helpful in some patients. Management of renal disease is difficult, as it tends not to respond to corticosteroids and azathioprine. Cyclophosphamide and mycophenolate have been used with variable results.

Further reading
Aletaha D, Neogi T, Silman AJ, et al. (2010). 2010 Rheumatoid arthritis classification criteria: an American College of Rheumatology/European League Against Rheumatism collaborative initiative. *Arthritis & Rheumatism*, **62**, 2569–81.

Bertsias G, Ioannidis JP, Boletis J, et al. (2008). EULAR recommendations for the management of systemic lupus erythematosus. Report of a task force of the EULAR standing committee for international clinical studies, including therapeutics. *Annals of the Rheumatic Diseases*, **67**, 195–205.

Bertsias GK, Tektonidou M, Amoura Z, et al. (2012). Joint European League Against Rheumatism and European Renal Association-European Dialysis and Transplant Association (EULAR/ERA-EDTA) recommendations for the management of adult and paediatric lupus nephritis. *Annals of the Rheumatic Diseases*, **71**, 1771–82.

British Society for Rheumatology (2000). National guidelines for monitoring second line drugs. <http://www.rheumatology.org.uk/guidelines>.

British Thoracic Society Standards of Care Committee (2005). BTS recommendations for assessing risk and for managing

Mycobacterium tuberculosis infection and disease in patients due to start anti-TNF-alpha treatment. *Thorax*, **60**, 800–5.

Coakley G, Mathews C, Field M, *et al.* (2006). BSR & BHPR, BOA, RCGP and BSAC guidelines for management of the hot swollen joint in adults. *Rheumatology*, **45**, 1039–41.

Hagen EC, Daha M, Hermans J, *et al.* (1998). Diagnostic value of standardized assays for anti-neutrophil cytoplasmic antibodies (ANCA) in idiopathic systemic vasculitis. EC/BCR project for ANCA assay standardization. *Kidney International*, **53**, 743–53.

Jennette JC, Falk RJ, Bacon PA, *et al.* (2013). 2012 revised International Chapel Hill Consensus Conference Nomenclature of Vasculitides. *Arthritis & Rheumatism*, **65**, 1–11.

Jordan KM, Cameron JS, Snaith M, *et al.* (2007). British Society for Rheumatology and British Health Professionals in Rheumatology. Guideline for the management of gout. *Rheumatology*, **46**, 1372–4.

Miyakis S, Lockshin MD, Atsumi T, *et al.* (2006). International consensus statement on an update of the classification criteria for definite antiphospholipid syndrome (APS). *Journal of Thrombosis and Haemostasis*, **4**, 295–306.

Moll JM and Wright V (1973). Psoriatic arthritis. *Seminars in Arthritis & Rheumatism*, **3**, 55–78.

National Institute for Health and Clinical Excellence (2010). Etanercept, infliximab and adalimumab for the treatment of psoriatic arthritis. Technology appraisals 104 and 199. <http://www.nice.org.uk/nicemedia/live/13110/50422/50422.pdf>.

Petri M, Orbai AM, Alarcón GS, *et al.* (2012). Derivation and validation of the Systemic Lupus International Collaborating Clinics classification criteria for systemic lupus erythematosus. *Arthritis & Rheumatism*, **64**, 2677–86.

Rudwaleit M, van der Heijde D, Landewé R, *et al.* (2009). The development of Assessment of SpondyloArthritis International Society classification criteria for axial spondyloarthritis (part II): validation and final selection. *Annals of the Rheumatic Diseases*, **68**, 777–83.

Rudwaleit M, van der Heijde D, Landewé R, *et al.* (2011). The Assessment of SpondyloArthritis International Society classification criteria for peripheral spondyloarthritis and for spondyloarthritis in general. *Annals of the Rheumatic Diseases*, **70**, 25–31.

Special Writing Group of the Committee on Rheumatic Fever, Endocarditis, and Kawasaki Disease of the Council on Cardiovascular Disease in the Young of the American Heart Association (1992). Guidelines for the diagnosis of rheumatic fever. Jones Criteria, 1992 update. *JAMA*, **268**, 2069–73.

Van der Linden SM, Valkenburg HA, Cats A (1984). Evaluation of diagnostic criteria for ankylosing spondylitis: a proposal for modification of the New York criteria. *Arthritis & Rheumatism*, **27**, 361–8.

Vitali C, Bombardieri S, Jonsson R, *et al.* (2002). Classification criteria for Sjögren's syndrome: a revised version of the European criteria proposed by the American-European Consensus Group. *Annals of the Rheumatic Diseases*, **61**, 554–8.

Chapter 17

Dermatological diseases and emergencies

Introduction

The skin provides a mechanical defence barrier against infection but is also important in thermoregulation. Loss of normal function of this crucial organ predisposes an individual to infection, fluid loss, and body temperature fluctuation.

In the acute setting, dermatological conditions present frequently. Many doctors are not confident at managing skin conditions; however, this knowledge is essential for the acute physician. Life-threatening conditions, such as toxic epidermal necrolysis and necrotizing fasciitis, have a high mortality, and many other skin presentations (and their associated underlying diseases) warrant prompt investigation. For example, the incidence of malignant melanoma is increasing, and early recognition can save lives.

Often a patient presents with an unrelated concern but may draw attention to a skin problem, or one may be identified during general examination, such as skin cancers or systematic manifestations of disease requiring investigation.

Advances in dermatology and immunotherapy bring new problems. The use of systemic agents, including biologics, mean that associated complications, such as immunosuppression, malignancy, infection, and blood dyscrasias, are now increasingly recognized in dermatology patients.

Erythroderma

Erythroderma is the term used to describe diffuse wide-spread erythema of the skin, involving more than 90% of the body surface area. It can be the manifestation of many cutaneous and systemic diseases.

Erythroderma must be treated aggressively, as the consequences of widespread changes to the skin can result in infection, fluid and electrolyte imbalance, thermodysregulation, high-output cardiac failure, and acute respiratory distress. Establishing the underlying cause is difficult, and erythroderma is often classified as idiopathic.

Epidemiology
The average reported age range is 41 to 61 years where most published studies have excluded children. The proportion of idiopathic cases ranges from 9 to 47%.

Aetiology
Common causes are psoriasis, eczema, and drug reactions. However, there is a wide range of possible underlying pathologies:
- Dermatoses:
  - Psoriasis (see Figure 17.1).
  - Atopic dermatitis (eczema).
  - Cutaneous T cell lymphoma.
  - Pityriasis rubra pilaris.
  - Superficial pemphigus.
  - Bullous pemphigoid.

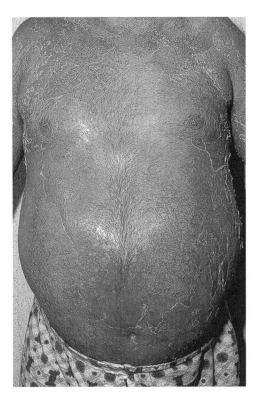

Figure 17.1 Erythrodermic psoriasis.

- Contact dermatitis.
- Infections:
  - Fungal.
  - Norwegian scabies.
  - HIV.
  - Tuberculosis.
- Systemic:
  - Subacute cutaneous lupus.
  - Dermatomyositis.
  - Acute graft versus host disease.
  - Post-operative transfusion-induced.
  - Sarcoidosis.
  - Thyrotoxicosis.
- Haematological:
  - Hodgkin's lymphoma.
  - B cell lymphoma.
  - Chronic lymphocytic leukaemia.
  - Myelodysplasia.
- Malignancies
  - Prostate, lung, thyroid, liver, breast, ovary.
- Drugs
  - Allopurinol, anticonvulsants, antibiotics.

Clinical features
Symptoms related to erythroderma include thermoregulatory disturbance, malaise, fatigue, and pruritus. In long-standing erythroderma, lichenification, diffuse alopecia, dermatopathic lymphadenopathy, keratoderma (skin thickening), nail dystrophy, and ectropion can all be seen. Pitting pretibial and pedal oedema is found in 50% of erythrodermic patients. Other clinical features depend on the underlying aetiology.

Common laboratory abnormalities include:
- High white cell count.
- Lymphocytosis.
- Anaemia.
- Eosinophilia.
- High ESR.
- High serum IgE.

Other abnormalities may include:
- Raised creatinine.
- Raised uric acid.
- Low serum protein.

Skin biopsy may prove helpful, and sometimes repeated biopsies over time are necessary to reach a diagnosis. HIV status should be considered.

Management
- Admit the patient.
- Nurse in a warm, humid environment.
- Assess the fluid and electrolyte balance.
- Assess the patient's nutritional requirements.
- Administer bland emollients.
- Prescribe low-potency topical corticosteroids (note increased absorption through the skin, with large body surface area involvement in erythroderma).
- Antihistamines may be required for pruritus.

- Prescribe systemic antibiotics for secondary infection.
- Discontinue all non-essential medications.
- If peripheral oedema is persistent and does not respond to leg elevation and skin care, consider treatment with diuretics.

Topical immunomodulators, tar preparations, and hydroxyl acid moisturizers are best avoided.

Further management depends on the underlying aetiology. Systemic corticosteroids are recommended for patients with systemic drug hypersensitivity reactions but should be avoided in patients with possible underlying psoriasis.

Complications

- Infections, including sepsis.
- Fluid and electrolyte losses.
- Protein loss (oedema, muscle wasting, hypoalbuminaemia, and high-output cardiac failure).
- Thermodysregulation.

Staphylococcal sepsis is a risk for patients with cutaneous T cell lymphoma and HIV-positive erythrodermic patients.

Prognosis

The natural course of the condition is dependent on underlying aetiology.

Further reading

Rothe MJ, Bernstein ML, Grant-Kels JM (2005). Life-threatening erythroderma: diagnosing and treating the 'red man'. *Clinics in Dermatology*, **23**, 206–17.

Drug eruptions

Cutaneous drug eruptions are relatively common, the incidence of which increases with the number of drugs taken, as well as the age of the patient. Viral infections, such as infectious mononucleosis, cytomegalovirus, and HIV, all increase the risk of a drug eruption.

Treatment in all cases involves stopping the offending drug. In most cases, topical and oral corticosteroids can help to resolve the condition. Antihistamines are used in urticarial drug eruptions.

The morphology of a drug eruption aids classification:
- Exanthematous.
- Urticarial.
- Blistering.
- Pustular.

Exanthematous eruptions

Exanthematous eruptions without systemic signs
These are also called maculopapular drug eruptions and represent around 95% of all cutaneous drug eruptions. Clinical features include:
- Widespread maculopapular pink or red lesions.
- Lesions usually start on the head, neck, or upper trunk and spread symmetrically downwards to the limbs.
- There may be pruritus.
- The rash usually begins within 1–2 weeks of starting the medication and gradually resolves 1–2 weeks after cessation.
- The eruption may progress to become an exfoliative dermatitis, or erythroderma, or develop into a drug hypersensitivity syndrome.
- Blood tests may demonstrate an eosinophilia.

Virtually any drug can cause this reaction. Beta-lactam antibiotics are commonly implicated.

Treatment is supportive, and the suspected drug must be stopped. Low to mild potency topical steroids, emollients, and oral antihistamines will help to relieve symptoms. In severe cases, a short course of oral corticosteroids may help to hasten resolution.

Exanthematous eruptions with systemic signs
Drug hypersensitivity syndrome (DHS) or drug eruption with eosinophilia and systemic symptoms (DRESS) is a serious condition. It is characterized by:
- Delayed-onset exanthematous skin rash, with or without pruritus.
- Fever.
- Lymphadenopathy (in a large number of cases).
- Internal organ involvement, commonly hepatitis, nephritis, or pneumonitis, but any organ can be involved.

These symptoms start 1 to 8 weeks after exposure to the drug and are not related to drug dosage. The rash can range from a maculopapular eruption to an exfoliative dermatitis or erythroderma. Facial oedema is characteristic.

Exfoliative dermatitis is a dangerous condition. It may develop from an exanthematous eruption or develop as erythema and exudation in the flexures and rapidly generalize, for example, as a result of ingestion of arsenicals and heavy metals (e.g. with poisoning). An exfoliative dermatitis may also result from autosensitization of a contact dermatitis. Drugs most commonly implicated include allopurinol, captopril, carbamazepine, isoniazid, and penicillin, amongst others.

Investigations may show:
- Atypical lymphocytosis.
- Eosinophilia.
- Elevated serum creatinine.
- Abnormal liver enzymes.
- Proteinuria.
- Hypothyroidism.

Mortality has been estimated at 10%. Anticonvulsants are a major cause of DHS, and other anticonvulsants within the same aromatic category should also be avoided.

Treatment involves rapid withdrawal of the suspected drug plus systemic corticosteroid, given at a dose of 0.5–1.0 mg/kg. Oral antipyretics and topical corticosteroids are helpful.

Urticarial eruptions

Urticaria without systemic signs
Drugs can cause acute urticaria and angioedema. Acute urticaria is a common, transient skin eruption, characterized by multiple raised, red oedematous papules and plaques (wheals) over the body, with associated pruritus. Single lesions last less than 24 hours. Pathophysiologically, angiooedema is the same reaction within the subcutaneous and deep dermal tissue.

Common causes include penicillin, codeine, morphine, radiocontrast media, pressure, exercise, water, and latex.

Symptoms of nausea, vomiting, diarrhoea, abdominal pain, cutaneous flushing, bronchospasm, hypotension, and syncope indicate an increased risk of anaphylactoid reaction if re-exposed to the offending drug.

Treatment is with oral antihistamines. For more serious reactions like angioedema or anaphylaxis, then adrenaline or systemic corticosteroids may be needed.

Urticaria with systemic symptoms
Serum sickness reaction (SSR) is an immune complex-mediated disease, usually caused by administering foreign proteins, e.g. streptokinase or antivenom. Clinical features include:
- Urticarial/morbilliform rash.
- Fever.
- Malaise.
- Arthralgia.
- Lymphadenopathy.
- Gastrointestinal disturbance.
- Proteinuria.

Serum sickness-like reaction (SSLR)—unlike SSR, is not an immune complex disease. There is a skin rash, with fever and arthralgia. The rash can be urticarial. SSLRs occur 1–3 weeks after starting the offending drug.

Treatment is to stop the causative drug and administer oral antihistamines and topical corticosteroids.

Pustular eruptions

Drug-induced acne
Clinical features include:
- Papules or pustules.
- Comedones (clogged hair follicles) are rare (unlike acne vulgaris).
- Eruption tends to be monomorphous (i.e. one form or structure, including during development).

- Atypical areas like the arms may be affected, with lesser involvement of the face.

Corticosteroids, lithium, isoniazid, phenytoin, and ciclosporin can all cause drug-induced acne.

Chloracne is a florid acneiform and scarring eruption seen in, for example, toxic exposure to dioxins, chlorinated aromatic hydrocarbons, insecticides, and herbicides.

Treatment is to stop the offending agent. Topical therapies, such as benzoyl peroxide, retinoids, and antibiotics, may help.

Acute generalized exanthematous pustulosis
This acute pustular eruption is usually accompanied by a fever. The main differential diagnosis is pustular psoriasis.

Clinical features include:
- Diffuse, oedematous erythema, followed by an eruption of hundreds of small non-follicular sterile pustules.
- Mucous membranes may be involved.
- Vesicles, blisters, or erythema multiforme-like lesions may form.
- Petechial purpura.
- Facial oedema.
- No internal organ involvement.

These changes last 1–2 weeks and resolve spontaneously, followed by desquamation.

Investigations show a neutrophilia and mild eosinophilia.

More than 90% of cases are drug-induced. Onset of eruption from when the drug was commenced can vary from 2 days to 2–3 weeks. Overall prognosis is good.

Treatment is to stop the drug. Systemic corticosteroids, at a dose of 1 mg/kg/day, can be used if severe and widespread.

Blistering eruptions
Fixed drug eruption
Clinical features include:
- A sharply demarcated round or oval, dusky, erythematous, and oedematous plaque that may have a central blister. It will resolve spontaneously without scarring after 2–3 weeks.
- The lesion will recur at the same anatomical site on repeated drug exposure.
- Mucosal surfaces can be involved.
- Associated constitutional symptoms, such as fever, malaise, nausea, and vomiting, can occur.

Treatment involves discontinuing the causative drug and applying topical corticosteroids.

Stevens–Johnson syndrome and toxic epidermal necrolysis
Stevens–Johnson syndrome (SJS) and toxic epidermal necrolysis (TEN) belong to a spectrum of severe cutaneous reactions, often caused by drugs. The main feature of the SJS/TEN spectrum is that of epidermal detachment. TEN is the more severe form whilst SJS is at the milder end of the spectrum. Late stages will demonstrate full-thickness epidermal necrosis, leading to subepidermal bullae. In SJS, less than 10% of the body surface area undergoes epidermal detachment, whereas, this may be greater than 30% in TEN. Essentially, in TEN, there is 'acute skin failure', and the patient is extremely unwell. SJS and TEN may overlap as SJS/TEN overlap syndrome. They are all rare. Among Europeans, the incidence is around 2 patients per million per year. TEN and other drug reactions have a higher incidence in HIV-infected individuals.

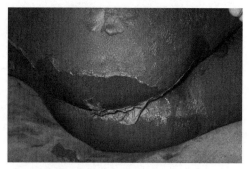

Figure 17.2 Toxic epidermal necrolysis. There is evidence of flaccid blisters, and the underlying dermis is visible under the epidermal detachment.

Clinical features include:
- Abrupt onset of fever.
- Systemic toxicity.
- Flat, atypical target lesions (not essential).
- Purpuric macules (not essential).
- Widespread, mainly central, distribution of a monomorphous skin rash.
- Flaccid blisters may develop (see Figure 17.2).
- Epidermal loss (Nikolsky's sign positive where slight pressure to the epidermis causes lateral displacement and sheet-like loss of epidermis).
- Mucositis of at least two areas (e.g. mouth, genital, eyes, gastrointestinal tract, respiratory disease).
- Skin is painful to touch.

The fever and mucositis generally appear several days before the onset of cutaneous lesions.

Although virtually always an idiosyncratic reaction to medication, there have been other triggers for SJS/TEN, such as vaccination (e.g. measles, mumps, rubella), exposure to industrial chemicals and fumigants, and infection, such as *Mycoplasma pneumoniae*.

Diagnosis of SJS/TEN is confirmed by histology of the skin lesions. Two biopsy specimens must be taken, one for routine formalin-fixed haematoxylin and eosin processing and one for immediate frozen section. Full-thickness epidermal necrosis is a pathognomonic finding of TEN.

Investigations may show anaemia and lymphopenia. Neutropenia indicates a poorer prognosis, and the risk of infection is significantly increased.

Differential diagnoses include:
- Staphylococcal scalded skin syndrome.
- Linear IgA dermatosis.
- Paraneoplastic pemphigus.
- Acute graft versus host disease.
- Drug-induced pemphigoid and pemphigus.
- Acute generalized exanthematous pustulosis.

The mortality of TEN is approximately 30%. SCORTEN (severity-of-illness score for toxic epidermal necrolysis) is a tool used to assess severity of illness and predicted mortality (see Table 17.1).

The score is the sum of seven clinical variables (1 point each), calculated within the first 24 hours and repeated at day 3 (the predicted mortality performance has been validated and remains good during this period):
- Age >40 years.
- Pulse >120/min.

Table 17.1 The SJS/SCORTEN score

SCORTEN	Mortality (%)
0–1	3.2
2	12.1
3	35.3
4	58.3
5 or greater	90.0

Reprinted by permission of Macmillan Publishers Ltd: *Journal of Investigative Dermatology*, Bastuji-Garin S et al., 'SCORTEN: A severity-of-illness score for toxic epidermal necrolysis', 115, 2, pp. 149–153, copyright 2000.

- Cancer/haematological malignancy.
- Epidermal detachment, involving body surface area >10% on day 1.
- Blood urea >10 mmol/L.
- Glucose >14 mmol/L.
- Bicarbonate <20 mEq/L.
  Predicted mortality increases with the total score.

  SJS/TEN both require rapid treatment.
- Admit to burns unit or ITU, and involve a multiprofessional team, including burns/plastics, dermatology, and ophthalmology.
- Manage in a clean environment, with an air mattress.
- Regulate the room temperature.
- Ensure IV access, catheterization and a NG tube for supportive management.
- Pierce blisters with a sterile needle.
- STOP the causative drug.
- Apply topical 50:50 white soft paraffin/liquid paraffin to denuded skin.
- Apply topical clobetasol propionate 0.05% ointment bd to blister unaffected skin and mucosae of body.
- Apply topical (clobetasone butyrate 0.05%) ointment bd to blister unaffected skin of face.
- Apply Trimovate® (clobetasone butyrate 0.05%, nystatin 100 000 IUg⁻¹, oxytetracycline 3%) cream bd to genital skin.
- Apply betamethasone 0.1% eye ointment to both eyes bd as severe conjunctivitis is common.
- Provide effective analgesia.
- Ensure affected skin is dressed to protect from infection and to prevent fluid and protein loss.
- Give antibiotics for identified infection.

  Adjuvant therapies can be used, although there is no conclusive evidence of their effectiveness. Therapy should be commenced as soon as possible. Adjuvant therapies include intravenous immunoglobulins, ciclosporin, granulocyte colony-stimulating factor, and plasmapheresis. The role of corticosteroids is controversial. Combination treatments can be used, and our current guidelines promote the use of:
- Intravenous immunoglobulin.
- Intravenous ciclosporin.
- Intravenous/subcutaneous G-CSF (granulocyte colony-stimulating factor)—to aid re-epithelialization.

  These treatments should be initiated and guided by specialist input.

  In the absence of infection or active disease, the skin can heal within a few days. Healing of mucosal surfaces is slower.

Complications include:
- Skin:
  - Vaginal, urethral, and anal strictures.
  - Nail loss.
  - Scarring.
  - Hypo- and hyperpigmentation.
  - Vulvar adenosis.
  - Phimosis.
- Eyes:
  - Synechiae (i.e. iris adheres to the cornea or lens).
  - Corneal ulcers.
  - Xerophthalmis (i.e. failure to produce tears).
  - Symblepharon (i.e. adhesion of the eyelid palpebral conjunctiva to the eyeball bulbar conjunctiva).
  - Meibomian gland dysfunction.
  - Panophthalmitis.
  - Blindness.
- Systemic:
  - Dyspnoea.
  - Sputum production.
  - Hypoxaemia.
  - Atelectasis.
  - Pulmonary oedema.
  - Bacterial pneumonia.
  - Sloughing of GI tract.
  - Fibrosis of trachea, oesophagus, and anogenital region.

Erythema multiforme (EM)

Erythema multiforme was thought to be part of the spectrum of SJS and TEN but is now considered a separate entity. EM is often a result of infectious agents, such as herpes simplex virus (HSV) or mycoplasma, rather than drugs, but, in up to 50% of cases, there is no provoking factor. It usually affects young and otherwise healthy people.

Clinical features:
- Typical or raised atypical target lesions, although a bullous version is recognized.
- Acral distribution (i.e. affecting body protrusions like elbows, knuckles, toes).
- Mucositis—usually oral mucosa, but rarely two sites can be affected.
- Triggers include:
  - HSV.
  - Mycoplasma.
  - Cytomegalovirus.
  - HIV.
  - Hepatitis B.
  - Infectious mononucleosis.
  - Bacterial infections.
  - Fungal infections.
  - Drug reactions.
  - Malignancy.
  - Pregnancy.
  - Sarcoid.

Polymerase chain reaction assays will reveal herpes simplex virus DNA in lesional skin of a majority of patients with EM.

Treatment is symptomatic in most cases, but, if very severe, admission to a burns unit may be indicated and the administration of oral prednisolone at 30–60 mg/day, decreased over 1–4 weeks.

Antiviral agents can be used prophylactically for recurrent cases caused by HSV.

Other drug-induced blistering conditions

Drugs can cause pemphigus vulgaris or a pemphigus foliaceus-like picture. Bullous pemphigoid and linear IgA bullous dermatosis can also be drug-induced.

Other cutaneous eruptions

These include lichenoid drug eruptions and drug-induced photosensitivity. In the latter, sunblock, topical corticosteroids, oral antihistamines, and discontinuation of the causative drug is the treatment.

Further reading

Abela C, Hartmann CE, De Leo A, et al. (2014). Toxic epidermal necrolysis (TEN): the Chelsea and Westminster Hospital wound management algorithm. *Journal of Plastic, Reconstructive & Aesthetic Surgery*, **67**(8):1026–32.

Breathnach SM (2004). Erythema Multiforme, Stevens-Johnson Syndrome and Toxic Epidermal Necrolysis. In Burns T, Breathnach S, Cox N, Griffiths C, eds. *Rook's Textbook of Dermatology*, 7th edn, Volume 4, pp. 74.1–74.20. Blackwell Science Ltd, Malden.

de Sica-Chapman A, Williams G, Soni N, Bunker CB (2010). Granulocyte colony-stimulating factor in toxic epidermal necrolysis (TEN) and the Chelsea & Westminster TEN protocol. *British Journal of Dermatology*, **162**, 860–5.

National Institute for Health and Care Excellence (2014). Drug allergy: diagnosis and management of drug allergy in adults, children and young people. NICE clinical guideline 183. <https://www.nice.org.uk/guidance/cg183>.

Nigen S, Knowles S, Shear N (2003). Drug eruptions: approaching the diagnosis of drug-induced skin disease. *Journal of Drugs in Dermatology*, **3**, 278–99.

Angioedema

Angioedema is a sudden-onset, but transitory, swelling of the skin and/or mucous membranes, including the upper respiratory and intestinal epithelial linings. Females are more frequently affected than males, and it commonly affects those aged 40 to 50 years old. Angioedema and urticaria often exist concomitantly.

Angioedema can be due to mast cell degranulation and increased levels of bradykinin, and this forms the basis of classification.

Clinical features include a predilection for lax, rather than taut skin, with the face and genitalia commonly affected. The skin may be warm and tender, and the swelling is non-pitting.

Mucosal oedema can involve the tongue, throat, and larynx, with associated anaphylaxis.

As the intestinal epithelial lining can be affected, there may be abdominal pain, diarrhoea, or vomiting. It is important to differentiate angioedema from urticaria (see Table 17.2).

Hereditary angioedema is a rare inherited condition due to a deficiency of the C1-esterase inhibitor (C1-INH) gene. The exact cause is unknown.

Classification of angioedema
See Table 17.3.

Table 17.2 Features differentiating angioedema from urticaria

Feature	Urticaria	Angioedema
Pathology	Papillary (upper) dermal. Vasodilatation +++, oedema +, sparse perivascular infiltrate of mainly neutrophils, eosinophils, monocytes, and T lymphocytes.	Reticular (deep) dermal, subcutaneous/submucosal, vasodilatation +/−, oedema +++, little or no cellular infiltrate, except in allergic angio-oedema where eosinophils may be seen.
Clinical		
Location	Skin only	Skin and mucosae
Duration	<24 h	24–48 h
Colour of lesions	Red	Pink or skin-coloured
Itch	Almost invariable	Variable
Pain, tenderness	Rare	Common

Table 17.3 Classification of angioedema

Type of angioedema	Comment
Mast cell-mediated	
Acute allergic	
Onset within 1–2 hours of exposure of allergen	More common in atopic patients. Usually accompanied by urticaria. Causes include foods (peanuts, shellfish, milk, eggs), drugs (penicillin, sulpha drugs), insect venom and radiocontrast media.
Non-steroidal anti-inflammatory-induced (NSAID-induced) Onset in minutes	Most commonly aspirin. Urticaria common.
Chronic idiopathic	Associated with autoimmune thyroid disease. Evidence for autoimmune basis in some cases. Can occur with or without urticaria.
Bradykinin-mediated	
Angiotensin-converting enzyme inhibitor-induced (ACE inhibitor-induced)	Onset within first week of taking drug or after months. Continued administration leads to more severe attacks. Patients with pre-existing angioedema are predisposed to developing angioedema from ACE inhibitors. No urticaria.
Hereditary angioedema (HAE)	Dominantly inherited. Type 1—quantitative defect in C1 inhibitor (C1 inh). Type 2—functional defect in C1 inhibitor. Type 3—normal C1 inhibitor level and function but occurs only in women with relationship to oestrogen activity. In types 1 and 2, patients will have low C4 level. Asymptomatic up to puberty. Precipitants include exercise, alcohol, stress, hormonal factors.
Acquired C1 inhibitor deficiency	Occurs in lymphoproliferative disease. Thought to be due to overconsumption of C1 inhibitor.
Angioedema due to unknown causes	
Viral infection	Parvovirus B19 infection in neonates. Infectious mononucleosis may precipitate angioedema in patients with HAE.
Association with physical, cholinergic, and allergic contact urticaria	
Angioedema with eosinophilia	There is hypereosinophilia. Responds to systemic steroids.
Associated with urticarial vasculitis	Urticarial vasculitis may present with angioedema. Swelling may last for several days and leave residual staining to affected skin.

The differential diagnosis includes facial cellulitis, acute contact allergic or photodermatitis, Crohn's disease, dermatomyositis, facial lymphoedema, or superior vena caval syndrome.

Investigations

- Full blood count, including eosinophils.
- Urea and electrolytes.
- C4 levels in suspected HAE.
- Thyroid autoantibodies and thyroid function.
- Skin biopsy, especially if concerned about possible urticarial vasculitis.

Treatment of acute allergic angioedema

- Ensure the airway is patent and secure.
- Commence oxygen therapy as required.
- Administer subcutaneous or intramuscular adrenaline at a dose of 0.3 mg, repeated every 10 minutes (0.3 mL of 1:1,000 dilution).
- For antihistamine treatment, give diphenhydramine (50 mg) IM or IV.
- 200 mg of hydrocortisone intravenously.
- If severe, admit and monitor for at least 24 hours.
- Prior to discharge, advise the patient to wear a 'medic alert bracelet', providing medical staff with vital information in an emergency.

If NSAID-induced, avoid NSAIDs and foods which may contain this class of drugs. If chronic idiopathic, avoid potential food allergens, aspirin, opiates, alcohol, overtiredness, or vigorous exercise. If ACE inhibitor-induced, avoid prescribing them, but angiotensin II receptor antagonists may be tolerated.

In chronic autoimmune or idiopathic angioedema, consider treatment with antihistamines and a short tapering course of corticosteroids for acute relapses. However, avoid prolonged corticosteroid therapy. Ciclosporin or methotrexate may be indicated in severe cases.

For the treatment of acute attacks of hereditary angioedema, administer an intravenous C1 inhibitor, or icatibant subcutaneously (a synthetic peptide which blocks the bradykinin-2 receptor). The choice of drug and dosage is based on medical assessment. Admit and monitor the patient, with advice on discharge regarding possible future home self-drug administration. Antihistamines and corticosteroids are ineffective. Very occasionally, subcutaneous adrenaline (0.3 mg every 10 minutes) may help.

For acquired C1 inhibitor deficiency, treat the underlying disease. Acute treatment is the same as that for HAE.

Further reading

Kaplan AP and Greaves MW (2005). Angioedema. *Journal of the American Academy of Dermatology*, **53**, 373–88.

NHS Commissioning Board Clinical Reference Group (2013). NHS Commissioning Board Clinical Commissioning Policy: Treatment of Acute Attacks in Hereditary Angioedema. Ref: NHSCB/B09/P/b.

Kawasaki disease

Kawasaki disease (KD) is an acute self-limiting vasculitis, of the small- and medium-sized arteries. The diagnosis is clinical and should be considered in the differential diagnosis of a childhood rash because of the potentially serious complications. Coronary complications are reduced by the use of intravenous immunoglobulin plus aspirin.

Epidemiology
Kawasaki disease is one of the commonest childhood vasculitides. The typical age at presentation is 6 months to 5 years of age. It is rare in adolescents, adults, and children younger than 6 months.

Aetiology
The aetiology is unknown. However, there are two current hypotheses. The first is that KD is caused by an infectious agent, such as *Propionibacterium acnes*, *Rickettsiae*, Epstein–Barr virus, or retrovirus. The second is that the patient is genetically or immunologically susceptible to generating an immune-mediated response to a superantigen of an infectious agent.

Clinical features
Diagnosis is made using the Centers for Disease Control and Prevention guidelines and must include, as the presenting symptom, a fever of 5 days or more without other explanation (which occurs in at least 95% of patients) *plus* at least four of five of the following:
- A widespread rash that may present with a variety of morphologies (polymorphic exanthem).
- Changes of peripheral extremities:
  - Acute phase: erythema and/or indurative oedema of the palms and soles.
  - Convalescent phase: desquamation from finger tips.
- Bilateral non-exudative conjunctival injection.
- Changes in the oropharynx, such as injected or fissured lips, a 'strawberry tongue', and an injected pharynx.
- Acute non-suppurative cervical lymphadenopathy (>1.5 cm in diameter).

The fever is of sudden onset and may spike several times a day. Usually, the polymorphous widespread rash is present at onset and occurs predominantly on the trunk and extremities. The rash may be scarletiniform (i.e. innumerable small red papules that are widely and diffusely distributed), a generalized erythema, a papular rash, or erythema multiforme-like. There may be fine pustules on the soles of the feet, with associated erythema and oedema. Fusiform swelling of the digits may be present.

Other clinical features include:
- General:
  - Swollen hands and feet, crusted lips.
- Cardiovascular:
  - Cardiac murmurs, gallop rhythm, cardiomegaly, ECG changes, pericardial effusion, coronary and peripheral artery aneurysms, angina, and myocardial infarction.
- Central nervous system:
  - Irritability, lethargy, meningism, and cranial nerve palsies.
- Gastrointestinal:
  - Vomiting, diarrhoea, abdominal pain, and paralytic ileus.

- Respiratory:
  - Cough, rhinorrhoea.
- Musculoskeletal:
  - Arthralgia and arthritis, usually large joints.

The differential diagnosis includes:
- Measles—Koplik's spots (white spots on buccal mucosa), exudative conjunctivitis, and cough. The rash starts behind the ears.
- Scarlet fever—streptococcal pharyngitis and rapid response to penicillin.
- Toxic shock syndrome—hypotension and renal impairment.
- Staphylococcal scalded skin syndrome—hypotension and renal impairment, responds to flucloxacillin.
- Erythema multiforme.
- Stevens–Johnson syndrome—mucosal involvement.
- Drug reactions.
- Juvenile rheumatoid arthritis—evanescent salmon-pink rash.
- Rocky Mountain spotted fever.
- Leptospirosis.

Investigations
Laboratory findings are non-specific. During the first week, the following may be present:
- Neutrophil leucocytosis.
- Mild normochromic normocytic anaemia.
- High ESR.
- Raised C reactive protein.
- Raised alpha-1-antitrypsin.
- Sterile pyuria.

A high platelet count develops in the second week and coincides with the highest risk of coronary artery thrombosis.

Patients with ECG abnormalities (PR-QT prolongation, abnormal Q, low voltage, ST-T changes, and dysrhythmias) require echocardiography to assess ventricular function and to detect any pericardial effusion.

Treatment
Intravenous gammaglobulin decreases the incidence and severity of coronary artery lesions. It is given as a single infusion of 2 g/kg body weight. Aspirin at a dose of 80–100 mg/kg per day during the acute febrile phase, can be reduced to 3–5 mg/kg per day when the fever subsides. Antibiotics and corticosteroids, as monotherapy are contraindicated, as they are associated with a worse cardiac outcome. Corticosteroids may be beneficial as an adjunctive treatment.

Prognosis
Most cases, if untreated, will resolve without sequelae. However, 25% develop coronary artery abnormalities, with a 1–2% mortality rate in the acute phase.

Further reading
Centers for Disease Control and Prevention (2013). Kawasaki Syndrome. <www.cdc.gov/kawasaki/index.html>.
Nasr I, Tometzki JP, Schofield OMV (2001). Kawasaki disease: an update. *Clinical and Experimental Dermatology*, **26**, 6–12.

Staphylococcal toxic shock syndrome

Toxic shock syndrome (TSS) is potentially fatal. Fever, a cutaneous eruption, hypotension, multiple organ involvement, and eventual desquamation are the signs that characterize this staphylococcal exotoxin-mediated disease (see also Chapter 6, section on 'Toxic shock syndrome').

Aetiology

There are a variety of potential sources of infection, including:

- Sanitary tampons.
- Barrier contraceptives.
- Gynaecological surgery.
- Post-partum allergic contact dermatitis.
- Respiratory tract infection.
- Skin infection.
- Visceral infection.
- Vascular infection.
- Odontological infection.

The disease is caused by staphylococcal exotoxins that act as superantigens, leading to massive cytokine release. Patients that develop the disease do not appear to produce neutralizing antibodies. The clinical features include:

- Fever.
- Diffuse erythematous macular eruption.
- Desquamation 1–2 weeks after the onset of the disease.
- Systemic involvement of at least three organs.

There should be negative cultures and an absence of high titres for other infectious agents. The detection of toxigenic strains of *S. aureus* in the absence of acute phase antibodies may aid diagnosis.

Differential diagnoses

- Streptococcal toxic shock syndrome.
- Meningococcaemia.
- Scarlet fever.
- Kawasaki disease.
- Rocky Mountain spotted fever.
- Viral exanthema.
- Adverse cutaneous drug eruptions.
- Lupus erythematoses.

Investigations

- Routine bloods.
- Cultures (blood, urine, and wound sites).
- Viral titres.
- Creatinine kinase (CK) (an elevated CK can indicate necrotizing fasciitis or myositis).
- Antibody titres to other infectious agents.

Treatment

Urgent treatment is necessary with:

- Intravenous antistaphylococcal antibiotics.
- Intravenous fluids.
- Remove the cause, e.g. sanitary tampon and immediately, irrigate and clean the vagina or wound.

Prognosis

Mortality from menstrual TSS is approximately 3%. Mortality from non-menstrual TSS is 2–3-fold higher.

Streptococcal toxic shock syndrome (streptococcal TSS)

In all patients with a high fever and inexplicably intense musculoskeletal pain, streptococcal TSS should be considered (see also Chapter 6, section on 'Toxic shock syndrome').

Streptococcal TSS is caused by a pyogenic exotoxin of *Streptococcus pyogenes* (*Streptococcus* group A). Although clinically similar to staphylococcal TSS, there is an earlier onset of shock and organ failure, and necrotizing fasciitis occurs in around 50% of cases. The skin is the source in about 80% of cases from cellulitis, necrotizing fasciitis, and wounds. Cases post-chickenpox, pharyngitis, peritonitis, phlebitis, and osteomyelitis have been reported.

Clinical features include presentation with the sudden-onset of intense pain. The erythema of streptococcal TSS is generally localized. Systemic manifestations develop within 48–72 hours of onset. Bacteraemia is more frequent than in staphylococcal TSS, and, therefore, blood culture is positive in over 50% of cases. Mortality is very high at 30–70% of cases.

Treatment

Urgent treatment is necessary.

- Benzylpenicillin and clindamycin are the preferred antibiotics. Penicillin may be less effective when high concentrations of group A *Streptococcus* are present.
- Intravenous fluids should be given.

The use of intravenous immunoglobulin in streptococcal TSS warrants further investigation.

Avoid non-steroidal anti-inflammatory drugs, as these can contribute to shock and cause more aggressive infection.

Further reading

Ramos-e-Silva M and Pereira AL (2005). Life-threatening eruptions due to infectious agents. *Clinics in Dermatology*, **23**, 148–56.

Staphylococcal scalded skin syndrome

Staphylococcal scalded skin syndrome (SSSS) is a superficial skin blistering disease.

Aetiology and pathogenesis
It is caused by the staphylococcal exotoxins known as exfoliative toxins type A and B. Histologically, there is intraepidermal cleavage at the granular layer of the skin, leading to superficial exfoliation of the skin.

Epidemiology
SSSS tends to affect children. It rarely affects adults, but the mortality is higher in adults Adults usually have predisposing factors, including renal insufficiency, immunosuppression (including HIV), alcoholism, and malignancy.

Clinical features
• Initial infection may be of the nasopharynx, ear, conjunctiva, urinary tract, or skin.
• Fever.
• Skin tenderness.
• Erythematous skin eruption, more prominent in the flexures.
• Flaccid bullae develop 24–48 hours later, generally around orifices and in the flexures. Nikolsky's sign is positive with desquamation of the skin.

Differential diagnosis includes toxic epidermal necrolysis, toxic shock syndrome, and Kawasaki syndrome.

Investigations
• Culture:
  • Potential sources of infection—*Staphylococcus aureus* will only be present at the infection site and will not be recovered from sites of sloughing skin or bullae.
  • Blood and urine.
• Tzanck smear (scrape base of lesion, and apply to dry slide and stain for rapid cytology).
• Skin biopsy.

Treatment
• Admit to hospital with strict isolation.
• Support with IV fluids.
• Commence IV antistaphyloccocal antibiotics with or without Gram-negative cover for secondary infection.
• Apply emollients 50:50 white soft paraffin/liquid paraffin regularly with semi-occlusive dressings.

Mortality is <5% in children but can be as high as 60% in adult populations and 100% in patients with some previous disease. Complications include secondary skin infection, surgical wound infection, pneumonia, sepsis, and endocarditis.

Further reading
Hay RJ, Adriaans BM (2010). Bacterial Infections. In Burns T, Breathnach S, Cox N, Griffiths C, eds. *Rook's Textbook of Dermatology*, 8th edn, pp. 30.26–30.65. Wiley-Blackwell Publishing Ltd, Chichester.

Necrotizing fasciitis

Necrotizing fasciitis (NF) is a life-threatening soft tissue infection. Rapidly progressive, widespread fascial necrosis occurs. The condition can be subdivided into type I (polymicrobial) and type 2 (group A streptococcal). Prompt diagnosis and treatment are essential. Missed or delayed diagnosis is an important cause of litigation.

Surgical debridement and antibiotic therapy are the mainstays of treatment.

Epidemiology
Approximately 500 to 1,500 cases of necrotizing fasciitis are diagnosed in the USA each year. There are a number of conditions and predisposing risk factors.

Conditions leading to NF include:
- Site of skin biopsy, insect bite, needle puncture, laceration.
- Herpes zoster.
- Surgical wound.
- Skin abscess.
- Areas affected with chronic venous leg ulcer.

Risk factors for NF include:
- Diabetes mellitus.
- Increasing age.
- Surgery.
- Trauma.
- Alcohol abuse.
- Renal failure.
- Peripheral vascular disease.
- Chronic skin infection.
- HIV and other immunosuppressive conditions.

However, one half of cases occur in young, previously healthy individuals.

Ten per cent of cases are caused by group A *Streptococcus* alone, but most cases are polymicrobial and commonly include:
- *Staphylococcus aureus*.
- *Escherichia coli*.
- *Bacteroides*.
- *Clostridium* species.
  Rare pathogens include:
- *Pseudomonas aeruginosa*.
- *Haemophilus influenzae* type b.
- *Aeromonas hydrophila*.
- *Vibrio vulnificus*.

Pathogenesis
The infectious organism proliferates and extends along superficial and deep fascial planes. Bacterial enzymes and toxins play a part in this process. NF is associated with streptococcal toxic shock syndrome (see earlier section in this chapter).

Clinical features
The patient is unwell, with pain disproportionate to the initial skin findings. The skin becomes swollen and erythematous, with the erythema spreading at a visibly alarming rate despite elevation and antibiotics. The skin changes from a shiny red-purple to a pathognomonic grey-blue. The skin may demonstrate ill-defined patches, and violaceous bullae

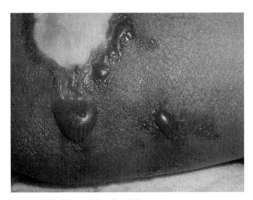

Figure 17.3 Necrotizing fasciitis.

formation can occur (see Figure 17.3). A malodorous fluid results from necrosis of the fascia and fat.

Later, due to cutaneous nerve destruction, the affected area becomes anaesthetized, and a hard wooden feel of the subcutaneous tissue may result. Ulceration may occur. Crepitus due to gas-forming organisms can result. However, this is not a feature of group A streptococcal necrotizing fasciitis.

The patient is usually extremely unwell, with fever, hypotension, altered mental state, leucocytosis, and tachycardia, and often requires intensive care. Fournier's gangrene refers to necrotizing fasciitis that affects the perineum and genitalia.

There is usually a marked leucocytosis with high inflammatory markers, including CRP, and an elevated creatinine kinase.

Diagnosis
Diagnosis is primarily clinical. CT, and preferably MRI, are used to identify soft tissue and fascial involvement, with or without evidence of subcutaneous gas.

A deep incisional tissue biopsy, along with cultures for aerobic and anaerobic organisms, is the gold standard for diagnosis of NF.

Blister fluid, pustular discharge, and discharge from open wounds should all be sampled for Gram staining as well as for aerobic and anaerobic cultures. Microscopy of the Gram-stained exudates may guide antibiotic choice. Rapid streptococcal diagnostic kits, polymerase chain reaction, and immunofluorescence tissue stains are all newer techniques to help diagnose streptococcal NF.

Management
- Urgent surgical exploration and ITU care.
- Excision debridement.
- Intravenous antibiotics—until the aetiology is known administer broad-spectrum therapy. Recommended antibiotics include a beta-lactam/beta-lactamase inhibitor, and clindamycin. In nosocomial infection or in the presence of meticillin (INN)-resistant *Staphylococcus aureus*, vancomycin with clindamycin, or a carbapenem or fluoroquinolone can be considered. Amend the antibiotic therapy to target the specific bacterial agents detected during investigation.
- Irrigate the wound.
- The wound should be kept open.

- Daily wound debridement (until there is no necrotic tissue).
- Nutritional support is crucial for wound healing.
- Hyperbaric oxygen has been suggested in the literature as an adjunct.

Intravenous immunoglobulin may be useful in NF associated with streptococcal infection.

Prognosis

NF is frequently fatal and has an overall mortality rate of 24–60%, regardless of treatment.

Further reading

Kihiczak GG, Schwartz RA, Kapila R (2006). Necrotizing fasciitis: a deadly infection. *Journal of the European Academy of Dermatology and Venereology*, **20**, 365–9.

National Institute for Health and Care Excellence (2015). Cellulitis - acute. Clinical knowledge summaries. <http://cks.nice.org.uk/cellulitis-acute>.

Public Health England (2013). Health protection – guidance. The characteristics, diagnosis, management and epidemiology of necrotising fasciitis (NF). <https://www.gov.uk/guidance/necrotising-fasciitis-nf>.

Psoriasis

Psoriasis is a chronic relapsing skin disease that can develop at any age. The pathogenesis is not certain, but tumour necrosis factor alpha, dendritic cells, and T cells are thought to contribute. At least nine chromosomal psoriasis susceptibility loci have been identified, and different subtypes of psoriasis exist. In the emergency setting, a patient may present acutely with severe presentations of different forms, and recognition of these is important.

Chronic plaque psoriasis is characterized by well-demarcated plaques, with loosely adherent silvery-white scales, with a predilection to the elbows, knees, lumbosacral area, natal cleft, and scalp. Nails are often affected in psoriasis (onycholysis or pitting). Early psoriatic lesions frequently start as small pinpoint papules that gradually show scaling. An inverse type of psoriasis appears in the intertriginous areas where scaling is minimal. Sometimes, psoriasis can predominate on the seborrhoeic areas of the scalp and face, and differentiating sebopsoriasis from seborrhoeic dermatitis is challenging.

During bouts of activity, plaque lesions may become more inflamed and expand centrifugally. Occasionally, pustular lesions may appear. Chronic plaque psoriasis is the most common variety of psoriasis, representing 70–80% of psoriatic cases.

Guttate psoriasis is the most common exanthematous form of psoriasis and is characterized by the acute onset of round, erythematous, slightly scaling papules over the trunk and extremities. The disease is self-limiting, resolving within 3 to 4 months. It is especially common in children or young adults with a family history of psoriasis and follows a streptococcal or viral infection. The risk of developing a more chronic form of psoriasis after the first episode of guttate psoriasis is estimated at 40%. There is a risk that guttate psoriasis may recur with greater severity.

Generalized pustular psoriasis may develop in patients with pre-existing plaque psoriasis or may develop after pustular episodes. Acute episodes may be triggered in patients with plaque psoriasis by irritating topical therapy or abrupt withdrawal of corticosteroids. At the onset of an attack of acute generalized pustular psoriasis, the skin becomes red and tender. There may be fever and systemic symptoms, such as anorexia and nausea. Within hours, numerous pinhead-sized pustules appear. The pustules may become confluent, producing large areas of pus. Oral lesions may be present, with pustules or acute geographic tongue (also known as benign migratory glossitis). Subungual (i.e. under a toe/finger nail) pustules may also appear. Remission of acute episodes may leave an erythrodermic state. See Figure 17.4.

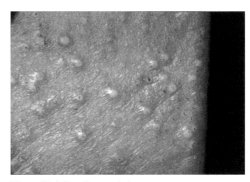

Figure 17.4 Pustular psoriasis.

Generalized pustular psoriasis may be associated with polyarthritis and cholestatis (neutrophilic cholangitis). It may also occur rarely during pregnancy and is called impetigo herpetiformis. Onset is usually before the sixth month of pregnancy.

The differential diagnosis includes acute generalized exanthematic pustulosis, a self-limiting febrile drug reaction resolving 2 weeks after withdrawal of the suspected agent. It is characterized by pinpoint non-follicular pustules on erythematous patches, mainly involving folds.

Unstable and erythrodermic psoriasis may develop from stable chronic plaque psoriasis. More extensive involvement is marked by the onset of an inflammatory phase, with predominantly erythema and limited scaling associated with itching and rapidly progressing lesions. The trigger factors are unknown. This unstable form may progress to whole body involvement. The erythrodermic phase is dominated by generalized erythema, loss of the characteristic features of psoriasis, and skin failure, that is, the inability to maintain homeostatic functions. For the management of erythrodermic psoriasis, see 'Erythroderma' earlier in this chapter.

Psoriatic arthritis

Psoriatic arthritis is a seronegative inflammatory arthritis that occurs in the presence of psoriasis. In approximately 10% of affected patients, the arthritis develops prior to the skin manifestations.

Further reading

Griffiths CE and, Barker JN (2007). Pathogenesis and clinical features of psoriasis. *Lancet*, **370**, 263–71.

Eczema and dermatitis

Atopic eczema (dermatitis)

Atopic eczema is a chronic relapsing skin disease, often present in infancy and early childhood, that can persist into adulthood. Patients with atopic dermatitis have alterations in cutaneous immunity and barrier function that may make them more susceptible to skin infection, including viruses, bacteria, and dermatophytic fungi. Patients with eczema and household contacts of patients with eczema should not be vaccinated with the smallpox vaccine because of the risk of eczema vaccinatum.

Acute atopic dermatitis presents with poorly defined erythematous patches and plaques without scale. There may be oedema and excoriation.

Infected atopic dermatitis results from secondary infection, and colonization with *Staphylococcus aureus* is common. Infected atopic dermatitis presents with oozing erosions and/or pustules that may crust. Treatment involves treating the underlying eczema and the use of appropriate oral antibiotics.

Eczema herpeticum

This can occur in patients with atopic dermatitis, even if mild, following a trivial herpetic infection on the lip or elsewhere.

Clinical features include:
- Erosions and vesicles.
- Painful tender skin.
- Fever.
- Malaise.
- Lesions in abnormal skin that may extend peripherally.

Differential diagnosis of eczema herpeticum
- Varicella.
- Disseminated varicella zoster virus (VZV) infection.
- Disseminated herpes simplex virus (HSV) infection.
- Wound infection.
- Eczema vaccinatum.

Investigations
- Tzanck smear—fluid from an intact vesicle is smeared thinly onto a microscope slide and stained. Positive direct microscopy demonstrates acantholytic keratinocytes or multinucleated giant acantholytic keratinocytes.
- Viral swabs from lesions:
  - Monoclonal antibodies specific to HSV-1 and HSV-2 antigens can be detected.
  - HSV cultures from the involved mucocutaneous site or tissue biopsy specimen.

Serology for antibodies to glycoproteins can differentiate past HSV-1 and HSV-2 infections. Polymerase chain reaction (PCR) can detect HSV DNA sequences in tissue, smears, or secretion.

Management
Immediately commence antiviral therapy, and treat any associated bacterial infection. Treat the underlying dermatosis with emollients and topical corticosteroids.

Erythroderma

Patients with an acute flare-up of their eczema are at risk of developing erythroderma. If erythroderma develops, this should be treated as an inpatient (see 'Erythroderma'), as the normal functional properties of the skin will be impaired.

Allergic contact dermatitis

Allergic contact dermatitis (ACD) is a type IV (cell-mediated or delayed) hypersensitivity reaction to a substance that has come into contact with the skin. The condition develops in individuals who have become sensitized to the offending agent. It is an immunological reaction that can potentially generalize and affect skin distant to the site of contact.

Clinical features include:
- Well-demarcated erythema, with oedema of the affected area.
- Superimposed non-umbilicated vesicles and/or papules.
- Bullae, erosions, and fever may be present in severe cases.

Management
- Topical corticosteroids.
- Patch testing may be indicated.
- Avoid the offending agent.
- Oral prednisolone, if severe.

Allergic phytodermatitis (APD)

Allergic phytodermatitis is a type of allergic contact dermatitis to a plant allergen that often presents in a linear arrangement.

Irritant contact dermatitis

Irritant contact dermatitis (ICD) is caused by exposure to a chemical or physical agent that is toxic to the skin. Common irritants include soap, detergents, acids and alkalis, industrial solvents, and plants. ICD can be chronic as a result of cumulative exposure to the offending agent.

Acute clinical features include:
- Burning/stinging.
- Sharply demarcated erythema.
- Oedema.
- Vesicles and bullae.
- Caustic burn.
- Erosions.
- Necrosis.
- Ulceration.
- Fever may occur, if severe.

Management
- Identify and remove the offending agent.
- Avoid future exposure.
- Cover with wet dressings.
- Large vesicles may be drained, but the roof of the lesions should not be removed.
- Apply potent topical corticosteroids.
- In severe cases, start oral prednisolone therapy.
- Use barrier emollients.

Phytophotodermatitis

Phytophotodermatitis (PPD) is a common inflammatory reaction of the skin to contact with certain photosensitizing chemicals found in some plant, fruit, and vegetable families, during exposure to sunlight. The phototoxic reaction occurs following contact of the skin to the sensitizing phototoxin and subsequent ultraviolet radiation.

Clinical features
- Erythema.
- Oedema.
- Vesicles and bullae.
- Affects areas at site of contact.

Differential diagnosis includes an acute irritant contact dermatitis. However, ICD is eczematous with papules and vesicles, whereas PPD is only vesicular.

Management is with topical corticosteroids. Wet dressings may be indicated in the acute vesicular stage.

Further reading

Rudikoff D, Akhavan A, Cohen SR (2003). Colour atlas: eczema. *Clinics in Dermatology*, **21,** 101–8.

Wolff K, Johnson RA, Suurmond D (2005). Eczema/dermatitis. In *Fitzpatrick's colour atlas and synopsis of clinical dermatology*, 5th edn, pp. 24–8. McGraw-Hill Medical, New York.

Cutaneous vasculitis

Vasculitis is an inflammatory cell-mediated pathology of blood vessels, with clinico-pathological findings seen in a variety of conditions, including systemic disease, malignancy, and infection (see also Chapter 16, section on 'Vasculitis').

Epidemiology
The annual incidence of biopsy-proven cutaneous vasculitis ranges from 39.6 to 59.8 per million. About 40% of all cases of cutaneous vasculitis are idiopathic. Most cases of cutaneous vasculitis are benign.

Clinical features
There may be both systemic and cutaneous features. Cutaneous involvement occurs in vasculitis of small and medium-sized vessels. Systemic features include fever, malaise, weight loss, arthralgia, and arthritis.

Cutaneous signs of vasculitis are variable, and the clinical presentation is dependent on the vessel size affected (see Figure 17.5).

Cutaneous small-vessel vasculitis may present with palpable or macular purpura, urticarial papules, pustules, vesicles, petechiae, or erythema multiforme-like lesions.

Medium-sized vessel vasculitis may present with livedo reticularis, retiform (i.e. net-like, reticular) purpura, ulcers, subcutaneous nodules, and digital necrosis.

Classification
A cutaneous vasculitis can be present in a variety of vasculitic syndromes. The clinical diagnosis usually warrants histological confirmation. Histology has to be considered in the context of the clinical history, clinical morphology, and laboratory findings.

Most accepted classification schemes are based on the size of the blood vessels involved (see also Chapter 16, section on 'Vasculitis'; Table 16.15).

Classification of vasculitis
- Cutaneous small-vessel vasculitis:
  - Idiopathic small-vessel cutaneous vasculitis.
  - Henoch–Schönlein purpura.
  - Essential mixed cryoglobulinaemia.
  - Waldenström's hypergammaglobulinaemic purpura.
  - Associated with collagen vascular disease.
  - Urticarial vasculitis.
  - Erythema elevatum diutinum.
  - Rheumatoid nodules.
  - Reactive leprosy.

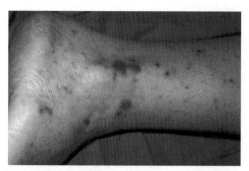

Figure 17.5 Cutaneous vasculitis.

- Septic vasculitis.
- Large-vessel necrotizing vasculitis:
  - Polyarteritis nodosa.
  - Granulomatous vasculitis (e.g. Wegener's granulomatosis).
  - Giant cell arteritis.
- Large-vessel vasculitis with collagen vascular disease.
- Nodular vasculitis.

In cases with a non-diagnostic biopsy, conditions that mimic vasculitis must be considered, for example, a pseudo-vasculitis, such as livedo reticularis, warfarin necrosis, infective endocarditis, amyloidosis, and scurvy.

Investigation
Although most cases of cutaneous vasculitis are benign, the possibility exists of an underlying systemic vasculitis with the risk of permanent organ damage and death.

A skin biopsy is required to confirm histological diagnosis for direct immunofluorescence, as this will be positive in immune complex-mediated vasculitic syndromes.

The choice and timing of the skin biopsy affect diagnostic yield. Early lesions, less than 48 to 72 hours old, are more likely to demonstrate a neutrophilic vasculitis than older lesions.

If a vasculitis is confirmed on biopsy, then a cause must be sought. Triggers, such as drugs, infection, malignancy, or concomitant disease, must be contemplated.

Investigations will include:
- Full blood count.
- Erythrocyte sedimentation rate.
- C-reactive protein.
- Urea and electrolytes.
- Liver function.
- Anti-hepatitis C antibody.
- Hepatitis B surface antigen
- Cryoglobulins.
- Complement.
- Antinuclear cytoplasmic antibody (ANCA).
- Antinuclear antibody (ANA).
- Rheumatoid factor.
- Anti-streptolysin O titre.
- HIV antibody.
- Serum and urine protein electrophoresis.
- Urinalysis.
- Chest X-ray.

Other more specific autoantibody tests may be necessary.

Treatment
The cutaneous vasculitis will be either primary or secondary to an underlying condition (infection, inflammatory disease, drug, or neoplasm). If secondary, treat the underlying cause or stop the offending drug.

Cutaneous small-vessel vasculitis often resolves without treatment, except avoiding the precipitant.

For mild disease, treatment is:
- Supportive:
  - Leg elevation, rest, and avoiding tight clothing.
- Symptomatic therapy:
  - Antihistamines.

- Non-steroidal anti-inflammatories.
- Topical corticosteroids and calcineurin.

More aggressive systemic treatment, for example with colchicine or dapsone, may be used in severe cutaneous disease or chronic disease of over 4 weeks duration. For severe ulcerating or progressive disease, rapid control of symptoms can be achieved with oral corticosteroids (prednisolone 1 mg/kg/day). A tapering dose is indicated to avoid the long-term side effects. Other immunosuppressive agents may be considered in recurrent disease as a steroid-sparing agent.

Further reading

Carlson JA, Cavaliere LF, Grant-Kels JM (2006). Cutaneous vasculitis: diagnosis and management. *Clinics in Dermatology*, **24**, 414–29.

Chung L, Kea B, Fiorentino DF (2008). Cutaneous vasculitis. In Bolognia JL, Lorizzo JL, Rapini RP. *Dermatology*, 2nd edn, pp. 347–67. Elselvier Limited, Philadelphia.

Jennette JC, Falk RJ, Bacon PA, *et al.* (2013). 2012 revised international Chapel Hill consensus conference nomenclature of vasculitides. *Arthritis & Rheumatology*, **65**, 1–11.

Lotti T, Ghersetich I, Comacchi C, Jorizzo JL (1998). Cutaneous small-vessel vasculitis. *Journal of the American Academy of Dermatology*, **39**, 667–89.

Immunobullous disorders

There are a group of primary blistering disorders that affect children and adults. These bullous dermatoses can be classified as genodermatoses (inherited, genetic skin conditions) or autoimmune disorders.

Blisters of the skin can also be a manifestation of a variety of skin conditions, including bacterial infections (e.g. impetigo), viral infections (e.g. herpes simplex and herpes zoster), insect bites, chemical or physical burns, or after necrosis of the skin due to thrombosis of cutaneous blood vessels (e.g. disseminated intravascular coagulation). Occasionally, blisters present secondary to other dermatological conditions, such as necrobiosis lipoidica diabeticorum, lichen planus, systemic lupus erythematosus, and mastocytosis.

The rest of this section covers the bullous dermatoses.

Bullous pemphigoid (BP)

Bullous pemphigoid is a chronic autoimmune bullous disorder, most commonly seen in the elderly.

The disease may present with erythema, urticarial plaques, and subepidermal tense blisters (see Figure 17.6). The blisters may develop subsequent to the urticaria and erythema. The patient will complain of a pruritus and have mucosal involvement. Onset may be gradual.

A skin biopsy should be taken for histology and direct immunofluorescence which will be positive with linear IgG deposits along the basement membrane zone. It may also be positive for C3, which can occur in the absence of IgG.

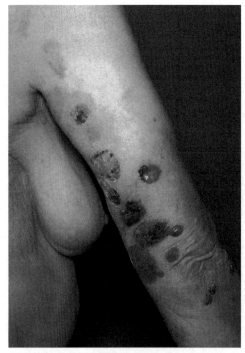

Figure 17.6 Bullous pemphigoid.

Blood should be sent for indirect immunofluorescence to identify circulating anti-basement membrane IgG antibodies present in 70% of these patients.

Treatment includes:
- Potent topical or intralesional corticosteroids.
- Oral prednisolone dose depends on severity:
  - Mild—20 mg/day or 0.3 mg/kg/day.
  - Moderate—40 mg/day or 0.6 mg/kg/day.
  - Severe—50–70 mg/day or 0.75–1 mg/kg/day.
- Bone prophylaxis.

Corticosteroids should be tapered over a few weeks. If new lesions develop, consider steroid-sparing agents, such as dapsone, systemic antibiotics, in combination with niacinamide, azathioprine, methotrexate, ciclosporin, cyclophosphamide, chlorambucil, and mycophenolate mofetil. Overall, BP is considered to have a better prognosis than other blistering diseases.

Bullous pemphigoid is associated with other conditions:
- Diabetes mellitus.
- Pernicious anaemia.
- Chronic inflammatory skin diseases (lichen planus, psoriasis).
- Malignancies (controversy exists over this association).

Drugs may mimic pemphigoid. These include furosemide, NSAIDs, captopril, phenacetin, penicillamine, and antibiotics.

Pemphigus vulgaris (PV)

Pemphigus is a rare group of autoimmune blistering diseases, affecting the skin and mucous membranes (except pemphigus foliaceus, in which there is no mucous membrane involvement). Pemphigus vulgaris is the most common subtype.

The disease is characterized by intraepithelial flaccid blisters, with a positive Nikolsky's sign, which following sloughing become painful sores. There can be painful mucosal involvement. The erosions tend to heal without scarring.

A skin biopsy should be sent for direct immunofluorescence staining. In pemphigus vulgaris it will be positive for IgG and often C3, which is deposited in lesions and paralesion skin in the intercellular substance of the epidermis and can also be detected from a serum sample (indirect immunofluorescence test).

Indirect immunofluorescence from a serum sample will identify IgG autoantibodies against desmoglein 3 located in desmosomes.

The treatment regime depends on age, severity, extent of progression, and subtype of pemphigus.
- Apply topical corticosteroids.
- Consider oral prednisolone 40–60 mg/day.

Once a clinical response is observed, the steroid dose can be tapered. A steroid-sparing agent may be needed to control disease, such as dapsone, azathioprine, cyclophosphamide, methotrexate, or mycophenolate mofetil.

Paraneoplastic pemphigus (PNP)

This is a rare form of pemphigus, mainly seen in patients over 60 years of age, that develops in association with neoplasia. Associated neoplasms include:
- Non-Hodgkin's lymphoma.
- Chronic lymphocytic leukaemia.
- Giant follicular hyperplasia (Castleman's tumour).

- Thymoma.
- Retroperitoneal sarcoma.
- Waldenström's macroglobulinaemia.
- Multiple myeloma.
- Cancer of the liver, lung, pancreas, and cervix.

There may be mucous membrane ulceration and a polymorphous skin eruption. Direct immunofluoresence of the skin biopsy is positive.

This condition is notoriously resistant to therapy, and prognosis is poor.

Other bullous disorders

Pemphigoid foliaceus is characterized by intraepithelial flaccid blisters without mucosal involvement. There are initially small bullae that erode easily and become chronic. Patients are usually not severely ill.

Pemphigoid gestationis is a rare autoimmune subepidermal bullous disease of pregnancy that is clinically, histologically, and immunologically similar to bullous pemphigoid.

Linear IgA bullous dermatosis is an idiopathic or drug-induced rare, blistering disorder of acute onset.

Further reading

Carr DR, Houshmand E, Heffernan MP (2007). Approach to the acute generalized blistering patient. *Seminars in Cutaneous Medicine and Surgery*, **26**, 139–46.
Wojnarowska F, Venning VA, (2010). Immunobullous Diseases. In Burns T, Breathnach S, Cox N, Griffiths C, eds. *Rook's Textbook of Dermatology*, 8th edn, pp. 40.1–40.21. Wiley-Blackwell Publishing Ltd, Chichester.

Pyoderma gangrenosum

Pyoderma gangrenosum (PG) is a destructive skin disorder, usually characterized by painful ulceration, often associated with underlying disease.

Epidemiology
The disease is rare.

Aetiology
Aetiology has not, as yet, been clearly determined. Although some cases are idiopathic, it can also be provoked by trauma ('pathergy') and drugs, such as propylthiouracil. It is a potential complication of surgery.

Pyoderma gangrenosum is associated with several conditions, including:
- Inflammatory bowel disease.
- Rheumatoid arthritis.
- Pregnancy.
- HIV.
- Hepatitis.
- Systemic lupus erythematosus.
- Monoclonal gammopathy.
- Haematological malignancy or paraproteinaemia.
- Malignancy.
- Behçet's disease.
- Sweet syndrome.
- Takayasu's arteritis.

Pathogenesis
This remains unclear. Inflammatory cytokines and neutrophil chemoattractant factors seem to have a role in generating a neutrophil-rich dermal inflammatory infiltrate.

Clinical features
The condition may start as sterile pustules but often presents with painful ulcers, with necrotic, undermined, violaceous, or bluish margins. The surrounding skin is oedematous and erythematous. The ulcers can develop a purulent cover and have a malodour due to secondary bacterial infection. The ulcers can recur over time. The legs are most commonly affected, but other areas, including mucous membranes, can be involved.

Extracutaneous manifestations include involvement of upper airway mucosa, eyes, genital mucosa, sterile pulmonary neutrophilic infiltrates, spleen infiltrates, and neutrophilic myositis.

Investigations
Diagnosis can be difficult and is based on the underlying disease and clinical features. Histopathology does not demonstrate any pathognomonic features. Other causes of ulcers must be excluded through biopsy, culture, and clinical acumen.

Once a diagnosis is made, it is important to investigate for a potential associated systemic disease.

Differential diagnosis
- Vascular occlusive or venous disease, including calciphylaxis (i.e. skin and fatty tissue necrosis, often seen in end stage kidney disease).
- Vasculitis.
- Malignancy.
- Infectious diseases—ecthyma (beta-haemolytic *Streptococcus*) and deep mycoses like sporotrichosis.
- Exogenous tissue injury—insect bites can cause necrotic ulcers.
- Factitious disease.
- Drug reactions

Management
Randomized, double-blinded, prospective, multicentre trials are not available, and there is no gold standard for treatment. Treatment is dependent on the extent of the lesions, associated disease, and comorbidities. Pain and signs of inflammation (extent of elevation and redness of the border) help to guide response to treatment.

Treatment includes:
- Analgesia, as pain can be severely debilitating.
- Topical wound management is important in healing the ulcers. In ulcers with heavy exudates, foam or laminate dressings are recommended. Moisture-retentive dressings are preferred to desiccated gauzes.
- Barrier cream or ointment (e.g. zinc oxide paste) around edge of wound to prevent further skin breakdown.
- Treat any underlying disease.
- Potent topical corticosteroids (such as clobetasol ointment) can be applied to the wound, although systemic absorption is a risk.

There is also some evidence for topical tacrolimus.

Systemic treatments have been used for severe pyoderma gangrenosum or if underlying disease is present. These include:
- Prednisolone (1–2 mg/kg/day). Rapid response but risk steroid side effects with long-term use.
- Ciclosporin—should be restricted to patients with idiopathic disease. Not appropriate for long-term treatment.
- Methotrexate—as adjunctive therapy.
- Mycophenolate mofetil.
- Dapsone.
- Infliximab in Crohn's disease has shown an effect on PG.
- Skin transplants and the application of bioengineered skin in selected cases as a complement to the immunosuppressive treatment.

Complications
Secondary bacterial infection can manifest as cellulitis or lymphangitis. Cultures from the ulcers often reveal a mixture of bacterial and fungal contaminants.

Scarring will result from the ulcerated lesion.

Prognosis
Despite advances in the treatment of PG, prognosis remains unpredictable.

Further reading
Wollina U (2007), Pyoderma gangrenosum—a review. *Orphanet Journal of Rare Diseases*, **2**, 19.

Scarring alopecia

Hair loss, or alopecia, can be managed in the outpatient dermatology department. However, there are dermatological conditions that present with a scarring alopecia, in which urgent management is required.

Scarring alopecia is also known as cicatricial alopecia which represents a heterogenous group of disorders, characterized by the permanent and pathologic destruction of the hair follicle, leading to irreversible hair loss. Scarring alopecia can be primary or secondary.

In primary alopecia, the hair follicle is the main target for destruction, and examples include discoid lupus erythematosus (DLE) and folliculitis decalvans (a bacterial folliculitis). In secondary cicatricial alopecia, non-follicular disease affecting the scalp inadvertently causes follicular destruction. The latter group may occur as a result of exogenous and endogenous factors, including inflammatory/autoimmune diseases (such as pemphigus vulgaris, follicular mucinosis, sarcoidosis, scleroderma, and morphoea (i.e. localised scleroderma)), infection (bacterial, viral, or fungal), neoplastic processes (such as primary and metastatic carcinoma), and physical agents (such as radiotherapy or burns).

Early diagnosis and treatment, depending on cause, will prevent permanent hair loss.

Further reading

Han A and Mirmirani P (2006). Clinical approach to the patient with alopecia. *Seminars in Cutaneous Medicine and Surgery*, **25**, 11–23.

Herpes simplex viruses 1 and 2

Herpes simplex viruses (HSVs) are enveloped, linear, double-stranded DNA viruses, whose only hosts are humans. There are two types, 1 and 2. They have different clinical manifestations and different epidemiologies. Aciclovir, valaciclovir, and famciclovir are antivirals used in treatment (see also Chapters 6 and 11).

Epidemiology

Herpes labialis (caused by HSV-1) and herpes genitalis (caused by HSV-2) are the most common HSV-induced diseases. More than 85% of the world's population is seropositive for HSV-1. Incidence of HSV-1 is influenced by socio-economic status, geographic location, and age.

Herpes genitalis is one of the most common sexually transmitted diseases in the world. Seroconversion for HSV-2 rarely occurs before the onset of sexual activity. The strongest predictor for HSV-2 infection is the lifetime number of sexual partners. Seroprevalence is higher among women than men.

Transmission

Herpes simplex viruses are transmitted during personal contact through exchange of saliva, semen, cervical fluid, or vesicle fluid from active lesions. The virus must contact mucosal surfaces or abraded skin.

Co-infection with HSV and HIV frequently occurs, probably because they potentiate each other's transmission (see also Chapter 13).

Clinical manifestations

A prodrome may occur, characterized by localized pain, tingling, burning, tenderness, paraesthesiae, lymphadenopathy, headache, fever, anorexia, or malaise.

With disease progression, papules, vesicles on an erythematous base, and erosions may appear over hours to days. The lesions crust, then re-epithelialize, healing without scarring within 7–10 days. Other presentations include oedema, fissures, ulcers, and pustules. Cystitis, meningitis, urethritis, or cervicitis may be the presenting condition in some cases.

Herpes labialis (HSV-1)

Affects the buccal and gingival mucosa during primary infection. Termed gingivostomatitis, it is a common presentation in children. Lesions frequently appear at the vermilion border of the lip and consist of 3 to 5 vesicles that often become pustular, ulcerative, or crusted within 72 to 96 hours. The pain resolves quickly afterwards. During an episode, there may be difficulty swallowing due to oedema of the oropharynx. Most patients have approximately two outbreaks per year. Topical antivirals are effective. Oral aciclovir for herpes labialis has mixed therapeutic value.

Herpetic whitlow

This is an infection of the distal phalanx, caused by HSV-1 (more commonly) or HSV-2, and characterized by pain, tingling, burning, swelling, erythema, and vesicles on an erythematous base.

Herpes gladitorium (HSV-1)

Athletes involved in contact sports, such as wrestling, may develop HSV-1 infection of the head or eye. The trunk or extremities may also be involved.

HSV folliculitis

A viral folliculitis of the beard (herpes sycosis) or other parts of the body present as painful, grouped, erythematous, perifollicular vesicles.

HSV keratoconjunctivitis

This is the commonest cause of corneal blindness in the USA.

Herpes genitalis (HSV-2)

This disease is sexually transmitted and is caused by HSV-2. In women, lesions may involve the vulva, cervix, vagina, or perianal skin and extra-genital areas, such as buttocks, thighs, or perineum. Women have more severe disease and higher complication rates from the primary infection than men. Inguinal adenopathy, dysuria, and retention may result.

Men develop vesicles (often 6–10) most commonly on the glans penis or penile shaft. Perianal infection with proctitis is more common in homosexual men, and extra-genital disease may occur.

Oral aciclovir is effective when started within 24 hours of lesion formation, shortening the viral shedding and hastening lesion healing. Aciclovir is also used for the treatment of recurrent genital herpes. Valaciclovir is as effective as aciclovir for recurrences.

Neonatal herpes

Neonatal herpes simplex infections can have devastating consequences. Infection can range from involvement of the skin, eyes, mouth, as well as encephalitis or disseminated disease.

Herpes simplex virus in the immunocompromised

This group of patients develop more severe HSV infection. Recurrent outbreaks occur with greater frequency, and lesions may be extensive or persistent.

Investigations

Gold standard for diagnosis is viral culture. An adequate sample requires vigorous swabbing of the base of the lesions. A rapid diagnostic method involves unroofing the vesicle, scraping the base of the lesion, and examining the sample under the microscope, using the Tzanck smear technique.

Further reading

National Institute for Health and Care Excellence (2012). Herpes simplex - oral. Clinical knowledge summaries. <http://cks.nice.org.uk/herpes-simplex-oral>.

National Institute for Health and Care Excellence (2012). Herpes simplex - genital. Clinical knowledge summaries. <http://cks.nice.org.uk/herpes-simplex-genital>.

Yeung-Yue KA, Brentjens MH, Lee PC, Tyring SK (2002). Herpes simplex viruses 1 and 2. *Dermatologic Clinics*, **20**, 249–66.

Varicella zoster virus infection

Varicella zoster virus (human herpesvirus 3) causes varicella (or chickenpox) and herpes zoster (or shingles) (see also Chapter 6). Herpes zoster infection represents reactivation of latent varicella infection and develops in up to 20% of healthy adults and 50% of immunocompromised patients. The most important complications are post-herpetic neuralgia and herpes zoster ophthalmicus. Rarely, herpes zoster infection can occur in children.

Incidence

In the UK, the average incidence rate of varicella and herpes zoster between 1991 and 2000 was 1,291 and 373 per 100,000 population per year, respectively.

Aetiology

On resolution of primary varicella infection, residual viral segments travel up sensory nerve fibres and lodge in cranial or dorsal root ganglia. Exactly what triggers reactivation is unclear. Risk factors for reactivation include:

- Age >50 years.
- Immunocompromised state.
- Immunosuppressive drugs.
- HIV/AIDS.
- Bone marrow or organ transplantation.
- Cancer.
- Chronic steroid therapy.
- Psychological stress.
- Trauma.

Clinical features of herpes zoster

Four days to 2 weeks prior to the development of the classic unilateral dermatomal vesicular rash (usually one to three adjacent dermatomes), there may be a prodrome of pain and paraesthesiae in the zoster-affected dermatomes. The pain can be throbbing, sharp, stabbing, burning, or shooting. The skin sensations may be abnormal, such as tingling or itching. Malaise and dysaesthesia are frequently seen in the prodrome.

The rash appears proximally, then spreads distally along the affected dermatome. The initial lesions, erythematous papules, develop into vesicles within 12 to 24 hours. The vesicles become pustules in 3 days and crust over 7 to 10 days later. New lesions generally appear over no more than 3 to 7 days. Increased duration of the rash has been correlated with increased patient age. Zoster affecting the first division of the trigeminal nerve causes herpes zoster ophthalmicus, with lesions over the forehead, periocular area, and nose. Ophthalmic complications are the major risk in this condition.

Diagnosis

Diagnosis is made clinically. Laboratory confirmation can be made from viral culture or direct immunofluorescence assay. More recently, polymerase chain reaction testing from skin lesions is rapid and highly sensitive. Laboratory tests allow differentiation from herpes simplex infection.

Complications

These include:

- Secondary infection of the rash area.
- Post-herpetic neuralgia.
- Meningoencephalitis.
- Transverse myelitis.
- Cranial nerve palsies.
- Motor paralysis—rare (less than 5% of patients).
- Ramsay–Hunt syndrome—hearing loss, vertigo, and facial paraesthesiae.
- Cerebral arteritis, leading to stroke, can occur months after the acute infection.
- Lid ulceration.
- Conjunctivitis, keratitis, uveitis.
- Optic nerve neuritis.
- Retinal necrosis.
- Secondary glaucoma.
- Pneumonitis.
- Myocarditis.
- Hepatitis.
- Oesophagitis.

Management

Treatment for acute zoster aims to accelerate healing, control pain, and, when possible, reduce the risk of complications. Early intervention with antivirals can accelerate rash healing, reduce rash severity, and reduce the risk of some complications. The addition of corticosteroids to antiviral medication may further alleviate short-term zoster pain but is associated with an increased risk of serious adverse effects, especially among older patients.

For post-herpetic neuralgia, gabapentin, pregabalin, opioids, tricyclic antidepressants, lidocaine patch 5%, and capsaicin may all be considered.

Further reading

Tyring SK (2007). Management of herpes zoster and postherpetic neuralgia. *Journal of the American Academy of Dermatology*, **57** (Suppl 1), S136–42.

Bacterial infections affecting the skin

Meningococcal disease

Neisseria meningitides causes a spectrum of clinical syndromes, such as meningococcal meningitis, meningococcal bacteraemia, meningococcaemia, and respiratory tract infection (see also Chapter 6, section on 'Meningococcal disease').

Acute meningococcaemia may present with pink macules and papules. Petechiae and purpura develop, representing disseminated intravascular coagulation. The petechiae can coalesce and form haemorrhagic bullae and ulceration. In fulminant disease, purpura, ecchymoses, and grey/black necrosis occur, associated with disseminated intravascular coagulation. See Figure 17.7.

Cellulitis

This is a bacterial infection of the dermis and subcutaneous tissue that presents with painful, erythematous, warm, oedematous skin. Cellulitis can be caused by a variety of organisms. It commonly occurs at skin breaks in the skin, such as at surgical wound sites, trauma, tinea infection, ulceration, but can occasionally occur in normal skin. The leg affected by venous stasis is a frequent site.

There may be a fever, and investigations will reveal raised inflammatory markers. Treatment with a penicillinase-resistant penicillin, first-generation cephalosporin, co-amoxiclav, macrolide, or fluoroquinolone (in adults only) is appropriate. If disease is extensive, admission and intravenous therapy are indicated. Swabs and an anti-streptolysin O titre should also be performed.

Antibiotics should continue for at least 3 days after the resolution of acute inflammation.

In patients with diabetes, immunocompromised patients, and those with unresponsive infections or young children, an intravenous second- or third-generation cephalosporin should be considered.

Prophylactic antibiotics are needed in patients with recurrent cellulitis (for example, where there is venous disease) or in patients undergoing surgery or lymph node dissection, as venous or lymphatic circulation can be compromised, causing dermal fibrosis, lymphoedema, and epidermal thickening.

Erysipelas

Whereas cellulitis involves infection of the dermis and subcutaneous tissue, erysipelas is primarily an infection of the deep dermis, with lymphatic involvement. It is most often caused by *Streptococcus pyogenes*. Erysipelas presents as an intensely erythematous infection with clearly demarcated raised margins. There will be fever, chills, malaise, and nausea. The area is hot, tense, tender, and indurated with non-pitting oedema. Regional lymphadenopathy is present, with or without lymphatic streaking. There may be pustules, vesicles, bullae, and areas of haemorrhagic necrosis.

Common sites are the legs and face. Influenza-like symptoms often precede each case, and most cases do not have an initial skin lesion or wounds.

Treatment is with oral or intravenous penicillin. Complications are the same as for cellulitis.

Impetigo

Impetigo mostly affects young children aged between 2 and 5 years of age. It can be spread directly from person to

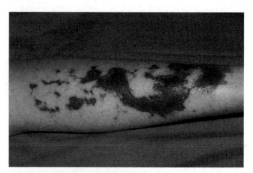

Figure 17.7 Meningococcal septicaemia.

person; therefore, hygiene is important to prevent spread. Nasal carriage may contribute to recurrent disease; therefore, a 2–5-day course of mupirocin nasally can reduce carriage.

Impetigo can be classified morphologically into a bullous and non-bullous variety. Both forms are thought to be caused by *Staphylococcus aureus*, with *Streptococcus* spp. usually involved in the non-bullous form.

The non-bullous form is the most common, and this presents as painful erosions, small vesicles, or pustules that have a honey-yellow crust. The bullous form presents with large, thin-walled blisters, 2–5 cm in size, containing serous yellow fluid. A mixture of morphologies can exist. Satellite lesions may be seen.

Treatment of impetigo is with topical and oral antibiotics. Complications include the small risk of a post-streptococcal glomerulonephritis, especially in children aged 2 to 6 years.

Carbuncles

These are an aggregate of infected hair follicles that create swollen, deep, painful, erythematous masses that open and drain through multiple tracts. There may be fever and malaise.

If the lesions are fluctuant or boggy, gentle incision and drainage is indicated. The wound may be packed to encourage further drainage. Caution is required not to incise deeper than the pseudocapsule that has developed at the site of infection.

In severe cases, intravenous antibiotics are indicated. Complications include the risk of gas-containing abscesses or necrotizing fasciitis (see section above).

Further reading

National Institute for Health and Care Excellence (2015). Cellulitis - acute. Clinical knowledge summaries. <http://cks.nice.org.uk/cellulitis-acute>.

Public Health England (2014). Guidance for public health management of meningococcal disease in the UK. <https://www.gov.uk/government/uploads/system/uploads/attachment_data/file/322008/Guidance_for_management_of_meningococcal_disease_pdf.pdf>.

Stulberg D, Penrod M, Blatny R (2002). Common bacterial skin infections. *American Family Physician*, **66**, 119–24.

Fungal infections affecting the skin

Fungal infections are generally divided into four types:

1. Superficial, including tinea versicolor, piedra, and tinea nigra.
2. Cutaneous, including onychomycosis, tinea capitis, tinea corporis, tinea barbae, tinea pedis, and candidiasis of skin, mucosa, and nails.
3. Subcutaneous, including mycetoma, sporotrichosis, and chromoblastomycosis.
4. Systemic, including North American blastomycosis and cryptococcosis.

The superficial fungal infections are caused by dermatophytes and *Candida* species.

Infections caused by dermatophytes include tinea pedis, tinea cruris, and tinea capitis, affecting the feet, groin, and scalp, respectively. Tinea can become secondarily infected by bacteria.

Tinea corporis affects the trunk and extremities. There are various clinical presentations. Infection spreads centrifugally, and there are typically annular lesions with a central clearing of the fungus. Most are scaly, although this is lessened if topical steroids have been used (tinea incognito). The lesions may also be vesicular, granulomatous, or verrucous. See Figure 17.8.

Pityriasis versicolor presents with multiple oval to round patches or thin plaques with mild scale. The patches can be brown, tan, or pink. The condition is asymptomatic and is caused by *Malassezia* spp.

The subcutaneous infections, with some exceptions, mainly occur in the tropics and subtropics. Amongst others, this group includes sporotrichosis, mycetoma, and chromoblastomycosis.

Sporotrichosis

This is caused by the dimorphic fungus *Sporothrix schenckii* found in decaying vegetation, soil, timbers, thorns, animal claws, and sphagnum moss. Florists, gardeners, vets, farmers, and laboratory workers are at risk. It can be classified into three forms:

- Lymphocutaneous sporotrichosis—the most common form, characterized by painless, hard, pink nodules, appearing 3 weeks to 6 months after infection. Lesions may undergo necrosis and ulcerate. Lymphatic spread occurs, and lesions occur following the lymphatic tract of the area.
- Fixed cutaneous sporotrichosis—presents as localized lesions involving the face, neck, trunk, and legs, without lymphatic involvement. Lesions manifest as ulcerated nodules, verrucous plaques, scaly patches, and/or acneiform eruptions.
- Disseminated sporotrichosis—occurs via haematogenous spread from a primary infection site or regional lymph node involved in primary infection. Kidneys, testes, bones, joints, lungs, and CNS can be affected. This form is rare and is usually in association with immunosuppression.

Cryptococcosis

Cryptococcus neoformans is a dimorphic fungus seen in pigeon droppings and nesting places, soil, and dust. After

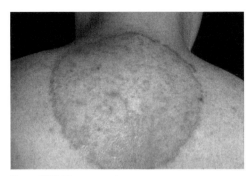

Figure 17.8 Tinea corporis.

exposure, immunosuppressed individuals or those with connective tissue disease are at increased risk for this disease. Cryptococcosis is the most common systemic mycotic infection in AIDS patients.

The condition can manifest as primary cutaneous and disseminated systemic disease. Primary cutaneous cryptococcosis results from direct infection from an object contaminated with *Cryptococcus*. This rare presentation would manifest as a single lesion at the site of infection.

Disseminated cryptococcosis begins as an infection in the respiratory tract that spreads haematogenously from the primary pulmonary site to the skin, prostate, liver, kidneys, bone, and peritoneum. Lesions mostly appear on the head and neck, first as painless papules or pustules, then developing into nodules that ulcerate. The condition may also present as vasculitic lesions or plaques. Secondary osteomyelitis may develop.

Histoplasmosis

This is caused by the dimorphic fungus *Histoplasma capsulatum*, found most often in contaminated soil enriched by bird and bat droppings. Clinical manifestations include primary pulmonary, disseminated, primary cutaneous, and African histoplasmoses. Patients with primary pulmonary disease frequently report erythema nodosum, erythema multiforme, and panniculitis, together with pulmonary symptoms.

Disseminated histoplasmosis spreads haematogenously to the skin, liver, spleen, bone marrow, and lymph nodes. It affects immunocompromised patients and is an AIDS-defining illness. It also affects patients with a genetic predisposition and psoriatic patients treated with methotrexate.

Lesions may first appear on the extremities and trunk as pink plaques which ulcerate and become infected. Other cutaneous manifestations include umbilicated nodules, abscesses, pustules, purpura, petechiae, exfoliative erythroderma, and eczematous lesions.

Further reading

Schwartz RA (2004). Superficial fungal infections. *Lancet*, **364**, 1173–82.
Trent JT and Kirsner RS (2003). Identifying and treating mycotic skin infections. *Advances in Skin & Wound Care*, **16**, 122–9.

Ectoparasitic disease

Ectoparasites are parasites that live on the outside of a host on the skin or hair and cause external infestation or act as a vector for disease.

Scabies

Scabies is an infestation caused by the mite *Sarcoptes scabiei var. hominis*. The infestation is spread directly from person to person and is highly contagious. It is seen worldwide. It can affect any age group but is commoner in the elderly and the immunosuppressed. Crusted scabies, or Norwegian scabies, is seen in the immunosuppressed where, rather than around 12 mites on an individual, thousands may be seen.

Symptoms are of a severe, generalized pruritus. The pruritus is worse at night. Symptoms may start 3 to 4 weeks after infestation or within a day or two of reinfestation. Immunosuppressed patients with crusted scabies may not itch. The patient may have family members who are also itchy.

Burrows present as short linear or serpiginous grey ridges on the skin surface. They are typically seen on the hands, feet, interdigital web spaces, and wrists and are pathognomonic of scabies.

Vesicles, pustules, papules, and nodules may be seen, especially in the genital and axillary regions. In men, itchy papules or nodules on the penis are pathognomonic of scabies. In babies and young children, scabies also affects the scalp, face, palms, and soles of the feet.

A widespread erythema or eczema may be seen.

Diagnosis is based on clinical findings and history. Diagnosis can be confirmed by skin scrapings of mites and eggs from the burrows viewed microscopically using a drop of potassium hydroxide on a slide. A dermatoscope may also be used to examine the burrows.

The treatment choice for scabies in the UK is permethrin 5% dermal cream, applied on two occasions 1 week apart. Wash the cream off 12 hours later. All members of a household should be treated at the same time as well as the patient's sexual partner.

In adults, apply the cream to the entire body, except the head and neck. Include under the fingernails, the interdigital web spaces, and genitalia. In children, the head, neck, face, and ears should also be treated.

Clothes and bed linen should be washed in temperatures greater than 50°C.

Other treatment options include topical malathion, benzyl benzoate, 10% crotamiton cream, and 2–10% sulphur in petroleum.

In multiresistant crusted scabies, a single oral dose of ivermectin 200 mcg/kg can be used.

Tungiasis

Tungiasis is caused by the gravid female sand flea *Tunga penetrans* that is endemic from Mexico to Northern Argentina, several Caribbean islands, sub-Saharan Africa, and Madagascar.

Characteristically, one may see periungual lesions as red/pink papules with an erythematous halo. The clinical manifestations depend on the stage of the sand flea life cycle.

- Over 24–48 hours, the gravid female sand flea swells, and the lesion becomes a white papule with a central dark spot (the rear cone of the flea).
- There may be desquamation around the edges.
- Shiny white eggs can be seen 2–21 days after penetration.

- 3–5 weeks later, the flea dies and leaves a black crust.
- A circular depression may remain for several months.

Symptoms include a foreign body sensation, pain, and sometimes intense itching. Although tungiasis resolves spontaneously, it is best to treat it initially to reduce the risk of potential complications, including cellulitis, lymphoedema, sepsis, tetanus, and chronic ulceration.

Treatment options include:

- Surgical removal, using scalpel and fine forceps, or a punch biopsy under sterile conditions and using a topical antiseptic afterwards.
- Oral ivermectin and oral thiabendazole have been used.

Myiasis

Bed bugs are nocturnal blood-sucking ectoparasites. The common bed bug *Cimex lectularius* is present in temperate and tropical climates and found in furniture, wallpaper, clothes, and luggage.

Clinically, insect bites will present in a variety of forms from urticated wheals to haemorrhagic blisters (see Figure 17.9). They form linear patterns or clusters and are often seen around the waist or axillae or on areas left uncovered by clothing.

Treatment is symptomatic and includes symptom relief with oral antihistamines and topical corticosteroids. The bed bugs are killed by heat; therefore, hot washing of clothes and bedding, along with steam cleaning of furniture or treatment with insecticides, is needed.

Tick-borne disease

Mediterranean spotted fever (endemic in Southern Europe, Africa, and India)

Mediterranean spotted fever is caused by *Rickettsia conorii* and transmitted by the brown dog tick.

Presentation is with high fever and a maculopapular rash, and there can be petechiae. In 70% of patients, there is a black eschar at the site of tick inoculation.

Treat with doxycycline.

Rocky Mountain spotted fever (endemic to parts of America)

This tick-borne infection is caused by *Rickettsia rickettsii*, transmitted by dog and wood ticks.

Symptoms include malaise, headache, nausea, vomiting, and fever. The macular exanthema begins acrally and

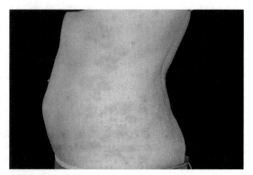

Figure 17.9 Insect bite reaction.

spreads centrally. Petechiae may coalesce to form ecchymoses and ulceration.

Treat with a tetracycline, such as doxycycline 100 mg bd for 5–7 days or until the patient is afebrile for 2–3 days. As there is a direct association between time delay from symptoms, to onset of treatment and subsequent mortality, commence treatment as soon as suspected.

Lyme disease (endemic to the USA and Europe)

Borrelia burgdorferi is transmitted by a deer tick and causes Lyme disease and is the most common tick-borne infection in the USA and Europe.

There may be constitutional symptoms, such as headache, arthralgia, malaise, fever, and headache, with 70% of cases developing erythema migrans, an indurated erythematous macule that often clears centrally, leaving an annular lesion (see also Chapter 6: Figure 6.1).

There may also be a borrelial lymphocytome, a purplish nodule that occurs on the earlobe, nipple, or nose. Cranial nerve palsies, radiculopathies, or meningitis can occur.

Investigations include specific IgG and IgM antibody testing to *B. burgdorferi*. ELISA and polymerase chain testing can be performed on tissue and spinal fluid if further conformation is needed.

Treatment of Lyme disease must not be delayed, pending results. Doxycycline is the drug of choice for early Lyme disease. Intravenous penicillin and ceftriaxone are used for neuroborreliosis.

HIV infection and the skin

The skin is always affected in HIV disease. Common dermatoses may present more frequently and with increased severity. Rare and atypical presentations are more common. It may be difficult to differentiate one clinical diagnosis from another, and skin biopsy is often indicated for histology and culture. Below is a summary of skin conditions that may present acutely in HIV-positive individuals.

Acute HIV seroconversion is an acute febrile illness, usually occurring 2–6 weeks after HIV exposure.

- Skin lesions can be seen in 75% of cases:
  - Acute urticaria.
  - Infectious exanthema.

The illness is similar to infectious mononucleosis or aseptic meningitis. The skin lesions consist of an erythematous maculopapular rash, with areas of confluence over the trunk, and can involve the palms and soles. Lesions can become keratotic or haemorrhagic. Oral-genital erosions may occur. Presentations also include urticaria or erythema multiforme.

Differential diagnosis is of other viral and bacterial infections, rickettsial infection, mycoplasma, strongyloides, and toxoplasma.

Inflammatory conditions

Seborrhoeic dermatitis is the most common dermatosis in HIV.

Psoriasis, although not increased in incidence, may flare severely or arise *de novo* such that it may be the first presentation of HIV disease.

Reiter's syndrome, consisting of the triad of non-gonococcal urethritis, arthritis, and conjunctivitis, is much more common. Cutaneous features include keratoderma blenorrhagicum, circinate balanitis, and oral ulceration.

Bacterial infections

Staphylococcus aureus infections are common and range from boils to staphylococcal scalded skin syndrome and toxic epidermal necrolysis. meticillin (INN)-resistant *Staphylococcal aureus* should be suspected.

Bartonella quintana and *Bartonella henselae* can cause bacillary angiomatosis, clinically characterized by angiomatous lesions. It occurs when the CD4 count is less than 200 cells/microlitre. History may include a preceding cat scratch or bite. Single and multiple red-purple papules present in varying sizes. The differential diagnosis includes pyogenic granuloma, Kaposi's sarcoma, and haemangiomas. Biopsy is indicated, and first-line treatment is erythromycin 500 mg four times daily for 8–12 weeks.

Mycobacterial infection rarely present with skin lesions. Acute forms can include miliary tuberculosis, in which crops of bluish papules, vesicles, pustules, or haemorrhagic lesions may occur. Treatment is a specialist area.

Viral infections

Herpes simplex virus infection is very common (see Section: 'Herpes simplex viruses 1 and 2'). Its usual characteristic features may not be seen, especially in advanced disease. The lesions may be more verrucous or vegetative, show deeper ulcers, and be more resistant to treatment.

Investigations include a Tsanck smear, direct fluorescent antibody staining or viral culture. Serologic tests have no value in diagnosing cutaneous HSV infection.

Treat with oral or intravenous aciclovir at a dose for immunocompromised individuals. For frequent relapses or slowly healing lesions, a continuous suppressive dose of 400 mg bd may be indicated.

Herpes zoster also has an increased incidence (see also Section: 'Varicella zoster virus infection', and Chapters 6 and 13). In advanced HIV disease, multi-dermatomal lesions are more common, and there may be widespread dissemination of lesions similar to primary varicella. The eruption may be vesicopustular or even haemorrhagic or necrotic. If the ophthalmic branch of the trigeminal nerve is involved, early ophthalmological assessment is mandatory.

Investigations include a Tsanck smear (from the base of the lesions) but will not differentiate between HSV and VZV. Viral culture and fluorescent antibody testing will help to identify the diagnosis.

Treat with 800 mg of oral aciclovir five times a day until the lesions are healed for uncomplicated infection. In complicated cases, admit to hospital, and use intravenous aciclovir at a dose of 10 mg/kg every 8 hours for 7–10 days.

Molluscum contagiosum is caused by a pox virus and occurs in up to 20% of patients with advanced HIV disease. Molluscum are characterized by 3–5 mm pink or skin-coloured papules with central umbilication.

Differential diagnosis includes disseminated cryptococcus and histoplasmosis. On the face, differentials include syringomas and comedones.

Treatment options include cryotherapy, electrocoagulation, curettage, shave excision, carbon dioxide laser, application of topical wart preparations, 5-fluorouracil, and imiquimod.

Human papilloma virus infection is common as verrucae and condylomata accuminata. They are often refractory to conventional topical treatment, and recurrence is common.

Cytomegalovirus infection rarely has skin manifestations but can include ulceration (especially perianal and oral), papulovesicular eruptions, purpura, nodules, and verrucous lesions.

Epstein–Barr virus infection can lead to oral hairy leukoplakia. These are usually asymptomatic and appear as corrugated white plaques, with hair-like projections on the lateral aspect of the tongue (see Figure 17.10). The lesions have no malignant potential. They do not require treatment unless unsightly or if causing dysphagia.

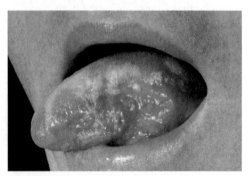

Figure 17.10 Oral hairy leukoplakia.

Fungal infections

Mucocutaneous candidiasis is common in HIV. Manifestations include:

- Onychomycosis (fungal nail infection).
- Acute and chronic paronychia, causing tenderness and fluctuance of the nail bed.
- Intertrigo (flexures become macerated, red, and tender, with characteristic satellite pustules).
- Oropharyngeal candidiasis.

Onychomycosis must be proven by mycology (microscopy and culture) and requires a prolonged course of systemic anticandidal treatment, whereas acute paronychia and intertrigo can respond to a topical agent, such as miconazole. Oropharyngeal candidiasis will require systemic treatment.

Dermatophyte infections in HIV may present with unusual morphology, and they often mimic inflammatory conditions, such as psoriasis or seborrhoeic dermatitis, but fungal infections have asymmetric lesions. Diagnosis is confirmed from fungal scrapings and hair plucks (if on the scalp). For tinea pedis, a broad-spectrum topical antifungal is sufficient; however, for most other forms of fungal infection, a systemic antifungal is likely to be required, such as an imidazole, triazole, or terbinafine, having proven the diagnosis mycologically.

Deep fungal infections, such as *Cryptococcus*, histoplasmosis, and sporotrichosis, may present with skin lesions which are investigated with biopsy for culture and histology.

Skin infestations

Scabies is caused by the mite *Sarcoptes scabiei*. Infection is through close contact. Characteristic signs and symptoms include:

- Generalized pruritus.
- Pink papules and large indurated nodules around axillae, periareolar regions, abdomen, buttocks, thighs, scrotum, and penis.
- Scabetic burrows in the interdigital web spaces.
- Excoriation.
- Secondary eczematous change may be seen.

In advanced HIV, there may be crusted scabies (Norwegian scabies), in which there are millions of mites infecting the skin. This is highly contagious and requires careful (barrier) nursing management.

Diagnosis is made clinically and confirmed by microscopy: a scabetic burrow is scraped with a blunt scalpel onto a microscopic slide and a drop of 10% potassium hydroxide is added to clear the keratin and identify the mites and eggs.

Treatment of scabies is with either topical permethrin or malathion over the entire body and treatment is repeated a week later. Close contacts should be treated. Crusted scabies may be resistant to topical treatment and may require a single dose of ivermectin 200 mg/kg. The crusts can be removed with warm bath soaks.

Neoplasia

Kaposi's sarcoma (KS) is the commonest malignancy of AIDS. This rare endothelial-derived multifocal tumour is seen in its classical form in immune-competent individuals and has a separate distinct form in HIV-infected individuals.

Although rarely fatal in HIV, there is an aggressive form that may progress rapidly and enlarge over weeks, causing death, often from lung involvement. Therefore, on suspecting KS, urgent referral to the HIV or dermatology team is indicated.

The disease usually affects the skin, gut, lungs, and lymphoreticular system. Clinically, early presentation is as asymptomatic pink, brown, or purple-coloured macules that can then enlarge to become firm or hard violaceous plaques, nodules, or tumours. There should be a low threshold for biopsy. Initially the lesions can be clinically difficult to differentiate from pigmented melanocytic naevi, angiomas, dermatofibroma, purpura, pyogenic granuloma, bacillary angiomatosis lesions, and lichen planus.

Kaposi's sarcoma will often resolve several months after the commencement of HAART. Specific treatment is generally reserved for persistent disease. This includes radiotherapy or surgical excision amongst others.

Lymphomas are also seen in HIV.

Drug eruptions

Cutaneous drug eruptions are more frequent in the presence of HIV. The most common form of drug eruption is the maculopapular ('morbilliform') rash, also described as 'toxic erythema'. Stevens–Johnson syndrome and toxic epidermal necrolysis are also thought to occur at increased frequency in HIV disease.

Further reading

Bunker CB, Gotch F (2010). HIV and the Skin. In Burns T, Breathnach S, Cox N, Griffiths C, eds. *Rook's Textbook of Dermatology*, 8th edn, pp. 35.1–35.10. Wiley-Blackwell Publishing Ltd, Chichester.

Malignant melanoma

Malignant melanoma is increasingly common and often not identified early. Missed diagnosis is an important cause of litigation. The incidence of melanoma in the UK is approximately 10 cases per 100,000 population per annum and is fatal unless identified early.

Malignant melanoma may be an incidental finding in patients who present as an emergency. Early identification will save lives.

Aetiology

High-risk individuals include those with fair complexions who burn easily, never tan, and have sunlight for short intense periods of time, especially in childhood. Other factors include multiple atypical melanocytic naevi, congenital melanocytic naevus, and those who have had a previous melanoma or have an immediate family member diagnosed with melanoma.

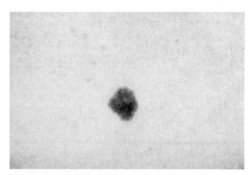

Figure 17.11 Superficial spreading melanoma.

History and clinical features

There are internationally described major and minor features:

- Major:
  - Change in size.
  - Irregular shape.
  - Irregular colour.
  - Duration of the lesion (as recommended by 2010 UK guidelines).
- Minor:
  - Largest diameter 7 mm or more.
  - Inflammation.
  - Oozing.
  - Change in sensation.

Lesions with any of the major features or three of the minor ones are suspicious of melanoma.

The ABCD acronym also aids clinical analysis.

- **A**—Asymmetry.
- **B**—Border and bleeding.
- **C**—Colour—melanoma lesions may constitute a variety of colours, such as brown, black, red, and blue. Most benign moles have a homogenous brown colour. Pigment variegation is suspicious.
- **D**—Diameter. Larger moles, generally greater than 0.6 mm, are more likely to be suspicious.

Some clinicians add an 'E' to the acronym for evolution of the mole or egregious signs or symptoms.

All patients presenting with suspected melanoma should have their lymph nodes examined and their abdomen palpated for organomegaly. Differential diagnoses include pyogenic granuloma (Figure 17.12). This is a benign vascular lesion occuring most commonly in children and young adults.

There are four major subtypes of melanoma.

1. Superficial spreading melanoma—the most common type of melanoma in fair-skinned individuals. It begins as a brown to black macule, with colour variegation and irregular notched borders. A papule or nodule may subsequently occur, with the development of the vertical growth phase. See Figure 17.11.
2. Nodular melanoma—these usually present as a blue to black or pink to red-coloured nodule which may be ulcerated or bleeding and have developed rapidly over months. See Figure 17.13.

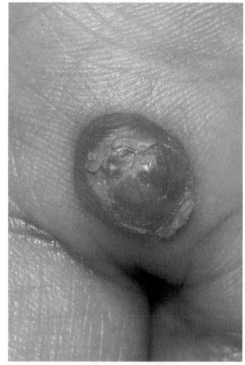

Figure 17.12 Pyogenic granuloma: another differential diagnosis of melanoma.

3. Lentigo malignant melanoma—this is diagnosed mainly in the seventh decade of life on chronically sun-damaged skin. It develops as a slow-growing, asymmetric brown to black macule, with colour variegation and an irregular indented border. It arises in a precursor lesion called a lentigo maligna. 5% of lentigo malignas progress to invasive melanoma.
4. Acral lentiginous melanoma—this tends to occur on palms or soles or in and around the nails. It represents a

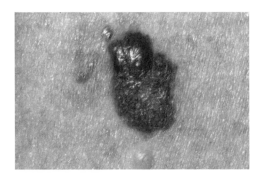

Figure 17.13 Nodular melanoma.

large proportion of melanomas in blacks and Asians. Amelanotic melanomas are an important consideration; the differential diagnosis of which includes a pyogenic granuloma. See Figure 17.12.

Preventing melanoma

All individuals should be advised to avoid sunburn and limit their total cumulative sun exposure throughout life. Sun protection with adequate clothing is preferred to topical sunscreens.

Investigations

Lesions suspicious of melanoma should be excised to full thickness to include the whole tumour, with a 2 to 5 mm clinical margin of skin laterally and a cuff of subdermal fat.

Treatment

On histological confirmation of melanoma, re-excision may be mandated by the Breslow thickness.

Follow-up

Five-year follow-up is recommended to monitor the scar, remaining naevi and to examine for enlarged lymph nodes and for organomegaly. Follow-up should be 3-monthly for the first 3 years and 6-monthly for the subsequent 2 years. All patients should be taught self-examination, as recurrence of the disease is often first noticed by the patient.

Further reading

Marsden JR, Newton-Bishop JA, Burrows M, et al., British Association of Dermatologists (2010). Revised UK guidelines for the management of cutaneous melanoma 2010. British Journal of Dermatology, **163**, 238–256.

National Institute for Health and Care Excellence (2015). Melanoma: assessment and management. NICE guideline 14. <https://www.nice.org.uk/guidance/ng14>.

Roberts DL, Anstey AV, Barlow RJ, et al., British Association of Dermatologists; Melanoma Study Group (2002). UK guidelines for the management of cutaneous melanoma. British Journal of Dermatology, **146**, 7–17.

Non-melanoma skin cancer

The term 'non-melanoma skin cancer' encompasses cutaneous lymphoma, Merkel cell carcinomas, and other neoplasms but is mainly used to define squamous cell and basal cell carcinomas. In the UK, the incidence of non-melanoma skin cancer is estimated at around 100,000 cases per year. The incidence of squamous cell carcinoma has risen annually since the 1960s.

Squamous cell carcinoma

Primary cutaneous squamous cell carcinoma (SCC) is a form of non-melanoma skin cancer that originates from epithelial keratinocytes or their appendages. It is the second most common skin malignancy. Although mortality is low, associated morbidity is high. SCC may be an incidental finding in patients presenting with other conditions, but early diagnosis will reduce morbidity.

Aetiology

Squamous cell carcinoma has multiple aetiologies. It may arise *de novo* or as a result of previous ultraviolet ionizing radiation, arsenic exposure, within chronic wounds or scars, or from pre-existing lesions, such as SCC *in situ*, Bowen's disease (intraepidermal SCC), bowenoid papulosis, or erythroplasia of Queyrat (SCC of the penis).

Factors associated with the development of squamous cell carcinoma include:

- Chronic UV exposure.
- Fair skin that burns easily.
- Geographic latitude.
- Genodermatosis.
- Human papillomavirus infection.
- HIV infection.
- Psoralen UV-A therapy.
- Chronic inflammatory conditions.
- Allogeneic transplant recipients.
- Smoking.
- Male gender age >50 years.

SCCs can occur in injured or chronically diseased skin, such as long-standing ulcers, sinus tracts, osteomyelitis, radiation dermatitis, or vaccination scars. They also occur in genital areas. Chronic inflammatory dermatoses that predispose to the development of squamous cell carcinoma include discoid lupus erythematosus, lichen sclerosis, lichen planus, dystrophic epidermolysis bullosa, and cutanous tuberculosis. SCCs arising from damaged skin appear to be more aggressive.

Clinical features

Most SCCs arise on sun-damaged skin of the head and neck. Fewer lesions arise on the extremities and on the trunk. Early lesions frequently present as erythematous, scaly papules. Later lesions may form nodules or firm plaques, either of which can ulcerate.

Bowen's disease (SCC *in situ* or intraepidermal carcinoma) presents as an asymptomatic, well-defined, erythematous scaly plaque on sun-exposed areas, in particular, the face and legs.

Squamous cell carcinomas typically metastasize 1 to 2 years after initial diagnosis. It tends to spread to local lymph

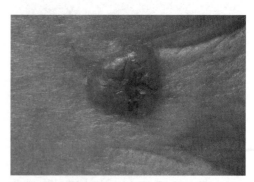

Figure 17.14 Basal cell carcinoma.

nodes before distant metastasis occurs. Certain parameters determine SCCs that are at high risk of metastasis:

- Size greater than 2 cm.
- Depth greater than 4 mm.
- Poorly differentiated histology or perineural invasion.
- Immunosuppressed patients.
- Previous radiotherapy.

Excision remains the treatment of choice.

Follow-up

Patients with histologically proven SCC should be followed up in a dermatology clinic.

Basal cell carcinoma

Basal cell carcinoma (BCC) is a tumour of proliferating basaloid keratinocytes. There are numerous subtypes, including nodular, superficial, morpheaform, cystic, and basosquamous (see Figure 17.14). It is locally invasive and can be aggressive and destructive. However, basal cell carcinomas rarely metastasize. The best treatment is excision.

Keratoacanthomas

These are fast-growing cutaneous neoplasms that usually show spontaneous regression. They usually present as flesh-coloured dome-shaped papules with a central keratin plug. The tumour grows to a rapid size (1 to 2 cm) over 2 months before spontaneously involuting after 3 to 6 months. Clinically, they can be difficult to differentiate from SCC. Histology is helpful, as the keratinocytes are well differentiated and cytological atypia is minimal. If hyperchromatic nuclei or abnormal mitoses are prominent, then a diagnosis of an ordinary invasive SCC is made.

Further reading

Madan V, Lear JT, Szeimies RM (2010). Non-melanoma skin cancer. *Lancet*, **375**, 673–85.

National Institute for Health and Care Excellence (2010). Improving outcomes for people with skin tumours including melanoma. NICE guideline CSGSTIM. <https://www.nice.org.uk/guidance/csgstim>.

Cutaneous T cell lymphoma

Cutaneous T cell lymphoma (CTCL) is a subset of non-Hodgkin's T cell lymphomas, in which patients present with a malignant lymphocytic infiltration of the skin. There are subtypes of CTCL which have different clinical features. Advanced disease can present with erythroderma, and the patient will be at risk of all the complications of erythroderma, such as electrolyte imbalance, fluid loss, and infection. Generalized erythroderma is often accompanied by pruritus, scaling, alopecia, and oedema.

Epidemiology
Two subtypes of CTCL include mycosis fungoides (MF) and Sézary syndrome (SS). MF and SS make up 65% of newly diagnosed CTCL cases. Men are more commonly affected than females.

Clinical features
CTCL manifests as patches, plaques, tumours, and generalized erythroderma. Early stages are sometimes mistaken for a contact dermatitis, atopic dermatitis, or psoriasis. Patients with early disease characteristically have erythematous flat patches that can involve all body surfaces but are typically on the trunk.

Over time, the patches become well demarcated and raised. As the disease progresses, the patches become increasingly infiltrated and ulcerate which increases the risk of infection.

Generalized erythroderma signals advanced disease and can be severely symptomatic, often with intense pruritus, scaling, alopecia, and oedema. These patients are at increased risk of peripheral blood involvement and of Sézary syndrome, in which there will be circulating atypical lymphocytes called Sézary cells.

Investigations
Diagnosis is made on the clinical findings and skin biopsy. Immunophenotyping of the infiltrate can aid diagnosis and further defines the clonal population.

Management
Treatment modalities for CTCL remain conservative and skin-directed in early disease. For acute presentation or deterioration of CTCL, admit the patient and manage as one would for all erythrodermic patients (see 'Erythroderma').

Topical agents for early disease have a good evidence base:

- Topical corticosteroids.
- Topical mechlorethamine.
- Topical carmustine.
- Topical retinoids.
- Psoralen plus UV-A irradiation.
- Total skin electron beam therapy.
- Superficial X-irradiation.

There is no cure, so palliation and symptom control comprise management. With disease progression, systemic therapy, such as chemotherapy and immunotherapy, may be indicated.

Prognosis
Patient prognosis and appropriate treatment options depend on the stage of the disease. End-stage disease has a 5-year survival estimate of 0–15%, whereas early disease has a 5-year survival of 96–100%.

Further reading
Bagot M (2008). Introduction: cutaneous T-cell lymphoma (CTCL) classification, staging, and treatment option. *Dermatology Clinics*, **26** (Suppl 1), 3–12.

Chapter 18

Disorders due to physical agents

Trauma

Trauma is the leading cause of death in young people (<40 years old). It is categorized as:

- **Blunt trauma** which is relatively common and usually due to road traffic accidents (RTA), falls, or assaults. It can be difficult to treat because injuries are often internal, multiple, and not easily recognized.
- **Penetrating trauma** from stabbing or gunshot wound, which is less common.

Initial triage aims to identify patients with acute life-threatening injuries. Severe (± multiple) trauma cases can be rapidly recognized by the presence of reduced consciousness, respiratory distress, and shock. Assessment, diagnosis, and treatment need to be concurrent, and lack of a definitive diagnosis must not delay appropriate therapy. Initial assessment can be made at the scene of the injury or on arrival in hospital. In any event, the Advanced Trauma Life Support (ATLS) programme recommends a structured approach to management by a well-organized trauma team. Treat the greatest risk to life first (i.e. ABC system), recognizing that airways obstruction is more rapidly fatal than inadequate ventilation, which is more serious than loss of circulating volume, followed by expanding intracranial mass lesions.

Although early resuscitation reduces morbidity and mortality, pre-hospital treatment is usually limited to ensuring adequate oxygenation, ventilation, and spinal immobilization. Fluid resuscitation should not delay transfer to hospital. Immobilization is recommended in most, if not all, multiple trauma patients, and the spine should be assumed to be vulnerable until cleared by an appropriate senior clinician (most often in the emergency department), surgeon, or radiologist. The sequence of management is as follows:

Primary survey and emergency resuscitation

Airway maintenance and cervical spine protection

Ensure a patent upper airway, and initiate oxygen therapy. Immobilize the cervical spine (see later text) with manual in-line stabilization (MILS; see Figure 18.1) and a hard cervical collar, with sandbags, tape, and rigid spinal board. If the airway is at risk, intubate the patient using rapid sequence induction, with MILS and cricoid pressure. Hypotension may occur during anaesthetic induction due to hypovolaemia.

Breathing

Treat immediate life-threatening chest injuries (see later text), and anticipate pneumothorax (± tension), especially in intubated patients. Head-injured patients at risk of hypoxia, hypercapnia, and shock (see later text) may need prophylactic mechanical ventilation (MV).

Circulation

Haemorrhage and the associated hypovolaemic shock are the main causes of avoidable post-injury death. Visible bleeding is stemmed with direct pressure. Occult or concealed bleeding occurs with fractures, haemothorax, retroperitoneal haematoma, and peritoneal cavity haemorrhage. Although less common, other causes of shock include sepsis, myocardial contusion (± tamponade), tension pneumothorax, and neurogenic shock (secondary survey). Clinical features associated with increasingly severe haemorrhage are reported in Table 18.1. In young patients, hypotension and shock may not be apparent until >30% loss of intravascular volume. Initially, establish intravenous access (i.e. large-bore cannulae), cross-match blood, and monitor the ECG and blood pressure. The appropriate resuscitation fluids are discussed in later text, but blood is indicated if the haematocrit is <0.3 or haemoglobin level <10 g/dL. Fluid replacement is guided by appropriate monitoring and aims to prevent ischaemia and organ dysfunction. Early surgical control of haemorrhage is essential when feasible.

Neurological status

Rapidly assess initial responsiveness (i.e. alert, verbal stimuli response, painful stimuli response, unresponsive), pupillary light responses, lateralizing signs, and potential spinal cord injury level. The Glasgow coma score (GCS; see Table 1.2 in Chapter 1) establishes conscious level and is predictive of patient outcome. Check for recent drugs and blood sugar or alcohol levels. Immobilization is vital if spinal cord or cervical injury is suspected. Log-roll, and move the patient as a single unit onto a rigid spine board, with cervical hard collar, sandbags, and tape to secure the head.

General management

Undress the patient to facilitate examination, but try to avoid aggravating hypothermia. Urine output should be monitored, but urethral injury must be excluded before catheterization. If a basal skull fracture is suspected, an orogastric, rather than nasogastric, tube is used to reduce the

Manual in-line cervical immobilization

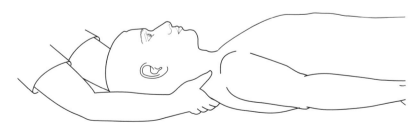

Figure18.1 Manual in-line cervical immobilization. Reproduced from Richard M. Leach, Acute and Critical Care Medicine at a Glance, second edition, Figure a, Chapter 52, page 110, Wiley, Copyright 2009, with permission.

Table 18.1 Classification of haemorrhage severity

Class	Blood loss	Approx volume loss (70 kg man)	Clinical signs
Class 1	<15%	<750 mL	Minimal signs
Class 2	15–30%	<1,500 mL	↑ HR + ↓ BP; sweating ↓ pulse pressure
Class 3	30–40%	<2,000 mL	Agitated, sweating, oliguria, ↑ HR (>120/min) ↓ BP (systolic ~90 mmHg)
Class 4	>40%	>2,000 mL	Preterminal, drowsy ↓ BP (systolic <90 mmHg)

Reproduced from *Advanced Trauma Life Support Program for Doctors*, Eighth Edition, Committee on Trauma, American College of Surgeons, Copyright 2008, with permission from American College of Surgeons.

risk of meningeal infection and also avoids placement in the cranial vault in mid-face trauma.

Adequate analgesia may be difficult to achieve, as the contracted circulating volume results in exaggerated haemodynamic responses. Trauma physicians recommend small incremental doses of intravenous opiate. Experienced anaesthetists may use nerve blocks as an opiate-sparing strategy, especially for lower limb fractures. Ketamine is useful in the shocked patient.

After basic initial X-rays, most trauma units rapidly progress to extensive CT scan surveys which may improve outcome and certainly saves hours of uncertainty. These patients need to be accompanied during imaging.

Secondary survey and definitive treatment

Following initial resuscitation, detailed clinical examination and referral for specialist therapy is required. If, at any time during the secondary survey, the patient deteriorates, the primary survey must be repeated.

Head and face

Examine for lacerations, haematomas, eye and orbit injuries, depressed fractures, and mobile mid-face or mandibular segments. Typical clinical features of basal skull fracture include racoon eyes, subhyloid haemorrhage, bruising over the mastoids (Battle's sign), CSF rhinorrhoea (or otorrhoea), and haemotympanum. Head injury is discussed in later text.

Chest

Life-threatening bronchial injuries, pulmonary or cardiac contusions, and aortic, oesophageal, or diaphragmatic ruptures must be detected and treated (see later text).

Abdomen

Suspect concealed intra-abdominal bleeding or viscus perforation if shock persists despite fluid resuscitation. Abdominal bruising, lacerations, tenderness, and distension may be detected. Rectal examination reveals bleeding due to bowel injury. A high prostate occurs with urethral injury, and reduced anal sphincter tone (± perianal sensation) suggests spinal injury. In the setting of major blunt trauma when patients may be unconscious, ventilated, or hypotensive, clinical examination of the abdomen is unreliable. Focused abdominal ultrasound scanning (FAST) and/or CT scan, and occasionally laparotomy, must be considered in all such patients. Diagnostic peritoneal lavage is rarely performed and is almost of historical interest.

Peripheral trauma (e.g. long bone fractures)

Occult haemorrhage and neurovascular injuries due to long bone or pelvic fractures must be detected and treated early. Many physicians fail to appreciate the amount of blood lost with a fractured femur or pelvis, even when closed. Pelvic and long bone fractures require appropriate splintage (traction or 'butt binder') in the emergency department, as part of the initial resuscitation, rather than fixation. A useful practical tip is that a compound leg fracture should be considered a high-energy injury, and consequently associated with internal organ damage (e.g. ruptured spleen), until actively excluded. Crush injuries initiate compartment syndromes that may require decompressive fasciotomy. Associated rhabdomyolysis causes hyperkalaemia and renal failure, unless preventative measures are instituted.

Skin care

As soon as reasonably feasible, transfer the patient from the rigid spine board to a firm mattress. This provides equivalent stability for potential spinal fractures whilst avoiding potential skin breakdown and discomfort.

Cervical and spinal injury

Cervical and spinal injury is discussed in later text.

Fluid resuscitation

Blood transfusion is necessary in most hypotensive, vasoconstricted trauma patients. Although uncross-matched group O Rh-negative blood may be indicated in the exsanguinating patient, other fluids are usually used whilst blood is cross-matched. Initially, isotonic (e.g. 0.9% saline) or balanced salt solutions (e.g. Hartmann's) are used. Shocked patients may require 2–3 L in the first few minutes. Although there is no proven benefit compared to crystalloids, colloid plasma expanders (e.g. Gelofusine®) may occasionally be used (see Chapter 2). By 20–30 minutes, cross-matched red cells should be available. Ideally, fluid should be warmed before administration, as hypothermia increases bleeding. Rapid infusion devices and in-line pumps may be required during extensive resuscitations.

In massively transfused patients (MTP), platelets and fresh frozen plasma (FFP) were previously reserved for suspected or documented coagulopathy (due to coagulation factor dilution from the use of fluids deficient in haemostatic factors or disseminated intravascular coagulopathy (DIC) during prolonged shock). Recent clinical trial data suggest that earlier administration of FFP and platelets in MTP improves survival. Current recommendations suggest administration of red blood cells, FFP, and platelets in a ratio of 1:1:1.

All resuscitation fluids have a high sodium concentration, similar to that of extracellular fluid. Hypertonic fluids may have some advantages, particularly in patients with head injuries, but their place in trauma resuscitation is still unresolved. Low sodium solutions (e.g. glucose 5%, glucose saline) are ineffective resuscitation fluids, are rarely necessary during the first 24 hours following trauma, and are contraindicated in head trauma patients.

Shocked patients have a reduced interstitial fluid volume, in addition to the depleted blood volume, and need resuscitation volumes greater than the actual volume of blood lost. With blunt injuries, volume loss may continue for 48 hours due to venous and capillary ooze that can only be partially controlled. In these patients, inadequate resuscitation and persistent hypotension lead to renal failure, ARDS, sepsis, and DIC, and may aggravate potentially disastrous cerebral ischaemia in head injury cases.

In contrast, in penetrating trauma, there is some evidence that extensive fluid resuscitation prior to haemostasis may be detrimental, presumably due to dilutional coagulopathy and because higher blood pressures potentiate bleeding. Consequently, the concept of '*damage control surgery*' has been widely adopted, in which partial or 'hypotensive' resuscitation (i.e. to achieve cerebral and cardiac perfusion) is followed by early surgery to control bleeding and exteriorize damaged viscera (i.e. achieve a degree of haemostasis), before proceeding to full 'aggressive' resuscitation. This strategy reduces bleeding from insecure vascular beds and avoids loss of temperature and coagulation control.

Spinal injury

Spinal cord injury (SCI) occurs in 3% of major trauma victims, and 50% of cases are due to RTA. The cervical region accounts for 50% of SCI, with 50% of these being unstable. The commonest sites are C5/6, C6/7, and T12/L1. Assessment requires that the patient is log-rolled to facilitate palpation of the spine for tenderness and 'step off' deformities. Detailed neurological examination, particularly of motor and sensory function below suspected cord lesions, is essential and has prognostic implications.

Cervical, thoracic, and lumbar imaging is necessary, although injury can occur without radiographic abnormality.

Cervical spine assessment

Cervical spine assessment requires anteroposterior, lateral, and open mouth X-ray views. The lateral must visualize from the occiput to the C7/T1 junction. Assess:

1. *Alignment (C0-C7/T1).* Loss of lordosis, increased anterior soft tissue shadows (>4 mm at C4; >15 mm at C6), increased interspinous distance, malaligned spinous processes, and cortical discontinuity indicate injury.
2. *Bony contours (+ cartilages)*, including vertebral bodies and spinous processes. Look for avulsion, burst, and wedge fractures (i.e. >3 mm height difference between front and back of the body).
3. *Disc spaces and soft tissues.* The distance from C3 or C4 to the back of the pharynx should be <4 mm and, if greater, suggests a haematoma.
4. *Odontoid peg assessment* requires open mouth and lateral views. The distance between the anterior arch of C1 and the peg should be <3 mm.

CT scans

CT scans assess injured regions not clearly visualized on X-ray.

MRI scans

MRI scans detect ligament and cord damage.

Management

Management aims to prevent secondary SCI by immobilizing the spine and reducing potential spinal cord ischaemia with aggressive resuscitation. If a cervical injury is suspected, the neck should be stabilized with manual 'in-line' cervical immobilization (see Figure 18.1). A semi-rigid hard collar should be applied without neck movement, although a head bolster is most often used these days, and, if pre-hospital (i.e. at the scene of the injury, not in hospital), the patient should be placed on a rigid spine board and the head secured with tapes and sandbags. Patients with suspected thoracolumbar spinal injuries should also be moved as a single unit and log-rolled, as necessary.

Spinal stability

Spinal stability should be assessed by an appropriately trained specialist. Fracture dislocations (distraction) or injuries, causing disruption of the posterior ligamentous complex, often cause spinal instability and may require early surgical fixation. Potentially unstable cervical fractures may be managed with a halo frame.

Respiration

Cord lesions above C4 inhibit diaphragmatic function and always require ventilatory support. The intercostal muscles are innervated by T2–T12, and patients with lesions above this level depend on diaphragmatic breathing, with reduced tidal volumes and impaired cough.

Circulation

Following the immediate hyperstimulation and hypertension that accompanies injury, there is subsequent loss of sympathetic control in cord lesions above T1–6. This limits the cardiovascular stress response, causing bradycardia, peripheral vasodilation, hypotension, and neurogenic shock. Acute pulmonary oedema may occur due to excessive volume expansion in the absence of CVP monitoring. In the first few weeks following severe cervical SCI, unopposed vagal activity (e.g. after bronchial suctioning) causes profound bradycardia (71%) and cardiac arrest (16%) but is prevented with atropine. Without prophylaxis, venous thromboembolism occurs in 40% of cases, and pulmonary embolism causes 15% of deaths in the first 12 months after SCI.

Neurology

Spinal shock refers to the temporary loss of somatic and autonomic reflex activity below the level of complete SCI. It lasts for 2–70 days after the injury and is associated with muscle flaccidity, vasodilation, areflexia, loss of bladder function, and paralytic ileus. Muscle contractures and spasms may follow resolution. Autonomic dysreflexia is associated with SCI above T6 (~65%). Stimulation below the level of the lesion (e.g. bladder distension) causes a sympathetic reflex, with flushing, sweating, severe hypertension, and bradycardia, that can precipitate seizures or strokes. Steroid therapy is no longer recommended for SCI.

General factors (and associated treatments)

- Hypothermia due to vasodilation (rewarming).
- Muscle wasting or contractures (physiotherapy).
- Psychological distress (psychological support).
- Gastric dilation (nasogastric tube drainage).
- Gastric stress ulcers (ulcer prophylaxis).
- Paralytic ileus and constipation (laxatives).
- Bladder atony (catheterization).
- Pressure sores (meticulous skin care).

Head injury

A third of all trauma deaths are due to head injury. It is a leading cause of death in young men and causes significant long-term morbidity in survivors. It is most commonly due to RTAs, falls, assaults, and gunshot wounds. Although the majority of head injuries (~75%) are minor, many have a poor functional outcome due to secondary insults (e.g. inadequately treated shock), missed injuries, and comorbidities. Moderate or severe head injury occurs in ~25% of cases, and most will need ICU admission.

Two types of neural tissue damage occur:

1. **Primary injury** is due to the initial trauma (e.g. brain lacerations, contusions, diffuse axonal injury caused by shear forces during deceleration). This is irreversible.

2. **Secondary injury** due to raised intracranial pressure (ICP) and poor cerebral perfusion causes 50% of deaths. Preventative therapy improves outcome. Causes are:

   • **Intracranial** and include cerebral oedema, hydrocephalus, space-occupying lesions (SOL; for example, extradural haematomas), cerebral ischaemia due to vasospasm or seizures, and inflammatory mediators.

   • **Systemic**, such as hypotension, hypoxia, anaemia, hyper-/hypoglycaemia, hyper-/hypocapnia, infection, hyper-/hyponatraemia, and hyperthermia.

Pathophysiology

The skull is a fixed-volume container, encasing brain, blood, and CSF. Cerebral oedema (or an SOL) initially displaces blood and CSF, with little effect on normal ICP (~5–10 mmHg). Further swelling increases ICP rapidly, which normally peaks at ~72 hours after trauma. The rise in ICP (>25 mmHg) reflects the severity of brain injury and may eventually cause cerebral herniation. However, reduced cerebral perfusion pressure (CPP; the difference between mean arterial pressure (MAP) and ICP) is more important, as this determines the decrease in cerebral blood flow (CBF) and associated ischaemia. Therapy aims to maintain a normal CPP (>60 mmHg). Neuronal failure and death occur at CPP <40 and <20 mmHg, respectively.

Normally, CBF is sensitive to PaO_2 and $PaCO_2$ but independent of BP. In injured brain, this BP autoregulation fails, and perfusion directly parallels CPP. In these patients:

• **Hypoxia or hypercapnia** vasodilates normal vessels and diverts blood flow away from damaged cerebral tissue. The associated increase in cerebral blood volume (CBV) raises ICP, reduces CPP and CBF, and further aggravates ischaemia in damaged brain tissue.

• **Hypocapnia** vasoconstricts normal vessels, reducing CBV and ICP. This increases CPP and improves CBF. In addition, vasoconstriction in normal tissue and failure of autoregulation in damaged brain tissue divert blood flow to injured brain, relieving ischaemia. Unfortunately, raised CPP eventually increases oedema and ICP in damaged brain, and excess vasoconstriction may cause ischaemia in normal tissue. Consequently a low normal $PaCO_2$ (~35–40 mmHg) is currently recommended in the management of ventilated head trauma patients.

Immediate management

Prompt resuscitation should include supplemental oxygen to correct hypoxaemia and respiratory support to prevent hypercapnia. In ventilated patients, sedation (± paralysis) prevents ICP elevation and reduces SCI in agitated patients. Fluid resuscitation and antiarrhythmics aim to maintain BP and haemodynamic stability and optimize CPP. Spinal immobilization is vital. It should be assumed that all head-injured patients have spinal injuries. Protect the airways in obtunded patients, and use manual in-line cervical stabilization during intubation. Chest and abdominal injuries may occur in up to 50% of head-injured patients and must be addressed.

Head injury assessment

Document the **Glasgow coma score** (GCS) at admission, and monitor at regular intervals. It is a prognostic, reproducible method of assessing patient responsiveness (see Table 1.2 in Chapter 1). Severe head injury is defined as: a GCS ≤8, post-resuscitation GCS ≤8 within 48 hours of injury, or any intracranial contusion, haematoma, or laceration.

Physical examination

Physical examination must detect head wounds and spinal cord damage. Basilar skull fractures cause CSF rhinorrhoea, bleeding behind the tympanic membrane, 'racoon eyes', and bruising behind the ears (Battle's sign). Papilloedema suggests an increase in ICP. Full neurological examination is essential.

Radiographic evaluation

Radiographic evaluation usually requires a CT scan. Skull radiographs are now rarely performed. An immediate CT scan is performed if the patient is comatose, has deteriorating consciousness, a GCS ≤8 or GCS 9–13 with skull fractures, and prior to planned surgery. Intracranial haematomas are ten times more common in patients with skull fractures.

Monitoring

GCS assessment is adequate in most mild to moderate injuries. In ventilated patients with severe head injuries, ICP monitoring, using extradural, subarachnoid space, or intracerebral (e.g. Camino bolt) pressure transducers, may be required. Unfortunately, infection risks and inaccuracy limit the value of these techniques. Alternatively, cerebral oxygen saturation (SjO_2) can be measured with a jugular venous bulb fibreoptic catheter. SjO_2 <55% suggests inadequate CBF. Blood sugar should be monitored, and, in some cases, EEG is required.

Ongoing management

Treatment aims to prevent secondary cerebral damage. General measures include resuscitation to optimize CBF, aiming for a MAP >70 mmHg, ICP <15–20 mmHg, CPP >60 mmHg, and good oxygenation (i.e. PaO_2 >90%, SjO_2 >55%). Techniques to reduce ICP include:

• **Optimizing cerebral venous drainage** by preventing hard collars, neck flexion, or tracheostomy ties impeding venous blood flow. Drainage is optimum when the head is in the midline position with 15–30° elevation. Suctioning, physiotherapy, and PEEP, which increase venous pressure and ICP, should be kept to a minimum.

• **Loop diuretics** (e.g. furosemide) and **osmotic agents** (e.g. mannitol) can effectively, but briefly (~6–8 hours), reduce ICP and may prevent early cerebral herniation. Mannitol increases intravascular osmotic pressure, encouraging fluid movement out of cells which reduces brain cell volume, and hence ICP.

• **Hyperventilation**, to lower $PaCO_2$ to 25–30 mmHg in MV patients, reduces ICP by ~25% in <1 min. However, routine use is not recommended (as previously described).

• **Ventriculostomy (CSF) drainage and decompressive surgery** (e.g. 'burr' holes) is occasionally required if other methods fail. CSF drainage is particularly useful in obstructive hydrocephalus.

• **Steroids** do not reduce ICP or improve outcome.

Reducing cerebral metabolism decreases oxygen requirements and alleviates ischaemia. For example:

• **Tight glycaemic control** (BS 4–7 mmol/L) reduces cerebral lactate production and may improve outcome.

- **Prophylactic anticonvulsants** prevent the seizures that complicate ~10–40% of severe head injuries.
- **Sedation (± paralysis)** decreases agitation and metabolism in ventilated cases. Propofol may have neuroprotective effects. Barbiturates (e.g. thiopental (INN)) reduce brain metabolic demand but cause haemodynamic instability. Benzodiazepines are a good alternative.
- **Antipyretic agents and cooling** reduce hyperthermia which can damage injured brain. Moderate hypothermia (33–34°C) may be neuroprotective.

Head injury-associated complications

Head injury-associated complications, e.g. neurogenic pulmonary oedema, ARDS, atelectasis, diabetes insipidus, pituitary deficiency, obstructive hydrocephalus, DIC (25%), DVT, decubitus pressure sores, must be addressed. Avoid nasogastric tubes in basilar skull fractures, and treat signs of meningitis with antibiotics.

Prognosis

Prognosis is determined by the severity of the injury, presentation GCS, age (>60 years), and comorbidities. Road safety measures, including helmets, drink-driving legislation, and safety belts have reduced head injury-associated RTA deaths. Nevertheless, in the USA, ~50,000 head-injured patients with a GCS ≤8 die before reaching hospital, and a further ~50,000 die in hospital. Outcome prediction is difficult because, despite severe initial impairment, young patients may make significant improvements over time. About a third of RTA survivors with an initial GSC ≤8 never regain independent function. However, the majority are active and self-reliant.

Chest trauma

Chest injuries are penetrating or blunt and are usually associated with multiple trauma. Initial cardiopulmonary resuscitation always takes precedence, as correction of initial hypoxaemia, hypercapnia, and hypotension prevents secondary organ damage. The chest X-ray is integral to the initial assessment, and a 12-lead electrocardiogram (ECG) aids exclusion of myocardial injury due to contusion. The secondary assessment aims to anticipate complications and detect missed injuries.

Penetrating chest trauma

Penetrating chest trauma is relatively uncommon but is usually due to stabbing with a knife or gunshot wound. The previous classification of gunshot wounds into 'low' (subsonic, e.g. handgun) or 'high' (supersonic, e.g. rifle) velocity wounds has been superseded with the realization that energy transfer is the important factor. Although high-velocity rounds have more 'kinetic' energy, the transfer of energy is dependent on the resistance of the tissues penetrated, impact on bone, and whether the round penetrated 'point first' or was unstable in flight. Thus, a 'low-velocity' handgun round at close range may cause extensive damage, and occasionally a high-velocity rifle round may pass through tissue, causing relatively little damage.

Stab (e.g. knife) and 'low-energy' gunshot wounds

Stab and 'low-energy' gunshot wounds into the chest often cause haemopneumothorax. In most cases, this is effectively managed with chest drainage alone. However, penetrating injuries to major intrathoracic organs (e.g. heart) and vital structures (e.g. aorta) may require urgent surgery. Indications for thoracotomy include cardiac tamponade, transmediastinal injury, initial blood loss from chest drains >1.5–2 L, or ongoing bleeding of >200–250 mL/h.

'High-energy' gunshot wounds

'High-energy' gunshot wounds may cause extensive tissue injury and cavitation due to kinetic energy release. Early surgery is required to control haemorrhage or air leaks, evacuate blood clots, and remove damaged lung, chest wall tissue, and clothing fragments. Air embolism is particularly common in 'high-energy' gunshot wounds, especially during MV. It should be suspected if neurological (e.g. stroke) or cardiac (e.g. arrhythmias) complications develop.

Non-penetrating blunt chest trauma

Non-penetrating blunt chest trauma is common but easily missed, as there may be few external clinical signs apart from bruising. A high index of suspicion is required to avoid delayed diagnosis of serious internal injury.

Three mechanisms cause intrathoracic injury:

1. **Rib fractures** damage local tissues (e.g. pneumothorax), causing pain, splinting, hypoventilation, and atelectasis. However, the chest wall is more flexible in the young, and intrathoracic damage can occur without rib fractures. Treatment involves chest drainage, physiotherapy, nerve blocks, and opioid (± epidural) analgesia.

2. **Abrupt intrathoracic pressure increases** can rupture air or fluid-filled structures. Resulting alveolar, oesophageal, and diaphragmatic damage causes pneumothorax, mediastinitis, and herniation of abdominal structures into the thoracic cavity.

3. **Shear stress** between tethered intrathoracic structures causes visceral or vascular tears (e.g. aortic rupture, tracheobronchial leaks, pulmonary haematoma).

Specific injuries

Lung, tracheobronchial, and diaphragmatic injuries

- **Pneumothorax and haemothorax** are common and may require intercostal tube drainage.
- **Pulmonary contusions** appear as ill-defined infiltrates at the site of trauma on CXR. Localized bleeding, oedema, and V/Q mismatch cause haemoptysis and hypoxaemia.
- **Flail chest** describes a 'free' or 'disconnected' section of chest wall (or sternum) that results from multiple rib fractures. The subsequent 'paradoxical' movement (i.e. in during inspiration and out during expiration) reduces ventilation, but it is the associated discomfort which is most likely to impede chest wall movement, cough, and secretion clearance. Effective oral analgesia and local anaesthetic nerve blocks are required, but thoracic epidurals are most effective. Underlying lung contusion is usually the determining factor in the need for respiratory support in flail chest. If respiratory failure develops, MV, and a subsequent tracheostomy, may be required for ~7–14 days to restore normal chest wall movement. External chest wall stabilization (e.g. fixation, taping) is of no benefit.
- **Tracheobronchial tears** must be suspected in patients with first or second rib fractures, bilateral pneumothorax, haemoptysis, mediastinal/subcutaneous emphysema, or if air leaks persist. Longitudinal tears occur in the posterior membranous portion of the lower trachea (~15%), and spiral tears in the main bronchi (~80%). Bronchoscopy confirms the diagnosis. Early surgical repair prevents atelectasis, infection, and late development of bronchial stenosis (± bronchiectasis). Occasionally, a main bronchus is completely severed. The 'drop' lung is easily recognized, and surgical repair is associated with no long-term complications.

- **Diaphragmatic injuries** occur in ~5–7% of blunt chest injuries. The left diaphragm is most commonly affected (~80%), as the right is protected by the liver. Mortality is high because of associated splenic or hepatic rupture.
- **Lung torsion** (i.e. rotation on the hilar axis) is rare.

Heart and arterial injuries

- **Cardiac contusion** describes oedema and microvascular haemorrhage at the site of cardiac impact and causes ischaemia, arrhythmias, heart block, and impaired contractility. Cardiac enzymes, ECG, echocardiography, and rarely angiography or perfusion scans establish the diagnosis. Treatment is non-specific, including management of arrhythmias and circulatory failure.
- **Traumatic heart damage** involves valves (aortic 55–65%, mitral 25–35%), papillary muscles, or heart wall. Transmural rupture is rapidly fatal in >80% of patients. Early surgery is often necessary.
- **Aortic tears and dissection** are due to shear stresses associated with abrupt deceleration (e.g. RTA). Most cases are fatal at the scene of the accident. Clinically, there may be no evidence of external trauma. Rib fractures are not always present. Tears usually occur just distal to **ligamentum arteriosum** (~80%). Aortic root tears (~15%) can damage the valve or coronary arteries. The diagnosis is suspected on CXR if there is a left-sided apical pleural fluid cap, indistinct aortic arch, depression of the left main bronchus, widened mediastinum, fractures of first and second ribs, and increased left-sided opacification or pleural effusion. Aortography or contrast CT scans confirm the diagnosis.
- **Pericardial tamponade** is due to aortic root disruption, coronary artery laceration, or rupture of the heart wall. It usually requires surgical drainage.

Other injuries

- **Oesophageal rupture** is suspected when haematemesis or subcutaneous emphysema occurs with a pleural effusion, pneumothorax, or mediastinitis. Aspirated pleural fluid may reveal food particles or a raised amylase. Diagnosis is confirmed by a gastrografin swallow. Endoscopy and/or CT scan can be unhelpful. Delayed diagnosis increases mortality which is high, even with early surgical repair.
- **Fat embolism syndrome** develops 1–72 hours after multiple long bone or pelvic fractures. Unsaturated fatty acids, liberated by lipases, cause lung toxicity and coagulopathy. In addition, small fat emboli pass through pulmonary capillaries to occlude retinal, skin, and CNS vessels. The characteristic clinical triad includes confusion, pulmonary dysfunction (e.g. cough, dyspnoea, pleurisy), and a petechial skin rash over the upper torso. Investigations reveal hypoxaemia, a normal early CXR, and lipase or fat globules in urine and serum.

Prognosis

Prognosis varies greatly. In patients with three unilateral or three bilateral rib fractures, chest-related deaths occur in 17% and 41%, respectively. Mortality due to unilateral lung contusion is 16–25%, but, if bilateral or combined with haemothorax or flail segment, mortality increases to 42–54%. In patients with multiple trauma, chest sepsis (~30%), head injury (~30%), and exsanguination (20%) are the commonest causes of death.

Further reading

American College of Surgeons (2012). Advanced Trauma Life Support Student Manual (9th edition). 12T–0001.

Fehlings MG and Tator CH (1999). An evidence-based review of decompressive surgery in acute spinal cord injury; rationale, indications and timings based on experimental and clinical studies. *Journal of Neurosurgery*, **91**, 1–11.

Feliciano DV and Rozycki GS (1999). Advances in the diagnosis and treatment of thoracic trauma. *Surgical Clinics of North America*, **79**, 1417–29.

Pape HC, Remmers D, Rice J, et al. (2000). Appraisal of early evaluation of blunt chest trauma: development of a standardized scoring system for initial clinical decision making. *Journal of Trauma*, **49**, 496–504.

Pretre R and Chilcott M (1997). Blunt trauma to the heart and great vessels. *New England Journal of Medicine*, **336**, 626–32.

PTSD UK. <http://www.ptsduk.co.uk>.

Shaz BH, Dene CJ, Harris R, MacLeod JB, Hillyers CD (2009). Transfusion management of trauma patients. *Anesthesia & Analgesia*, **108**, 1760–8.

Stiell IG, Nesbitt LP, Pickett W, et al. (2008). The OPALS Major Trauma Study: impact of advanced life support on survival and morbidity. *Canadian Medical Association Journal*, **178**, 1141–52.

The Brain Trauma Foundation, the American Association of Neurological Surgeons (2000). Management and prognosis of severe traumatic brain injury. *Journal of Neurotrauma*, **17**, 449–604.

The Primary Trauma Care Foundation. <http://www.nda.ox.ac.uk/research/the-primary-trauma-care-foundation/>.

The Trauma Center Association of America. <http://www.trauma-foundation.org>.

Trauma.org. <http://www.trauma.org>.

Thermal burns

A thermal burn is defined as an injury to, or destruction of, cells in the skin due to hot liquids (scalds), hot solids (contact burns), or flames (flame burn). Injuries to skin and other organic tissues due to radiation, electricity, or chemical contact are also identified as burns (see 'Electrical and chemical injury').

In the UK, 250,000 people are treated annually by primary care teams for minor burns, scalds, and smoke inhalation. The young and elderly (<5 and >75 years old) are most at risk, with 50% of episodes occurring in the kitchen. Serious burns cause ~10,000 hospital admissions and ~200 deaths annually in the UK. Hospital mortality and cosmetic outcomes have improved, largely due to management in specialized burns units. Burns to >80% of total body surface area (TBSA) are now associated with a reasonable chance of survival.

Pathophysiology

Thermal injury causes local and systemic effects. At the site of the burn, there is immediate vasodilation, increased vascular permeability, plasma protein leakage, and local oedema, although, in severe burns, oedema is more generalized. Hypovolaemic shock occurs without adequate resuscitation. Microthrombosis and later infection extend wound necrosis beyond the area of thermal damage.

Systemic circulatory effects

Systemic circulatory effects affect burns >15% TBSA and are proportional to the burn size. Initially, cardiac output (CO) falls, and systemic and pulmonary vascular resistance increase due to vasopressor release (e.g. epinephrine), myocardial depressant factors, hypovolaemia, and wound fluid loss. CO recovers on the second post-burn day (PBD) and becomes supranormal by the third PBD.

Hypermetabolic state

A hypermetabolic state extends from the third PBD until wound healing. It is a manifestation of the systemic inflammatory response and energy expenditure related to evaporative loss, pain, anxiety, and wound infection.

Infection

Infection complicates most burns. The moist, protein-rich, avascular environment encourages bacterial growth, reduces systemic antibiotic penetration, and impairs immune cell migration and response. Risk factors for infection include burns >30% TBSA, full-thickness or open burns, age (<5 or >75 years old), pre-existing disease (e.g. diabetes), bacterial antibiotic resistance, failed skin grafts, and inadequate burn care.

Drug pharmacokinetics

Drug pharmacokinetics are altered due to altered absorption, cardiovascular (± renal) effects, drug absorption and loss through burn wounds (e.g. topical antibiotics), and the 'third space' effects of oedema fluid.

Classification

Burn depth is the most significant determinant of mortality, final cosmetic appearance, and functional outcome. Superficial burns do not destroy epithelial-lined appendages in surviving dermis, including sweat glands, hair follicles, and sebaceous glands. When the dead dermal tissue is removed, epithelial cells migrate from these appendages to form a new, fragile epidermis on the residual dermal bed. With deeper burns, fewer appendages survive, and healing takes longer and scarring is more severe.

First-degree or epidermal/superficial

First-degree or epidermal/superficial burns involve only the epidermis. They are red and painful but do not blister. Over 2–3 days, erythema and pain subside, and, on day 4–5, the injured epithelium peels away from the newly healed epidermis below, a process commonly seen following sunburn. As blistering is often delayed for several hours, burns that initially appear epidermal are reclassified as partial thickness 12–24 hours later.

Second-degree or partial-thickness

Second-degree or partial-thickness burns involve the epidermis and dermis. Fibrinous exudate and necrotic debris accumulate on the burn surface, predisposing to bacterial colonization, delayed healing, and difficulty assessing wound depth. These burns are subclassified as:

- **Superficial partial-thickness** burns and affect the superficial dermis (papillary layer). They are characterized by blisters between the epidermis and dermis and are red, oedematous, wet, and extremely painful, even to air currents. Most heal spontaneously within <3 weeks with minimal scarring.
- **Deep partial-thickness** burns extend into the lower dermis (reticular layer), affecting hair follicles and sweat glands. If infection is prevented, they heal in 3–9 weeks. Hypertrophic scarring and joint contractures are common despite physiotherapy. A partial-thickness burn that fails to heal within 3 weeks is functionally and cosmetically equivalent to a full-thickness burn and best treated by excision and grafting.

Third-degree or full-thickness

Third-degree or full-thckness burns destroy all layers of the dermis (± underlying adipose tissue). The burn may appear 'waxy' white (and be mistaken for normal skin) or charred, and is indurated, firm, dry, and painless (anaesthetic) due to dead, denatured dermis, described as 'eschar'. Over many weeks, the eschar separates from underlying viable tissue, leaving a bed of granulation tissue that heals by contraction and marginal epithelialization. Even after surgery and grafting, scarring and functional limitation are common. Although not an official classification, 'fourth-degree burn' is often used to describe a burn involving fascia, muscle, and bone.

Assessment of burns

Establish the following:

Cause

It may be dry (e.g. flame), moist (e.g. hot liquids), blast, electrical, or chemical. Consider non-accidental injury, especially in children.

Depth

This determines healing time, scarring, and appropriate therapy (e.g. grafting). The important decision is whether a burn is full or partial thickness. This can be difficult, even for an experienced burns specialist.

Burn size

This aids assessment of fluid loss and inflammatory response. For adults, apply the 'rule of nines', which divides the body into anatomical regions that represent 9% of TBSA (see Figure 18.2). The palmar surface of the hand and

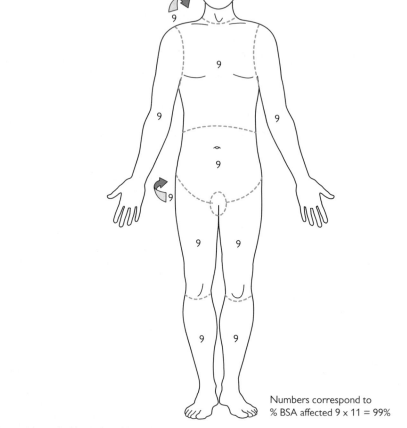

Figure 18.2 **Assessment of BSA.** 'Wallace's rule of 9s'. Reprinted from *The Lancet,* 257, 6653, Wallace AB, 'The exposure and treatment of burns', pp. 501–504, Copyright 1951, with permission from Elsevier.

fingers represents 1% TBSA. In children, body surface areas are different (use Lund and Browder charts). For example, in a child <1 year old, the head is 18% (not 9%) of TBSA.

Time of the burn
This is important, as fluid is replaced from the time of the burn, not admission.

Site affected
Face (e.g. eyelids), perineum, hands, feet, and circumferential burns require specialist attention.

Smoke inhalation and associated injuries
Smoke inhalation is more likely in enclosed spaces and increases mortality. Blasts and injuries caused by escaping a fire include fractures and internal injury. (See 'Toxic inhalation injury'.)

Review tetanus immunization
Human tetanus immunoglobulin (HTI) is required if immunization has not occurred within the last 5 years.

Pre-existing illness
Pre-existing illness, including diabetes mellitus, obesity, and cardiovascular disease can be important barriers to burn wound healing.

Management of major burns
Specialist treatment of direct thermal injury, smoke inhalation, and carbon monoxide poisoning improves survival and cosmetic outcome. Box 18.1 suggests indications for hospital and/or specialist burns centre admission. Immediate management should address the following:

Stop the burning process
Rinse the involved body surface with large amounts of clean, cool tap water. However, great care is required, as excessive cooling causes hypothermia, especially in children and those with extensive burns. This worsens shock and exacerbates the lethal triad of hypothermia, coagulopathy, and acidosis. Initially, remove clothing, and cover the patient

Box 18.1 Indications for hospital and/or burns unit referral

Second-degree burn (SDB) >20–25% BSA
Third-degree burn (TDB) >5–10% BSA
Any SDB or TDB if >60 or <5 years old
Burns affecting the hands, feet, face, eyes, or perineum
Burns affecting major joints or circumferential burns
Inhalational or airways burn injury
Chemical or electrical burns
Comorbid conditions or coexisting trauma

Data from Hettiaratchy S, Papini, 'Initial management of a major burn: 1-overview', *British Medical Journal*, 2004, 328, pp. 1555–1557.

with clean, warm, dry linens to prevent hypothermia. Adherent synthetic clothing and tar is cooled with tap water but left in place to await formal debridement.

Resuscitation
Large-calibre intravenous access must be established immediately. Patients with burns >15–20% TBSA (>10% with smoke inhalation) require immediate fluid replacement to maintain organ function and preserve viable skin tissue by restoring perfusion. If vasoactive agents are required, avoid alpha-adrenergic agonists (e.g. norepinephrine) which reduce blood flow to burnt skin.

- **In the first 24 hours**, crystalloid fluid regimes, calculated from the time of injury, are recommended. Neither colloid nor hypertonic solutions improve outcome. The Parkland formula recommends 3–4 mL of Ringer's lactate (Hartmann's) solution per kilogram of body weight per per cent of TBSA with second- or third-degree burns in the first 24 hours, with 50% given in the first 8 hours. The Gaveston formula is more accurate in children (5 L/m^2 x % burn TBSA plus 2 L/m^2/24 h of maintenance). However, formulae are guidelines, and fluid replacement should also be guided by clinical response, aiming to maintain a good blood pressure, CO, and urine output >0.5–1 mL/kg/h. Excessive fluid can be harmful, but only specialists should consider using hypertonic solutions to reduce tissue oedema.
- **After 24 hours**, sodium requirements and vessel permeability decrease, and fluid replacement is tailored to requirements. Lower sodium solutions, including 5% dextrose as supplemental water, are used to maintain circulating volume and electrolyte balance.

Upper airways damage
This is associated with early death in major burns injuries. Hot gases (e.g. steam) and toxic chemicals in smoke cause rapid upper airways obstruction. Patients with second or third degree facial burns require early intubation, as it may be impossible later due to oedema. Monitor pulmonary function tests, and give humidified supplemental oxygen and nebulized bronchodilators (± ephedrine) in non-intubated patients. Steroids do not reduce oedema and increase infection risks.

Presentation of toxic inhalation injury (TII) can be delayed for 12–24 hours. It must be considered in patients with facial or neck burns, oropharyngeal swelling, cough, carbonaceous sputum, eyebrow singeing, involvement in explosions or confinement in enclosed spaces, hoarseness, stridor, or respiratory distress. Hyperventilation and hypercapnia due to increased metabolism may also cause respiratory failure. Baseline arterial blood gases and carboxyhaemoglobin levels should be measured and high-dose supplemental oxygen started. Management of TII,

including carbon monoxide and cyanide poisoning, is discussed in Toxic inhalation injury.

Metabolism and nutrition
Fever (~38.5°C) and hypercapnia reflect an increase in basal metabolic rate, which peaks at ~7 days. The increase is proportional to burn size and associated infection. A 60% burn doubles calorie requirements and CO_2 production, and the increased ventilation required to clear CO_2 can lead to respiratory failure. High humidity and environmental temperatures (30–32°C) reduce heat and water loss from burns and lower calorie expenditure. Start enteral feeding early. Calorie requirements are calculated from burn size. Prophylaxis (e.g. ranitidine) prevents gastric stress ulcers.

Burn wound care and skin grafts
Initially, following cooling cover the burn using cling film. Partial-thickness burns can then be protected with biological or synthetic dressing. Early excision and split-skin grafting of full thickness burns improves survival and decreases infection, pain, and healing time. Transplant or biosynthetic skins are often used in burns >60% TBSA. Topical antibiotics (e.g. silver sulfadiazine) reduce early staphylococcal and later pseudomonal colonization.

Infection
Isolation, burn wound microbiological surveillance, early detection of sepsis, and judicious antibiotic therapy improve outcome.

Analgesia
Initially, intravenous opioids (e.g. morphine) are required. Ketamine provides analgesia for dressing changes when combined with a benzodiazepine. Monitor drug levels due to altered renal and hepatic clearance.

Complications
Circumferential contraction of neck, chest, and limb burns can cause life-threatening ventilatory impairment or distal limb ischaemia requiring immediate escharotomy. Other potential complications include renal impairment due to rhabdomyolysis or haemoglobinuria, shock, sepsis, respiratory failure or poisoning from smoke inhalation, thrombosis, and scarring.

Further reading
American Burn Association (2009). American Burn Association White Paper. Surgical management of burn wounds and use of skin substitutes. <http://www.ucdenver.edu/academics/colleges/medicalschool/departments/surgery/divisions/GITES/burn/Documents/American%20Burn%20Association%20White%20Paper.pdf>.

Hettiaratchy S and Papini R (2004). Initial management of a major burn: 1—overview. *BMJ*, **328**, 1555–7.

McIndoe Burns Support Group. <http://www.mcindoeburnssupport.org>.

National Network for Burns Care (2012). <www.specialisedservices.nhs.uk>.

Papini R (2004). Management of burns of various depths. *BMJ*, **329**, 158–60.

Patient.co.uk. Burns—assessment and management. <http://www.patient.co.uk/doctor/Burns-Assessment-and-Management.htm>.

Public Health England (2014). The Green Book: Immunisation against infectious disease. <https://www.gov.uk/government/collections/immunisation-against-infectious-disease-the-green-book>.

RAFT (Restoration of Appearance & Function Trust). <http://www.raft.ac.uk>.

The Healing Foundation. <http://www.thehealingfoundation.org>.

Toxic inhalation injury

The majority of toxic inhalation injury (TII) follows smoke inhalation. Fire smoke is composed of many toxic compounds, depending on the fuel burnt (see Table 18.2), and exposure occurs in both enclosed urban (e.g. house fires) and outdoor (e.g. bush fires) spaces. However, TII due to specific gases may follow accidental occupational exposure or occur during military or crowd control situations.

Smoke inhalation

Smoke inhalation is associated with increased mortality in burns and trauma patients and requires specialist management (e.g. burns centre). It should be suspected in patients with facial, eyebrow, or neck burns, oropharyngeal swelling, cough, carbonaceous sputum, respiratory distress, or stridor. Hot, toxic inhaled gases cause three distinct types of injury which often occur together.

Upper airway heat-induced injury
Inhalation of hot gases (e.g. steam), in conjunction with the toxic chemicals in smoke, can cause upper airways burns with airways obstruction due to oropharyngeal or facial oedema. Heat-induced damage rarely extends beyond the larynx. Early intubation is recommended in patients with second or third degree facial burns, as this may be impossible later due to the development of oropharyngeal oedema over 12–72 hours. If intubation can be avoided, monitor pulmonary function tests and treat with humidified oxygen and nebulized bronchodilators. Simple measures, such as elevating the head of the bed, may reduce oedema formation. Nebulized epinephrine may alleviate oedema but should not delay intubation in patients with symptomatic obstruction or hypoxaemia. Steroids do not reduce oedema and may increase the risk of infection.

Tracheobronchial and lung damage
Many chemicals in smoke are highly reactive and can cause irritation, inflammation, or damage to the tracheobronchial tree and alveolar tissue. In severe cases, mucosal epithelial cell sloughing, with associated oedema, airways narrowing, and cast formation, occurs at 48–72 hours, and the mucosa requires 7–14 days to regenerate. Extensive small airways closure (e.g. bronchiolitis obliterans) causes hypoxaemia and respiratory failure. Secondary infection and pneumonitis are common. Extensive burns increase the risk of acute respiratory distress syndrome (ARDS).

Highly soluble gases (e.g. sulphur dioxide (SO_2), chlorine) dissolve in upper airway secretions to form potent acids which cause mucosal inflammation, ulceration, and bronchospasm. Less soluble toxins (e.g. nitrogen dioxide (NO_2), phosgene) penetrate to the lower respiratory tract, causing alveolar damage and pulmonary oedema.

Cough, breathlessness, wheeze, stridor, and oropharyngeal soot suggest the diagnosis. Mild cases are managed with supplemental oxygen alone, but severe cases require intubation, ventilatory support, positive end expiratory pressure (PEEP) to maintain airways patency, and regular bronchial toilet to clear debris. Early detection of airway infection and antibiotic therapy improve outcome, but prolonged respiratory support may be required.

Systemic effects of inhaled toxic gases
Any inhaled gas can be a lethal asphyxiant when it displaces oxygen to produce a hypoxic gas mixture. In addition, inhaled smoke contains many toxic gases and compounds that may be absorbed and cause serious systemic toxicity (see Table 18.2). The most important of these are:

Carbon monoxide (CO) poisoning
This is the principal cause of death in 75% of fire fatalities. Affinity of CO for Hb is ~250 times that of oxygen. Even low CO concentrations (e.g. 0.1%) displace oxygen to produce non-functional carboxyhaemoglobin (COHb). Symptoms of CO poisoning are those of tissue hypoxia and correlate with COHb levels (see Table 18.3). Co-oximeters with multi-wavelength spectroscopy differentiate between COHb and oxyhaemoglobin, but pulse oximeters cannot do this and incorrectly report high saturations. Treatment with 100% oxygen decreases the elimination half-life of COHb from 180 to 30 minutes and is continued until the level of COHb is <10%. Hyperbaric oxygen therapy reduces neuropsychiatric sequelae if COHb levels are >30%, but practical issues usually outweigh benefits.

Cyanide (CN)
This is produced by the combustion of wood, nylon, or polyurethane. Histotoxic hypoxia follows inhalation, as CN binds to tissue cytochrome enzymes, impairing oxygen metabolism. Exposure is often unrecognized, as a diagnostic test for CN is not available. However, in smoke inhalation, lactic acid levels correlate well with CN levels. Mild poisoning is treated with oxygen and inhaled amyl nitrite, more severe poisoning with sodium thiosulphite which speeds metabolism, or hydroxocobalamin which forms inactive complexes.

Occupational (± environmental) toxic inhalation injury
There are many occupational toxins, but the following have relevance because of their frequency and toxicity:

Chlorine products
These are potent toxins used and associated with accidents during water purification (e.g. swimming pools) and with cleaning agents (e.g. bleach).

Oxides
Oxides of nitrogen (NO_2), ozone, and sulphur (SO_2) and acid aerosols (e.g. hydrofluoric acid) cause acute lung injury.

Table 18.2 Toxic components of smoke

Material	Products	Effects
Plastic	Phosgene, chlorine, benzene, hydrochloric acid, SO_2	Acute lung injury, airways irritation
Wood/paper	Acrolein, formaldehyde, acetaldehyde, acetic acid	Bronchospasm, mucosal sloughing
Synthetic goods (e.g. nylon)	Nitrogen oxides (e.g. NO_2), HCN, ammonia (NH_3), SO_2	Tissue hypoxia, pulmonary oedema
All the above	Carbon monoxide	Tissue hypoxia

Table 18.3 Symptoms in carbon monoxide (CO) poisoning

COHb level	Symptoms
<15%/15–20%	Usually none/headache, confusion
20–40%	Disorientation, nausea, visual impairment
40–60%	Hallucinations, coma, shock
>60%	Death

Classically, NO_2 exposure occurs in farmers (silo-fillers disease), welders, during use of combustion engines in enclosed spaces, or following decomposition of organic matter. SO_2 exposure occurs in mining and ore refining.

Metal fumes

Metal fumes, commonly cadmium or mercury, cause acute pneumonitis, typically during welding processes.

Crowd control agents

Crowd control agents (e.g. tear gas, smoke bombs) can cause pulmonary oedema at high concentrations.

Further reading

Blanc PD (2000). Acute pulmonary responses to toxic exposures. In JA Nadel, JF Murray, RJ Mason, VC Bouchey, eds. *A textbook of respiratory medicine*, 3rd edn, pp. 1903–15. WB Saunders, Pennsylvania.

Palmiere TL (2009). Inhalation injury consensus conference. *Journal of Burn Care & Research*, **30**, 141–91.

Electrical and chemical injury

Injury can be caused not only by thermal burns and trauma, but by a wide variety of substances and external sources, including exposure to electricity, chemicals, radiation, friction, and extreme cold.

Electrical injury and burns

Electrocution causes 1,000 deaths annually in the USA and occurs mainly in young adults at work (~60%) and young children at home (~30%). Extension cable misuse is a common cause. The extent of the injury depends on the amount of current (I), measured in amperes (A), that passes through the body and the duration of, and resistance of tissues traversed by the current. Body resistance is mainly provided by the skin, with a resistance (R) of 10^5 Ohms (Ω) when dry but 10^3 Ω when wet. From Ohm's law, Voltage (V) = I x R, dry skin contact with a 240 V mains supply will produce a 0.24 mA current through the body, whereas wet skin will result in a 240 mA current.

The amperage correlates best with injury severity, but often only the voltage is known. In general, lower voltages cause less injury. The clinical effect of increasing the level of electrical current is as follows:

- <0.5 mA causes tingling or harmless microshocks.
- >1 mA results in pain and withdrawal.
- >10–20 mA causes tetanic skeletal muscle contraction, which may prevent the voluntary release of the source of electrocution or cause long bone or spinal vertebrae fractures. The threshold is especially low with alternating currents at household frequencies of ~50 Hz.
- >100 mA, alternating current, can cause ventricular fibrillation (VF), and >5 A will cause asystole, myocardial damage, and potential left ventricular failure.
- >1 A generates sufficient heat energy to cause skin burns and occult thermal injury to internal tissues and organs. Blood vessels and nerves are most susceptible.
- >1,000 A causes severe burns due to heat generation.

Further injuries associated with electrical current passing through the body include:

- **Acute renal failure** due to rhabdomyolysis, following myoglobin release associated with muscle necrosis.
- **Compartment syndrome** follows tissue ischaemia and necrosis and may require limb amputation.
- **Vascular thrombosis** due to thermal injury.
- **Neurological injuries**, including peripheral nerve paralysis (e.g. median nerve), coma, spinal cord damage with para- or tetraplegia, respiratory centre failure and autonomic dysfunction with vasospasm, and late sympathetic dystrophy. Late complications include epilepsy, encephalopathy and parkinsonism.

Lightning strikes
Lightning strikes generate electrical currents of 10^4–20^5A. Victims may be thrown many feet due to violent muscle contraction. Entrance site burns and blistering have a characteristic 'spider-like' appearance, but exit wounds over the hands, knees, or feet can be more severe and may be overlooked at initial evaluation. Patients are initially comatose, and immediate death is usually due to asystole. Internal tissue damage may be extensive, with little external evidence of injury. Bone and muscle injury are common. Nevertheless, many victims survive, and good recovery is reported despite initial neurological unresponsiveness (i.e. fixed dilated pupils).

Management of electrical burns is mainly supportive. Rescuers must first ensure safety (i.e. turn electricity off). In young patients, prolonged cardiopulmonary resuscitation can be successful, even if the situation appears hopeless. Protect the neck/spine in view of the risk of fractures.

Investigations aim to detect organ, nerve, and spinal damage and include serum creatine kinase and creatinine, urine myoglobin, ECG, echocardiography, spinal and limb X-rays, nerve conduction studies, and head CT scan. Check tetanus vaccination status, and monitor for arrhythmias and myocardial injury.

Management is directed to treatment of burns, necrotic tissue, and damaged organs. Extensive debridement of electrical burns is often required to reduce the risk of sepsis and renal failure. If urine is dark, check for myoglobin, and start treatment for myoglobinuria immediately. Fluid administration should aim to achieve a urine output of 100 mL/h, and urine alkalinization with sodium bicarbonate should be considered. Arteriograms may aid with the decision to amputate a limb, and fasciotomies are often required to prevent compartment syndrome.

Chemical burns

Chemical burns account for 2–8% of burns centre admissions in the USA. Domestic chemical burns have increased whereas industrial chemical burns have decreased due to improved health and safety policies. Injury is due to direct skin contact, inhalation or ingestion of strong alkalis (e.g. sodium hydroxide, silver nitrate), acids (e.g. sulphuric, hydrofluoric), petroleum products, and some chemical weapons (e.g. vesicants like mustard gas). Alkali burns tend to be deeper and more serious than acid burns. Copious irrigation with clean water for 20–30 minutes (longer for alkali burns), preferably in a shower, is the primary treatment for all chemical burns. Alkali eye burns require continuous irrigation for 8 hours after the injury. Dry chemical powders must be carefully brushed off the skin or burn prior to irrigation. Avoid further burns by removing contaminated clothing and by preventing the patient from lying in contaminated flush solution. Avoid the use of neutralizing solutions in acid or alkali burns, as these may cause exothermic reactions and risk further thermal damage. After flushing, chemical burns are treated as thermal burns.

Radiation burns

Protracted ultraviolet (UV) light exposure from strong sunlight, sunlamps, tanning booths, cancer radiation therapy, or during X-rays can cause radiation burns. Sun exposure is, by far, the most common radiation burn and is due to two specific wavelengths of light, UVA and UVB, the latter being more dangerous.

Cold burns, frostbite

Cold burns occur when skin is in contact with cold objects. It can be caused by prolonged exposure to moderately cold objects like snow or brief contact with very cold objects like liquid nitrogen or dry ice. Heat transfers from the skin (± organs) to the external object. Freezing, necrosis, and permanent damage occur in affected tissues.

Further reading

Murphy JV, Banwell PE, Roberts AH, McGrouther DA (2000). Frostbite: pathogenesis and treatment. *Journal of Trauma*, **48**, 171–8.

Spies C and Trohman RG (2006). Narrative review: electrocution and life-threatening electrical injuries. *Annals of Internal Medicine*, **145**, 531–7.

Sykes RA, Mani MM, Hiebert JM (1986). Chemical burns: retrospective review. *Journal of Burn Care & Rehabilitation*, **7**, 343–7.

Thermal disorders

Body temperature is normally tightly controlled at $37 \pm 1°C$ through a complex feedback mechanism, involving afferent input from 'A' fibre cold sensors and unmyelinated 'C' fibre heat sensors, and the thermoregulatory centre in the hypothalamus which controls a series of behavioural and autonomic efferent responses to maintain temperature. Extremes of age, exogenous pyrogens in infective illness, cytokine release, and immune complexes (e.g. malignancy, drugs, connective tissue disorders) can impair hypothalamic temperature regulation, causing both hyperthermia and hypothermia.

In general, altered temperature regulation is harmful, however, it may be beneficial in some situations. For example, mild hyperthermia enhances resistance to infection and improves survival in Gram-negative bacteraemia (whilst hypothermia is associated with a poorer outcome). In contrast, mild hypothermia may be beneficial in situations associated with cerebral hypoxia.

Hyperthermia

Hyperthermia is defined as a core temperature $>37.5°C$ (99°F) and occurs when there is excessive heat production, impaired heat loss, an altered hypothalamic 'setpoint' (e.g. infection), or hypothalamic damage (e.g. stroke). It is associated with a number of deleterious physiological effects, including increases in metabolic rate, CO_2 production, oxygen consumption (10%/1°C temperature rise), cardiac output, and energy expenditure. Sweating and vasodilation may result in hypovolaemia. Metabolic acidosis, epilepsy, neurological impairment, acute renal failure, rhabdomyolysis, and myocardial ischaemia may all follow. Severe hyperthermia ($>42°C$) is potentially lethal, and even short periods may cause permanent cerebral damage.

Sweating and active precapillary vasodilation are the two autonomic responses to heat stress. Sweating is often extremely effective and can dissipate up to ten times the heat associated with basal metabolic rate, provided the environmental conditions, including temperature, humidity, and wind speed, are optimal.

Table 18.4 lists the causes of hyperthermia. About 50% are non-infective in origin. Infective causes are discussed in later chapters. Important non-infectious causes of hyperthermia that require immediate recognition and treatment include the following:

Heatstroke

Heatstroke causes about 1,500 deaths a year in the USA. About 80% of deaths occur in patients >50 years old because of the diminished ability of the older body to compensate for increased core temperatures. Heat stroke is suggested when hyperthermia is associated with neurological abnormalities. Rectal temperature is usually $>42°C$. Factors predisposing to heatstroke include increasing age, environmental causes (e.g. heat waves, poor ventilation), behavioural issues (e.g. dehydration, obesity), underlying illness (e.g. diabetes, alcoholism, hyperthyroidism, impaired sweating), and drugs (e.g. anticholinergics, anti-Parkinson's, phenothiazines, tricyclic antidepressants, diuretics).

Heatstroke is a medical emergency and is associated with electrolyte abnormalities (e.g. hypokalaemia), dehydration ($\pm$ hypovolaemia), organ dysfunction (e.g. acute kidney injury, confusion), coagulation abnormalities, and rhabdomyolysis.

Table 18.4 Causes of hyperthermia

Infection and pyrogens
- Sepsis, burns, allergy, transfusion reactions

Increased heat production
- Hypothalamic injury (e.g. stroke)
- Disease-related (e.g. arthritis, malignancy, vasculitis)
- Muscular activity (e.g. exercise, rigidity, seizures, agitation)
- Drug-related (e.g. salicylates, thyroxine, cocaine, sympathomimetics, amphetamines, tricyclic antidepressants, serotonin reuptake inhibitors)
- Endocrine (e.g. hyperthyroidism, phaeochromocytoma)

Reduced heat loss
- Cooling mechanism failure (e.g. elderly, neonates)
- Heat stroke (e.g. insulating garments)
- Drug-related (e.g. anticholinergics)

Malignant hyperthermia

Neuroleptic malignant syndrome

The principal therapeutic objectives are to reduce temperature below 40°C, correct fluid and electrolyte imbalance, and maintain organ function. Two distinct forms are recognized and compared in Table 18.5:

Exertional heatstroke

This is the result of prolonged intense exercise in warm, humid environments. It often affects athletes, military recruits, or firefighters and those wearing garments that restrict heat loss. It presents with hyperthermia, altered mental status, hypotension, and tachypnoea, followed by shock, rhabdomyolysis, and renal failure.

Classical (non-exertional) heatstroke

This usually affects sedentary, elderly, inner city dwellers, with underlying illness during heatwaves. Patients with thermoregulatory disorders (e.g. hypothalamic strokes), inability to dissipate heat (e.g. heart failure, skin disease with decreased sweating), and those using drugs that impair heat loss (e.g. anticholinergics, phenothiazines, diuretics) or generate heat (e.g. cocaine, tricyclics) are at most risk. Classical heatstroke presents with hyperthermia, hot (dry) skin, and altered mental status, followed by shock and organ failure. Table 18.5 lists the metabolic effects. Volume depletion and rhabdomyolysis occasionally cause acute kidney injury. About 80% of deaths occur in those >50 years old. Mortality is ~10–15%, even with rapid cooling.

Drug-induced hyperthermia

Several drugs cause hyperthermia usually due to failure of heat dissipation, rather than resetting of the thermoregulatory centre.

- Mild to severe hyperthermia may be associated with all centrally acting sympathomimetics (e.g. cocaine, amphetamine derivatives like methylene dioxy-methamphetamine (MDMA; 'ecstasy')), which increase synaptic concentrations of dopamine and serotonin. Other potential drug-induced mechanisms include serotonin reuptake inhibitors (e.g. fluoxetine, imipramine) or serotonin agonists (e.g. lithium).

Table 18.5 Comparison of classical and exertional heatstroke

	Classical heatstroke	Exertional heatstroke
Usual age (y)	Over 60	Any age
Common causes	Pre-existing disease, diuretics, tricyclics, anticholinergics	Hot environment, exercise, confining garments
Arterial gases	Respiratory alkalosis; later metabolic acidosis correlates with prognosis	Severe metabolic acidosis
Serum electrolytes	Normal Na$^+$, K$^+$, Mg^{2+}, Ca^{2+}, hypophosphataemia	Hyperkalaemia, hypocalcaemia, hyperphosphataemia
Blood sugar	Hyperglycaemia	Hypoglycaemia
Creatinine kinase	Some elevation	Marked elevation
Hepatic enzymes	Marked elevation	Some elevation
Acute phase proteins	Marked elevation	Some elevation

• Anticholinergic drugs block muscarinic acetylcholine receptors and cause an anticholinergic syndrome. Central toxicity results in confusion, agitation, tremor, and myoclonus. Peripheral features include dry mucous membranes, mydriasis, reduced sweating, blurred vision, tachycardia, and urinary retention. The combination of muscular hyperactivity with impaired sweating may result in severe hyperthermia, rhabdomyolysis, and organ damage.

Malignant hyperthermia
Malignant hyperthermia (MH) is a rare autosomal dominant trait that causes excessive skeletal muscle heat production due to altered calcium kinetics during, or up to 12 hours after, anaesthetic drug exposure. Halothane and succinylcholine precipitate 80% of cases. The incidence is ~1/60,000 with succinylcholine and ~1/250,000 with volatile agents alone.

Clinical features include muscle rigidity, sudden hyperpyrexia (41–45°C), tachycardia, metabolic acidosis (pH as low as 6.8), hypercarbia, prolonged bleeding, cyanosis, and oliguria. The electrocardiogram shows peaked T waves.

Treatment involves stopping anaesthetic drugs and administering intravenous dantrolene, the only specific therapy which acts by inhibiting the release of calcium from the sarcoplasmic reticulum. An initial dose of 2.5 mg/kg is repeated at 5–10 minute intervals (max 10 mg/kg) until the metabolic derangements of MH have been reversed. Further doses of 1–2 mg/kg may be given at 4-hourly intervals for 1–3 days and then orally, if still required. Arrange cooling of the patient; correct fluid and electrolyte imbalance, and address potential arrhythmias and acute kidney injury. Early recognition has reduced mortality from 70% in the 1960s to <10% at present.

Neuroleptic malignant syndrome
Neuroleptic malignant syndrome (NMS) is an idiosyncratic reaction to neuroleptic drugs (e.g. haloperidol, phenothiazines, metoclopramide). It may be due to hypothalamic dopamine receptor blockade. Confusion, agitation, muscle rigidity, encephalopathy, catatonia, extrapyramidal symptoms, and autonomic effects (e.g. sweating, labile hypertension, tachycardia) are common. Organ failure (e.g. acute kidney injury, cardiovascular collapse, and neurological impairment), rhabdomyolysis, and death (10–15%) may occur. Withdrawal of precipitating drugs may be all that is required. However, cooling, fluid and electrolyte correction, renal protection, or replacement therapy may be required. The role of dantrolene in the treatment of NMS has not been established, but it may be beneficial. Other potential therapies include bromocriptine and amantadine.

Thyrotoxic crisis (thyroid storm)
Thyrotoxic crisis is a life-threatening hypermetabolic emergency which affects <2% of thyrotoxic patients. It has a mortality of 20%. Precipitants include infection, surgery, diabetes, labour, radio-iodine therapy, and iodinated contrast media. Thyroxine overdose and eclampsia are rare causes.

Clinical features include those of hypermetabolism and severe hyperthyroidism, including hyperthermia, anxiety, weight loss (>15 kg in ~50%), confusion, and tachycardia. High-output cardiac failure complicates ~50% of cases. Differential diagnosis includes sepsis, phaeochromocytoma, drug abuse, and malignant hyperthermia.

Treatment may be required before diagnostic confirmation (i.e. T3, T4 levels). Treat the precipitating cause, and correct dehydration, electrolyte disturbances, and hypoglycaemia. Institute cooling techniques (e.g. tepid sponging, fans), but avoid aspirin which displaces T4 from binding protein. Sedation controls agitation, and dantrolene may reduce pyrexia due to extreme muscle activity. High-dose beta-blockers (e.g. propranolol) are the mainstay of therapy. They inhibit the peripheral effects of thyroid hormone, reducing fever, heart rate, hypertension, and tremor. Antithyroid drugs block T4 synthesis and should be given immediately. Propylthiouracil is preferred because it blocks T4 to T3 conversion, but it must be given enterally. Alternatively, carbimazole can be given by rectal suppository. This has a slow onset, but long duration of action. White cell suppression occurs with both drugs, and therapy is stopped if sore throat develops. Intravenous hydrocortisone (100 mg 6-hourly) also inhibits T4 to T3 conversion. Iodine also prevents T4 release from the thyroid gland, but antithyroid drugs should be given 2 hours before iodine which inhibits their thyroid uptake.

General management of hyperthermia
Early recognition of hyperthermia can be lifesaving. Initial management includes stopping precipitating drugs, replacing fluids, and correcting electrolyte imbalance. Renal protection against rhabdomyolysis using alkaline diuresis and mannitol may reduce myoglobin-induced renal damage. Renal replacement therapy and seizure prophylaxis may be required.

Cooling is best achieved by spraying unclothed skin with tepid water and using a fan to encourage evaporation. Ice packs in the axilla or groin are often advocated. Cold water immersion is occasionally used but causes cutaneous vasoconstriction and may prevent heat loss. Additional measures include cold intravenous fluids, iced gastric or peritoneal lavage, and haemofiltration.

Temperature-reducing drugs like paracetamol and non-steroidal anti-inflammatory drugs are usually ineffective.

Specific therapies are rarely indicated. However, intravenous dantrolene, a muscle relaxant that uncouples excitation-contraction mechanisms by inhibiting calcium release from sarcoplasmic reticulum is effective in MH and may be beneficial in NMS and MDMA. Bromocriptine and amantadine are useful in NMS. Anticholinergics and muscle relaxants may be helpful.

Hypothermia

Hypothermia is defined as a core temperature <35°C. It accounts for about 3% of hospital admissions in elderly patients and about 1% of winter hospital admissions in the UK. Mild hypothermia is defined as 32–35°C, moderate 28–32°C, and severe <28°C. Mortality varies, according to severity and cause. For example, hypothermia at 28–32°C alone has a mortality of about 20% but, with an underlying cause (e.g. sepsis or trauma), is >60%.

Potential causes and predisposing factors for accidental hypothermia, which is usually multifactorial, include:

- Extremes of age.
- Exposure to low environmental or water immersion temperatures (e.g. near-drowning).
- Poor living conditions, malnutrition, alcohol intoxication.
- Strokes and other primary neurological insults.
- Trauma and surgery (i.e. exposure, anaesthetic drugs, impaired shivering).
- Thermoregulatory compromise (e.g. due to spinal cord injury), burns, dermatitis.
- Endocrine factors (e.g. hypoglycaemia, hypopituitarism). Hypothyroidism, which depresses heat production, impairs temperature perception and blunts shivering, is an aetiological factor in ~10% of cases.
- Predisposing factors (e.g. brain tumours, mental illness, Alzheimer's and Parkinson's disease).
- Drugs that alter cold perception cause vasodilation, inhibit heat generation (e.g. barbiturates, phenothiazines), or prevent shivering (e.g. anaesthetic drugs).

Therapeutic hypothermia during cardiac, vascular, and neurosurgery has been used to provide cerebral protection. There is also increasing evidence that therapeutic mild hypothermia is beneficial, following cardiac arrest and traumatic head injury. In near-drowning cases with severe hypothermia and prolonged cardiac arrest, remarkable recoveries have been reported, following rewarming and resuscitation (especially in children). Death should not be assumed in these cases until resuscitation has failed in an adequately rewarmed patient (i.e. >35°C).

Clinical features

Hypothermia initially stimulates protective peripheral vasoconstriction, shivering, and increased metabolism. However, as core body temperature falls, progressive physiological dysfunction and organ failure follow, including cardiorespiratory and neurological depression, tissue hypoperfusion, metabolic derangement, and renal diuresis.

- Basal metabolic rate falls by 6% for every 1°C fall in temperature. At below 28°C, it is less than 50%. Below 30°C, shivering stops.
- Cardiac conduction and pacemaker activity are progressively impaired, and myocardial irritability increases, with atrial fibrillation and heart block common below 33°C. Ventricular fibrillation, resistant to cardioversion, is precipitated by rough handling (due to cardiac irritability and susceptibility to arrhythmias) and by cardiopulmonary resuscitation (CPR) below 28°C. Asystole occurs when the core temperature falls below 20°C. Cardiac output

falls by 50% at 28°C due to reduced heart rate and contractility.
- The ECG shows prolongation of PR, QRS and QT intervals, and J (or Osborn) waves below 33°C.
- Respiratory depression with reduced respiratory rate and minute ventilation occurs below 33°C, with subsequent abolition of cough and respiratory arrest at <20°C. Blood gases show a falsely high PaO_2 and a falsely low pH.
- Blood sugar is initially high due to suppression of insulin secretion and peripheral resistance. Hypoglycaemia develops later.
- Other effects include impaired clotting, disseminated intravascular coagulation, and venous thrombosis.
- Hypothermia is associated with generalized cerebral depression, and both cerebral blood flow and oxygen consumption halve during a 10°C temperature fall. This response may be neuroprotective, increasing the chance of survival, even after prolonged hypothermic arrest. Initial neurological responses include reduced respiratory drive, lethargy, and confusion; coma and fixed pupils occur below 28°C. Cerebral electrical activity ceases below 20°C.

Management

General management includes oxygen therapy, gentle handling (to avoid precipitating arrhythmias), close monitoring, prevention of further heat loss, and treatment of underlying causes. Fluid resuscitation often requires central access due to intense peripheral vasoconstriction.

Arrhythmias and heart block usually respond to rewarming alone. Prolonged CPR is often successful in hypothermic patients. Although resuscitation is performed as normal, cardioversion is often ineffective below 30°C. Consequently, rewarming to >35°C is essential before death is declared.

Rewarming

The type of rewarming is determined by the severity and physiological response to hypothermia.

Passive external rewarming

This uses a warm environment (>30°C) and insulating covers and is usually adequate in mild (i.e. >33°C) hypothermia without circulatory compromise.

Active external rewarming

This utilizes warming blankets, radiant heat, and immersion techniques. Convective, forced air warming (e.g. Bair Hugger) at 43°C has been shown to increase body temperature by 2–3°C/h. Active external rewarming is recommended in moderate to severe hypothermia, with no evidence of circulatory collapse. However, caution is required, as rapid peripheral vasodilation may increase organ hypoperfusion and mortality.

Active core rewarming

This is required in moderate to severe hypothermia with poor physiological tolerance, circulatory failure, or cardiac arrest (i.e. when rapid rewarming is necessary). Techniques include:

- Warm intravenous fluids or inhaled gas (40°C) increases body temperature by about 1°C/h. Warm fluid rewarming is limited by the volume of fluid that can be given.
- Bladder or pleural lavage with warm sterile saline (40–42°C) or peritoneal lavage with heated dialysate are equally effective and rewarm at 2–3°C/h.
- Haemodialysis is extremely effective in raising body temperature and rewarms at 5°C/h.

- Cardiopulmonary bypass rewarms rapidly (10°C/h) and may be very effective in patients with haemodynamic instability or cardiac arrest but is rarely necessary.

Further reading

Argaud L, Ferry T, Le QH, *et al.* (2007). Short- and long-term outcomes of heatstroke following the 2003 heat wave in Lyon, France. *Archives of Internal Medicine*, **167**, 2177–83.

Aslam AF, Aslam AK, Vasavada BC, Khan IA (2006). Hypothermia: evaluation, electrocardiographic manifestations and management. *American Journal of Medicine*, **119**, 297–301.

Bouchama A, Dehbi H, Mohamed G, *et al.* (2007). Prognostic factors in heat wave related deaths: a meta-analysis. *Archives of Internal Medicine*, **167**, 2170–6.

Center for Disease Control (1995). Heat related illness and deaths 1994-95. *MMWR Recommendations and Reports*, **44**, 465–8.

Gordon L, Paal P, Ellerton J, *et al.* (2015). Delayed and intermittent CPR for severe accidental hypothermia. *Resuscitation*, **90**, 46–9.

Hopkins PM (2000). Malignant hyperthermia: advances in clinical management and diagnosis. *British Journal of Anaesthesia*, **85**, 118–28.

Polderman KH (2009). Mechanisms of action, physiological effects and complications of hypothermia. *Critical Care Medicine*, **37**, S186–202.

Rosenberg MR and Green M (1989). Neuroleptic malignant syndrome: a review of response to therapy. *Archives of Internal Medicine*, **149**, 1927–31.

Soar J, Perkins GD, Abbas G (2010). European Resuscitation Council Guidelines for Resuscitation 2010 Section 8. Cardiac arrest in special circumstances: electrolyte abnormalities, poisoning, drowning, accidental hypothermia, hyperthermia, asthma, anaphylaxis, cardiac surgery, trauma, pregnancy, electrocution. *Resuscitation*, **81**, 1400–33.

Varon J (2010). Therapeutic hypothermia: implications for acute care practitioners. *Postgraduate Medical Journal*, **122**, 19–27.

Allergy and anaphylaxis

Allergy is due to:

- Antigen-mediated triggering of specific IgE antibodies on mast cell surfaces which causes rapid release of pre-formed mediators (e.g. histamine, chemokines) stored in cell granules.
- Direct activation of mast cells by irritants or activated complements (e.g. C3a, C5a), with the synthesis of new mediators (e.g. prostaglandins, leukotrienes).

These mediators cause vasodilation, smooth muscle constriction (e.g. bronchospasm) and increase capillary permeability, resulting in oedema.

Severity of an allergic reaction depends on the dose and site of allergen exposure, individual characteristics, current medication (e.g. beta-blockers, angiotensin-converting enzyme (ACE) inhibitors), and previous exposure or sensitization.

Specific disorders include pollen-induced allergic rhino-conjunctivitis (hayfever), perennial rhinitis, atopic eczema, allergy to foods and drugs, oral allergy syndromes, allergy to bee stings and stinging insects, anaphylaxis, urticaria, or angio-oedema.

Forearm skin prick tests, using standardized solutions of allergen extracts, are a useful method to assess allergy in patients without skin disease. Antihistamines and some drugs (e.g. calcium channel inhibitors) should have been stopped for at least a week before testing. The response is compared with positive (i.e. histamine) and negative (i.e. saline) controls. A wheal more than 2 mm greater than the negative control is a positive test. Great care is required in patients with previous anaphylaxis. Specific IgE to certain antigens (e.g. inhalant allergens, nuts) can be tested in blood samples and are a good alternative to skin prick testing when not available. They are less useful for drug allergies and foods with labile allergens (e.g. fruits).

Anaphylaxis

Anaphylaxis is an acute, generalized, life-threatening allergic reaction. It causes about 1,500 deaths annually, and up to 41 million people are at risk in the USA. About a third of cases are due to venoms (e.g. bee, wasp or hornet stings, ant or snake bites), a third to food allergy (e.g. peanuts, shellfish), and the remaining third to drugs (e.g. penicillins, opiates, non-steroidal anti-inflammatory drugs (NSAIDs)) and non-ionic radiocontrast media. Occasionally, the anaphylaxis may be idiopathic or due to exercise or latex allergy.

Mechanism

Anaphylaxis occurs when an allergen reacts with specific, pre-sensitized surface, mast, or basophil cell IgE antibodies, causing rapid, often massive, release (degranulation) of biologically active preformed mediators (e.g. histamine, tryptase, chymase) and the production of newly formed mediators (e.g. prostaglandins, leukotrienes).

Clinical features

The onset is usually rapid (i.e. within minutes of exposure), although it may be delayed for several hours, depending on the route of exposure, the quantity of antigen, and rate of administration. In addition, beta-blockers, alcohol, tricyclic antidepressants, and cocaine potentiate the reaction.

The initial response is mainly due to histamine release. Patients present with a feeling of impending doom, followed by generalized pruritus, nausea, abdominal pain, rhinitis, conjunctivitis, tachyarrhythmias, erythema/urticaria (50%), and bronchospasm. Severe reactions cause laryngeal oedema, with stridor, angio-oedema, hypotension, and sometimes cardiac arrest. The response is sometimes biphasic, and symptoms recur after several hours. These late phase reactions are due to the de novo synthesis of leukotrienes, which have similar properties to histamine, by mast cells. This late reaction can be inhibited by early steroid therapy. Therefore, all patients should be observed for at least 6 hours after an anaphylactic reaction.

Management

Anaphylaxis is a medical emergency and requires immediate treatment.

- Secure the airway, and administer high-flow oxygen. If respiratory obstruction is imminent (e.g. laryngeal oedema), intubate and ventilate. Consider emergency cricothyroidotomy if the airway is obstructed.
- Check the circulation, and obtain intravenous access.
- Early administration of intramuscular adrenaline (0.3–1 mL of 1/1,000 solution) is essential, repeated at 5–10 minute intervals, according to response. Do not await intravenous access before giving adrenaline. Subcutaneous adrenaline is poorly absorbed. In the seriously ill patient, intravenous adrenaline can be given slowly (preferably as a continuous infusion) as a dilute solution (1/10,000) into a central vein, with appropriate monitoring, and titrated according to the response. Patients on beta-blockers who fail to respond may require an intravenous salbutamol infusion.
- Corticosteroid. Give 100–300 mg hydrocortisone intravenously. This prevents late reactions.
- Antihistamines. Give chlorphenamine 10–20 mg IV (although this is not of proven value), followed by 4 mg 4-hourly orally for 24–48 h or until urticaria and pruritus resolve.
- Fluid resuscitation should aim to restore normal blood pressure. Occasionally, inotropic support may be necessary.
- Treat bronchospasm with nebulized beta-agonists (e.g. salbutamol).
- Local wound care, with cleaning, antibiotics, and tetanus inoculation, should not be neglected.
- Observe for at least 6 hours before discharge, and ensure appropriate follow-up with an allergist for investigation.

Prevention

An adrenaline auto-injector for self-administration of adrenaline should be considered in patients with previous severe anaphylaxis, although avoidance of the potential trigger is the mainstay of ongoing management. Commercially available beesting kits containing pre-filled adrenaline syringes and chewable chlorphenamine tablets are available. Occasionally, desensitization programmes with graded concentrations of allergens are used to reduce the risk of further reactions.

Anaphylactoid reactions

Anaphylactoid reactions are due to non-specific degranulation of mast cells by drugs, chemicals, or venoms, and they are indistinguishable from anaphylactic reactions. Clinical differentiation is unimportant, as management is identical. However, differentiating IgE from non-IgE-mediated disease may aid identification of the precipitating agent.

Angio-oedema

Angio-oedema can occur alone or with urticaria and describes deep tissue swelling which is non-itchy. It is triggered by bradykinin. Two types are recognized:

Hereditary angio-oedema

This is a rare autosomal dominant deficiency of the complement regulatory protein C1 esterase inhibitor. Urticaria is never present, but abdominal pain is common. Angio-oedema may affect the face, lips, larynx, and neck. The finding of normal C3 with undetectable levels of C4 makes the diagnosis. C1 esterase inhibitor levels may also be measured. Androgens (e.g. stanozolol) or anti-fibrinolytics (e.g. tranexamic acid) may be useful prophylactically, and purified C1 esterase inhibitor during an attack or during surgery.

Acquired angio-oedema

This is caused by stress, infection, food, and drug allergies and rarely due to the formation of antibodies against the C1 esterase inhibitor in elderly patients with lymphoma, myeloma, or autoimmune disease (e.g. SLE). In some cases, an identifiable trigger may not be identified in idiopathic nocturnal angio-oedema. The commonest drugs causing angio-oedema are ACE inhibitors (which prevent the breakdown of bradykinin), NSAIDs, and statins. Most acute attacks require steroid therapy, and occasionally adrenaline may be required for laryngeal oedema. Tranexamic acid may be useful prophylactically in idiopathic angio-oedema. Antihistamines are not effective in most cases.

Urticaria (hives)

Urticaria is common. The typical itchy red rash is a wheal and flare response (i.e. nettle rash), with swelling due to leaky capillaries caused by a histamine-induced type 1 hypersensitivity, following degranulation of mast cells.

Causes

Causes include stress, infection, allergy (e.g. food, pollen, drugs), and physical factors (e.g. heat, cold, sun, pressure, vibration, or water). It also occurs in association with thyroid disease and haematinic deficiency. However, 70% of patients have idiopathic urticaria. When severe, it can affect the subcutaneous tissue, producing angio-oedema. It often presents acutely with generalized hives or rash, and the patient feels systemically unwell. Chronic urticaria (>6 weeks) is rarely due to allergy.

Management

Management aims to exclude an underlying cause, remove the precipitant, and provide effective symptomatic treatment.

- Acute urticaria is treated with high-dose, non-sedating, oral antihistamines (e.g. cetirizine 10–20 mg daily) and oral corticosteroids (e.g. prednisolone 20–30 mg daily for 2–3 days). Occasionally, the addition of high doses of anti-H2 receptor inhibitor, such as cimetidine, may be helpful.
- Chronic urticaria is treated with high-dose antihistamine. Tricyclic antidepressants like doxepin have potent anti-H1 and H2 blocking activity and, like montelukast (10 mg daily), may also be effective. Prolonged steroid therapy should be avoided, as side effects outweigh the benefit.

Food allergy

Anaphylaxis represents the severe end of a spectrum of IgE-mediated food allergy presentations and occurs with some nuts and shellfish. Urticaria and angio-oedema represent less severe manifestations. In children, eczema is associated with dairy and wheat food allergies, whereas adult eczema is less often helped by dietary changes. Milk intolerance can cause excessive catarrh in some cases. Occasionally, it may be necessary to undertake elimination diets, with subsequent re-introduction of foods to identify the foods causing symptoms

Many symptoms are attributed to 'food allergy', not all of which are due to true IgE-mediated food allergy. In addition, there is no evidence that irritable bowel syndrome is associated with food allergy.

Oral allergy syndrome

Oral allergy syndrome describes the association of patients sensitized to aeroallergens (e.g. tree, grass pollen), who subsequently develop localized lip and tongue angio-oedema after ingestion of specific fruit (e.g. peaches, almonds) that share cross-reactive epitopes with the pollen allergens. The allergens are heat-labile and destroyed by cooking, and anaphylaxis rarely occurs. Birch pollen cross-reacts with apple, hazelnut, and potato, whereas ragwort pollen shares the same epitopes as melon and banana.

Inhalant allergy

Allergy to aeroantigens, such as pollen (e.g. grass, tree), house dust mite, animal danders (e.g. cat), will trigger allergic rhinoconjunctivitis (hayfever), sinusitis, and asthma.

Typical clinical features include sneezing, rhinitis, headache, conjunctivitis with red, itchy eyes, sinus pain, and bronchospasm with wheeze and breathlessness. Onset is usually rapid after allergen exposure, but symptoms may be chronic if contact cannot be avoided. The history often identifies the trigger, but skin prick or RAST tests are helpful in some cases.

Management includes:

- Oral antihistamines, such as the potent non-sedating agents like cetirizine (10 mg once daily), fexofenadine, and levocetirizine.
- Topical eye agents, including sodium cromoglicate or nedocromil sodium eye drops.
- Nasal steroid sprays, such as mometasone, fluticasone, and betamethasone.
- Asthma therapy, including inhaled bronchodilators like salbutamol, and inhaled steroids, including betamethasone, fluticasone, and budesonide.
- Upper airways allergy uncontrolled by medical therapy may improve after desensitization with immunotherapy.

Bee and wasp stings

These cause local reactions or anaphylaxis, requiring prompt treatment. At presentation, it is important to establish whether there have been previous reactions (in particular, whether there is a history of urticaria, angio-oedema, bronchospasm, or anaphylaxis, although most patients with anaphylaxis have no previous history). Carefully examine the wound, and remove the sting. Observe the patient for several hours for signs of evolving reactions, and treat individual responses, as described previously.

Further reading

Allergy & Anaphylaxis Australia. <http://www.allergyfacts.org.au>.
Allergy UK. <https://www.allergyuk.org>.
Anaphylaxis Campaign. <https://www.anaphylaxis.org.uk>. Tel: 01252 546100.
Asthma and Allergy Foundation of America. <http://www.aafa.org>. Tel: 1 800 727 8462.

Choo KJ, Simon FE, Sheikh A (2010). Glucocorticoids for the treatment of anaphylaxis. *Cochrane Database of Systematic Reviews*, **3**, CD007596.

Craig T, Riedl M, Dykewicz MS, *et al.* (2009). When is prophylaxis for hereditary angio-oedema necessary? *Annals of Allergy, Asthma & Immunology*, **102**, 366–72.

Kemp SF and Lockey RF (2002). Anaphylaxis: a review of causes and mechanisms. *Journal of Allergy and Clinical Immunology*, **110**, 341–8.

Kids with Food Allergies. <http://www.kidswithfoodallergies.org>.

Neugut AI, Ghatak AT, Miller RL (2001). Anaphylaxis in the United States: an investigation into its epidemiology. *Archives of Internal Medicine*, **161**, 15–21.

National Institute for Health and Care Excellence (2014). Drug allergy: diagnosis and management of drug allergy in adults, children and young people. NICE clinical guideline 183. <guidance.nice.org.uk/cg183>.

Pumphrey RS and Roberts IS (2000). Postmortem findings after fatal anaphylactic reactions. *Journal of Clinical Pathology*, **53**, 273–6.

Resuscitation Council UK (2008). Emergency treatment of anaphylactic reactions. <resus.org.uk>.

Simon FE (2009). Anaphylaxis: recent advances in assessment and treatment. *Journal of Allergy and Clinical Immunology*, **124**, 625–36.

UK National Poisons Information Service. Tel: 0844 892 0111. <https://npis.org/> or <https://www.toxbase.org/>.

Envenomation, stings, and bites

Envenomation, stings, and bites from snakes, spiders, scorpions, bees, wasps, ants, ticks, wild animals, jellyfish, cone shell snails, and octopuses are rare, but potentially life-threatening injuries. Although less common in Europe and North America than in many other parts of the world, travellers are at risk, and the acute physician should be aware of the clinical features and basic principles of management of these injuries and anaphylaxis.

Snakebites

Snakes are found on every continent, except Antarctica, and most snakebites are caused by non-venomous species. Only 15% of the 3,000 snake species are considered dangerous to man, and only 1/1,000 snakebites is fatal. Snakes avoid human contact and rarely attack without provocation. Venom production requires considerable energy expenditure and is rarely wasted on a species or prey that cannot be eaten. Even aggressive or territorial species (e.g. black mamba) often inflict a venom-free 'dry bite' (~25–50% of cases), although an angry or frightened snake may increase the amount of venom injected in a defensive, compared to a predatory, bite.

Estimates suggest 1.2–5.5 million snakebites, 0.5–1.8 million envenomations, and 20,000–125,000 deaths worldwide annually. Envenomations and fatalities vary geographically, and most occur in tropical or subtropical regions and in agricultural areas where large numbers of people have to coexist with numerous snakes. South and South East Asia and sub-Saharan Africa are most affected, with the highest frequency in India where an estimated 81,000 envenomations and 11,000 deaths occur annually. In comparison, there are about 45,000 snakebites, 8,000 evenomations, and 10 deaths annually in the USA.

Snakes are divided into three main families, of which two account for most venomous snakes dangerous to humans.

The elapid family
This includes the cobras (e.g *Naja*) of Asia and Africa, the mambas (*Dendroaspis*) of Africa, the kraits (*Bungarus*) of Asia, coral snakes (*Micrurus*) of the Americas, and Australian elapids, like the coastal taipan, tiger and eastern/king brown snakes, and the death adder, all of which are highly venomous. Although Australian snakes are amongst the most venomous in the world, deaths are rare due to wide access to antivenom, with ~60% of fatalities due to the eastern brown snake. Poisonous sea-snakes found in the Indian and Pacific oceans are related to Australian elapids. Most are non–aggressive, and over 50% of bites occur in fishermen attempting to free snakes tangled in fishing nets. Bites are managed in the same way as other elapids.

The viper family
This includes the puff adder (*Bitis arietans*) and Gaboon viper (*Bitis gabonica*) of Africa, the rattlesnakes (*Crotalus*), moccasins (*Agkistrodon*), and lance-headed vipers (*Bothrops*) of the Americas, and the Russell and saw-scaled vipers of Asia. In sub-Saharan Africa, the puff adder is responsible for most fatalities. Most bites occur on industrial plantations which harbour many types of snake prey. Palm and rubber plantations tend to attract elapids, including cobras and mambas, whilst banana plantations are associated with vipers like the night adder. In Europe, 30 deaths occur annually, mainly due to venomous vipers.

The colubrid family
This is the largest, and most diverse, snake family. They are largely harmless and lack venom that is dangerous to humans. However a few highly venomous species, including the boomslang (*Dispholidus typus*), brown tree and twig snakes, and the Japanese garter snake, can be dangerous.

Snake venom contains numerous proteins and enzymes produced in modified parotid glands, produced teliologically to aid capture and digestion of prey. They vary in strength (i.e. the most potent snake venom occurs in the Australian inland taipan), volume (i.e. the Gaboon viper delivers 5–7 mL of venom in a single bite), and composition between species and families of snake, resulting in a wide variety of clinical presentations. Types of snake venom toxins can be classified into:

- Cytotoxins that increase vascular permeability and can cause extensive local tissue destruction.
- Haemotoxins. Venom contains anticoagulants, haemolytic agents, and prothrombin activators with pro-coagulant and consumptive effects (e.g. disseminated intravascular coagulation). Haemoglobinuria may cause renal impairment.
- Neurotoxins that act as pre- or post-synaptic neuromuscular blockers may cause limb/respiratory muscle paralysis.
- Myotoxins that cause heart muscle damage, rhabdomyolysis, and myoglobulinuria, with associated renal impairment.

Symptoms
The effects of venomous snakebites range from simple puncture wounds, with local inflammation, to life-threatening illness and death. Onset can be delayed with no initial symptoms, followed several hours later by sudden onset of severe illness, respiratory failure, and shock.

- **Local effects** are minor in 90% of snakebites. 'Dry bites' may become infected (e.g. septic arthritis, tetanus) and occasionally cause anaphylaxis. Bites from vipers and some cobras may be painful, with swelling, blistering, and bleeding. In contrast, coral or rattlesnake bites are often painless despite being serious injuries. Some cobra venoms can cause severe local tissue necrosis.
- **Initial symptoms** include fear, lethargy, tiredness, weakness, nausea, abdominal discomfort, vomiting, transient hypotension and tachycardia, and local tender lymphadenopathy. Some victims describe a 'rubbery' or metallic taste after being bitten by a rattlesnake. Spitting cobras and rinkhalses can spit venom into the eyes of their victims, causing pain, ophthalmoplegia, and occasionally blindness.
- **Coagulopathy** follows most viper and some Australian elapid bites. Spontaneous bleeding can occur from the mouth (e.g. after brushing teeth), nose, and puncture sites, with internal haemorrhage into the brain or intestines and unexpected bruising.
- **Neurotoxins** found in many elapid, viper, and sea-snake venoms can cause visual disturbance (e.g. diplopia, ophthalmoplegia), dysphonia, dysphagia, paraesthesiae, and dyspnoea. Cobra and mamba venoms may cause rapid respiratory and limb paralysis which can last several days, resulting in rapid death, unless lifesaving mouth-to-mouth resuscitation and subsequent mechanical ventilation are

started immediately. However, onset may be delayed for several hours before progressing rapidly.

- **Rhabdomyolysis**, with widespread muscle necrosis, including cardiac muscle, follows envenomation by most vipers and sea-snakes and some elapids. Myoglobin and other muscle debris, with associated hypotension, can cause renal impairment or failure.

Management

Assessment of the severity and likely outcome of a snakebite can be difficult. It depends on the type of snake, the area of the body bitten, the amount of venom injected, the age and premorbid health of the victim, and the time it takes for the patient to find, and quality of, subsequent treatment.

Snake identification

Snake identification can be important in planning treatment. In some areas of the world it is not always possible, although knowledge of the local snake population and symptoms associated with envenomation by individual snakes may be helpful. In countries (e.g. USA) where polyvalent antivenoms are available, snake identification is less of a priority.

First aid

Recommendations vary according to the type of venom injected by the local snake populations, and the regional first aid guidelines should be followed. If the venom causes:

- Few local effects but results in life-threatening systemic illness, containing the venom in the region of the bite by pressure immobilization is preferred.
- Severe localized tissue damage, immobilization may increase the damage in the bitten area.

Most guidelines recommend the following:

- Call for help, and arrange transport to the nearest hospital emergency room as soon as possible, where antivenom for snakes common to that region will often be available.
- Protect the patient from further bites. Do not risk further bites by attempting to capture the snake.
- Keep the patient still, and remain calm, as movement and stress increase blood flow and aid dissemination of venom.
- Keep the bitten limb in a functional position and below heart level to minimize blood return to the heart and subsequent transport of venom to the organs.
- Remove items that may constrict the bitten limb if it swells (e.g. rings, bracelets, footwear).
- Clean the bite site, but this may prevent swabs being taken for venom identification at a later stage. If venom has been sprayed into the eyes, copious washing with sterile (or at least clean) water is required, followed by application of a sterile ophthalmic antibiotic ointment.

The following first aid treatments are outdated, ineffective, and often harmful.

- Tourniquet application is not recommended. Cutting off the circulation can lead to gangrene and death, a tragedy in non-threatening snakebites (e.g. dry bites). A compression bandage (see later text) is more effective and safer.
- Incision of the bitten area, often prior to suction, causes more damage and increases the risk of infection.
- Suction at the site of the bite by mouth or pump is ineffective and risks poisoning the medical attendant due to absorption through the mouth mucosa and infection of

the bite wound due to mouth bacteria. After 3 minutes, less than one thousandth of the venom will be extracted.

- Anecdotal remedies, including immersion in sour milk, snake stones, potassium permanganate, and electroshock therapy, do not work and delay transport and early antivenom therapy.

Sutherland's pressure immobilization

As 95% of snakebites occur on the arms or legs, the object of pressure immobilization is to contain venom within a bitten limb. Most snakebite venom is injected into subcutaneous tissues, and gentle pressure inhibits normal lymphatic drainage and subsequent transport to vital organs, whilst immobilization inhibits the pumping action of skeletal muscle which normally aids limb fluid drainage. Pressure is applied with an elasticized (or any) bandage, starting 2–4 inches above the site of the bite, initially winding up around the limb in overlapping turns, towards the heart, then returning down over the bite and towards the hand and foot. The bandage must be as tight as when strapping a sprained ankle (i.e. it must not cut off blood flow or be uncomfortable) and must be applied as soon as possible after the bite for maximum benefit. The limb should be immobilized with a sling or splint. The location of the bite should be marked on the outside of the bandage.

The combination of pressure and immobilization may effectively contain venom in the limb and delay symptoms for up to 24 hours. However, removing the bandage releases the venom, with rapid and potentially fatal consequences. Only remove the bandage when antivenom is available or has been administered and facilities for resuscitation are available.

The Australian National Health Service formally adopted pressure immobilization as the preferred method of first aid treatment of snakebites in 1979. Evidence for efficacy is relatively limited, and it is only attempted by a third of snakebite victims in Australia. It is probably most effective against neurotoxins, such as those released by many Australian elapids, but is not appropriate for cytotoxic bites, such as those inflicted by most vipers. Although not validated for African or American snakes, pressure immobilization has been cautiously adopted by other regions and probably does no harm, provided that the bandage is not applied too tightly and limb swelling is allowed for by slowly releasing tension, as needed.

Venom detection kits

An *in vitro* sensitive enzyme immunoassay venom detection kit, using rabbit antibodies, can identify snake venom in swabs of secretion from the site of the bite, blood, and urine. This allows use of specific antivenoms which are more effective, reduce side effects, and are less likely to cause severe anaphylactic or serum sickness reactions.

Antivenom

Antivenom is still the only effective treatment for some snake evenomations. They are made by injecting small amounts of venom into an animal, usually a horse or sheep and harvesting the resulting antibodies from the animal's blood. Prior to their advent, bites from some species of snake were usually fatal. They are often expensive and available from local poisons units (see next paragraphs).

- **Specific antivenoms**, if available, are more effective and may cause less side effects if the type of snake is known (e.g. Australian tiger snake or Boomslang antivenom) or the results of venom detection tests can be awaited.

- **Polyvalent antivenoms**, effective against numerous snake species, are used in severe envenomations when delay may be harmful, or when the type of snake is unknown. Polyvalent antivenoms are usually specific to the types of snake found in a specific region. Organizations that assist in locating these antivenoms include CSL Ltd, Parkville, Australia (polyvalent Australian antivenom) and The South African Institute for Medical Research (polyvalent snake antivenom).

Slow intravenous infusion of antivenom, diluted in crystalloid solution, neutralizes venom enzymes and reduces anaphylactic reactions. Treatment should be as early as possible, as it is difficult to reverse established damage (i.e. myonecrosis, binding to presynaptic neuromuscular receptors).

The dose of antivenom required varies. One ampoule of specific antivenom neutralizes the average yield from milking the snake involved. However, the dose required depends on the severity of the envenomation. After a large mamba or cobra bite, the initial dose may be as high as ten ampoules, given over a few minutes and guided by the response.

Australian guidelines recommend adult premedication with 0.25 mg of subcutaneous epinephrine, which is the only effective method of reducing the incidence and severity of adverse reactions which occur in 8–13% of cases. This is because treating iatrogenic anaphylaxis, as it occurs, has a high mortality despite early expert resuscitation. During severe anaphylaxis, antihistamines are of relatively little benefit, and steroids are limited by their slow onset of action. In any event, facilities should be available for immediate resuscitation, following antivenom administration.

However, mild adverse reactions, including headache, rash, arthralgia, abdominal discomfort, vomiting, and pyrexia, may be treated with antihistamine and steroids. Steroids may also reduce delayed hypersensitivity reactions (i.e. serum sickness), which often occur several days after antivenom administration.

General therapy
Fluid resuscitation is essential, following initial antivenom therapy, in patients with severe local tissue damage and massive tissue oedema due to vascular endothelial permeability, following viper bites (e.g. puff adder, Gaboon viper). Elevate, and immobilize the limb. Combination of paracetamol and opioid analgesia may be required, but avoid non-steroidal anti-inflammatory agents due to potential renal impairment associated with haemolysis and rhabdomyolysis.

Coagulation defects (e.g. after Boomslang snakebites) may require correction with fresh frozen plasma or platelets. Ventilatory failure due to neurotoxins (e.g. elapids) may require support with mechanical ventilation for many days.

Larger snakes can inflict nasty wounds with their many strong fangs/teeth. The physical damage and secondary infection (e.g. cellulitis, septic arthritis) can cause severe damage. Tetanus is a real danger, and human tetanus immunoglobulin (HTI) should be given as for any animal bite (see further text). The wound may need surgical cleaning and antibiotics.

Spiders

Most spiders are venomous, but few are able to penetrate skin and inject venom. Only a few of the Australian and South American species that can envenomate humans produce neurotoxins requiring antivenom. The vast majority of spider bites are non-fatal, but some can produce severe and painful local injury. Harmful species of spider include:

Australian funnel web spiders
These (*Atrax* or *Hadronyche*) are potentially lethal. The Sydney funnel web spider is a large aggressive spider that lives around Sydney and is responsible for several deaths annually. The male is more dangerous than the female. It often enters houses after rainfall and shelters in bedding or among clothes, giving a painful bite when disturbed. Envenomation, which presents with nausea, vomiting, sweating, salivation, and abdominal pain, may be rapidly fatal (i.e. within 90 minutes to several hours) but does not always occur. Venom contains a polypeptide that stimulates the release of acetylcholine at neuromuscular junctions and release of catecholamines. Muscle fasciculation around the bite rapidly progresses to distant muscle groups, followed by central hypoventilation, coma, hypertension, tachycardia, vasoconstriction, bronchorrhoea, pulmonary oedema, and finally respiratory failure. It should be treated like a snakebite with pressure immobilization (as previously described), antivenom, and support of vital functions, including mechanical ventilation. Deaths are unlikely after administration of antivenom.

The fiddle spider or brown recluse spider
This is from North Africa, the Mediterranean, and the Americas. Its bite can be fatal, but deaths are rare. However, the bite which is initially painless can cause severe localized tissue damage, with severe scarring.

Australian red back spider
This has a 1 cm body with a characteristic red or orange strip on its abdomen. It is found in gardens and rural areas. Following a relatively painless bite, the site becomes inflamed, with severe pain which spreads up the limb, and is associated with headache, vomiting, fever, hypertension, profuse sweating, and rashes. Untreated, progressive muscle paralysis which may require mechanical ventilation can occur. A pressure bandage is not recommended for red back spider bites as this aggravates the pain. It is the commonest cause of antivenom administration in Australia, and there have been no deaths since its introduction. However, a current study is assessing antivenom versus opioid plus paracetamol/NSAID analgesia.

Black widow spiders
These are found in the Americas, Africa, Southern Europe, Australia, and Asia. Its bite can cause painful muscle spasms, lasting several days.

Banana spiders
These spiders, from South America, are quite aggressive, with painful bites that are rarely fatal.

Wolf spiders
These are found in South America and Europe. The bite causes local tissue death and scarring.

Painful bites with local skin damage should be immobilized and a cold/ice compress applied to the bite site. Antihistamines and analgesics alleviate associated symptoms.

Bites from poisonous spiders are treated in a similar manner to snakebites. The spider should be killed, if possible, and taken to the emergency room for identification. The patient should be transported to hospital as quickly, and as passively, as possible. Pressure immobilization may impede venom distribution. Appropriate antivenom may be lifesaving.

Scorpions

Scorpions are found in dry, arid regions. They hide in dark, shady places (e.g. shoes, cupboards). They use their tail sting in self-defence, causing painful, rather than life-threatening, stings. However, potentially lethal scorpions whose sting envenomations cause neurotoxicity, with visual blurring, respiratory paralysis, and myocardial damage are found in South America, India, Mexico, North Africa, and the Middle East. All scorpion stings require medical review. If possible, kill and take the scorpion to the emergency room for identification. Initially, wash the sting area, and apply a cold compress. Immobilize the patient, and seek immediate medical advice. Antihistamines and analgesics alleviate local pain and swelling. Antivenoms are available for the more dangerous species but must be given quickly.

Jellyfish, stinging fish, and octopuses
Many marine and freshwater species are able to deliver severe, or potentially fatal, envenomations. However, in UK waters, most jellyfish are harmless, and minor stings are treated with vinegar (5% acetic acid) to neutralize the toxin. Weeverfish spines produce a heat-labile toxin, neutralized by immersion in hot water for 30 minutes. However, tiny spine sections can cause long-term irritation and require expert removal.

Box jellyfish (Chironex fleckeri)
This is probably the most venomous species in the world. The semi-transparent cuboid bell, which is 30 cm across, and the numerous tentacles that trail for several metres are difficult to see in shallow water. The tentacles contain millions of nematocysts which discharge poisoned barbs which can pierce subcutaneous tissue on contact and cause severe pain, envenomation, and potentially death within minutes. The venom is both neurotoxic, causing potentially fatal apnoea, and cardiotoxic, causing rapidly fatal hypotension. Survivors may have severe skin scarring. Avoidance or prevention with the use of wetsuits or baggy clothing in potentially affected waters is essential. Immediate treatment requires acetic acid application to adherent tentacles to inactivate undischarged nematocysts prior to removal. Ovine antivenom is available.

Irukandji jellyfish (Carukia barnesi)
This jellyfish which has a small square-shaped bell a few centimetres across, with single tentacles from the corners, and some other jellyfish cause a mild sting but stimulate massive catecholamine release. Typical general symptoms include hypertension, limb, abdominal, and back pain, chest tightness, and occasionally cardiogenic pulmonary oedema which may require mechanical ventilation and inotropic therapy.

Venomous fish
These carry venom in stinging spines. The stonefish is most dangerous, releasing venom when trodden on. Initial excruciating local pain is followed by venom-induced cardiovascular, neuromuscular and myotoxicity, and potential death. Antivenom is available, and nerve blocks may be required to control the pain.

Gastropod molluscs (cone shells)
These may release a venom-laden harpoon from their beautiful shells that causes rapid neurotoxicity and potential death. There is no antivenom, and mechanical ventilation is required until spontaneous recovery occurs.

Octopuses
Octopuses may bite and inject a neurotoxin, tetrodotoxin, which causes a flaccid paralysis and potential death. Mechanical ventilation is required whilst awaiting recovery.

Insect bites
Minor local reactions are common. These can be treated with cold compresses, rest, elevation, analgesia, and antihistamines (e.g. chlorphenamine 4 mg tds, loratadine 10 mg od). Prophylactic antibiotic therapy is not usually required but may be considered in immunosuppressed patients (e.g. diabetics, high-dose steroids). However, occasionally, secondary infection/cellulitis and ascending lymphangitis may require treatment. Patients can usually be discharged with instructions to return if they develop breathlessness, wheeze, rash, generalized pruritus, or oropharyngeal swelling. Patients with previous systemic reactions should be admitted for observation.

Ticks can be acquired from domestic animals or whilst walking in undergrowth or woodland. Some ticks (e.g. Ixodes holocyclus) in America and Australia can inject a toxin that causes a flaccid paralysis, tick paralysis, similar to Guillain–Barré syndrome after 3–5 days. The tick must be carefully and fully removed. An antitoxin is available. Ticks may also transmit infections like typhus, Lyme disease, and Rocky Mountain spotted fever.

Lyme disease
Lyme disease is caused by a sheep, mouse, or deer tick-borne spirochaete Borrelia burgdorferi. It occurs in the UK, Europe, North America, and parts of Asia, China, Russia, and Australia. It usually occurs in summer or early autumn and 2–40 days after the initial tick bite which is only detected in 20% of cases.

• Initially, there is local inflammation and redness around the site of the bite, with central clearing (erythema migrans) and mild systemic symptoms.

• Blood-borne disseminated disease follows over the next few weeks or months and manifests as a fluctuating, acute febrile illness, with secondary skin lesions and subsequent development of large joint, often monoarticular, arthritis in 60%, neurological symptoms in 15% (e.g. meningitis, encephalitis, cranial, or peripheral nerve palsies), and myocarditis in 10%.

• Late persistent symptoms develop (if the early disease is not treated) with chronic, recurrent autoimmune arthritis, peripheral neuropathy, encephalopathy, and skin changes.

Diagnosis is confirmed by serology. Early treatment is with amoxicillin or doxycycline for 2–3 weeks or cephalosporins for arthritis and neurological features. Late disease does not respond to antibiotics.

Bee and wasp stings
These cause local reactions or anaphylaxis, requiring prompt treatment. At presentation, it is important to establish whether there have been previous reactions, in particular, whether there is a history of urticaria, angio-oedema, bronchospasm, or anaphylaxis (although most patients with anaphylaxis have no previous history). Carefully examine the wound, and remove the sting. Observe the patient for 2–3 hours for signs of evolving reactions.

Contact with other wild animals
Contact with rat's urine may cause leptospirosis (Weil's disease). It is caused by the spirochaete Leptospira interrogans and is spread by contact with infected rat's urine in canals, rivers or sewers. The spirochaete enters the body through small breaks in the skin or via the mucous membranes of the eyes, nose, or mouth. This is followed ten days later by fever, headache, vomiting, diarrhoea,

haemorrhagic rash, conjunctivitis, jaundice, and renal failure. Treatment is with a penicillin or doxycycline, with haemodialysis if necessary. Consider prophylactic penicillin in patients who inadvertently fall into potentially infected waterways. Mortality is 1%.

Unusual bites present specific hazards and require expert advice from infectious disease specialists. For example, monkey bites may cause herpes simplex infection, requiring prophylactic aciclovir, and bats may carry rabies.

Bite wounds

Contaminated puncture wounds and crush injuries follow bites and carry a high risk of bacterial, and occasionally viral, infection. Bacterial infection with streptococci, *Staphylococcus aureus*, *Clostridium tetani*, *Bacteroides*, *Eikenella corrodens* (human bites), and *Pasteurella multocida* (cat bites or scratches) is common, following puncture wounds due to cat or human bites, in hand wounds over 24 hours old, and in diabetics, alcoholics, or the immunocompromised.

Septicaemia is uncommon after bite injuries. It can occur with the Gram-negative bacillus *Capnocytophaga canimorsus* which causes a severe illness with disseminated intravascular coagulation, usually in immunocompromised subjects (e.g. alcoholics or following splenectomy).

Management
Local treatment
Initially, clean the wound thoroughly with normal saline; debride under anaesthetic, and remove foreign material. Obtain radiographs if fracture, joint involvement, or foreign bodies (e.g. teeth) are suspected. Facial, tendon, and joint injuries must be referred to a specialist. Primary or delayed primary closure depends on the site (e.g. cosmetic considerations may take precedence in facial wounds), and expert advice should be sought.

Prophylactic antibiotic treatment
This is controversial. Some departments recommend antibiotics for all bite wounds; others suggest treatment for immunocompromised individuals, puncture wounds, hand bites, and bites from humans, cats, and rats. Co-amoxiclav is an effective broad-spectrum agent against streptococci, *Bacteroides*, *Staphylococcus aureus*, *Pasturella*, and *Eikenella*. Erythromycin is given in penicillin-allergic individuals.

Tetanus prophylaxis
This is essential. Tetanus causes many adult deaths in the developing world and occasional fatalities in the UK, particularly in drug addicts using the subcutaneous or intramuscular routes. *Clostridium tetani* is an anaerobic, spore-forming Gram-positive bacillus that proliferates in contaminated, often devitalized, wounds and produces an exotoxin tetanospasmin that interferes with neurotransmission. Any wound, including burns, is at risk. Most adults in the UK will have been fully immunized with five doses of tetanus toxoid (three initial doses of tetanus toxoid in early childhood and then at 4 and 14 years of age). Inadequate immunity may occur in immigrants, immunocompromised, and elderly patients. The need for tetanus prophylaxis depends on immune status and whether the wound is tetanus-prone. Heavily contaminated wounds (e.g. soil), those with devitalized tissue, and puncture wounds or bites are considered tetanus-prone.

* If the patient is fully immunized (i.e. five previous vaccine doses), do not give further vaccine. Only give human tetanus immunoglobulin if the risk is especially high.

* If the vaccination programme is incomplete, consider giving the next dose of vaccine early.
* If the patient is not up to date with the vaccination programme or is unvaccinated, give combined tetanus/diphtheria and polio vaccine, and refer for completion of the vaccination course. Give human tetanus immunoglobulin if the risk is especially high.

Rabies prophylaxis
This should be considered, following bites from potentially rabid animals. It is transmitted in saliva through puncture wounds or mucous membranes. The long incubation period of rabies (14–90 days) allows successful post-exposure prophylaxis at a relatively late stage.

Hepatitis and HIV infection
This should be considered, following human bites, and treated as 'needle-stick injuries'

Needle-stick injury

A needle-stick injury is a specialized puncture wound that may follow failure to follow universal precautions in the clinical setting. A vast number of organisms have been transferred by needle-stick injuries, including *Staphylococcus aureus*, tuberculosis, syphilis, gonorrhoea, streptococci, hepatitis, HIV, diphtheria, toxoplasmosis, typhus, leptospirosis, malaria, rickettsial infections, and many more.

In practice, the main dangers are from hepatitis B and C and HIV. The risk of acquiring hepatitis B or C from a carrier after a needle-stick injury is 20–40% and 3–10%, respectively. All hospital workers should be vaccinated against hepatitis B and antibody levels checked at regular intervals. The risk of acquiring HIV from a HIV-positive patient after a needle-stick injury is less at 0.2–0.5%, unless significant volumes are injected. Post-exposure prophylaxis reduces the risk further if treatment is given as soon as possible. There is a very small risk (~0.05%) of HIV transmission after mucocutaneous exposure (e.g. through cuts/abrasions, eye splashes, etc.).

Management of needle-stick injuries
* Prevention of needle-stick injuries is essential.
* Wash the wound with soap and water.
* Give tetanus cover, if necessary.
* Take blood for storage (serology for future testing), and, in the case of a possible HIV source patient, also check routine bloods.
* Obtain consent from the source patient prior to taking blood to check hepatitis and HIV status. If the patient cannot give consent, follow local guidelines or obtain specialist advice from a virologist or infection control specialist.
* Assess hepatitis B cover. If previously vaccinated, check antibody levels. If low, give a booster vaccine; if very low, give immunoglobulin and a booster vaccine; if satisfactory, take no further action. If not immunized, give hepatitis B immunoglobulin, and start an active immunization course. Do not withhold hepatitis B prophylaxis if there is difficulty obtaining consent from source patient or if there is any doubt.
* If the patient is HIV-positive or suspected to be HIV-positive, follow local guidelines and/or contact a virologist or infectious disease specialist to discuss the need for post-exposure prophylaxis. Combined prophylactic therapy with zidovudine 250 mg twice daily, lamivudine 150 mg

twice daily, and nelfinavir 1,250 mg twice daily is most effective and should be started within 1 hour of exposure but may be effective for up to 2 weeks after exposure. However, prophylaxis has side effects, affecting mainly the gastrointestinal system, and the decision to start prophylaxis must be taken in consultation with a local expert. Until seroconversion has been ruled out, advise the patient to use barrier contraception and avoid blood donation.

- No proven post-exposure prophylaxis exists for hepatitis C, and prevention of needle-stick injuries is, therefore, essential in these patients.
- Arrange follow-up counselling.
- Inform occupational health if the incident occurred in hospital, and review policy and procedures.

Further reading

Australian Venom Research Unit Advisory Unit. Tel: 03 9483 8204.

Campbell JA and Lamar WW (2004). *The venomous reptiles of the western hemisphere*. Cornell University Press, Ithaca.

Clinical Management Guidelines (2013). Snakebite and spiderbite. <www0.health.nsw.gov.au>.

Health Protection Agency (2012). Eye of the needle: 2012. <http://www.hpa.org.uk/Publications/InfectiousDiseases/BloodBorneInfections/EyeOfTheNeedle/1212EyeoftheNeedle2012Report/>.

Gold BS, Dart RC, Barish RA (2002). Bites of venomous snakes. *New England Journal of Medicine*, **347**, 347–56.

Kasturiratne A, Wickremasinghe AR, de Silva N (2008). The global burden of snakebite: a literature analysis and modeling based on regional estimates of envenoming and deaths. *PloS Medicine*, **5**, e218.

Little M , Mulcahy RF, Wenck DJ (2001). Life threatening cardiac failure in a healthy young female with Irukandji syndrome. *Anaesthesia and Intensive Care*, **29**, 178–80.

Public Health England (2014). Blood borne viruses: Eye of the needle. <www.gov.uk>.

Public Health England (2014). The Green Book: Immunisation against infectious disease. <https://www.gov.uk/government/collections/immunisation-against-infectious-disease-the-green-book>.

Thorpe RS, Wuster W, Malhotra A (1996). *Venomous snakes: ecology, evolution, and snakebite*. Oxford University Press, Oxford.

Tibballs J, Williams D, Sutherland SK (1998). The effects of antivenom and verapamil on the haemodynamic actions of *Chironex fleckeri* (Box jellyfish) venom. *Anaesthesia and Intensive Care*, **26**, 40–5.

UK National Poisons Information Service. Tel: 0844 892 0111. < www.npis.org/> or <https://www.toxbase.org/>

Venom Supplies Ltd, Tanunda, South Australia. Tel: 08 8563 0001.

Virus Reference Department, London UK. Tel: 020 327 6017.

Warrell DA (2009). Management of exotic snakebites. *QJM*, **102**, 593–601.

Fitness to fly and effects of altitude

In excess of 1.5 billion people per year travel by air. Whilst pilots are screened for their capacity to tolerate the stresses of flight, passengers are not. Up to 5% of airline passengers have pre-existing medical conditions, and the incidence of serious medical incidents in-flight is 1 in 10,000 passengers. With increasing frequency and duration of air travel and increasing population age, these figures are predicted to rise.

The role of physicians in maximizing air safety is predominantly in pre-flight assessment and preparation. It is essential physicians consider the following:

1. Will the flight environment exacerbate the medical condition of the passenger?
2. Will the medical condition affect the comfort or safety of other passengers or the operation of the aircraft?

The flight environment

Oxygenation

With increasing altitude, there is a reduction in atmospheric pressure and in the partial pressure of oxygen. The standard cruising altitude for commercial aircraft is 30,000 ft. Aircraft are pressurized to a cabin altitude around 8,000 ft. At 8,000 ft, atmospheric pressure is reduced by 75%, and the inspired partial pressure of oxygen is reduced from 21 kPa to 15 kPa. This corresponds to a PaO_2 around 8–10 kPa in an individual with normal respiratory function and oxygen saturation around 90–94%.

The acute response to a fall in PaO_2 is driven by peripheral chemoreceptors to produce hyperventilation and mild tachycardia. These physiological adjustments are well tolerated by most travellers but may lead to compromise in passengers with cardiopulmonary disease.

Gas expansion

Reduced atmospheric pressure within the aircraft cabin is associated with an increase in the volume of any gas present. At 8,000 ft, the volume increase is around 30%.

This commonly results in symptoms of ear discomfort in passengers unable to equalize the pressures between their middle and outer ears, abdominal discomfort in passengers with excess bowel gas, and tooth pain in passengers with fillings.

Volume expansion is potentially hazardous when gas is trapped within a contained space as may occur with penetrating eye injury, depressed skull fracture, pneumothorax, or post-surgery.

Humidity

Reduction in the partial pressure of water vapour and air temperature at altitude results in a fall in relative humidity. Relative cabin humidity is 10%, compared with 40–50% in buildings. There is no evidence that low humidity causes passengers to become dehydrated, but irritation of mucous membranes does occur.

Passenger immobility

In susceptible passengers, prolonged immobility is the main contributor to in-flight deep venous thrombosis. The risk of thrombosis increases with travel longer than 4 hours' duration. Passengers at high risk should receive prophylactic heparin. All other passengers should be encouraged to ambulate and consider anti-embolism stockings. There is no role for aspirin in thrombosis prevention.

Circadian rhythm disruption

Circadian desynchronosis (jet lag), also termed circadian dysrhythmia by the UK Civil Aviation Authority, occurs when there is loss of agreement between an individual's body clock and environmental cues, occurring with rapid, long-distance, east-west, or west-east travel. This may complicate the timing of medication within a regular dosing regime.

Pre-existing medical conditions

Cardiovascular disease

The tachycardic response to hypobaric hypoxia increases myocardial oxygen demand. Passengers with cardiovascular disease may require supplementary oxygen to minimize the risk of cardiac decompensation.

Oxygen supplementation

In-flight oxygen is recommended in passengers with congestive cardiac failure (NYHA III–IV), angina (Canadian Cardiovascular Society grading of angina; (CCS) III–IV), cyanotic congenital heart disease, pulmonary hypertension, and baseline hypoxaemia (PaO_2 <9 kPa).

Ischaemic heart disease

Passengers with stable angina pectoris usually tolerate flight but should carry their medication in the cabin. Unstable angina is a contraindication to flight. Passengers with uncomplicated myocardial infarction should not fly for at least 3 days (10 days if the LV ejection fraction is <45%). Passengers with myocardial infarction complicated by failure of flow restoration on angiography, dysrhythmia, or cardiac failure, should not fly.

Cardiothoracic surgery

Passengers undergoing uncomplicated percutaneous coronary intervention can fly after 2 days. Those undergoing coronary artery bypass grafting or other thoracic surgery are safe to fly once any residual air in the chest has resorbed. This usually occurs within 10–14 days and should be confirmed by chest X-ray.

Other

Uncontrolled hypertension and uncontrolled dysrhythmia are contraindications to air travel. Symptomatic valvular heart disease is a relative contraindication. Modern pacemakers and implantable defibrillators are compatible with aircraft systems. Following a cerebrovascular accident, passengers should not fly for 10 days. Supplemental oxygen is advised in known cerebral artery insufficiency.

Respiratory disease

Fitness to fly with respiratory disease should be judged pragmatically, based upon previous flight experience, flight duration, and the stability of the patient's underlying respiratory condition. Complex patients can be assessed in a hypobaric chamber under medical supervision. If PaO_2 falls below 6kPa after breathing the equivalent of 15% inspired oxygen for 20 minutes then supplemental oxygen is indicated in flight.

Oxygen supplementation

Any passenger with baseline hypoxaemia or using long-term oxygen should be considered for in-flight oxygen. Flow rates may need to be increased at altitude. Sea level oxygen requirements exceeding 4 L/min are a contraindication to air travel.

Pneumothorax

Closed pneumothorax with a persistent air leak is a contraindication to air travel due to the risk of expansion and progression to tension. Passengers with treated pneumothorax should have complete resolution confirmed by chest X-ray; thereafter, it is advisable to wait a further 14 days before flight.

Pleural effusion

Pleural effusions, especially if large, should be drained pre-flight. A post-drainage chest X-ray should be taken to exclude recurrence or pneumothorax, and flight should be delayed for 14 days.

Obstructive airway disease

Passengers with asthma and COPD should have their treatment regime optimized pre-flight. They should carry their regular inhalers in the cabin and consider an emergency supply of prednisolone. Nebulizers are not routinely available in-flight.

Other

Passengers with bronchiectasis and cystic fibrosis should maintain adequate hydration and consider carrying antibiotics and mucolytics. Those with interstitial lung disease may also wish to carry antibiotics and corticosteroids. Passengers with severe neuromuscular disease should be considered for non-invasive ventilation in-flight.

Infectious disease

Individuals with active or contagious infection should not fly. Passengers with pulmonary tuberculosis require three smear-negative sputum samples on separate days. Immunosuppressed patients, including those with HIV, may be at risk of acquiring infection in flight. Pre-flight vaccination should be considered.

Haematology

Anaemia should be considered for correction at levels less than 8 g/dL. Neutropenic passengers should be informed of the infection risk arising from proximity to other passengers.

Surgical

Post-operative patients are in a state of increased oxygen consumption, and post-operative anaemia also contributes to reduced oxygen-carrying capacity. It is advisable to delay flight for several days post-operatively or to consider supplemental oxygen. Gas expansion with altitude has implications for all types of surgery.

Gastrointestinal

Abdominal surgery predisposes to ileus. Intra-abdominal gas expansion may result in mucosal stretching with haemorrhage and ultimately rupture of anastomoses. Flight should be delayed for 10 days post-laparotomy and for 24 hours post-endoscopy or laparoscopy.

Neuro/ophthalmic

Post-neurosurgery passengers should not fly for 7 days to avoid complications of increased intracranial pressure. Post-ophthalmic surgery passengers should not fly for 6 weeks if intraocular gas has been introduced.

Trauma/orthopaedics

Expansion of air trapped beneath plaster casts may lead to discomfort and neurovascular compromise. Most airlines restrict flying for 24–48 hours following cast application, or insist casts are bi-valved.

Obstetric

Airline travel is not considered hazardous to a normal pregnancy. Despite maternal hypobaric hypoxia, fetal oxygena-tion is maintained by the favourable oxygen-binding affinity of fetal haemoglobin and high fetal haematocrit. Pregnant women should be encouraged to ambulate and wear anti-embolism stockings. To minimize the risk of delivery in-flight, most airlines do not allow women to travel after 36 weeks for a single pregnancy or 32 weeks for a multiple pregnancy.

Neuropsychiatric

Passengers with controlled epilepsy should be informed of the seizure threshold-reducing effects of altered circadian rhythm, sleep deprivation, and hypoxia. Flight should be delayed for 24 hours following a seizure. Individuals with the potential for unpredictable, aggressive, or disruptive behaviour should not travel by air. Stable psychiatric passengers may travel with an escort.

In-flight medical emergencies

Most in-flight medical problems can be dealt with by cabin crew or by liaison with ground-based medical advice centres. When physicians are called upon to assist, GMC guidance states, 'In an emergency, wherever it arises, you must offer assistance, taking account of your own safety, your competency, and the availability of other options for care'.

Medical equipment

All airlines carry medical equipment, though the contents vary significantly. International aircraft usually carry first aid kits, a medical kit for advanced life support, and an automated external defibrillator. Oxygen is invariably available, although supply may be limited and flow rates are restricted to 4 L/min.

Passengers wishing to bring their own medical equipment on board must seek permission from the airline. Equipment must be certified airworthy. This restricts the use of some types of oxygen cylinder and electrically powered equipment which may interfere with aircraft systems.

Medication

Passengers requiring prescription medication should carry this with them in the aircraft cabin and maintain routine dosing schedules. Diabetics may need to make minor adjustments to long-acting insulin doses if there is a greater than 2-hour difference in time zone between their departure and arrival destinations. A physician's letter is required for passengers carrying greater than 100 mL of liquid medication, controlled medication, needles, and syringes. The NHS website advises patients to check the rules for all countries being visited and to carry medicines and medical equipment in the original labelled packages, in hand luggage, with a copy of the prescription and physician letter.

Medical documentation

The majority of airlines adhere to standardized procedures for acceptance and handling of passengers with medical requirements. The Incapacitated Passengers Handling Advice (INCAD) form, completed by a travel agent, details flight schedules, mobility and seating requirements, and medical requirements, such as modified diet, oxygen, and equipment. The Medical Information Form (MEDIF) is used to supplement the INCAD and is completed by a physician. INCAD and MEDIF forms are valid for a single flight. Incapacitated passengers who fly frequently can apply to individual airlines for a Frequent Traveller Medical Card (FREMEC) which is an enduring record of their specific needs.

Altitude sickness

Altitude sickness encompasses a spectrum of disorders which typically onset at altitudes exceeding 8,000 ft (i.e.

greater than cabin altitude). Risk factors are rapid rate of ascent, altitude attained, physical activity at altitude, and individual susceptibility. The pathophysiology is thought to relate to hypobaric hypoxia.

Acute mountain sickness (AMS), the most benign disorder, is usually self-limiting. It is characterized by headache, nausea, anorexia, lethargy, and sleep disturbance. High-altitude pulmonary oedema (HAPE) and high-altitude cerebral oedema (HACE) are potentially fatal. HAPE is characterized by dyspnoea at rest, cough, frothy blood-stained sputum, cyanosis, raised JVP, and pulmonary crepitations. Features of HACE are severe headache, ataxia, confusion, altered behaviour, hallucinations, reduced conscious level, and papilloedema.

Prevention, predominantly altitude acclimatization, is the key to managing altitude sickness. Acetazolamide, taken prior to ascent, induces mild acidosis and facilitates hyperventilation but is not recommended routinely. AMS may be treated with hydration, analgesia, and avoidance of further ascent. Severe altitude sickness must prompt urgent descent from altitude. Supplemental oxygen and portable hyperbaric chambers are beneficial but should not delay descent. Nifedipine is used in HAPE to reduce pulmonary artery pressure, and dexamethasone reduces cerebral oedema in HACE.

Further reading

Aerospace Medical Association Medical Guidelines Taskforce (2003). Medical guidelines for airline travel: 2nd edn. *Aviation, Space and Environmental Medicine*, **74** (5 Suppl), A1–19.

Ahmedzai S, Balfour-Lynn I, Bewick T, *et al.* (2011) Managing passengers with respiratory disease planning air travel: British Thoracic Society recommendations. *Thorax*, **66**, i1–i30.

Aviation Health Unit, UK Civil Aviation Authority (2012). Assessing fitness to fly: guidelines for medical professionals.

Smith D, Toff W, Joy M, *et al.* (2010). Fitness to fly for patients with cardiovascular disease. *Heart*, **96**, ii1–16.

Chapter 19

Practical procedures
and monitoring

Practical procedures and monitoring

Practical procedures are usually performed to confirm the diagnosis (e.g. lumbar puncture, aspiration of pleural fluid), to facilitate monitoring (e.g. blood or central venous pressure monitoring), or as therapeutic procedures (e.g. chest drainage). Some procedures may be multifunctional (e.g. central venous catheterization aids diagnosis, monitoring, and therapeutic interventions). Practical and monitoring procedures are associated with potentially severe risks, and appropriate precautions (e.g. INR), discussions with patients (and/or relatives), and consents are essential.

Monitoring in acute medicine

Monitoring ensures early detection of change in clinical parameters and accurate assessment of progress and response to therapy. However, the following principles always apply:

- **Monitoring aids assessment**, but regular clinical examination is essential. Simple physical signs like appearance (e.g. pallor), peripheral perfusion, and conscious level are as important as parameters displayed on a monitor. When clinical signs and monitored parameters disagree, **assume that clinical assessment is correct**, until potential errors from monitored variables have been excluded (e.g. blocked CVP lines, incorrect calibration). Trends are generally more important than single readings.
- **Use non-invasive techniques whenever possible**, as invasive monitoring is associated with risks (e.g. line infection) and complications (e.g. pneumothorax). Review 'invasive techniques' regularly, and replace as soon as possible. Alarms are a crucial safety feature (e.g. ventilator disconnection). They are set to physiological safe limits and should never be disconnected.

Haemodynamic monitoring

- **Blood pressure (BP)** is usually measured intermittently, using an automated sphygmomanometer. However, in severely ill patients, continuous intra-arterial monitoring is preferred, using an intra-arterial catheter attached to a pressure transducer. It must be appreciated that BP does not reflect cardiac output (CO). Thus, the BP can be normal or high but CO low if peripheral vasoconstriction raises systemic vascular resistance (SVR). Conversely, vasodilated 'septic' patients with low SVR may be hypotensive despite a high CO.

- **Electrocardiogram (ECG).** Rate and rhythm are displayed by standard single-lead ECG monitors, but ST segment changes can be monitored in patients with IHD.

- **Central venous pressure (CVP)** reflects right atrial pressure (RAP) and is measured, using internal jugular (see Figures 19.1 and 19.2) or subclavian vein catheters. It is a useful means of assessing circulating blood volume and determining the rate at which fluid should be administered. However, increased venous tone can act to maintain CVP and mask volume depletion during hypovolaemia or haemorrhage. In this situation, CVP is not as important as the response to a fluid challenge (see 'Circulatory assessment'). A high CVP indicates 'fluid overload', impaired myocardial contractility, or high right ventricular afterload, and management depends on the underlying cause.

- **Pulmonary artery wedge/occlusion pressure (PAWP/PAOP)** reflects the left atrial pressure (LAP). Normally, the LAP is ~5–7 mmHg greater than RAP, but, in ischaemic heart disease or severe illness, there is often 'disparity' between left and right ventricular function. Thus, the LAP may be high, despite a low RAP in left ventricular dysfunction, and a small increase in RAP can cause a large increase in LAP which may precipitate pulmonary oedema. In these patients, PAWP (i.e. LAP) is monitored, using a pulmonary artery catheter (see Figure 19.3). PAWP is normally 6–12 mmHg but may be >25–35 mmHg in left ventricular failure. Provided the pulmonary capillary membranes are intact (i.e. not 'leaky'), a PAWP of ~15–20 mmHg ensures good left ventricular filling and optimal function without risking pulmonary oedema. Pulmonary artery catheters also measure CO, mixed venous saturation, and right ventricular ejection fraction.

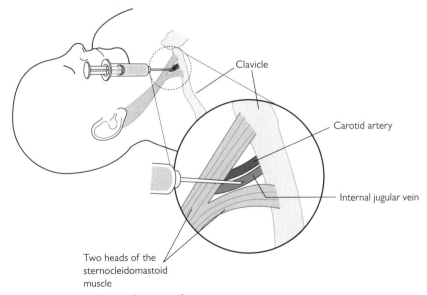

Clavicle

Carotid artery

Internal jugular vein

Two heads of the sternocleidomastoid muscle

Figure 19.1 Internal jugular vein central venous catheter.

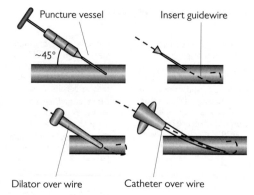

Puncture vessel

Insert guidewire

~45°

Dilator over wire

Catheter over wire

Figure 19.2 Insertion of catheter over a guidewire (Seldinger technique).

Sternal head

Sternal
head

Sternocleidomastoid
muscle

Clavicular
head

External jugular
vein

(a) Surface anatomy of external and internal jugular veins

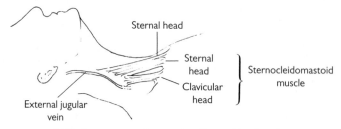

(b) Anterior approach: the chin is in the midline and the skin puncture
is over the sternal head of SCM muscle (and the needle
should subsequently be directed lateral to the palpable,
pulsatile carotid artery)

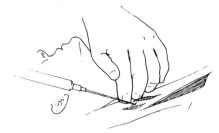

(c) Central approach: the chin is turned away and the skin puncture is
between the two heads of SCM muscle

Figure 19.3 Internal jugular vein cannulation. Reproduced from Punit S. Ramrakha, Kevin P. Moore, and Amir Sam, Oxford
Handbook of Acute Medicine, third edition, 2010, Figure 15.3, page 745, copyright Punit S. Ramrakha and Kevin P. Moore, with permission.

- **Cardiac output.** Thermodilution techniques for CO measurement (e.g. PA catheter (see further text), pulsion continuous cardiac output monitor (PiCCO)) are considered the 'gold standard', but error is at least 10%. Non- (or less) invasive techniques of CO monitoring utilize dye/lithium dilution, transoesophageal Doppler ultrasonography, echocardiography, or impedance methods.

Respiratory monitoring

- **Arterial oxygen saturation (SaO$_2$)** is determined by spectrophotometric analysis of the ratio of saturated to desaturated haemoglobin. Oxygenation is usually adequate if SaO$_2$ is >90%. Finger and earlobe probes may be unreliable if peripheral perfusion is poor.
- **Arterial blood gases** monitor PaO$_2$, PaCO$_2$, and acid-base balance. Measurement aids diagnosis and allows adjustment of ventilation to achieve optimum gas exchange.
- **Mixed venous oxygen saturation (SvO$_2$)** is measured using fibreoptic pulmonary artery catheters or pulmonary artery/right atrial blood sampling and co-oximetry. It is normally >65–70%. A low SvO$_2$ (<55–60%) may indicate inadequate tissue O$_2$ delivery, even if SaO$_2$ or PaO$_2$ are normal (e.g. anaemia).
- **Lung function.** Alveolar-arterial PO$_2$ gradient and PaO$_2$/FiO$_2$ ratio measure gas exchange. Arterial and end-tidal CO$_2$ (see further text) reflect alveolar ventilation (VA). Thus, PaCO$_2$ is inversely proportional to alveolar ventilation (PaCO$_2 \propto 1/VA$). Peak expiratory flow rate (PEFR) and spirometry (e.g. FEV$_1$, VC) are useful for monitoring airways obstruction and lung volumes in self-ventilating patients. In intubated patients, maximum inspiratory pressure (MIP) is normally ~100 cmH$_2$O. An MIP <25 cmH$_2$O indicates muscle weakness and that spontaneous ventilation, following extubation, is unlikely.
- **Lung compliance (LC)** reflects lung 'stiffness' or ease of inflation and is reduced in damaged lungs. It is calculated by dividing tidal ventilation (Tv; mL) by the pressure (cm/ H$_2$O) required to achieve Tv. High airways pressures during ventilation indicate reduced LC.
- **Capnography.** Inspired air contains virtually no CO$_2$. At the end of expiration, end-tidal CO$_2$ concentration mirrors arterial PaCO$_2$ and reflects alveolar ventilation, provided the distribution of ventilation is uniform.

Organ and tissue oxygenation

- **Global measures (e.g. SvO$_2$, lactate)** reflect total tissue perfusion but may be normal despite severe regional perfusion abnormalities. Raised serial lactate levels and metabolic acidosis suggest anaerobic metabolism and inadequate tissue oxygenation, although lactate may increase in the absence of hypoxia (e.g. liver failure). An SvO$_2$ <55% indicates global tissue hypoxia.
- Organ-specific measures include:
  - **Urine flow** which is a sensitive measure of renal perfusion, provided that the kidneys are not damaged (e.g. acute tubular necrosis) or affected by drugs (e.g. diuretics). Hourly urine output is normally ~1 mL/kg.

- **Core peripheral temperature**, the gradient between peripheral (e.g. skin temperature over the dorsum of the foot) and core temperature (e.g. rectal) is often used as an index of peripheral perfusion.
- **Gastric tonometry** which is occasionally used to detect shock-induced splanchnic ischaemia by measuring gastric luminal PCO$_2$ and subsequently deriving mucosal pH.
- **Neurological monitoring** which utilizes the Glasgow coma score, intracranial pressure measurement, and jugular venous bulb saturation.

Further reading

Anderson ID (1997). Care of the critically ill surgical patient courses of the Royal College of Surgeons. *British Journal of Hospital Medicine*, **57**, 274–5.

BTS Pleural Disease Guideline (2010). *Thorax*, **65**, (supplement 2), 1–82.

Chappell D, Jacob M, Hofmann-Kiefer K, Conzen P, Rehm M (2008). A rational approach to perioperative fluid management. *Anaesthesiology*, **109**, 723–40.

Dellinger RP, Carlet JM, Masur H, et al. (2008). Surviving Sepsis Campaign guidelines for management of severe sepsis and septic shock. *Critical Care Medicine*, **32**, 858–73.

Department of Health (2008). The National Archives: competencies for recognising and responding to acutely ill patients in hospital. <http://webarchive.nationalarchives.gov.uk/+http://www.dh.gov.uk/en/Consultations/Closedconsultations/DH_083630>.

Hemmila MR and Napolitano LM (2006). Severe respiratory failure: advanced treatment options. *Critical Care Medicine*, **34**, S278–90.

Millar AC, Harvey JE, on behalf of Standards of Care Committee, British Thoracic Society (1993). Guidelines for the management of spontaneous pneumothorax. *BMJ*, **307**, 114–16.

National Institute for Health and Clinical Excellence (2007). Recognition of and response to acute illness in adults in hospital. <http://guidance.nice.org.uk/CG50>.

National Patient Safety Agency (2007). Safer care for the acutely ill patient: learning from serious incidents. <http://www.npsa.nhs.uk/easysiteweb/gatewaylink.aspx?alid=6241>.

O'Driscoll BR, Howard LS, Davison AG (2008). British Thoracic Society guideline for emergency oxygen use in adults. *Thorax*, **63** (Suppl 6), vi1–68.

Royal College of Physicians (2012). National early warning score (NEWS). Standardizing the assessment of acute illness. <http://www.rcplondon.ac.uk/sites/default/files/documents/national-early-warning-score-standardising-assessment-acute-illness-severity-nhs.pdf>.

Royal College of Physicians (2013). Acute care toolkit 6. The medical patient at risk: recognition and care of the seriously ill or deteriorating medical patient. <http://www.rcplondon.ac.uk/sites/default/files/acute_care_toolkit_6.pdf>.

Smith GB, Osgood VM, Crane S (2002). ALERT™—a multiprofessional training course in the care of the acutely ill adult patient. *Resuscitation*, **52**, 281–6.

Task Force of the American College of Critical Care Medicine. Practice parameters for haemodynamic support in adult patients with sepsis. *Critical Care Medicine*, **27**, 639–60.

Vincent JL and Gerlach H (2004). Fluid resuscitation in severe sepsis and septic shock; an evidence-based review. *Critical Care Medicine*, **32**, S451–4.

Vascular and haemodynamic practical procedures

Central venous catheters

In the past, central venous catheter insertion has relied on anatomical surface landmarks to locate the position of the underlying vein. However, there is normally significant variation in the relationship between such landmarks and the actual vein position. Consequently, failure to achieve cannulation is common, and there is a significant incidence of serious complications (e.g. pneumothorax, arterial puncture). Recent advances in portable ultrasound equipment and increasing availability and training have now made it possible to insert central venous catheters under 2D ultrasound guidance.

For medical practitioners in England and Wales, the National Institute for Health and Clinical Excellence guidelines (September 2002) state: 'Two-dimensional imaging ultrasound guidance is recommended as the preferred method for insertion of central venous catheters into the internal jugular vein (IJV) in adults and children in elective situations'.

Advantages of this technique include identification of the vein and its relationship to other structures (e.g. arteries), confirmation of vein patency, and identification of anatomical variations.

Equipment needed

- Sterile dressing pack and gloves.
- 10 mL and 5 mL syringes.
- Green (21G) and orange (25G) needles.
- Saline flush.
- Local anaesthetic (e.g. 1% lidocaine).
- Central line, usually a standard Seldinger-type kit (16G long Abbocath® or Seldinger catheter).
- Silk suture, scalpel blade.
- Sterile occlusive dressing.
- Ultrasound equipment:
  - Ultrasound probe: transducer which emits and receives ultrasound information to be processed for display. Marked with arrow or notch for orientation. Use a sterile sheath of PVC or latex to cover the probe and the connecting cable to ensure sterility is maintained (a rubber band secures the sheath to the probe).
  - Screen: displays 2D ultrasound image of anatomical structures.
  - Sterile gel that transmits ultrasound and provides good interface between patient and probe is required.

Potential risks

- Arterial puncture (remove and apply local pressure).
- Infection (local cellulitis, septicaemia, endocarditis).
- Pneumothorax/haemothorax (insert chest drain or aspirate, if required).
- Chylothorax (mainly left subclavian lines).
- Arrhythmias (e.g. right atrial stimulation).
- Brachial plexus/cervical root damage (overenthusiastic infiltration with local anaesthetic).

Preparation

- An assistant is always essential when inserting central lines to ensure sterility is maintained.
- Initially, perform a preliminary non-sterile scan to access the central vein size and patency, and mark the approximate site for local anaesthesia and subsequent cannulae insertion.
- Lie the patient supine. Ensure optimal positioning. For example, when performing an internal jugular vein cannulation, the patient's head should be slightly turned away from the site of insertion. Excessive rotation or extension of the head may decrease the diameter of the vein. If tolerated, place the patient with head-down tilt or leg elevation to increase internal jugular filling and size of the internal jugular vein. It is easier, and safer, to cannulate a central vein with the patient supine or head down. There is an increased risk of air embolus if the patient is semi-recumbent.
- Sterile precautions should be taken and adequate drapes placed to maintain a sterile field.
- Ensure that the ultrasound scan display can be seen.

Procedure

- The Seldinger technique (i.e insertion over a guidewire) is the same, irrespective of the vein cannulated (i.e. internal jugular, femoral, subclavian: see Figure 19.2). Ensure a fully sterile technique with mask, gown, and gloves. Clean the skin with 2% chlorhexidine from the angle of the jaw to the clavicle for internal jugular vein (IJV) cannulation, and from the midline to axilla for the subclavian approach. The entire inguinal area should be cleaned for femoral line insertions.
- Check the central line; flush the lumens with saline, and apply 3-way tap hubs on all ports, except on the lumen through which the guidewire will pass. Clamp or apply caps to the lumens of the central venous catheter (CVC). Ensure the insertion needle (and attached syringe for aspiration of blood from the penetrated vessel), scalpel, tissue dilator, guidewire (and associated applicator), needle and thread (i.e. to secure the inserted catheter), along with the checked and prepared central line are easily accessible and can be reached whilst using the ultrasound probe. Draw up the 1% lidocaine for skin anaesthesia.
- Infiltrate the skin and subcutaneous tissues at the previously marked insertion site with 1% lidocaine.
- Whilst awaiting anaesthesia, the ultrasound sheath is opened by the operator, and sufficient gel is inserted by the assistant to ensure good contact and air-free contact between the probe tip and sheath. Insufficient gel may compromise image quality.
- The probe and connecting cable are lowered into the sheath by the assistant. A rubber band secures the sheath to the connecting cable or probe.
- Smooth out the sheath over the detector surface of the probe, as wrinkles will degrade image quality. Apply liberal amounts of gel to the sheathed probe tip for good ultrasound transmission and increased patient comfort during movement.
- Scanning is usually in the transverse plane during internal jugular vein catheter placement. The probe tip is gently applied to the neck, lateral to the carotid pulse at the cricoid level or in the sternomastoid-clavicular triangle. The probe should be perpendicular at all times, with the tip flat against the skin. Orientate the probe so that movement to the left ensures that the display looks to the left (and vice versa). Probes are usually marked to help orientation. By convention, the mark should be to the patient's

right (i.e. transverse plane) or to the head (i.e. longitudinal scan). The marked side appears on the screen as a bright dot.

If the vessels are not immediately visible, keep the probe perpendicular, and gently glide the probe medially or laterally until the vein (and associated artery when inserting an internal jugular or carotid central venous line) is found. Watch the screen, not your hands, when moving the probe. The parallel vein and artery in the carotid and femoral regions can be differentiated by applying gentle pressure over the site. The vein will rapidly collapse, whilst the artery will require greater pressure to occlude. After identification of the vein, position the probe so that the vein is shown at the display's horizontal midpoint.

- When the vein has been clearly identified, and whilst keeping the probe immobile, direct the needle (bevel towards the probe) caudally under the marked midpoint of the probe tip at approximately 60° to the skin. The needle bevel faces the probe to help direct the guidewire down the vein later. Advance the needle towards the vein. Needle passage causes a 'wavefront' of tissue compression. This is used to judge the progress of the needle and position. Absence of visible tissue reaction indicates incorrect needle placement. Just before entering the vessel, 'tenting' of the vein is usually observed. Needle pressure may oppose vein walls, resulting in vein transfixion. Slow withdrawal of the needle with continuous aspiration can help result in lumen access. One of the 'difficult' aspects of learning this technique is the initial steep needle angulation required, but this ensures that the needle enters the vein in the ultrasound beam and takes the shortest, and most direct, route through the tissues. Aspirate blood from the vein to confirm the correct position of the needle.
- Remove the syringe from the inserted needle (blood should flow back freely), and pass the guidewire through the inserted needle into the vein, using the guidewire applicator (which is designed for one-handed insertion, whilst the other hand secures the needle's position). The guidewire should pass freely. If there is resistance, remove the wire and reposition the needle, checking that blood can be easily aspirated, and then re-try inserting the guidewire. Re-angling the needle from 60° to a shallower angle (e.g. 45°) may aid guidewire passage. When the wire has been inserted, remove the needle over the guidewire which is left in the vein. Use a sterile swab to maintain gentle pressure over the site of venepuncture to prevent excessive bleeding.
- Nick the skin with the scalpel blade at the site of guidewire skin penetration to ease passage of the dilator and to facilitate dilatation of the subcutaneous tissues. Pass the dilator over the guidewire into the vein and then remove, leaving the guidewire *in situ*, whilst applying gentle pressure over the insertion site to avoid excessive blood loss. It is rarely necessary to insert more than a few centimetres of the dilator. Finally, pass the CVC over the guidewire into the vein. Remove the guidewire through the CVC. Attach a syringe to the lumen of the CVC through which the guidewire was removed, and aspirate blood to confirm placement in the vein. Attach a 3-way tap to the CVC lumen, and then inject saline before 'clamping' to prevent blood clotting in, and occluding, the lumen.
- Secure the CVC to the skin with silk sutures. Apply a transparent plastic dressing to allow daily assessment of the skin for development of potential cellulitis.

- Scanning the vein in the longitudinal plane may demonstrate the catheter in the vessel, but, after securing and dressing the central venous catheter (CVC), an X-ray should still be obtained to confirm the CVC position and exclude pneumothorax.
- Measurement of central venous pressure is most often compromised by partial or complete occlusion, particularly in CVCs which have been in place for some time. Therefore, with the manometer connected, always ensure the line is free-flowing. Measure the CVP at the mid-axillary line, with the patient supine. CVP falls with upright or semi-upright recumbency, regardless of the reference point. If the CVP is high, lift the stand that holds the manometer so that the apparent CVP falls by 10 cm or so, and replace the CVP stand to ground level. If the saline or manometer reading rises to the same level, then the CVP reading is accurate. In other words, one ensures that the CVP manometer level both falls to and rises to the same level.

Specific central vein cannulation

The insertion of a central venous catheter should be performed under ultrasound guidance whenever possible. However, on occasions (e.g. in an emergency), it may be necessary to insert a catheter using anatomical landmarks to determine the position of the underlying central vein despite the associated risks and morbidity (as previously described).

Internal jugular vein cannulation

The internal jugular vein (IJV) runs posterolateral to the carotid sheath and lies medial to the sternocleidomastoid (SCM) muscle in the upper part of the neck, between the two heads of the SCM in its medial portion, and enters the subclavian vein near the medial border of the anterior scalene muscle (see Figures 19.1 and 19.3).

There are three basic approaches to IJV cannulation: medial to the SCM, between the two heads of the SCM, or lateral to the SCM. The approach used varies and depends on the experience of the operator and the institution.

- Locate the carotid artery between the sternal and clavicular heads of the SCM at the level of the thyroid cartilage; the IJV lies just lateral and parallel to it.
- Keeping the fingers of one hand on the carotid pulsation, infiltrate the skin with local anaesthetic (e.g. lidocaine (INN) 1%), aiming just lateral to this and ensuring that you are not in a vein (intravenous lidocaine (INN) can cause seizures).
- Ideally, initially locate the vein with a blue or green needle. Approach the vein at 45° to the skin, with gentle negative suction on the syringe, aiming for the ipsilateral nipple, lateral to the pulse (see Figure 19.2). Once you have located the vein with a green needle, remove this needle but bear in mind the depth and angle of approach to the vein. Now, change to a syringe connected to the guidewire introducer needle, taking care not to release your fingers from the pulse; they may be distorting the anatomy slightly, making access to the vein easier, and, if released, it may prove difficult to relocate the vein. Approach the vein in the same manner remembering the angle and depth used earlier with the green needle.
- If you initially fail to find the vein, withdraw the needle slowly, maintaining negative suction on the syringe (you may have inadvertently transfixed the vein). Aim slightly more medially, and try again. Venous blood is dark, and arterial blood is pulsatile and bright red!

- Once you have identified the position of the vein, advance the guidewire introducer needle very slightly to ensure the bevel is within the lumen of the vein and check you can still withdraw venous blood into the syringe. Detach the syringe from the needle leaving the introducer needle in the vein (there will be some initial bleeding until the guidewire is inserted) and then pass the guidewire through the introducer needle into the vein (see Figure 19.2). The guidewire should pass freely down the needle and into the vein. With the left IJV approach, there are several acute bends that need to be negotiated. If the guidewire keeps passing down the wrong route, ask your assistant to hold the patient's arms out at 90° to the bed, or even above the patient's head, to coax the guidewire down the correct path.
- In intubated patients requiring respiratory support, it may be difficult to access the head of the bed. The anterior approach may be easier (see Figure 19.3) and may be done from the side of the bed (the left side of the bed for right-handed operators, using the left hand to locate the pulse and the right to cannulate the vein).
- The IJV may also be readily cannulated with a long Abbocath®. No guidewire is necessary, but, as a result, misplacement is commoner than with the Seldinger technique. When using an Abbocath®, on cannulating the vein, remember to advance the sheath and needle 1–2 mm to allow the tip of the plastic sheath (~1 mm behind the tip of the bevelled needle) to enter the vein. Holding the needle stationary, advance the sheath over it into the vein.
- Arrange for a chest X-ray (CXR) to confirm the position of the line.

Subclavian vein cannulation
The axillary vein becomes the subclavian vein (SCV) at the lateral border of the first rib and extends for 3–4 cm, just deep to the clavicle (see Figure 19.4). It is joined by the ipsilateral IJV to become the brachiocephalic vein behind the sternoclavicular joint. The subclavian artery and brachial plexus lie posteriorly, separated from the vein by the scalenus anterior muscle. The phrenic nerve and the internal mammary artery lie behind the medial portion of the SCV and, on the left, lies the thoracic duct.

- Select the point 1 cm below the point of maximum curvature of the clavicle (just lateral to the junction of the medial third and middle third of the clavicle). If possible, place a bag of saline between the scapulae to extend the spine.
- Clean the skin with 2% chlorhexidine. Infiltrate the skin and subcutaneous tissue and periosteum of the inferior border of the clavicle with local anaesthetic up to the hilt of the green (21G) needle, ensuring that it is not in a vein.

- Insert the introducer needle with a 10 mL syringe, guiding gently directly under the clavicle, aiming slightly upwards (i.e. away from the lung apex). It is safest to initially hit the clavicle and 'walk' the needle under it until the inferior border is just cleared. In this way, you keep the needle as superficial to the dome of the pleura as possible. Once it has just skimmed underneath the clavicle, advance it slowly towards the contralateral sternoclavicular joint, aspirating as you advance. Using this technique, the risk of pneumothorax is small, and success is high.
- Once the venous blood is obtained, rotate the bevel of the needle towards the heart. This encourages the guidewire to pass down the brachiocephalic vein, rather than up the IJV.
- The guidewire should pass easily into the vein. If there is difficulty, try advancing during the inspiratory and expiratory phases of the respiratory cycle.
- Once the guidewire is in place, remove the introducer needle, and pass the dilator over the wire. When removing the dilator, note the direction that it faces; it should be slightly curved downwards. If it is slightly curved upwards, then it is likely that the wire has passed up into the IJV. The wire may be manipulated into the brachiocephalic vein under fluoroscopic control, but, if not available, it is safer to remove the wire and start again.
- After removing the dilator, pass the central venous catheter over the guidewire; remove the guidewire, and secure, as described previously.
- A CXR is mandatory after subclavian line insertion to exclude a pneumothorax and to confirm satisfactory placement of the line, especially if fluoroscopy was not employed.

Femoral vein cannulation
The femoral vein passes under the medial aspect of the inguinal ligament at the junction of the upper leg and groin and lateral to the femoral artery. It is a relatively easy cannulation, as the site is readily accessed and is less intimidating for the patient. However, it may be associated with a slightly higher risk of line infection.

- Following careful skin cleansing and under sterile conditions, the skin lateral to the femoral pulse is anaesthetized with 1% lidocaine (INN), whilst ensuring it is not in a blood vessel, about 6–9 cm below the inguinal ligament.
- The easily palpable femoral artery is marked with the opposite hand. The introducer needle and syringe are introduced at an angle of 45° to the skin, aiming towards the head and parallel and lateral to the femoral artery, whilst applying constant suction until venous blood is aspirated.

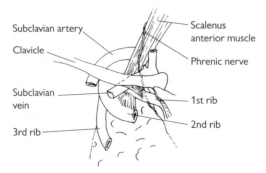

Subclavian artery
Clavicle
Subclavian vein
3rd rib
Scalenus anterior muscle
Phrenic nerve
1st rib
2nd rib

Figure 19.4 The subclavian vein and surrounding structures. Reproduced from Punit S. Ramrakha, Kevin P. Moore, and Amir Sam, *Oxford Handbook of Acute Medicine*, third edition, 2010, Figure 15.4, page 746, copyright Punit S. Ramrakha and Kevin P. Moore, with permission.

- The guidewire is inserted into the vein, followed by the dilator, and finally the central venous catheter. The line is secured as described previously.

Measuring the central venous pressure
Problem solving and potential pitfalls
When asked to see a patient at night on the wards with an abnormal CVP reading, it is important to re-zero the manometer and check the reading.
- Always do measurements with the mid-axillary point as the zero reference. Sitting the patient up will drop the central filling pressure (i.e. due to pooling in the veins).
- Fill the manometer line, being careful not to soak the cotton ball stop. If this gets wet, it limits the free-fall of saline or dextrose in the manometer line.
- Look at the rate and character of the venous pressure. It should fall to its value quickly and swing with respiration. If it fails to fall quickly, consider whether the line is open (i.e. saline running in), blocked with a blood clot, positional (i.e. abutting a vessel wall; ask the patient to take some deep breaths), or is it an arterial pressure measurement due to accidental cannulation of an artery (i.e. blood tracks back up the line). Raise the drip-stand, and ensure that the level falls. If it falls when the whole stand is elevated, it may be that the CVP is very high.
- In many high dependency units, the CVC is connected to a pressure transducer which provides continuous monitor readout.
- When clinical signs and monitored parameters disagree, **assume that clinical assessment is correct**, until potential errors from monitored variables have been excluded (e.g. blocked CVP lines, transducer failure, incorrect calibration).

Pulmonary artery catheterization
Pulmonary artery (PA; or Swan–Ganz catheters®) catheters allow direct measurement of haemodynamic parameters that aid clinical decision-making in severely ill patients. In particular, they facilitate assessment of right and left ventricular function, guide treatment, and provide prognostic information. However, the PA catheter has no intrinsic therapeutic benefit, and several studies have shown increased mortality (and morbidity) with their use.

Insertion of a PA catheter in critically ill patients should only be considered if the measurements will influence decisions on therapy and should not delay treatment of the patient. Thorough clinical assessment of the patient should always accompany measurements.

General indications for PA line insertion
- Management of complicated myocardial infarction.
- Management of left ventricular failure.
- Assessment and management of shock.
- Assessment and management of respiratory distress (e.g. cardiogenic vs non-cardiogenic pulmonary oedema).
- Evaluating effects of treatment in unstable patients (e.g. inotropes, vasodilators, mechanical ventilation, etc.).
- Delivering therapy (e.g. thrombolysis for pulmonary embolism, epoprostenol for pulmonary hypertension, etc.).
- Assessment of fluid requirements in critically ill patients (e.g. with sepsis, acute respiratory distress syndrome).
(This is not a comprehensive list.)

Preparation and equipment required
- Resuscitation facilities should be available, and the patient's ECG should be continuously monitored.
- Bag of heparinized saline for flushing the catheter.
- Transducer set for pressure monitoring. Before you start, ensure that your assistant is able to set up the transducer system.
- 8F introducer kit. Ideally, use a pre-packaged kit that contains the introducer sheath and all the equipment required for central venous cannulation.

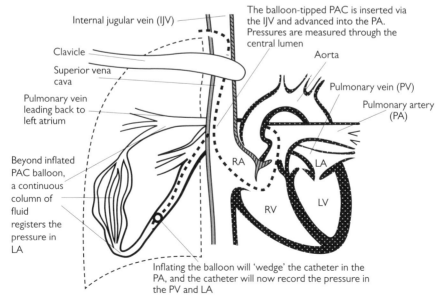

Internal jugular vein (IJV)

Clavicle

Superior vena cava

Pulmonary vein leading back to left atrium

Beyond inflated PAC balloon, a continuous column of fluid registers the pressure in LA

The balloon-tipped PAC is inserted via the IJV and advanced into the PA. Pressures are measured through the central lumen

Aorta

Pulmonary vein (PV)

Pulmonary artery (PA)

RA

LA

RV

LV

Inflating the balloon will 'wedge' the catheter in the PA, and the catheter will now record the pressure in the PV and LA

Figure 19.5a Pulmonary artery catheter (PAC). Reproduced from Richard M. Leach, Acute and Critical Care Medicine at a Glance, second edition, Figure d, Chapter 3, page 16, Wiley, Copyright 2009, with permission

- Pulmonary artery catheter: commonly a triple-lumen catheter, that allows simultaneous measurement of right atrial pressure (proximal port) and pulmonary artery pressure (distal port) and incorporates a thermistor for measurement of cardiac output by thermodilution (see Figure 19.6). Check your catheter before you start.
- Fluoroscopy may aid insertion but is not essential.

General technique for insertion

- This procedure should only be performed by an experienced clinician with appropriate training. It should not be attempted without supervision if you are inexperienced.
- Strict aseptic technique (e.g. sterile drapes, masks, gowns, gloves, available assistants, etc.) is essential.
- Insert the introducer sheath (at least 8F in size) into either the internal jugular or subclavian vein in the standard way (as described previously). Flush the sheath with saline, and secure to the skin with sutures.
- The plastic sterile expandable sheath for the introducer is not attached at this point. Keep it sterile for use once the catheter is in position. During initial insertion, the catheter is easier to manipulate without the plastic covering.
- Flush all the lumens of the PA catheter, and attach the distal lumen to the pressure transducer. Check the transducer is zeroed (i.e. this is conventionally to the mid-axillary point). Check the integrity of the balloon by inflating it with air, using the 2 mL syringe provided, and then deflate the balloon.

Pulmonary artery catheterization

See Figure 19.5a.

- Locate the selected vein (i.e. jugular or subclavian), and insert the guidewire into the vein, as described previously.

Pass the dilator over the guidewire to produce a suitable tract for the sheath to enter the vein. Then remove the dilator, and press at the site of insertion to prevent excessive blood loss. Pass the sheath over the guidewire into the vein.

- The guidewire is then removed. The sheath has a haemostatic valve at the end, preventing leakage of blood.
- The PA catheter is then inserted through the introducer sheath into the vein.
- Before inserting the PA catheter, re-check that all the lumens of the PA catheter have been flushed, the distal lumen is attached to the pressure transducer, the transducer is zeroed (conventionally to the mid-axillary point), and the balloon is intact (as described previously).
- Pass the tip of the PA catheter through the plastic sheath, with the sheath compressed. The catheter is easier to manipulate without the sheath. However, once the PA catheter is in position, the sheath is extended over the catheter to maintain sterility.
- With the balloon deflated, advance the tip of the catheter 10–15 cm from the insertion site of the right internal jugular vein (IJV) or subclavian vein (SCV) and 15–20 cm from left-sided insertions. The markings on the side of the catheter are at 10 cm intervals: two lines = 20 cm. Check that the pressure tracing is typical of the right atrial pressure (see Figure 19.5b).
- Inflate the balloon, and advance the catheter gently. The flow of blood will carry the balloon (and catheter) across the tricuspid valve, through the right ventricle and into the pulmonary artery. The position of the catheter can be determined from the pressure transducer readout (see Figure 19.5b) and measured pressures. Normal right heart pressures and flows are reported in Table 19.1.

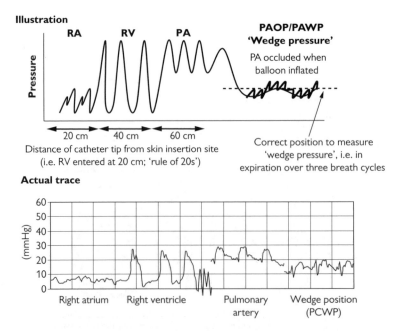

Figure 19.5b Pulmonary artery catheter trace passing from the right atrium to pulmonary artery. Reproduced from Punit S. Ramrakha, Kevin P. Moore, and Amir Sam, Oxford Handbook of Acute Medicine, third edition, 2010, Figure 15.6, page 755, copyright Punit S. Ramrakha and Kevin P. Moore, with permission.

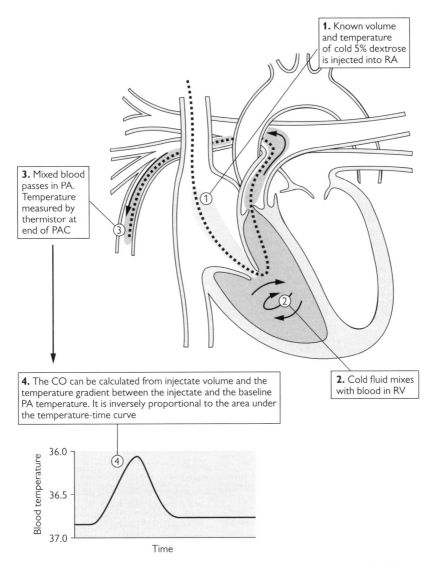

1. Known volume and temperature of cold 5% dextrose is injected into RA

3. Mixed blood passes in PA. Temperature measured by thermistor at end of PAC

4. The CO can be calculated from injectate volume and the temperature gradient between the injectate and the baseline PA temperature. It is inversely proportional to the area under the temperature-time curve

2. Cold fluid mixes with blood in RV

Figure 19.6 Thermodilution cardiac output (CO). Reproduced from Richard M. Leach, *Acute and Critical Care Medicine at a Glance*, second edition, Figure f, Chapter 3, page 16, Wiley, Copyright 2009, with permission.

- Watch the ECG tracing closely whilst the catheter is advanced. The catheter commonly triggers runs of ventricular tachycardia (VT) when crossing the tricuspid valve and passing through the right ventricle (RV). The VT is usually self-limiting but should not be ignored. Deflate the balloon; pull back, and try again.
- If more than 15 cm of catheter is advanced into the RV without the tip entering the PA, this suggests the catheter is coiling in the RV. Deflate the balloon, and withdraw the catheter into the RA; reinflate the balloon, and try again, using clockwise torque, while advancing in the ventricle, or flushing the catheter with cold saline to stiffen the plastic. If this fails repeatedly, stop and arrange for the radiologists to try again under fluoroscopic guidance.

- As the tip passes into a distal branch of the PA, the balloon will impact and not pass further than the pulmonary capillary wedge (PCW) position, and the pressure tracing will change (see Figure 19.5b).
- Deflate the balloon, and check that a typical PA tracing is obtained (see Figure 19.5b). If not, try flushing the catheter lumen. If this fails, withdraw the catheter until the tip is within the main PA, and then advance into a distal PA again.
- Reinflate the balloon slowly. If the PCW pressure is seen before the balloon is fully inflated, it suggests the tip has migrated further into the PA. Deflate the balloon, and withdraw the catheter 1–2 cm and try again.

- If the pressure tracing flattens and then continues to rise, you have 'overwedged'. Deflate the balloon; pull back the catheter 1–2 cm, and start again.
- When a stable position has been achieved, extend the plastic sheath over the catheter, and secure it to the introducer sheath. Clean any blood from the skin insertion site with antiseptic, and secure a coil of the PA catheter to the patient's chest to avoid inadvertent removal.
- The balloon must always be left deflated (i.e. when measurements are not being taken) to avoid causing pulmonary artery infarction.
- Perform a CXR to check the position of the catheter. The tip of the catheter should ideally be in a right lower lobe distal PA, no more than 5–10 cm from the midline.

Pulmonary artery tips and pitfalls
- Never withdraw the catheter with the balloon inflated.
- Never advance the catheter with the balloon deflated.
- Never inject liquid into the balloon.
- Never leave the catheter with the balloon inflated, as pulmonary infarction may occur.
- The plastic of the catheter softens at body temperature, and the tip of the catheter may migrate further into the PA branch. If the pressure tracing with the balloon deflated is 'partially wedged' (and flushing the catheter does not improve this), withdraw the catheter 1–2 cm and reposition.
- Sometimes, it may be impossible to obtain a wedged trace. In this situation, use the PA diastolic pressure as a guide. In health, there is about 3–5 mmHg difference between PA diastolic pressure and PCWP (see Table 19.1). Any condition which causes pulmonary hypertension (e.g. ARDS, severe lung disease, valvular heart disease) will alter this relationship.
- Consult a cardiologist prior to inserting a PA catheter in patients with **valvular lesions, ventricular septal defects, prosthetic valves, and pacemakers**. For example, the risk of developing subacute bacterial endocarditis may outweigh the benefit of a PA catheter.
- Positive end expiratory pressure (PEEP; see further text) affects measurement and interpretation of the PCW pressure and depends on the position of the PA catheter. Ensure the catheter is below the level of the left atrium on a lateral CXR. Removing PEEP during measurement causes marked fluctuations in haemodynamics

Table 19.1 Normal right heart pressures and flows

Right atrial pressure	0–8 mmHg
Right ventricular pressure	
Systolic pressure	15–30 mmHg
End diastolic	0–8 mmHg
Pulmonary artery pressure	
Systolic/diastolic pressure	15–30/4–12 mmHg
Mean	9–16 mmHg
Pulmonary capillary wedge pressure	2–10 mmHg
Cardiac index	2.8–4.2 L/min/m^2

and oxygenation and does not reflect the situation during normal ventilation.

Pulmonary artery complications
- **Arrhythmias.** Monitor the ECG closely during PA catheter insertion, as VT may be triggered whilst crossing the tricuspid valve and passing through the RV (as described previously).
- **Pulmonary artery rupture** (~0.2%). Damage may occur if the balloon is overinflated in a small branch. Risk factors include mitral valve disease, pulmonary hypertension, multiple inflations, or hyperinflation of the balloon. Haemoptysis is an early sign. It is safer to follow PA diastolic pressures if these correlate with the PCWP.
- **Pulmonary infarction.**
- **Knots.** Usually occur at the time of initial placement in patients where there has been difficulty in traversing the RV. Signs include loss of pressure tracing, persistent ectopy, resistance to catheter manipulation. Knots may be visible on chest radiography. If this occurs, stop manipulation, and seek expert radiologcal or surgical help.
- **Infection.** Risks increase with length of time the catheter is left *in situ*. The pressure transducer may occasionally be a source of infection. Remove the catheter and introducer, and replace, only if necessary.
- **Other complications** include those associated with central line insertion: thrombosis and embolism, balloon rupture, intracardiac damage.

Arterial blood sampling

Arterial blood samples are used to measure arterial oxygen tension (PaO$_2$), carbon dioxide tension (PaCO$_2$), acidity (pH), and bicarbonate/base excess levels. Arterial oxyhaemoglobin saturation (SaO$_2$) can also be determined.

Before taking the ABG sample, familiarize yourself with the location and the use of the blood gas machine. Arterial blood is obtained either by percutaneous needle puncture or from an indwelling arterial line (see further text).

Procedure
- Ensure the required equipment is easily accessible, including a blue needle, heparin-coated syringe, cleaning solution, and anaesthetic agent, if required. A heparin-coated syringe is vital to prevent the aspirated arterial blood clotting and subsequently damaging the arterial blood gas analyser.
- Locate a palpable artery. Common sites include:
  - **The radial artery** which is accessible and more comfortable for the patient. It is best palpated between the bony head of the distal radius and the tendon of the flexor carpi radialis, with the wrist dorsiflexed.
  - **The brachial artery** is best palpated medial to the biceps tendon in the antecubital fossa, with the arm extended and the palm facing up. The needle is inserted just above the elbow crease.
  - **The femoral artery** is palpated just below the midpoint of the inguinal ligament, with the leg extended. The needle is inserted below the inguinal ligament at a 90° angle.
- Clean the chosen puncture site with 2% chlorhexidine or equivalent.
- Consider local analgesia. This has been shown to prevent pain, with no adverse effect on the success of the procedure.

- Use one hand to palpate the artery and the other hand to advance the heparin-coated syringe and needle (22–25G) at 60–90° angle to the skin.
- A flush of bright red blood indicates successful puncture. Remove about 2–3 mL of blood; withdraw the needle, and apply pressure to the puncture site for 5 minutes.
- Air bubbles should be removed, as these can cause a falsely high PaO_2 and a falsely low $PaCO_2$.
- The sample is ideally placed on ice and must be analysed within 15 minutes to reduce oxygen consumption by leucocytes, which can result in a falsely low PaO_2.

Complications
- Persistent bleeding.
- Bruising.
- Injury to the blood vessel.
- Impaired circulation distal to the puncture site (presumably due to thrombosis at the puncture site).

Arterial line

Arterial cannulation allows real-time blood pressure measurement, assessment of beat-to-beat variation and waveform (i.e. the wide pulse pressure of aortic regurgitation, slow upstroke of aortic stenosis, or pulsus paradoxus in spontaneously breathing patients), and regular arterial blood sampling. Most arterial lines are inserted into the radial or femoral arteries, although brachial, posterior tibial, and dorsalis pedis arteries can be used, without increasing the complication profile.

The radial artery is generally preferred, as it is easily accessible and, to a lesser extent, because the hand has a dual arterial supply (i.e. radial and ulnar arteries). About 10% of patients do not have an ulnar artery, and the ulnar collateral circulation can be tested clinically, using the Allen test, in which pressure is exerted over the medial and lateral aspects of the wrist to occlude both the ulnar and radial arteries, respectively. The patient then clenches and unclenches the hand for about 30 seconds. If the hand flushes, following release of pressure over the medial aspect of the wrist (i.e. ulnar artery), the presence of an ulnar artery is confirmed. Alternatively, the ulnar artery can be imaged by Doppler ultrasound. In practice, necrosis or hand amputation, following radial artery occlusion, is rare, occurring in less than 1 in 2,000 cases, and is not predicted by the Allen test or Doppler ultrasonography.

It is often recommended that end arteries, such as the brachial artery, are avoided because of the theoretical risk of distal ischaemia, infarction, and potential loss of the limb in the event of arterial occlusion. However, in practice, it has not been demonstrated to be the case, and the complication profile is unaffected (see further text).

The main indications for an arterial catheterization are:
- Continuous monitoring of arterial blood pressure in critically ill patients with haemodynamic instability.
- Repeated arterial blood sampling (e.g. respiratory failure, acidosis).
Relative contraindications to arterial line insertion include:
- Coagulopathy.
- Raynaud's phenomenon.
- Thromboangiitis obliterans.
- Advanced atherosclerosis.

Procedure
- Locate a palpable artery. Common sites include the radial and femoral arteries.

- Prior to radial artery catheterization, the modified Allen test can be performed to assess collateral flow.
- Position the hand in moderate dorsiflexion with the palm facing up (to bring the artery closer to the skin).
- The site should be cleaned with a sterile preparation solution (e.g. 2% chlorhexidine) and draped appropriately.
- Sterile technique is essential, including appropriate drapes and sterile gloves.
- Use local anaesthetic (1% lidocaine (INN)) in a conscious patient.

Over-the-wire technique
- Palpate the artery with the non-dominant hand (1–2 cm from the wrist between the bony head of the distal radius and the flexor carpi radialis tendon).
- The catheter and needle are advanced towards the artery at a 30–45° angle until a blood 'flash-back' is seen (e.g. into an attached syringe or the dedicated chamber in commercial devices).
- The catheter and needle are then advanced into the vessel by a few millimetres, and the needle is removed.
- The catheter is slowly withdrawn until pulsatile blood flow is seen, at which point the wire is advanced into the vessel.
- The catheter is then advanced over the wire into the vessel.
- With pressure over the artery, the wire is removed and the catheter is connected to a transduction system.
- Secure the catheter, using suture or tape.
- Check perfusion to the hand after insertion of the arterial line and at frequent intervals. Remove the catheter if there are any signs of vascular compromise or as soon as it is no longer needed.

Over-the-needle technique
- Locate and palpate the artery with the non-dominant hand (1–2 cm from the wrist between the bony head of the distal radius and the flexor carpi radialis tendon).
- The catheter and needle are advanced towards the artery at a 30–45° angle until a blood 'flash-back' is seen.
- Fractionally advance the catheter and needle, before lowering the angle to 10–15° and advancing the catheter over the needle into the artery.
- Apply pressure to the artery; remove the needle, and connect the catheter to the transduction system.
- Secure the catheter in place, using suture or tape, and check perfusion of the hand at frequent intervals.

Complications
- Local and systemic infection.
- Distal ischaemia (risk factors include sepsis, shock, air or clot emboli, vasculitis, female sex, intra-arterial drug injection, prothrombotic states).
- Bleeding, haematoma, bruising.
- Vascular complications: blood vessel injury, pseudoaneurysm, thromboembolism, and vasospasm.
- Compartment syndrome.
- Arteriovenous fistula.
- Damage to neighbouring structures (e.g. nerves).
- Arterial spasm may occur after multiple unsuccessful attempts at arterial catheterization. If this is suspected, try an alternative site.
- There may be difficulty in passing the wire or catheter despite the return of pulsatile blood. Adjustment of the angle, withdrawal of the needle, or a slight advance may be helpful.

Pericardial aspiration and catheter placement

Echocardiography-directed pericardial drainage is required for cardiac tamponade due to excess pericardial fluid and to obtain samples of pericardial fluid for the purposes of investigation.

Preparation and equipment required

Establish peripheral venous access, and check that full facilities for resuscitation are available. Pre-prepared pericardiocentesis sets may be available. You will need:

- A dressing trolley with iodine or chlorhexidine for skin cleansing, dressing pack, sterile drapes, local anaesthetic (lidocaine (INN) 1%), syringes (including a 50 mL), needles (25G and 22G), no. 11 blade, and silk sutures.
- Pericardiocentesis needle (15 cm, 18G) or similar Wallace cannula.
- J-guidewire (≥80 cm, 0.035 diameter), dilators (up to 7F), and a pigtail catheter ≥60 cm long with multiple side holes (a large Seldinger-type CVP line can be used if no pigtail catheters are available).
- Drainage bag and connectors.
- Facilities for echocardiography and occasionally fluoroscopy screening.

Pericardial aspiration technique

See Figure 19.7.

- Position the patient at about 30°. This allows the effusion to pool inferiorly within the pericardium.
- Sedate the patient lightly with midazolam (2–5 mg intravenously) and fentanyl (25–100 mcg intravenously), if necessary. Beware a fall in blood pressure in patients with cardiac tamponade who are already compromised by the effusion.
- Sterile technique is essential, including sterile gown, masks, gloves, and drapes. Clean the skin from the midchest to mid-abdomen, and place the sterile drapes on the patient.
- Infiltrate the skin and subcutaneous tissues with local anaesthetic, starting 1–1.5 cm below the xiphisternum and just to the left of midline, aiming for the left shoulder and staying as close to the inferior border of the rib cartilages as possible.
- The pericardiocentesis needle is introduced into the angle between the xiphisternum and the left costal margin, angled at about 30° to the skin. Advance towards the left shoulder slowly whilst aspirating gently and injecting lidocaine (INN).
- As the parietal pericardium is pierced, the needle may 'give' and fluid is aspirated. Remove the syringe, and introduce the guidewire through the needle if a catheter is to be placed.
- Check the position of the guidewire with the echocardiograph (or screening). It should loop within the cardiac silhouette only and not advance into the superior vena cava or pulmonary artery.
- Remove the needle, leaving the wire in place. Enlarge the skin incision slightly, using the blade, and dilate the track.
- Insert the pigtail catheter over the wire into the pericardial space, and remove the wire.
- Take specimens for microscopy; culture, cytology, and haematocrit if bloodstained. Also inoculate a sample into blood culture bottles.
- Aspirate the pericardial space to dryness, watching the patient carefully. Symptoms and haemodynamics (e.g.

blood pressure) often improve with the removal of as little as 100 mL of pericardial fluid. If the aspirated fluid is heavily bloodstained, suggesting the catheter is in the right ventricle, withdraw fluid cautiously, as sudden withdrawal of blood may cause cardiovascular collapse. Arrange measurement of an urgent haemoglobin/haematocrit.

- Leave the catheter on free drainage and attached to the drainage bag. Suture the pigtail to the skin securely, and cover with a sterile occlusive dressing.

Pericardial catheter aftercare

- Closely observe the patient for recurrent tamponade (e.g. due to obstruction of drain), and repeat ECHO.
- Discontinue anticoagulants.
- Remove the catheter after 24 hours or when the drainage stops.
- Consider the need for surgery (biopsy or pericardial window) or specific therapy (chemotherapy if malignant effusion, antimicrobials if bacterial, dialysis if renal failure, etc.).

Management tips and pitfalls

- Whenever possible, use echocardiographic guidance.
- If during insertion, the **needle touches the heart's epicardial surface**, you may feel a 'ticking' sensation transmitted down the needle: withdraw the needle a few millimetres; angulate more superficially, and try again, aspirating as you advance.
- **If you do not enter the effusion** and the heart is not encountered, withdraw the needle slightly and advance again, aiming slightly deeper, but still towards the left shoulder. If this fails, try again, aiming more medially (e.g. mid-clavicular point). Echocardiographic guidance aids positioning.
- An apical approach (starting laterally at cardiac apex and aiming for right shoulder) may be considered if the echocardiogram confirms sufficient fluid at the cardiac apex.
- If available, **intrathoracic ECG** can be monitored by a lead attached to the needle, as it is advanced, but is rarely clinically useful. Penetration of the myocardium results in ST elevation, suggesting the needle has been advanced too far.
- **Difficulty in inserting the pigtail** may be due to insufficient dilatation of the tract and requires use of a larger dilator. Holding the wire taut (by gentle traction), while pushing the catheter, may help; take care not to pull the wire out of the pericardium.
- Differentiating haemorrhagic effusions from intracardiac blood. This can be achieved by:
  - Comparing the haemoglobin content of pericardial fluid with that of venous blood.
  - Alternatively, place the aspirated fluid in a clean container, and observe whether it clots. Intracardiac blood clots, whereas haemorrhagic effusion does not because the 'whipping' action of the heart defibrinates it.
- If it is still unclear whether the catheter is in the pericardial space or the heart, positioning can be confirmed by:
  - Injecting contrast (~10–20 mL) and assessing whether it remains intrapericardial, using fluoroscopy or radiology.
  - Using echocardiography to detect 'microbubble contrast' in the pericardium, following injection of 5–10 mL saline. This is aided by injecting 20 mL saline into a

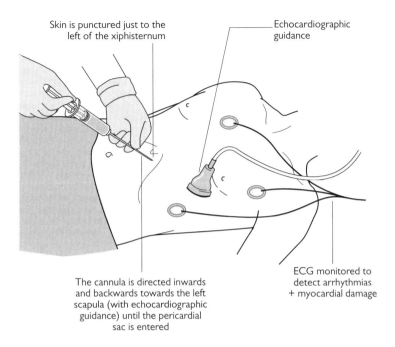

Skin is punctured just to the left of the xiphisternum

Echocardiographic guidance

The cannula is directed inwards and backwards towards the left scapula (with echocardiographic guidance) until the pericardial sac is entered

ECG monitored to detect arrhythmias + myocardial damage

Figure 19.7 Needle pericardiocentesis (aspiration of a pericardial effusion).

peripheral vein which produces 'contrast' in the right atrium and ventricle, distinguishing them from the pericardial space.
• Connecting a pressure transducer to the catheter; a characteristic waveform confirms right ventricular penetration.

Complications of pericardiocentesis
• Penetration of a cardiac chamber (usually right ventricle).
• Laceration of an epicardial vessel.
• Arrhythmia (e.g. atrial arrhythmias as the wire is advanced, ventricular arrhythmias if the RV is penetrated).
• Pneumothorax.
• Perforation of abdominal viscus (e.g. liver, stomach, colon).
• Ascending infection.

Temporary pacing wire placement
Indications for temporary pacing include:
Those related to acute myocardial infarction (MI)
• Asystole.
• Symptomatic complete heart block (CHB) in any territory.
• Symptomatic secondary heart block in any territory.
• Trifascicular block.
  • Alternating left bundle branch block (LBBB) and RBBB.
  • Primary heart block + RBBB + left axis deviation (LAD).
  • New RBBB and left posterior hemiblock.
  • LBBB and long PR interval.
• After an anterior MI.
  • Asymptomatic CHB.
  • Asymptomatic second-degree (Mobitz II) block.

• Symptomatic sinus bradycardia unresponsive to atropine.
• Recurrent VT for atrial or ventricular overdrive pacing.

Unrelated to myocardial infarction
• Symptomatic sinus or junctional bradycardia unresponsive to atropine (e.g. carotid sinus hypersensitivity).
• Symptomatic secondary heart block or sinus arrest.
• Symptomatic complete heart block.
• Torsades de pointes tachycardia.
• Recurrent VT for atrial or ventricular overdrive pacing.
• Bradycardia-dependent tachycardia.
• Drug overdose (e.g. verapamil, beta-blockers, digoxin).
• Permanent pacemaker box change in a patient who is pacing-dependent.

Before general anaesthesia
• The same principles as for acute MI (as described previously).
• Sinoatrial disease, secondary (Wenckebach) heart block only need prophylactic pacing if there are symptoms of syncope or presyncope.
• Complete heart block.

Transvenous temporary pacing
This is the most commonly used technique in emergency situations. The mode of choice for life-threatening bradyarrhythmias is ventricular demand pacing (VVI), with a single bipolar wire positioned in the right ventricle. In patients with impaired cardiac pump function and symptomatic bradycardia (e.g. after right ventricular infarction), cardiac output is increased by up to 20% by maintaining atrioventricular synchrony (see section on atrioventricular sequential pacing).

Epicardial temporary pacing
Following cardiac surgery, **epicardial wires** (attached to the pericardial surface of the heart) may be left in for up to a week after surgery in case of post-operative heart block or bradyarrhythmia. These are used in the same way as the more familiar transvenous pacing wires, but the threshold may be higher.

Atrioventricular sequential pacing
In critically ill patients with impaired cardiac pump function and symptomatic bradycardia (especially those patients with right ventricular infarction), cardiac output may be increased by up to 20% by maintaining atrioventricular synchrony. This requires two pacing leads, one atrial and one ventricular, and a dual pacing box. Patients most likely to benefit from AV sequential pacing include:
- Acute MI (especially RV infarction).
- 'Stiff' left ventricle (e.g. aortic stenosis, hypertrophic cardiomyopathy, hypertensive heart disease, amyloidosis).
- Low cardiac output states (e.g. cardiomyopathy).
- Recurrent atrial arrhythmias.

Technique of temporary cardiac pacing
Ventricular pacing
- **Cannulate a central vein.** The pacing wire is easiest to manipulate, using the right internal jugular vein (IJV) approach, but is more comfortable for the patient when the right subclavian vein (SCV) is used. The left IJV approach is best avoided, as several acute bends must be negotiated with the pacing wire, and a stable position is difficult to achieve. Avoid the left subclavicular area, as this is the preferred area for permanent pacemaker insertion. The femoral vein can be used, but the incidence of DVT and infections is high.
- **Insert a sheath** (as for PA catheterization), through which the pacing wire can be fed. Pacing wires are commonly 5F or 6F, and a sheath at least one size larger is necessary. Most commercially available pacing wires are pre-packed with an introducer needle and sheath and a sterile plastic wire cover that can be removed after wire insertion, leaving the bare wire entering the skin once a stable position has been achieved. This reduces the risk of wire displacement but makes repositioning difficult if this becomes necessary, and the risk of infection is higher.
- Pass the wire through the sterile plastic cover, and pass the wire through the newly inserted introducer sheath. Advance the wire into the upper right atrium, but do not unfurl the cover yet. The wire is much easier to manipulate with gloved hands, without the additional hindrance of the plastic cover.
- Advance the wire, with the tip pointing towards the right ventricle (the wire tends to retain a curl associated with packaging). It may cross the tricuspid valve easily. If it fails to pass across the valve, twist the wire so that the tip points to the lateral wall of the atrium and forms a loop. Then, rotate the wire again, and the loop should fall across the tricuspid valve and pass into the right ventricle.
- Advance and rotate the wire so that the tip points inferiorly and is as close to the apex of the right ventricle (laterally) as possible. If the wire does not rotate down to the apex easily, it may be because it is in the coronary sinus, rather than the right ventricle. In this situation, the tip of the wire points to the left shoulder. Withdraw the wire, and re-cross the tricuspid valve.
- Leave some slack in the wire; the final appearance should be like the outline of a sock, with the 'heel' in the right atrium, the 'arch' over the tricuspid, and the 'big toe' at the tip of the right ventricle.
- Connect the wire to the pacing box, and check the threshold. The ventricular pacing thresholds should be less than 1.0 volt (V), but a threshold of up to 1.5V is acceptable if another stable position cannot be achieved.
- Check for positional stability. This is performed by setting the pacing rate higher than the intrinsic heart rate and asking the patient to take some deep breaths, to cough forcefully, and to sniff. Watch for failure of pacing capture on the ECG, and, if so, reposition the wire.
- Set the pacemaker box output to 3 V and the mode to 'demand'. If the patient is in sinus rhythm and has an adequate blood pressure, set the pacing box rate just below the patient's own heart rate. If there is complete heart block or bradycardia, set the rate at 70–80/min.
- Cover the wire with the plastic sheath, and suture sheath and wire securely to the skin. Loop the rest of the wire, and fix to the patient's skin with adhesive dressing.
- When the patient returns to the ward, obtain a CXR to confirm satisfactory positioning of the pacing wire and to exclude a pneumothorax.

Atrial pacing
The technique of inserting an atrial temporary wire is similar to that of ventricular pacing. Advance the atrial wire until the 'J' is re-formed in the right atrium. Rotate the wire, and withdraw slightly to position the tip in the right atrial appendage. Aim for a threshold of <1.5 V. If atrial wires are not available, a ventricular pacing wire may be passed into a similar position or passed into the coronary sinus for left atrial pacing.

Complications of temporary pacing include:
- Complications associated with central line insertion.
- Ventricular ectopics.
- Non-sustained VT.
- Perforation.
- Pericarditis.
- Diaphragmatic pacing.
- Infection.
- Pneumothorax.
- Cardiac tamponade.

Ventricular ectopics or VT
- Non-sustained VT is common as the wire crosses the tricuspid valve (especially in patients receiving an isoprenaline infusion) and does not require treatment.
- Try to avoid long runs of VT, and, if necessary, withdraw the wire into the atrium and wait until the rhythm has settled.
- If ectopics persist after the wire is positioned, try adjusting the amount of slack in the wire in the region of the tricuspid valve (either more or less).
- Pacing the right ventricular outflow tract may provoke runs of VT.

Failure to pace and/or sense
- It is difficult to achieve a low pacing threshold (<1.0 V) in patients with extensive myocardial infarction (especially of the inferior wall), cardiomyopathy, or who have received class I antiarrhythmic drugs. In these patients, accept a slightly higher value if the position is otherwise stable and satisfactory.
- If the position of the wire appears satisfactory and yet the pacing thresholds are high, the wire may be in a left

hepatic vein. Pull the wire back into the atrium and try again, looking specifically for the ventricular ectopics as the wire crosses the tricuspid valve.

- The pacing threshold commonly doubles in the first few days due to endocardial oedema.
- If the pacemaker suddenly fails, the most common reason is usually wire displacement.
  - Increase the pacing output of the box.
  - Check all wire connections and the pacing box battery.
  - Try moving the patient to the left lateral position until arrangements can be made to reposition the wire.

Cardiac perforation
Presentation is typically with pericardial chest pain, breathlessness, falling blood pressure, an enlarged cardiac silhouette on CXR, signs of cardiac tamponade, and left diaphragmatic pacing (see next paragraph) at low output. A pericardial rub may be present in the absence of perforation (especially post-MI). Management includes urgent echocardiography and pericardial drainage if there are signs of cardiac tamponade. Reposition the wire, and monitor the patient carefully over the next few days, with repeat echocardiograms to detect incipient cardiac tamponade.

Diaphragmatic pacing
High-output pacing (10 V), even with satisfactory position of the ventricular lead, may cause pacing of the left hemidiaphragm. At low voltages, this suggests perforation (as described previously). Right hemidiaphragm pacing may be seen with atrial pacing which stimulates the right phrenic nerve. Consider repositioning the wire if symptomatic (e.g. painful twitching, dyspnoea).

Checklist for pacing wire insertion
- Check screening equipment and defibrillators are working.
- Check the type of pacing wire: atrial pacing wires have a pre-formed 'J' that allows easy placement in the atrium or atrial appendage and is very difficult to manipulate into a satisfactory position in the ventricle.
- Ventricular pacing wires have a more open, gentle 'J'.
- Check the pacing box (single vs dual or sequential pacing box) and the leads that attach to the wire(s). Ensure you have familiarized yourself with the pacing box controls before starting. You may need to connect up in a hurry if the patient's intrinsic rhythm slows further.
- Remember to put on the lead apron before wearing the sterile gown, mask, and gloves.

DC cardioversion
DC cardioversion is an essential skill in cardiopulmonary resuscitation and the management of cardiac arrhythmias.

Relative contraindications
- Digoxin toxicity.
- Electrolyte disturbance (Na^+, K^+, Ca^{2+}, Mg^{2+}, acidosis).
- Inadequate anticoagulation and chronic AF.

Checklist for DC cardioversion
See Table 19.2.

Table 19.2 Checklist for DC cardioversion

Defibrillator	Ensure this is working. A fully equipped arrest trolley should be available.
Informed consent	(Unless a life-threatening emergency.)
12-lead ECG	Atrial fibrillation (AF) or flutter, supraventricular tachycardia (SVT), VT, signs of ischaemia, or digoxin. If ventricular rate is slow, have an external (transcutaneous) pacing system nearby in case of asystole.
Nil by mouth	For at least 4 hours.
Anticoagulation	Does the patient need anticoagulation? Is the INR >2.0 and has it been so for over 3 weeks?
Potassium	Check this is >3.5 mmol/L.
Digoxin	Check there are no features of digoxin toxicity. If taking >250 mcg/day, check that renal function and a recent digoxin level are normal. If there are frequent ventricular ectopics, give intravenous Mg^{2+} 8 mmol.
Thyroid function	Treat thyrotoxicosis or myxoedema first.
IV access	Peripheral venous cannula.
Sedation	Short general anaesthesia (propofol) is preferable to sedation with benzodiazepine and fentanyl. Bag the patient with 100% oxygen.
Select energy	(See Table 19.3.)
Synchronization	Check this is selected on the defibrillator for all shocks (unless the patient is in VF or haemodynamically unstable). Adjust the ECG gain so that the machine is only sensing QRS complexes, and not P or T waves
Paddle placement	Conductive gel pads should be placed between the paddles and the skin. Position one just to the right of the sternum, and the other to the left of the left nipple. Alternatively, place one anteriorly just left of the sternum, and one posteriorly to the left of midline. There is no convincing evidence for superiority of one position over the other.
Cardioversion	Check no one is in contact with the patient or with the metal bed. Ensure your own legs are clear of the bed! Apply firm pressure on the paddles.
Unsuccessful	Double the energy level, and repeat up to 360 J. Consider changing paddle position (see above). If prolonged sinus pause or ventricular arrhythmia during an elective procedure, stop.
Successful	Repeat ECG. Place in recovery position until awake. Monitor for 2–4 h, and ensure effects of sedation have abated. Patients should be accompanied home by a friend or relative if being discharged.

Complications of DC cardioversion
- Asystole/bradycardias.
- Ventricular fibrillation.
- Thromboembolism.
- Transient hypotension.
- Skin burns.
- Aspiration pneumonitis.

Initial energy levels for DC shock in elective cardioversion
See Table 19.3.

If the initial shock is unsuccessful, increase the energy (50, 100, 200, 360 J), and repeat.

If still unsuccessful, consider changing paddle position, and try 360 J again. It is inappropriate to persist further with elective DC cardioversion.

Anticoagulation in DC cardioversion
The risk of thromboembolism in patients with chronic atrial fibrillation (AF) and dilated cardiomyopathy is 0–7%, depending on the underlying risk factors (see Table 19.4).

Patients at risk of thromboembolism should be anticoagulated with warfarin for at least 3–4 weeks. For recent-onset AF (1–3 days), anticoagulate with intravenous heparin for at least 12–24 hours, and, if possible, exclude intracardiac thrombus with a transoesophageal echocardiogram before the cardioversion. If there is thrombus, anticoagulate with warfarin, as described previously. For emergency cardioversion of AF (<24 h), heparinize prior to the DC shock.

The risk of systemic thromboembolism with cardioversion of atrial flutter and other tachyarrhythmias is very low, provided there is no ventricular thrombus, because coordinated atrial activity prevents clot formation. In these cases, routine anticoagulation with warfarin is not necessary. However, heparin is recommended before DC shocks, as the atria are often rendered mechanically stationary for several hours after the shock, even though there is coordinated electrical depolarization.

After successful cardioversion, if the patient is on warfarin, continue anticoagulation for at least 3–4 weeks. Consider indefinite anticoagulation if there is intrinsic cardiac disease (e.g. mitral stenosis) or recurrent AF.

Table 19.3 Initial energy levels for DC shock in elective cardioversion

Sustained VT	200 J	Synchronized
Atrial fibrillation	50–100 J	Synchronized
Atrial flutter	50 J	Synchronized
Other SVTs	50 J	Synchronized

Table 19.4 Risk factors for thromboembolism during DC cardioversion

Increased risk	Low risk
Prior embolic event	Age <60 years
Mechanical heart valve	No previous heart disease
Mitral stenosis	Recent onset AF (<3 days)
Dilated left atrium	

Special situations
Pregnancy
DC shock during pregnancy appears to be safe. Auscultate the fetal heart before and after DC cardioversion, and, if possible, fetal ECG should be monitored.

Pacemakers
There is a danger of damage to the pacemaker generator box or at the junction between the tip of the pacing wire(s) and endocardium. Position the paddles in the antero-posterior position, as this is theoretically safer. Facilities for backup pacing (external or transvenous) should be available. Check the pacemaker post-cardioversion, as both early and late problems have been reported.

Intra-aortic balloon (IAB) counterpulsation
This is a specialist procedure and should only be performed by trained specialists. It is presented to aid understanding of when it should be employed in general medical practice.

Indications
- Cardiogenic shock post-MI.
- Acute severe mitral regurgitation.
- Acute ventricular septal defect.
- Preoperative (ostial left coronary stenosis).
- Weaning from cardiopulmonary bypass.
  Rarely:
- Treatment of ventricular arrhythmias post-MI.
- Unstable angina (e.g. as a bridge to CABG).

Contraindications
- Aortic regurgitation.
- Dilated cardiomyopathy (if patient not a candidate for transplantation).
- Aortic dissection.
- Severe aorto-iliac atheroma.
- Bleeding diathesis.

Complications
- Aortic dissection.
- Thrombocytopenia.
- Arterial perforation.
- Peripheral embolism.
- Limb ischaemia.
- Balloon rupture.

Mechanism of action
See Figure 19.8.

The device consists of a catheter with a balloon (40 mL in size) at its tip which is positioned in the descending thoracic aorta. The balloon inflation/deflation is synchronized to the ECG. The balloon should inflate just after the dicrotic notch (in diastole), thereby increasing pressure in the aortic root and increasing coronary perfusion. The balloon deflates just before ventricular systole, thereby decreasing afterload and improving left ventricular performance.

Arterial balloon counterpulsation has a number of beneficial effects on the circulation.
- Increased coronary perfusion in diastole.
- Reduced left ventricular end diastolic pressure.
- Reduced myocardial oxygen consumption.
- Increased cerebral and peripheral blood flow.

The IAB cannot assist the patient in asystole or ventricular fibrillation. It requires a minimum cardiac index of 1.2–1.4 L/min/m^2 and may require additional inotropes.

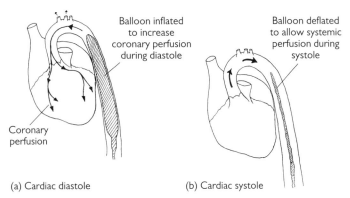

Balloon inflated to increase coronary perfusion during diastole

Balloon deflated to allow systemic perfusion during systole

Coronary perfusion

(a) Cardiac diastole   (b) Cardiac systole

Figure 19.8 Intra-aortic balloon counterpulsation. Reproduced from Punit S. Ramrakha, Kevin P. Moore, and Amir Sam, *Oxford Handbook of Acute Medicine*, third edition, 2010, Figure 15.10, page 774, copyright Punit S. Ramrakha and Kevin P. Moore, with permission.

The technique
Balloon insertion
Previous experience is essential. Formerly, a cut-down to the femoral artery was required, but newer balloons come equipped with a sheath which may be introduced percutaneously. Under fluoroscopic control, the balloon is positioned in the descending thoracic aorta, with the tip just below the origin of the left subclavian artery. The patient must be fully anticoagulated with intravenous heparin. Some units routinely give intravenous antibiotics (e.g. flucloxacillin) to cover against staphylococcal infections.

Triggering and timing
The balloon pump may be triggered either from the patient's ECG (R wave) or from the arterial pressure waveform. Slide switches on the pump allow precise timing of inflation and deflation during the cardiac cycle. Set the pump to 1:2 to allow you to see the effects of augmentation on alternate beats.

Troubleshooting
- Seek help from an expert! There is usually an on-call cardiac technician, senior cardiac physician, or surgeon.
- Counterpulsation is inefficient with heart rates over 130/min. Consider antiarrhythmics or 1:2 augmentation instead.
- Triggering and timing. When using ECG triggering, select a lead with the most pronounced R wave. Ensure that the pump is set to trigger from the ECG and not the pressure. Permanent pacemakers may interfere with triggering. Select a lead with negative and smallest pacing artefact. Alternatively, set the pump to be triggered from the external pacing device. A good arterial waveform is required for pressure triggering. The timing will vary slightly, depending on the location of the arterial line (slightly earlier for radial artery line, compared with a femoral artery line). Be guided by the haemodynamic effects of balloon inflation and deflation, rather than the precise value of delay.
- Limb ischaemia is exacerbated by poor cardiac output, adrenaline, noradrenaline, and peripheral vascular disease. Wean off, and remove the balloon (as described in the next section).

- Thrombocytopenia is common. It does not require transfusion, unless there is overt bleeding, and returns to normal once the balloon is removed. Consider prostacyclin infusion if platelet counts fall below 100×10^9/L.

Removal of the intra-aortic balloon
The patient may be progressively weaned by gradually reducing the counterpulsation ratio (1:2, 1:4, 1:8, etc.) and/or reducing the balloon volume and checking that the patient remains haemodynamically stable. Stop the heparin infusion, and wait for the ACT (activated clotting time) to fall <150 s (APTT <1.5 normal). Using a 50 mL syringe, have an assistant apply negative pressure to the balloon. Pull the balloon down until it abuts the sheath; **do not attempt to pull the balloon into the sheath**. Withdraw both balloon and sheath, and apply firm pressure on the femoral puncture site for at least 30 minutes or until the bleeding is controlled.

Further reading
Bellomo R and Pinsky MR (2006). Invasive monitoring. In J Tinker, D Browne, W Sibbald, eds. *Critical care standards, audit and ethics*, pp. 82–104. Arnold Publishing Co., London.

Dellinger RP, Carlet JM, Masur H, et al. (2008). Surviving Sepsis Campaign guidelines for management of severe sepsis and septic shock. *Critical Care Medicine*, **32**, 858–73.

Kumar A, Anel R, Bunnell E, et al. (2004). Pulmonary artery occlusion pressure and central venous pressure fail to predict ventricular filling volume, cardiac performance, or the response to volume infusion in normal subjects. *Critical Care Medicine*, **32**, 691–9.

Lynn-McHale Wiegand D (2011). *AACN procedure manual for critical care*. Elsevier Saunders, Philadelphia.

Magder S (2005). How to use central venous pressure measurements. *Current Opinion in Critical Care*, **11**, 264–70.

Scheer B, Perel A, Pfeiffer UJ (2002). Clinical review: complications and risk factors of peripheral arterial catheters used for haemodynamic monitoring in anaesthesia and intensive care medicine. *Critical Care*, **6**, 199–204.

Shah MR, Hasselblad V, Stevenson, LW, et al. (2005). Impact of the pulmonary artery catheter in critically ill patients: meta-analysis of randomized clinical trials. *JAMA*, **294**, 1664–70.

The American College of Critical Care Medicine (2004). Practice parameters for haemodynamic support in adult patients with sepsis. *Critical Care Medicine*, **32**, 1928–48.

Vincent JL and Gerlach H (2004). Fluid resuscitation in severe sepsis and septic shock; an evidence-based review. *Critical Care Medicine*, **32**, S451–4.

Respiratory practical procedures

The aim of respiratory therapy is to relieve hypoxia and maintain or restore a normal $PaCO_2$ for the individual. Relative indications for mechanical ventilation are discussed in the appropriate chapters. This section discusses some of the principles involved.

Oxygen therapy

The therapeutic aims of oxygen therapy depend on the risk of developing hypercapnic respiratory failure (HCRF):

• **In normal patients** (i.e. at low risk of developing HCRF): aim to achieve SaO_2 of 94–98% if aged <70 years and 92–98% if aged >70 years (i.e. wider normal range in the elderly). These ranges are on the plateau of the oxygen-haemoglobin dissociation curve where haemoglobin is fully saturated. Consequently, increasing PaO_2 has no impact on oxygen delivery, as little oxygen is dissolved in plasma.

• **In patients at risk of developing hypercapnic respiratory failure** (e.g. neuromuscular disease, COPD): the target saturation should be 88–92%, pending arterial blood gas (ABG) analysis. A higher SaO_2 has few advantages but results in hypoventilation, hypercapnia, and respiratory acidosis in patients dependent on hypoxaemic respiratory drive.

Initial oxygen dose and delivery method depends on the underlying cause. Ideally, oxygen should be administered by mask systems that deliver a defined percentage, between 28% and 100%, according to the patient's requirements (e.g. Venturi masks). Figure 19.9 illustrates the important features of oxygen delivery systems.

• **High-dose supplemental oxygen (>60%)** is delivered through a non-rebreathing reservoir mask at 10–15 L/min. It is given during cardiac or respiratory arrests, shock, major trauma, sepsis, carbon monoxide (CO) poisoning, and other critical illness. When clinical stability has been restored, oxygen dose is reduced, whilst maintaining SaO_2 at 92–98%. As with seriously ill patients, patients at risk of HCRF are initially treated with high-dose oxygen, pending ABG analysis.

• **Moderate-dose supplemental oxygen (40–60%)** is given in many serious illnesses (e.g. pneumonia), usually through nasal cannulae (2–6 L/min) or simple oxygen face masks (5–10 L/min), aiming for SaO_2 of 92–98% (as described previously). A reservoir mask is substituted if target saturations are not achieved.

• **Low-dose (controlled) supplemental oxygen (24–28%)** is delivered through a fixed performance Venturi mask. It is indicated in patients at risk of HCRF, including COPD, neuromuscular disease, chest wall disorders, morbid obesity, and cystic fibrosis. Long-term smokers, >50 years old, with exertional dyspnoea, and without another obvious cause for breathlessness should be suspected of having, and treated for, COPD. In these patients, the target saturation is 88–92% whilst awaiting ABG results. If $PaCO_2$ is normal, SaO_2 is adjusted to 92–98% (except in patients with previous HCRF), and ABG are re-checked after 1 hour on higher-dose oxygen therapy.

If an air compressor is not available, nebulizers are driven with oxygen, but only for 6 minutes to limit the risk of HCRF. A raised $PaCO_2$ and bicarbonate with normal pH suggests long-standing hypercapnia, and the target SaO_2 should be 88–92%, with repeat ABG at 1 hour.

If the patient is hypercapnic ($PaCO_2$ >6 kPa) and acidotic (pH <7.35), consider using non-invasive ventilation (NIV), especially if the acidosis has persisted for >30 min despite appropriate medical treatment.

Venturi masks are replaced with nasal cannulae (1–2 L/min) when the patient is stable. An oxygen alert card and Venturi mask are issued to patients with previous HCRF to warn future emergency staff of the potential risk.

Additional notes on oxygen delivery systems

• Nasal prongs only deliver FiO_2 of 30% at flows of 2 L/min and become less efficient at higher flow rates (~35% at 3 L/min, with little further increase with increasing flow). Higher flow rates require humidification.

• Combining nasal prongs and a high-flow mask can achieve an FiO_2 of ~80–90%.

• In practice, it is rarely possible to consistently deliver >60% unless using CPAP or mechanical ventilation.

• Where sudden deterioration in oxygenation occurs, always check the delivery system for empty cylinders, disconnected tubing, etc.

Indications for oxygen therapy

Table 19.5 lists indications for initiating oxygen therapy. It should be prescribed on the drug chart (i.e. dose, delivery method, duration, target saturation), signed for by the doctor, and documented by the nursing staff at each drug round. Initial oxygen saturation (SaO_2) and associated FiO_2 should be recorded. Table 19.6 reports the risks of oxygen therapy.

Monitoring

Arterial oxygen saturation (SaO_2), measured by oximetry, should be measured regularly in all breathless patients and in those on oxygen therapy. It should be recorded on the observation chart, with the associated oxygen dosage. In unstable patients and in high dependency areas, SaO_2 is monitored continuously. SaO_2 should be observed for 5 minutes after starting or changing oxygen dose and adjusted to achieve the target saturation. If possible, an ABG is measured before, and within 1 hour of starting oxygen therapy, especially in those at risk of HCRF, and then at intervals to assess therapeutic response.

Although oximetry is an invaluable aid, it has some limitations. In certain situations (e.g. Guillain–Barré syndrome), falling oximetry is a late marker of impending respiratory failure, and CO_2 accumulation (e.g. in COAD) is clearly not monitored by oximetry. A SaO_2 of 90% correlates very approximately with a PaO_2 of 8 kPa, and, below 88%, the PaO_2 may fall disproportionately quickly.

Table 19.5 Indications for acute oxygen therapy

1. **Cardiac and respiratory arrest**
2. **Hypoxaemia (PaO_2 <8 kPa, SaO_2 <90%)**
3. **Hypotension (systolic BP <100 mmHg)**
4. **Low cardiac output**
5. **Metabolic acidosis (bicarbonate <18 mmol/L)**
6. **Respiratory distress (respiratory rate >24/min)**
7. **Respiratory failure**
8. **Carbon monoxide poisoning**
9. **Cluster headaches**

1. Variable performance devices

- Air is entrained during breathing whilst oxygen is delivered from a reservoir (i.e. mask, reservoir bag, nasopharynx).

- The FiO_2 delivered to the lungs depends on the oxygen flow rate, the patient's inspiratory flow, respiratory rate, and the amount of air entrained.

- e.g. (a) 'Low-flow face masks': O_2 flows at ~2–10 L/min into the mask and is supplemented by air drawn into the mask. The FiO_2 achieved depends on ventilation.

- Ventilation = 5 L/min
  O_2 flow = 2 L/min; air (21% O_2) flow = 3 L/min
  FiO_2 = (2 + 0.21 × 3) / 5 × 100 = 53%

- Ventilation = 25 L/min
  O_2 flow = 2 L/min; air (21% O_2) flow = 23 L/min
  FiO_2 = (2 + 0.21 × 23) / 25 × 100 = 27%

- These devices cannot be used if accurate control of FiO_2 is desirable, e.g. COPD with hypercapnia.

- Examples of variable performance devices are nasal cannulae (b), 'low-flow' face masks, and non-rebreathing with reservoir bags (c).

2. Fixed performance devices

- Are independent of the patient's pattern of breathing and inspiratory volume.

- Figure (d) illustrates that a fixed O_2 flow through a Venturi valve entrains the correct proportion of air to achieve the required O_2 concentration.

- This system delivers more gas than is inspired (i.e. >30 L/min). Consequently, FiO_2 is less affected by the breathing pattern. The resulting masks are high flow, low concentration, and fixed performance.

- Used in patients with COPD and respiratory failure to avoid CO_2 retention.

(a) 'Low-flow face masks'.

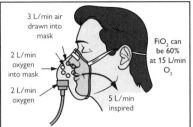

- O_2 flows at ~2–15 L/min into the mask and is supplemented by air drawn into the mask.
- Flow rate must be >5 L/min to prevent CO_2 rebreathing.

(b) Nasal prongs.

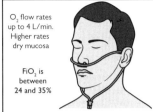

- The O_2 flow is constant, so FiO_2 varies with ventilatory volume.
- More comfortable and not removed during eating or coughing.
- O_2 inhaled, even when mouth breathing.

(c) Non-rebreathing and anaesthetic masks.

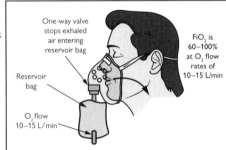

- High (10–15 L/min) flow rates of O_2 provide high FiO_2 >60% and up to 100%.

- Non-rebreathing masks have a reservoir bag which should be filled before use. They increase FiO_2 by preventing O_2 loss during expiration.

(d) 'High-flow' (Venturi), low-concentration face mask.

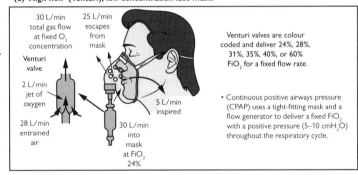

Venturi valves are colour coded and deliver 24%, 28%, 31%, 35%, 40%, or 60% FiO_2 for a fixed flow rate.

- Continuous positive airways pressure (CPAP) uses a tight-fitting mask and a flow generator to deliver a fixed FiO_2 with a positive pressure (5–10 cmH$_2$O) throughout the respiratory cycle.

Figure 19.9 Oxygen delivery systems are either variable or fixed performance devices. Reproduced from Richard M. Leach, Acute and Critical Care Medicine at a Glance, second edition, Figure d, Chapter 12, page 32, Wiley, Copyright 2009, with permission.

Table 19.6 Risks associated with high-dose oxygen therapy

1. **Carbon dioxide retention:**
   ~10% of breathless patients, mainly COPD, have type II respiratory failure (RF). ~40–50% of COPD patients are at risk of type II RF

2. **Rebound hypoxaemia:**
   Occurs if oxygen is suddenly withdrawn in type II RF

3. **Absorption collapse:**
   O_2 in poorly ventilated alveoli is rapidly absorbed, causing collapse, whereas N_2 absorption is slow

4. **Pulmonary oxygen toxicity:**
   FiO_2 >60% may damage alveolar membranes, causing ARDS if inhaled for >24–48 h (chapter 26). Hyperoxia can cause coronary and cerebral vasospasm

5. **Fire:**
   Deaths and burns occur in smokers during O_2 therapy

6. **Paul–Bert effect:**
   Hyperbaric O_2 can cause cerebral vasoconstriction and epileptic fits

Stopping oxygen therapy
When the patient is clinically stable on low-dose oxygen (e.g. 1–2 L/min) and SaO_2 is within the desired range on two consecutive occasions, oxygen therapy can be stopped. Monitor SaO_2 for 5 min after stopping oxygen, and re-check at 1 h. If SaO_2 remains within the desired range, oxygen has been safely discontinued.

Lung expansion techniques

- Periodic 'sighs' are a normal part of breathing and reverse microatelectasis. Lung expansion techniques are indicated for patients who cannot or will not take periodic large breaths (e.g. post-abdominal or chest surgery, neuromuscular chest wall weakness).
- Post-operative techniques, used commonly by physiotherapists, include incentive spirometry, coached maximal inspiration with cough, combined with postural drainage and chest percussion.
- Volume-generating devices, such as 'the BIRD', are triggered by the patient initiating inspiration and deliver a preset tidal volume to augment the patient's breath. Liaise with your physiotherapist.
- 'Pressure-generating' techniques (such as CPAP, NIPPV, and BiPAP) have the advantage that, even if a leak develops around the mask, the ventilator is able to 'compensate' to provide the patient with the prescribed positive pressure (see following section).
- For both volume- and pressure-generating techniques, the patients must be able to protect their airway and generate enough effort to trigger the machine.

Non-invasive ventilation

Non-invasive ventilation (NIV) provides respiratory support, aids alveolar recruitment, and reduces work of breathing (WoB), without the need for endotracheal intubation (ETI), laryngeal mask ventilation, or tracheostomy. Negative and positive pressure techniques are available.

Negative pressure ventilation (NPV) works by 'sucking' out the chest wall. It was initially developed to support victims of poliomyelitis-induced respiratory paralysis and has also been used in patients with chronic hypoventilation (e.g. kyphoscoliosis, muscle disease). Tank ventilators, often called 'iron lungs', are the best recognized of this type of ventilator. Lowering the pressure in the tank ventilator expands the chest, causing inspiration. Expiration is passive. However, inadequate nursing access, poor carbon dioxide (CO_2) clearance, and secretion retention with airways obstruction (± pneumonia) limit the use of these ventilators.

Current techniques include jacket (cuirass) ventilators which localize external negative pressure to the chest region, and rocking beds that utilize gravity to enhance diaphragmatic movement.

NPV has been superseded by positive pressure ventilation (PPV) and is now largely limited to specialist centres for rehabilitation (e.g. spinal injury) or chronic hypoventilation (e.g. kyphoscoliosis).

Non-invasive positive pressure ventilation (NIPPV) is particularly effective in acute respiratory failure. It is most successful in alert, cooperative, haemodynamically stable patients who can protect and clear their airways. It is delivered through the upper airway, using full face masks or helmets. Nasal masks are more comfortable in stable patients (see Figure 19.10). Table 19.7 lists the benefits and disadvantages.

- **Non-invasive ventilation (NIV)** usually refers to PPV which assists inspiration. Pressure-controlled (PC) modes of ventilation compensate for mask leaks and have largely replaced volume-controlled modes (see 'Mechanical ventilation'). Tidal volume is determined by lung (± chest wall) compliance and circuit resistance.
  - **Pressure support mode (PS).** In this mode of NIV, the patient determines breath timing and frequency of ventilation, as respiratory effort 'triggers' the ventilator on and off (i.e. assisted spontaneous breathing). Only the pressure (~10–30 cmH_2O) is adjusted to support inspiration. However, most PS ventilators incorporate a back-up breath rate of 6–8/min to ensure ventilation in patients who make no respiratory effort.

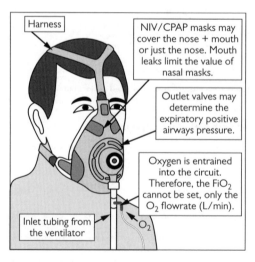

Figure 19.10 NIV/CPAP mask. Reproduced from Richard M. Leach, Acute and Critical Care Medicine at a Glance, second edition, Figure b, Chapter 14, page 36, Wiley, Copyright 2009, with permission.

Table 19.7 Benefits and limitations of positive pressure NIV

Benefits	Limitations

• Avoids complications associated with MV
  - Pulmonary infection
  - Pressure induced damage
• Avoids ETT complications
  - Mini-aspiration
  - Upper airway trauma
• Allows rest periods
• Preserves cough
• Allows oral nutrition
• Speech (+ decision-making)
• Allows earlier mobilization
• Allows time to decide if MV is appropriate
	• Lack of airways protection
	• No endotracheal suction
	• Less complete correction of blood gases than with MV
	• Mask discomfort; eye damage
	  - Prolonged use difficult
	• Ulceration over nasal bridge
	• Gastric dilation + vomiting
	  - May need NG tube
	• Limits ventilatory capacity
	• Increases nursing time
	• Needs patient reassurance
	• Intolerance + distress
	• Impedes sputum clearance

• **Bilevel pressure support** combines inspiratory positive airways pressure (IPAP; typically ~20–30 cm/H_2O) to aid inspiration (i.e. reduce WoB) with expiratory positive airways pressure (EPAP; typically ~5 cm/H_2O) to recruit underventilated lung and prevent airways collapse. EPAP also offsets intrinsic positive end expiratory pressure (PEEP) which aids ventilator triggering. These ventilators are simple to use and are cheap.

  • **Pressure-controlled ventilation (PCV).** The decelerating flow of a pressure-controlled breath improves the distribution of ventilation. In this mode of NIV, inflation pressure, frequency, and inspiratory time (Ti) are selected, according to patient requirements (e.g. Ti is usually set at ~0.8–1.2 s in acute hypercapnic COPD). A preset number of mandatory breaths are delivered in the absence of patient effort. Although patient triggering can occur, delivered breaths are identical to mandatory breaths. Triggered breaths delay the next machine-determined breath (i.e. synchronization), the spontaneous/timed (S/T) mode on NIV machines.

• **Continuous positive airways pressure (CPAP).** In this mode of NIV, a continuous pressure is maintained throughout inspiration and expiration (e.g. 5–10 cm/H_2O) by a flow generator. Consequently CPAP does not assist inspiration. Resulting alveolar recruitment (i.e. inflation of collapsed lung) reduces V/Q mismatch and improves oxygenation.

  CPAP is most successful in cardiogenic pulmonary oedema or acute lung injury (ALI). In obstructive sleep apnoea (OSA), it prevents upper airways collapse during sleep. Although CPAP is not usually considered respiratory support, the increase in functional residual capacity reduces WoB by making the lungs easier to inflate (i.e. the steep upstroke of the lung pressure-volume relationship). In patients with hyperinflation due to airways obstruction, further increases in lung volume may be detrimental, but, by offsetting intrinsic PEEP (e.g. in COPD), CPAP can reduce WoB, increase ventilation, and reduce $PaCO_2$.

Indication for NIV and CPAP
NIV is most beneficial in patients with respiratory acidosis (pH <7.35; H^+> 45 nmol/L). Arterial blood gas (ABG) measurement is usually required in patients with acute breathlessness, neuromuscular disease, chest wall deformity, obesity, or acute confusional states. Before starting, decide whether NIV will be the ceiling of treatment (e.g. end-stage COPD) or a therapeutic trial leading to endotracheal intubation (ETI) in the event of failure. A trial of NIV is required if ABG does not improve with oxygen and medical therapy in patients with:

1. **Acute hypercapnic respiratory failure:**
   • **COPD exacerbations.** Mortality, ETI rates, and complications (e.g. pneumonia) are substantially reduced with early NIV. In addition, pH, $PaCO_2$, and respiratory rate usually improve within 1 hour.
   • **Neuromuscular disease and chest wall deformity (e.g. kyphoscoliosis).** NIV is the treatment of choice in acute decompensation. In chronic respiratory failure, home NIV achieves 80% 5-year survival, depending on bulbar involvement and severity.

2. **Cardiogenic pulmonary oedema.** CPAP reduces mortality and ETI rates in patients who are hypoxaemic despite maximal medical treatment. NIV is less effective and used when CPAP is unsuccessful.

3. **Obstructive sleep apnoea.** CPAP and NIV are equally effective in decompensated OSA. BIPAP is required in patients with respiratory acidosis.

4. **Weaning.** NIV may aid weaning of COPD patients from invasive ventilation.

5. **Other conditions.** NIV is used with varying success in chest wall trauma, ALI, post-operative respiratory failure, and pneumonia. It should only be used in critical care units in patients for ETI if NIV fails.

6. **When ETI is considered inappropriate** (e.g. end-stage respiratory disease).

Contraindications to NIV
• Facial trauma/burns/surgery.
• Oesophageal surgery.
• Severe hypoxaemia.
• Haemodynamic instability.
• Coma/confusion/claustrophobia.
• Active TB/epistaxis.
• Vomiting/bowel obstruction.
• Copious respiratory secretions.
• Fixed upper airway obstruction.
• Focal consolidation on CXR.
• Undrained pneumothorax.

Setting up NIV
- **Ensure correct mask size** to reduce leaks. Use a circuit filter, either bacterial or bacterial/viral.
- **Set NIV mode.** For example, CPAP, pressure support, or pressure control.
- **Set inspiratory positive airway pressure (IPAP).** This improves ventilation, increases PaO_2, and decreases $PaCO_2$.
- **Set expiratory positive airway pressure (EPAP).** This improves PaO_2 but may cause CO_2 retention.
- **Set timed inspiratory phase (Ti).** This is only necessary in pressure control modes. In acute hypercapnic COPD exacerbations, Ti is set at 0.8–1.2 s.
- **Set trigger sensitivity** in pressure control.
- **Set low flow alarm.** This detects circuit occlusion (e.g. sputum plugs).
- **Set high-flow alarm.** This indicates excess leakage (e.g. circuit disconnection).
- **Set backup rate for apnoea.**
- **Check ABGs** before, and within 1 hour of starting NIV.

Problem solving in NIV
- **If $PaCO_2$ remains elevated.** Increase IPAP or decrease EPAP.
- **If PaO_2 remains low.** Increase EPAP or IPAP or both, and increase FiO_2.
- **If patient-ventilator synchronization is poor.** Adjust trigger sensitivity or EPAP. Also check mask size and fit.
- **If the machine is cycling at the backup rate.** Check if the patient has stopped breathing or is not triggering breaths.
- **Factors that indicate NIV has failed.** Failure of $PaCO_2$ to decrease by 4–6 h; failure of PaO_2 to increase by 4–6 h; reducing conscious level.

Monitoring
Monitoring of NIV and CPAP should include clinical evaluation (e.g. comfort, conscious level, respiratory rate, chest wall motion), continuous oximetry (i.e. SaO_2), and ABG measurements 1 hour after starting NIV and at 4–6 h if the earlier sample showed little improvement.

Factors associated with NIV success and failure
See Table 19.8.

Table 19.8 Factors associated with success and failure in NIV

Success
- High $PaCO_2$
- Low A-a O_2 gradient
- pH 7.3–7.35
- Improvement in pH, $PaCO_2$, and respiratory rate within 1 h of NIV
- Good conscious level

Failure
- Pneumonia on CXR
- pH <7.25–7.3
- Copious respiratory secretions
- Edentulous/mask leak
- Poor patient-ventilator synchrony
- Poor nutritional status
- Impaired consciousness/confusion
- High APACHE score

Patients who benefit from NIV are ventilated as much as possible during the first 24 hours, with breaks for meals, drugs, and physiotherapy. A nasogastric tube prevents gastric distension and reduces aspiration risk. Benefit is usually evident at 1 hour and certainly after 4–6 hours of NIV.

The point at which treatment is considered to have failed and should be withdrawn, or ETI considered, depends on the severity of respiratory failure, patient wishes, and whether other factors (e.g. secretions) could be better managed, following ETI.

Follow-up spirometry and ABG are measured before discharge in those who benefit from NIV. Patients with chronic hypercapnic hypoventilation (e.g. obesity) should be referred for home NIV assessment.

Mechanical ventilation
Mechanical ventilation (MV) is usually delivered through an endotracheal tube or tracheostomy and provides complete or partial respiratory support, usually in critically ill or anaesthetized patients who are no longer able to maintain spontaneous ventilation. In contrast, non-invasive ventilation aids spontaneous ventilation and avoids the need for endotracheal intubation and MV.

Indications for mechanical ventilation
The main indication for MV, excluding surgical procedures, is respiratory failure (see Table 19.9). However, its value in the support of other organs, especially during shock or cardiac failure, is increasingly being recognized. Apart from in emergencies (e.g. cardiac arrest), the difficult decision is when, and whether to, ventilate a deteriorating patient.

Table 19.9 Indications for mechanical ventilation

Lung disease
- ARDS, pneumonia, acute asthma, COPD
- Aspiration, smoke inhalation

Respiratory centre depression
- Head injury + raised intracranial pressure
- Severe hypercapnia; $PaCO_2$ >7–8 kPa
- Drug overdose, e.g. opiates, barbiturates
- Status epilepticus, encephalitis, meningitis, tumours

Circulatory
- Cardiac arrest, pulmonary oedema, shock

Trauma
- Cervical cord trauma above C4; neck fractures

Neuromuscular disorders
- Guillain–Barré, myasthenia gravis, poliomyelitis

Chest wall disorders
- Kyphoscoliosis; traumatic flail segment

Other factors
- Poor nutrition causing respiratory muscle weakness
- Abdominal distension/pain which splints the diaphragm

Surgical
- General anaesthesia; post-operative

There are no simple guidelines, but important indicators suggesting the need for MV include:

- Hypoxaemia (PaO$_2$ <8 kPa on FiO$_2$ >0.4).
- Hypercapnia (PaCO$_2$ >7.5 kPa).
- Respiratory/metabolic acidosis (pH <7.2).
- Physical factors (e.g. confusion, exhaustion, poor cough).

Trends in these variables are often more helpful than absolute values. In general, MV is only appropriate when there is a reasonable chance of survival. If ventilation is anticipated to be needed for more than a week, consider a tracheostomy. In terminal illness, support is often limited to NIV, after discussion with the patient and/or relatives.

Mechanical ventilators

There are two basic types of mechanical ventilator.

- **Pressure-cycled ventilators** deliver gas into the lungs until a prescribed pressure is reached when inspiratory flow stops, and, after a short pause, expiration occurs by passive recoil. This has the advantage of reducing the peak airway pressures without impairing cardiac performance in situations, such as ARDS. However, if the airway pressures increase or compliance decreases, the tidal volume will fall, so patients need to be monitored closely to avoid hypoventilation.
- **Volume-cycled ventilators** deliver a preset tidal volume into the lungs over a predetermined inspiratory time, usually about 30% of the breathing cycle, then hold the inspiratory phase for about 10% of the breathing cycle, and then allow passive expiration as the lungs recoil.

Ventilator set-up

- **Initially, set FiO$_2$ (O$_2$)**, aiming for PaO$_2$ >8 kPa.
- **Set the mode** (see 'Ventilatory mode'; e.g. IPPV, SIMV, PSV).
- **If full support, set the respiratory rate (RR: ~8–14/min), and then set one of the two following parameters:**
  - Tidal volume (Tv: 6–8 mL/kg or ~4–600 mL).
  - Minute ventilation (Mv: ~6 L/min).
  - (The third parameter is a function of the other two: Mv = RR x Tv.)
- **Set PEEP** ≥5 cmH$_2$O.
- **Set inspiratory:expiratory time.** The normal I:E ratio is ~1:2.
- **Set ventilator alarms.** These are essential to detect disconnection, hypoventilation, airway obstruction, etc.

Typical initial adult intermittent positive pressure ventilation (IPPV) settings are: tidal volume (Tv) ~6-8 mL/kg; respiratory frequency (f) ~8–14 breaths/min; and minute ventilation (Mv = Tv x f) ~6 L/min. FiO$_2$ and Mv are adjusted to maintain PaO$_2$ >8 kPa and PaCO$_2$ <7 kPa, respectively, but acceptable values depend on individual diseases. Initially, PEEP is set at ≥5 cmH$_2$O.

The inspiratory:expiratory time (I:E ratio) is normally set at ~1:2. The relative proportions of time spent in inspiration and expiration can be altered. Thus, in acute asthma, where air trapping is a problem, a longer expiratory time is needed to reduce air trapping. In ARDS, where the lung compliance is low, a longer inspiratory time is beneficial (inverse ratio ventilation). Disease-specific ventilatory strategies are discussed in individual chapters.

Ventilatory mode

The mode of ventilation describes whether a breath is:

- Fully or partially supported.
- Volume- or pressure-controlled (as described previously).
- Mandatory (delivered by the ventilator, regardless of patient respiratory effort) or spontaneously triggered.

Duration of a breath may be fixed (i.e. timed) or variable (i.e. dependent on Tv delivery). Modern ventilators with microprocessor controls provide considerable flexibility, allowing a change from mandatory full-support modes to partial-support modes that minimize sedation requirements and allow patients to be conscious but comfortable.

Specific ventilatory modes include:

- **Full (mandatory) support modes** (e.g. IPPV). Controlled mechanical ventilation (CMV) is uncomfortable and may require full sedation, as no allowance is made for spontaneous respiration. Patients capable of spontaneous breaths who are ventilated with full-support modes (e.g. CMV) can get 'stacking' of breaths when the present ventilator cycle may give a breath on top of one which the patient has just taken. This leads to overinflation of the lungs, a high peak inspiratory pressure, and the risk of pneumothorax.

  Full-support modes are used in severe respiratory disease, in circulatory instability, or when respiratory drive is absent. Prolonged use of these modes can result in respiratory muscle atrophy; this may complicate subsequent 'weaning', especially in combination with a proximal myopathy from steroids (e.g. in acute asthma).

  Volume- or pressure-controlled (VC, PC) modes are available, but the pattern of gas flow in PC ventilation achieves better gas exchange.

  - **Volume-controlled IPPV/CMV** is often used postoperatively. Each breath is delivered at a preset volume over a fixed time. Airway pressure varies with lung compliance.
  - **Pressure-controlled IPPV/CMV** delivers preset pressures, and there is no direct control of Tv, which depends on inspiratory time, lung compliance, and airways resistance. PC ventilation protects lungs by limiting peak inspiratory pressures (PIP) and encourages alveolar recruitment.

- **Partial-support modes** allow the patient to breathe spontaneously, whilst supporting effective ventilation, and allows gradual transfer of the work of breathing to the patient. These modes of ventilation are preferable, as they reduce sedation requirements. Breaths are patient-initiated and detected by sensitive flow/pressure triggers in the ventilator, which then provide inspiratory support.

  - **Assist control.** The ventilator delivers a breath when triggered by inspiratory effort or independently if the patient does not breathe within a certain time.
  - **Synchronized intermittent mandatory ventilation (SIMV)** delivers a set number of mechanically imposed breaths to achieve a minimum Mv, but also allows pressure-supported spontaneous breathing. Imposed breaths are reduced, as the patient becomes ventilator-independent during weaning.
  - **Pressure support.** A preset pressure supports each spontaneous breath. The patient determines breath rate. Gradual pressure reductions make it a comfortable and effective mode of weaning.

Positive end expiratory pressure

Positive end expiratory pressure (PEEP) is a positive pressure, maintained throughout expiration, that increases functional residual capacity (i.e. alveolar recruitment), prevents alveolar collapse at end expiration, reduces V/Q mismatch, and decreases alveolar oedema by increasing lymphatic drainage. PEEP improves oxygenation for any given mode of ventilation. However, the trade-off is an increase in intrathoracic pressure which can significantly decrease venous return and hence cardiac output. There is also an increased risk of pneumothorax.

In general, PEEP should be kept at a level of 5–10 cm H_2O, where required, and the level adjusted in 2–3 cm H_2O intervals every 20–30 minutes, according to a balance between oxygenation and cardiac performance.

'Auto-PEEP' (intrinsic PEEP) is seen if the patient's lungs do not fully empty (i.e. air trapping, hyperinflation) before the next inflation (e.g. asthma, COPD). This results in the need for increased effort to trigger breaths when mechanically ventilated, increasing the work of breathing. In these patients, increasing the ventilator-applied PEEP to match this intrinsic PEEP reduces the effort required to trigger breaths and consequently reduces work of breathing.

Physiological responses to mechanical ventilation
- **Cardiovascular responses** are due to alveolar overdistension and two effects of increased intrathoracic pressure:
  - **Right ventricular preload reduction** is due to increased right atrial pressure which reduces venous return and right ventricular cardiac output. However, fluid infusion rapidly restores venous return and cardiac output.
  - **Left ventricular afterload reduction** is due to reduced left ventricular transmural pressure, which decreases left ventricular work. In the normal heart, any beneficial effect of left ventricular afterload reduction is offset by reduced venous return. However, in the failing heart, cardiac output is relatively insensitive to preload changes but very sensitive to afterload reduction. Consequently, mechanical ventilation may increase cardiac output in heart failure, a useful therapeutic effect.
  - The overall response to raised intrathoracic pressure depends on the state of the heart, vasomotor tone, and fluid status (e.g. hypovolaemia). Mechanical ventilation also increases lung volumes, but overinflated alveoli compress alveolar blood vessels, increasing pulmonary vascular resistance and causing pulmonary hypertension. Subsequent right ventricular distension displaces the septum into the left ventricular cavity, reducing left ventricular filling and cardiac output, an effect known as interventricular dependence.
- **Respiratory effects.** Mechanical ventilation reduces work of breathing which increases the proportion of cardiac output going to potentially ischaemic organs. Re-expansion of collapsed alveoli also improves oxygenation. Unfortunately, supine position, reduced surfactant, and ventilation of poorly perfused lung increases V/Q mismatch.
- **Fluid retention** is due to antidiuretic hormone secretion.

Complications of mechanical ventilation
- **'Barotrauma'** refers to pressure-induced lung damage (e.g. pneumothorax). High PIP (>35 cmH_2O) due to reduced lung compliance (e.g. ARDS) may cause airways disruption and interstitial gas formation.
- **'Volutrauma'** describes damage to healthy alveoli due to overdistension (i.e. excessive Tv). **'Protective' ventilation strategies** use low Tv (~6 mL/kg) to avoid

volutrauma, keep PIP <35 cmH_2O, and maintain alveolar recruitment with PEEP >5 cmH_2O.
- Risks associated with ETT or tracheostomy.
- Oxygen toxicity.
- Impaired cardiac output.
- Ventilator-associated pneumonia due to microaspiration.
- Stress ulceration.
- Bronchopulmonary dysplasia.
- Ventilator failure/disconnection.

Endotracheal intubation

Endotracheal intubation (ETI) may be necessary to support failing ventilation, to maintain a clear airway, to protect against aspiration, and for routine surgery. Occasionally, a physician may be called upon to undertake an emergency ETI, most commonly at a cardiac arrest, but, whenever possible, this procedure should be performed by an appropriately trained clinician, skilled in airways management.

However, in order to assist during emergencies, acute physicians should be familiar with basic airways management, ETI techniques, and failed intubation drills. The description below is not intended as a substitute for practice under the supervision of a skilled anaesthetist.

Indications for endotracheal intubation
- **Clinical indications** include routine surgical procedures, respiratory failure, decreased conscious level (Glasgow coma score ≤8), sputum clearance, airways protection from aspiration of oral secretions or gastric contents, and upper airways obstruction.
- **Objective measures**, indicating the need for ventilatory support and ETI (if non-invasive ventilation is not possible), include a respiratory rate >35/min, vital capacity <15 mL/kg, PaO_2 <8 kPa on >40% O_2 and $PaCO_2$ >7.5 kPa (except in patients with chronic carbon dioxide retention).

Preparation and equipment required
- **Airways assessment** only predicts ~50% of difficult intubations (incidence ≤1:65). When feasible, the anaesthetic notes should be reviewed and the patient asked about previous difficult intubations. Clinical examination should assess cardiorespiratory status and oxygen requirements. Problems may arise in obese patients and those with short necks, distorted neck anatomy (e.g. goitres), reduced neck movement, beards, or pregnancy.
- **Airway examination** should assess features that are known to be associated with difficult intubation, including:
  - Absence of key anatomical landmarks during oropharyngeal inspection with tongue protrusion (e.g. faucial pillars, soft palate, uvula), as described in Mallampati's modified classification (see Figure 19.11).
  - Short thyromental distance (i.e. <3 fingerbreadths or 6 cm from thyroid cartilage to chin).
  - Restricted mouth opening (i.e. <4 cm).
  - Reduced neck extension.
  - Oral factors (e.g. large tongue, buck teeth).
- **Decide on the most appropriate route for intubation.** Oral intubation is preferred in most circumstances. Oral endotracheal tubes are wider which reduces airways resistance and improves secretion clearance. Nasotracheal intubation is rarely undertaken, except for ENT surgery (e.g. oral trauma).

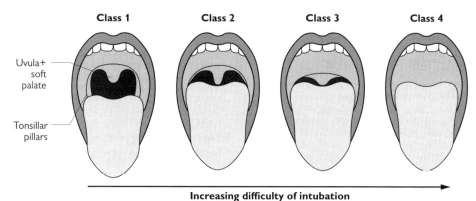

Increasing difficulty of intubation

Figure 19.11 Mallampati's (modified) oropharyngeal classification for assessment of the relative difficulty of endotracheal intubation. Reproduced from Samsoon, GL, and Young, JR, 'Difficult tracheal intubation: a retrospective study', Anaesthesia, 42, 5, pp. 487–490, Copyright © 2007, John Wiley and Sons, with permission from Wiley and The Association of Anaesthestists of Great Britain & Ireland.

- **Preparation for endotracheal intubation.** All equipment and drugs must be immediately available and easily accessible.
  - **Establish intravenous access.**
  - **Place a nasogastric tube, if necessary.**
  - **Remove dentures.**
  - **Position the patient correctly**, with the neck flexed (one pillow) and head extended ('sniffing the morning air').
  - **Resuscitate** and correct electrolyte balance, if required. In emergencies, full resuscitation may not be feasible.
  - **Preoxygenation.** This increases the time to desaturation fivefold and is achieved using tight-fitting face masks to deliver 100% oxygen therapy.
  - **Ventilation.** A well-fitting anaesthetic face mask, breathing circuit, oxygen source, and ventilator will be required.
  - **Suction apparatus**, with rigid (Yankauer) and long, flexible catheters, is required to clear oropharyneal secretions.
  - **Laryngoscopes** (long and short blades) enable laryngeal visualization. In adults, curved Macintosh blades are most popular.
  - **Endotracheal tubes** should be available in a number of sizes. The usual tube size in adult males is 8–9 mm (internal diameter in mm), and 7–8 mm in adult females. Most endotracheal tubes have low-pressure, high-volume cuffs to limit tracheal mucosal damage.
  - **Drugs** include anaesthetic, analgesic, muscle relaxant, and vasoactive agents (e.g. atropine, ephedrine, metaraminol), as most anaesthetic agents are vasodilators.
  - **Monitoring equipment** should include capnography for end-tidal CO_2 measurement.
  - **Syringes** for cuff inflation and clamp to prevent air escaping from the cuff once inflated.
  - **Scissors and tape or bandage** to secure the tube.
  - **Lubricating jelly.**
  - Magill forceps, bougies, flexible stylet.

Procedure

All patients requiring emergency intubations are assumed to be at high risk of aspiration (i.e. full stomach) because fasting status is either unknown or less than 6 hours and/or gastric emptying may be impaired (e.g. obstruction, diabetic, or opiate-induced gastric paresis). These patients require rapid sequence, rather than normal, induction. In acute emergencies, in which the patient is deeply unconscious, anaesthesia may not be necessary, and the sequence of intubation must be more rapid.

- **Emergency intubation** (e.g. unconscious cardiac arrest).
  - Place the patient with the neck slightly flexed and the head extended. Take care if cervical injury is suspected.
  - Pre-oxygenate the patient with ≥85% oxygen for 15–30 seconds, using a tight-fitting face mask and self-inflating bag. Open the mouth, and clear the airway with suction.
  - With the laryngoscope in your left hand, insert the blade on the right side of mouth. Advance to base of tongue, identifying the tonsillar fossa and the uvula. Push the blade to the left, moving the tongue over. Advance the blade until the epiglottis comes into view. Insert the blade tip between the base of the tongue and the epiglottis (into the vallecula), and pull the whole blade (and larynx) upwards along the line of the handle of the laryngoscope to expose the vocal cords (see Figure 19.12). Brief suction may be necessary to clear the view.
  - The oesophagus can be occluded by applying cricoid pressure and compressing the cricoid cartilage posteriorly against the vertebral body at C6. This prevents passive regurgitation into the trachea but not active vomiting. Ask your assistant to maintain pressure until the endotracheal tube is in place and the cuff inflated.
  - Insert the endotracheal tube between the vocal cords, and advance it until the cuff is just below the cords and no further. Inflate the cuff with air.
  - Intubation should not take longer than 30 seconds; if there is any doubt about the position, remove the tube; reoxygenate, and try again.

- With the tube in place, listen to the chest during inflation to check that both sides of the chest are ventilated. If the tube is in the oesophagus, chest expansion will be minimal, though the stomach may inflate; air entry into the chest will be minimal.
- Tie the endotracheal tube in place, and secure to prevent it from slipping up or down the airway. Ventilate with high concentration oxygen.

- **Rapid sequence induction** (RSI: see Figure 19.13) is used for emergency intubations in conscious patients who require anaesthetic induction but who have not been adequately starved prior to the procedure. It rapidly secures the airway after anaesthetic-induced loss of consciousness, reducing the risk of aspiration. The procedure differs in a number of aspects from that described above.
  - Following 10–15 minutes pre-oxygenation with high-flow oxygen, an induction agent (e.g. propofol) is administered, quickly followed by a rapidly acting muscle relaxant (e.g. suxamethonium).
  - Simultaneously, an assistant applies anterior pressure to the cricoid cartilage (as described previously), which closes the oesophagus, preventing gastric regurgitation.
  - The patient is positioned, with the neck flexed (i.e. one pillow beneath the occiput) and head extended ('sniffing the morning air'), to align the glottis, pharynx, and oral cavity which achieves the best view on laryngoscopy (see Figure 19.12). Intubation rapidly follows (i.e. **without the normal mask ventilation used in a normal intubation** (see further text)). Cricoid pressure is released only after confirmation of correct tube placement and cuff inflation.
  - A modified rapid sequence induction, using a non-depolarizing muscle relaxant (e.g. rocuronium), is rec-ommended in situations where suxamethonium is contraindicated (i.e. hyperkalaemia in renal failure, neuromuscular disorders, trauma).

- **Normal intubation** differs from RSI in that the patient is usually stable (i.e. haemodynamically, metabolically), and has fasted for >6 h to ensure an empty stomach. These patients do not require cricoid pressure during intubation, and mask ventilation is established before giving the muscle relaxant, which is then continued for 2–3 min to ensure complete paralysis before intubation.

Potential problems during intubation

- Certain anatomical variations (e.g. receding mandible, short neck, prominent incisors, high arched palate) as well as stiff neck or trismus may complicate intubation.
- Vomiting may require suction and, occasionally, cricoid pressure to protect the airway.
- Cervical spine injury. Immobilize the head and neck in line with the body. Avoid extending the head during intubation.
- Facial burns or trauma may make orotracheal intubation impossible. Consider nasal intubation or cricothyroidotomy.
- **Difficult intubation aids** include gum elastic bougies/flexible stylets which aid endotracheal intubation when the tracheal opening is anterior to the visual axis (see Figure 19.12). Fibreoptic endoscopy and video laryngoscopes allow direct visualization of the larynx during intubation. Specialist laryngoscope blades (e.g. McCoy blade) lift the epiglottis, improving the laryngoscopic view.

Failed intubation drill

Initial intubation attempts fail in ≤1:300 intubations. The failed intubation drill is as follows:

- Summon experienced help. Consider waking the patient, but this may not be an option in emergencies.
- Mask-ventilate the patient or, if this is not possible, consider laryngeal mask ventilation, until senior help arrives.
- If ventilation is inadequate with these methods, consider an emergency cricothyroidotomy (see 'Cricothyroidotomy').
- Experienced personnel may consider alternative approaches to intubation (e.g. fibreoptic endoscopy).

Complications

Endotracheal intubation complications include:

- Intubation failure, oesophageal intubation.
- Hypoxaemia.
- Gastric aspiration.
- Bronchospasm.
- Arrhythmias.
- Trauma (e.g. lips, teeth, vocal cords, cervical spine).

Tracheostomy

Despite the low-pressure, high-volume cuffs used in modern endotracheal tubes, prolonged intubation risks damage to the vocal cords and/or tracheal stenosis. Tracheostomy is usually advisable after 7–14 days mechanical ventilation, or earlier, if it is evident that a patient will require prolonged intubation.

Advantages and potential risks of tracheostomy

- **General advantages** include comfort, reduced sedation, decreased dead space, with earlier and easier weaning, improved mouth care, and less accidental extubations. There is also the potential for speech when the cuff is deflated and with special speaking tubes.

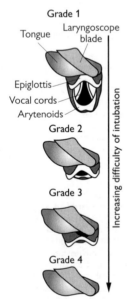

Figure 19.12 Laryngoscopy assesses difficulty of intubation.

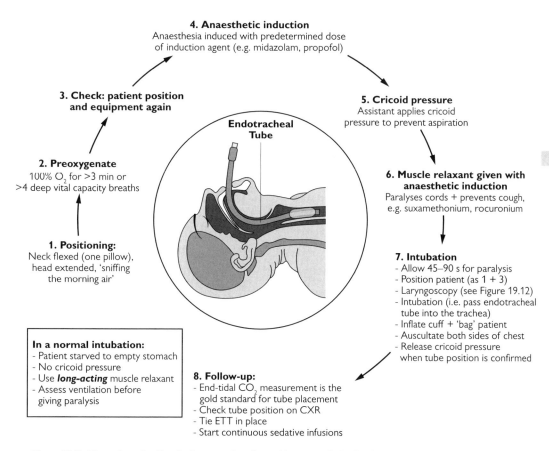

4. Anaesthetic induction
Anaesthesia induced with predetermined dose
of induction agent (e.g. midazolam, propofol)

**3. Check: patient position
and equipment again**

**Endotracheal
Tube**

5. Cricoid pressure
Assistant applies cricoid
pressure to prevent aspiration

2. Preoxygenate
100% O$_2$ for >3 min or
>4 deep vital capacity breaths

**6. Muscle relaxant given with
anaesthetic induction**
Paralyses cords + prevents cough,
e.g. suxamethonium, rocuronium

1. Positioning:
Neck flexed (one pillow),
head extended, 'sniffing
the morning air'

7. Intubation
- Allow 45–90 s for paralysis
- Position patient (as 1 + 3)
- Laryngoscopy (see Figure 19.12)
- Intubation (i.e. pass endotracheal
  tube into the trachea)
- Inflate cuff + 'bag' patient
- Auscultate both sides of chest
- Release cricoid pressure
  when tube position is confirmed

In a normal intubation:
- Patient starved to empty stomach
- No cricoid pressure
- Use *long-acting* muscle relaxant
- Assess ventilation before
  giving paralysis

8. Follow-up:
- End-tidal CO$_2$ measurement is the
  gold standard for tube placement
- Check tube position on CXR
- Tie ETT in place
- Start continuous sedative infusions

Figure 19.13 The endotracheal intubation procedure for rapid sequence induction. Reproduced from Richard M. Leach, Acute and Critical Care Medicine at a Glance, second edition, Figure b, Chapter 15, page 38, Wiley, Copyright 2009, with permission.

- **General disadvantages** include the need for theatre time with surgical tracheostomies; there are insertion complications, including haemorrhage, false tract formation, and tracheal wall damage. Secondary skin infections occur (~10%). Longer-term complications include tracheal stenosis and erosion into the oesophagus.
- **Percutanoeus tracheostomy** has the advantages of simplicity, reduced cost, saved theatre time, and fewer complications (e.g. infection, tracheal stenosis), compared to surgical tracheostomy.

Tracheostomy tubes (± cuffs) are available in a variety of sizes and types. Some have inner tubes that facilitate cleaning, reduce obstruction, and allow less frequent tube changes (i.e. ~30 days). Others have long flanges for obese necks.

Removal follows a period of cuff deflation and tube capping to ensure respiratory independence. The remaining stoma is covered with an airtight dressing and heals within a few days.

Minitracheostomy. A small tube (~5 mm) is inserted through the cricothyroid membrane, through which a suction catheter can be passed. Minitracheostomies may be useful for short-term secretion clearance when cough or conscious level is temporarily impaired in high dependency areas.

Cricothyroidotomy

This is an emergency procedure which is used to bypass the upper airway and larynx when obstruction (e.g. an inhaled foreign body like a marble, sweet, food) prevents adequate ventilation of the lower respiratory tract. It should only be attempted as a last resort after other less invasive procedures (e.g. the Heimlich manoeuvre) have failed to clear the obstruction.

Indications

- To bypass upper airway obstruction (e.g. trauma, infections, neoplasms, post-operative, burns, and corrosives) when oral or nasotracheal intubation is contraindicated.
- In situations when endotracheal intubations fail (e.g. massive nasopharyngeal haemorrhage, structural deformities, obstruction due to foreign bodies, etc.).
- As an elective procedure in select patients to provide a route for suction of airway secretions (e.g. patients in neuromuscular disease). This should be converted to a tracheostomy if required for prolonged periods or if infection or inflammation occurs.

Procedure

This should **not** be attempted, except in a life-threatening emergency, without appropriate training from an experienced upper airway specialist (e.g. anaesthetist). If there is time to obtain assistance, this should be considered.

The aim of the procedure is to open a tract into the trachea through the cricothyroid membrane which is just under 1 cm in its vertical dimension. The membrane lies between the thyroid and cricoid cartilages and can be felt just below the 'Adam's apple'. The cricothyroid artery runs across the midline in the upper portion of the membrane. The technique is determined by the urgency of the situation.

- **Emergency cricothyroidotomy.** This procedure may be required in hyperacute situations (e.g. in a restaurant), with few, if any, medical facilities available. It is usually due to acute aspiration (e.g. 'café coronary' due to food aspiration), with occlusion of the larynx that cannot be cleared with simple manoeuvres, and rapidly leads to severe hypoxaemia. Usually, the patient is unconscious by the time this procedure is attempted.
    - Locate the thyroid and cricoid cartilages.
    - If a wide-bore needle is available, this is passed through the cricothyroid membrane to establish an airway (give 100% oxygen through the needle, if available).
    - If a needle is not available, a penknife, kitchen knife, or other sharp implement is passed through the skin and cricothyroid membrane in the horizontal plane just above the cricoid cartilage. The use of biros is extremely difficult, as these are not usually sufficiently strong or sharp to pass through the tough anterior neck tissues.
    - Once inserted, the horizontal penknife/knife/implement is then twisted into the vertical plane, opening a tract into the upper trachea and allowing immediate ventilation.
    - If available, a tube (e.g. biro case) may then be used to hold the tract open.

- **Percutaneous cricothyroidotomy** is used for less acute situations (e.g. to aid sputum clearance) and employs the Seldinger technique. It is quicker and generally safer than surgical procedures (see further text) and may be performed by non-surgeons at the bedside (see Figure 19.14).
    - Clean the skin with iodine, and isolate the area with sterile towels.
    - Infiltrate the skin and the area around the cricothyroid space with local anaesthetic.
    - After anaesthetizing the area, a needle is used to puncture the cricothyroid membrane, and, through this, a guidewire is introduced into the trachea. Over this, a series of dilators and the tracheostomy tube can be safely positioned.

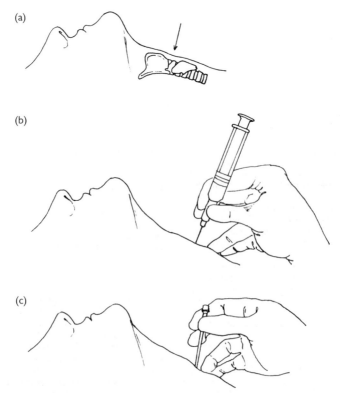

(a)

(b)

(c)

Figure 19.14 Emergency cricothyroidotomy. Reproduced from Punit S. Ramrakha, Kevin P. Moore, and Amir Sam, *Oxford Handbook of Acute Medicine*, third edition, 2010, Figure 15.11, page 783, copyright Punit S. Ramrakha and Kevin P. Moore, with permission.

- **Surgical cricothyroidotomy.** May be performed in less urgent situations.
  - Locate the cricothyroid space. This is just under 1 cm in its vertical dimension. The cricothyroid artery runs across the midline in the upper portion.
  - Clean the skin with iodine, and isolate the area with sterile towels.
  - Infiltrate the skin and the area around the cricothyroid space with local anaesthetic.
  - Make a 3 cm vertical midline incision through the skin, taking care not to cut the membrane.
  - Palpate the cricothyroid membrane through the incision. Stabilize the larynx by holding between the index finger and thumb. Make a short transverse incision in the lower third of the cricothyroid membrane, just scraping over the upper part of the cricoid cartilage (preferably using the tip of a no. 11 blade to go through the membrane). This minimizes the risk of cutting the cricothyroid artery.
  - Dilate the membrane with forceps; insert the minitracheostomy or small tracheostomy tube (4–6 mm internal diameter) through the incision into the trachea, and secure.

Complications of cricothyroidotomy
- Haemorrhage—often due to cricothyroid artery damage.
- Tube misplacement occurs in up to 15% of cases.
- Subglottic stenosis.
- Hoarseness.
- Laryngotracheal-cutaneous fistula.

Aspiration of a pneumothorax
Figure 19.15 illustrates British Thoracic Society Guidelines for the management of spontaneous pneumothorax in haemodynamically stable patients. In primary spontaneous pneumothorax with a >2 cm rim (i.e. the distance from the lung edge to chest wall at the level of the hilum) or a small (1–2 cm rim) secondary pneumothorax, it is reasonable to attempt aspiration of the pneumothorax in the first instance.

Preparation and equipment
- Syringes (10 and 50 mL) and needles (green (18G) and orange (25G)).
- Dressing pack (sterile drapes, antiseptic).
- Mask, gown, and sterile gloves.
- 16–18 Venflon® or alternative large-bore cannula.
- Local anaesthetic (e.g. 1% lidocaine (INN)).
- Three-way tap.

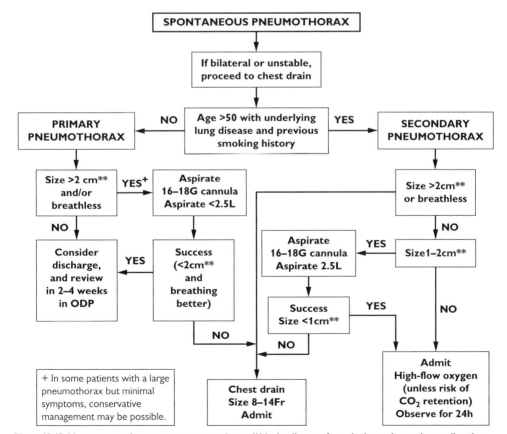

Figure 19.15 Management of spontaneous pneumothorax.(is the distance from the lung edge to chest wall at the level of the hilum)** Reproduced from *Thorax*, M Henry, *et al.*, 'BTS guidelines for the management of spontaneous pneumothorax', 58, Suppl 2, pp. ii39–ii52, copyright 2003, with permission from BMJ Publishing Group Ltd.

Procedure

- Ensure an assistant is available to help during this procedure.
- Sit the patient up, propped against pillows, with his/her hands behind his/her head; ensure you are comfortable and on a similar level.
- Select the space to aspirate; usually this is the second intercostal space in the mid-clavicular line. Confirm on the chest radiograph that you are aspirating the correct side (a surprisingly common cause of disasters is aspirating the normal side).
- Clean the skin, and ensure asepsis with drapes and aseptic technique.
- Connect a 50 mL syringe to a 3-way tap, and ensure that the port which will be 'connected' to the patient is turned 'off' to prevent air entering the pleural cavity when connecting it to the inserted drainage cannula.
- Infiltrate 1% lidocaine (INN) from skin to pleura, just above the upper border of the rib in the space you are using. Confirm the presence of air by aspirating approximately 5 mL via a green needle.
- Insert a 16–18G intravenous cannula (e.g. Venflon®) into the pneumothorax, preferably whilst aspirating the cannula with a syringe, so that entry into the pleural space is confirmed. Allow the tip of the cannula to enter the space by approximately 1 cm.
- Ask the patient to hold their breath, and remove the needle. Swiftly connect the 3-way tap with attached 50 mL syringe. Aspirate 50 mL of air/fluid, and void it through the expiration port through a cannula attached to an underwater seal.
- Repeat the aspiration until resistance to suction is felt, the patient coughs excessively, or ≥2.5 L of air has been aspirated.
- Withdraw the cannula, and cover the site with a dressing plaster (e.g. Band-aid).
- Check a post-procedure CXR. Aspiration is successful in 60–80% of primary spontaneous pneumothorax (PSP) and 35–60% of secondary pneumothorax (SP) and is confirmed by complete or near lung re-expansion on repeat CXR. Although the ideal time for a repeat CXR is unknown, it should be several hours in order to detect slow air leaks. Successfully aspirated SP should be observed in hospital for at least 24 h before discharge (see 'Pneumothorax' in Chapter 5).
- Simple aspiration should not be repeated, unless there were technical difficulties. Compared to intercostal tube drainage, aspiration is associated with less recurrence. If there is significant residual pneumothorax, insert a chest drain.

Aspiration of a pleural effusion

Pleural aspiration (thoracentesis) is the primary means of evaluating a pleural effusion and is used to guide further investigation and management. It may be diagnostic or therapeutic (i.e. relieves breathlessness), depending on the volume of fluid removed.

The basic procedure is similar to that for a pneumothorax, but the site of aspiration (drainage) differs, as fluid is located in the lower pleural cavity due to gravitational forces. Fluid is usually aspirated from the posterior chest wall, one or two intercostal spaces below the level at which dullness is detected.

In England and Wales, recent guidelines have recommended that real-time ultrasound guidance should be used to guide aspiration of most pleural fluid collections.

Ultrasound scans confirm the level of the effusion and ensure that the diaphragm is not higher than anticipated due to underlying pulmonary collapse. The previous practice of marking the aspiration or drainage site on the chest wall at earlier ultrasound scanning is now discouraged, especially with small effusions. Complications have occurred (e.g. liver laceration, bowel perforation) due to later changes in fluid and anatomical relationships with changes in position at the time of aspiration.

Procedure

- Position the patient leaning forward over a table, with the arms resting just below shoulder height on a pillow. Clean the skin, and infiltrate with local anaesthetic.
- Determine the site of the effusion on real-time ultrasound, and use the image to guide the aspiration needle and cannula (e.g Venflon®) into the effusion.
- Remove the needle, leaving the cannula in the effusion. Attach a 3-way tap and 50 mL syringe to the cannula, and aspirate the effusion, voiding it through the 3-way tap. Repeat the aspirations until resistance is felt and the tap is dry.
- The appearance of the fluid should be recorded and samples placed in sterile containers for protein, lactate dehydrogenase (LDH), and microbiology (e.g. Gram stains, culture, acid-fast bacilli stains and culture). A 20 mL fresh sample is sent to cytology to examine for malignant cells and differential cell counts. Use of a 3.8% sodium citrate tube may aid cell preservation in cytology samples. Blood culture bottle samples should also be sent for microbiology. A non-purulent, heparinized sample is processed in the arterial blood gas analyser for pH (without exposure to air or lidocaine (INN)). Measurement with pH litmus paper or pH meters is not reliable. Purulent samples should never be examined, as they may damage the analyser.
- A CXR should be ordered post-procedure to exclude pneumothorax.

Insertion of a chest drain

Chest drains can be inserted using either the:

- **Seldinger technique** (insertion over a guidewire). This is a relatively simple technique, and this is the only method practised by a generation of young physicians. It has the advantage of being less uncomfortable and invasive for the patient, as the drainage catheter and tract are generally smaller (12–16Fr), with the associated limitations of a narrow-gauge catheter for large air leaks and the thick viscid secretions associated with empyema. However, it is the technique of choice for pneumothorax.

  Unfortunately, this method involves the use of a 'sharp, pointed' dilator (to open a tract for the drain) which has resulted in a series of serious complications and several fatalities. These include impalement of the heart, liver, and bowel due to incorrect positioning and inappropriately deep insertion of the dilator. Consequently, recent guidelines have strongly recommended the use of real-time ultrasound guidance when using this technique, particularly in complex pneumothoraces or if pleural fluid is present. This requirement has limited its use to daytime practice in many hospitals where ultrasound facilities and appropriately trained ultrasonographers are not readily available overnight.

- **Blunt dissection technique**. This technique is more complex and less comfortable for the patient, as the tract for drain insertion is larger and involves blunt dissection between the ribs and into the thoracic cavity. However, it facilitates the insertion of much larger chest drains for complex situations, including the drainage of empyema. It is also considerably safer, as sharp trocars are not introduced into the thoracic (or abdominal) cavity, although there is greater risk of infection and haemorrhage (from intercostals vessels). Consequently, it is a safer procedure than the Seldinger technique when performed without ultrasonography, which is a significant advantage out of hours. Unfortunately, few young physicians, the main providers of emergency overnight treatment in many health systems, have been appropriately trained over recent years.

Preparation and equipment required

- Dressing pack (sterile gauze, gloves, drapes, 2% chlorhexidine or povidone iodine).
- Local anaesthetic (20 mL 1% lidocaine (INN)), 10 mL syringe, green (18G) and orange (25G) needles.
- Scalpel and no. 11 blade for skin incision; two packs silk sutures (1–0).
- Two forceps (Kelly clamps), scissors, needle holder (often pre-packaged as a 'chest drain set').
- **Seldinger technique:** pre-packed chest drain kit with introducer needle, guidewire, dilator, and chest drain 10–16Fr.
- **Blunt dissection technique:** mosquito forceps and a pair of larger forceps to introduce the chest drain through the chest wall into the pleural space, chest drains with the trocars removed; selection of 24, 28, 32, and 36Fr.
- Chest drainage bottles, tubing, and sterile water for underwater seal.
- An assistant will be required.

Procedure

- Position the patient leaning forward over the back of a chair or table. If possible, premedicate the patient with an appropriate amount of opiate ~30 minutes before.
- For a pneumothorax, the drain should be inserted in the fifth intercostal space in the 'safe triangle' demarcated anteriorly by the lateral border of the pectoralis major muscle, posteriorly by the mid-axillary line, and inferiorly by the nipple line. When draining an effusion, the drain is inserted under ultrasound guidance below the level of the effusion in the mid-axillary.
- Clean the skin (e.g. with 2% chlorhexidine), and position sterile drapes.
- Use gown, mask, and sterile gloves.
- Infiltrate the skin, subcutaneous tissues, and pleura with 15–20 mL of lidocaine (INN) 1%, and aspirate air/fluid with a green needle.
- Check that the underwater seal bottle is ready.
- Check the length of the tube against the patient's chest to confirm how much needs to be inserted into the patient's chest. Aim to get the tip of the chest drain to the lung apex for a pneumothorax or the base of the pleural space when trying to drain pleural fluid.
- Insert two sutures across the insertion site or incision (or a purse-string). These will gently tighten around the tube once inserted to create an airtight seal, but do not knot—these sutures will be used to close the wound after drain removal.

Seldinger technique

- Insert the introducer needle through the chest wall whilst applying suction on the syringe into the pneumothorax/

effusion which will be confirmed when air/fluid is aspirated.

- Pass the guidewire through the needle into the pleural space. It should pass freely. If there is any resistance, remove the guidewire and re-aspirate through the needle to confirm the position within the pneumothorax or effusion. Then reintroduce the guidewire.
- When the guidewire is in position, nick the skin with a scalpel at the point it enters the chest wall.
- Pass the dilator over the wire into the pleural space, using a gentle twisting motion to move it through the chest wall tissue. There may be a 'giving' sensation as it enters the pleural cavity. It is not necessary to pass the whole dilator which may be >20 cm into the chest (as it may damage underlying lung/heart). Remove the dilator.
- Pass the chest drain (10–16Fr) over the wire into the pleural space, and remove the wire through the drain, leaving the drain *in situ*.
- Connect to the tubing of the pre-prepared underwater seal. Bubbling confirms it is in the pneumothorax, or fluid drainage that it is in the effusion.
- Secure the drain with stitches and tape.

Blunt dissection technique

- Select a chest tube: small (24Fr) for air alone, medium (28Fr) for serous fluid, or large (32–36Fr) for blood/pus. The trocar must be removed.
- Blunt-dissect a short subcutaneous tunnel, using the mosquito forceps for the chest tube, before it enters the pleural space (see Figure 19.16). Anaesthetize the periosteum on the top of the rib. Check that you can aspirate air/fluid from the pleural space.
- Make a horizontal 2 cm incision in the anaesthetized skin of the rib space. Use the mosquito forceps to blunt-dissect through the fat and intercostal muscles to make a track large enough for your gloved finger down to the pleural space. Stay close to the upper border of the rib to avoid the neurovascular bundle.
- Clamp the end of the chest tube with large forceps, and gently pass the tube through the chest wall into the pleural space. Rotating the forceps 180° directs the tube to the apex (see Figure 19.16). Condensation in the tube (or fluid) confirms the tube is within the pleural space. Check that all the holes are within the thorax, and connect to the underwater seal.
- Tighten the skin sutures (as described previously), but do not knot. The drain should be secured with several other stitches and copious amounts of adhesive tape. They are very vulnerable to accidental traction and removal.
- Wrap adhesive tape around the join between the drain and the connecting tubing.

Finally, for both techniques:

- Prescribe adequate analgesia for the patient for when the anaesthetic wears off.
- Arrange for a CXR to check the position of the drain.
- Do not drain off more than 1–1.5 L of pleural fluid/24 hours to avoid re-expansion pulmonary oedema.
- Heimlich valves are an increasingly popular alternative to underwater bottle drainage, as they allow mobilization and, occasionally, outpatient management.

Tips and pitfalls

- **Infection.** The chest drain should only be left in place while air or fluid continues to drain. The risk of ascending

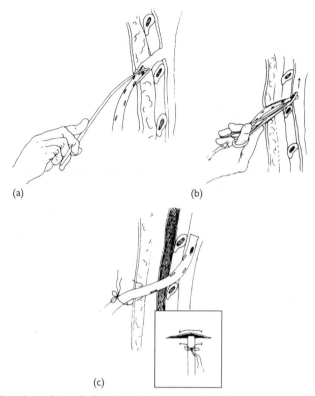

(a)   (b)

(c)

Figure 19.16 Blunt dissection technique for insertion of a chest drain. (a), (b) Chest drain lifted into the pleural space through the tract dissected through the chest wall with forceps, and (c) secured with sutures.
Reproduced from Punit S. Ramrakha, Kevin P. Moore, and Amir Sam, *Oxford Handbook of Acute Medicine*, third edition, 2010, Figure 15.13, page 789, copyright Punit S. Ramrakha and Kevin P. Moore, with permission.

infection increases with time. Prophylactic antibiotics are not usually indicated.

- **Malpositioned tube.** Obtain a CXR post-procedure (and daily) to check the position of the drain and examine the lung fields. If the drain is too far out, there will be an air leak and the patient may develop subcutaneous emphysema. Ideally, remove the drain, and replace with a new drain at a new site; the risk of ascending infection is high if the 'non-sterile' portion of the tube is just pushed into the chest.

  If the drain is too far in, it may be uncomfortable for the patient and impinge on vital structures (e.g. thoracic aorta). Pull the tube out the appropriate distance, and resuture.

- **Obstructed tube.** Check the water column in the chest drain bottle swings with respiration. This will stop if the tube is obstructed. Check the drains and tubing are free of bends and kinks. Blood clots or fibrin may block the tube and may be 'milked' cautiously. If the lung is still collapsed on CXR, replace the chest drain with a new tube at a new site.

- **Lung fails to re-expand.** This is either due to an obstructed system or persistent air leak (e.g. tracheo-bronchial fistula). If the chest drain continues to bubble, apply suction (5–20 cmH$_2$O) to the drain to help expand the lung. Consider inserting further drains or surgical

repair of leak. If the chest drain is obstructed (as described previously), replace the drain.

Removing the chest drain

- Chest drains should not be clamped before removal.
- Remove the dressings, and release the sutures holding the drain in place. Leave the skin incision sutures (purse-string) in position to close the wound once the drain is removed.
- Remove the drain in a gentle motion, either in inspiration or in expiration with Valsalva.
- Tighten the skin sutures. These should be removed after 3–4 days and a fresh dressing applied. Alternatively, apply an airtight dressing.
- Residual pneumothorax is treated, according to symptoms, with a fresh chest drain, if necessary.

Complications

- Bleeding (intercostal vessels, laceration of lung, spleen, liver).
- Pulmonary oedema (e.g. due to rapid lung expansion).
- Empyema.
- Subcutaneous emphysema.
- Residual pneumothorax or effusion (malpositioned or obstructed chest drain).

Further reading

Boldrini R, Fasano L, Nava S (2012). Non-invasive mechanical ventilation. *Current Opinion in Critical Care*, **18**, 48–53.

Davies RJO, Gleeson FV, Ali N, *et al.* (2003). BTS guidelines for the management of pleural disease. *Thorax*, **58** (Suppl II), ii1–59.

Girard TD and Bernard GR (2007). Mechanical ventilation in ARDS: a state-of-the-art review. *Chest*, **131**, 921–9.

Hemmila MR and Napolitano LM (2006). Severe respiratory failure: advanced treatment options. *Critical Care Medicine*, **34**, S278–90.

Kirsch TD and Mulligan JP (2004). Tube thoracostomy. In JR Roberts and JR Hedges, eds. *Clinical procedures in emergency medicine*, 4th edn, pp. 187–211. Saunders, Philadelphia.

Laws D, Neville E, Duffy J (2003). BTS guidelines for the insertion of a chest drain. *Thorax*, **58**, ii53.

MacDuff A, Arnold A, Harvey J, on behalf of the BTS Pleural Disease Guideline Group (2010). Management of spontaneous pneumothorax. *Thorax*, **65**:ii18–ii31.

McConville JF and Kress JP (2012). Weaning patients from the ventilator. *New England Journal of Medicine*, **367**, 2233–9.

O'Driscoll BR, Howard LS, Davison AG (2008). British Thoracic Society guideline for emergency oxygen use in adults. *Thorax*, **63** (Suppl 6), vi1–68.

Gastrointestinal practical procedures

Ascitic tap

An ascitic tap may be performed for diagnostic purposes or as a therapeutic procedure for patient comfort or fluid overload. Table 19.10 illustrates the characteristics of an ascitic transudate and exudate. Table 19.11 reports the causes of transudative and exudative ascites.

- *Diagnostic indications:*
  - Diagnose or exclude spontaneous bacterial peritonitis (SBP).
  - Ascitic protein and albumin.
  - Ascitic cytology (may require 100 mL fluid).
  - Ascitic amylase (pancreatic ascites).
  - Stain and culture for AFBs; lymphocyte count (N <500 cells/mm^3).
- *Therapeutic indications:*
  - To drain cirrhotic ascites.
  - To drain malignant ascites.

Procedure for an ascitic tap

- Lie patient supine and tilted slightly to the left or right.
- Select the site (level with the umbilicus, and 3–4 cm lateral to a line passing to the mid-inguinal point), and clean the area with 2% chlorhexidine, iodine, or equivalent. Ensure the bladder is empty, and avoid any scars.
- Use a 20 mL syringe with an 18G (green) needle to aspirate the ascites. In an obese patient, use a longer needle (e.g. 18G Abbocath®). If you plan to use a larger needle, infiltrate the area with local anaesthetic before proceeding.
- Insert the needle slowly into the abdomen whilst aspirating until fluid is obtained.
- In cirrhotic patients, inoculate 5 mL of ascitic fluid into each bottle of a set of blood culture bottles to exclude spontaneous bacterial peritonitis. Further samples should be sent in a Sterilin® container and a plain bottle for microscopy and protein.

Table 19.10 Characteristics of an ascitic transudate and exudate

	Transudate	Exudate
Total protein	<30 g/L	≥30 g/L
Ascitic protein:serum protein	<0.5	>0.5
Serum-ascitic albumin gradient	>11 g/L	<11 g/L

Table 19.11 Causes of transudative and exudative ascites

Transudative ascites	Exudative ascites
Cirrhosis	Cirrhosis (rarely)
Nephrotic syndrome	Pancreatic
	Tuberculous peritonitis
	Budd–Chiari syndrome (i.e. hepatic vein thrombosis)
	Malignancy
	Heart failure

Most causes of transudates can give rise to exudates.

- Add 2 mL of ascitic fluid to an EDTA tube, and send for blood count to haematology.
- Remove the needle, and apply a sterile plaster over the puncture site.

Total paracentesis

Daily small-volume paracentesis is time-consuming and unnecessary, as it increases the risk of infection and ascitic leakage. It is also hazardous to leave a peritoneal tap catheter in place for more than a few hours, as the risk of infection is significant. It is safer to drain the ascites to dryness.

The rate of ascitic fluid drainage should be as fast as possible. During the first 3–6 hours of paracentesis, there is a significant increase in cardiac output, a decrease in systemic vascular resistance, and a modest fall of ~5–10 mmHg in mean arterial pressure. The right atrial pressure (RAP) in patients with tense ascites may be artificially elevated by transmitted intra-abdominal pressure and may fall acutely by ~3–5 cmH$_2$O during ascitic fluid drainage. Early fluid replacement is essential.

To prevent the omentum occluding catheter drainage, some companies produce special catheters with pre-formed side holes, and these should be used if available. However, total paracentesis is often performed with a Kuss needle (if available), a large 14G long Abbocath® (used for central lines), a peritoneal dialysis (PD) catheter, or alternatively a Swan–Ganz introducer (8.5F) (which is rather too large for this purpose). Although additional drainage ports are often made in the side of non-specialist catheters prior to insertion, this is not recommended by manufacturers, as it risks the catheter fracturing and being left in the abdomen on withdrawal. If the catheter is to be modified, the introducer must be removed under strict aseptic conditions, and the small side perforations, made with a green or blue needle, should not be too close together. Great care must be exercised when re-inserting the introducer to avoid tearing the cannula.

Take a 'drip set' (intravenous fluid 'giving set'), and, with a sterile blade, cut off the reservoir, leaving the tubing, luer locking device, and rate control mechanism. If a PD cannula or other device is used, then some form of tubing needs to be attached to facilitate drainage.

Procedure

- Position the patient supine and slightly tilted to one side. Select, clean, and anaesthetize the site with 1% lidocaine (INN), as for an ascitic tap.
- The selected cannula, attached to a 20 mL syringe, is inserted and advanced whilst continuously aspirating. When ascitic fluid is obtained, introduce the needle a further 75 mm. Finally, advance the plastic cannula, holding the metal introducer to prevent it going any deeper (as for inserting a Venflon®). Remove the metal introducer, and attach the drainage tube (modified 'giving set').
- Strap the introducer to the abdominal wall with Elastoplast. It is not necessary to suture the cannula in place, as it will be removed within 3–4 hours.
- Drain the ascites as rapidly as possible into an appropriate container. When the ascites stops draining or slows down, move the patient from side to side and lie towards the drainage site.

- When drainage is complete, remove the catheter; apply a plaster, and lie the patient with the drainage site uppermost for at least 4 hours.

Percutaneous liver biopsy

Most liver biopsies are now performed under ultrasound guidance by a gastroenterologist. Before the procedure, the following will be required:

- **Patient consent.** The patient must be warned about the risk of bleeding, pneumothorax, gall bladder puncture, shoulder tip pain, which may last several hours, and failed biopsy.
- **Coagulation screen.** Ensure the prothrombin time is <3 seconds prolonged, compared to the control, and the platelet count is >80 x 10⁹/L, and that there is no other bleeding diathesis (e.g. severe renal failure in which platelet function is impaired).
- **Exclude other contraindications**, including ascites and potential tumour, because of the risk of tumour seeding (depending on planned management).

Preparation and equipment
You will need the following:

- Biopsy needle (Tru-Cut or Menghini).
- 1% lidocaine (INN).
- Orange (25G) and green (18G) needles and 5 mL syringes.
- No. 11 scalpel blade.
- 2% chlorhexidine, iodine, or equivalent.
- Sterile towels, a plaster, sterile gloves, and a dressing pack.
- A bottle of formalin for the biopsy sample.
- Ultrasound guidance should always be used if available, particularly if the liver is small and cirrhotic.

Procedure

- Premedicate the patient with an appropriate amount of analgesia (e.g. 30–60 mg dihydrocodeine) 15–30 minutes before the procedure.
- Lie the patient supine, with the right hand behind their head. Percuss the upper border of the liver in expiration (and mark with a pen). Select a site two intercostal spaces below the upper border laterally, making sure it is not too close to the costal margin (and adjacent gall bladder).
- Clean the skin with antiseptic, and infiltrate with lidocaine (INN) as far as the liver capsule. Always go just above a rib (to avoid the neurovascular bundle), and make a skin incision with the scalpel to facilitate the larger biopsy needle passing through the skin.
- The capsule is felt as a grating feeling and, if the syringe is allowed to float on the palm of the hand, will be seen to move with gentle respiration when the tip of the needle has penetrated the capsule. Allow the needle to move with respiration, as this reduces the risk of tearing the capsule. Do not ask the patient to breathe deeply with the needle in this position.
- Remove the needle. Rehearse the patient, asking them to breathe in, then out, and stop in expiration. Emphasize to the patient that they must not breathe in until told to do so. It is imperative during the actual biopsy that they do not take a sudden gasp of breath. Rehearse it several times.

- It is useful to keep saying 'stop, stop, stop' until the biopsy has been completed. Avoid saying 'hold' since many patients will then breathe in at the crucial moment.
- Make a small skin incision with the scalpel, and insert the biopsy needle into the liver when the patient is at end expiration.
- After the biopsy (do not attempt more than two passes), place a plaster over the site, and ask the patient to lie on their right side for 4 hours.
- Arrange for nursing observations of pulse and blood pressure every 15 minutes for 1 hour, every 30 minutes for 2 hours, hourly for 3 hours, and finally every 2 hours for 8 hours. Avoid evening or late afternoon biopsies.

Plugged liver biopsy technique

This technique is used if there is a mild bleeding diathesis and can be performed when the prothrombin time is up to 6 s prolonged, with a platelet count of >40,000 mm³. The biopsy is done through a sheath and the tract embolized using Gelfoam® to try to prevent bleeding. This procedure should be performed by an interventional radiologist or experienced gastroenterologist.

Transjugular liver biopsy

This technique is often performed in patients in whom the risk of bleeding after percutaneous biopsy (e.g. bleeding diathesis) is particularly high. It is based on the assumption that, by taking the biopsy through the hepatic vein, any bleeding will occur into circulation.

It is usually performed under fluoroscopic guidance by interventional radiologists or experienced gastroenterologists. It is not without risk and should not be undertaken simply to obtain histology for completeness. The biopsy should assist diagnosis and subsequent management.

Procedure

- A large introducer is placed into the internal jugular vein or femoral vein.
- A catheter is introduced through this and manipulated into the hepatic vein under fluoroscopic guidance.
- The catheter is removed, leaving a guidewire *in situ*.
- A metal transjugular biopsy needle is passed over the wire and advanced into the hepatic vein. One has to avoid being too peripheral because of the risk of capsular puncture.
- The wire is removed and the needle advanced whilst suction is applied.
- A biopsy is obtained by the 'Menghini' technique. The biopsies obtained are usually smaller and of poorer quality than those obtained by conventional techniques.

Insertion of a Sengstaken–Blakemore or Minnesota tube

Sengstaken–Blakemore (SBT) or Minnesota tubes are inserted to control variceal bleeding when other measures, including injection sclerotherapy, intravenous vasopressin, or octreotide have failed. It should not be used as the primary treatment of bleeding varices since it is unpleasant and increases the risk of oesophageal ulceration. In addition, if they are inserted into an unintubated patient, there is a very real risk of aspiration.

Seek experienced or specialist help early. Balloon tamponade is not a definitive procedure, and it is essential to make arrangements for variceal injection or oesophageal transection once the patient is stable. Continue infusions of vasopressin or octreotide (see Chapter 8).

Preparation and equipment
You will need the following:

• Sengstaken or Minnesota tube.
• Sphygmomanometer.
• Bladder syringe (for balloons).
• X-ray contrast (diluted).

Procedure
See Figure 19.17.

• It is assumed that the patient is already being resuscitated and is receiving intravenous glypressin.
• The patient should ideally be intubated and ventilated. If not, there is an increased risk of aspiration. This risk may be reduced in the unintubated patient by injecting 10 mg metoclopramide immediately before insertion. This can cause temporary cessation of haemorrhage and reduce the aspiration risk.
• The unintubated patient should have a low threshold for sedation, endotracheal intubation, and ventilation.
• The SBT or Minnesota tube should be stored in the fridge, which increases its 'stiffness', and removed just before use. Familiarize yourself with the various parts

before insertion, if necessary. Check the integrity of the balloons before you insert the tube.

• Place an endoscope protection mouth-guard in place to prevent the patient biting the tube. Cover the end of the tube with lubricating jelly, and, with the patient in the left semi-prone position, push the tube down, asking the patient to swallow (if conscious). If the tube curls up in the mouth, try again or try another cooled tube.
• Insert at least 50 cm, and inflate the gastric balloon with 200 mL water containing gastrografin which enables the balloon to be visualized on a CXR or an abdominal x-ray (AXR). Clamp the balloon channel. Then gently pull back on the tube until the gastric balloon abuts the gastro-oesophageal junction (i.e. resistance felt). Then pull gently until the patient is beginning to be tugged by pulling. Note the position at the edge of the mouthpiece, and mark with a pen. Attach the tube to the side of the face with Elastoplast. Weight contraptions should not be necessary.
• In general, the oesophageal balloon should never be used. Virtually all bleeding varices occur at the oesophagogastric junction and are controlled using this technique.
• If the bleeding continues, inflate the oesophageal balloon. Connect this to a sphygmomanometer via a 3-way tap to monitor the balloon pressure. Inflate to 40 mmHg, and

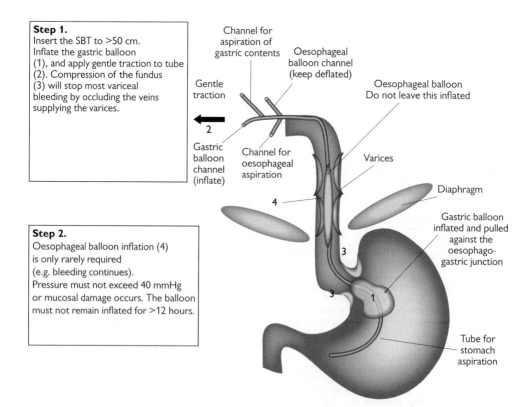

Step 1.
Insert the SBT to >50 cm.
Inflate the gastric balloon
(1), and apply gentle traction to tube
(2). Compression of the fundus
(3) will stop most variceal
bleeding by occluding the veins
supplying the varices.

Step 2.
Oesophageal balloon inflation (4)
is only rarely required
(e.g. bleeding continues).
Pressure must not exceed 40 mmHg
or mucosal damage occurs. The balloon
must not remain inflated for >12 hours.

Channel for aspiration of gastric contents
Oesophageal balloon channel (keep deflated)
Gentle traction
Oesophageal balloon Do not leave this inflated
2
Gastric balloon channel (inflate)
Channel for oesophageal aspiration
Varices
4
Diaphragm
3
Gastric balloon inflated and pulled against the oesophago-gastric junction
3
1
Tube for stomach aspiration

Figure 19.17 Use of the Sengstaken–Blakemore tube (SBT) to control variceal bleeding when other measures have failed (e.g. octreotride). Reproduced from Richard M. Leach, *Acute and Critical Care Medicine at a Glance*, second edition, Figure c, Chapter 42, page 92, Wiley, Copyright 2009, with permission.

close the 3-way tap. Check the pressure in this balloon every 1–2 hours. Do not deflate every hour.
- Do NOT leave the balloons inflated for more than 12 hours since this increases the risk of oesophageal ulceration.
- Obtain a CXR to check the position of the tube.
- The gastric channel should be aspirated continuously.
- If facilities for variceal injection are available, remove the SBT or Minnesota tube immediately prior to endoscopy. If not, discuss the patient with your regional hepatology centre, and transfer, if appropriate.

Transjugular intrahepatic portosystemic shunt (TIPSS)

This is a procedure that is only performed in few specialist centres by interventional radiologists and hepatologists. It is presented here only to aid understanding of when the technique should be used.

The aim is to lower the portal pressure acutely by introducing a shunt between a hepatic vein and a portal vein tributary. As a result, blood flows from the high pressure portal system to the lower pressure hepatic venous system which drains into the inferior vena cava. The lowered portal pressure makes bleeding from the oesophageal or gastric varices less likely.

It is technically quite difficult, but it does not require a general anaesthetic. Consequently, the risk is lower than for a formal portacaval or mesocaval shunt procedure, and it does not hinder future liver transplantation.

Contact your regional hepatology centre for advice if you feel this procedure may be appropriate for a specific patient. UK centres carrying out these procedures include the Royal Free Hospital London, Newcastle Royal Infirmary, Edinburgh Royal Infirmary, and Addenbrookes Hospital Cambridge.

Indications
- Uncontrolled or recurrent bleeding from oesophageal or gastric varices.
- Diuretic-resistant ascites

Method
- The internal jugular vein is catheterized and a cannula passed through the right atrium into the inferior vena cava (IVC) and into a hepatic vein.
- The portal vein is localized by USS and a metal transjugular biopsy needle advanced through the liver substance into one of the portal vein tributaries (usually right portal vein).
- A wire is then passed into the portal vein and the metal needle withdrawn, leaving the wire joining the hepatic vein and portal vein.
- An expandable stent is then passed over the wire and expanded by balloon inflation. A typical stent size is 8–12 mm.

Complications
- Hepatic encephalopathy occurs in about 20%.
- Mortality is ~3% and is usually due to capsular puncture.
- Failure to reduce portal pressure may occur if there are large extrahepatic shunts. These may need to be embolized.

Further reading

Becker G, Galandi D, Blum HE (2006). Malignant ascites: systematic review and guideline for treatment. *European Journal of Cancer*, **42**, 589–97.

British Society of Gastroenterology. Endoscopy clinical guidelines. <http://www.bsg.org.uk/clinical-guidelines/endoscopy/index.html>.

British Society of Gastroenterology. Guidelines on the use of liver biopsy in clinical practice. <http//:www.bsg.org.uk/pdf_word_docs/liver_biopsy.pdf>.

Mittal R and Dangoor A (2007). Paracentesis in the management of ascites. *British Journal of Hospital Medicine (London)*, **68**, M162–5.

Moore KP and Aithal GP (2006). Guidelines on the management of ascites in cirrhosis. *Gut*, **55** (Suppl 6), vi1–vi12.

Other practical procedures

Neurological procedures
Lumbar puncture
All physicians involved with acute medical admissions or emergencies must be able to perform a lumbar puncture. If bacterial (e.g. meningococcal, pneumococcal) meningitis is suspected, antibiotics should be given before the lumbar puncture. In general, a CT scan should **always** be carried out prior to a lumbar puncture to exclude raised cranial pressure due to an obstructed cerebrospinal fluid (CSF) system or a space-occupying lesion (SOL).

Contraindications to lumbar puncture
- Raised intracranial pressure characterized by a falling level of consciousness, with reduced pulse rate, increasing blood pressure, vomiting, focal neurological signs, and papilloedema.
- Coagulopathy.
- Reduced platelets ($<50 \times 10^9$/L).

Preparation and equipment
You will need the following:
- Dressing pack (sterile gauze, drapes, antiseptic, gloves, plaster).
- Local anaesthetic (e.g. 1% lidocaine (INN)), 5 mL syringes, orange (25G) and blue (22G) needles.
- A spinal needle.
- Three sterile bottles for collecting CSF and a glucose bottle.
- Manometer and 3-way tap for measuring the opening CSF pressure.

Procedure
- Explain the procedure to the patient, and obtain consent.
- Position the patient carefully, as this is crucial to success. Lie the patient on their left side (or right side if you are left-handed), with their back on the edge of the bed and fully flexed (i.e knees pulled up to the chin), with a folded pillow between their legs and keeping the back perpendicular to the bed. Flexion separates the interspaces between the vertebrae, making access to the spinal canal easier (see Figure 19.18).
- The safest site for lumbar puncture is the L4–L5 intervertebral space, as the spinal cord ends at L1–L2. An imaginary line drawn between the iliac crests intersects the spine at the L4 process or L4–L5 intervertebral space exactly.

(a)

L3–4 Inter-vertebral space

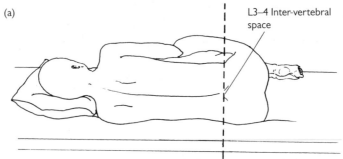

Position the patient so that the line joining the iliac crests is perpendicular to the bed.

(b)

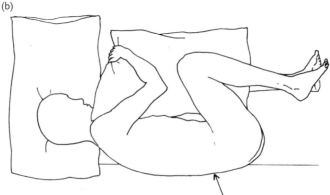

Ask the patient to curl up with a pillow between the knees to open the interspace. Point the needle cranially and advance gently.

Figure 19.18 Positioning and the angle of approach to perform a lumbar puncture. Reproduced from Punit S. Ramrakha, Kevin P. Moore, and Amir Sam, *Oxford Handbook of Acute Medicine*, third edition, 2010, Figure 15.15, page 807, copyright Punit S. Ramrakha and Kevin P. Moore, with permission.

Mark the L4 to L5 intervertebral space (e.g. with a ball-point pen).

- Clean the skin with 2% chlorhexidine, and isolate the access point with sterile drapes.
- Anaesthetize the surrounding skin and deep structure with lidocaine (INN). Inject 0.25–0.5 mL 1% lidocaine (INN) under the skin with a 25G needle at the access point for the spinal lumbar puncture needle. Anaesthetize the deeper structures with a 22G needle. Use the anaesthetic sparingly, as it may distort the surrounding anatomy, making the procedure more difficult and unnecessarily longer.
- Insert the spinal needle, with its stylet in place, in the mid-line, aiming slightly cranially (i.e. towards the umbilicus) and horizontal to the bed. Do not advance the needle without the stylet in place.
- With experience, the resistance of the spinal ligaments and dura is recognized followed by a 'give' as the needle enters the subarachnoid space. Alternatively, entry into the subarachnoid space can be tested for by periodically removing the stylet and examining for the escape of CSF. Always replace the stylet before advancing.
- When the subarachnoid space has been entered, measure the CSF pressure with a manometer and 3-way tap. The normal opening pressure is 7–20 cm CSF, with the patient in the lateral position. CSF pressure increases with anxiety, subarachnoid haemorrhage (SAH), infection, space-occupying lesions, benign intracranial hypertension, and congestive cardiac failure.
- Collect 0.5–1.5 mL fluid in three serially numbered bottles, and remember to fill the glucose bottle.
- Send specimens promptly for microscopy, culture, protein, and glucose (with a simultaneous plasma sample for comparison). When appropriate, also send fluid and blood for virology, syphilis serology, cytology for malignancy, AFB, oligoclonal bands in suspected multiple sclerosis, cryptococcal antigen testing (e.g. in immunocompromised patients), India ink stains, and fungal culture.
- Remove the needle, and apply a plaster over the puncture site.
- The patient should lie flat for at least 6 hours after the procedure and should have hourly neurological observations and blood pressure measurements. Encourage fluid intake.

Complications of lumbar puncture

- **Headache** is common and occurs in up to 25% of cases. Typically, it occurs when the patient is upright and improves when supine. It may last for several days. It is thought to be due to intracranial traction due to CSF depletion caused by a persistent leak from the lumbar puncture site. Some cases may be prevented by using finer spinal needles, keeping the patient supine for 6–12 hours

after the lumbar puncture and encouraging fluid intake. Treat with simple analgesia, fluids, and reassurance.
- **Trauma to nerve roots.** This is rare but seen if the needle deviates from the midline. The patient experiences a sharp, stabbing pain or paraesthesiae down the leg. The needle should be withdrawn, and, if the symptoms persist, stop the procedure and seek expert help.
- **Bleeding.** Minor bleeding may occur with a 'traumatic spinal tap' when a small spinal vein is cut. The CSF appears bloody (see CSF analysis section), but the bleeding stops spontaneously and does not require specific therapy. Coagulopathy, severe liver disease, or thrombocytopenia carries the risk of subarachnoid/subdural bleeding and paralysis.
- **Coning.** Herniation of cerebellar tonsils with compression of the medulla is very rare, unless the patient has raised intracranial pressure (ICP). Always obtain and review a CT brain scan prior to lumbar puncture. Mortality is high, but the patient may respond to reducing ICP using standard measures (e.g. mild hyperventilation, mannitol).
- **Infection.** This is rare if proper sterile technique is used.

CSF analysis

- **Normal CSF** is a clear fluid, with an opening pressure <200 mm CSF. Examination reveals:
  - Lymphocytes <4/mm^3.
  - Polymorphs 0/mm^3.
  - Protein <0.4 g/L.
  - Glucose >2.2 mmol/L (or >70% plasma level).
- **Abnormal CSF.** The features of CSF obtained in bacterial, viral, and tuberculous meningitis are shown in Table 19.12.
- **Bloody tap.** Artefact is indicated when fewer red cells are seen in successive bottles and no yellowing of the CSF (xanthochromia) is detected. The true WBC count may be estimated by:

True CSF WBC = CSF WBC – (blood WBC × CSF RBC)/blood RBC

(i.e. if the patient's blood count is normal, subtract approximately one white cell for every 1,000 RBCs.)
To estimate the true protein level, subtract 10 mg/L for every 1,000 RBCs/mm^3 (be sure to do the count and protein estimation on the same bottle).
- **Subarachnoid haemorrhage** is associated with xanthochromia (yellow CSF) and equal numbers of red cells in all bottles. The RBCs will excite an inflammatory response (with an increase in CSF WCC), most marked after 48 h.
- **Increased CSF protein** is associated with acoustic neuroma and spinal tumours and Guillain–Barré syndrome.

Table 19.12 CSF features with specific infections

	Bacterial	Viral	TB meningitis
Appearance	Turbid	Clear	Clear
Cells (mm^3)	5–2,000	5–500	5–1,000
Main cell type	Neutrophils	Lymphocyte	Lymphocyte
Glucose (mmol/L)	Very low	Normal	Low
Protein (g/L)	Often >10	0.5–0.9	Often >1.0
Other tests	Gram stain	PCR	Ziehl–Neelsen
	Bacterial antigen		Fluorescent test
			PCR

Intracranial pressure monitoring

Invasive intracranial pressure monitoring is mainly limited to neurological and trauma intensive care units. Insertion of these devices is performed in specialist units. Presentation here is to aid understanding of the mechanisms and indications for use of these techniques.

Indications

- Cerebral trauma:
  - GCS ≤8.
  - Compression of basal cistern on brain CT scan.
  - Midline shift >0.5 mm on brain CT scan.
  - Raised ICP not requiring surgery.
- After intracranial haemorrhage (SAH or intracerebral).
- Acute liver failure (grade 4 coma with signs of raised ICP).
- Metabolic diseases with raised ICP (e.g. Reye's syndrome).
- Post-operative oedema (after neurosurgery).

Intracranial pressure monitoring in patients who are at risk of unexpected rises in ICP should ideally be started before secondary brain injury has occurred (see Chapters 8 and 18) and where it can influence the management of the patient. As facilities in neurosurgical centres may be limited, it has been suggested that these patients may be effectively managed in general intensive care units.

Contraindications

- Uncorrectable coagulopathy.
- Local infection near placement site or meningitis.
- Septicaemia.

Method

There are many intracranial pressure devices available, including subdural, extradural, parenchymal, and intraventricular monitors. Parenchymal and intraventricular monitors are more accurate but associated with greater risk than extradural monitors. They should be implanted by experienced persons only.

Pre-packaged kits are available (e.g. Codman® subdural bolt). This monitor is inserted in the prefrontal region, and the kit contains the necessary screws for creating a burr-hole and spinal needles to perforate the dura.

The ICP waveform obtained is a dynamic real-time pressure recording that looks superficially similar to the pulse waveform. It is created by the pulsations of the cerebral blood vessels within the confined space of the cranium, with the effects of respiration superimposed.

Cerebral perfusion pressure = mean arterial pressure − ICP.

The normal resting mean ICP measured in a supine patient is less than 10 mmHg (<1.3 kPa). The level which requires treatment depends, to some extent, on the disease or trauma.

- **In benign intracranial hypertension**, values of ~40 mmHg may not be associated with neurological symptoms.
- **In cerebral trauma**, treatment should be initiated with a mean ICP >25 mmHg, though this value is debated.

Several types of pressure wave are described, of which the most significant are '**A waves**'. These are sustained increases of the ICP of up to 50–100 mmHg (6–13 kPa), lasting 10–20 minutes. They are associated with a poor prognosis.

The readings of the ICP monitors should always be accompanied by careful neurological examination. Treatment of raised ICP is discussed in Chapters 8 and 18.

Complications of intracranial pressure monitoring

These include:

- Infection (up to 5%).
- Bleeding (e.g. local, subdural, extradural, intracerebral).
- Seizures.
- CSF leakage.
- Misreading of ICP pressures.

Rheumatological procedures

Joint aspiration

Many synovial joints can be safely aspirated by an experienced operator. Knee effusions are common, and aseptic aspiration can be safely performed in the emergency department. The risk of inducing a septic arthritis is less than 1 in 10,000 aspirations but is dependent on:

- Identification of anatomical landmarks.
- The skin is cleaned with 2% chlorhexidine or iodine.
- A no-touch technique is essential.

Indications for synovial fluid aspiration

- Suspected septic arthritis.
- Suspected crystal arthritis.
- Suspected haemarthrosis.
- Relief of symptoms by removal of effusion in degenerative arthritis.

Contraindications to joint aspiration

- Overlying sepsis.
- Bleeding diathesis.

Procedure

1. **Knee joint.** The patient lies with the knee slightly flexed and supported. The joint space behind the patella, either medially or laterally, is palpated, the skin cleaned, and a needle (18G, green) inserted horizontally between the patella and femur, using a no-touch technique. There is a slight resistance as the needle goes through the synovial membrane. Aspirate on the syringe until fluid is obtained.
2. **Elbow joint.** Flex the elbow to 90°, and pass the needle between the proximal head of the radius which is located by rotating the patient's hand and the lateral epicondyle, or the needle can be passed posteriorly between the lateral epicondyle and the olecranon.
3. **Ankle joint.** Plantarflex the foot slightly; palpate the joint margin between the extensor hallucis longus (lateral) and tibialis anterior (medial) tendons, just above the tip of the medial malleolus.

When synovial fluid is obtained:

- Note the colour, and assess viscosity.
- Microscopy for cell count and crystals.
- Gram stain and culture.
- Measure synovial fluid glucose (compared with blood glucose in sepsis).

Analysis of the features of synovial fluid from normal, osteoarthritic, rheumatoid and crystal arthropathies, and sepsis are reported in Table 19.13.

Renal procedures

Absolute indications for renal replacement therapy (RRT) are listed in Table 19.14. Three main methods of fluid and

Table 19.13 Synovial fluid analysis

	Viscosity	Opacity	Lymphocyte count (per mm^3)
Normal	High	Clear	<200
Osteoarthritis	High	Clear	1,000 (<50% PMN)
Rheumatoid	Low	Cloudy	1–50,000 PMN
Crystal	Low	Cloudy	5–50,000 PMN
Sepsis	Low	Cloudy	10–100,000 PMN

solute removal are used in acute kidney injury (AKI). In haemodynamically unstable patients, continuous forms of RRT, e.g. haemofiltration, are usually better tolerated.

Intermittent renal haemodialysis
During dialysis, blood flows down one side of a semi-permeable membrane, and a solution of crystalloids (dialysis fluid) is pumped in the opposite direction along the other side of the membrane. Small molecules and toxic waste diffuse across the membrane, according to the imposed concentration gradients.

Dialysis fluid composition is designed to normalize plasma. Small molecules, such as urea (60 Da), are efficiently removed, whereas larger molecules like creatinine (113 Da) less so. Hyperphosphataemia occurs due to poor clearance of phosphate ions. Dialysis corrects biochemical abnormalities and removes excess extracellular fluid within a relatively short period of 2–4 hours. However, it may cause hypokalaemia and intravascular hypovolaemia. In haemodynamically unstable patients, life-threatening hypotension or cardiac arrhythmias may occur.

Practical aspects of the procedure
A blood flow of ~250–300 mL/min is needed across the dialysis membrane. The equivalent clearance obtained is approximately 20 mL/min.

- **Vascular access.** Vascular access may be obtained by fashioning an arteriovenous (AV) shunt, using the radial artery or, more commonly, by using a Vascath which uses venous, rather than arterial, blood. This involves cannulation of the internal jugular, subclavian, or femoral vein.
- **Anticoagulation.** Heparin is normally used. If contraindicated (e.g. recent haemorrhage), prostacyclin may be used but can cause hypotension and abdominal cramps.
- **Haemodynamic stability.** Patients with multiorgan failure commonly develop hypotension during haemodialysis. This may be ameliorated with high sodium dialysate and priming the circuit with 4.5% human albumin solution.

Complications of haemodialysis

1. **Hypotension.** This usually occurs within the first 15 minutes of commencing dialysis. It probably involves the activation of circulating inflammatory cells by the membrane, osmotic shifts, and possibly loss of fluid. It is treated with cautious fluid replacement and inotropes. Watch for pulmonary oedema if overtransfused.

Table 19.14 Absolute indications for renal replacement therapy in acute kidney injury

1. Fluid overload
2. Uncontrolled hyperkalaemia
3. Metabolic acidosis
4. Uraemic pericarditis
5. Raised creatinine (no specific value but usually >700 micromoles/L in acute kidney injury)
6. Encephalopathy

Risk factors or exacerbating factors for hypotension are:
- Multiorgan failure.
- Arrhythmias.
- Autonomic neuropathy.
- Pericardial tamponade.
- Valvular lesions (e.g. mitral, myocardial infarction, poor left ventricular function, regurgitation, aortic stenosis).
- Sepsis.

2. **Line infection.** Central lines are often infected. Fever of >38°C in a dialysis patient should be assumed to be due to line infection, even when an alternative septic focus is a possibility. Blood cultures should be taken both peripherally and from the central line. The line should be removed and re-inserted at a new site. Empirical antibiotic treatment is given over an hour at the end of dialysis, using intravenous vancomycin 750 mg–1 g in 100 mL normal saline. Vancomycin should be given slowly or severe vasodilatation may cause 'red man syndrome'. An alternative is intravenous teicoplanin 400 mg, followed by 200 mg daily. Both drugs are poorly removed by dialysis, and a single dose will ensure therapeutic levels for several days. Infection is due to *Staphylococcus aureus* or *S. epidermidis* in up to 90% of cases. Right-sided endocarditis may occur.

3. **Dialysis disequilibrium** tends to occur frequently during initial dialysis in patients with severe uraemia. It is also more common in patients with pre-existing neurological disease. Clinical features include headache, nausea and vomiting, fits, and cerebral oedema. It is prevented by short or slow initial dialyses. Cerebral oedema is treated as normal.

4. **Dialyser reaction** is caused by an allergic IgE or complement-induced response to ethylene oxide (sterilizing agent) or cellulose components. Use of 'biocompatible' membranes (e.g. polysulfone, polyacrylonitrile (PAN)) or dialysers sterilized by steam or G-irradiation prevent further reactions.

The circuit should also be rinsed with normal saline. Clinical features are those of an allergic reaction with itching, urticaria, cough, and wheeze. Severe reactions may cause anaphylaxis. This response is managed by stopping the dialysis and treating the anaphylaxis with intravenous antihistamines (e.g. chlorphenamine (INN) 10 mg) and hydrocortisone (e.g. 100 mg) and bronchodilators (i.e. salbutamol 5 mg by nebulizer) and, if severe, adrenaline (1 mg intramuscularly).

5. **Air embolism** is rare but potentially fatal. Symptoms vary, depending on the patient's position. If sitting, air may pass directly to the cerebral veins, causing coma, fits, and death. If lying, air may pass into the right ventricle and then to the pulmonary vessels, causing breathlessness, cough, and chest tightness. If an air embolism is suspected, clamp dialysis lines; lie the patient head-down on the left side, and administer high-flow (>60%) oxygen by mask.

Aspiration of air with an intracardiac needle may be attempted in extreme circumstances.

6. Other complications of dialysis include cramps and potential haemorrhage.

Haemofiltration

During haemofiltration, plasma water and water-soluble substances (<50 kDa) pass across a highly permeable membrane by convective flow (e.g. similar to the process of glomerular filtration). In contrast to dialysis, urea, creatinine, and phosphate are cleared at similar rates. Hypophosphataemia may occur if phosphate is not supplemented. Molecules like heparin are also efficiently cleared.

The filtrate is discarded, and a physiological 'plasma' solution is replaced into the circulation. Low-flow rates make haemofiltration less efficient at removing uraemic toxins, but continuous use allows clearance of any amount of fluid and nitrogenous waste. Haemofiltration is usually performed continuously or over longer periods than haemodialysis. The relative ease of use of haemofiltration in haemodynamically unstable patients is its main advantage.

Haemodiafiltration (CHDF) involves the pumping of dialysate across the other side of the membrane.

Continuous venovenous haemofiltration (CVVH) or haemodiafiltration (CVVHD) are the most frequently used techniques. They involve pumping blood from a venous access port (e.g. internal jugular or femoral Vascath) to the dialysis membrane at about 150–200 mL/min. The equivalent glomerular filtration rate (GFR) obtained is about 15–30 mL/min. These techniques are most commonly used in intensive care.

Continuous arteriovenous haemofiltration (CAVHF) or haemodiafiltration (CAVDF) is less commonly used due to the need for arterial cannulation. In both arteriovenous haemofiltration and haemodiafiltration, arterial blood, driven by arterial pressure, is continuously filtered at a relatively low flow rate of 50–100 mL/min. Both arteriovenous and venovenous techniques cause less haemodynamic instability and are particularly useful in patients with multiorgan failure.

Acute peritoneal dialysis

Peritoneal dialysis uses hypertonic dialysate to draw fluid and solutes across the peritoneum, following insertion of a peritoneal catheter. The dialysate (1–3 L) dwells in the abdominal cavity for ~4–5 hours before drainage. It is rarely used in modern practice but does not require vascular access or anticoagulation. However, it produces insufficient dialysis in hypercatabolic patients, as the creatinine clearance rate is only ~10 mL/min.

The technique requires:

- A peritoneal dialysis catheter (may be inserted under local anaesthetic on the ward).
- An intact peritoneal cavity free of infection, herniae, and adhesions. Abdominal pathology, infection risks, and interference with ventilation limit use.

Complications of peritoneal dialysis

Peritonitis. The commonest complication of continuous acute peritoneal dialysis (CAPD) is infection (0.8 episodes/patient/year). Infection occurs through the lumen of the catheter, along the catheter tract, transmurally from the gastrointestinal tract, or haematogenously (rare).

Assessment

- Clinical features include cloudy peritoneal dialysate (PD) bags (99%), abdominal pain (95%), and abdominal tenderness (80%). Other features include fever (33%), nausea and vomiting (30%), leucocytosis (25%), diarrhoea or constipation (15%).
- Investigations should include PD effluent cell counts (e.g. peritonitis if >100 neutrophils/mm^3), PD fluid culture (inoculate a blood culture bottle), Gram stain of PD fluid, FBC (for leucocytosis), and blood cultures.

Management

- All patients require antibiotics, but some may be treated as outpatients. Antibiotic use depends on the Gram stain and culture results. A typical protocol may include a cephalosporin, ciprofloxacin, or vancomycin with metronidazole. Patients who have a high fever with leucocytosis, and/or who are systemically unwell, warrant intravenous antibiotics.
- Gram-negative infection, in particular, *Pseudomonas*, is associated with severe infections. Ileus may occur, whatever the organism.
- If pain is a prominent feature, give opiate analgesia, and consider intermittent peritoneal dialysis, instead of PD.
- Patients may lose up to 25 g protein/day in severe cases and should receive adequate nutritional support.
- If the infection is resistant to treatment, consider removal of the Tenckhoff (peritoneal dialysis) catheter and atypical organisms (e.g. fungi).
- Consider the possibility of another underlying gastrointestinal pathology, especially if the infection is due to multibacterial, Gram-negative organisms, or is associated with other symptoms.

Fluid overload

Mild cases may respond to hypertonic exchanges (6.36% or 4.25% glucose (INN)) fluid restriction (1 L/day), and large doses of diuretics (e.g. furosemide 500 mg bd). In patients with pulmonary oedema, fluid removal is best achieved by rapid cycle intermittent peritoneal dialysis (e.g. 4.25% glucose (INN) 60-minute cycle time).

Poor exchanges

- Constipation may cause malposition of the peritoneal dialysis catheter.
- Malpositioning of the catheter. The catheter should sit in the pelvis but occasionally flips upwards to lie against the diaphragm, causing shoulder tip pain and poor drainage. If the patient is constipated, try laxatives, but surgical repositioning may be required.
- Omentum may wrap around the tip of catheter. This can be prevented by performing an omentectomy at time of insertion.
- Fibrin debris that may block the catheter can be seen as white deposits in effluent. Treat by addition of heparin (1,000 U/litre) to bags.

Hyperglycaemia

A significant amount of the dextrose in peritoneal dialysis solutions is absorbed (especially with 'heavy' 4.26% glucose (INN)). Renal failure induces insulin resistance, so an elevated blood glucose may occur as well as hypercholesterolaemia. Diabetic patients require special attention to insulin therapy.

Plasmapheresis

Plasmapheresis is used to remove circulating high molecular weight compounds not removed by dialysis. It is often used to remove plasma antibodies or lipoproteins.

Indications for use
- Myasthenia gravis.
- Guillain–Barré syndrome.
- Goodpasture's syndrome.
- Thrombotic thrombocytopenic purpura (TTP).
- Haemolytic uraemic syndrome (HUS).
- Severe hyperlipidaemia.
- Multisystem vasculitis.
- Hyperviscosity syndrome (e.g. Waldenström's macroglobulinaemia).
- HLA antibody removal.

Technique
Plasmapheresis requires central venous access with a large-bore, dual-lumen cannula. Usually five treatment sessions are given on consecutive days. Plasma is removed and is usually replaced with 2 units of fresh frozen plasma (FFP) and 3 L of 4.5% albumin. Intravenous calcium (10 mL 10% calcium gluconate) is given with the FFP. As with other blood products, febrile reactions may occur.

Plasmapheresis has no effect on the underlying rate of antibody production. However, it is a useful treatment in acute situations, such as Goodpasture's syndrome and myasthenia gravis. In HUS and TTP, only fresh frozen plasma is used (preferably cryodepleted), usually a minimum of 3 L/day. For hyperviscosity syndrome, a centrifugation system is required, rather than a plasma filter. Finally, in lipopheresis, there may be a severe reaction if the patient is on an ACE inhibitor.

An alternative to plasmapheresis is immunoabsorption. This may be used in the removal of HLA antibodies, anti-GBM disease, or multisystem vasculitis.

Renal biopsy
Renal biopsies should only be performed by renal specialists and interventional radiologists. It is presented here to aid understanding of when the technique should be used. Do not attempt this if you have not been fully trained.

Indications for renal biopsy
- Cause is unknown.
- Heavy proteinuria (>2 g/day).
- Immune-mediated acute renal failure (ARF).
- Features of systemic disease (e.g. SLE).
- Suspected interstitial nephritis (e.g. drug-induced).
- Active urinary sediment.
- Prolonged renal failure (>2 weeks).

Contraindications
- Bleeding diathesis—unless correctable prior to biopsy.
- Urinary tract obstruction.
- Solitary functioning kidney.
- Uncontrolled hypertension, i.e. diastolic >100 mmHg.
- Small kidneys, since it is unlikely to reveal any treatable condition but has significant risks.
- If the patient is unable to comply with procedure (consider biopsy under general anaesthetic).

Preparation and equipment needed for renal biopsy
- Check haemoglobin, clotting screen.
- Group and save serum.
- Ensure intravenous pyelogram or ultrasound has been carried out to determine the presence and size of the two kidneys.

- Consent patient, and report a 1% risk of bleeding requiring transfusion.
- You will need a Tru-Cut or other biopsy needle (e.g. Bioptigun®). Ensure you are familiar with the workings of the needle.
- Dressing pack, sterile drapes, gown, and gloves.
- Real-time ultrasound guidance.

Technique
- Position the patient prone on the bed, with pillows under the abdomen.
- Visualize lower pole of either kidney with the ultrasound (right kidney lies more inferiorly and may be easier to image).
- Sterilize the skin, and drape the area with towels.
- Infiltrate local anaesthetic (10 mL 1% lidocaine (INN)) under the skin and to the depth of the kidney.
- Make a small skin incision with a scalpel to facilitate entry of the biopsy needle. Insert the biopsy needle as far as the renal capsule under real-time ultrasound guidance.
- Ask the patient to hold their breath at the end of inspiration which displaces the kidneys inferiorly. Take the biopsy from lower pole.
- Apply a sterile dressing.
- Bed rest for 24 hours to minimize the risk of bleeding.
- Monitor blood pressure and pulse half-hourly for 2 hours, 1-hourly for 4 hours, and then 4-hourly for 18 hours.
- Send the renal biopsy tissue for light microscopy, immunofluorescence, electron microscopy, and special stains (e.g. Congo red), if indicated.

Complications
- **Bleeding.** Microscopic haematuria is usual. Macroscopic haematuria occurs in 5–10%, and bleeding requiring transfusion in 1%.
- **Formation of an intrarenal arteriovenous fistula** may occur but is rarely of significance. If bleeding occurs from this, angiography and embolization may be needed.
- **Loin pain** if severe suggests bleeding.
- **Pneumothorax** is now rare.
- **Ileus** rarely.
- **Organ laceration** (e.g. liver, spleen, bowel rarely).
  Renal transplant biopsies may be needed if there is a decline in transplant function, or in primary non-function post-transplant.

Procedure
In principle, the technique is similar to native renal biopsy, though the transplanted kidney lies more superficially in the iliac fossa. Ultrasound localization is useful. Biopsies may be taken from either the upper or lower pole. Some centres find fine needle aspiration biopsy (FNAB) useful in the diagnosis of transplant rejection.

Occupational procedures
Needle-stick injuries
Occupational exposures to blood-borne viruses (BBVs) in healthcare workers are divided into two groups:
- Percutaneous (needle-stick) injuries.
- Mucocutaneous exposure through broken skin or via splashes into the eyes.

High-risk body fluids include blood, saliva (in dentistry), semen, vaginal secretions, pericardial fluid, pleural fluid, peritoneal fluid, pericardial fluid, cerebrospinal fluid, synovial fluid, amniotic fluid, human breast milk, and unfixed tissues and organs. In addition, vomit, faeces, and urine are a potential risk when contaminated with blood.

The major pathogens associated with needle-stick injuries and mucocutaneous exposures are:

- Hepatitis B virus (HBV).
- Hepatitis C virus (HCV).
- Human immunodeficiency virus (HIV).

Occupational exposures to BBVs can be caused by certain work practices, such as:

- Not properly disposing of used needles.
- Recapping needles.
- Not using protective equipments, e.g. eye protection.

Prevention

Always assume that every patient is potentially infected with a blood-borne infection. Therefore, the same precautions should be taken for every patient and every procedure.

- Cover skin cuts and abrasions with waterproof dressings.
- Never recap needles.
- Never leave sharps to be cleared up by others.
- Never guide needles with your fingers.
- Never pass sharps hand to hand.
- Always dispose of used needles promptly in appropriate sharps disposal containers. A significant proportion of needle-stick injuries occur after procedures.
- Always use eye protection. Ordinary spectacles offer inadequate protection, so safety spectacles, which can fit over prescription lenses and frames, should be used.
- Double gloving. In needle-stick injuries, 80% of visible blood is removed by the latex in a surgical glove. With double gloving, the inner glove will remove 80% of the remaining blood on the needle.

Management of exposure incidents

- If the mouth or eyes are involved, they should be washed thoroughly with water.
- If the skin is punctured, let the wound bleed, and wash it with soap or 2% chlorhexidine and running water. Avoid scrubbing or sucking the injury.
- Report to the occupational health department to arrange immediate assessment, or, if out of hours, attend the emergency department in accordance with the local policy.

Assessment of the risk of blood-borne virus transmission

Estimated seroconversion risks are:

- 30% for percutaneous exposure of a non-immune individual to HBsAg and HBeAg positive source.
- 0.5–1.8% for percutaneous exposure to HCV-infected blood with detectable RNA.
- 0.3% for percutaneous exposure to HIV-infected blood.

Factors that increase the risk, following an incident, include:

- Percutaneous injury poses a higher risk than mucous membrane or broken skin exposure.
- Injury with a device directly from the source patient's artery/vein.
- Injury from hollow bore and wide gauge needles.
- Deep injury.
- Visible blood on the device.

- High HIV viral load, or detectable HCV RNA or HBeAg in the source patient.
- Staff member inadequately immunized against hepatitis B.

Approaching source patients for blood-borne virus testing

- Due to the sensitivity of the issue, the source patient should not be approached by the exposed member of staff.
- Occupational health (or A&E if out of hours) will arrange this test in accordance with local policies.

Post-exposure prophylaxis (PEP) for HIV

- Risk assessment is carried out by occupational health (emergency department if out of hours).
- If indicated, PEP ideally should be started within an hour. However, it can be started up to 2 weeks after exposure.
- Follow-up is carried out by the occupational health department.

Further reading

British HIV Association. <http://www.bhiva.org>.

British Infection Association. <http://www.britishinfection.org>.

Coakley G, Mathews C, Field M, et al. (2006). BSR & BHPR, BOA, RCGP and BSAC guidelines for management of the hot swollen joint in adults. *Rheumatology*, **45**, 1039–41.

Deibel M, Jones J, Brown M (2005). Best evidence topic report: reinsertion of the stylet before needle removal in diagnostic lumbar puncture. *Emergency Medicine Journal*, **22**, 46.

National Institute for Health and Clinical Excellence (2010). Bacterial meningitis and meningococcal septicaemia. <http://www.nice.org.uk/CG102>.

National Institute for Health and Clinical Excellence (2012). Infection: prevention and control of healthcare-associated infections in primary and community care. <http://www.nice.org.uk/CG139>.

National Institute for Health and Clinical Excellence (2013). Acute kidney injury: Prevention, detection and management of acute kidney injury up to the point of renal replacement therapy. NICE clinical guideline 169. <https://www.nice.org.uk/guidance/cg169/resources/guidance-acute-kidney-injury-pdf>.

National Institute for Health and Clinical Excellence (2014). Chronic kidney disease: early identification and management of chronic kidney disease in adults in primary and secondary care. NICE clinical guideline 182. <https://www.nice.org.uk/guidance/cg182/resources/guidance-chronic-kidney-disease-pdf>.

NHS Employers. Needlestick injury. <http://www.nhsemployers.org/Aboutus/Publications/Documents/Needlestick%20injury.pdf>.

Public Health England (2013). Immunisation. <https://www.gov.uk/government/organisations/public-health-england/series/immunisation>.

Rifat SF and Moeller JL (2001). Basics of joint injection. General techniques and tips for safe, effective use. *Postgraduate Medical Journal*, **109**, 157–60, 165–6.

Steiner T, Juvela S, Unterberg A, et al. (2013). European stroke organization guidelines for the management of intracranial aneurysms and subarachnoid haemorrhage. *Cerebrovascular Diseases*, **35**, 93–112.

Tang S, Li JH, Lui SL, et al. (2002). Free-hand, ultrasound-guided percutaneous renal biopsy: experience from a single operator. *European Journal of Radiology*, **41**, 65–9.

The Brain Trauma Foundation, The American Association of Neurological Surgeons (2000). Management and prognosis of severe traumatic brain injury. *Journal of Neurotrauma*, **17**, 449–604.

The Renal Association (2011). Acute kidney injury. <http://www.renal.org/clinical/guidelinessection/AcuteKidneyInjury.aspx>.

Emergencies in the elderly

Delirium

Definition

Delirium is a clinical syndrome with the following characteristic features (Diagnostic and Statistical Manual of Mental Disorders–IV).

- Disturbance of consciousness, with reduced ability to focus, sustain, or shift attention.
- A change in cognition or the development of a perceptual disturbance that is not better accounted for by a pre-existing, established, or evolving dementia.
- The disturbance develops over a short period of time (usually hours to days) and tends to fluctuate during the course of the day.
- There is evidence from the history, physical examination, or laboratory findings that the disturbance is caused by a medical condition, substance intoxication, or medication side effect.

Delirium is important, as it is associated with poor outcomes (higher mortality and increased length of stay) during inpatient care, is often misdiagnosed, and is frequently preventable. It is also a marker of underlying dementia, a predictor of the development of future dementia, and can, in itself, contribute to the development of progressive cognitive impairment.

Although multiple clinical precipitants are recognized, the precise pathophysiological cause is uncertain. Current hypotheses include neurotransmitter imbalance (cholinergic deficiency and dopaminergic excess), effects of TNF and other inflammatory cytokines, and direct neuronal injury (for example, hypoxia or hypoglycaemia).

Delirium can occur in patients of any age but is most commonly encountered in the elderly, in whom even relatively minor intercurrent illness may precipitate significant cognitive change. The higher prevalence of dementia and the overlap of the clinical features of dementia and delirium can cause particular diagnostic difficulty in older age groups.

Predisposing factors, other than increased age, include male gender, pre-existing cognitive impairment, polypharmacy, and visual impairment.

Clinical subtypes

Delirium may be hyperactive ('agitated'), hypoactive ('quiet'), or mixed. The prognosis of hypoactive delirium is poorest, as rates of misdiagnosis are higher.

Clinical approach

Diagnosis

Prompt diagnosis of delirium is hindered by the use of imprecise terms to describe patients who exhibit features of possible delirium or dementia (e.g. 'muddled' or 'poor historian'), and the terms 'confusion' or 'cognitive impairment' are to be preferred.

'Confused' patients are unable to think with normal speed, clarity, or coherence. Communication problems may be misdiagnosed as confusion, and particular care should be taken to exclude dysphasia.

Confusion is under-recognized in acute hospital settings, and detection is enhanced by objective mental state testing with screening tools, such as the mini-mental state examination (MMSE, a 30-point questionnaire that examines; orientation in time and place, ability to repeat lists of words and undertake simple arithmetic (e.g. serial sevens), use of and comprehension of language, and performance of basic motor skills) or the abbreviated mental test (AMT; see Chapter 14, Box 14.1). The routine use of objective scales,

for example, in all inpatients aged over 85 years, also aids assessment of cognitive function on future healthcare contacts. Alternative shorter-form tests may be used; the choice of specific test is of secondary importance.

When confusion is identified, the differential diagnosis typically lies between dementia and delirium, although depression or other psychiatric disorders are alternative possibilities. Distinguishing between dementia and delirium can be difficult, as they may coexist, but key features suggesting that delirium is present include:

- Evidence of change in cognitive function.
- The presence of delirium-specific features, such as poor attention or disturbed consciousness.
- The presence of identifiable precipitants of delirium.

History: key points

It may be difficult to take a history from the patient. It is, therefore, vital that a detailed collateral history be taken from a family member or carer and available medical records reviewed.

The history should establish:

1. Usual level of cognitive function.
2. Evidence of change in cognitive function.
3. Evidence of a precipitating factor, commonly:

    - Any acute medical illness (commonly, metabolic disturbance and infection).
    - Introduction or cessation of drugs, and/or change of drug dosages.
    - Recent surgery.

Examination: key points

Physical examination should aim to identify evidence of possible precipitants or conditions that can mimic delirium, such as:

- Deafness or dysphasia.
- Focal neurological signs.
- Fever and/or signs of focal infection.
- Evidence of urinary retention or injury (abnormal pain behaviour in patients with dementia may mimic delirium). Tongue biting or other injury could also suggest a recent seizure.
- Assessment of mental state.

The MMSE or AMT (see Chapter 14, Box 14.1) are simple screening tests that should be compared with any previous recordings that are available in the medical record. In patients with confusion, the use of an objective tool, such as the confusion assessment method (CAM) (see Figure 20.1) facilitates detection of delirium and is highly sensitive and specific.

Investigations

Initial investigations should be utilized to identify common underlying precipitants. Remember that disease often presents atypically in the older person and that the differential diagnosis of precipitants is broad. Common precipitants are covered by the acronym **MIND**.

- Metabolic—urea, potassium, sodium, magnesium, calcium, glucose.
- Infective—C-reactive protein, white cell count and differential, urinalysis (nitrites are most specific for urinary infection), chest X-ray, blood cultures. Although urinary and chest infections are the commonest precipitants, think routinely of less common sources, such as septic arthritis (is there a hot or tender joint?), cholangitis (are the liver function tests abnormal?), prosthetic joint or

device infection (does the patient have a prosthetic hip or knee joint, or a pacemaker?).

- Neurological—consider CT scan or LP (see next paragraphs).
- Drugs—review the admission drugs or inpatient prescription carefully.

Drugs commonly causing delirium include anticholinergics, benzodiazepines, and opioids. Many other drugs can, however, be implicated, and the current prescription should be critically reviewed on a frequent basis and careful comparison made for recent changes.

Other conditions, such as NCSE (non-convulsive status epilepticus), post-ictal states, and space-occupying lesions, such as subdural haematoma, may produce a clinical picture that mimics delirium. In cases of delirium (or 'confusion') without a clear cause, these conditions should be specifically sought and excluded.

Which patients require neuroimaging?
Patients with a recent fall or head injury; focal neurological signs; seizures without clear precipitant; or delirium with no clear cause should have a cerebral CT scan.

Which patients require a lumbar puncture?
Patients with fever or evidence of infection without good alternate peripheral source, seizures without clear precipitant, or focal neurological signs (if CT fails to demonstrate causative pathology and shows no contraindication) should be considered for lumbar puncture.

Which patients require psychiatric review?
If there is clinical suspicion of depression or psychotic illness, doubt about the differentiation between dementia and delirium, no clear cause for a delirium, or if advice is required regarding drug treatment or the possible detention of patients who lack capacity to consent to treatment, psychiatric input should be requested.

Treatment
The emphasis in treatment should be on the identification and management of precipitants and the use of non-pharmacological measures, such as reality orientation, nursing in a well-lit, quiet, side-room, one-to-one care, and correction of sensory impairment (e.g. batteries for hearing aids).

If patients are at risk of harming themselves or others, short-term pharmacological treatment should be considered.

All drugs used to treat delirium can cause harm. Patients who cannot consent to receive treatment should be managed under the terms of relevant mental health legislation. Proxy decision-makers should contribute to decision-making, regarding the use of such treatment. Family members or carers who have no formal decision-making capacity should be informed of all such treatment. Emergency treatment may, at times, be necessary without such involvement and should be carefully documented.

Acute units should establish an agreed treatment protocol, specifying preferred drugs, dosages, routes, frequency

Confusion Assessment Method for the ICU (CAM-ICU) Flowsheet

1. Acute Change or Fluctuating Course of Mental Status:
- Is there an acute change from mental status baseline? OR
- Has the patient's mental status fluctuated during the past 24 hours?

— NO → CAM-ICU negative NO DELIRIUM

↓ YES

2. Inattention:
- "Squeeze my hand when I say the letter 'A'."
  Read the following sequence of letters:
  S A V E A H A A R T or C A S A B L A N C A or A B A D B A D A A Y
  ERRORS: No squeeze with 'A' and Squeeze on letter other than 'A'
- If unable to complete Letters → Pictures

0–2 Errors → CAM-ICU negative NO DELIRIUM

↓ > 2 Errors

3. Altered Level of Consciousness
Current RASS level

RASS other than zero → CAM-ICU positive DELIRIUM Present

↓ RASS = zero

4. Disorganized Thinking:
1. Will a stone float on water?
2. Are there fish in the sea?
3. Does one pound weigh more than two?
4. Can you use a hammer to pound a nail!

Command: "Hold up this many fingers" (Hold up 2 fingers)
         "Now do the same thing with the other hand" (Do not demonstrate)
    OR   "Add one more finger" (If patient unable to move both arms)

> 1 Error → CAM-ICU positive DELIRIUM Present

0–1 Error → CAM-ICU negative NO DELIRIUM

Figure 20.1 reproduced with permission. In cases where the differentiation between dementia and delirium remains difficult, it is preferable to regard the patient as having delirium and seek treatable precipitants.

of administration, and triggers for involving senior colleagues and/or psychiatric input. Doses of any drug used should start low and be uptitrated slowly.

The antipsychotic haloperidol (adverse effects: extrapyramidal syndromes, QT prolongation) is currently the drug of choice, as there is RCT evidence of efficacy. It should be avoided in patients with known Lewy body dementia because of a higher risk of adverse effects in comparison to patients with other forms of dementia. Starting dose should be 0.5 mg to 1.0 mg orally or IM. Starting dose frequency should ideally be no less than 4-hourly, although more frequent administration may be needed in emergency situations.

Alternative second-line agents include the benzodiazepine lorazepam (adverse effects: possible paradoxical agitation, oversedation) or second-generation, atypical antipsychotics, such as quetiapine and olanzapine (adverse effects: extrapyramidal syndromes, QT prolongation), and there is current interest in the use of cholinesterase inhibitors, such as donepezil.

Prevention

Interventions demonstrated to prevent delirium are complex and multidisciplinary but cost-effective. The HELP programme is the most established of such interventions and combines targeted multiprofessional geriatric assessment with input from care volunteers who support daily orientation, early mobilization, assistance with feeding, therapeutic activities, a non-pharmacological sleep protocol, and adaptations to support hearing and vision. Implementation of a complex intervention of this sort is challenging in many current national healthcare settings including the NHS in the UK. Attention should, therefore, be directed to the reduction of modifiable risk factors in the most vulnerable patients with multiple predisposing factors for delirium, such as advanced age, frailty, pre-existing cognitive impairment, multiple morbidities, and polypharmacy, who are inpatients because of acute illness or the need for acute surgical intervention. Preventive actions should include verbal and visual orientation cues (e.g clocks), early mobilization, sleep routines, maintaining hydration, avoiding pain, and minimizing moves within and between wards.

Further reading

American Psychiatric Association (2000). DSM-IV Criteria for Delirium. In: Diagnostic and Statistical Manual of Mental Disorders, 4th edn. Washington, DC, USA.

Anthony JC, LeResche L, Niaz V, Von Korff MR, Folstein MF (1982). Limits of the 'MMSE' as a screening test for dementia and delirium among hospital patients. *Psychological Medicine*, **12**, 397–408.

British Geriatrics Society (2006). The prevention, diagnosis and management of delirium in older people. Summary of guidelines to prevent and treat delirium in hospital. <http://www.bgs.org.uk/index.php/clinicalguides/170-clinguidedeliriumtreatment>.

Davis D and Maclullich A (2009). Understanding barriers to delirium care: a multicentre survey of knowledge and attitudes amongst UK junior doctors. *Age and Ageing*, **38**, 559–63.

Fleet J, Ernst T (2013). The prevention, recognition and management of delirium in adult in-patients. GTi Clinical Guidance Database. <http://www.guysandstthomas.nhs.uk/resources/our-services/acute-medicine-gi-surgery/elderly-care/delirium-adult-inpatients.pdf>.

Fong TG, Tulebaev SR, Inouye SK (2009). Delirium in elderly adults: diagnosis, prevention and treatment. *Nature Reviews Neurology*, **5**, 210–20.

Inouye SK, Bogardus ST Jr, Charpentier PA, et al. (1999). A multi-component intervention to prevent delirium in hospitalized older patients. *New England Journal of Medicine*, **340**, 669–76.

Inouye SK, Bogardus ST Jr, Baker DI, Leo-Summers L, Cooney LM Jr (2000). The Hospital Elder Life Program: a model of care to prevent delirium and functional decline in hospitalized older patients. *Journal of the American Geriatrics Society*, **48**, 1697–706.

Inouye SK, van Dyck CH, Alessi CA, Balkin S, Siegal AP, Horwitz RI (1990). Clarifying confusion: the Confusion Assessment Method. A new method for detection of delirium. *Annals of Internal Medicine*, **113**, 941–8.

Jitapunkul S, Pillay I, Ebrahim S (1991). The abbreviated mental test: its use and validity. *Age and Ageing*, **20**, 332–6.

National Institute for Health and Clinical Excellence (2010). Delirium: Diagnosis, prevention and management. NICE clinical guideline 103. <https://www.nice.org.uk/guidance/cg103>.

O'Keeffe ST, Mulkerrin EC, Nayeem K, Varughese M, Pillay I (2005). Use of serial Mini-Mental State Examinations to diagnose and monitor delirium in elderly hospital patients. *Journal of the American Geriatrics Society*, **53**, 867–70.

Siddiqi N, House AO, Holmes JD (2006). Occurrence and outcome of delirium in medical inpatients: a systematic literature review. *Age and Ageing*, **35**, 350–64.

Tabet N, Hudson S, Sweeney V, et al. (2005). An educational intervention can prevent delirium on acute medical wards. *Age and Ageing*, **34**, 152–6.

The Hospital Elder Life Program (HELP). <http://hospitalelderlife-program.org>.

Young J and Inouye SK (2007). Delirium in older people. *BMJ*, **334**, 842–6.

Incontinence

Introduction

Incontinence is a common symptom in all age groups, particularly in elderly and institutionalized patients. Urinary incontinence (UI) is more prevalent in females, with 5–15% in the 15–65 age group and 10–20% in the over 65s, compared with 3% and 7–10%, respectively, in men. The rate in residential homes for both sexes is 25%, nursing homes 40%, and hospital care 50–70%. The prevalence of faecal incontinence (FI) is less well known, with a range of 2.2–2.5%.

Although incontinence is rarely life-threatening, it has a marked effect on the physical and psychological well-being of the affected individual, leading to embarrassment and social exclusion. It is easy to miss in acute settings where other clinical parameters take priority and patients rarely admit to symptoms. A prompt, high-quality, comprehensive continence service is an essential part of healthcare; however, assessment of continence is often overlooked and managed predominantly by containment. Catheter use in secondary care is particularly high despite the high incidence of catheter-associated UTI (one of the commonest hospital-acquired infections).

Risk factors

These vary, depending on age, sex, and frailty. The presentation, diagnosis, and treatment also vary, according to these groups. There may be situational or environmental factors which can result in incontinence in someone who is normally continent, such as poor access to toilet facilities or reduced mobility as a result of intercurrent illness. Acute presentations of UI/FI need urgent investigation to exclude acute neurological lesions.

UI in women is more common with increasing age, obesity, parity, diabetes, hysterectomy, drugs (see Table 20.1), moderate to severe dementia, and reduced physical function. Possible associations include smoking, depression, constipation, and UTIs.

In men, UI is associated with increasing age, UTIs, lower urinary tract symptoms, drugs (see Table 20.1), functional and cognitive impairment, neurological disorders, and post-prostatectomy.

FI is more common in nursing home residents, increasing age, obesity, neurological disease, GI disorders (irritable bowel syndrome and inflammatory bowel disease), obstetric factors (e.g. birth trauma), foods/dietary supplements, drug therapy (see Table 20.2), and sequelae of surgical procedures.

Normal function

The lower urinary and bowel tracts have similar developmental origins and lie in close communication, sharing the muscular structures of the pelvic floor and innervated by autonomic and somatic nerves. They are autonomic organs with a central control regulated to necessary social requirements.

The function of the bladder can be divided into storage and voiding phases. As the bladder fills, the urethral sphincter contracts tonically while the detrusor remains relaxed. Afferent impulses are transmitted to the brainstem until a trigger level is reached, resulting in excitation of an indirect inhibitory pathway in the sacral cord, causing sphincter relaxation, detrusor contraction, and bladder emptying. This pathway can be suppressed by higher brain centres, giving voluntary control over voiding. The frontal lobes play a major role in sensing bladder filling, but other areas are also implicated in higher control. Voluntary contraction of the pelvic floor can help to maintain closure of the urethral sphincter and indirectly relax the detrusor.

Enteric reflexes in the lower bowel tract generate the peristaltic reflex and relaxation of the internal anal sphincter. Rectal distension activates a pathway, alerting the higher brain of the need to pass stool; in IBS and other functional disorders, hypervigilance leads to an increased awareness and need to defecate. The external anal sphincter is under voluntary control and maintains continence until it is safe and convenient to pass stool. A vesico-ano-rectal reflex allows bladder voiding without defecation, if required.

The consequences of neurological lesions depend on the level affected in both UI and FI:

- **Lesions above the pons.** The reflex contractions of the detrusor remain, but cerebral regulation is lost, resulting in UI secondary to bladder overactivity. Similarly, reflex contraction and bowel movement continue in the lower bowel, but cerebral regulation is lost.
- **Lesions above the conus medullaris** (most distal bulbous part of the spinal cord)**.** Result in urethral sphincter dyssynergia; UI may be due to detrusor overactivity or retention with overflow incontinence. In the lower bowel, this results in an overactive bowel, with increased anal

Table 20.1 Drugs that cause/worsen urinary incontinence

Drug	Effect
Alpha-adrenergic agonists	Outlet obstruction in men
Alpha-adrenergic blockers	Stress incontinence in women
ACE inhibitors (cough)	Stress urinary incontinence
Anticholinergics	Impaired emptying, retention, delirium, sedation, faecal impaction
Antipsychotics	Rigidity, immobility, anticholinergic effects
Calcium channel blockers	Impaired detrusor contractility, pedal oedema (nocturnal enuresis)
Loop diuretics	Polyuria, frequency, urgency
Narcotic analgesics	Urinary retention, faecal impaction, sedation, delirium
Sedative hypnotics	Sedation, delirium, immobility

Table 20.2 Drugs that cause/worsen faecal incontinence

Effect	Drug
Altering sphincter tone	Nitrates, calcium channel antagonists, beta-blockers, sildenafil, selective serotonin reuptake inhibitors (SSRIs)
Multiple mechanisms	Cephalosporins, penicillins, erythromycin
Reduction in anal pressure	Glyceryl trinitrate ointment, diltiazem gel, bethanechol cream, botulinum toxin A injection
Profuse loose stools	Laxatives, metformin, orlistat, SSRIs, digoxin, magnesium-containing antacids
Constipation	Loperamide, opioids, tricyclic antidepressants, aluminium-containing antacids, codeine
Reduced alertness	Benzodiazepines, tricyclic antidepressants, SSRIs, antipsychotics

tone. Central control of the external anal sphincter is lost, leaving it shut tight. Reflex coordination and stool propulsion remain, resulting in faecal impaction and overflow.

- **Lesions in the cauda equina/peripheral nerves.** As with lesions above the conus, damage to pudendal nerve nuclei (Onuf's nuclei; a distinct group of neurons located in the ventral anterior horn of the sacral region of the spinal cord) causes pelvic floor paralysis, with reduced outflow resistance and stress incontinence. For the lower bowel, loss of pelvic nerve function results in lack of spinal cord-mediated peristalsis and a non-contractile external anal sphincter, causing constipation and FI.

Symptoms

Storage symptoms

- **Overactive bladder (OAB).** Results in urgency (sudden compelling desire to pass urine which is difficult to defer). This is usually due to detrusor overactivity and can be associated with or without UI and normally causes frequency and nocturia.
- **Urinary incontinence.** Any involuntary leakage of urine should be further described, according to type, severity, precipitating factors, social impact, and whether acute or chronic.
- **Stress urinary incontinence (SUI).** An involuntary leakage on effort, exertion, sneezing, coughing, or laughing due to failure of the urethral sphincter or pelvic floor weakness.
- **Urge urinary incontinence (UUI).** Involuntary leakage, immediately preceded or accompanied by urgency. Can be small volumes or catastrophic leaks with complete emptying. Often associated with trigger events.
- **Mixed urinary incontinence.** Involuntary leakage associated with both stress and urgency.

Voiding symptoms
(due to bladder outflow obstruction or detrusor failure)

- **Slow or intermittent stream.**
- **Hesitancy:** difficulty initiating micturition.
- **Straining:** muscular effort to initiate/maintain stream.
- **Terminal dribble:** prolonged final part of micturition.
- **Post-micturition dribble:** involuntary loss of urine after leaving toilet due to urine not expelled from the bulb.

Faecal incontinence
(involuntary loss of faecal material)

- **Urgency/urge incontinence:** due to damage/weakness in the external anal sphincter.
- **Passive soiling:** due to damage/weakness of internal anal sphincter.

- **Frequency/urgency:** due to intestinal hurry from IBS/IBD, infections, or drugs.
- **Impaction/overflow:** due to immobility, drugs, cognitive impairment, neurological disease.

Diagnosis/evaluation

In younger patients, the aetiology is usually a specific condition of the lower urinary tract or its neurological control. In the elderly, it is more likely to be part of a geriatric syndrome with additional risk factors (polypharmacy, comorbidity, functional and cognitive impairment) and is associated with greater morbidity, risk of falls, functional decline, and institutionalization. In addition, the elderly are more susceptible to the side effects of pharmacological treatment.

All patients should be asked about urinary or bowel symptoms, and the severity, duration, and impact on the patient should be sought. Certain red flags (see Box 20.1) should alert the clinician to more serious underlying pathology and need for further investigation and onward referral (haematuria, rectal bleeding, acute onset, pain, sensory loss, or change in bowel habit).

Assess any previous conservative, medical, or surgical treatment (including radiotherapy) or coexisting disease that may impact on incontinence (asthma/COPD in SUI; comorbid conditions in elderly) or prolapse, including past obstetric history and visual or physical impairment (can render a patient incontinent as they are unable to reach the bathroom or toilet). Drug history should include over-the-counter and herbal remedies. Examine lifestyle issues (smoking, fluid, and food intake, including type and amount), as well as the desire for treatment by the patient and what treatment they would accept. Patient's goals, expectations, and support mechanisms available should be explored.

General examination should take account of the mental status, obesity, and physical dexterity/mobility of the patient; the presence of abdominal masses and scars, and

---

Box 20.1 Red flags in incontinence

Pain (particularly back pain)
Haematuria
Rectal bleeding
Acute neurological presentation (including gait disturbance; beware patients labelled 'off legs' or with 'psychiatric/hysterical' faecal incontinence)
Unexplained change in bowel habit or weight loss
Acute urinary retention
Abdominal or pelvic mass
Nocturnal diarrhoea
New-onset faecal incontinence

bladder palpation for distension. Pelvic examination (with a chaperone) should always include examination of the external genitalia (tissue quality and sensation), vaginal examination (half speculum for prolapse; bimanual for pelvic masses and function), and a digital rectal examination (for masses and stool impaction). Neurological examination should look for underlying neurological disease, in particular, an assessment of sensation (especially perianal sensation), anal tone, sensory level, and gait.

Investigations

Should include standard biochemistry (diabetes or renal failure); urine dipstick test (cytology/microscopy and MSU); post-void residual volume (PVR) assessment (preferably with a bladder scanner) and a frequency/volume chart (see Figure 20.2) or bladder diary. Further imaging is not routinely required unless indicated from the history or examination. Consider endoscopy if the history is suggestive (e.g. Crohn's, ulcerative colitis, or haematuria); all cases of FI should undergo proctoscopy/flexisigmoidoscopy.

Management

The assessment should identify patients requiring referral for specialist management. Basic treatment depends on the underlying diagnosis and the patient group but should include discussion and joint decision with the patient. The least invasive treatment should be tried first and most invasive last, allowing sufficient time to assess response. Initial lifestyle

Name: _____   **Date:** _____

Time	Day 1			Day 2			Day 3			Day 4		
	F	U	W	F	U	W	F	U	W	F	U	W
6 a.m.												
7 a.m.												
8 a.m.												
9 a.m.												
10 a.m.												
11 a.m.												
12 md												
1 p.m.												
2 p.m.												
3 p.m.												
4 p.m.												
5 p.m.												
6 p.m.												
7 p.m.												
8 p.m.												
9 p.m.												
10 p.m.												
11 p.m.												
12 mn												
1 a.m.												
2 a.m.												
3 a.m.												
4 a.m.												
5 a.m.												
Total												

Measure and record the amount of fluid taken in column marked F.   Tea cup = 150 mL
Measure and record the amount of urine passed in the column marked U.   Coffee mug = 200 mL
Put a cross in the W column every time you wet yourself before reaching the toilet.

Figure 20.2 Bladder record chart—frequency and volume.

Table 20.3 Antimuscarinic agents for treatment of UUI (level 1 evidence)

Drug	Dose/formulations
Oxybutynin	Immediate-release: 2.5–5 mg bd Extended-release: 5 mg od Transdermal: 3.9 mg twice weekly
Tolterodine	Immediate-release: 1–2 mg bd Extended-release: 2–4 mg od
Solifenacin	5–10 mg od
Darifenacin	7.5–15 mg od
Trospium	20 mg od–bd
Fesoterodine	4–8 mg od

All metabolized via cytochrome P450, except trospium.

advice (reduce caffeine, smoking, and weight loss), change of medication, if possible, and treatment of associated comorbidity (e.g. faecal impaction or symptomatic UTI), is followed by reassessment for ongoing incontinence.

Treatment of asymptomatic bacteriuria should be avoided, as it is not beneficial. Scheduled voiding regimens can maintain continence in cognitively impaired or neurogenic patients; these can be guided by information from a fluid/volume chart.

Continence products, such as clean intermittent self-catheterization/indwelling catheters, should be considered for retention but not routinely for management of incontinence. Assisted toileting devices (commodes, bottles, bedpans, etc.) or improved access to toilet facilities are helpful where mobility problems undermine the ability to maintain independent continence. Containment products (e.g. pads or sheaths) should be reserved for those awaiting treatment or its response, where treatment is unsuccessful/inappropriate, or patient preference.

Supervised pelvic floor muscle training is the treatment of choice in SUI and bladder retraining in OAB; both are used for mixed UI. These treatments should also be considered in elderly patients who are willing and able to try them.

Antimuscarinics (see Table 20.3) are used in OAB/mixed UI, in addition to bladder retraining, if still symptomatic or in those unable to perform them (can worsen UI due to retention). These target detrusor muscarinic receptors and increase bladder capacity but may also result in worsening cognitive impairment, blurred vision, constipation, and dry mouth. Alpha blockers (tamsulosin, alfuzosin, and doxazosin) and 5-alpha-reductase inhibitors (finasteride and dutasteride) are used in benign prostatic outflow to reduce lower urinary tract symptoms (LUTS) and increase success of catheter removal in men but are not effective in reducing concomitant UI or urgency. Patients should be reassessed after 8–12 weeks and referred to a specialist if still symptomatic.

FI management, once local or systemic pathology has been excluded, depends on the symptom presentation and is often made worse in the presence of loose stool. Urgency associated with FI is usually a symptom of external anal sphincter dysfunction or intestinal hurry; passive stool loss may indicate internal anal sphincter dysfunction. Provide diet and fluid advice to ensure ideal stool consistency, establish a regular bowel habit with complete evacuation, and encourage simple exercises to strengthen and enhance awareness of the anal sphincter. Antidiarrhoeal medication can be considered in the presence of loose stool. If no improvement occurs after 8–12 weeks, referral should be made to a specialist.

Further reading

Abrams P, Andersson KE, Birder L, et al. (2010). Fourth International Consultation on Incontinence Recommendations of the International Scientific Committee: evaluation and treatment of urinary incontinence, pelvic organ prolapse, and fecal incontinence. Neurourology and Urodynamics, 29, 213–40.

Age UK. Advice on incontinence. Tel: 0800 169 65 65.

Bladder and Bowel Foundation. <http://www.bladderandbowel-foundation.org>. Nurse helpline: 0845 345 0165. General enquiries: 01536 533255.

Department of Health (2000). Good practice in continence services. Department of Health, London. <http://webarchive.national-archives.gov.uk/+/www.dh.gov.uk/en/Publicationsandstatistics/Publications/PublicationsPolicyAndGuidance/DH_4005851>.

Drake MJ, Fowler CJ, Griffiths D, Mayer E, Paton JF, Birder L (2010). Neural control of the lower urinary and gastrointestinal tracts: supraspinal CNS mechanisms. Neurourology and Urodynamics, 29, 119–127.

Du Beau CE (2009). Therapeutic/pharmacologic approaches to urinary incontinence in older adults. Clinical Pharmacology & Therapeutics, 85, 98–102.

National Institute for Health and Clinical Excellence (2013). Urinary incontinence. The management of urinary incontinence in women. NICE clinical guideline 171. <https://www.nice.org.uk/guidance/cg171>.

National Institute for Health and Clinical Excellence (2007). Faecal incontinence: the management of faecal incontinence in adults. NICE clinical guideline 49. <http://www.nice.org.uk/nicemedia/live/11012/30548/30548.pdf>.

National Institute for Health and Clinical Excellence (2012). Urinary incontinence in neurological disease: Management of lower urinary tract dysfunction in neurological disease. NICE clinical guideline 148. <https://www.nice.org.uk/guidance/cg148>.

Norton C, Whitehead WE, Bliss DZ, et al. (2010). Management of fecal incontinence in adults. Neurourology and Urodynamics, 29, 199–206.

Patient.co.uk. Urinary incontinence. <http://www.patient.co.uk/pdf/4278.pdf>.

Royal College of Physicians (1995). Incontinence. Causes, management and provision of services. A Working Party of the Royal College of Physicians. Journal of the Royal College of Physicians London, 29, 272–4.

Royal College of Physicians (2005). National audit of continence care for older people. Royal College of Physicians, London.

The Cochrane Library. Urinary incontinence. <http://www.thecochranelibrary.com/view/0/browse.html?cat=ccochgynaeurinaryincontinence>.

The Cystitis & Overactive Bladder Foundation. <http://www.cob-foundation.org/>. Tel: 01908 569 169.

Thirugnanasothy S (2010). Managing urinary incontinence in older people. BMJ, 341, c3835.

Thuroff J, Abrams P, Andersson KE (2011). EAU guidelines on urinary incontinence. European Urology, 59, 387–400.

Vasavada SP (2013). Urinary Incontinence, Medscape. <http://emedicine.medscape.com/article/452289-overview>.

Wing RR, Creasman JM, West DS, et al. (2010). Improving urinary incontinence in overweight and obese women through modest weight loss. Obstetrics & Gynecology, 116, 284–92.

Falls and syncope

Falls and syncope are common presentations to acute medical services. Clear evidence-based guidelines are available to healthcare professionals for the evaluation and management of these problems and are summarized in the next paragraphs. Further reading is listed at the end of this chapter.

Falls

Around one-third of people aged over 65 years old fall each year. The incidence of falls is higher in institutionalized older people. Half of falls in older people occur in the home, with no obvious environmental hazard. Falls lead to loss of confidence and limitation of activities, and around 5% of falls result in a fracture. Hip fractures cost the NHS around £1.7 billion per year.

Falls in older people are common, but they are rarely 'mechanical' (i.e. accidental). Older people fall because of medical problems, **many of which are treatable**, and there is good evidence that simple interventions can prevent falls. Most falls are multifactorial in origin, and multifactorial interventions have been shown to be most successful.

Why do older people fall?

A fall can be the presenting complaint for a wide range of acute illnesses in an older person. Sepsis is the most common, but haemorrhage, acute coronary syndromes, and metabolic disturbances are other examples. So the first assessment should address whether there is any acute illness.

If there is no acute illness, several risk factors for falls have been identified. Table 20.4 summarizes these in six categories. These risk factors are synergistic, so the risk of falling rises significantly with the number of risk factors.

Evaluation of a person who has fallen

Any older person who has fallen should have a multifactorial risk assessment performed. This starts with a history:

Table 20.4 Risk factors for falls

1 Social:
  • Advanced age.
  • Living alone.
  • Previous falls.
  • Limited in activities of daily living.
2 Age-related changes:
  • Reduced proprioception.
  • Reduced ability to discriminate edges.
  • Slower reaction times.
  • Muscle weakness.
3 Poor gait and balance.
4 Medical problems:
  • Cerebrovascular disease.
  • Eye diseases.
  • Complications of diabetes.
  • Arthritis.
  • Incontinence.
5 Medications:
  • Being on four or more medications.
  • Psychiatric medication.
  • Cardiovascular medication.
6 Environmental factors:
  • Wearing bifocals.
  • Ill-fitting footwear.

'How did you come to fall?' Vague answers, such as 'I don't know, I must have tripped,' often point to cognitive impairment or syncope (see the next sections). Dizziness requires further evaluation. Medications, past medical history, alcohol intake, bladder problems, and an abbreviated mental test score are other key parts of the history, along with information about social circumstances and activities of daily living.

The examination should include an assessment of vision (fields, acuity, and type of spectacles), cardiovascular examination, including lying and standing blood pressure, and a neurological examination that includes the 'get-up-and-go test'.

The 'get-up-and-go test' is a key screening test for gait and balance abnormalities. The person is asked to rise from a chair (without using his arms, if possible), walk 3 metres, turn around, and sit down again. A normal person should be able to do this within 10 seconds. An abnormal gait and/or balance should be further evaluated.

A 12-lead electrocardiogram should be performed in all cases.

Management of falls

The most important components of the multifactorial risk assessment are:

1. Making a medical diagnosis.

2. Assessment of vision.

3. Identifying side effects of medications.

4. Muscle strength and balance training.

5. Assessment of 'home hazards'.

This is why the assessment should be performed by a multidisciplinary team, either in hospital or in a specialist falls clinic.

While some problems may not be treatable (e.g. diabetic peripheral neuropathy), other problems will be—for example, bifocal use or cataracts, the wrong walking aid, postural hypotension caused by medication, an unstable bladder, and so on. Many 'untreatable' medical problems can be helped considerably by simple interventions, often after evaluation by another member of the multidisciplinary team, such as a physiotherapist or occupational therapist.

It is important to ask about previous fractures as a result of a fall. Osteoporosis and other metabolic bone diseases are common in older people. If treatment for osteoporosis is indicated (see Further reading), this should be started without delay.

The overlap between falls and syncope

Many older people live alone, may have cognitive impairment, or are found lying on the floor with no eyewitness to account for how they got there. Retrograde amnesia is common in some types of syncope (for example, carotid sinus hypersensitivity). An older person may deny they lost consciousness when they had. Therefore, some syncope presents as 'unexplained falls'—the person seems to 'just go down' **without** loss of consciousness, but the mechanism is, in fact, syncope.

Unexplained falls (i.e. normal gait and balance, no obvious explanation on multifactorial risk assessment) should be evaluated as syncope.

Syncope

Syncope (which means 'interrupt') accounts for up to 5% of emergency department visits and is considerably more common in people over the age of 65 years old. Even though most syncope has a benign cause, recurrent syncope impacts considerably on people's lives.

There are many causes of transient loss of consciousness. Syncope is one of the most common causes and is always the result of **transient global cerebral hypoperfusion**. There is a relatively rapid onset of loss of consciousness and loss of voluntary muscle tone, with usually spontaneous, complete, and prompt recovery. In simple terms, syncope is due to either a blood pressure that is too low or a heart rate that is too fast or too slow.

Classification of syncope

There are four main types of syncope, and the investigation and management of each are different, so it is important to classify the type of syncope your patient has after an initial evaluation.

Cardiac causes only account for around 20% of all syncope. Neurally mediated syncope is the most common type, accounting for around 50%. Orthostatic syncope accounts for one-third of syncope in the over 70s but is uncommon in young people. Structural problems account for only 3% of syncope overall. A significant proportion of syncope, around 20%, remains unexplained after a thorough evaluation, and this has a good prognosis.

The four main types of syncope are shown in Table 20.5.

Initial evaluation of a person with syncope

The first, and most important, factor in establishing a diagnosis of syncope is **an eyewitness account**. A person who has suffered transient loss of consciousness cannot tell you whether they had a seizure or syncope, but an eyewitness can.

Careful history taking is required, as people can jerk during syncope or be incontinent of urine if they lose muscle tone when their bladder is full. The overall picture—from both the patient and the eyewitness—is most important in terms of diagnosis, particularly if there have been previous episodes.

The '3 Ps' are strongly suggestive of vasovagal syncope: upright Posture, Provoking factors, and a typical Prodrome before losing consciousness (feeling warm, light-headed, with blurred vision).

Older people experience vasovagal or orthostatic syncope without any prodrome because of their impaired sympathetic response to a falling blood pressure. The presence or absence of a prodrome does not help in deciding whether a person's syncope is due to a cardiac arrhythmia.

Because patients are asymptomatic at the time of the initial evaluation, the purpose of the evaluation is to look for 'circumstantial evidence'—problems that could be the cause of the syncope. Clues are gleaned from the history, but the physical examination (focusing on the heart and neurological system), 12-lead electrocardiogram, and a lying and standing blood pressure are also key.

After the initial evaluation, it should be easy to decide if there is an obvious culprit for the cause of syncope and also whether the person has a normal heart or not. The patient is then classified into one of three groups before deciding what to do next:

1. Obvious diagnosis.
2. Suspected diagnosis.
3. Unexplained syncope.

Further investigations depend on whether the person has a normal heart or not. A normal heart is defined as: no cardiac history, a normal cardiac examination, normal 12-lead electrocardiogram, and no history of sudden death in the family or 'red flags' (e.g. syncope during exercise). These people should be referred for tests for neurally mediated syncope if they have recurrent or unexplained syncope.

Further investigations

Tests for neurally mediated syncope include the head-up tilt test, carotid sinus massage, and sometimes an implantable loop recorder. Tests for possible arrhythmias (in people with abnormal hearts) include ambulatory cardiac monitoring, echocardiography, stress testing, and sometimes electrophysiology and an implantable loop recorder. A CT scan of the head is not a test for syncope.

Management of syncope

The management of syncope depends on the cause. For neurally mediated and orthostatic syncope, this often includes a medication review, general advice, and sometimes medication to increase blood pressure. In the UK, whether a person can drive after syncope is governed by the Driving and Vehicle Licensing Agency rules.

Table 20.5 The four main types of syncope

1. Neurally mediated:
   - Vasovagal ('simple faint').
   - Carotid sinus hypersensitivity.
   - Situational:
     - Unpleasant stimuli.
     - Cough.
     - Micturition.
2. Orthostatic:
   - Medication-induced.
   - Autonomic failure (primary or secondary).
   - Endocrine (eg Addison's).
3. Cardiac arrhythmias:
   - Sick sinus syndrome.
   - AV blocks.
   - Supraventricular or ventricular tachycardias.
   - Long QT interval.
4. Structural:
   - Aortic stenosis.
   - Hypertrophic obstructive cardiomyopathy.

Further reading

Benditt DG, Blanc JJ, Brignole M, Sutton R, eds. (2006). *The evaluation and treatment of syncope*, 2nd edn. European Society of Cardiology guidelines. Blackwell, Oxford.

Cooper N, Forrest K, Mulley G, eds. (2009). *ABC of geriatric medicine*. Wiley-Blackwell, Oxford.

National Institute for Health and Clinical Excellence (2013). Falls. Assessment and prevention of falls in older people. NICE clinical guideline 161. <https://www.nice.org.uk/guidance/cg161>.

Multiprofessional teamwork and assessment of complex needs

Complex needs patients: a definition. These patients present with impairment of physical and/or cognitive systems that may be complicated by disability. As a result, they have impairment of their personal and domestic activities of daily living.

- This is a result of multisystem chronic pathology.
- Patients are usually, but not exclusively, older.
- They have formal or informal carer involvement.
- Are taking four or more prescribed medications.
- They may have significant psychological and social dysfunction.
- They may have chronic mental health problems.

The admission and readmission rates for >75-year-old patients continues to rise, and most will have complex needs. Often these patients have a relatively minor acute illness, but, for them, this results in physical or mental deterioration, with a disproportionate impact on functional ability. Admission to the acute care setting may be with a defined acute illness but is often as a result of diagnostic doubt and concern regarding the patient's functional ability.

Admission to acute care for this vulnerable group of patients is associated with poorer patient outcomes and with:

- Hospital-acquired infection.
- Increased falls risk.
- Suboptimal nutrition.
- Drug errors.

Rapid physical and cognitive deconditioning can lead to increased patient dependency and institutionalizaton. This results in prolonged hospital stays and placement difficulties at discharge.

To deliver high-quality care for complex needs patients, a multiprofessional team approach is mandatory. In addition to medical and nursing teams, allied health professionals are required to address key issues, including mobility, continence, and communication needs. In light of the negative impact admission can have, it is vital that this assessment is provided as early as possible in the inpatient journey. This facilitates rapid and safe placement into the optimal care setting for the patient's needs. Ideally, this should be the patient's own home if the acute illness and any other associated functional change can be managed in primary care.

To achieve an accurate assessment, the information obtained from primary care at admission is key. Ideally, the patient's own general practitioner should have been involved in the admission and will have provided the required information. In the UK, however, the present out-of-hours arrangements mean this is often not the case. It is important to gain a clear reason for admission from the patient, and, where a clear reason is not determined, a collateral history from those involved in the care and/or admission process must be sought. There needs to be a clear understanding of the primary care concerns and related clinical questions to ensure these are addressed in the acute care setting. The patient's usual functional ability must be determined to identify changes required to allow safe discharge.

This patient group are often labelled as an 'inappropriate admission' group. This is, however, an unhelpful label and can lead to a lower standard of clinical care.

These patients are often assessed in the community by clinicians unfamiliar with their case. In this situation, admission is often the only safe decision to make. A clean, smiling patient in a hospital bed, following a short period of inpatient observation, investigation, and functional assessment, may not seem to have needed to be admitted. However, this does not reflect the domestic situation until accurately assessed by the multiprofessional team liaising with primary and community care.

In assessing patients from this vulnerable group, the cognitive state of the patient must be recorded. An example is the AMT (abbreviated mental test) which is a well-known, but limited, screening tool for cognitive impairment (see Chapter 14, Box 14.1). A score of less than 7 is significant.

In addition, delirium should be identified (see 'Delirium' earlier in this chapter, and Chapter 14). Furthermore, the physician should be aware that a change in functional state can be an atypical presentation of organic disease. This may include iatrogenic illness associated with drug therapy or the use of alcohol or other substance misuse.

The initial nursing assessment ideally records change in ADL (activities of daily living). These are bathing, dressing, toileting, continence, feeding, and transferring.

The input from the rest of the multiprofessional team should be tailored to the individual patient.

Most complex needs patients will need a physiotherapy and occupational therapy assessment.

In providing this multiprofessional input, there are key desirable elements. These include:

- Seven days a week provision.
- Continual multiprofessional review of patient progress and management plan.

Rapid access to diagnostics and multiprofessional assessment at the point of entry to care is, therefore, vital to ensure such patients do not have prolonged hospital stays.

Physiotherapy

Patient assessment, with mobilization and advice, constitutes the majority of the workload of the physiotherapist. Early active mobilization is key to enable patients to regain balance and confidence. Prompt provision of the required walking aid within the acute care setting helps to facilitate safe and early discharge.

Rapid assessment of a patient's mobility is important. It allows patients requiring longer term inpatient rehabilitation to move out of the acute medicine setting into the appropriate downstream ward. This allows the therapist to focus on the remaining patients who may have a better prognosis for mobilization. These patients should be kept in the acute medical setting to allow continuity of care over a short stay of approximately 24–48 hours. This maximizes the efficiency of care, reduces patient transfers, and avoids the risk of increasing patient dependency.

Occupational therapy

Occupational therapists provide social status verification, functional assessment, provision of aids, and discharge planning—all of which are vital to optimize care for this patient group.

For social status verification, a comprehensive overview of the patient's pre-existing services and function is obtained. This is achieved through patient interview and includes collateral information from the family and members of the primary care team.

Ideally, the occupational therapy service has ready access to a suitable assessment suite that enables the observation of the patient performing activities of daily living relevant to the individual.

The ability to augment and/or restore care packages is vital to facilitate safe discharge, and is a significant part of the occupational therapist's role, and must start at point of entry to care. Communication with the appropriate primary care services is essential when discharge home is being planned.

Pharmacy

Active medicines management is of paramount importance. Pharmacists working in acute medical units are essential and contribute to:

- Medicines reconciliation at presentation and discharge.
- Liaising with primary care pharmacists and general practice, as indicated.
- Ensuring patient safety for all existing prescribing and new prescribing.

This involves close liaison between all members of the multiprofessional group who are involved in the prescription and dispensing of medicines to this patient group.

General practice

A general practitioner who works closely within the multiprofessional team may have a variety of roles:

- Involvement in the medical management of the patient, with a focus on the aspects of care that may be complementary in the secondary care setting.
- A generalist skill mix, with primary care sensibilities and the knowledge of local primary care service provision.
- Primary role as a member of the 'complex needs' multiprofessional assessment team.
- Using multiple sources across the primary/secondary care interface to achieve a true holistic patient assessment.
- Liaising with specialty and primary care teams to develop patient-specific management plans to facilitate patient movement in both directions across the primary/secondary care interface.
- Utilizing chronic disease management skills.
- Risk management, including working with diagnostic uncertainty and appropriate investigation rationalization, but also recognition of the patients who are best managed in the community.
- Strategic role between primary and secondary care, developing appropriate patient pathways for locality and need.

Exact roles will vary, depending on the individual, the needs of the service, and individual competences, but it is an area for potential development. The minimum is that the AMU has good links with primary care.

Specific specialty input

Medicine for the elderly
Proactive in-reach to the acute medical setting is desirable to promptly identify patients who are most likely to benefit from specialist medicine for the elderly input, including comprehensive inpatient assessment.

This may be achieved with input from a specialist nurse or consultant and close liaison with the multiprofessional team.

Psychiatry
Early access to adult and older care specialty psychiatry services is critical to enable the management of patients who have acute or subacute psychiatric needs. Often the general practitioner working within acute medicine is best placed to refer the patient to the most suitable secondary or primary care-based service.

Discharge planning

There is evidence to suggest that early assessment of patients from this vulnerable group facilitates a greater proportion being discharged directly home from the acute medical unit. Discharge planning is critical to a safe return home.

Prompt and accurate communication within the multiprofessional team and between primary and secondary care is vital. In addition, clear communication with the patient and their carers is of paramount importance.

This communication must include:

- Diagnosis.
- Management plan.
- Follow-up plans.
- Medication list and changes, including rationale for change.
- Care package restarted and/or augmented.
- Referral to community-based services, e.g. day hospital, day centre community psychiatry services, allied health professionals.

Conclusion

The assessment process, therefore, commences at the 'front door', utilizing information obtained from primary care, patients, and carers, and must not be deferred until transfer to downstream medical wards. The aim is to provide prompt holistic multiprofessional assessment, including investigation, to reach an accurate diagnosis with subsequent management, and an emphasis on maintaining function and independence.

This approach permits safe placement in the appropriate care setting, with a significant proportion returning directly home to the care of the primary care team. Understanding, and close liaison with, the primary healthcare team is required to promote high-quality, seamless patient care across the primary-secondary care interface.

Further reading

Crosswaite AG, Dougall H, Duguid I, Mearns N, Jones M, Bell D (2009). Providing better care for patients with complex needs in acute medicine. *Acute Medicine*, **8**, 80–4.

The Royal College of Physicians (2007). Acute medical care, the right person, in the right setting—first time. Report of the Acute Medicine Task Force, October 2007, The Royal College of Physicians, London.

Obstetric emergencies

Obstetric emergencies

Introduction

Maternal deaths are rare in developed countries. The UK confidential maternal death enquiry (MDE) identified 252 women, who died from causes directly, or indirectly, related to their pregnancy, of 2 million mothers who gave birth between 2009 and 2011. From these figures, the all-cause maternal mortality rate (MMR) was 10.63 per 100,000 maternities. However, most countries derive official statistics from death certificates alone. Although the MMR is greater in less developed economies, it is decreasing with improved healthcare.

- Direct deaths describe those that could only be due to the pregnancy (e.g. eclampsia, haemorrhage), and the MDE maternal mortality rate for these was 3.49 per 100,000 maternities or 82 deaths. The commonest cause of direct death was thromboembolism (see Table 21.1).
- Indirect deaths refer to those due to pre-existing, or new, medical or mental health conditions aggravated by pregnancy (e.g. heart disease). The mortality rate for these was 7.15 per 100,000 maternities or 170 deaths. Over the last 10 years, indirect deaths have consistently outnumbered direct deaths. Cardiac disease is the commonest cause (see Table 21.1) and reflects the increasing incidence of acquired heart disease in younger women due to obesity, poor diet, smoking, and alcohol. Over 50% of women who die in pregnancy or the puerperium are overweight or obese, and 15% are morbidly obese.

Life-threatening obstetric emergencies may occur antepartum, in labour, or post-partum. Emergency medical personnel must be able to manage these conditions and should be familiar with techniques used to resuscitate pregnant women. Unfortunately, avoidable deaths continue to occur, and sub-standard care was reported in >50% of direct and ~40% of indirect maternal deaths.

Table 21.1 Causes of maternal deaths (2009–2012)

Medical condition	Rate/million pregnancies	Number of deaths in the UK
Direct pregnancy-related causes	19.4	82
Venous thromboembolism	12.6	30
Pre-eclampsia and eclampsia	4.2	10
Genital tract sepsis	6.3	14
Amniotic fluid embolism	2.9	7
Obstetric haemorrhage	5.9	14
Indirect causes	71.5	170
Cardiac	21.4	51
Suicide and overdose	5.5	13
Other indirect causes	30.3	72
Neurological	12.6	30

Data from Knight M, Kenyon S, Brocklehurst P, Neilson J, Shakespeare J, Kurinczuk JJ (eds.) on behalf of MBRRACE-UK (2014). Saving Lives, Improving Mothers' Care - Lessons learned to inform future maternity care from the UK and Ireland Confidential Enquiries into Maternal Deaths and Morbidity 2009–12. Oxford: National Perinatal Epidemiology Unit, University of Oxford, pp. 81–87.

Physiological changes related to pregnancy

Pregnancy is associated with physiological changes that modify the presentation and management of subsequent medical problems. Blood pressure falls by 5–15%; heart rate and cardiac output increase by 15% and 45%, respectively, and total blood volume rises by 40%. Increases are also seen in respiratory rate (10%), tidal and minute ventilation (40–50%), PaO_2 (~1 kPa), and oxygen consumption (~20%). Most of these changes revert to normal within a few days of delivery. Aortocaval compression by the gravid uterus may impede uterine perfusion after 20 weeks' gestation and is best prevented by positioning the expectant mother in the left lateral position or displacing the uterus manually. Venous stasis due to the gravid uterus and procoagulant changes predispose to thromboembolic disease, and prophylactic heparin must not be neglected. Restriction of diaphragmatic movement by the enlarging uterus may impair ventilation. Delayed gastric emptying, increased oxygen consumption, and oedema may complicate endotracheal intubation.

In pregnancy, both the mother and fetus are influenced by disease and treatment. Ensuring the mother's survival takes precedence over the fetus. Fetal survival is dependent on optimal maternal management. Fetal surveillance will assist in assessing preterm labour, placental perfusion, oxygenation, and the effects of placental transfer of drugs.

Pre-eclampsia

Pre-eclampsia is a syndrome specific to pregnancy. It is usually diagnosed when hypertension and proteinuria develop after 20 weeks' gestation of pregnancy. It may present intrapartum or post-partum. Diagnostic criteria vary internationally, and proteinuria is not always a mandatory feature. Pre-eclampsia affects 3–5% of pregnancies, usually at 32–38 weeks' gestation, and often resolves 2–3 days after delivery. It may be superimposed on pre-existing hypertension. Eclampsia is diagnosed if tonic clonic convulsions also occur. Maternal mortality for pre-eclampsia and eclampsia is 0.42 per 100,000 maternities in the UK but is much greater in less developed countries. Factors associated with increased maternal risk include onset at <32 weeks' gestation, greater maternal age and parity, Afro-Caribbean ethnicity, pre-existing medical disease, and HELLP syndrome (haemolysis, elevated liver enzymes, low platelets) which is often associated with epigastric pain or vomiting and raised serum creatinine. Neonatal mortality in eclampsia is about 7%.

Aetiology

Aetiology is unknown, but there is a genetic predisposition. It is more frequent in those with pre-existing hypertension, renal disease, diabetes, or hydatiform mole and is twice as common in primigravid women. Placental hypoperfusion and ischaemia have been proposed as potential triggers for the associated systemic hypertension, widespread vasoconstriction, decreased intravascular volume, impaired organ perfusion, and proteinuria.

Clinical features

Hypertension is usually the main clinical feature, but some cases present with malaise, abdominal pain, or convulsions. Pre-eclampsia is defined as systolic and diastolic arterial blood pressures >140 and >90 mmHg, respectively, with proteinuria ≥300 mg/24h.

Features of severe pre-eclampsia, as defined by the American College of Obstetricians and Gynaecologists include:

- **Blood pressure.** Systolic and diastolic arterial blood pressure >160 and >110 mmHg, respectively. Characteristic haemodynamic changes include increased systemic vascular resistance, decreased intravascular volume, and reduced cardiac output.
- **Renal.** Proteinuria >2 g/24 h (+3/+4 on urinary dipstix), oliguria <0.5 L/24 h, or serum creatinine >0.09 mmol/L. Glomerular filtration and renal plasma flow are reduced.
- **Cardiac.** Iatrogenic fluid load, impaired ventricular function, and increased capillary permeability predispose to pulmonary oedema which often occurs after delivery in older, multiparous women with pre-existing hypertension.
- **Neurological.** Visual disturbance, persistent headaches, cerebral oedema (± raised intracranial pressure), convulsions, and stroke.
- **Hepatic.** Epigastric or right upper quadrant discomfort, raised bilirubin, and abnormal liver function tests. Life-threatening intrahepatic or subcapsular bleeding and rupture may rarely require emergency surgery in severe pre-eclampsia.
- **Haematological.** Thrombocytopenia is most common; haemolysis and deranged coagulation also occur.

The main causes of maternal death in pre-eclampsia/eclampsia are intracerebral haemorrhage (ICH), pulmonary oedema, and liver damage.

Management
Management aims to control BP, prevent seizures (± end-organ damage), and maintain uterine perfusion. However, only delivery of the fetus and placenta is curative. In mild cases, disease control and delayed delivery aid fetal maturation. Ideally, more severe cases should be transferred to a tertiary centre, and the most severe cases should be managed in a high dependency or intensive care unit before, and for 48–72 h, after delivery.

General management
General management should include nursing in the lateral or semi-lateral position, with fetal heart rate monitoring. Prophylactic steroids should be given, if gestation is <34 weeks, to aid fetal lung maturation. Ranitidine reduces gastric acid and associated reflux oesophagitis. Monitoring should include blood pressure, oximetry, fluid balance (± central venous pressure), urine output, and serial measurement of renal and liver function tests and platelet count to assess disease progression.

Specific management
Specific management includes blood pressure control, fluid management, prevention or treatment of seizures, and a decision regarding the optimal timing for delivery of the baby.

1. **Antihypertensive therapy** aims to reduce BP and prevent complications (e.g. ICH, abruptio placentae, heart failure), without impairing uterine perfusion. Acute treatment is indicated if the blood pressure is >160–170 mmHg systolic or >105–110 mmHg diastolic, aiming to reduce systolic pressure by 20–30 mmHg and diastolic by 10–15 mmHg, whilst monitoring the fetus. Labetalol, nifedipine, and hydralazine are the most frequently used antihypertensive agents.

- **Labetalol**, a non-selective beta-blocker with alpha-blocking effects, reduces blood pressure rapidly without impairing uterine perfusion. It is given intravenously as an infusion at a rate of 1–2 mg/min, reducing to 0.5 mg/min when the blood pressure is controlled. It does not cause reflex tachycardia, headache, nausea, nor fetal bradycardia or hypoglycaemia, although it does cross the placental barrier. It is contraindicated in patients with asthma and heart failure.
- **Nifedipine**, a calcium channel blocker that relaxes arterial smooth muscle, causes a steady decrease in blood pressure in pre-eclamptic patients over 30 minutes. It is given orally (i.e. 10 mg modified release, repeated after 30 min, as required). Sudden hypotension has been reported when given to patients receiving magnesium. It is associated with an increase in maternal heart rate and cardiac index and can cause uterine muscle relaxation which increases the risk of post-partum haemorrhage.
- **Hydralazine**, a direct arteriolar vasodilator with a long history of use in pre-eclampsia, is associated with more maternal and perinatal adverse effects than labetalol or nifedipine. It has a slow onset of action, and infusions can be difficult to titrate, causing hypotension (± fetal distress). Judicious plasma expansion reduces the risk of sudden hypotension due to vasodilation of the depleted intravascular compartment.
- **Sodium nitroprusside** rapidly reduces blood pressure but causes fetal cyanide poisoning if used for >4 h.
- **Nitrates** may be useful in pulmonary oedema.
- **Methyldopa** is used in mild cases, but its slow onset of action makes it unsuitable for acute therapy.

Antihypertensive agents that should be avoided include angiotensin-converting enzyme inhibitors (which impair fetal renal function, and are associated with neonatal abnormalities and intrauterine deaths), diuretics (which may precipitate hypotension due to reduced intravascular volume), and diazoxide (which risks profound hypotension).

2. **Fluid management** is controversial in pre-eclampsia because, despite intravascular depletion, pulmonary oedema is a leading cause of morbidity and mortality in these patients. Fluid loading has been advocated in the past to improve urine and cardiac output and to reduce systemic vascular resistance and blood pressure, but, unfortunately, the CVP is an unreliable guide to fluid filling, and overhydration with pulmonary oedema is not uncommon. A maintenance fluid regime of 85 mL/h, aiming for a urine output of >0.5 mL/kg/h, is reasonable. However, if oliguria persists or there are signs of poor perfusion, consider invasive monitoring, and assess the response to a fluid challenge (250 mL crystalloid) whilst monitoring saturation for early signs of pulmonary oedema.

3. **Anticonvulsant therapy** is used in conjunction with antihypertensive therapy to prevent and terminate convulsions in eclampsia and severe pre-eclampsia.

- **Magnesium sulfate** is the drug of choice. In eclampsia, the efficacy of magnesium sulfate to treat and prevent recurrent seizures is well established. In pre-eclampsia, the benefit is less clear, although it is often advocated in severe cases. The mechanism of action is not established, but it appears to have CNS depressant effects, has mild antihypertensive actions, and antagonizes intracellular and membrane channel calcium, causing cerebral vasodilation. The intravenous loading dose is 4 g over 20 minutes, followed by an infusion of 1 g/h, aiming for a serum concentration of 2–3.5 mmoL/L (4.8–8.4 mg/dL). Magnesium is rapidly excreted by the kidneys, and monitoring of levels is not usually required if tendon reflexes are checked and present (toxicity is unlikely if tendon reflexes are normal). In renal impairment, doses should be reduced and serum levels monitored. In overdose, magnesium causes muscle weakness with respiratory paralysis (>7.5 mmoL/L), impaired conduction and heart block (>7.5 mmoL/L), increased susceptibility to pulmonary oedema, bleeding, and neonatal flaccidity (± respiratory depression). Magnesium toxicity is treated with small doses of calcium gluconate.

- **Other anticonvulsants (e.g. diazepam, phenytoin)** should be considered if convulsions are refractory to therapeutic magnesium levels.

4. **Early fetal delivery** may be required in severe pre-eclampsia or eclampsia. If the pregnancy is <34 weeks, betamethasone aids fetal lung maturation, with best results if delivery can be delayed for 48 h. After delivery, patients with pre-eclampsia should be closely monitored for at least 48 h, as ~40% have their first seizure after delivery, and the risk of pulmonary oedema and maternal death is greatest at this time. Magnesium should be continued for at least 24 h and antihypertensives adjusted, according to the blood pressure. Full recovery of organ dysfunction is expected within 6 weeks.

HELLP syndrome

HELLP syndrome is a form of severe pre-eclampsia, characterized by **h**aemolysis due to microangiopathic haemolytic anaemia, **e**levated **l**iver enzymes, and **l**ow **p**latelets. It is more common in white, multiparous women and usually presents preterm. Presentation is insidious, with right upper quadrant discomfort, nausea, and features of pre-eclampsia, although not all patients have hypertension or proteinuria. About 30% present post-partum, with no pre-delivery features of pre-eclampsia. Frequent complications include disseminated intravascular coagulation (DIC), acute kidney injury (AKI), pulmonary oedema, abruptio placentae, and ascites. Platelet counts and liver function tests continue to deteriorate for about 36 h after delivery, followed by gradual resolution and recovery if complications can be avoided. Following resuscitation and physiological stabilization, management usually requires early delivery, but, in some cases, expectant treatment improves neonatal and maternal outcome.

Eclampsia

Eclampsia may occur without marked hypertension or proteinuria. During seizures, protect the airway; ensure oxygenation, and terminate and prevent further fitting. Magnesium 4 g IV (no faster than 1 g/min, with further boluses to a maximum of 8 g total for repeated seizures) can be given to control seizures. Following control of seizures, maintenance magnesium should be started to prevent recurrence. Ongoing seizures may require endotracheal intubation, paralysis, and heavy sedation. A CT brain scan excludes other causes of persistent seizures (e.g. ICH, cerebral oedema), but, if present, the aim is to maintain cerebral perfusion and reduce intracranial pressure. Following maternal stabilization, early fetal delivery should be considered.

Amniotic fluid embolism (AFE)

AFE has an incidence of 1.7 per 100,000 births, with a maternal mortality of 19%. About 25–50% of deaths occur within the first hour. However, there may be many more asymptomatic mild cases. It is more common in older (>35 years old), multiparous mothers with large babies, with placenta praevia, abruptio placentae, Caesarean or forceps delivery, and during oxytocin-driven labour.

AFE occurs when amniotic fluid (± fetal matter, meconium) enters the maternal circulation. It is thought to enter through uterine or cervical lacerations or uterine veins at the site of placental separation. Factors associated with AFE include amniotomy, insertion of intrauterine pressure catheters, and placental abruption. Uterine tetany often occurs concomitantly. Prostaglandins, fetal debris, and endothelins cause inflammatory mediator and complement activation, with pulmonary vasoconstriction and occlusion.

Initial AFE diagnosis is clinical. Patients classically present with severe dyspnoea, cyanosis, hypotension (± cardiac arrest), coma, and convulsions that typically occurs during labour, delivery, or immediately post-partum, although it can occur at other times in pregnancy (e.g. amniocentesis, termination of pregnancy, abdominal trauma). Some patients present with bleeding, and most develop a coagulopathy. The early phase of the presentation lasts <30 min and is characterized by severe hypoxia and right heart failure due to pulmonary hypertension. About 50% of patients die during this early period. Patients surviving this initial phase develop seizures (~20%), DIC with bleeding (~40%), left ventricular failure and pulmonary oedema (~75%) due to the release of inflammatory mediators and tissue factors in response to amniotic fluid. Detection of squamous cells and fetal debris in pulmonary artery blood supports the diagnosis but is not specific. The differential diagnosis includes pulmonary embolism, sepsis, anaphylactic or haemorrhagic shock, air embolism, eclampsia, ICH, or local anaesthetic toxicity.

No specific therapy is available, and management is symptomatic and supportive. Immediate cardiopulmonary resuscitation with high-flow oxygen is required. This is followed by aggressive management of acute respiratory distress syndrome (ARDS), with appropriate invasive monitoring and treatment of massive obstetric haemorrhage. Early diagnosis is essential, as urgent delivery (by Caesarean section under GA if undeliverable vaginally) improves resuscitation and prevents further AFE. Patients who survive the initial resuscitation phase are at risk of ARDS and DIC and may require ongoing ventilatory support and blood component therapy to manage coagulopathy. Survivors of AFE regain normal cardiopulmonary function but may have neurological sequelae. Women who died or had permanent neurological injury were more likely to present with cardiac arrest (83% versus 33%), be from ethnic minority groups (adjusted odds ratio [OR] 2.85), have had a hysterectomy (unadjusted OR 2.49), had a shorter time interval between the AFE event and when the hysterectomy was performed, and were less likely to receive cryoprecipitate.

Severe obstetric haemorrhage

Blood loss of greater than 40% of intravascular volume (~2 L) is life-threatening. Good intravenous access is required and prompt resuscitation with warmed fluids, blood, and clotting factors. Unfortunately, underestimation of blood loss has contributed to many deaths. In life-threatening haemorrhage, compression of the aorta against the vertebral column by applying pressure above the umbilicus allows time to institute resuscitation and definitive surgical therapy. Obstetric intervention depends on the cause.

Antepartum haemorrhage (APH)

APH is bleeding from the birth canal after 20 weeks of pregnancy. The commonest causes are placental abruption (~25%) and placenta praevia (~20%). Both are managed by delivery. Uterine rupture and placental abnormalities (e.g. vasa praevia) are less common causes. Diagnosis is usually determined by ultrasound scan.

- **Placental abruption** occurs when the placenta separates from the uterine wall. Precipitating factors include hypertension, trauma, or sudden changes in uterine size, but usually there is no obvious cause. The incidence is 0.5–1.5% of pregnancies, and it is more common in smokers and older, multiparous women. Perinatal mortality can be as high as 50%. Bleeding may be concealed or revealed, and, with increasing placental separation, there is abdominal pain and tenderness. Several litres of blood may be concealed in the uterus as a retroplacental clot. Retroplacental bleeding >500 mL can cause fetal death, and >1 L results in serious maternal sequelae, with shock and DIC. Bleeding may continue after delivery due to uterine atony, placenta accreta, DIC, and traumatic lacerations.

- **Placenta praevia (PP)** affects ~1% of pregnancies, but severe haemorrhage is relatively rare. It is due to placental encroachment on the lower uterine segment (LUS); the more severe, the higher maternal morbidity and mortality. If the placenta lies over the cervical os, it is a major praevia; otherwise, it is a minor praevia. This has superseded the original clinical I–IV grading system. The LUS endometrium is less well developed, and placental attachment to underlying muscle (PP accreta) impairs separation during third stage of delivery. PP classically presents with painless vaginal bleeding in the second or third trimester of pregnancy. Significant APH may require hospitalization in later pregnancy, but management is conservative to allow fetal maturation. Delivery by Caesarean section (CS) is usually required.

Primary post-partum haemorrhage (PPH)

PPH describes blood loss of more than 500 mL within 24 h of delivery. PPH is considered severe if greater than 1 L/24 h. Table 21.2 reports risk factors for PPH, and the common causes are listed as follows:

- **Retained products of conception** complicate 4–5% of deliveries and require uterine evacuation.
- **Uterine rupture** occurs in multiparous women with previous Caesarean deliveries, fetal malpresentations, operative trauma, breech delivery, PP accreta, and those requiring oxytocin use.

Table 21.2 Risk factors for, and causes of, post-partum haemorrhage (PPH)

Risk factors	Causes
Placenta praevia	Retained products of conception
Placental abruption	Uterine atony
Pre-eclampsia	Trauma
Caesarean section	DIC
Operative delivery	Birth canal lacerations
HELLP syndrome	Uterine rupture
Previous PPH	Bleeding diathesis
Obesity	Trauma
Chorioamnionitis	

- **Uterine atony** may be due to multiparity, prolonged labour, uterine sepsis, bladder distension, or drugs (e.g. calcium antagonists). Treatments include uterine massage, bimanual compression, uterotonic drugs, and insertion of intrauterine compression balloons. Severe haemorrhage may require uterine artery embolization or surgical intervention with insertion of a uterine compression suture, internal iliac artery ligation, or, occasionally, hysterectomy. Uterotonic drugs initially administered are ergometrine (maximum 500 mcg but avoided in women with hypertension or cardiac disease) and a oxytocin infusion (40–50 IU in 500 mL normal saline over 4 hours). Second-line agents are carboprost, a prostaglandin F_2-alpha (0.25 mg intramuscularly every 15–30 min, up to a maximum of 2 mg, avoided in asthmatics), and misoprostol 600 mcg orally or rectally.

- **Coagulation defects** with PPH follow massive loss of blood, pre-eclampsia or eclampsia, amniotic fluid embolism, and intrauterine death or sepsis.

Secondary PPH

Secondary PPH describes severe bleeding >24 h post-partum until the end of the puerperium. It is often due to infected retained products of conception and is treated with antibiotics and uterine evacuation.

Sheehan's syndrome is panhypopituitarism, following pituitary hypoperfusion, due to severe obstetric haemorrhage. Failure of lactation and amenorrhoea are early features. Adrenal and thyroid gland failure follows.

Further reading

Abenhaim HA, Azoulay L, Kramer MS, Leduc L (2008). Incidence and risk factors of amniotic fluid embolisms: a population-based study on 3 million births in the United States. *American Journal of Obstetrics & Gynecology*, **199**, 49.e1–8.

Department of Health (2007). Maternity matters: choice, access and continuity of care in a safe service. Department of Health, London. <http://www.familieslink.co.uk/download/july07/Maternity%20matters.pdf>.

Duley L, Henderson-Smart DJ (2001). Magnesium sulphate versus phenytoin for eclampsia (Cochrane review). In *The Cochrane Library*, Oxford.

Fitzpatrick K, Tuffnell D, Kurinczuk J, Knight M (2015). Incidence, risk factors, management and outcomes of amniotic-fluid embolism: a population-based cohort and nested case control study. *BJOG*, Feb 12. doi: 10.1111/1471-0528.13300. [Epub ahead of print.]

Knight, M, on behalf of UKOSS (2007). Eclampsia in the United Kingdom 2005. *BJOG*, **114**, 1072–1078.

Knight M, Kenyon S, Brocklehurst P, Neilson J, Shakespeare J, Kurinczuk JJ (eds.) on behalf of MBRRACE-UK (2014). Saving Lives, Improving Mothers' Care - Lessons learned to inform future maternity care from the UK and Ireland Confidential Enquiries into Maternal Deaths and Morbidity 2009–12. Oxford: National Perinatal Epidemiology Unit, University of Oxford, pp. 81–87.

National Institute for Health and Care Excellence (2010). Hypertension in pregnancy: The management of hypertensive disorders during pregnancy. NICE clinical guideline 107 <http://publications.nice.org.uk/hypertension-in-pregnancy-cg107/>.

Royal College of Obstetricians and Gynaecologists (2015). Thromboembolic Disease in Pregnancy and the Puerperium: Acute Management. Guideline no. 37b. RCOG Press, London.

World Health Organization (2004). Beyond the numbers—reviewing maternal deaths and complications to make pregnancy safer. World Health Organization, Geneva. <http://whqlibdoc.who.int/publications/2004/9241591838.pdf>.

Medical emergencies in pregnancy

Introduction

Obstetric patients may present with a full range of medical and surgical problems (see Table 21.3). It is important that women with pre-existing medical disease are counselled before pregnancy because the risk to both them and their fetus may be considerable. Nevertheless, acute physicians must be familiar with the specific requirements pertinent to the management of medical disorders in pregnancy. The golden rules are:

- The mother must take priority over the baby.
- Remember to tilt the mother on her side to reduce aortocaval compression.
- Trust your medical instincts, but remember that pulmonary hypertension from whatever cause is extremely dangerous in pregnancy.
- Never withhold essential investigations. Chest X-rays, V/Q scans, CT pulmonary angiograms, and MRIs are safe.
- Do not withhold lifesaving treatments. Steroids, thrombolysis, and most drugs are safe (see Table 21.4). The dose of low molecular weight heparin (LMWH) is higher (1 mg/kg twice daily; equivalent to the acute coronary syndrome (ACS) dose). However, first-trimester exposure to angiotensin-converting enzyme (ACE) inhibitors is associated with an increased risk of major congenital malformation (odds ratio (OR) 2.7), especially of the cardiovascular (OR 3.7) and central nervous (OR 4.4) systems.
- If in doubt about a drug or investigation, ask an obstetrician.
- Work in multidisciplinary teams with the obstetrician and obstetric anaesthetist.

Table 21.3 Medical problems in pregnancy

Pre-existing	Pregnancy-specific
Asthma	Pre-eclampsia/eclampsia
Epilepsy	Thromboembolism
Hypertension	Gestational diabetes
Diabetes	Obstetric cholestasis
Thyrotoxicosis	Hyperemesis gravidarum
Renal	Acute fatty liver of pregnancy
Cardiac	

Table 21.4 Drugs that are safe and not safe in pregnancy

Safe	Not safe
Asthma drugs (e.g. prednisolone, salbutamol, theophyllines)	Non-steroidal anti-inflammatory drugs (but safe in 1st and 2nd trimesters)
Anti epileptic drugs (teratogenic)	Tetracycline
Antithyroid drugs	ACE inhibitors
Diabetic drugs (insulin, sulfonylureas, and metformin)	Angiotensin II receptor blockers
Most antibiotics (e.g. penicillins, cephalosporins, gentamicin)	Statins
LMWH	Cyclophosphamide
Antiemetics	Mycophenolate mofetil
Some antihypertensives (eg. Ca²⁺ antagonists, beta-blockers)	Sirolimus (INN)
Immunosuppressants (e.g. ciclosporin, tacrolimus, azathioprine)	Warfarin

Cardiac disease in pregnancy

Heart disease is the commonest cause of all maternal deaths. In some pre-existing cardiac conditions (e.g. Eisenmenger syndrome), the mortality associated with pregnancy can be 25–40%, even with optimal management. The important physiological changes of pregnancy that impact on patients with cardiac disease are the increased blood volume (40%) and cardiac output (45%) by the 20th week of gestation, with a further 50% increase in cardiac output during labour, the reduction in systemic vascular resistance (SVR), and the susceptibility to aortocaval compression. Heart failure ensues in patients unable to achieve these changes. Similarly, the fall in SVR encourages blood to bypass the lung in patients with right-to-left shunts, and, when combined with the associated fetal demands and reduced maternal pulmonary reserve, there is a significant risk of severe hypoxaemia.

Antepartum management of pre-existing heart disease aims to reduce cardiac workload by reducing physical activity in severe heart disease, optimizing afterload reduction, and treating arrhythmias. Echocardiography is the mainstay of serial assessment. Antithrombotic prophylaxis with LMWH is particularly important in those at increased risk of thromboembolism, even without enforced bed rest. Peripartum, a well-controlled vaginal delivery, with regional low-dose epidural analgesia (0.1% bupivacaine ± fentanyl), is considered less stressful and is preferred to Caesarean section unless indicated for obstetric indications. Bolus oxytocin, which has marked cardiovascular effects and may cause tachycardia, increased shunt, and catastrophic hypotension, is best avoided in these patients. If oxytocin is required a slow dilute, low dose infusion is preferred. Peripartum complications, including bleeding, drug-induced hypotension (e.g. oxytocin), arrhythmias, infection, pulmonary oedema, and increased pulmonary vascular resistance are particularly poorly tolerated by these patients.

In the post-partum period, cardiac patients are at particular risk of pulmonary embolism and PPH if oxytocin has been withheld. Patients with significant pulmonary hypertension are typically at risk of death within the first week after delivery. Potential chest and wound infections should be detected and treated early.

Cardiac arrest

Cardiac arrest affects 1 in 30,000 pregnancies. In late pregnancy, the role of obstetric emergencies (e.g. AFE), drug toxicity (e.g. magnesium sulphate), and fetal viability must be considered. During resuscitation, the advanced life support (ALS) drug and defibrillation protocols should be followed. However, after 20 weeks' gestation, it becomes increasingly important to alleviate aortocaval compression which impairs venous return during basic life support. Consequently, chest compressions are performed, with a wedge (~25° angle) below the right hip or manual uterine displacement to prevent caval compression. Early intubation prevents hypoxaemia due to the associated diaphragmatic splinting and increased oxygen consumption. In advanced gestation, both maternal and fetal survival during cardiac arrest may depend on immediate fetal delivery by Caesarean section to relieve the effects of aortocaval compression. In addition, if there is no immediate maternal response to ALS, perimortem Caesarean delivery should be considered to aid maternal resuscitation. However, the decision must be made promptly, as the baby should be delivered within 5 minutes of the onset of the arrest, and resuscitation should be continued until after delivery. Gastric compression makes aspiration a significant risk during resuscitation.

Myocardial infarction/acute coronary syndrome (MI/ACS)
MI/ACS is rare during pregnancy. Nevertheless, not all chest pain and breathlessness in pregnancy is due to pulmonary embolism, and the diagnosis of MI/ACS should be considered and excluded, especially in pregnant women with risk factors (especially smoking and diabetes) and chest discomfort. In these cases, the aetiology is more likely (than outside pregnancy) to be non-atherosclerotic coronary artery thrombosis or dissection. Aspirin, clopidogrel, beta-blockers, and LMWH can be used as normal. Thrombolysis (intravenous, intracoronary), percutaneous coronary angioplasty, and stents are also safe in pregnancy. In contrast, statins and glycoprotein IIb/IIIa receptor inhibitors should be avoided. MI/ACS is rare in pregnancy, with an incidence of 6.2 per 100,000 deliveries and a maternal mortality of 5.1–7.3%. It is more common in older women (>30 years old) with diabetes mellitus, hypertension, eclampsia, and a previous smoking history.

Pulmonary thromboembolism (PTE)
PTE causes 12% of maternal deaths and affects ~1 in 1,000 pregnancies. Pregnancy is associated with a fivefold increase in thromboembolism due to venous stasis, hypercoagulability, and injury to the blood vessels during delivery. Caval compression by the gravid uterus also predisposes to antepartum lower limb and pelvic vein thrombosis, and mobilization immediately after delivery may subsequently precipitate pulmonary embolism (PE). Deep venous thrombosis (DVT) during pregnancy affects the left leg in 85%, and the iliofemoral veins in 72%, of cases (55% and 9%, respectively in non-pregnant patients).

Accurate diagnosis of suspected DVT and PE is essential in patients with chest pain, breathlessness, or swollen calves, in view of the need for prolonged therapy. D-dimers are of little or no use in pregnancy, and DVT diagnosis is best achieved using Doppler ultrasound. Perfusion lung scanning and CT pulmonary angiography may be required to establish the diagnosis of PE and should not be avoided, if necessary.

LMWH has replaced unfractionated heparin for the prophylaxis and treatment of DVT and PE in pregnancy due to a low incidence of side effects, ease of administration, and reduced need for monitoring. Warfarin is best avoided in pregnancy. Pregnant patients with proven DVT or PE or who require anticoagulation (e.g. metal cardiac valves) should be given LMWH (e.g. enoxaparin 1 mg/kg twice daily) throughout pregnancy (i.e. higher than the usual dose of 1.5 mg/kg once daily and equivalent to an ACS dose). Heparin is continued until labour begins and restarted in the post-partum patient for at least 6 weeks. Patients at high risk of thrombosis (e.g. thrombophilia and previous thrombosis on long-term warfarin) are treated with LMWH 0.5 mg/kg twice daily. Prophylaxis in low-risk patients of normal weight is with LMWH 40 mg once daily.

Thrombolysis is required during pregnancy for massive life-threatening PTE with haemodynamic compromise. It was previously thought to be contraindicated due to the risk of maternal and fetal haemorrhagic complications. However, reviews of cases of thrombolytic therapy in pregnancy report bleeding rates similar to those in the non-pregnant population.

Pulmonary hypertension (PHT)
PHT is associated with approximately 25% maternal mortality. The fixed pulmonary vascular resistance results in an inability to increase pulmonary blood flow and refractory hypoxaemia. Most deaths in patients with PHT are attributed to PTE, hypovolaemia, or pre-eclampsia. Non-alienating pre-pregnancy counselling about pregnancy avoidance and the need for effective contraception is essential in these at-risk PHT patients. The possibility of termination should be seriously considered if pregnancy occurs.

Respiratory disease in pregnancy
The physiological effects of pregnancy on the respiratory system include diaphragmatic splinting, reduced functional residual capacity, increased oxygen demand, and the stimulus to hyperventilate. These add an extra burden to ventilation that may precipitate respiratory failure in pregnant patients with pre-existing respiratory impairment. Pneumonia and asthma are the commonest respiratory problems in pregnancy. Cystic fibrosis is rare but is more likely to be associated with a poor outcome due to the risks of infection, respiratory failure, and poor nutrition. In mild cystic fibrosis, mortality is not increased during pregnancy but is 5% at 2 years and 10–20% within 5 years.

Regional analgesia is indicated in patients with significant respiratory impairment, as this reduces the demands of labour and may decrease the risk of pulmonary complications after Caesarean section. However, ventilation and the ability to cough may be impaired if epidural anaesthesia extends too high or if post-operative pain limits inspiration. Non-invasive ventilation (NIV) may be considered in patients with respiratory fatigue or failure to avoid the need for endotracheal intubation and mechanical ventilation. The respiratory benefits of delivery on oxygenation and ventilation are usually immediate, although post-operative pain, following Caesarean section, may limit inspiration and encourages atelectasis.

Asthma
Asthma improves in one-third of pregnant asthmatic women, deteriorates in one-third, and is unchanged in a third. Severe asthma is more likely to deteriorate than mild asthma, but the course is similar in successive pregnancies. Suggested causes for this variation in asthma control include changes in maternal hormones and beta-2-adrenoreceptor responsiveness and alterations in immune function.

The risk of low birthweight babies increases twofold in mothers with asthma exacerbations during pregnancy (i.e. similar to smoking during pregnancy), but rates of preterm delivery or pre-eclampsia do not increase. The risk factors for acute exacerbations during pregnancy are severe asthma prior to pregnancy, inappropriate discontinuation of inhaled corticosteroid (ICS) therapy, and increased susceptibility to viral infection. Exacerbations can occur at any time but predominantly late in the second trimester. Acute attacks are rare during labour due to endogenous steroid production.

The British Thoracic Society guidelines (2014) advise the normal use of beta-2-agonists, theophyllines, ICS, and oral steroids in stable and acute exacerbations of asthma. The maternal and fetal risks of poorly controlled asthma outweigh the small risks from therapy. Unfortunately, many expectant mothers reduce their ICS (~23%), beta-agonists (~13%), and rescue oral steroids (~54%) during pregnancy.

In addition, clinicians undertreat acute exacerbations and are less likely to provide appropriate oral steroid therapy, resulting in persistent poor asthma control. Oral steroids and nebulized bronchodilators are used at standard doses. Leukotriene antagonists should be continued in those who have failed to achieve control with other agents in the past.

Acute asthma is unusual during labour due to the associated high sympathetic drive. Patients on more than 7.5 mg of oral steroid daily, for longer than 2 weeks prior to delivery, should be given intravenous hydrocortisone 50–100 mg 8-hourly during labour. Prostaglandin E_2 can be safely used to induce labour, but prostaglandin F_2-alpha for post-partum haemorrhage may induce bronchospasm. Regional anaesthetic blockade (e.g. epidural anaesthesia) is preferable to general anaesthesia in women with asthma.

Breastfeeding may reduce the incidence of atopy in the children of asthmatic mothers and should be strongly encouraged. Even when the mother is on high-dose prednisolone, which is secreted in breast milk, the infant is only exposed to small, and clinically irrelevant, doses.

Acute lung injury

Acute respiratory distress syndrome (ARDS), due to gastric acid aspiration, is a particular risk in pregnancy due to reduced gastric emptying, increased intra-abdominal pressure, and increased gastric acidity. Chemical pneumonitis and pulmonary oedema develop over several hours, and patients present with breathlessness, hypoxaemia, bronchospasm, and progressive chest X-ray infiltrates. Treatment is supportive, with supplemental oxygen, ventilatory support, antibiotic therapy that covers gastric anaerobes (e.g. co-amoxiclav) and, occasionally, bronchoscopy to remove particulate matter. Steroids are not beneficial.

Neurological disease in pregnancy

Intracranial bleeding

Intracranial bleeding causes ~10% of maternal deaths. It is associated with pre-eclampsia and eclampsia, uncontrolled hypertension, primary cerebrovascular accidents, and subarachnoid haemorrhage.

Epilepsy

Epilepsy now causes more maternal deaths than eclampsia. The differential diagnosis of seizures in pregnancy includes eclampsia, epilepsy, cerebrovascular accidents, subarachnoid haemorrhage, ICH, cerebral venous thrombosis, meningitis, drug (or alcohol) withdrawal, hypoglycaemia and thrombotic thrombocytopenic purpura. A first seizure during pregnancy that cannot readily be attributed to eclampsia or epilepsy warrants investigation with CT or MRI scan of the brain. Poor gestational control of epilepsy is thought to be due to poor concordance with therapy and altered pharmacokinetics of anticonvulsant drugs during pregnancy.

Myasthenia gravis

Myasthenia gravis may be associated with respiratory problems and requires regular medication throughout labour and after delivery. This can be difficult, as gastric emptying is decreased during labour and further impaired with opioid analgesia. Alternative routes of drug administration should be considered. Equivalent doses of 15 mg oral neostigmine are 1 mg when given intramuscularly and 0.5 mg when given intravenously. Similarly, 60 mg oral pyridostigmine equates to 4 mg via the intramuscular and 2 mg via the intravenous routes. Epidural analgesia limits maternal fatigue during

labour, but careful observation is required for 7–10 days post-partum for signs of increasing weakness.

Psychiatric disease and drug addiction

Suicide, parasuicide, violence, and drug addiction are all common causes of maternal morbidity and mortality. Pregnant patients are more susceptible to psychiatric disease during, and particularly after, pregnancy when postnatal depression can be a serious issue and requires early involvement of psychiatric support. Drug abuse raises the same issues as in the non-pregnant population, with the additional problems of HIV, hepatitis B and C infection, fetal addiction, and growth restriction.

Cocaine abuse

Cocaine abuse during pregnancy is a significant problem in the USA and may affect 5% of expectant mothers in some populations. Cocaine causes maternal hypertension, tachycardia, increased cardiac output, and ACS. It also reduces uterine blood flow and increases uterine contractility. Patients frequently present with placental abruption and fetal distress. Acute toxicity may mimic pre-eclampsia by presenting with convulsions and ICH. Labetalol is the antihypertensive treatment of choice, although hydralazine, calcium antagonists, and nitrates have also been advocated.

Systemic and metabolic disease in pregnancy

Diabetes mellitus

Diabetes mellitus is the most important pre-existing metabolic disease in pregnancy and increases both maternal and fetal morbidity. Regular review by diabetic physicians and tight glycaemic control improves outcome. Gestational diabetes has a similar pathophysiology to type 2 diabetes mellitus and usually occurs in the last trimester of pregnancy. Not surprisingly, 30–50% of these patients develop overt type 2 diabetes within 10 years.

Biochemical thyrotoxicosis

Biochemical thyrotoxicosis (i.e. raised free T3 and free T4 and suppressed TSH) occurs in hyperemesis gravidarum (HG) due to human chorionic gonadotrophin (hCG) mediated stimulation of the thyroid. Abnormal thyroid function tests occur in 60% of patients with HG and correlate with the severity of the HG and hCG levels. Oestradiol levels are also increased in HG, compared to controls. It does not require antithyroid drug treatment and resolves with treatment of the HG. True hyperthyroidism is suggested by a history preceding pregnancy, eye signs, goitre, and positive thyroid receptor antibodies.

Abnormal liver function tests (LFTs)

Abnormal LFTs are detected in ~25% of patients with HG, with a moderate increase in transaminases (<200 IU/L). Bilirubin is slightly raised, and jaundice is rare. Raised LFTs are a marker of severe HG, but the differential diagnosis includes other pregnancy-induced liver diseases, including obstetric cholestasis, pre-eclampsia, HELLP syndrome, and acute fatty liver of pregnancy. Incidental causes of liver disease in pregnancy include viral hepatitis, drug hepatotoxicity (e.g. methyldopa), sepsis, cholelithiasis, and exacerbation of pre-existing liver disease, including chronic active hepatitis, primary biliary cirrhosis, and sclerosing cholangitis.

Sepsis and septic shock

Sepsis and septic shock are rare complications of maternal infections (e.g. urinary tract infections, pyelonephritis, pneumonia, septic abortion, post-partum endometritis). Increased susceptibility to endotoxin in pregnancy increases the risk of cardiovascular collapse. The commonest organisms are Gram-negative coliforms, but streptococci and bacteroides may be involved. Appropriate antibiotics in pregnancy include ampicillin, amoxicillin, co-amoxiclav, cefuroxime, clarithromycin, gentamicin, imipenem, vancomycin, and clindamycin. Tetracyclines and quinolones should not be used.

Connective tissue disease
Connective tissue disease (e.g. systemic lupus erythematosus, systemic sclerosis) patients may be less well due to the increased cardiac and pulmonary demands during pregnancy. The risk of obstetric complications is also increased in these patients.

Trauma in pregnancy
Trauma occurs in 5–7% of pregnancies, but hospital admission is rarely required. Less than 1% of all trauma admissions are in pregnant women. Nevertheless, head injuries and haemorrhagic shock, often due to road traffic accidents, are leading causes of non-obstetric maternal mortality. Traumatic placental abruption and maternal death are the commonest cause of fetal death. Initial post-traumatic resuscitation follows the same protocols as in non-pregnant patients but with the mother on a tilt. Hypotension does not occur until >35% blood loss due to pregnancy-associated increase in blood volume, but, because uterine blood flow is not autoregulated, uterine underperfusion may occur despite normal maternal haemodynamics. Consequently, overhydration is preferable to underhydration in these cases. Abdominal trauma with pelvic fractures carries increased risk of uterine injury and retroperitoneal bleeding in pregnancy. Herniation of abdominal contents through a ruptured diaphragm should also be excluded.

Radiological investigations must be performed, as necessary, as the radiation risk to the fetus is small, except in the first trimester when exposure to >100 mGy is a cause for concern. A chest X-ray delivers <0.05 mGy to the lungs and even less to the shielded abdomen. A pelvic X-ray is 1 mGy and an abdominal pelvic CT scan 10–20 mGy. Ultrasound is often used initially. When necessary, diagnostic peritoneal lavage is performed through an incision above the fundus.

In pregnant patients with thoracic trauma and injury, chest drains are placed slightly higher than normal in the third and fourth intercostal spaces. Ideally, the fetus should be monitored with cardiotocography intermittently if appropriate, for 6–24 h to detect potential preterm labour and placental abruption. Anti-D Rh immune globulin (500 mcg) should also be considered and given within 72 h of the injury in Rh D-negative women.

Further reading
Aherne GS, Hadjiliadis D, Govert JA, Tapson VF (2002). Massive pulmonary embolism during pregnancy successfully treated with recombinant tissue plasminogen activator: a case report and review of treatment options. *Archives of Internal Medicine*, **162**, 1221–7.

Asthma in Pregnancy (2014). In: British Thoracic Society (BTS)/ Scottish Intercollegiate Guideline Network (SIGN) guidelines on Asthma. *Thorax*, **69**, i1–i192.

Bedard E, Dimopoulos K, Gatzoulis MA (2009). Has there been any progress made on pregnancy outcomes among women with pulmonary arterial hypertension? *European Heart Journal*, **30**, 256–65.

Cooper WO, Hernandez-Diaz S, Arbogast PG, et al. (2006). Major congenital malformations after first trimester exposure to ACE inhibitors. *New England Journal of Medicine*, **354**, 2443–51.

Cydulka RK, Emerman CL, Schreiber D, Molander KH, Woodruff PG, Camargo CA (1999). Acute asthma among pregnant women presenting to the emergency department. *American Journal of Respiratory and Critical Care Medicine*, **160**, 887–92.

Department of Health (2007). Maternity matters: choice, access and continuity of care in a safe service. Department of Health, London. <http://www.familieslink.co.uk/download/july07/ Maternity%20matters.pdf>.

Edenborough FP, Borgo G, Knoop C, et al. (2008). Guidelines for the management of pregnancy in women with cystic fibrosis. *Journal of Cystic Fibrosis*, **7**, (Suppl 1), S2–S32.

ESC Guidelines on the management of cardiovascular diseases during pregnancy: The Task Force on the Management of Cardiovascular Diseases during Pregnancy of the European Society of Cardiology (ESC). *Eur Heart J*, **32**, 3147–3197.

Kiely DG, Condliffe R, Wilson VJ, Gandhi SV, Elliot CA (2013). Pregnancy and pulmonary hypertension. *Obstetric Medicine*, **6**, 144–154.

Knight M, Kenyon S, Brocklehurst P, Neilson J, Shakespeare J, Kurinczuk JJ (eds) on behalf of MBRRACE-UK (2014). Saving Lives, Improving Mothers' Care - Lessons learned to inform future maternity care from the UK and Ireland Confidential Enquiries into Maternal Deaths and Morbidity 2009–12. Oxford: National Perinatal Epidemiology Unit, University of Oxford, pp. 81–87.

Royal College of Obstetricians and Gynaecologists (2015). Reducing the Risks of Thrombosis and Embolism During Pregnancy and the Puerperium. Guideline no. 37a. RCOG Press, London.

Royal College of Obstetricians and Gynaecologists (2015). Thromboembolic Disease in Pregnancy and the Puerperium: Acute Management. Guideline no. 37b. RCOG Press, London.

Shah KH, Simons RK, Holbrook T, et al. (1998). Trauma in pregnancy: maternal and fetal outcomes. *Journal of Trauma*, **45**, 83–6.

The Task Force on the Management of Cardiovascular Diseases during Pregnancy of the European Society of Cardiology (ESC) (2014). ESC Guidelines on the management of cardiovascular diseases during pregnancy. *European Heart Journal*, **32**, 3147–3197.

World Health Organization (2004). Beyond the numbers—reviewing maternal deaths and complications to make pregnancy safer. World Health Organization, Geneva. <http://whqlibdoc.who. int/publications/2004/9241591838.pdf>.

Chapter 22

Ethics and
end of life issues

Ethics and end of life issues

Ethics is the science of moral behaviour and examines theories that attempt to determine right from wrong. Medical ethics usually refers to decisions regarding patient care but also applies to individual behaviour ('professionalism') and the management of medical practice. The international code of medical ethics, a modern day Hippocratic oath, is documented in Box 22.1.

Medical ethics is increasingly important because of rapid medical advances, escalating costs, the impact of 'rationing', with restricted availability of some therapies, and an increasingly knowledgeable and demanding public.

Ethical and moral principles
The primary aim of medicine is the welfare of the patient. It is achieved by maintaining the highest standards of clinical management, teaching, and research. However, these goals may, at times, conflict with personal beliefs, financial interests, and workload pressure. Ethical principles provide a framework for reasoning and analysis which help the physician in making difficult decisions.

- **Respect for autonomy** is the right of the patient to make informed choices and to decide on their subsequent medical treatment. It contrasts with paternalism in which 'the doctor knows best'.
- **Beneficence** is the principle of doing good and acting in the best interest of the patient. This implies an obligation to preserve life or to strive to cure the patient, moderated by the need to relieve pain and suffering.
- **Non-maleficence** is the duty not to do harm to patients or members of the healthcare team.
- **Professional virtue or fidelity** is the requirement to fulfil duties and obligations, ensure patient care, maintain confidentiality, be compassionate, preserve integrity, tell the truth, and keep up with medical knowledge (i.e. continued professional development).
- **Social justice** is the right of patients to be fairly treated and entitled to medical care, according to medical need.
- **Utility** describes the fair allocation of medical resources. It aims to achieve the maximum benefit for the largest number of people and society, without wasting resources.

These basic principles have continued to evolve and be refined to improve modern healthcare. The multidisciplinary 'Tavistock principles' are the most recent proposals and were developed to encompass all healthcare professionals and to encourage individual professions to work together in addressing ethical issues (see Box 22.2).

Duty of care
The **'duty of care'** expected from medical professionals has been documented by many statutory bodies, including the American Medical Association and the General Medical Council (UK). However, legal requirements, which vary between states, are often entangled with ethical issues and guidelines, and, in some circumstances, the law may take precedence. These conflicts often occur during decisions related to consent, confidentiality, and withdrawal of life-maintaining therapy.

Where doubt exists, the physician should seek the advice of trusted colleagues, institutional ethical committees, and professional bodies. The physician's personal beliefs and values should be assessed in relation to the often diverse

---

Box 22.1 International code of medical ethics

I solemnly pledge myself to consecrate my life to the service of humanity.
I will give my teachers the respect and gratitude which is their due.
I will practise my profession with conscience and dignity.
The health of my patient will be my first consideration.
I will respect the secrets which are confided in me, even after the patient has died.
I will maintain by all means in my power, the honour and the noble traditions of the medical profession.
My colleagues will be my brothers and sisters.
I will not permit considerations of age, disease or disability, creed, ethnic origin, gender, nationality, political affiliation, race, sexual orientation, or social standing to intervene between my duty and my patient.
I will maintain the utmost respect for human life from its beginning even under threat and I will not use my medical knowledge contrary to the laws of humanity
I make these promises solemnly, freely and upon my honour.

Reproduced with permission from WMA Declaration of Geneva available at http://www.wma.net/en/30publications/10policies/g1/. Accessed 21st May 2014. Copyright, World Medical Association. All Rights Reserved.

Box 22.2 The Tavistock principles

Rights. People have right to health and health care
Balance. Care of individual patients is central, but the health of populations is also our concern
Comprehensiveness. In addition to treating illness, we have an obligation to ease suffering, minimize disability, prevent disease and promote health
Cooperation. Healthcare succeeds only if we cooperate with those we serve, each other, and those in other sectors
Improvement. Improving health care is a serious and continuing responsibility
Safety. Do no harm
Openness. Being open, honest, and trustworthy is vital in health care

Reproduced from British Medical Journal, Berwick D et al., 'Redefining and implementing the Tavistock Principles for everybody in health care', 323, pp. 616–620, Copyright 2001, with permission from BMJ Publishing Group Ltd.

---

views held about these issues in multicultural societies. Consultation with the family, nurses, and other healthcare personnel is always good practice. It may help to refer to state legislation, case-based consensus outcomes, and the guidelines set out by professional bodies like the General Medical Council in the UK. In difficult cases, seeking a legal opinion is usually a wise precaution.

Principles of consent
During all medical care, 'consent' is a legal and moral requirement and underpins the relationship between physician and patient. The basic principles of consent are that:
- Consent must be obtained on every occasion that a physician wishes to initiate treatment, except in emergencies.
- The physician must provide sufficient information about the intervention, including both the risks and benefits, such that the patient can make an informed choice.
- Patient consent must be voluntary and without pressure.

- 'Consent forms' provide the written evidence of consent discussions. Ideally, consent is a two-part process, in which the intervention is discussed in advance to allow the patient time to consider, discuss, and question potential options. At this stage, the use of pamphlets, which report the potential benefits and risks of the procedure, describe the intervention (including type of sedation) and indicate the pre- and post-procedure requirements (e.g. fasting prior to bronchoscopy, endoscopy, or surgery and the potential need for a relative to accompany the patient home afterwards), is recommended. The final written document is completed by the physician or healthcare professional delivering the intervention after further discussion and when outstanding queries have been addressed.
- Consent does not always need to be in writing unless required by a local authority. Nevertheless, verbal consent should always be recorded in the notes.
- Competent patients may refuse consent to treatment, even if doing so may result in death.
- Consent is required when testing for hepatitis B and C, HIV, and some other conditions (e.g. genetic tests), depending on jurisdiction. Consent is required, even in the unconscious patient or if a member of staff has sustained a needle-stick injury.
- In emergencies, when a patient is unable to give consent or if the healthcare giver is unaware of previous 'consent' decisions (e.g. advance directives), treatment should be provided that is necessary to save life or prevent deterioration.
- Incompetent patients may be treated without consent in some circumstances and jurisdictions if this is in the patient's best interests. For example, a proxy or surrogate may give consent on behalf of an incompetent adult patient. However, the surrogate cannot demand treatment that is judged not to be in the patient's best interests. Surrogates, in order of priority, are partners, adult children, parents, and nearest living relatives.
- An enduring power of attorney can make decisions on a patient's financial affairs but normally has no legal right to consent to treatment.
- Consent is required for teaching (i.e. photographs, practical procedures) and research purposes. Research consent forms and protocols should be used.
- Competent minors may, or may not, have the right to consent to, or refuse, treatment, and legal age varies, depending on the jurisdiction. Otherwise, parents or a person of local authority with parental responsibility may give consent. Although parental involvement should be encouraged, a competent minor's request for confidentiality should be respected.

Confidentiality

Patient confidentiality is a legal and moral responsibility for all healthcare staff. Stored information should be accurate, updated, and protected against unauthorized access. Recorded patient information should be necessary for patient care and may only be used or disclosed for the purpose for which it was collected. Disclosure of information to a third party requires patient consent. In the case of information relating to incompetent adult patients or minors, consent should be obtained from an authorized third party. Use of patient information for research, audit, or quality assurance requires consent, unless the data are anonymous.

Advance directives

Some competent patients may choose to state their preferred treatment choices in the event of subsequent incapacity in an advance directive. This may be a written document, witnessed oral statement, or recorded discussion. For example, an advance directive may give clear instructions on refusing blood transfusion or 'life support' (e.g. mechanical ventilation). Inevitably, these so-called 'living wills' are made without knowing the nature of future illness or whether such events will transpire. As a consequence, they are often imprecise and may have unintended consequences. For example, refusal of 'life support' may prevent lifesaving therapy in potentially reversible conditions like sepsis or diabetic ketoacidosis. Nevertheless, all physicians must be aware that:

- They may be legally liable if they disregard an advance directive, except in cases where refusal may harm others (e.g. spread of infection) or conflicts with local jurisdiction.
- Relatives and surrogates cannot overrule an advance directive.
- Preferences that do not refuse treatment should be respected but are not legally binding.
- Demands for futile treatment have no legal force.
- An advance directive can be superseded by a contemporaneous decision by a competent patient.

End of life decisions

Acute medicine is often lifesaving, and, although some cases do not make a complete recovery, they achieve a quality of life which, although impaired, is tolerable for that patient. Unfortunately, in some cases, treatment prolongs the dying process or results in an unacceptable long-term quality of life, with unnecessary suffering, loss of dignity, and undue emotional distress.

In emergency situations, it is often impossible to identify individuals who will not benefit from therapy. In these patients, humane and cost-effective management requires a willingness to limit or withdraw therapy when it becomes clear that the prognosis is poor and that ongoing therapy is not in the patient's best interests. These decisions are often difficult and based on the accepted ethical, moral, and legal principles described previously. Nevertheless, interpretation of these principles varies, according to an individual's political, personal, and religious beliefs, and is subject to the influence of organizations with fixed ideals (e.g. voluntary euthanasia, right-to-life groups), irresponsible public media, and public misconceptions, all of which can make these decisions exceptionally difficult. End of life decisions can be considered in terms of the following:

Euthanasia

Euthanasia is defined as 'a direct action, in which the primary intent is to terminate life'. There are three categories of euthanasia: 'voluntary euthanasia' (i.e. deliberate killing of a patient who has made a competent decision to end their life), physician-assisted suicide, and 'non-voluntary euthanasia' (i.e. by agreement of all parties, except the patient).

In most jurisdictions, euthanasia of all types is illegal, although some countries sanction 'voluntary euthanasia'. It is important to recognize that withholding or withdrawal of therapy is not considered euthanasia, as a 'direct action' does not occur and the primary intent is not to kill. In the same way, liberal doses of opioid in the terminally ill patient may hasten death due to respiratory depression, but this is not considered euthanasia, as the primary intent is to alleviate suffering and pain, rather than to kill (i.e. the 'double effect' doctrine).

Euthanasia is the subject of considerable debate. Advocates argue that it is morally justified, as the ultimate outcome is in the best interests of the patient (i.e. reduced suffering), respects the autonomy of the patient, and because there is no moral difference between allowing a patient to die on request and killing on request. Opponents of euthanasia fear that, if society allows euthanasia, it may be unable to protect against 'non-voluntary euthanasia' in the elderly and those with end-stage debilitating disease. There is also the potential concern that the trust between patient and doctor may be damaged.

Withholding and withdrawal of treatment

When death is inevitable, allowing a patient to die by withholding therapy that will not confer benefit or withdrawing failed treatment is not considered euthanasia, as the primary intent is not to cause death. The public, some clinicians, and local jurisdiction may differentiate between withdrawing and withholding therapy, but there is no moral difference. Patients with brainstem death (BSD) are legally dead, and the prognostic certainty of death relieves anxiety associated with treatment discontinuation.

However, the situation can be more complex when death is not imminent. Prolonged self-ventilated survival without cognitive function is possible when the brainstem is intact, but cortical function ceases due to ischaemic damage (e.g. prolonged cardiac arrest) or diffuse cerebral injury (e.g. head trauma). This situation is termed 'persistent vegetative state'. In these patients, withholding or withdrawing therapy decisions may be difficult because there is often prognostic uncertainty. Previous ethical and medico-legal deliberations recommend that decision-making should focus on 'the likelihood of return to cognitive function' and suggest that life-sustaining therapy should be withdrawn when it is clear that the patient is 'unlikely to regain cognitive behaviour, the ability to communicate, or purposeful environmental interaction'. In these circumstances, most authorities agree that treatment, other than basic medical and nursing care, is inappropriate.

In severely disabled patients, ethical dilemmas can be particularly complicated. It is important to appreciate that a rational patient, or legal surrogate, has the right to refuse treatment, even if this includes discontinuation of mechanical ventilation. Conversely, patients cannot demand lifesaving therapy when clinicians consider it inappropriate.

In practice, many patients cannot discuss treatment. In these cases, the senior physician is responsible for the decision to withdraw or withhold therapy and must review any such judgements made by other staff. These decisions are usually made in consultation with the family, taking into account prognosis, benefits, expected quality of life, the opinions of the wider medical team (e.g. nursing staff), and the patient's previously expressed views (e.g. advance directives). It should be recognized that medical staff often underestimate a patient's willingness to undergo treatment, independent of age or prognosis. Where doubt exists, it is often wise to obtain legal or independent ethical advice. All discussions with the patient, relatives, and other representatives should be documented

When the patient has no next of kin and is unable to communicate, it is good practice, and a legal obligation in some jurisdictions, to appoint a lay 'advocate' to represent the patient's best interests. The patient's dignity, comfort, cultural and religious beliefs must always be respected.

Withholding and withdrawing therapy is common in North America, Europe, and Australasia, particularly in high dependency and intensive care units, where it may be the commonest cause of death. It fulfils ethical principles by putting the welfare of the patient first, avoiding harm from ongoing treatment, and ensuring equity of use of medical resources.

Treatment withdrawal protocols

Once a decision to withdraw treatment is made, management plans or protocols ensure patient comfort and dignity, reduce stress, and reiterate the support required by relatives and junior staff. Use of colloquial terms, such as 'terminal weaning', may cause confusion and should be avoided.

Physicians must decide which interventions to withdraw, recognizing that this will influence the rapidity, comfort, and dignity of the patient's death. However, there are no moral differences between the protocols used. Immediate removal of an endotracheal tube in a mechanically ventilated patient may be the preferred first step. However, it is often less distressing for the patient, relatives, and staff if the process is sequential, rather than a single step. The usual preference for the order of withdrawal of therapy is: renal replacement therapy, inotropic support, antibiotics, mechanical ventilation, feeding, and finally intravenous fluids. Unfortunately, withdrawal biases can prolong dying, causing unnecessary suffering. To prevent this, protocols must be regularly updated. Liberal opiate and sedative therapy may be required to relieve discomfort, particularly when ventilation is discontinued.

Further reading

Berwick D, Davidoff F, Hiatt H, Smith R (2001). Redefining and implementing the Tavistock Principles for everybody in health care. *BMJ*, **323**, 616–20.

Boyd KM (2005). Medical ethics: principles, persons, and perspectives: from controversy to conversation. *Journal of Medical Ethics*, **31**, 481–6.

British Medical Association. <http://www.bma.org.uk>. Tel: 0870 6060 828.

British Medical Asssociation (1995). Advanced statements about medical treatment. Report of the Working Party 1995. British Medical Association, London.

British Medical Association (1999). Confidentiality and disclosure of health information. Report of the Working Party 1999. British Medical Association, London.

British Medical Association (2001). Consent. Report of the Working Party 2001. British Medical Association, London.

Brody HML, Campbell ML, Faber-Langendoen K, Ogle KS (1997). Withdrawing intensive life-sustaining treatment—recommendations for compassionate clinical management. *New England Journal of Medicine*, **336**, 652–7.

Chafe R, Levinson W, Sullivan T (2009). Disclosing errors that affect multiple patients. *Canadian Medical Association Journal*, **180**, 1125–8.

Coulter A, Entwistle V, Gilbert D (1999). Sharing decisions with patients: is the information good enough? *BMJ*, **318**, 318–22.

General Medical Council. <http://www.gmc-uk.org>. Tel: 0161 923 6602.

General Medical Council (1995). Duties of a doctor: guidance from the General Medical Council. General Medical Council, London.

Gillon R (1994). Medical ethics: four principles plus attention to scope. *BMJ*, **309**, 184–8.

Limentani AE (1999). The role of ethical principles in health care and the implications for ethical codes. *Journal of Medical Ethics*, **25**, 394–8.

Medical Defence Union. <http://www.the-mdu.com>. Tel: 0207 202 1500 or 0800 716 646.

Medical Protection Society. Tel: 0113 243 6436. Email: info@mps.org.uk or querydoc@mps.org.uk.

Royal College of Physicians. <http://www.rcplondon.ac.uk>. Tel: 020 3075 1649.

World Medical Association (1994). International code of medical ethics. Declaration of Geneva: World Medical Association.

Subject index

Notes

Abbreviations used in the index may be found on pages xxi to xxx. *vs.* indicates a differential diagnosis or comparison
Page numbers suffixed with *f* refer to material found in figures, *t* tables and *b* boxed material.

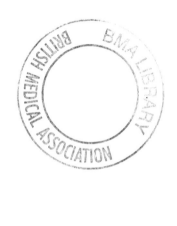